The Basic Science
of Oncology

The Basic Science of Oncology

Third Edition

Editors

Ian F. Tannock, M.D., Ph.D., F.R.C.P.C.

Daniel E. Bergsagel Professor of Medical Oncology
Princess Margaret Hospital/Ontario Cancer Institute
Professor, Departments of Medicine and Medical Biophysics
University of Toronto
Toronto, Ontario, Canada

Richard P. Hill, Ph.D.

Senior Scientist, Division of Experimental Therapeutics
Ontario Cancer Institute/Princess Margaret Hospital
Professor, Departments of Medical Biophysics and Radiation Oncology
University of Toronto
Toronto, Ontario, Canada

McGraw-Hill
Health Professions Division

New York   St. Louis   San Francisco   Auckland
Bogotá   Caracas   Lisbon   London   Madrid
Mexico City   Milan   Montreal   New Delhi
San Juan   Singapore   Sydney   Tokyo   Toronto

McGraw-Hill

A Division of The McGraw·Hill Companies

4 5 6 7 8 9 0   MALMAL   0 9 8 7 6 5 4 3 2 1

ISBN 0-07-105484-7

This book was set in New Baskerville by Digitype.
The editors were James Morgan III and Muza Navrozov.
The production supervisor was Richard C. Ruzycka.
The cover was designed by Marsha Cohen/Parallelogram.
The index was prepared by Irving Conde Tullar.
Malloy Lithographing, Inc. was printer and binder.

This book is printed on acid-free paper.

Library of Congress Cataloging-in-Publication Data

The basic science of oncology / editors, Ian F. Tannock, Richard P. Hill.—3rd ed.
    p. cm.
  Includes bibliographical references and index.
    1. Cancer. 2. Oncology. I. Tannock, Ian. II. Hill, Richard P.
    [DNLM: 1. Neoplasms. QZ 200 B3115 1998]
  RC261.B37   1998
  616.99'4—dc21
  DNLM/DLC
  for Library of Congress

Contents

Contributors vii

Preface xi

1. Introduction to Cancer Biology 1
   Richard P. Hill and Ian F. Tannock

2. Epidemiology of Cancer 6
   John R. McLaughlin and Norman F. Boyd

3. Methods of Genetic Analysis 26
   Jeremy A Squire and Robert A. Phillips

4. Genetic Basis of Cancer 48
   Jeremy A. Squire, Gordon F. Whitmore, and Robert A. Phillips

5. Viruses, Oncogenes, and Tumor Suppressor Genes 79
   Sam Benchimol and Mark D. Minden

6. Growth Factors and Intracellular Signaling 106
   Brent W. Zanke

7. Cell Proliferation and Cell Death 134
   Joyce M. Slingerland and Ian F. Tannock

8. Chemical and Radiation Carcinogenesis 166
   Allan B. Okey, Patricia A. Harper, Denis M. Grant, and Richard P. Hill

9. The Extracellular Environment and Cancer 197
   Shoukat Dedhar, Gregory E. Hannigan, Janusz Rak, and Robert S. Kerbel

10. Tumor Progression and Metastasis 219
    Ann F. Chambers and Richard P. Hill

11. Immunology Related to Cancer 240
    David Spaner, Laszlo Radvany, and Richard G. Miller

12. Hormones and Cancer 263
    Paul E. Goss and Lesley M. Tye

13. Molecular and Cellular Basis of Radiotherapy 295
    Robert G. Bristow and Richard P. Hill

14. Experimental Radiotherapy 322
    C. Shun Wong and Richard P. Hill

15. Cellular and Molecular Basis of Chemotherapy 350
    Michael J. Boyer and Ian F. Tannock

16. Pharmacology of Anticancer Drugs 370
    Malcolm J. Moore and Charles Erlichman

17. Drug Resistance and Experimental Chemotherapy 392
    Ian F. Tannock and Gerald G. Goldenberg

18. Biological Therapy of Cancer 420
    Neil L. Berinstein

19. Hyperthermia and Photodynamic Therapy 443
    Fei-Fei Liu and Brian C. Wilson

20. Guide to Studies of Diagnostic Tests, Prognostic Factors and Treatments 466
    Martin R. Stockler, Norman F. Boyd, and Ian F. Tannock

Glossary 493

Index 511

Contributors*

Sam Benchimol, Ph.D. [5]
Senior Scientist and Head, Division of Cellular and
  Molecular Biology
Ontario Cancer Institute/Princess Margaret Hospital
Professor, Department of Medical Biophysics
University of Toronto
Toronto, Ontario, Canada

Neil L. Berinstein, M.D., Ph.D., F.R.C.P.C. [18]
Staff Oncologist, Department of Medical Oncology/
  Hematology
Toronto-Sunnybrook Regional Cancer Centre
Associate Professor, Departments of Medicine
  and Immunology
University of Toronto
Toronto, Ontario, Canada

Norman F. Boyd, M.D., F.R.C.P.C. [2, 20]
Senior Scientist and Head, Division of Epidemiology
  and Statistics
Ontario Cancer Institute/Princess Margaret Hospital
Professor, Department of Medicine
University of Toronto
Toronto, Ontario, Canada

Michael J. Boyer, M.D., Ph.D., F.R.C.P. [15]
Head, Department of Medical Oncology
Royal Prince Alfred Hospital
Senior Lecturer, Department of Medicine
University of Sydney
Sydney, Australia

Robert G. Bristow, M.D., Ph.D., F.R.C.P.C. [13]
Staff Radiation Oncologist, Department of Radiation
  Oncology
Ontario Cancer Institute/Princess Margaret Hospital
Assistant Professor, Department of Radiation
  Oncology
University of Toronto
Toronto, Ontario, Canada

Ann F. Chambers, Ph.D. [10]
Senior Scientist, London Regional Cancer Centre
Professor and Head, Experimental Oncology
  Division, Oncology Department
University of Western Ontario
London, Ontario, Canada

Shoukat Dedhar, Ph.D. [9]
Senior Scientist, Cancer Control Agency
  of British Columbia
Professor, Department of Biochemistry
  and Molecular Biology
University of British Columbia
Vancouver, British Columbia, Canada

Charles Erlichman, M.D., F.R.C.P.C. [16]
Director of Phase I Programs, Mayo Cancer Center
Mayo Clinic, Rochester, Minnesota
Professor of Oncology, Mayo School of Medicine
Rochester, Minnesota U.S.A.

Gerald J. Goldenberg, M.D., Ph.D., F.R.C.P.C. [17]
Director, Interdepartmental Division of Oncology
Professor, Departments of Medicine
  and Pharmacology
University of Toronto
Toronto, Ontario, Canada

Paul E. Goss, M.D., Ph.D., F.R.C.P.C. [12]
Head, Breast Group, The Toronto Hospital
  and Ontario Cancer Institute/Princess Margaret
  Hospital
Associate Professor, Department of Medicine
University of Toronto
Toronto, Ontario, Canada

---

*Numbers in brackets refer to chapters written or co-written by
the contributor.

Denis M. Grant, Ph.D. [8]
Senior Scientist, Research Institute
The Hospital for Sick Children
Associate Professor, Departments of Pediatrics,
    Pharmacology and Pharmacy
University of Toronto
Toronto, Ontario, Canada

Gregory E. Hannigan, Ph.D. [9]
Scientist, Department of Pediatric Laboratory
    Medicine, Division of Molecular Diagnostics
    Research Institute
The Hospital for Sick Children
Assistant Professor, Department of Laboratory
    Medicine and Pathobiology
University of Toronto
Toronto, Ontario, Canada

Patricia A. Harper, Ph.D. [8]
Scientist, Research Institute
The Hospital for Sick Children
Associate Professor, Departments of Pediatrics,
    Pharmacology and Pharmacy
University of Toronto
Toronto, Ontario, Canada

Richard P. Hill, Ph.D. [1,8,10,13,14]
Senior Scientist, Division of Experimental
    Therapeutics
Ontario Cancer Institute/Princess Margaret Hospital
Professor, Departments of Medical Biophysics and
    Radiation Oncology
University of Toronto
Toronto, Ontario, Canada

Robert S. Kerbel, Ph.D. [9]
Director, Cancer Biology Research
    and Biological Sciences
University of Toronto and Sunnybrook Health
    Science Centre
Professor, Department of Medical Biophysics
University of Toronto
Toronto, Ontario, Canada

Fei-Fei Liu, M.D., F.R.C.P.C. [19]
Senior Scientist, Division of Experimental
    Therapeutics
Ontario Cancer Institute/Princess Margaret Hospital
Associate Professor, Departments of Medical
    Biophysics and Radiation Oncology
University of Toronto
Toronto, Ontario, Canada

John R. McLaughlin, Ph.D. [2]
Associate Professor, Department of Public
    Health Sciences
University of Toronto
Toronto, Ontario, Canada

Richard G. Miller, Ph.D. [11]
Senior Scientist, Division of Cellular
    and Molecular Biology
Ontario Cancer Institute/Princess Margaret Hospital
Professor, Departments of Immunology
    and Medical Biophysics
University of Toronto
Toronto, Ontario, Canada

Mark D. Minden, M.D., Ph.D., F.R.C.P.C. [5]
Senior Scientist, Division of Cellular
    and Molecular Biology
Ontario Cancer Institute/Princess Margaret Hospital
Professor, Departments of Medicine
    and Medical Biophysics
University of Toronto
Toronto, Ontario, Canada

Malcolm J. Moore, M.D., F.R.C.P.C. [16]
Staff Oncologist, Department of Medical Oncology
    and Hematology
Associate Scientist, Division
    of Experimental Therapeutics
Ontario Cancer Institute/Princess Margaret Hospital
Associate Professor, Departments of Medicine
    and Pharmacology
University of Toronto
Toronto, Ontario, Canada

Allan B. Okey, Ph.D. [8]
Chairman and Professor
Department of Pharmacology
University of Toronto
Toronto, Ontario, Canada

Robert A. Phillips, Ph.D. [3,4]
Executive Director
National Cancer Institute of Canada
Professor, Department of Medical Biophysics
University of Toronto
Toronto, Ontario, Canada

Laszlo Radvany, Ph.D. [11]
Senior Scientist, Department of Immunology
Scripps Research Institute
La Jolla, California, U.S.A.

Janusz Rak, Ph.D. [9]
Research Associate, Cancer Biology Research
    and Biological Sciences
University of Toronto and Sunnybrook Health
    Science Centre
Toronto, Ontario, Canada

Joyce M. Slingerland, M.D., Ph.D., F.R.C.P.C [7]
Senior Scientist, Division of Cancer Biology
    Research and Staff Oncologist
Department of Medical Oncology
Toronto-Sunnybrook Regional Cancer Centre
Assistant Professor, Department of Medicine
University of Toronto
Toronto, Ontario, Canada

David Spaner, M.D., F.R.C.P.C. [11]
Senior Scientist, Division of Cancer Biology Research
Staff Oncologist, Department of Medical
    Oncology/Hematology
Toronto-Sunnybrook Regional Cancer Centre
Assistant Professor, Department of Medicine
University of Toronto
Toronto, Ontario, Canada

Jeremy A. Squire, Ph.D. [3,4]
Staff Scientist, The Hospital for Sick Children
Senior Scientist, Division of Cellular
    and Molecular Biology
Ontario Cancer Institute/Princess Margaret Hospital
Associate Professor, Department of Pathology
University of Toronto
Toronto, Ontario, Canada

Martin R. Stockler, M.B.B.S., M.Sc., F.R.A.C.P. [20]
Senior Lecturer in Cancer Medicine
University of Sydney
Coordinator of Medical Education and Clinical
    Academics in Medical Oncology
Royal Prince Alfred Hospital
Sydney, NSW, Australia

Ian F. Tannock, M.D., Ph.D., F.R.C.P.C. [1,7,15,17,20]
Daniel E. Bergsagel Professor of Medical Oncology
Princess Margaret Hospital/Ontario Cancer Institute
Professor, Departments of Medicine
    and Medical Biophysics
University of Toronto
Toronto, Ontario, Canada

Lesley M. Tye, Ph.D. [12]
Clinical Research Scientist
The Toronto Hospital and Ontario Cancer Institute/
    Princess Margaret Hospital
Toronto, Ontario, Canada

Gordon F. Whitmore, Ph.D. [4]
Senior Scientist Emeritus, Research Department
Ontario Cancer Institute/Princess Margaret Hospital
Professor Emeritus,
    Department of Medical Biophysics
University of Toronto
Toronto, Ontario, Canada

Brian C. Wilson, Ph.D. [19]
Senior Scientist and Head,
    Division of Medical Physics
Ontario Cancer Institute/Princess Margaret Hospital
Professor, Department of Medical Biophysics
University of Toronto
Toronto, Ontario, Canada

C. Shun Wong, M.D., F.R.C.P.C. [14]
Senior Scientist,
    Division of Experimental Therapeutics
Ontario Cancer Institute/Princess Margaret Hospital
Associate Professor,
    Department of Radiation Oncology
University of Toronto
Toronto, Ontario, Canada

Brent W. Zanke, M.D., Ph.D., F.R.C.P.C. [6]
Staff Oncologist,
    Department of Medical Oncology and Hematology
Senior Scientist,
    Division of Experimental Therapeutics
Ontario Cancer Institute/Princess Margaret Hospital
Assistant Professor, Departments of Medicine
    and Medical Biophysics
University of Toronto
Toronto, Ontario, Canada

Preface

The first two editions of *The Basic Science of Oncology* described basic aspects of the science underlying the treatment of cancer in a manner suited to both clinical and scientific trainees. The wide acceptance of these two editions of the book and the many positive comments that we received from members of the oncology community have prompted us to produce this third edition. Enormous advances have taken place in the scientific basis of oncology since the second edition was published in early 1992. The current edition, therefore, has undergone substantial changes. All the chapters have been thoroughly revised, and we have added several new authors. As in the first two editions, almost all contributors are drawn from among our colleagues at the University of Toronto, and as previously, the chapters underwent considerable editing to provide complete but succinct coverage of a broad field, using a common style of presentation.

Some of the more important changes in the current edition are as follows. The initial part of the book describing molecular oncology has been reorganized and rewritten to reflect the convergence of our knowledge of the various topics covered. The separate chapter that describes the principles underlying the molecular technology which is now used routinely in research on basic and clinical oncology has been retained and updated. A new chapter describing the rapid progress in the understanding of intracellular signaling has been added (Chapter 6). Our increasing understanding of molecular aspects of cell and cancer biology is apparent in many other chapters, particularly those related to the control of cell proliferation (Chapter 7), to the malignant phenotype and metastasis (Chapter 10), to the immunology of cancer (Chapter 11), and in a new chapter on the extracellular environment (Chapter 9). Approaches to the biological therapy of cancer, including gene therapy, are now described in a new chapter (Chapter 18), and the chapter on hormones and cancer has also been completely revised with new authors. Other chapters describing the biological basis of cancer treatment have undergone extensive changes to include major advances in experimental radiotherapy, new drugs, and the rapid increase in knowledge about drug resistance. To maintain the book at a manageable length, we have deleted, most notably, the chapter on tumor markers and combined in Chapter 8 (with new authors) the previous chapters on chemical and radiation carcinogenesis.

We are grateful to many people for their assistance in producing the third edition: to the reviewers who indicated areas in need of updating, to our authors, particularly the new ones, who responded to our many requests for alterations with forbearance, to our publishers who have encouraged us and accepted with good grace our failure to meet our initially unrealistic deadline, to our students and clinical trainees who provided us with helpful and constructive criticism of earlier drafts of each chapter; and, of course, to our families who have again provided support and encouragement during the several phases of writing and rewriting.

The preparation of this edition has been tinged with sadness because of the tragic and untimely death of Ron Buick in July 1996, one of our colleagues and an author in the previous two editions. Ron was the Research Director of the Ontario Cancer Institute/Princess Margaret Hospital; he was a close friend of ours and of many of the contributors to this book. Ron had a distinguished career both in laboratory-based research and as the leader of one of the largest cancer research institutes in North America. We dedicate this edition to his memory.

I. F. Tannock
R. P. Hill

The Basic Science
of Oncology

1

Introduction to Cancer Biology

Richard P. Hill and Ian F. Tannock

1.1 PERSPECTIVE

1.2 CANCER AS A GENETIC DISEASE

1.3 CANCER AS A CELLULAR DISEASE

1.4 CANCER AND THE EXTRACELLULAR ENVIRONMENT

1.5 CONCLUSIONS

1.1 PERSPECTIVE

Although cancer has become increasingly prominent as a disease in modern times, it is not a modern disease. Malignant tumors were described in pictures or writings from many ancient civilizations, including those of Asia, South America, and Egypt, and bone cancers (osteosarcomas) have been diagnosed in Egyptian mummies. Cancer also occurs in all known species of higher animals. Early cultures attributed the cause of cancer to various gods, and this belief was held generally until the Middle Ages. Hippocrates, however, described cancer as an imbalance between the black humor (from the spleen) and the three bodily humors: blood, phlegm, and bile. Although incorrect, the theory was the first (~400 B.C.) to attribute the origin of cancer to natural causes. The suggestion that cancer might be an inherited or environmental disease appeared later: writings from the Middle Ages made reference to "cancer houses," "cancer families," and "cancer villages."

One of the first scientific enquiries into the cause of cancer dates from 1775, when Sir Percival Pott, an English physician, carried out an epidemiological study. At that time young boys were used as chimney sweeps in London, since they were small enough to climb inside the chimneys. Pott observed that young men in their twenties who had been chimney sweeps as boys had a high rate of death due to cancer of the scrotum. He suggested that the causative agent might be chimney soot (now known to be tar) and recommended frequent washing and changing of clothing that trapped the soot so as to reduce exposure to the "carcinogen." Not only did Pott's study identify a putative carcinogenic agent but it also demonstrated that a cancer may develop many years after exposure to the causative agent—that is, that there can be an extended latent period. Pott's deductions about the origin of scrotal cancer in chimney sweeps were made with little knowledge of the biological properties of tumors. The recognition that the growth of cancer results from a disordered proliferation of cells followed the development of the microscope. Microscopic examination of tumors allowed Virchow, the eminent nineteenth-century pathologist, to declare that "every cell is born from another cell." Thus, cancer was established as a cellular disease.

Epidemiological studies have identified major environmental causes of cancer, such as tobacco smoke and various occupational exposures. Such studies raise the possibility of prevention through changes in lifestyle and diet, as has already happened through decreased rates of smoking in some western countries.

Recently, the most important advances in knowledge about the biology of cancer have come from our increased understanding of molecular genetics. However, many of these advances were dependent on prior information from epidemiological studies of the incidence of cancer in populations. Studies of relatively inbred populations, such as the Mormons in Utah, have shown that many types of cancer depend on relatedness—that is, on the sharing of genes. Studies of families that have a high incidence of certain types of cancer have assisted in the identification of genetic defects that can lead to malignancy, such as mutations of the retinoblastoma gene (*Rb*) in children with that disease or of the *p53* gene in the Li-Fraumeni syndrome and of the *BRCA1* and *BRCA2* genes, which are associated with familial breast and ovarian cancer. Studies of cancer incidence in families that have inherited genetically based defects in DNA repair have also demonstrated the involvement of DNA repair genes in preventing malignancy. This and other evidence have established cancer as a genetic disease.

The rapid evolution of techniques of molecular biology has led to the characterization, cloning, and sequencing of a variety of genes where mutation can lead to malignant transformation. Thus the current model of initial cancer development envisions cells undergoing a series of genetic mutations and/or alterations, brought about in various ways, which result in their inability to respond normally to intracellular and/or extracellular signals that control proliferation, differentiation, and, ultimately, death. The number of required genetic alterations apparently varies from as little as two to at least six for different types of cancer, and it is likely that further changes occur during progression to increased malignancy. These genetic alterations may arise directly or indirectly from such factors as inherited gene mutations, chemical- or radiation-induced DNA damage, incorporation of certain viruses into the cell, or random errors during DNA synthesis.

While clinical observation has divided tumor development into a number of discrete categories of increasing severity (benign, malignant, metastatic), the underlying biology is better conceptualized as a process of many small changes similar to evolution. Thus, genetic changes that can affect the cell's growth potential may occur, and cells with such changes are selected for (or against) by the conditions that they are exposed to at that particular time. Increasing knowledge of signal-transduction pathways in cells has demonstrated that many aspects of cell function, including growth, are controlled by a balance of positive and negative signals received from inside and outside the cell. Thus, lack of ability or increased ability to respond to a specific signal may allow the cell to proliferate in the face of other signals that would normally prevent such proliferation. Cancer treatment can be thought of as adding negative signals to the cellular environment. The process of genetic change, however, may give rise to subpopulations of cells that have evolved varied mechanisms of resistance, particularly for drug treatments, and these cells may survive and regrow the tumor. The genetic evolution of cancer cells and the signals that the cells receive from their extracellular environment thus play a critical role in the growth and treatment of cancer.

1.2 CANCER AS A GENETIC DISEASE

Cancer is a disease in which malignant cells proliferate to produce progeny that are also malignant. This inheritance of the malignant trait, or *phenotype*, provides strong evidence that fundamental properties of malignancy are encoded in the genes of the cancer cell. Studies of genetic markers—such as expression of unique immunoglobulin molecules in lymphomas or myelomas; the common translocation of chromosomes 9 and 22, which generates the Philadelphia chromosome in chronic myelogenous leukemia; and the study of genes linked to the X chromosome, such as glucose-6-phosphate dehydrogenase (G6PD) in heterozygous females—provide strong evidence that cells of human tumors are derived clonally from a single precursor cell. However, the clonal origin of a tumor does not imply homogeneity among cancer cells, since further genetic changes as well as microenvironmental influences occur during tumor growth. These lead to heterogeneity in a wide variety of the properties of the individual tumor cells; these can affect many aspects of tumor development, including invasiveness, metastatic properties, and resistance to therapeutic agents (i.e., tumor progression).

Much of current cancer research is directed to the identification, characterization, and cloning of genes whose protein products are involved in the transformation of a normal cell into a malignant cell. Historically, one line of investigation involved the transfer of genes from a malignant cell to a normal cell (usually a fibroblast) and subsequent identification of the genes that could cause malignant transformation of the normal cell. This procedure led to the identification of genes, known as *dominantly acting oncogenes*, where a mutation caused a change in a normal cellular protein that could lead to malignant change in an appropriate recipient cell. Many of these genes are involved in the normal transmission of growth-promoting signals from the cell surface to the nucleus (e.g., *ras, src*) or are transcription factors (e.g., *myc, fos*). A second line of investigation, which included the characterization of genetic changes in inherited retinoblastoma, led to the identification of normal cellular genes that suppress malignant transformation, known as *tumor suppressor genes*. For malignant transformation, both copies of the gene (e.g., *Rb*, *p53*, *BRCA1* or *BRCA2*) must be either lost, mutated, or inactivated. Identification of tumor suppressor genes has been facilitated by the study of sites in the genome where there is commonly loss of heterozygosity between the genes (alleles) on the two corresponding chromosomes in malignant tumors. Such sites may indicate the presence of a mutated tumor suppressor gene where the corresponding normal allele has either been deleted or lost by a variety of mechanisms.

As noted earlier, many aspects of cell function are controlled by a balance of positive and negative signals received from inside and outside the cell. In normal tissues, there is a balance between cell proliferation and cell death. In tumors, this balance is disturbed, perhaps because of genetic defects that lead to faulty cell signaling or to an imbalance of molecules that stimulate [e.g., cyclins and cyclin-dependent kinases (cdks)] or inhibit (cdk inhibitors) the movement of cells around the cell cycle. It is not surprising, therefore, that some of the approaches described above led to the identification of genes involved in these fundamental processes, where mutation or other change (deletion, amplification, chromosomal translocation, etc.) led to malignancy. The identification of new putative oncogenes and tumor suppressor genes has followed the elucidation of the metabolic pathways associated with control of cell growth. The ability to direct specific site-directed mutations to target genes and to generate mice that either contain a mutated gene (transgenic mice) or lack a fundamental gene (knockout mice) has greatly facilitated study of the function of these genes and their role in malignant transformation.

1.3 CANCER AS A CELLULAR DISEASE

Tumors grow because of the proliferation of constituent cells and metastasize as a result of the spread of malignant cells from the primary tumor to other sites. Tumors tend to grow exponentially, with the implication that, even without considering the time taken for a normal cell to develop into a cancer cell, it takes longer for a tumor to grow to a size that can just be detected clinically (1 to 10 g) than it would for this just-detected tumor to grow to a size that will kill the host (1 to 10 kg) if no treatment is given. A tumor of 1 g contains 10^8 to 10^9 cells and would require about 30 doublings in volume to grow from a single cell; another 10 doublings in volume would produce a very large tumor of about 1 kg. With a typical volume doubling time of 2 months for common adult human tumors (childhood tumors usually grow faster), the latent period of growth would be about 5 years. The overall latent period from initiation of the carcinogenic process to clinical detection of a tumor may be much longer (10 to 20 years). Characterization of cell proliferation and cell death in tumors has provided the information that, contrary to general belief, tumor cells usually proliferate more slowly than cells in normal tissues, such as the intestine or bone marrow. Furthermore, tumors contain quiescent (i.e., nonproliferating) cells; they have a high rate of cell differentiation and ultimately cell death. A relatively small proportion of tumor cells may retain the capacity for unlimited proliferation, and these stem cells are the important targets of therapy. Cell death may occur because of limited supply of nutrient metabolites to tumors, leading to necrosis, and/or through the process of programmed cell death or apoptosis, which maintains homeostasis in nongrowing normal tissues.

There is evidence that tumors contain some molecules differing from those in normal cells, such as the products of mutated oncogenes and proteins that are normally expressed in fetal tissue. These "non-self" proteins can be presented on antigen-presenting cells and may elicit an immune rejection response. It has been argued that this immune response might eradicate some tumors prior to their clinical detection in a process known as *immune surveillance* and thus that tumors that do grow either do not express such non-self antigens or have mechanisms allowing them to evade the immune rejection response. Recent work has provided information about the complex molecular basis underlying activation and control of the immune response. This information has led to renewed efforts to use mechanistically based approaches to devise biological and immune therapies that might induce tumor rejection by the host.

The effectiveness of cancer therapy with radiation, chemotherapy, hormonal approaches, or more experimental approaches using biological agents, heat, or light all depend on reducing the number of tumor stem cells. The likely effectiveness of therapy is best assessed, therefore, by treating a population of tumor cells and assessing their reproductive potential by using a colony-forming (or *clonogenic*) assay. While other assays such as exclusion of dye from cells or assays of apoptosis may also indicate cell death, they may not detect lethal damage in cells that appear morphologically viable but have lost their ability to remain stem cells (i.e., their ability to regenerate a tumor). More important than the absolute sensitivity of tumor cells to a given therapeutic agent is their relative sensitivity in comparison to that of normal cells, which will limit the dose that can be given to a patient. Much of current research into experimental cancer therapy is directed to understanding the relative sensitivities of cells from tumors and normal tissues, of factors that lead to therapeutic resistance, and of methods for overcoming resistance in tumor-cell populations. Various genetic factors that may influence cellular sensitivity to radiation are under intense study, and several laboratories are trying to individualize treatment by studying the sensitivity of cells from tumors and normal tissues in predictive assays.

The responses of cells to anticancer drugs are more variable than those following treatment with radiation. In general, rapidly proliferating cells are more sensitive to chemotherapeutic agents, and some drugs act at only one phase in the cell cycle; these observations correlate with the clinical experience that it is toxicity to normal tissues that contain rapidly proliferating cells—such as the bone marrow or intestine—which usually limits the dose of drug that can be given. A variety of mechanisms allow malignant cells to become resistant to multiple anticancer drugs: these include the export of drugs from the cytoplasm via molecular pumps expressed in the cell membrane (e.g., P-glycoprotein, multidrug-resistance protein); increases or decreases in target enzymes such as DNA topoisomerases; increased binding of drugs, detoxification, and export from cells by glutathione and associated enzymes; and increased DNA repair. There is also evidence that some cells develop resistance to a variety of therapeutic agents through failure to activate pathways leading to cell death. The expanding knowledge about important molecular pathways in cancer cells has allowed the design of new drugs with different mechanisms of action. Promising experimental drugs include those that inhibit *ras*-mediated cell signaling or the enzyme telomerase, which may allow cancer cells to avoid the process of shortening chromosomes at their telomeres and thereby to escape from senescence.

A major barrier to effective therapy of human cancer arises because of the ability of tumor cells to metastasize. Metastasis involves a number of steps including detachment of cells from the primary tumor, invasion of lymphatics or blood vessels, survival of tumor cells in the circulation, and extravasation and establishment of a new growth. The process is (fortunately) inefficient, with a low probability that any cell that detaches from the primary tumor will establish a secondary growth. Molecular studies of the determinants of metastases are establishing that properties of both the tumor cell (i.e., the turning on or off of specific genes) and the microenvironment of the tissue in which metastases are established influence the efficiency of the metastatic process. Although some therapeutic approaches may inhibit the metastatic process, their clinical utility is limited by the probability that metastasis may have occurred (at a microscopic level) prior to detection of the primary tumor.

1.4 CANCER AND THE EXTRACELLULAR ENVIRONMENT

Some properties of cancers, and of therapeutic agents used to treat them, can be explained by study of their action on dispersed tumor cells. The application of these studies is limited, however, because a solid tumor represents a society in which there are important interactions between the constituent cells and between the cells and the extracellular matrix. These interactions may be mediated by growth factors and hormones, which interact with specific receptors and thereby propagate a signal to the nucleus and influence gene expression, or by cellular adhesion molecules, which can interact with components of the extracellular matrix and initiate intracellular signaling. This, in turn, can control properties such as cell shape, cell movement, and cell proliferation or death. The extracellular matrix provides both a surface for cell attachment (e.g., the basement membrane) and a barrier to cell movement, but the constituent molecules can also bind many growth factors, limiting their interaction with cells. Thus breakdown of components of the extracellular matrix through secretion of proteolytic enzymes, such as matrix metalloproteinases, which is thought to be an important mechanism in the generation of metastases, may assist both invasion and growth of cancer cells. Tissue inhibitors of metalloproteinases may act thus as metastasis suppressor genes.

The microenvironment of solid tumors is remarkably heterogeneous with respect to the delivery of nutrient metabolites such as oxygen and glucose and the removal of catabolites. In order to grow larger than a size of ~1 mm in diameter, tumors must elicit proliferation of blood vessels to provide nutrition to the cancer cells. This process of angiogenesis is stimulated by release of several growth factors from tumor cells (and sometimes by surrounding normal cells). The most important of these appears to be vascular endothelial growth factor (VEGF), whose synthesis and release is stimulated by the presence of a hypoxic microenvironment. Several experimental approaches to cancer therapy are using agents that inhibit the process of angiogenesis.

The vascular supply to solid tumors is often much poorer than that to normal tissues; patent vessels are relatively far apart, and stasis or interruptions of blood flow are common. This leads to marked variation in local concentration of metabolites, and many solid tumors contain regions of hypoxia that convey resistance to ionizing radiation. Cell death and necrosis are observed to occur in tumor regions that are distant from functional blood vessels, presumably as a result of nutrient deprivation and/or the presence of toxic catabolites. Exposure to such conditions may be one of the factors that helps to select for tumor cells with more aggressive phenotypes during the process of tumor progression.

The limited blood supply in tumors also poses problems for the delivery of anticancer drugs: limited penetration of drugs from tumor blood vessels and the slow proliferation of tumor cells in nutritionally deprived regions of tumors may both convey therapeutic resistance. Even the generation of resistance to anticancer drugs may depend on the environment to which the cells are exposed; several types of malignant cells have been found to be highly resistant when treated as solid tissue but quite sensitive to the same drugs when treated as a dispersed cell suspension. The environment within solid tumors is both complex and heterogeneous and plays an important role in the growth and development of tumors and in their response to therapy.

1.5 CONCLUSIONS

Currently, evaluation of diagnostic or screening tests, prognostic factors, and the efficacy of cancer therapy depends on the study of populations of patients. These studies recognize the presence of heterogeneity among patients with tumors of a given histological type but allow prediction of the probability of certain outcomes (e.g., survival as a function of time) based on properties of the tumor and host and on the treatment applied. A major challenge for the next generation of therapeutic studies will be to apply knowledge about the heterogeneity of individual tumors at the molecular, cellular, and tissue levels to design treatment strategies that will target the different properties of different tumors, even those of similar histopathologic type, to produce overall improvements in treatment outcome with acceptable levels of toxicity.

2

Epidemiology of Cancer

John R. McLaughlin and Norman F. Boyd

2.1 INTRODUCTION
  2.1.1 The Scope of Epidemiology
  2.1.2 General Principles

2.2 METHODS OF EPIDEMIOLOGIC INVESTIGATION
  2.2.1 Epidemiologic Measures
  2.2.2 Generation and Testing of Hypotheses about Cancer Causation
  2.2.3 Cohort Studies
  2.2.4 Case-Control Studies
  2.2.5 Random Error
  2.2.6 Bias
  2.2.7 Confounding and Effect Modification
  2.2.8 Criteria for Inferring That Epidemiologic Associations Are Causal

2.3 DESCRIPTIVE EPIDEMIOLOGY OF HUMAN CANCER
  2.3.1 Data Sources and Trends
  2.3.2 Geographic Distribution
  2.3.3 Age Distribution

2.4 RISK FACTORS FOR CANCER
  2.4.1 Tobacco
  2.4.2 Alcohol
  2.4.3 Diet
  2.4.4 Occupational Exposures
  2.4.5 Hormonal and Reproductive Factors
  2.4.6 Other Environmental Exposures

2.5 SPECIFIC TYPES OF CANCER
  2.5.1 Lung Cancer
  2.5.2 Breast Cancer
  2.5.3 Melanoma

2.6 SUMMARY

REFERENCES

BIBLIOGRAPHY

2.1 INTRODUCTION

2.1.1 The Scope of Epidemiology

Epidemiology is defined as the study of the distribution and determinants of disease in human populations (Last, 1988). The subject is concerned with explaining, in Acheson's phrase, why "this patient developed this disease at this time," as well as with explaining why different populations of individuals are at different risks for different diseases. In addition to being the focus for those concerned with population health, epidemiology is also of concern to clinicians, clinical researchers, and laboratory scientists.

Clinicians must advise patients about any risk of cancer that is associated with their lifestyle and with medical procedures or treatments. Thus, they need to understand how data describing such risks are generated in order to assess the quantitative importance of the risks described and to appraise critically the credibility of reports of cancer risk.

Cancer epidemiologists seek ultimately to identify the causes of cancer and thus share this goal with clinical researchers and laboratory scientists. Epidemiologic descriptions of the distribution of cancer, and the identification of groups of individuals at different risks for the development of cancer, provide basic information that is required to test hypotheses concerning the causes of cancer.

Laboratory and clinical science, by developing improved methods of measuring exposure to potential causes of cancer or the biological consequences of such exposure, can also contribute substantially to the epidemiologic study of disease. Some of the most striking examples of progress in understanding the causes of cancer have come from such collaborative work, where markers of exposure or biologic effect were applied in studies of human populations. Research that has defined the relationship between smoking and lung cancer is an example of this collaboration (see Sec. 2.5.1).

An important ultimate application of epidemiologic findings is in the planning and evaluation of cancer-control strategies, such as in the primary prevention or early detection of cancer. Epidemiologic methods can be applied to study the determinants of a wide range of adverse outcomes. Although the scope of cancer epidemiology is broad, a primary concern is the search for causes of cancer that may facilitate the identification of high-risk populations and ultimately the prevention of cancer. Thus, epidemiologic principles and methodology relevant to the study of cancer etiology are the focus of this chapter.

2.1.2. General Principles

There are two phases in the general approach taken by cancer epidemiologists. First, *descriptive epidemiology* provides an indication of how frequently cancer occurs in terms of rates, risks, and number of cases. Second, *analytic epidemiology* is used to study cancer etiology, whereby comparisons of cancer risks are made between subgroups of the population.

The unique contribution of epidemiology in the study of cancer etiology is its ability to elucidate the determinants of disease that are actually found in human populations. To achieve this, epidemiology predominantly employs *observational* rather than experimental research methods, in part because it is unethical to intentionally expose people to potential carcinogens. There are potential limitations of observational research, such that epidemiologists must carefully consider the design, methods, and interpretation of their studies.

Analytic epidemiologic studies search for causes of cancer by determining whether a particular trait or exposure is associated with the risk of developing a particular type of cancer. Traditionally, the associations considered in epidemiologic studies were between readily identifiable states, such as potential risk factors measured by questionnaire, and a clearly defined outcome, such as cancer. However, subdisciplines have evolved that focus on particular risk factors, as in "nutritional epidemiology" or "environmental epidemiology." Recent developments in basic sciences now make it possible to incorporate molecular and cellular measurements of exposures and underlying biologic processes in "molecular epidemiologic" studies of cancer (Schulte, 1993). "Genetic epidemiologic" studies focus on the determinants of disease in families and on inherited causes of cancer in populations (Last, 1988). Each branch of epidemiology shares a common set of methods and basic principles.

Other chapters in this volume give detailed accounts of specific etiologic associations; no attempt is made in this chapter to provide a comprehensive description of the epidemiology of all cancers. Rather, the general principles used in the epidemiologic study of cancer are described. Examples of the epidemiology of selected cancers are cited to illustrate these general principles or particular issues in methodology.

2.2 METHODS OF EPIDEMIOLOGIC INVESTIGATION

2.2.1 Epidemiologic Measures

The *frequency* of cancer in a population can be measured in several ways. The total number of cases in the population is particularly relevant in the planning of health services. Incident cancers and prevalent cases are distinguished when measuring disease frequency. *Incidence* refers to the number of new events, such as deaths or newly diagnosed disease, occurring in a defined population within a specified period of time. *Prevalence* is defined as the number of instances of a given disease (or other condition), both newly and previously diagnosed, in a defined population at a designated time.

Rates are measures of disease frequency that allow comparisons between populations or their subsets. An *incidence rate* is obtained by dividing the number of incident cases over a fixed time interval by the number of people in the population during that time. Incidence rates provide an estimate of disease *risk*, which is the probability that an individual will develop the disease in a specified period of time. Given that cancer rates vary substantially with age, the validity of comparisons between populations is further enhanced by calculating *age-standardized* rates, which account for differences in age distribution as well as population size.

Figure 2.1 presents examples of two measures of disease frequency. In Canada, the number of incident cases for all cancers combined (excluding non-melanoma skin cancer) increased from 74,000 in 1980 to 104,000 in 1990, while age-standardized incidence rates remained relatively stable. Given the

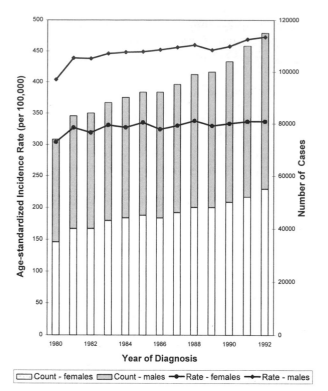

Figure 2.1. Age-standardized incidence rates (per 100,000) and the number of incident cases in Canada, for all types of cancer combined, by year and sex (figures exclude non-melanoma skin cancer; rates standardized to the 1991 Canadian census population). (Adapted from the National Cancer Institute of Canada, 1997)

stability of the rates, this change in the number of cancer cases can be attributed largely to an increase in, and aging of, the population. Figure 2.1 also demonstrates the convention of referring to a large denominator of fixed size when expressing rates of rare diseases; for example, cancer incidence rates in 1990 were 458 per 100,000 males and 246 per 100,000 females.

Prevalence is a function of both the incidence and duration of a disease or trait. Thus, for cancers with a favorable prognosis (i.e., high survival rate), prevalence is much higher than incidence, whereas prevalence is much lower for cancers with poor prognosis. Examples of prevalence rates are the number of individuals surviving with cancer at a point in time per 100,000 in the population and the proportion of individuals in a population who smoke at a point in time. Studies of disease etiology generally use incidence rather than prevalence as the measure of disease frequency because this is not affected by what happens after diagnosis.

The above measures are used in descriptive epidemiology to depict the frequency of cancer in terms of its geographic distribution (place), the age and sex distributions of the affected individuals (person), and any temporal associations such as changes in frequency of disease that occur over time. Analytic epidemiologic studies of cancer etiology use measures of association to compare cancer risks between different groups of individuals. The ratio of risks (or rates) in two comparable groups provides a *relative risk* estimate, which is a simple summary measure of whether cancer risk is associated with the traits that distinguish the groups. In interpreting a relative risk estimate, a value of 1.0 is indicative of equal risks for the groups being compared (i.e., no association). For example, the relative risk estimate of 1.86, obtained by taking the ratio of age-standardized incidence rates for Canadian males and females in 1990 (Fig. 2.1), indicates that cancer risk was 1.86 times greater for males than for females.

2.2.2 Generation and Testing of Hypotheses about Cancer Causation

The epidemiologic approach to the study of the causes of cancer is based on the comparison of cancer risks. The risk of cancer among individuals exposed to some factor that is suspected to cause (or protect against) cancer is compared with the risk of cancer in individuals not so exposed. These comparisons involve several scientifically distinct steps.

The first of these steps involves the *generation of hypotheses* about cancer etiology. Ideas about the causes of cancer may come from several sources. Alert clinical observers frequently have been the first to draw attention to etiologic associations. Examples include scrotal cancer, which was noted by Sir Percival Pott in 1775 to be common in chimney sweeps; the association of lung cancer and smoking; and clear-cell vaginal carcinoma in the daughters of mothers exposed to diethylstilbestrol. Other hypotheses may be developed from epidemiologic data collected for purely descriptive purposes. For example, descriptions of the geographic distribution of malignant melanoma led to the observation that the frequency of the disease was associated with latitude and to the hypothesis that the disease might be caused by exposure to the ultraviolet components of sunlight (Sec. 2.5.3).

For many types of cancer there is insufficient information to formulate prior hypotheses about causative factors, and epidemiologic studies may be conducted to generate leads requiring further investigation. In such exploratory studies, populations or groups at high and low risk for a particular cancer may be contrasted, in the first instance, for as many attributes as it is feasible to examine. In analyzing the collected data, these attributes will be compared in a search for differences between the groups that might be causally related to their different risks for developing cancer. Such exercises, while necessary and important in the preliminary search for the causes of cancer, can do no more than generate hypotheses, as they do not distinguish between causative factors and factors that are merely associated with the development of cancer.

The second step in the epidemiologic approach to study the causes of cancer involves the *testing of hypotheses* generated by the above methods. Hypothesis testing is done by comparing cancer risks for groups that differ in their level of exposure to a suspected causal factor to determine the extent to which exposure to the factor has altered the risk. This can be accomplished, first, by specifying a null hypothesis such as that the true relative risk due to exposure is 1.0 (i.e., no association). A statistical test can then be applied to assess whether the relative risk estimated from the data differs significantly from 1.0, or, in other words, whether the null hypothesis can be rejected. While testing for statistical significance, a distinction must be made between the test of a specific a priori hypothesis and exploratory analyses of numerous potential risk factors because the latter could give rise to a statistical association by chance alone (e.g., because of multiple comparisons). If a statistical association is found, the final step of epidemiologic research then involves its interpretation, by taking into consideration the potential for biases given the study design and by considering the criteria used in causal inference (see Sec. 2.2.8).

The most important methods available for assembling the information required to make these comparisons of risk are cohort and case-control studies. The design of such studies and their major variants are described in the following sections.

2.2.3 Cohort Studies

In cohort studies, subsets of a given population are defined on the basis of whether (or not) individuals are exposed to a factor suspected of increasing or decreasing the risk of cancer. These subsets are followed forward in time and observed to detect the development of cancer. After a period of time sufficient for a number of cancers to develop, cancer risks in the exposed and nonexposed groups are

compared and the relative risk due to exposure can then be calculated directly (Fig. 2.2). The major types of cohort studies are randomized controlled (experimental) trials and observational studies.

Randomized controlled trials provide the strongest possible evidence about etiologic relationships, but they can be applied only rarely in cancer epidemiology. Randomized trials have the advantage that the exposure under investigation can be allocated randomly, and the process of randomization should, on average, make the groups to be compared similar at the start of the study. Ethical considerations limit the use of randomized trials to the investigation of exposures that may be protective against cancer, such as trials that examine the influence of dietary modification, vitamin supplements, and other possible means of reducing cancer risk.

Observational cohort studies differ from experimental trials in that the allocation of the primary exposure is not under the control of the investigator. Genetic influences, occupational exposure, habits such as cigarette smoking, medical treatments, and exposure to atomic explosions are among the many types of exposures that have been investigated in cohort studies.

In observational cohort studies, the investigator can characterize baseline risk factors for the development of the outcome (e.g., development of a particular type of cancer) and can arrange for regular surveillance for outcome detection in the same way as in an experimental trial. The inability to control the allocation of exposure in an observational cohort study means that the results may be open to more than one interpretation. Given that exposure is self-selected for many potential causes of cancer—such as occupation, cigarette smoking, and dietary practices—the finding of an association with cancer risk may mean either that these exposures are related causally or, alternatively, that some other

Initial Classification	Subsequent Classification	
	Diseased	Nondiseased
Exposed	A	B
Nonexposed	C	D

Risk of Disease with Exposure $= A/(A + B)$
Risk of Disease with Nonexposure $= C/(C + D)$
Relative Risk due to Exposure $= A/(A + B) \div C/(C + D)$

Figure 2.2. The general design of cohort studies and the measures of risk and relative risk that are calculated.

attribute both determined the decision to be exposed and influenced independently the risk of cancer. For example, it was at one time argued that a genetic factor influenced both the risk of lung cancer and the decision to smoke cigarettes. Studies in identical twins, discordant for smoking habits, later showed this suggestion to be incorrect and that smoking and not genetic makeup is the major determinant of lung cancer risk. However, data from the original cohort studies linking cigarette smoking and risk of lung cancer were open to both interpretations.

Observational cohort studies can be conducted either prospectively, as described above, or retrospectively. A historical cohort study is possible if the exposure status can be determined retrospectively for members of the population, sufficient time has elapsed after exposure, and the development of cancer has occurred in some subjects. It is not possible with this approach to arrange for the population to be examined with a predetermined frequency, as can be done in experimental trials or prospective observational cohort studies. This is a shortcoming for those diseases in which investigation is required to detect the presence of disease; however, many types of cancer can be expected to declare their presence even when not sought deliberately; in these circumstances, the historical approach to cohort studies may give valid estimates of risk.

The major advantage of cohort studies is that they address directly the etiologic sequence of cause preceding effect. When such studies are carried out prospectively, it is feasible to measure exposure accurately, characterize baseline cancer risk, and follow the population for the development of cancer. A limitation of the cohort design is that because most human cancers occur infrequently, these studies often need very large numbers of subjects to have a good chance of finding an increase in risk associated with a particular exposure. Table 2.1 shows the required number of subjects according to the incidence of cancer in the nonexposed group and the magnitude of the relative risk that the investigator aims to detect. If a specific type of cancer occurred at a rate of 1 per 10,000 in the nonexposed during the course of the study and an investigator wished to determine that a tripling of risk (i.e., a relative risk of 3) was not due to chance variation, then there would need to be 67,000 individuals in the nonexposed group and an equal number in the exposed group. Table 2.1 also shows how sample size requirements decline with increasing relative risk and as the outcome becomes more common. The prevalence of exposure, which affects the relative sizes of exposed and nonexposed groups, is another important determinant of the required size of a cohort study (Breslow and Day, 1987). The rarity of cancer creates the need for most cohort studies to be large, time-consuming, and expensive, which has motivated the development of the more economical case-control design for the investigation of etiologic relationships.

2.2.4 Case-Control Studies

Whereas a cohort study follows individuals from exposure to the development of disease, a case-control study begins with individuals who are either dis-

Table 2.1. Sample Sizes Required in Cohort Studies, by Level of Detectable Relative Risk and for Varying Levels of Baseline Risk in the Nonexposed Group[a]

Relative Risk	Number or Events Required in Nonexposed Group	Number of Subjects Required in Nonexposed Group for Various Levels of Baseline Cancer Risk		
		If risk = 1/10,000	If risk = 1/1,000	If risk = 1/100
2	20.0	200,000	20,000	2,000
3	6.7	67,000	6,700	670
4	3.7	37,000	3,700	370
5	2.5	25,000	2,500	250
10	0.92	9,200	920	92

[a]Table lists the number in each of the comparison groups. Estimates are based on the selection of two groups (exposed and nonexposed) of equal size, and standard statistical parameters (alpha = 0.05, beta probability = 0.2).

Source: Adapted from Breslow and Day, 1987.

Subsequent Classification	Initial Classification	
	Diseased (Cases)	Nondiseased (Controls)
Exposed	A	B
Nonexposed	C	D
Odds of exposure in cases:	A/C	
Odds of exposure in controls:	B/D	
Odds ratio:	A/C÷B/D = AD/BC	

Figure 2.3. The general design of case-control studies and the measures of risk (odds) and relative risk (odds ratio) that are calculated.

eased (cases) or not diseased (controls) and then assesses these individuals for their previous exposure (Fig. 2.3). Cases may be drawn from several sources, including hospital diagnostic indexes, cancer registry files, or files of one or more physicians. Controls may also be selected from hospitals, outpatient facilities, or the general population using random-sampling techniques. In designing a case-control study, careful consideration must be given to the selection of cases and appropriate controls (Schlesselman, 1982) because there are many ways of introducing bias into the assessment of the relationship between exposure and disease (see Sec. 2.2.6). The measurement of exposure in case-control studies depends on the type of information that is sought, with the most frequently used method being a questionnaire to assess factors such as occupational history, diet, or personal habits (e.g., smoking). In some circumstances assessment of exposure can be enhanced by referring to existing records or databases, as may be possible for medical history or occupational exposures. Other factors, such as prior exposure to viruses or the influence of some aspect of the individual's phenotype on disease risk, may be assessed by direct examination or biomarkers.

Relative risk cannot be calculated directly in case-control studies, but it can be approximated by a measure called the *odds ratio* (Fig. 2.3). This approximate relationship is valid if the disease is uncommon in the population, which is true of even the most common human cancers. Thus, in Fig. 2.2, if A and C are much smaller than B and D, respectively, then relative risk (RR) can be determined as follows:

$$RR = A/(A + B) \div C/(C + D)$$

$$\approx A/B \div C/D$$

$$\approx AD/BC$$

Thus, under these circumstances, the odds ratio shown in Fig. 2.3 is a valid estimate of relative risk.

To detect a given level of cancer risk, case-control studies can be performed more quickly and involve fewer subjects than can cohort studies. For example, under the conditions described in the previous section, which required a cohort study to be based on 134,000 individuals (relative risk = 3, prevalence of exposure = 50 percent, baseline risk = 1/10,000), a case-control study would require only 33 cases and 132 controls for a total of 165 individuals (Breslow and Day, 1987). The case-control design achieves this increased efficiency by focusing on the most informative individuals (i.e., all of the cases in the population) but only a small random sample of the large number of healthy individuals (controls). Case-control studies are particularly useful in the investigation of diseases that are rare or those that have a long interval between exposure and the development of disease. This applies to essentially all types of human cancer.

A limitation of the case-control design is that exposure must often be measured by the recollection of the subjects, and there is frequently no means available to check the accuracy of this information. Also, as discussed in Sec. 2.2.6, there are many types of potential bias in the selection of subjects and measurement of exposure that are often easier to avoid or detect in cohort than in case-control research. Despite these disadvantages, case-control studies are frequently the only feasible means of assessing, in human populations, the validity of new claims about the determinants of cancer risk.

The design selected for an epidemiologic study may also be a hybrid or specialized application of the two basic designs. One hybrid design is when a case-control study is undertaken within a cohort. If the cost of measuring exposure on all cohort members is prohibitively high (e.g., laboratory analysis of biomarkers in stored specimens), cost-effectiveness can be enhanced by measuring exposure for selected individuals, including the individuals who develop the cancer (cases) and a random sample of other cohort members who do not develop the cancer (controls). Specialized applications of the standard designs are also used in genetic epidemiology, as in a cohort study where, instead of being selected from the general population as in more traditional studies, the cohort is selected from family members. By comparing disease risk in families that differ in their genetic traits while accounting for measured differences in environmental exposures, it is possible in genetic epidemiology to detect the relative contribution of both genetic and environmental risk factors (Khoury et al, 1993).

2.2.5 Random Error

In common with other forms of scientific enquiry, the results of epidemiologic studies can be distorted by features in their design. The common sources of distortion are random error, bias, and confounding: an understanding of the origins and effects of these factors will help in the interpretation of epidemiologic data.

Random error is a deviation that arises by chance between an observed value and a true value. The concept of random error, or chance variation, is important in epidemiology because it is central to the statistical analysis of data, as in the assessment of whether or not an observed association (e.g., an increase in relative risk estimates) may have arisen by chance. This can be accomplished by testing for statistical significance, whereby a p value is calculated to determine whether the null hypothesis should be rejected. Confidence intervals for estimates of relative risk or odds ratio provide further information as they indicate the range of values with which the data are consistent.

In epidemiologic studies, errors may occur through the random misclassification of subjects according to either exposure or disease status. Exposure status is often determined by questioning subjects about events that took place many years earlier, and some inaccuracies in the classification of exposure are inevitable. The determination of disease status, even when based on histologic material, is also subject to error; thus, some incorrectly classified diseased and nondiseased individuals may be included in a study. The careful development, pretesting, and validation of questionnaires and the use of independent assessments of disease status are important components of epidemiologic research.

The usual effect on study results of random error in exposure measurement is to conceal or reduce the magnitude of true associations rather than to give rise to associations that are spurious (Rothman, 1986). For example, if there is random misclassification of smokers and nonsmokers, then a study of whether smoking is associated with lung cancer will result in an underestimation of the relative risk due to smoking.

2.2.6 Bias

A study is biased if its results deviate from the truth. This could occur due to systematic error introduced by measurement, study design, data collection, or analysis. In contrast to random error, which is likely to conceal true associations, bias distorts the truth by giving rise to results that systematically either overestimate or underestimate associations. Bias, therefore, can create associations where none exist or magnify or diminish associations that are genuine.

Studies must be designed in such a way that bias is either prevented or, if this is impossible, checked to determine whether it has occurred and to estimate its influence on the results. A full discussion of the problem is beyond the scope of this chapter; details should be sought in standard epidemiologic texts (e.g. Rothman, 1986; Breslow and Day, 1987).

Many varieties of bias have been described (Sackett, 1979, Last, 1988); these can be classified into two general groups—those that affect the selection of subjects and those that affect the measurement of exposure (Rothman, 1986). A *selection bias* may occur if there are systematic differences in traits between those who are selected for study and those who are not.

Berkson's (or admission rate) *bias* is a type of selection bias that may arise in a case-control study of hospitalized individuals if differential rates of admission apply to those with cancer who were exposed to a putative risk factor as opposed to those with cancer who had no such exposure. The result of the bias is that subjects with cancer who are in hospital may have a higher (or lower) frequency of exposure than subjects with the same disease who are not in hospital. For example, a case-control study of lung cancer could underestimate the adverse effect of smoking in the population if it compared lung cancer cases to hospitalized controls because smoking is associated with many reasons for hospitalization (e.g., cardiovascular diseases). In this situation, the prevalence of smoking among controls would be higher than the true value in the general population. To overcome this potential bias, which may affect any hospital-based study, population-based designs are selected for many epidemiologic studies.

Prevalence-incidence (or length) bias refers to a distortion in the estimation of effect that would arise if exposure and survival after diagnosis were related. Neyman (1955) first recognized this bias as a possible explanation for the association observed between smoking and lung cancer, reasoning that if smokers with lung cancer had a better survival after diagnosis than did nonsmokers with the same disease, then smokers would be overrepresented in the population of subjects with lung cancer. Studies of patients with newly diagnosed lung cancer ultimately showed that the association with smoking persisted and thus was not explained by better survival among smokers. Nevertheless, the possibility that exposure might influence survival is important and is the reason that newly diagnosed (i.e., incident) cases are selected for case-control studies of disease etiology (Sackett, 1979).

Detection bias is a type of selection bias that occurs if there are systematic differences in the way cases are identified or assessed. If an exposure gives rise to clinical symptoms or signs that resemble those of cancer, it could cause clinicians to initiate a search for cancer. For example, drugs like stilbestrol can cause endometrial bleeding, and it has been suggested that the association found between estrogens and endometrial cancer may have arisen because estrogens caused endometrial bleeding, which then caused occult cancers to be detected. Detection bias is important in the epidemiology of diseases that have a long preclinical course and that may escape detection in the absence of a diagnostic search.

Information bias is defined as a distortion of study results due to differential accuracy of information relating to exposure or outcome between the comparison groups. *Recall bias,* which is a potentially important type of information bias in case-control studies, arises because diseased subjects are more likely to think about and recall previous exposure than are nondiseased controls. In genetic epidemiology there may be bias in information about illnesses in other family members, since family members who are themselves diseased are more likely to know about disease in other members of the family than are those who are not diseased.

2.2.7 Confounding and Effect Modification

Confounding is defined as a distortion of the effect of an exposure on risk that arises because of an association with other factors that affect risk (Last, 1988). Confounding, like bias, can cause a study to find spurious associations or can mask associations that are real. A confounding variable must satisfy two criteria: (1) it must be related to the risk of disease under study and (2) it must be associated with the exposure of interest (but not be a consequence of exposure). It is possible to control for confounding variables during data analysis, whereas other sources of bias can be averted only in the design or conduct of the study.

One example of a confounding variable is ingestion of alcohol when the risk of oropharyngeal cancer following exposure to cigarettes is under investigation. Both alcohol ingestion and smoking are risk factors for this disease. In addition, smokers are more likely than nonsmokers to ingest alcohol. Thus, confounding leads to uncertainty as to how much risk is due directly to smoking and how much is attributable to associated alcohol use.

Confounding can be dealt with either in the design or in the analysis of a study. Selection of matched cases and controls that are alike with respect to the confounder ensures that any difference between them in the exposure of interest is not due to confounding. However, matching may cause an increase in both the cost and the difficulty of doing the study, and it prevents an examination of the relationship between the confounder and the disease. In the statistical analysis of an etiologic study, confounding can be examined by assessing the frequency of exposure in cases and controls, among those with and without the potential confounding variable. In the above example, the effect of smoking on risk for oropharyngeal cancer could be distinguished from the effect of alcohol by examining the association between smoking and risk separately for groups defined according to alcohol consumption.

Effect modification, which is sometimes referred to as *interaction,* occurs when the effect of a putative causal factor differs according to the level of another factor (Last, 1988). For example, age modifies the effect of exposure to ionizing radiation on breast cancer risk, as the risk per unit dose varies with the age at which the exposure occurred (Howe and McLaughlin, 1996). In the example of oropharyngeal cancer, effect modification would be indicated if the relative risk for smoking differed between categories of alcohol consumption. Epidemiologic studies often collect information on numerous potential risk factors, which would result in many potential combinations; thus an unfocused search for statistical interactions would be subject to artifact because of spurious associations from multiple significance testing. Accordingly, the search for effect modifiers in a statistical analysis should be restricted to variables for which a biologic or theoretical model can first be justified. Examples of interactions between environmental and genetic factors on the risk of lung cancer are presented in Sec. 2.5.1.

2.2.8 Criteria for Inferring That Epidemiologic Associations Are Causal

Epidemiologic research that detects an association between an exposure and the risk of cancer must be interpreted carefully before it can be inferred that the association is causal. Guidelines that are used to distinguish causal from noncausal associations were first proposed by Hill (1971) and are listed below in descending order of importance.

Evidence from True Experiments in Humans Although randomized trials provide the strongest evidence of causality, for ethical reasons they cannot be performed to study putative causes of cancer in humans. Randomized studies of potential protective factors are feasible and trials on the role of vitamins and other dietary factors are likely to provide the most convincing epidemiologic evidence on the effect of these agents on cancer risk.

Strength of Association The stronger an association between an exposure and the risk of cancer, the less likely is it to be due to confounding or bias. The quantitative magnitude of a relative risk or odds ratio is thus a rough indication of whether the observed relationship is causal.

Consistency Associations between an exposure and cancer that are demonstrated repeatedly, by different investigators using different research methods, are more likely to be causal than those where different methods have generated different results. However, the same result obtained repeatedly from one research method does not necessarily strengthen it, because the same mistake may occur repeatedly. The absence of consistency does not rule out a causal role, because some studies may be better done and some effects may arise only under unusual circumstances

Temporality For an association to be causal, the exposure must precede the disease. This rather obvious requirement is always met in cohort studies by virtue of their design but is often difficult to establish in case-control studies. Increasing risk with increasing duration of exposure can be examined in case-control studies.

Gradient of Effect Exposure to possible causes of cancer is seldom an all-or-none phenomenon, and the incidence of cancer can usually be related to the level of exposure. Finding a relationship between increasing level of exposure and increasing risk strengthens a causal interpretation (e.g., the association between smoking and risk of lung cancer discussed in Sec. 2.4.1).

Biological Plausibility Associations between exposure and disease that agree with present knowledge about the reaction of cells and tissues to the expo-

sure make it more plausible that the association is causal. Thus, the results of animal experiments showing that estrogen induces hyperplasia followed by carcinoma in situ and invasive cancer of the endometrium make it more likely that the association between estrogen use and endometrial cancer in humans is causal. While the existence of supporting biologic information adds to the credibility of causal arguments, the absence of such support may arise from the incomplete state of available information and does not necessarily detract from causal interpretations. This limitation is illustrated by the difficulties experienced in demonstrating, in the laboratory, the teratogenic effects of thalidomide and the carcinogenic effects of cigarette smoke—both exposures whose causal association with human disease has been amply demonstrated.

Coherence The existence of supporting evidence, including epidemiological observations on the distribution of the causes of disease, makes causal interpretations of associations more likely to be correct. For example, the observed association between obesity and endometrial cancer gains credibility because of the independent associations between obesity and both diabetes and hypertension—disorders that are also associated with endometrial cancer.

Specificity An association between a single type of exposure and one disease may make it easier to infer causality. This only contributes to causal reasoning when it is present, as, for example, in the association between maternal exposure to diethylstilbestrol and clear-cell carcinoma of the vagina in offspring. The absence of specificity is of no importance at all, as is shown by the multitude of diseases that have been found to be associated with cigarette smoking.

2.3 DESCRIPTIVE EPIDEMIOLOGY OF HUMAN CANCER

2.3.1 Data Sources and Trends

Cancer incidence data are available in many countries from registries that monitor cancer occurrence in defined populations. The primary resource for international comparisons of incidence rates is *Cancer Incidence in Five Continents* (Parkin et al, 1992), which contains data from cancer registries around the world. In the United States, an important data source is the Surveillance, Epidemiology and End Results (SEER) program, which maintains cancer registries covering approximately 10 percent of the population. Incidence, mortality and survival data from the SEER program are published regularly in detailed statistical reports (Ries et al., 1994) and at a "web" site (www.seer.ims.nci.nih.gov). In Canada, one of the few countries with total coverage of its population by a national cancer registry, an overview of cancer incidence (e.g., Fig. 2.1), mortality, and survival data is published annually by the National Cancer Institute of Canada (NCIC 1997; www.cancer.ca/stats) and more detailed reports are published periodically (e.g., Statistics Canada, 1992).

Data from cancer registries can be used to describe the cancer burden in terms of person, place, and time. For example, Fig. 2.4 shows trends for the most frequently diagnosed cancers in Canada (excluding nonmelanoma skin cancer), which are breast cancer among women, prostate cancer among men, and lung cancer for women and men combined. The steady increase over time in age-standardized incidence rates for prostate cancer can be attributed partly to detection of occult cancer through use of a screening test based on serum levels of prostate-specific antigen (see also Chap. 20, Sec. 20.2.4), whereas the increase in lung cancer among women follows the increase in tobacco use by women. The patterns depicted in Fig. 2.4 for Canada are similar to those seen in the United States (Ries et al., 1994).

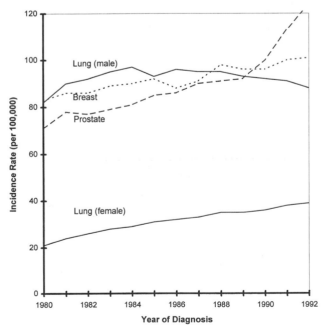

Figure 2.4. Trends in age-standardized incidence rates for the leading types of cancer in Canada, standardized to the 1991 Canadian population. (Adapted from National Cancer Institute of Canada, 1997.)

2.3.2 Geographic Distribution

Epidemiologic observations show a striking international variation in the frequency of specific types of cancer. Figure 2.5 uses data from *Cancer Incidence in Five Continents* to show examples of this variation. Breast cancer and prostate cancer have incidence and mortality rates that are generally low in Asian countries but high in Europe and North America. For example, there is a fivefold variation in breast cancer incidence between North America and Japan. In contrast, there can also be wide variation in risk within broad geographic regions, as for lung cancer, for which rates are much higher in Hong Kong than in Japan or China (Fig. 2.5A).

International differences in cancer incidence are due to a combination of genetic (inherited) and environmental factors. Evidence for genetic predisposition is summarized in Chap. 4, Sec. 4.2: the risk of developing several types of cancer is increased if other family members have been afflicted. Strong evidence for the importance of environmental factors comes from the study of migrant populations. Migrants who move from countries where the incidence of cancers such as breast and colon is low to countries where the incidence of these tumors is high eventually acquire the cancer incidence of the country to which they have moved. An example of this phenomenon is seen in breast cancer among Japanese migrants, where Japanese women born in Hawaii have an age-adjusted incidence of breast cancer that is about three times higher than that for women born and resident in Japan (Fig. 2.6). The rate at which this change in frequency of cancer takes place varies according to the type of cancer and the migrant group. Japanese migrants to North America acquire, within one generation, an incidence of colon cancer typical of North America but take two generations to show a substantial change in the incidence of breast cancer. These differences may be related to the rate at which migrant groups abandon their old culture, assimilate in the population, and adopt the culture of their new country. The implication of these migrant studies is that the international variation in cancer rates, while being due partly to genetic differences between *populations* of each country, is also due to some feature of life in those countries. Genetic differences between *individuals* may also influence the variation in cancer rates within countries. Further evidence in support of the importance of environmental factors is provided by observed changes in cancer rates within countries that have experienced rapid changes in their diet or lifestyle. An example is the rapid rise in

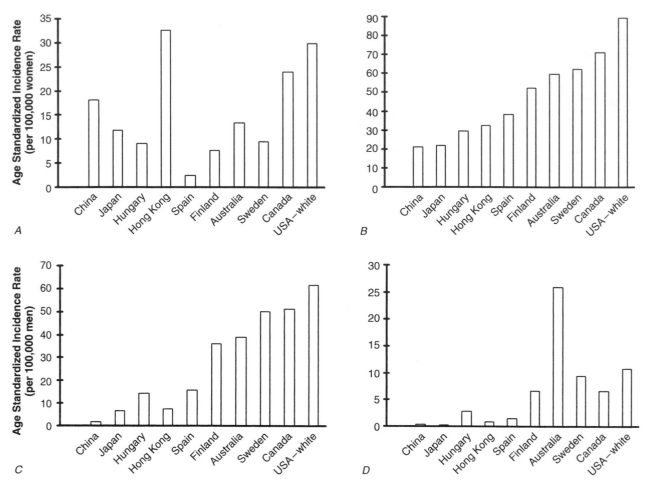

Figure 2.5. International variation in the incidence of selected types of cancer. *A.* Lung cancer in women. *B.* Breast cancer in women. *C.* Prostate cancer in men. *D.* Melanoma in men. (Adapted from Parkin et al., 1992.)

breast cancer incidence, and the adoption of a more "westernized" diet that has occurred in Japan since World War II.

2.3.3 Age Distribution

Age exerts a strong influence on the incidence of most common cancers. Figure 2.7 shows the relation between age and incidence of cancers of the lung, breast, prostate, and colon and rectum in Canada. For each type of cancer, the frequency of disease rises sharply with increasing age. In contrast to prostate and colorectal cancer, lung and breast cancer have an earlier age of onset and increase in incidence up to a certain age, after which age-specific rates decline. Analyses of these age-incidence curves have suggested implications for their causation. For example, the shape of these age-incidence curves was noted more than 40 years ago to be consistent with a multistage model of carcinogenesis (Armitage

and Doll, 1954), which was postulated subsequently to involve distinct mutational events (Knudson, 1973; see also Chap. 4, Secs. 4.2.1 and 4.5.1).

2.4 RISK FACTORS FOR CANCER

Analytic epidemiologic studies have identified a wide range of environmental and genetic factors that are determinants of cancer risk in the population. Some of the many environmental factors that have been associated with an increased risk of cancer are shown in Table 2.2. Reviews of these factors led to the conclusion that a large proportion of common cancers in the western world are potentially avoidable (Doll and Peto, 1981; Tomatis et al., 1990). The proportion of all cancer deaths in the United States that was attributable to specific environmental factors was estimated by Doll and Peto (1981) to be 30 percent for tobacco products, 35 percent for dietary factors, 3 percent for alcohol, and

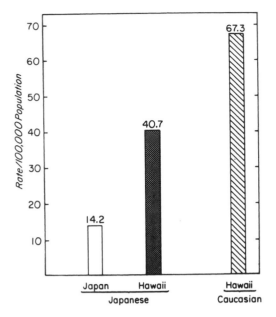

Figure 2.6. The incidence of breast cancer in Japanese women born in Japan, Japanese women born in Hawaii, and Caucasians born in Hawaii. (Adapted from Reddy et al., 1980.)

4 percent for occupational exposures. The evidence linking the most important environmental exposures to cancer risk is reviewed briefly in the following sections.

2.4.1 Tobacco

Tobacco use is the environmental exposure most widely known to be associated with an increased risk of cancer as well as several nonmalignant diseases. The associated cancers include lung, larynx, pharynx, esophagus, bladder, pancreas, kidney, and cervix (Table 2.2) (Tomatis et al., 1990). There is overwhelming evidence that active smoking causes cancer in humans (IARC, 1986), based in part on the consistent findings of significant associations in epidemiologic studies, the presence of strong dose-response relationships, and established biologic mechanisms of carcinogens found in tobacco smoke. The risk of lung cancer is 10- to 15-fold greater in smokers than nonsmokers (Doll et al., 1994) and increases dramatically with the amount smoked (Fig. 2.8).

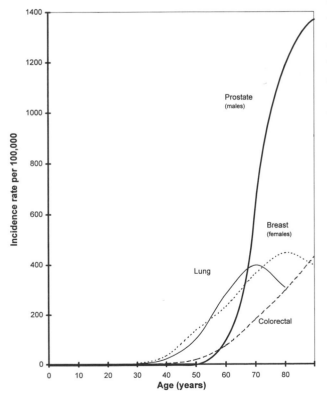

Figure 2.7. Relationship between age and cancer incidence rates in Canada for four types of cancer. (Adapted from National Cancer Institute of Canada, 1997.)

Table 2.2. Selected Environmental Causes of Cancer

Agent	Type of Cancer
Aflatoxin	Liver
Alcohol	Mouth, pharynx, larynx, esophagus, liver
Alkylating agents (e.g., cyclophosphamide)	Leukemia (myeloid)
Estrogens	Endometrium
Ionizing radiation	Leukemia, lung, skin, breast (and many other sites)
Polycyclic aromatic hydrocarbons (e.g., benzo[a]pyrene in tobacco smoke)	Skin, lung
Tobacco smoking	Lung, lip, mouth, pharynx larynx, esophagus, bladder, pancreas, kidney cervix
UV light	Skin, lip
Virus	
Hepatitis B	Liver (hepatoma)
Human papillomavirus	Cervix
Epstein-Barr virus	Nasopharynx, Hodgkin's disease, Burkitt's lymphoma

Source: Adapted from Schottenfeld and Fraumeni, 1996.

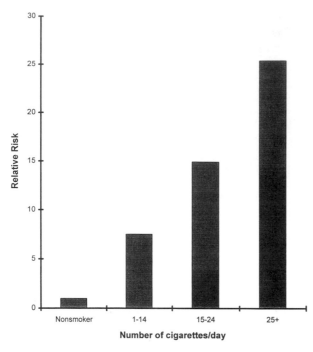

Figure 2.8. The increase in the relative risk of lung cancer in males according to number of cigarettes smoked. (Adapted from Doll et al., 1994.)

More than 30 case-control studies have examined the risk of lung cancer that is associated with environmental tobacco smoke (passive smoking). Many studies did not detect statistically significant associations, partly because sample sizes were not sufficient to detect small differences in risk. However, when data from existing studies were combined in meta-analyses, it was found that high exposures to second-hand smoke increased the risk of lung cancer, with a relative risk of approximately 1.3 to 1.5 (Blot and Fraumeni, 1989; EPA, 1992).

There is strong evidence that the risk of lung cancer associated with tobacco smoking is also influenced by an interaction with other exposures. The relative increase in risk due to smoking differs according to the level of exposure to certain genetic factors (see Sec. 2.5.1 regarding lung cancer), asbestos, radon (e.g., in uranium miners), nickel, and dietary factors (e.g., vitamin A intake; Saracci and Boffetta 1994).

2.4.2 Alcohol

Alcohol is associated with many cancers of the upper respiratory and digestive tracts but, more importantly, shows evidence of an interaction with tobacco in the etiology of these cancers. An interaction is in-

ferred from evidence that the combined effects of tobacco and alcohol on the risk of these cancers exceed the separate additive effects of these agents and that there is a dose-response relationship for each of them (Fig. 2.9).

There is also evidence that alcohol consumption may increase the risk of breast cancer. A meta-analysis of published studies that examined this relationship concluded that the data strongly supported an association between alcohol use and an increased risk of breast cancer and that there was evidence of a dose-response relationship (Longnecker et al., 1988). The combined relative risk was 1.24 (95 percent confidence interval = 1.15 to 1.34) for alcohol intake of two versus zero drinks per day.

2.4.3 Diet

Experiments in animals indicate that dietary variables—including dietary fat, total calories, and several micronutrients—influence carcinogenesis. Epidemiologic data suggest that some of this evidence is relevant to human cancer. For example, there are large differences between countries in dietary fat intake, and these correlate with the incidence of cancer of the breast (Fig. 2.10), colon, ovary, prostate, endometrium, and pancreas. These correlations do not necessarily imply cause and effect and might be due to other differences in lifestyle between countries of high and low incidence (Willett, 1989).

Prentice et al. (1988) showed that the association of breast cancer with dietary fat cannot be explained by international differences in the intake of total calories, weight, or parity. A pooled reanalysis of 12 case-control studies by Howe et al. (1990) showed strong evidence of a gradient of increasing risk of breast cancer with increasing intake of di-

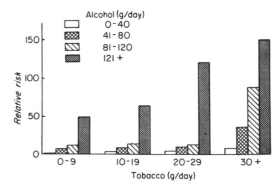

Figure 2.9. The relative risk of esophageal cancer, showing an interaction between alcohol and tobacco use. (Adapted from Doll and Peto, 1981.)

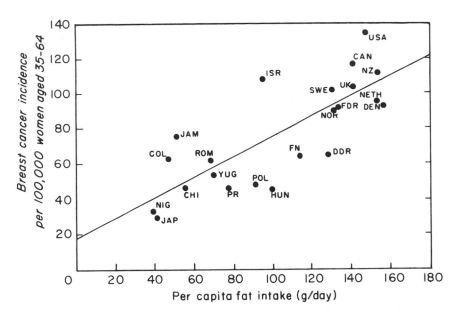

Figure 2.10. International variation in breast cancer incidence and per capita fat intake. (Adapted from Goodwin and Boyd, 1987.)

etary fat, whereas cohort studies had inconsistent results (Goodwin and Boyd, 1987). The limited range of fat intake in western populations combined with errors in estimating fat intake make it unlikely that observational epidemiology will be able to show major effects of dietary fat on breast cancer risk, even if the large international differences in disease rates are due entirely to fat. Experimental trials of dietary modifications that may protect against cancer are feasible, and several have been initiated, including trials of supplementation with beta carotene and fiber and trials of dietary fat reduction. Even though there was a strong prior expectation that beta carotene supplementation would reduce cancer risk, two of the three trials reported to date found that risk actually increased, while the other study found no effect (Omenn et al., 1996, Rowe 1996). It remains to be seen what will result from the trials of dietary fiber and dietary fat reduction.

The possible risks of cancer associated with chemicals that are added to food as preservatives or that contaminate food have been a source of widespread concern. Despite intensive investigation, there is little evidence to suggest that food additives are an important cause of human cancer. Some food additives, including antioxidants and other preservatives, minerals, and vitamins may inhibit the formation of carcinogenic compounds or otherwise block the process of carcinogenesis. Nitrites, which are used as food preservatives, are known to be converted in the body to nitroso compounds that are potent carcinogens in animals (see Chap. 8, Sec. 8.2.2); however, epidemiologic investigations have not found a major role for nitrites in the causation of human cancer. Studies of the potential effect of food contamination by chemicals have been stimulated by reports of associations between the risk of breast cancer and blood levels of metabolites from the insecticide DDT (Wolff et al., 1993). Although the biologic plausibility of such an association derives from the estrogen-mimicking effect of these organochlorine compounds, a causal role has not been established.

2.4.4 Occupational Exposures

Several occupational exposures are associated with an increased risk of cancer, and some of the occupations and agents known or suspected of causing cancer are listed in Table 2.3 (see also Chap. 8, Secs. 8.2 and 8.3). Important examples of industrial exposure include asbestos, which increases the risk of mesothelioma and lung cancer, and vinyl chloride, which increases the risk of angiosarcoma of the liver.

2.4.5 Hormonal and Reproductive Factors

Reproductive and sexual behavior influence risk for cancer of the breast, cervix, endometrium, and prostate. The risk of cervical cancer is increased by the number of sexual partners and by the early onset of sexual activity. These features suggested that a

Table 2.3. Selected Occupational Exposures That Influence Cancer Risk

Occupation	Agent	Type of Cancer
Dye manufacturers, rubber works	Aromatic amines (e.g., benzidine, napthylamine)	Bladder
Asbestos mining and handling	Asbestos	Lung, mesothelioma
Uranium miners	Ionizing radiation	Lung
Coal gas manufacturers, asphalters	Polycyclic aromatic hydrocarbons (e.g., coal tar)	Skin, lung
Farmers	UV light	Skin, lip
	Pesticides	Lymphoma
PVC manufacturers	Vinyl chloride	Liver (angiosarcoma)

Source: Adapted from Monson, 1996.

transmissible etiologic agent was involved and there is now strong evidence that human papillomavirus is a cause of cervical cancer (see Chap, 5, Sec. 5.2.3). The risk of breast cancer (see Sec. 2.5.2) and endometrial cancer is reduced in women who have had several pregnancies. In breast cancer, this influence appears to be due to a protective effect of a pregnancy resulting in a live birth early in a woman's life. Prostate cancer risk was found to be elevated among men who had a greater number of sexual partners, an earlier age at first intercourse or marriage, and a previous venereal disease; however, these associations have not been observed consistently (reviewed by Ross and Schottenfeld, 1996).

The relationship between cancer risk and levels of endogenous hormones—as well as the demonstrated relevance of hormones to carcinogenesis in some animal models (see Chap. 12, Sec. 12.3)—has prompted extensive investigation of the cancer risk associated with exogenous hormones. Both oral contraceptives and postmenopausal estrogens have been associated sometimes but not consistently with an increased risk of breast cancer (IARC, 1987; Vessey, 1985). A recently completed metanalysis found that breast cancer risk was increased slightly for 10 years after using oral contraceptives (Collaborative Group on Hormonal Factors in Breast Cancer, 1996). Conversely, there is more conclusive evidence that the use of oral contraceptives protects against ovarian cancer (IARC, 1987). In the 1970s an increased risk of endometrial cancer was seen in women who used oral contraceptives or estrogen replacement therapies containing unopposed estrogens, whereas the subsequent use of combinations that contained progestogen resulted in significantly

reduced risks (Grady et al., 1995; Weiss and Sayvetz, 1980).

2.4.6 Other Environmental Exposures

Exposure to ionizing radiation of any type is a rare but widely recognized cause of cancer. Risk estimates have been generated from large cohort studies of survivors of atomic bomb explosions in Japan and from individuals who received occupational or medical exposures to ionizing radiation. Many types of cancer are known to be caused by radiation, with the most firmly established dose-response relationships being for leukemia and cancers of the thyroid, breast, lung, stomach, colon, bladder, esophagus, and ovary (see Chap. 8, Sec. 8.5). Although for high doses the excess risk may be substantial, it is small or even undetectable for the low levels of exposure that occur most frequently in the population. There is no convincing evidence for the existence of a "threshold" of carcinogenic effect; thus, it is prudent to regard any exposure to ionizing radiation as potentially damaging (see Chap. 8, Sec. 8.5). Exposure to ultraviolet light is known to increase the risk of skin cancer of all types (basal cell, squamous cell, and melanoma), whereas the effects of electromagnetic fields have been inconsistent in epidemiologic studies (Tomatis et al., 1990).

The role of viruses in the etiology of cancer is discussed in Chap. 5. Despite substantial evidence from animals that viruses cause cancer, a definitive causal relationship between viruses and human cancer has been shown for only a few diseases, such as cervical cancer (human papillomavirus), hepatocellular carcinoma (hepatitis B virus) and Burkitt's lymphoma (Epstein Barr virus). The association of disease with serologic evidence of prior viral infection and with molecular evidence of viral genome or protein also provides strong evidence for a role for Epstein Barr virus as an etiologic agent in nasopharyngeal cancer.

In summary, many environmental factors may influence the risk of cancer. Detailed evaluations of the carcinogenic risk to humans for numerous agents are available in an extensive series published by the International Agency for Research on Cancer (e.g., IARC, 1987). A major task of health and environmental protection agencies is to evaluate the role of these factors and to set guidelines that are socially acceptable and will lead to a reduction in cancer incidence in the population.

2.5 SPECIFIC TYPES OF CANCER

A description of the epidemiology of three types of human cancer is presented in this section to illustrate some of the previously described epidemiologic methods and risk factors.

2.5.1 Lung Cancer

Lung cancer is the most common cause of cancer death for both men and women in the United States and Canada (Ries et al., 1994; NCIC, 1997). There is wide international variation in incidence rates, with Europe and North America having higher rates than Asia. Incidence rates continue to increase steadily among women in most western countries, whereas the much higher rates among men have remained stable or declined slightly in recent years (Fig. 2.4). These trends in incidence and the geographic distribution are largely attributable to tobacco use; for example, the increase in incidence among women follows the steady increase in the number of women who smoke.

The relationship between cigarette smoking and lung cancer is the most extensively documented etiologic relationship in cancer epidemiology. It is estimated that approximately 80 percent of lung cancer is due to tobacco smoke (Doll and Peto, 1981; Tomatis et al., 1990). Other risk factors include ionizing radiation and certain occupational exposures, such as organic chemicals, heavy metals, and asbestos. Smoking is more prevalent and carries a higher relative risk than other common exposures. For example, smokers have a 10- to15-fold greater risk of lung cancer than nonsmokers (Doll et al., 1994), whereas uranium miners who are exposed to radiation in the form of radon have a 2- to 5-fold in-

creased risk (Lubin et al., 1995) Several dietary risk factors have been identified, such as low intake of vitamins A, C, and E; however, the protective effects of these vitamins have not been consistently observed in dietary intervention trials (Omenn et al., 1996, Rowe et al., 1996).

Recent research has focused on the role of genetic susceptibility as a determinant of lung cancer risk. Case-control studies found that lung cancer risk was two- to fourfold greater among individuals with a family history of lung or other cancer (Tokuhata and Lilienfeld 1963, Shaw et al., 1991) — a pattern which could be due to either genetic or shared environmental factors. A genetic-epidemiologic analysis indicated that the familial pattern of lung cancer risk was consistent with Mendelian inheritance of an unknown susceptibility gene, the effect of which is expressed only in the presence of tobacco smoke (Sellers et al., 1992).

In the search for susceptibility genes, recent molecular-epidemiologic studies have focused on genes involved in the metabolism (e.g., cytochrome P-450 enzymes coded by CYP1A1, CYP2D6) and elimination (e.g., glutathione S-transferases) of carcinogens in tobacco smoke (see also Chap. 8, Sec. 8.2.3). In early studies of susceptibility, which relied on phenotypes such as the ability to metabolize debrisoquine, an increased risk of lung cancer was found among extensive metabolizers in some (Caporaso et al., 1990, Ayesh et al., 1984) but not all studies (Shaw et al., 1995, Wolf et al., 1992). It is now possible to determine the metabolic genotype, such as polymorphisms in the gene (CYP2D6) responsible for the metabolism of debrisoquine and certain chemicals contained in tobacco smoke (Gough et al., 1990). This has given more direct evidence of a "gene-environment interaction," as the association between metabolic genotype and risk of lung cancer was seen to differ according to smoking status. For example, while all smokers had an increased risk of lung cancer in the case-control study by London et al. (1995), smokers who had a CYP2D6 polymorphism (presumed to prevent formation of genotoxic activated metabolites) had a significantly lower risk (odds ratio for CYP2D6 = 0.57) than smokers who had the normal genotype.

Primary prevention is more feasible for lung cancer than for most other cancers, as the cause of the majority of cases is known and modifiable. Current research on genetic susceptibility may elucidate underlying mechanisms of carcinogenesis, but the reduction of tobacco use has the greatest potential for reducing the burden of lung cancer.

2.5.2 Breast Cancer

The incidence of breast cancer varies from 50 to 90 per 100,000 per year in high-risk areas such as Northern Europe, North America, and Australia (where it is the most common cancer in women) to less than 20 per 100,000 in low-risk areas such as Asia (Fig. 2.5*B*) (Ries et al., 1994; NCIC, 1997). Incidence rates for breast cancer have increased steadily in North America (Fig. 2.4), whereas mortality rates have remained relatively constant. Table 2.4 shows the major demographic and reproductive variables known to be associated with the risk of breast cancer. Most of the variables listed are associated with only a modest increase in risk and do not appear to explain the considerable international variation in the incidence of disease.

Several studies show that benign breast disease, in which there is hyperplasia associated with atypia in breast epithelium, increases the risk for subsequent breast cancer. As described in Sec. 2.4.3, there is a strong international correlation between dietary fat consumption and breast cancer incidence and mortality. Although studies have been somewhat inconsistent, a meta-analysis of published reports found that dietary fat intake was associated with a modest, but significant increase in risk (Boyd et al., 1993). Diet influences several risk factors, including hormone levels, age at menarche, age at menopause, and obesity. Support for a causal role of dietary fat has also been obtained from studies in experimental animals, where fat may promote the activity of carcinogens.

Family history is one of the strongest risk factors for breast cancer. It has been estimated that approximately 10 percent of breast cancer cases may be due to an inherited predisposition, and recent research has identified genes involved in breast cancer susceptibility (e.g., BRCA1 and BRCA1; see Chap. 4, Sec. 4.5.5). The risk associated with BRCA1 mutations has been shown to be modified by nongenetic risk factors such as parity, which in turn affects hormonal status (Narod et al., 1995). This observation is consistent with a general model of carcinogenesis, whereby breast cancer is thought to occur through the interaction of multiple biologic and environmental risk factors.

Epidemiologic studies of breast cancer provide the basis for a range of cancer-control initiatives. Intervention trials are in progress to assess whether breast cancer risk can be reduced by dietary changes. The high risk among women with a strong family history of breast cancer has led to proposals for genetic screening programs in which women who carry a susceptibility gene would be offered close follow-up or prophylactic surgery. Given the uncertain benefits of genetic testing for breast cancer susceptibility in terms of cancer incidence, mortality, and psychological impact, such programs must include in-depth genetic counseling and objective evaluation. At present, the greatest potential for reducing mortality due to breast cancer continues to be through mammographic screening, which enables the early detection of tumors.

2.5.3 Melanoma

Malignant melanoma of the skin is relatively rare, being about the tenth most common type of cancer in the United States and Canada, but incidence rates have been increasing steadily for many years (Ries et al., 1994; NCIC, 1997). There is more than a 20-fold international variation in incidence rates, with higher risks in Australia, New Zealand, and

Table 2.4. Demographic, Reproductive, and Other Risk Factors for Breast Cancer

Risk Factor	Higher-Risk Group	Lower-Risk Group	Relative-Risk Estimate
Age	Older	Younger	5–7
Country of residence	N. America, Europe	Asia, Africa	5–7
Age at first birth	Older	Younger	2–3
Number of births	None	Some	2–3
Age at menarche	Earlier	Later	1.5–2
Age at menopause	Later	Earlier	1.5–2
Oophorectomy	None	At young age	1.5–2
Body weight	Increased	Decreased	1.5–3
Height	Increased	Decreased	1.5–3

South Africa but low risks in Japan (Fig. 2.5*D*). There is an international gradient in incidence and mortality, with increasing risk closer to the equator. A similar gradient can be seen within the United States, where rates are up to twofold higher in the southern states. These observations led to the suggestion that exposure to the sun was a major determinant of risk. There are, however, anomalies in the distribution of disease that cannot be explained simply on the basis of exposure to sunlight, such as the observation that melanoma is more common in some parts of northern Europe than in the south.

An increased risk of melanoma has also been associated with host factors, including light hair or skin color, and the tendency to burn when exposed to the sun. The major environmental risk factors are exposure to sunlight, particularly when this is intermittent rather than continuous, as well as exposure to other sources of ultraviolet irradiation (Chap. 8, Sec. 8.5.5; Armstrong and English, 1992). A potential mechanism for the effects of ultraviolet light is seen in xcroderma pigmentosum, which is a rare hereditary disease characterized by deficient DNA repair after ultraviolet damage and ultimately predisposes to melanoma (see Chap. 4, Sec. 4.4.1). Further evidence for genetic predisposition is provided by the increased risk among individuals who have a family history of melanoma or who have a tendency to develop dysplastic nevi (Armstrong and English, 1992; Bale et al., 1992). This genetic susceptibility may be due partly to a tumor suppressor gene, such as *p16* (see Chap. 5, Sec. 5.5.3, and Chap. 7, Sec. 7.2.3), which is mutated in some patients with a strong family history of melanoma (Liu et al., 1995).

Preventive strategies applicable to the general population and high-risk subsets arise from the above epidemiologic observations. Population-based strategies that promote reduced sun exposure or increased protection from the sun (e.g., clothing, sunscreens) may reduce the frequency of disease. For individuals in high-risk families, there may be a role for genetic screening and clinical follow-up; however, the predictive value of such tests and the benefits of such programs remain to be demonstrated.

2.6 SUMMARY

Epidemiology is concerned with explaining the distribution of disease in individuals and populations. Descriptive epidemiology gives an account of the distribution of disease in terms of its frequency (incidence, prevalence, or mortality) in different geographic regions, the age and sex of affected individuals, and any associations with time. Analytic epidemiology attempts to explain observed variations in disease risk by identifying factors that are associated with the development of disease. The fundamental research designs for analytic epidemiology are the observational cohort study, case-control studies, and, occasionally, randomized trials. The application of these methods to the study of human cancer has shown large variations throughout the world in the incidence and mortality of most common cancers. This variation is due both to inherited differences between populations and to environmental factors: cancer rates change in migrant groups because of changes in diet, lifestyle, and other environmental factors. Analytic epidemiologic studies have identified several features of the environment that are associated with the risk of most common cancers, which are therefore, in principle, potentially avoidable. Once modifiable risk factors are known, primary prevention programs may be feasible; otherwise, prevention strategies need to focus on the detection of high-risk subsets of the population (e.g., as in genetic screening), or the early detection of disease (e.g., by mammography). Because of the widespread use of tobacco products and their strong association with many types of cancer, the control of tobacco use continues to have great potential to reduce the burden of disease and should be the first priority in cancer prevention.

REFERENCES

Armitage P, Doll R: The age distribution of cancer and a multi-stage theory of carcinogenesis. *Br J Cancer* 1954; 8:1–15.

Armstrong BK, English DR: Epidemiologic studies. In: Balch CM, Milton GW, Soong S (eds). *Cutaneous Melanoma*. Philadelphia: Lippincott; 1992:12–26.

Ayesh R, Idle JR, Ritchie JC, et al: Metabolic oxidation phenotypes as markers for susceptibility to lung cancer. *Nature* 1984; 312:169–170.

Bale SJ, Dracopoli NC, Tucker MA: The genetics of human malignant melanoma. In Balch CM, Milton GW, Soong S, eds. *Cutaneous Melanoma*. Philadelphia: Lippincott; 1992:93–100.

Blot WJ, Fraumeni JF: Passive smoking and cancer. In: DeVita VT, Hellman S, Rosenberg SA, eds. *Cancer Prevention*. Baltimore: Williams & Wilkins; 1989:1–10.

Boyd NF, Martin LJ, Noffel M, et al: A meta-analysis of studies of dietary fat and breast cancer risk. *Br J Cancer* 1993; 68:627–636.

Breslow N, Day N: *Statistical Methods in Cancer Research*: Vol II. *The Design and Analysis of Cohort Studies*. Lyon, France: International Agency for Research on Cancer; 1987.

Caporaso NE, Tucker MA, Hoover R, et al: Lung cancer and the debrisoquine metabolic phenotype. *J Natl Cancer Inst* 1990; 85:1264–1272.

Collaborative Group on Hormonal Factors in Breast Cancer. Breast cancer and hormonal contraceptives: Collaborative reanalysis of individual data on 53,297 women with breast cancer and 100,239 women without breast cancer from 54 epidemiological studies. *Lancet* 1996;347:1713-1727.

Doll R, Peto R: *The Causes of Cancer: Quantitative Estimates of Avoidable Risks of Cancer in the United States.* Oxford, England: Oxford University Press; 1981.

Doll R, Peto R, Wheatley K, et al: Mortality in relation to smoking: 40 years' observations on male British doctors. *Br Med J* 1994; 309:901–911.

EPA (Environmental Protection Agency): *Respiratory Health Effects of Passive Smoking: Lung Cancer and Other Disorders.* Washington, DC: US-EPA; 1992.

Goodwin P, Boyd NF: A critical appraisal of the evidence that dietary fat intake is related to breast cancer risk in humans. *J Natl Cancer Inst* 1987; 79:473–485.

Gough AC, Miles JS, Spurr NK, et al: Identification of the primary gene defect at the cytochrome P450 CYP2D locus. *Nature* 1990; 347:773–776.

Grady D, Gerbretsadik T, Kerlikowske K, et al: Hormone replacement therapy and endometrial cancer risk: A meta-analysis. *Obstet Gynecol* 1995; 85:304–313.

Hill BA: *Principles of Medical Statistics,* 9th ed. New York: Oxford University Press; 1971.

Howe GR, McLaughlin JR: Breast cancer mortality between 1950 and 1987 following exposure to fractionated dose rate ionizing radiation in the Canadian Fluoroscopy Study and a comparison with breast cancer mortality in the Atomic Bomb Survivors Study. *Radiat Res* 1996; 145:694–707.

Howe GR, Hirohata T, Hislop TG, et al: Dietary factors and risk of breast cancer: Combined analysis of 12 case-control studies. *J Natl Cancer Inst* 1990; 82:561–569.

IARC (International Agency for Research on Cancer): *IARC Monographs on the Evaluation of Carcinogenic Risks to Humans:* Vol 38. *Tobacco Smoke.* Lyon, France: IARC; 1986.

IARC (International Agency for Research on Cancer): *IARC Monograph on the Evaluation of Carcinogenic Risks to Humans:* Supple 7. *Overall Evaluations of Carcinogenicity: An Updating of IARC Monographs Volumes 1–42.* Lyon, France: IARC; 1987.

Khoury MJ, Beaty TH, Cohen BH: *Fundamentals of Genetic Epidemiology.* New York; Oxford University Press, 1993.

Knudson AG, Jr: Mutation and human cancer. *Adv Cancer Res* 1973; 17:317–352.

Last JM, ed: *A Dictionary of Epidemiology.* New York; Oxford University Press; 1988.

Liu L, Lassam N, Slingerland J, et al: Germline p16^{INK4A} mutation and protein dysfunction in a family with inherited melanoma. *Oncogene* 1995; 11:405–412.

London SJ, Daly AK, Leathart J, et al: Lung cancer risk and genetic polymorphism of CYP2D6 among African-Americans and Caucasians. *Proc AACR* 1995; 360:280.

Longnecker MP, Berlin JA, Orza MJ, et al: A meta-analysis of alcohol consumption in relation to breast cancer risk. *JAMA* 1988; 260:652–656.

Lubin J, Boice J, Edling C et al: Lung cancer in radon-exposed miners and estimation of risk from indoor exposure. *J Natl Cancer Inst* 1995; 87:817–827.

Monson R. Occupation. In: Schottenfeld D, Fraumeni JF Jr, eds. *Cancer Epidemiology and Prevention.* New York: Oxford University Press; 1996:373–405.

Narod S, Goldgar D, Cannon-Albright L, et al: Risk modifiers in carriers of BRCA1 mutations. *Int J Cancer* 1995; 64:394–398.

NCIC (National Cancer Institute of Canada): *Canadian Cancer Statistics—1997.* Toronto: NCIC; 1997.

Neyman J: Statistics: Servant of all sciences. *Science* 1955; 122:401–406.

Omenn G, Goodman G, Thornquist M, et al: Effects of combination of beta carotene and vitamin A on lung cancer and cardiovascular disease. *N Engl J Med* 1996;334:1150–5.

Parkin DM, Muir CS, Whelan SL, et al, eds: *Cancer Incidence in Five Continents:* Vol VI. Lyon, France: International Agency for Research on Cancer; 1992.

Prentice RL, Kakar F, Hursting S, et al: Aspects of the rationale for the women's health trial. *J Natl Cancer Inst* 1988; 80:802–814.

Reddy BS, Cohen LA, McCoy GD, et al: Nutrition and its relationship to cancer. *Adv Cancer Res* 1980; 32:237–345.

Ries LAG, Miller BA, Hankey BF, et al, eds: *SEER Cancer Statistics Review, 1973–1991: Tables and Graphs.* Bethesda; MD: National Cancer Institute; 1994.

Ross RK and Schottenfeld D. Prostate cancer. In: Schottenfeld D, Fraumeni JF Jr, eds: *Cancer Epidemiology and Prevention.* New York: Oxford University Press; 1996: 1180–1206.

Rothman K: *Modern Epidemiology.* Boston: Little Brown; 1986.

Rowe PM: Beta-carotene takes a collective beating. *Lancet* 1996; 347:249.

Sackett DL: Bias in analytic research. *J Chronic Dis* 1979; 32:51–63.

Saracci R, Boffetta P: Interaction of tobacco smoking with other sources of lung cancer. In: Samet JM, ed. *Epidemiology of Lung Cancer.* New York; Marcel Dekker; 1994:465–493.

Schottenfeld D, Fraumeni JF Jr; eds: *Cancer Epidemiology and Prevention.* New York: Oxford University Press; 1996.

Schlesselman JJ: *Case-Control Studies—Design, Conduct and Analysis.* New York: Oxford University Press, 1982.

Schulte P. A conceptual and historical framework for molecular epidemiology. In: Schulte PA, Perera FP: eds. *Molecular Epidemiology: Principles and Practices.* San Diego, CA: Academic Press; 1993.

Sellers TA, Bailey-Wilson JE, Potter J, et al: Effect of cohort differences in smoking prevalence on models of lung cancer susceptibility. *Genet Epidemiol* 1992; 9:261–271.

Shaw GL, Falk RT, Deslauriers J, et al: Lung cancer risk associated with cancer in relatives. *Cancer Epidemiol Biomed Prev* 1995; 4:41–49.

Shaw GL, Falk RT, Pickle LW, et al: Lung cancer risk associated with cancer in relatives. *J Clin Epidemiol* 1991; 44:429–437.

Statistics Canada: Cancer in Canada 1988. *Health Reports* 1992; 4(Suppl 8).

Tokuhata GK, Lilienfeld AM: Familial aggregations of lung cancer in humans. *J Natl Cancer Inst* 1963; 30: 289–312.

Tomatis L, Aitio A, Day N, et al, eds: *Cancer: Causes, Occurrence and Control.* Lyon, France: International Agency for Research on Cancer; 1990.

Vessey MP: Exogenous hormones. In: Vessey MP, Gray M, eds. *Cancer Risks and Prevention.* Oxford, England: Oxford University Press; 1985:166–194.

Weiss N, Sayvetz T: Incidence of endometrial cancer in relation to the use of oral contraceptives. *N Engl J Med* 1980; 302:551–554.

Willett WC: The search for the causes of breast and colon cancer. *Nature* 1989; 338:389–394.

Wolf CR, Smith CA, Gough AC et al: Relationship between debrisoquine hydroxylase polymorphism and cancer susceptibility. *Carcinogenesis* 1992; 13:1035–1038.

Wolff MS, Toniolo PG, Lee EW, et al: Blood levels of organochlorine residues and risk of breast cancer. *J Natl Cancer Inst* 1993; 85:648–652.

BIBLIOGRAPHY

DeVita VT, Hellman S, Rosenberg SA, eds: *Cancer Prevention.* Philadelphia: Lippincott; 1989.

Doll R, Peto R: *The Causes of Cancer: Quantitative Estimates of Avoidable Risks of Cancer in the United States.* Oxford, England: Oxford University Press; 1981.

Khoury MJ, Beaty TH, Cohen BH: *Fundamentals of Genetic Epidemiology.* New York: Oxford University Press; 1993.

Morton NE, Chung CS, eds: *Genetic Epidemiology.* New York: Academic Press; 1978.

Rothman K: *Modern Epidemiology.* Boston: Little Brown; 1986.

Schottenfeld D, Fraumeni JF Jr, eds: *Cancer Epidemiology and Prevention.* New York: Oxford University Press; 1996.

Schulte PA, Perera FP, eds: *Molecular Epidemiology: Principles and Practices.* San Diego: Academic Press; 1993.

3

Methods of Genetic Analysis

Jeremy A. Squire and Robert A. Phillips

3.1 INTRODUCTION

3.2 CHROMOSOMAL ANALYSIS OF CANCER CELLS
    3.2.1 Overview of Conventional Cytogenetic Techniques

3.3 MOLECULAR ANALYSIS
    3.3.1 Hybridization of Nucleic Acid Probes
    3.3.2 Restriction Enzymes
    3.3.3 Manipulation of Genes and Generation of a "Cloned" Probe or DNA Library
    3.3.4 Southern Blots
    3.3.5 Restriction Fragment Length Polymorphisms
    3.3.6 Sequencing of DNA
    3.3.7 Polymerase Chain Reaction
    3.3.8 Identification of Mutations in Tumors
    3.3.9 Specialized Application of the Polymerase Chain Reaction in Tumor Analysis

3.3.10 Putting New Genes into Cells
3.3.11 Site-Directed Mutagenesis
3.3.12 Transgenic and Knockout Mice

3.4 GENE MAPPING AND TUMOR ANALYSIS
    3.4.1 Linkage Analysis
    3.4.2 Somatic Cell Hybrids
    3.4.3 Electrophoretic Mapping Methods
    3.4.4 Fluorescence in situ Hybridization
    3.4.5 Comparative Genomic Hybridization
    3.4.6 Analysis of Tissue Sections and Single Cells

3.5 SUMMARY

REFERENCES

BIBLIOGRAPHY

3.1 INTRODUCTION

The level of understanding of any scientific phenomenon depends on the sophistication of the technology available for its investigation. In recent years, advances in the analysis of chromosomes and genes have occurred rapidly and have played a central role in the development of a conceptual understanding of cancer. Initial genetic analysis of tumors was limited to analyzing gross chromosomal abnormalities, but in recent years impressive progress in molecular biology has provided a diversity of molecular methods to understand the genetic processes that underlie chromosomal changes in cancer. This progress has resulted in the development of specific molecular tests to assay rapidly for genetic change in tumors. This chapter reviews the molecular and cytogenetic methods used in developing an initial understanding of the genetic basis of cancer, and highlights methodologies that are likely to affect cancer management in the future.

3.2 CHROMOSOMAL ANALYSIS OF CANCER CELLS

Cancer arises as a result of the accumulation of genetic changes that confer a selective advantage to the cells in which they occur. These changes consist of mutations together with numerical and structural chromosomal aberrations. They usually occur in somatic cells, but some of the genetic changes are heritable and cause a predisposition to cancer (see Chap. 4). While molecular techniques can identify the DNA mutations present in a tumor, cancer cytogenetics provides an overall description of chromosome number and the extent and nature of any cytogenetic abnormalities.

Chromosomes are recognized in preparations of metaphase cells by their size and shape and by the pattern of light and dark bands observed after staining by specific procedures. Methods for improving yields of dividing cells and for high-resolution banding of elongated chromosomes, developed in the

1980s, allowed precise definition of chromosomal aberrations in tumors as well as the identification of previously undetected rearrangements. With the use of these techniques, most tumor cells can now be shown to have chromosomal defects (reviewed in Heim and Mitelman, 1995).

Many different techniques are used to obtain dividing tumor cells for cytogenetic analysis. Leukemias and lymphomas are easily dispersed into single cells suitable for chromosomal analysis, and therefore, more data are available for these diseases than for solid tumors. Cells from lymphoid tumors can be obtained from peripheral blood, bone marrow, or lymph node biopsies. Because one property of malignant cells is their ability to proliferate autonomously, it is usually not necessary to stimulate them to divide or to incubate the cells in tissue culture prior to analysis.

In contrast to leukemias and lymphomas, cytogenetic analysis of solid tumors presents several difficulties. First, the cells are tightly bound together and must be dispersed by mechanical means or by digestion with proteolytic enzymes. These procedures can damage cells. Second, the mitotic index in solid tumors is often low, making it difficult to find enough mitotic cells to obtain good-quality cytogenetic preparations. Third, lymphoid and myeloid cells often infiltrate solid tumors as part of an inflammatory or immune response against the tumor, leading to chromosomal preparations that may not have originated from the malignant cell population. Despite these difficulties, cytogenetic analyses of cells from solid tumors have identified a large number of specific chromosomal aberrations. Subsequent studies have allowed some of the oncogenes involved to be recognized and cloned (see Chaps. 4 and 5). More recently, the study of solid tumors has been facilitated by new analytic approaches that combine elements of conventional cytogenetics with molecular methodologies. This new hybrid discipline is called *molecular cytogenetics,* and its application in tumor analysis usually involves the use of a powerful technique called *fluorescence in situ hybridization* (FISH—described in Secs. 3.4.4 to 3.4.6).

3.2.1 Overview of Conventional Cytogenetic Techniques

Chromosomes are conventionally examined during or just prior to the metaphase stage of mitosis, when they become condensed and have a defined, reproducible appearance under the microscope (Verma and Babu, 1995). DNA replication occurs before mitosis, so that each chromosome consists of two identical sister chromatids held together at the centromere. In making chromosome preparations, exposure of the tumor cells to colcemid or a related agent arrests them in metaphase by disrupting the formation of the mitotic spindle fibers that normally separate the chromatids. The cells are then swollen in a hypotonic solution, fixed in methanol-acetic acid, and metaphase "spreads" are prepared by dropping the fixed cells onto microscope slides.

Chromosomes are identified by one of several staining techniques, which produce a characteristic series of bands along the chromosomes. The most popular way of generating banded chromosomes is by a brief proteolytic digestion with trypsin, followed by exposure to Giemsa stain. The number of detectable dark-stained "G bands" depends on the quality of the chromosome spread and the stage of the cell in mitosis. Cells spread at prophase can have over 800 identifiable bands. However, a typical metaphase spread prepared using conventional methods (Fig. 3.1) has approximately 550 bands (reviewed in Verma and Babu, 1995). Analysis of G-banded chromosome preparations is performed using bright-field microscopy and photography. Modern cytogenetics laboratories usually use electronic cameras and analyze metaphase chromosomes with the help of computers attached to the microscope. The end result of cytogenetic analyses is a karyotype, which, in written form, describes the chromosomal complement using the internationally accepted cytogenetic nomenclature summarized in Table 3.1. An example of a high quality G-banded karyotype from a leukemic cell is shown in Fig. 3.1. A more detailed description of the accepted international nomenclature for describing chromosomes can be found in Heim and Mitelman (1995).

3.3 MOLECULAR ANALYSIS

The advances in technology that allow an analysis of genes at the nucleotide level have revolutionized the study of genetics, including the analysis of genetic changes in tumor cells. It has become possible to identify and isolate specific genes, and it is often easier to isolate a gene than its protein product. The nucleotide sequence can be determined from an isolated gene, and from the nucleotide sequence one can deduce the amino acid sequence of its putative product. It is possible to synthesize small peptides corresponding to the proposed amino acid sequence of the product and to make antibodies against this peptide sequence. Often the antibodies will react with the complete protein, allowing the subsequent isolation and purification of the gene

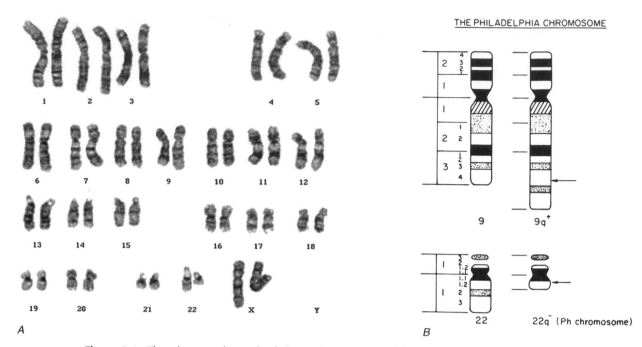

THE PHILADELPHIA CHROMOSOME

9   9q⁺

22   22q⁻ (Ph chromosome)

A

B

Figure 3.1. The photograph on the left (A) shows a typical karyotype from a patient with chronic myelogenous leukemia. By international agreement, the chromosomes are numbered according to their appearance following G-banding. Note the loss of material from the long arm of one copy of the chromosome 22 pair (*the chromosome on the right*) and its addition to the long arm of one copy of chromosome 9 (*also the chromosome on the right of the pair*). B. A schematic illustration of the accepted band pattern for this rearrangement. The arrows indicate the precise position of the break points that are involved. The karyotypic nomenclature for this particular chromosomal abnormality is t(9;22)(q34;q11). This description means that there is a reciprocal translocation between chromosomes 9 and 22 with break points at q34 on chromosome 9 and q11 on chromosome 22. The rearranged chromosome 22 is sometimes called the *Philadelphia chromosome* (or Ph chromosome), after the city of its discovery (adapted from Nowell et al.,1960, and Rowley, 1973). The molecular consequences of this abnormality are discussed in Chap. 5, Sec. 5.4.4.

product. The following sections concentrate on those techniques commonly used for the genetic analysis of tumors. For additional information, the reader is referred to comprehensive reviews on molecular genetics (e.g., Ausubel et al., 1996).

3.3.1 Hybridization of Nucleic Acid Probes

The ability of single-stranded complementary nucleic acids to hybridize, or renature, is fundamental to the majority of techniques currently used in molecular genetic analysis. The DNA of most organisms is double-stranded; that is, it is composed of two complementary strands of specific sequences of four nucleotide bases. When double-stranded DNA is heated, the complementary strands separate (denature) to form single-stranded DNA. Given suitable conditions, the separated complementary regions of DNA can join together to re-form a double-stranded molecule. This renaturation process is called *hy-*

Table 3.1. Nomenclature for Describing Chromosome Abnormalities

Description	Meaning
− 1	Loss of one chromosome 1
+ 7	Gain of extra chromosome 7
2q− or de12q	Deletion of part of long arm of chromosome 2
4p +	Addition of material to short arm or chromosome 4
t(9;22)(q34;q11)	Reciprocal translocation between chromosomes 9 and 22 with break points at q34 on chromosome 9 and q11 on chromosome 22
iso(6p)	Isochromosome with both arms derived from the short arm of chromosome 6
inv(16)(p13q22)	Part of chromosome 16 between p13 and q22 is inverted

bridization. The process is highly faithful, and when extensive hybridization has occurred, the resulting DNA duplex is very stable. DNA strands that are not highly complementary will not hybridize to one another or interfere with complementary strand hybridization. Duplexes can form between complementary single-stranded DNA molecules or between one DNA molecule and one RNA molecule.

The fidelity of base pairing in DNA replication is determined by the DNA polymerase enzymes that usually add only the correct base specified by the template strand in elongating a new strand. Commercial DNA polymerases are isolated and purified from *Escherichia coli* bacteria. The most frequently used polymerase enzyme is the large fragment of DNA polymerase I, often referred to as the *Klenow fragment*. This enzyme adds nucleotides to the 3'-hydroxyl end of an oligonucleotide hybridized to a template (Fig. 3.2), leading to synthesis of a complementary new strand of DNA. By including radionucleotides in the reaction mixture, the complementary copy of the template can be generated and used as a highly sensitive radioactive probe in techniques that depend on DNA hybridization, such as blotting (Sec. 3.3.4) or screening bacteria to isolate "cloned" DNA probes (Sec. 3.3.3). The success of most of the molecular biology–based techniques described in the following sections results from the extraordinary sensitivity of the hybridization process and the fidelity of nucleic acid synthesizing enzymes.

3.3.2 Restriction Enzymes

Restriction enzymes are endonucleases that have the ability to cut DNA only at specific sequences of nucleotides and that always cut the DNA at exactly the same place within the designated sequence. Restriction enzymes were first discovered in bacterial cells, where their functions include protection

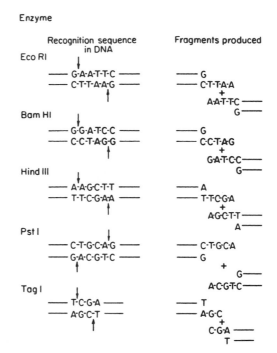

Figure 3.3. The nucleotide sequences recognized by five different restriction endonucleases are shown. On the left-hand side, the sequence recognized by the enzyme is shown; the sites where the enzymes cut the DNA are shown by the arrows. On the right side, the two fragments produced following digestion with that restriction enzyme are shown. Note that each recognition sequence is a palindrome; i.e., the first two or three bases are complementary to the last two or three bases. For example, for EcoR1, GAA is complementary to TTC. Also note that following digestion, each fragment has a single-stranded tail of DNA. This tail is useful in allowing fragments cut with the same restriction enzyme to anneal with each other.

against infecting viruses and perhaps participation in DNA repair and DNA recombination. Similar enzymes probably exist in mammalian cells, but few have been characterized. Figure 3.3 lists some commonly used restriction enzymes together with the sequence of nucleotides that they recognize and the position at which they cut the sequence.

The importance of restriction enzymes is that they allow DNA to be cut into reproducible segments that can be analyzed with great precision. For example, Fig. 3.4 presents a study of the *myc* gene using Southern blotting of DNA (see Sec. 3.3.4) from a number of human cell lines. After DNA is cut with EcoR1, this gene is found on a DNA fragment of 13 kilobase (kb) pairs. In contrast, an identical analysis of the cell line "Ramos" yields a much smaller fragment, indicating either mutation or rearrangement near this gene.

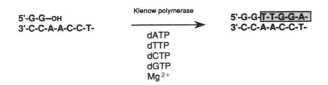

Figure 3.2. Synthesis of a complementary strand of DNA (*stippled*) using the "Klenow fragment" of DNA polymerase I. The substrate is a 3'-hydroxyl end of a primer hybridized to a single-stranded template. The primer is usually a short, synthetic, single-stranded oligonucleotide. All four nucleotides and magnesium ions are also required for DNA polymerases.

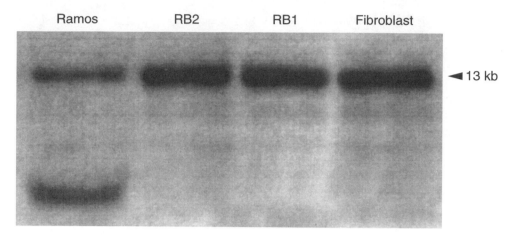

Figure 3.4. In the experiment shown, DNA was extracted from a normal fibroblast and from cells from two different retinoblastoma tumors (RB1, RB2); in addition, DNA was extracted from a Burkitt's lymphoma (Ramos). The DNA was digested with the restriction enzyme EcoR1 and probed with a DNA fragment specific for the c-*myc* oncogene. As shown in the figure, all of the samples have the usual germline-sized piece of DNA at 13 kb. However, in the Ramos tumor in which the t(8;14) translocation occurs in the middle of this oncogene, there is a new fragment of smaller size. Such an analysis illustrates the ease with which abnormalities in DNA can be detected by restriction endonuclease digestion and the Southern blot technique.

An important feature of many restriction enzymes is that they create "sticky ends." These ends occur because the DNA is cut in a different place on the two homologous strands. When the DNA molecule separates, the cut end has a small single-stranded portion that can hybridize to other fragments having compatible sequences (i.e., fragments prepared by digestion with the same restriction enzyme). The presence of sticky ends allows investigators to "cut and paste" pieces of DNA together, as described in Sec. 3.3.3.

3.3.3 Manipulation of Genes and Generation of a "Cloned" Probe or DNA Library

A gene contains DNA sequences that carry all of the information necessary to specify the amino acid sequence in the corresponding protein. In the chromosomes of higher organisms, the gene consists of coding and noncoding regions. These coding regions, called *exons*, are usually interrupted by noncoding transcribed regions, called *introns*. After the mRNA is synthesized on the DNA template, the sequences complementary to the introns are removed (spliced out), so that the mRNA is complementary only to the coding sequence. A complementary DNA strand (cDNA) can be synthesized using mRNA as the template and the enzyme reverse transcriptase. The cDNA then contains only the coding sequences (exons) of the gene from which the mRNA was transcribed.

Once a gene has been identified, the DNA segment of interest is usually inserted into a bacterial virus or plasmid to facilitate its manipulation and propagation. Figure 3.5 indicates schematically how a restriction fragment of DNA containing the coding sequence of a gene can be inserted into a bacterial plasmid that confers resistance against the drug ampicillin to the host bacterium. The plasmid or virus is referred to as a *vector* carrying the "passenger" DNA sequence from the gene of interest. The plasmid vector DNA can be cut with the same restriction enzyme used to prepare the cloned gene, so that all the fragments will have compatible sticky ends and can be spliced back together. The spliced fragments can be sealed with the enzyme DNA ligase, and the reconstituted molecule can be introduced back into bacterial cells. Because bacteria that take up the plasmid are resistant to the drug, they can be isolated and propagated to large numbers (Schaffner, 1980). In this way, large quantities of a gene can be obtained (i.e., "cloned") and labeled with radioactivity for use as a DNA probe for analysis in Southern blots (see Sec. 3.3.4), or labeled with biotin for use as a nonradioactive probe (see Sec. 3.4.4). Cloned DNA can be used directly for nucleotide sequencing (see Sec. 3.3.6), for transfer into other cells (see Sec. 3.3.10). Alternatively, the starting DNA may be a complex mixture of different restriction fragments derived from human cells. Such a mixture could contain enough DNA so

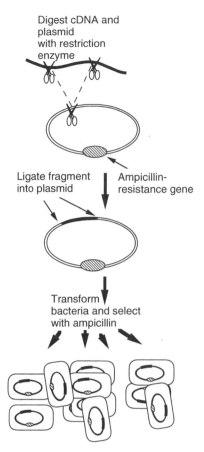

Digest cDNA and plasmid with restriction enzyme

Ligate fragment into plasmid

Ampicillin-resistance gene

Transform bacteria and select with ampicillin

Figure 3.5. Insertion of a human cDNA restriction fragment into a plasmid vector. The cDNA probe (*black line*) is digested with a restriction endonuclease (depicted by scissors) to generate a defined fragment of cDNA with "sticky ends." The circular plasmid DNA is cut with the same restriction endonuclease to generate single-stranded ends that will hybridize and circularize with the cDNA fragment under optimal ligation conditions. The recombinant DNA plasmid can be selected for growth using antibiotics because the ampicillin gene (*hatched*) is included in the construct. In this way large amounts of the human cDNA probe can be obtained

(1975), which involves the "blotting" of DNA onto a supporting matrix. The *Southern blot* technique is outlined schematically in Fig. 3.6. The DNA to be analyzed is cut into defined lengths using a restriction enzyme, and the fragments are separated by electrophoresis through an agarose gel. Under these conditions the DNA fragments are separated according to size, with the smallest fragments migrating farthest in the gel and the longest remaining near the origin. Pieces of DNA of known size are electrophoresed at the same time and act as a molecular weight scale. A piece of nitrocellulose or a nylon membrane is then laid on top of the gel and paper towels are placed on top of the nitrocellulose to draw fluid through the gel into the nitrocellulose paper. This blotting technique causes the DNA to migrate from the gel to the nitrocellulose paper, where it is immobilized and cannot diffuse further.

A common application of Southern blots is to determine the size of the fragment in the DNA that

that the entire human genome is represented in the passenger DNA inserted into the vector. When a large number of different DNA fragments have been inserted into a vector population and then introduced into bacteria, the result is a *DNA library* which can be plated out and screened by hybridization with a specific probe. In this way an individual *recombinant DNA clone* can be isolated from the library and used for most of the other applications described in the following section.

3.3.4 Southern Blots

A widely used method for analyzing the structure of DNA is the technique described by Southern

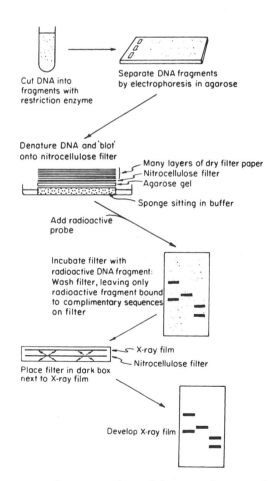

Cut DNA into fragments with restriction enzyme

Separate DNA fragments by electrophoresis in agarose

Denature DNA and 'blot' onto nitrocellulose filter

Many layers of dry filter paper
Nitrocellulose filter
Agarose gel
Sponge sitting in buffer

Add radioactive probe

Incubate filter with radioactive DNA fragment. Wash filter, leaving only radioactive fragment bound to complimentary sequences on filter

X-ray film
Nitrocellulose filter

Place filter in dark box next to X-ray film

Develop X-ray film

Figure 3.6. Schematic outline of the procedures involved in analyzing DNA fragments by the Southern blotting technique. The method is described in more detail in the text. A typical Southern blot is shown in Fig. 3.4.

carries a particular gene. For such an analysis, a cloned gene, propagated in a plasmid as described previously, can be isolated and made radioactive. The nitrocellulose filter containing all the fragments of DNA cut with a restriction enzyme is incubated in a solution containing the radioactively labeled gene. Under these conditions, the gene, usually called a *probe*, will anneal with homologous DNA sequences present on the nitrocellulose filter paper. Gentle washing will remove the single-stranded, unbound probe; hence the only DNA fragments remaining on the filter paper containing radioactively labeled material will be those homologous sequences that hybridized with the labeled probe. To detect the region of the filter paper containing the radioactive material, the filter is simply placed on top of a piece of x-ray film, enclosed in a dark container, and placed at $-70°C$ for several hours to expose the film. The film is then developed and the places where the radioactive material is located show up as dark bands. An alternative to conventional autoradiography is to use solid-state scintillation (phosphoimaging) to detect the location of radioactivity on blots. Phosphoimagers convert the energy released by radioactive molecules to visible light, which can be captured, digitized, and visualized using computer software. As discussed above, Fig. 3.4 shows a conventional autoradiogram of a Southern blot using a probe for one of the known oncogenes, c-*myc;* it shows that, after application of the restriction enzyme EcoR1, the gene is usually located on a piece of DNA 13 kb long.

An almost identical procedure can be used to characterize messenger RNA. In this case, RNA is separated by electrophoresis, transferred to nitrocellulose; and probed with a labeled, cloned fragment of DNA. The technique is called a *Northern blot* and is used to evaluate gross expression patterns of genes. An analogous procedure, called *Western blotting*, has also been devised to characterize proteins. Following separation by electrophoresis, the proteins are immobilized by transfer to nitrocellulose. To identify specific proteins, the nitrocellulose filter is incubated in a solution containing a specific antibody labeled with iodine 125 (^{125}I). The antibody will bind only to the region of the filter containing the protein used to induce the antibody, and the region of radioactivity can be located by the exposure of x-ray film. Proteins can also be detected by chromogenic or luminescent assays such as enhanced chemiluminescence (ECL) (Ausubel et al., 1996). This technique uses a second antibody coupled to horseradish peroxidase (HRP) to detect filter-bound antibodies. The bound second antibody is then visualized by the ECL light emissions that fol-

low the HRP substrate reaction, and the image is captured on film. The technique is more convenient to use than ^{125}I labeling because it requires autoradiographic film exposure of only minutes rather than days and it also avoids the use of radioactivity.

3.3.5 Restriction Fragment Length Polymorphisms

Restriction enzymes recognize specific sequences in DNA. Thus any mutation within a recognition sequence will prevent that sequence from being recognized by that restriction enzyme. Mutations at sites recognized by restriction enzymes therefore lead to changes in the length of the fragments that are obtained after digestion of DNA with such enzymes. Such mutations can occur as polymorphisms (i.e., changes in DNA that do not alter gene function), and when a polymorphism is present at a defined restriction enzyme site, it can be very useful for genetic analysis. Because such polymorphism leads to a difference in length of the fragments carrying the piece of DNA used for analysis, they are referred to as restriction fragment length polymorphisms (RFLPs).

The way RFLPs can be used for genetic analysis is illustrated in Fig. 3.7. In a normal cell, there are two copies of each piece of DNA, one derived from the maternal chromosome (M) and one from the paternal chromosome (P). The restriction sites for a specific restriction enzyme (designated by the arrows) are shown for each chromosome. Suppose that, in a given individual, the first restriction site to the right of a unique DNA sequence on the paternal chromo-

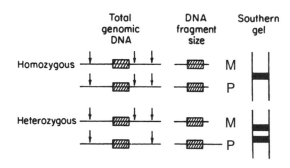

Figure 3.7. The principle of the method of detection and analysis of restriction fragment length polymorphisms (RFLPs) is illustrated. The individual labeled as homozygous contains two identical chromosomes with respect to the specific fragment of cloned DNA. In the individual labeled as heterozygous, one of the restriction enzyme sites has mutated; this results in the cloned DNA fragment appearing on a larger piece of DNA in that individual. It is important to note that with this technique, it is unnecessary to know the function of the fragment of DNA used in the analysis. The only requirement for RFLP analysis is that the cloned DNA fragment be unique—i.e., be present in only a single copy at a single location in the human genome.

some has mutated and is missing. The result of this mutation is that the gene will be found on a smaller fragment of DNA from the maternal chromosome than from the paternal chromosome. Thus, a Southern blot of DNA from the cells will show two bands, one identifying the maternal chromosome and one identifying the paternal chromosome. Mutations at restriction sites are inherited like any other genetic trait and can be used for linkage analysis (see Sec. 3.4.1) or can identify submicroscopic chromosomal deletions in tumors (see Chap. 4; Sec. 4.3.3).

3.3.6 Sequencing of DNA

The primary method for characterizing genes and the proteins that they encode is to determine the sequence of the DNA. The most frequently used method is dideoxy-chain termination, developed by Sanger (1981). This method is described here and is shown diagrammatically in Fig. 3.8. For other methods of DNA sequencing, see Ausubel et al. (1996).

Initially the DNA fragment to be sequenced must be isolated, as described in Sec. 3.3.3. To obtain single-stranded DNA for sequencing, one often takes advantage of a bacterial phage called M13. The fragment to be sequenced can be inserted into the DNA of the replicative form of this virus, as shown in Fig. 3.8. The unique feature of the M13 virus is that the virus particles released by an infected bacterium contain only single-stranded DNA. Thus, isolation of a plaque derived from recombinant phage will contain single-stranded DNA, including the fragment to be sequenced.

Sequencing is achieved by the method shown in Fig. 3.8 and involves the generation of a complementary DNA strand using DNA polymerase and the M13 primer. In brief, four different reaction mixtures are prepared. Each mixture contains the DNA polymerase enzyme and all the deoxynucleotide triphosphates (dATP, dCTP, dTTP, and dCTP); one nucleotide precursor will be labeled with radioactive sulfur or phosphorus. In addition, each of the four reaction mixtures will contain a limiting amount of one dideoxy nucleotide. For example, in the mixture containing dideoxy CTP (ddCTP), synthesis will occur as usual, with a "C" being inserted wherever there is a "G" in the template. Occasionally, the enzyme will choose ddCTP instead of dCTP. When ddCTP is incorporated into the new polynucleotide strand, DNA synthesis terminates because ddCTP lacks the 3'-hydroxyl group required for further chain elongation. Thus, termination will occur only at positions opposite a G, but because proportionally more dCTP is present than ddCTP, a set of fragments of different lengths are generated.

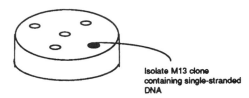

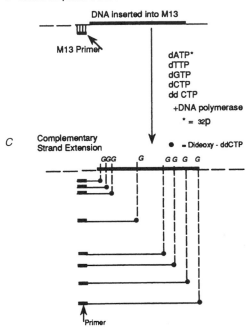

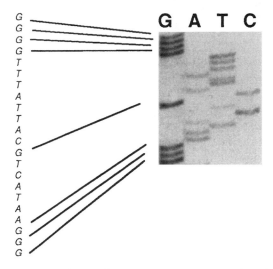

Figure 3.8. Dideoxy-chain termination sequencing showing an extension reaction to read the position of the nucleotide guanidine (see text for details). (Part D courtesy of Lilly Noble, University of Toronto, Toronto.)

Thus, in the mixture containing ddCTP, all of the fragments will initiate at the primer and terminate at one of the G positions in the DNA.

Separation of the newly synthesized radioactive DNA on polyacrylamide gels allows visualization of each fragment produced in the sequencing reaction. The use of polyacrylamide gels allows fragments differing by a single base to be separated (see Fig. 3.8D). When the four different reaction mixtures are run side by side on an acrylamide gel, one obtains a characteristic sequencing ladder that can be used to read the sequence of the DNA directly as shown in the figure. Usually a sequence of 200 to 500 bases can be read from a single gel.

When the sequence of a gene has been determined, it is entered into an international computer-based data bank. Genes can be recognized as regions of DNA that are in the register and can encode an amino acid sequence. Genes usually have characteristic sequence elements at the 5' initiating promoter region of DNA and also have specific sequence configurations at the 3' termination region. Once the region of DNA containing a gene has been characterized, comparisons are made with the sequences of genes that have been recorded previously to determine whether there may be regions of homology. This method has permitted the classification of some genes into families, such as the immunoglobulin supergene family (see Chap. 11, Sec. 11.2.6). Genes within these families have homologies ranging from 65 to 100 percent similarity and probably evolved from a common ancestral gene.

The human genome project is an international collaboration that aims to sequence the entire human genome. One of the challenges of this project has been to find ways to improve the cost, speed, and accuracy of DNA sequencing. The fastest current method involves sequence analysis by *capillary electrophoresis,* utilizing fluorescent nucleotides and a computerized sequence reader. Parallel tiny fiber-optic glass tubes containing a special polyacrylamide sieving medium replace conventional polyacrylamide gels. The sequence ladder is labeled with fluorescent nucleotides and it is "read" directly by the computer as each fragment migrates past an optical reader. Under experimental conditions, a four-color detection array has been shown to sequence with 97 percent accuracy at a rate of approximately 150 bases in 10 min (Woolley et al.,1995). In the future it is likely that there will be improvements in the resolution and sensitivity of capillary microsequencers.

3.3.7 Polymerase Chain Reaction

One of the major limitations of blotting techniques is that a large number of cells is required to produce enough DNA or RNA for conventional hybridization analysis, and signals obtained are often so weak that visualization requires several days of autoradiography. The polymerase chain reaction (PCR) addresses this problem of sensitivity. A unique DNA polymerase enzyme called *Taq* (which is resistant to denaturation at high temperatures) and specific oligonucleotide primers are used to increase the amount of target DNA for analysis. Analysis by PCR requires precise knowledge of the sequences flanking the region of interest. Usually DNA of about 200 to 1000 base pairs is amplified. Two short oligonucleotides homologous to the flanking regions can then be synthesized or obtained commercially, and these are used as primers for *Taq* polymerase. To amplify DNA, all components of the reaction—target DNA, primers, deoxynucleotides, and *Taq* polymerase—are placed in a small tube. The reaction sequence is accomplished by simply changing the temperature of the reaction mixture (see Fig. 3.9A). A typical PCR reaction would be as follows:

1. Incubation at 94°C denatures (separates) the DNA duplex and creates single-stranded DNA.
2. Incubation at 53°C allows hybridization of new primers that are in vast excess (this temperature may vary depending on the sequence of the primers).
3. Incubation at 72°C allows *Taq* polymerase to synthesize new DNA from the primers.

Repeating this cycle permits another round of amplification (Figure 3.9B). Each cycle takes only a few minutes, the precise time depending on the nature of the primers and the length of DNA to be amplified. Generally, 25 to 40 cycles can be completed in 2 to 5 h. Twenty cycles can theoretically produce a millionfold amplification that can usually be visualized as a bright ethidium bromide-stained band after a short period of gel electrophoresis (Fig. 3.9C). The products of PCR can then be sequenced or subjected to any of the conventional methods of genetic analysis. PCR has improved and greatly simplified many of the early, more cumbersome techniques of molecular biology required for isolating and analyzing cloned genes. Recently, polymerase proteins with greater heat stability and copying fidelity have been developed, allowing for long-range amplification using primers separated by as much as 15 to 30 kb of intervening target DNA (Ausubel et al., 1996).

The polymerase chain reaction is exquisitely sensitive and its applications include the detection of minimal residual disease in hemopoietic malignancies and of circulating cancer cells from solid tumors. Experiments have shown that as few as one

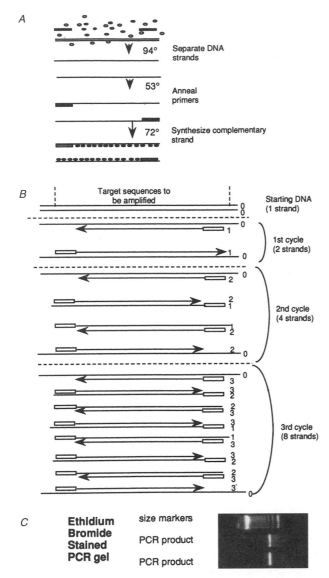

Figure 3.9. *A.* Reaction sequence for one cycle of PCR. Each line represents one strand of DNA; the small rectangles are primers and the circles nucleotides. *B.* The first three cycles of PCR shown schematically. *C.* Ethidium bromide–stained gel after 25 cycles of PCR. (See text for further explanation.)

leukemic cell in 10^5 to 10^6 normal cells can be detected with the appropriate PCR conditions.

With a slight modification, PCR can also be used to study gene expression or screen for genetic mutations in RNA. It is first necessary to use reverse transcriptase to make a complementary single-strand DNA copy (cDNA) of an mRNA prior to performing the PCR. The cDNA is used as a template for a PCR reaction as described above. This technique, which is usually called *reverse transcriptase PCR* (RT-PCR), allows amplification of cDNA corresponding to both abundant

and rare RNA transcripts, thereby providing a convenient source of DNA that can be screened for mutations. The RT-PCR technique can also provide approximate quantitation of expression of a particular gene (Ausubel et al., 1996). It is ideal for the detection of tumors with reciprocal chromosome translocations, since the fusion transcript generated by the rearrangement (see Chap. 4, Sec. 4.3) is present only in tumor cells and thus provides a unique substrate for RT-PCR detection. The PCR technology is used increasingly to detect gene rearrangements and molecular markers for use in diagnosis and prognosis (reviewed in Sheer and Squire, 1996).

3.3.8 Identification of Mutations in Tumors

Molecular mutations of DNA may be as small as a single base-pair substitution or can involve deletion or substantial rearrangement of thousands of base pairs of DNA. Smaller mutations present the biggest challenge, since identification of a single nucleotide change among thousands of nucleotides may be required. Most methods depend on identifying mismatched bases formed when complementary strands of a mutant and its normal sequence are allowed to hybridize to form a heteroduplex (double-stranded DNA, where each strand originates from a different source). Heteroduplexes will form when the PCR products from a heterozygous individual are denatured and cooled to allow single mutant strands amplified from one chromosome to base-pair with complementary strands from the normal chromosome. The electrophoretic mobility of a heteroduplex in polyacrylamide gels is less than that of homoduplexes, and this method for detection of mutation is referred to as a *heteroduplex mobility shift assay*. Detecting homozygous mutations in a tumor using a heteroduplex mobility shift assay requires addition of some normal DNA to the DNA under test (Keen et al., 1991).

Single-stranded DNA has a tendency to adopt complex conformational structures stabilized by weak intramolecular hydrogen bonds, and the electrophoretic mobility of such structures under nondenaturing conditions will depend on their shape. When a mutation is present in the DNA, different electrophoretic mobilities will arise. The technique that allows detection of these different forms of DNA is called *single-strand conformational polymorphism analysis* (SSCP). In typical SSCP experiments, PCR primers are radiolabeled and the DNA samples are amplified and then heated to make the PCR product single-stranded before it is subjected to nondenaturing polyacrylamide gel electrophoresis. Control samples must be run on the same gels so that differences from the wild-type electrophoretic pattern can be detected. Although SSCP is rapid and easy to perform, it does not reveal the nature or position of any mutation detected (Sheffield et al., 1993). Mutations of the *p53* gene (see Chap. 4, Sec. 4.5.3, and Chap. 5, Sec. 5.5.2) are frequently assayed by SSCP.

The technique of *RNase protection* allows for the accurate detection and quantitation of mutations in a gene. Radiolabeled RNA probes (Sec. 3.3.1) covering the coding region of the gene of interest are hybridized to total RNA from the cell or to the cDNA that has been amplified by PCR (Sec. 3.3.7). These hybridized molecules are then exposed to RNase enzymes, which cut single- but not double-stranded RNA. If there is a mismatch in nucleotide sequence between the radiolabeled RNA and the cellular RNA or the cloned cDNA, the RNase will cut within the radiolabeled RNA, and when the strands are denatured, two labeled fragments will result. These fragments can be detected by electrophoresis, as illustrated in Fig. 3.10.

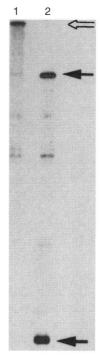

Figure 3.10. Detection of a molecular mutation in the RNA of the RB1 gene by RNase protection. Lane 1 is the expected size-protected fragment of the normal gene (*916 base pairs, open arrow*). Lane 2 contains RNA from a retinoblastoma tumor which only produces RNA containing a mutation. Because this mutation results in failure to hybridize to a part of the normal RB1 RNA, the RNase enzyme is able to cut the RNA and produce two fragments of 646 (*upper solid arrow*) and 270 (*lower solid arrow*) basepairs. The presence of a small deletion was confirmed by sequencing this region of RB1. (Courtesy of Dr. J Dunn, Visible Genetics Inc., Toronto)

The *protein truncation assay* (Roest et al. 1993) is a specific test to identify any mutations in a gene that lead to a shortened protein product. The method provides an indication of the type and position of a mutation and also confirms the nature of the functional defect. It is particularly useful for identification of frameshift, splice site, or nonsense mutations in a gene. The procedure involves making a cDNA copy of mRNA from the cells of interest by RT-PCR, using a special primer that includes a promoter and sequences that allow initiation and translation as well as sequences specific to the gene of interest. The cDNA PCR product is then placed in a transcription-translation system that makes mRNA and then translates the mRNA transcript into a protein product (Ausubel et al., 1996). The polypeptide product is run on a gel with normal control material and the size of truncated products indicates the position of the gene mutation. Two disadvantages of this approach are that some mutations do not alter the reading frame of the protein and will go undetected. Other mutations lead to unstable mRNA, making it difficult to obtain sufficient mutant cDNA for subsequent analysis (Dunn et al., 1989).

3.3.9 Specialized Application of the Polymerase Chain Reaction in Tumor Analysis

A major goal of cancer research is to isolate the unknown genes that characterize malignant cells. Old methods of distinguishing mRNA derived from differentially expressed genes relied mainly on differential hybridization or *subtraction hybridization*. For example, a subtracted cDNA library was used to isolate T-cell antigen receptor cDNAs. By repeatedly hybridizing T-cell cDNA to B-cell mRNA and selecting the nonhybridizing single-stranded cDNA molecules, it was possible to make a subtracted library in which a large percentage of the clones were T cell-specific (Yanagi et al., 1984). Such methods, while sometimes successful, are technically demanding and have largely been superseded by more convenient PCR-based approaches.

Differential display mRNA (Liang and Pardee, 1992) is a form of RT-PCR in which the reverse transcriptase initiates cDNA synthesis at the very end of a gene. Because the mRNA transcripts of nearly all mammalian genes have a tract of adenine residues at their 3' end, it is possible to use an oligonucleotide containing several thymidine residues to hybridize to the majority of expressed genes in a population of mRNAs. If the oligonucleotide GATTTTTTTTTTTT is used as a primer, it will preferentially prime cDNA synthesis

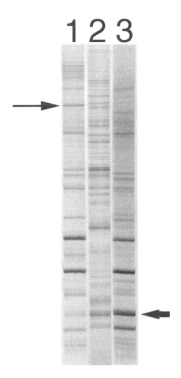

Figure 3.11. Electrophoretic pattern following differential display PCR analysis of mRNA. Radioactive DNA fragments generated by RT-PCR are size-fractionated by polyacrylamide gel electrophoresis and x-ray film is placed on top of the dried gel to display the "bar code" profiles of the expressed genes in the mRNA pool. In this experiment the profiles of two different muscle tumors (*lanes 1 and 3*) are compared with the pattern generated by a related embryonal tumor of the liver (*lane 2*). Notice that some bands are common to all three tumors and that the pattern in the two muscle tumors is similar in contrast to the pattern generated by the liver tumor display analysis. One band (*short arrow*) is very dark, indicating that it is highly expressed in one of the muscle tumors; another band (*long arrow*) is unique to the muscle tumor in lane 1.

from the polyadenine tail of any mRNA whose 3' end sequence is CT-poly A. The second primer is an arbitrary decamer sequence that can bind to a random subset of sequences. The resulting amplification pattern produces a complex ladder of cDNA bands when separated using high-resolution denaturing polyacrylamide gel electrophoresis (see Fig. 3.11). Some applications of differential display analysis compare gene expression under different physiologic conditions. Other approaches have studied expression at different developmental stages or have compared expression in normal and malignant tissue (Liang et al., 1992). These studies have identified a subset of genes whose expression patterns are different between the cell types. By isolating specific bands from the gel, performing further cycles of PCR, and then checking the differential expression of the genes in the original cell populations, cDNA clones of differentially expressed genes can be obtained rapidly.

3.3.10 Putting New Genes into Cells

The function of a gene can often be studied most effectively by placing it into a cell different from the one from which it was isolated. For example, one may wish to place a mutated oncogene, isolated from a tumor cell, into a normal cell to determine whether it causes malignant transformation (see Chap. 5, Sec. 5.4.1). A number of transfection protocols have been developed for efficient introduction of foreign DNA into mammalian cells, including calcium phosphate or DEAE-dextran precipitation, spheroplast fusion, lipofection, electroporation, and transfer using viral vectors (Ausubel et al., 1996). For all methods, the efficiency of transfer must be high enough for easy detection, and it must be possible to recognize and select for cells containing the newly introduced gene.

The standard method for introducing DNA into cells for experimental manipulations is the *calcium phosphate precipitation* technique (Graham and van der Eb, 1973). In this method, calcium phosphate is used to precipitate DNA in large aggregates; for unknown reasons, some cells take up large quantities of such DNA. The mechanism by which *DEAE-dextran transfections* allow for introduction of foreign DNA into cells is similar. It is believed that the positive charge of the DEAE-dextran polymer neutralizes the negative charge of the DNA polymer, forming a fine precipitate that can come into contact with the plasma membrane of the host cell. The DEAE-dextran/DNA complex is then internalized by pinocytosis. Other delivery systems involve the use of *viral vectors*, since they can be targeted to a variety of cell types, persist, and can infect nondividing cells (see also Chap. 18, Sec. 18.2.2). Retroviruses are very stable, since their complementary DNA integrates into the host mammalian DNA, but only relatively small pieces of DNA (up to 10 kb) can be transferred. Adenovirus vectors take larger inserts (~36 kb) and have a very high efficiency of transfer. Nonviral vectors, such as liposomes, are often used for transient expression of introduced DNA. For *lipofection*, plasmid DNA is complexed with a liposome suspension in serum-free medium. This DNA/liposome complex is added directly to cells grown in tissue culture plates, and after a 3- to 5-h incubation period, fresh medium containing serum is added. The cells are incubated to allow expression of the transfected gene. Whichever method is used to introduce the DNA, it is often necessary to select for retention of the transferred genes before assaying for expression. For this reason, a selectable gene, such as the gene encoding resistance to the antibiotic neomycin or to the anticancer drug methotrexate, can be introduced simultaneously by taking advantage of the fact that frequently cells that can take up one gene will also take up another.

3.3.11 Site-Directed Mutagenesis

The large increase in the number of genes being cloned without any knowledge of their function means that methods of studying protein function and secondary structure have become increasingly important. Sometimes important clues concerning the function of a new gene are provided by the occurrence of regions of similarity in the amino acid sequence that can lead to similarities in secondary structure. For example, many of the transcription-factor proteins have a characteristic sequence in which DNA-binding takes place (e.g., leucine-zipper or zinc-finger domain; see Chap. 6, Sec. 6.3.6). One way of testing the putative function of such a sequence is to see whether a mutation within the critical site causes loss of function. In the example of transcription factors, a mutation might result in a protein that failed to bind DNA appropriately. Because naturally occurring mutations are random, a large number must be screened to find one at a site of interest. Site-directed mutagenesis permits the introduction of mutations at a precise point in a cloned gene, resulting in specific changes in the amino acid sequence and hence secondary structure of an encoded protein.

By site-directed mutagenesis, amino acids can be deleted, altered, or inserted, but for most experiments, the changes do not alter the reading frame and disrupt protein continuity. There are two main ways of introducing a mutation into a cloned gene (Ausubel et al., 1996). The first method relies on the chance occurrence of a restriction enzyme site in a region one wishes to alter. Typically, the gene is digested with the restriction endonuclease, and a few nucleotides may be inserted or deleted at this site by ligating a small oligonucleotide complementary to the sticky end of the restriction enzyme (see Fig. 3.12A). The second method is more versatile but requires more manipulation. The gene is first obtained in a single-stranded form by cloning into a vector such as M13 (see Sec. 3.3.3). A short oligonucleotide is synthesized containing the desired nucleotide change but otherwise complementary to the region to be mutated. The oligonucleotide will anneal to the single-stranded DNA but contains a mismatch at the site of mutation (see Fig. 3.12B). The hybridized oligonucleotide-DNA duplex is then exposed to DNA polymerase I (plus the four nu-

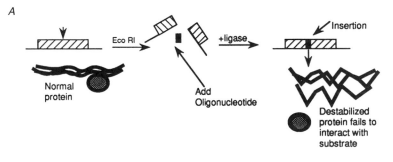

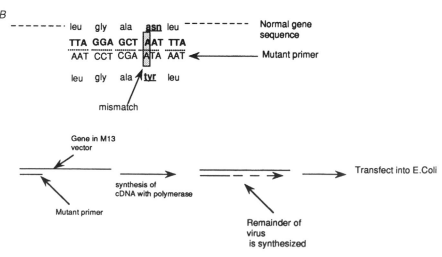

Figure 3.12. Methods for site-directed mutagenesis. *A.* Insertion of a new sequence at the site of action of a restriction enzyme by ligating a small oligonucleotide sequence within the reading frame of a gene. *B.* Use of a primer sequence that is synthesized to contain a mismatch at the desired site of mutagenesis.

cleotides and buffers), which will synthesize and extend a complementary strand with perfect homology at every nucleotide except at the site of mismatch in the primer used to initiate DNA synthesis. The double-stranded DNA is then transfected into bacteria, and because of the semiconservative nature of DNA replication, 50 percent of the M13 phage produced will contain normal DNA and 50 percent the DNA with the introduced mutation. Several methods allow easy identification of the mutant M13 virus. Using these techniques, the effects of artificially generated mutations can be studied in cell culture systems or in transgenic mice (see Sec. 3.3.12).

Another approach to studying a gene by functional inactivation is to introduce a DNA or RNA sequence that will specifically inactivate the expression of a target gene. This can be achieved by introducing DNA or RNA molecules with a sequence that is homologous to that contained within a target gene but where the order of the bases is opposite to that of the usual complementary strand (i.e., 3'→5' instead of 5'→3'). Several investigators have demonstrated that *antisense RNA or DNA* molecules can combine in vitro specifically with their homologous sequences in mRNA and interfere with the expression of that gene (reviewed in Crooke and Lebleu, 1993). An extension of antisense technology is *DNA triple helix formation,* in which a short oligonucleotide binds to *double-stranded DNA* by Hoogsteen hydrogen bonds and sterically hinders gene expression. Such approaches have potential for therapy of tumors—for example, by inhibiting expression of an oncogene. A limitation of all current antisense techniques is that once the antisense nucleic acids enter a cell, they are vulnerable to a variety of cellular nucleases. To be biologically effective, a high concentration of molecules is required inside the cells for a prolonged period of time.

3.3.12 Transgenic and Knockout Mice

One way to investigate the effects of gene expression in specific cells on the function of the whole organism is to transfer genes directly into the germline and generate transgenic mice (Palmiter and Brinster, 1985). For example, inappropriate expression of an oncogene in a particular tissue can provide clues about the possible role of that oncogene in normal development and in malignant transformation. Usually a cloned gene with the desired regulatory elements is microinjected into the male

pronucleus of a single-cell embryo so that it can integrate into a host chromosome and become part of the genome of the growing organism. If the introduced gene is incorporated into the germline, the resulting mouse will become a founder for breeding a line of mice, all of which carry the newly introduced gene. Such mice are called *transgenic mice,* and the inserted foreign gene is called a *transgene.* Its expression can be studied in a variety of different cellular environments in a whole animal. Each transgene will have a unique integration site in a host chromosome and will be transmitted to offspring in the same way as a naturally occurring gene. However, the site of integration often influences the expression of a transgene, possibly because of the activity of genes in adjacent chromatin. Sometimes the integration event also alters endogenous gene expression (insertional mutation), producing a recognizable phenotype. This observation led to the development of gene-targeting approaches, so that specific genes could be inactivated or "knocked out" as potential murine models of human diseases.

Site-directed in vivo mutagenesis is the method by which a mutation is targeted to a specific endogenous gene. Instead of introducing a modified cloned gene at a random position as described in the previous section, a cloned gene fragment is targeted to a particular site in the genome by a procedure called *homologous recombination* (reviewed in Zimmer, 1992). This technique relies on the ability of a cloned mammalian gene or DNA fragment to preferentially undergo homologous recombination in a normal somatic cell at its naturally occurring germline position, thereby replacing the endogenous gene. The introduced mutation may result in the "knocking out" of gene expression, thus facilitating the study of gene function (Fig. 3.13). The same approach can be used to correct a disease mutation in the mouse and restore normal function, thereby allowing murine models for gene therapy to be developed.

In typical targeting experiments, the desired genetic modification is either generated in cloned DNA by techniques described in Sec. 3.3.11 or, more usually, the gene is disrupted by insertion of a drug resistance gene into the middle of an endogenous gene, making it impossible to produce the normal protein product. Initially the modified DNA is introduced into pluripotent stem cells derived from a mouse embryo (called *ES* cells). The frequency of homologous recombination is low (less than one in a million cells) but is greatly influenced by a variety of factors such as the vector being used, the method

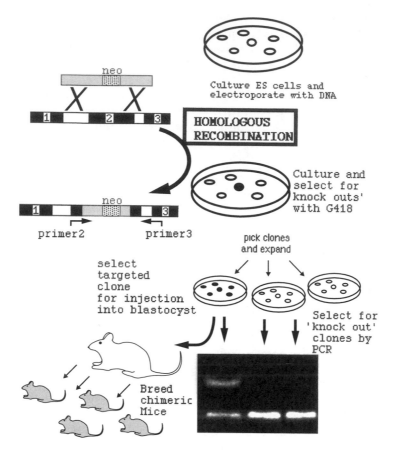

Figure 3.13. Disruption of a gene by homologous recombination in embryonic stem (ES) cells. Exogenous DNA is introduced into the ES cells by electroporation or by one of the methods described in Sec. 3.3.10. The homologous region on the exogenous DNA is shown in gray, the selectable gene neomycin (neo) is speckled, and the target exons are black. The two recombination points are shown by X's and the exogenous DNA replaces some of the normal DNA of exon 2, thereby destroying its reading frame by inserting the small "neo" gene. ES cells that have undergone a successful homologous recombination are selected as colonies in G418 because of the stable presence of the neo gene. PCR primers for exons 2 and 3 are used to identify colonies in which a homologous recombination event has taken place. ES cells from such positive cells (*dark colony*) are injected into blastocysts, which are implanted into foster mothers (*white*). If germ line transmission has been achieved, chimeric mice are bred to generate homozygotes for the "knocked out" gene.

of DNA introduction, the length of the regions of homology, and whether the targeted gene is expressed in ES cells. Homologous recombination with cloned sequences creates predictable novel DNA junctions in the genome, which can be conveniently detected by PCR. Oligonucleotide primers flanking the chosen site of recombination will generate the correct larger-sized PCR product only if the modified DNA fragment is present at the site of insertion. The ES cells that contain the modified gene are selected by growth in medium containing the drug G418, for which resistance is programmed by the modified gene, and these cells are cloned and tested with PCR for homologous recombination. Once an ES cell line with the desired modification has been isolated and purified, ES cells are injected into a normal embryo, where they often contribute to all the differentiated tissues of the chimeric adult mouse. If gametes are derived from the ES cells, then a breeding line containing the modification of interest can be established. Recent technologic advances in gene targeting by homologous recombination in mammalian systems enable the production of mutants in any desired gene.

3.4 GENE MAPPING AND TUMOR ANALYSIS

Once a gene or gene function has been identified, it is necessary to map it to a specific chromosome. Mapping of genes provides clues about which genes are affected by chromosome breaks or other abnormalities. For example, the observation that the *abl* oncogene was located on chromosome 9 near the region of the breakpoint in the Ph chromosome stimulated investigators to examine the tumor cells for possible involvement of the *abl* oncogene in this rearrangement (Heisterkamp et al., 1983).

Many methods allow localization of the genes that constitute the human genome. At the time of writing (spring 1997), it is estimated that 10 to 20 percent of the human genes have been sequenced and mapped and that mapping of the whole human genome will be completed soon after the turn of the century. The following sections describe methods used for mapping a specific gene or gene function to a specific chromosome that are being applied to the analysis of tumors.

3.4.1 Linkage Analysis

Linkage analysis of human genes has utilized DNA from large families with a high incidence of a specific disease. If two genes are close together on a chromosome, they tend to be inherited as a single unit (i.e., they appear "linked" together). Any two markers on a single chromosome can segregate (i.e., separate) through the phenomenon of meiotic recombination, but the closer the two genes are together on a chromosome, the less likely they are to be separated by a crossover during meiosis. Thus, one can attempt to map a new gene by looking for its linkage with other previously mapped genes. If several large families are available for analysis, one can also look for meiotic recombination and obtain an estimate of the distance of separation of two linked genes. The distance between genes in a linkage map is given in recombination units or centimorgans (1 cM = a meiotic recombination frequency of 1 percent in offspring).

The assignment of the retinoblastoma gene to chromosome 13 was confirmed by its close linkage to an enzyme, esterase D (ESD), which had been mapped previously to chromosome 13. Esterase D exists as isozymes that may be separated by electrophoresis, and many individuals are heterozygous

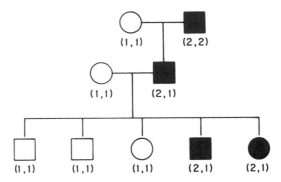

Figure 3.14. This pedigree shows the segregation of retinoblastoma (*solid symbols*) and esterase D isozymes (*indicated in parentheses below each symbol*). It is obvious that the chromosome with the retinoblastoma mutation must be linked to the chromosome containing isozyme type 2. In the second generation, the male with retinoblastoma is heterozygous for the ESD isozymes. In the third generation, only the children inheriting chromosome 13 with the type 2 isozyme developed retinoblastoma. This family illustrates the linkage of the retinoblastoma phenotype with the ESD locus.

for the type 1 and type 2 isozymes. Figure 3.14 shows a family in which both the retinoblastoma genes and the esterase D genes can be followed. This small family shows the close linkage between retinoblastoma and ESD. There has only been a single observation of a recombination between the two loci, indicating that they are approximately 1 cM or about 1 million base pairs of DNA (see Table 3.2) apart. If the assays for the genes being investigated are simple and if there are several families or a very large family available for investigation of linkage, this technique can provide rapid and accurate information about gene localization. However, reliable results require the examination of many members of several families. DNA polymorphisms have recently been recognized in which a large number of

Table 3.2. Size of Components of the Human Genome

Size of haploid genome	3.3×10^9 DNA base pairs
Estimated genetic constitution	40,000–100,000 genes
Size of average chromosome band	3×10^6 DNA base pairs
1 cM[a] (1% recombination)	1×10^6 DNA base pairs
Size of average gene	5×10^4 DNA base pairs[b]

[a]cM = centimorgan.

[b]An estimate of the proportion of the genome occupied by an average-size gene.

Source: Based on Lewin, 1994.

different alleles for a variety of genes can be readily assayed by PCR (Dracopoli, 1996). These are the best markers to obtain initial information on linkage of a novel genetic trait such as the familial clustering of cancer.

3.4.2 Somatic Cell Hybrids

The first method for mapping genes involved the use of somatic cell hybrids. A hybrid cell can easily be formed by fusing a rodent cell, such as a mouse fibroblast, and a human cell, such as a human fibroblast. The hybrid cells usually express most of the genes expressed by the two parent lines. As the human-rodent hybrid cells are propagated in tissue culture, the hybrids tend to lose human chromosomes and retain the rodent chromosomes. Shortly after fusion, loss of chromosomes occurs rapidly, but the hybrid cell becomes more stable after many human chromosomes have been lost. If a series of subclones are derived from an original hybrid cell line after the period of maximum chromosome loss, the cells in these clones will contain close to a full complement of mouse chromosomes and a random sample of human chromosomes. The individual human chromosomes in the somatic cell hybrid can be identified by PCR screening with sets of chromosome-specific primers. By collecting hybrid cell lines with different sets of human chromosomes, it is possible to generate a panel of hybrid cells that can be used to map any human DNA sequence to an individual chromosome (reviewed in Verma and Babu, 1995).

Use of somatic cell hybrids as described simply locates the gene somewhere on the chromosome, but refinements can allow a more precise localization of the gene. For example, it is possible to make a series of hybrid cells beginning with parental lines that have chromosomal deletions or translocations. After loss of human chromosomes, some of the hybrids will contain only a portion of one or more human chromosomes. The use of high-dose irradiation to disrupt chromosomes allows the generation of hybrid cells containing specific chromosomal fragments that can be screened by PCR or Southern blotting to produce a high-resolution ordered linear map for a region of interest (Walter et al., 1994).

3.4.3 Electrophoretic Mapping Methods

Conventional analysis of chromosomal DNA using Southern blotting (see Sec. 3.3.4) utilizes restriction mapping with resolutions limited by the frequency of the recognition sites and by the resolution of con-

ventional electrophoresis (~20 kb). The common restriction endonucleases listed in Fig. 3.3 cut DNA once every few thousand base pairs. The recognition sequences for the rare-cutter restriction endonucleases are more complex, typically 6 to 8 bp long, which are rare in DNA. As a result, they generate fragments that are several hundred kilobases in size. A new method of electrophoresis called *pulsed-field gel electrophoresis* (PFGE) is capable of separating such fragments of DNA (reviewed in Ausubel et al., 1996); it conveniently bridges the resolution gap between conventional Southern blot analysis and FISH chromosomal mapping methods (see below). Because a single chromosome band contains approximately 3 million base pairs of DNA, PFGE permits analysis of the component pieces of DNA. The technique has been useful in characterizing hybrid cells derived after irradiation of one of the cell types used in fusion and in physical mapping of deletion and translocation break points in tumors.

3.4.4 Fluorescence in situ Hybridization

Fluorescence in situ hybridization (FISH) has become an essential tool for mapping of genes and for characterization of chromosome aberrations (Verma and Babu, 1995). DNA probes—specific for a gene, chromosome segment, or whole-chromosome—are labeled, usually by incorporation of biotin and/or digoxigenin, and are then hybridized to metaphase chromosomes. Just prior to hybridization, metaphase chromosome spreads (Sec. 3.2) are heated briefly to ~75°C with 70% formamide in buffered isotonic saline to denature the chromosomal DNA and the slides are incubated with the labeled DNA probe from the gene to be studied. The DNA probe will reanneal to the denatured piece of DNA at its precise location on the chromosome. After the unbound probe is washed off, the hybridized sequences are detected using avidin, which binds strongly to biotin, and/or antibodies to digoxigenin, coupled to fluorescein isothiocyanate (FITC), Texas red, or another fluorochrome. The sites of hybridization are clearly visualized as fluorescent points of light where the probe is bound to chromatin. The advantage of FISH for gene mapping is that information is obtained directly about the positions of probes in relation to chromosome bands or to other previously mapped reference probes (Lichter et al., 1990).

By careful observation, it is possible to order genes and DNA segments that are 2 to 3 Mb or more apart using FISH with longer prophase chromosome preparations. However, many of the deletions and other rearrangements in the chromosomes of tumors are submicroscopic. To overcome these difficulties, a number of different high-resolution chromatin-based FISH methods have been developed (reviewed in Dracopoli et al., 1996). The resolution obtained with these FISH techniques (from a few kilobases to more than 10 Mb) is an extremely useful range for the physical ordering of genes on normal and abnormal chromosomes. An example of the power of high-resolution FISH analysis is shown in Fig. 3.15E in which a homogeneously staining region (HSR) in a neuroblastoma cell line with amplification of the N-*myc* gene (discussed below and in Chap. 5, Sec. 5.4.3) is shown in "stretched" or extended form.

FISH can be performed on interphase nuclei from tumor biopsies or cultured tumor cells, which enables cytogenetic aberrations to be visualized without the need for obtaining good quality metaphase preparations. Gene amplification as a mechanism of oncogene activation is discussed in Chap. 5, Sec. 5.4.3. In Fig. 3.15A and B, the cytogenetic changes present when gene amplification has taken place are shown. However, by using FISH with the N-*myc* probe against neuroblastoma cells, it is easy to detect massive copy number changes per cell (Fig. 3.15C through E). Numerical chromosome aberrations can also be detected using specific centromere probes that give two signals from normal nuclei but one signal when there is only one copy of the chromosome (monosomy) or three signals when there is an extra copy (trisomy) (Fig. 3.15F). Chromosome deletions can also be detected by using probes from the deleted region and counting the signals. If the probes used for FISH are close to specific translocation break points on different chromosomes, they will appear joined as a result of the translocation generating a "color fusion" signal (Fig. 3.15G). These procedures are particularly useful for rapid detection of aberrations such as the *bcr-abl* rearrangement in chronic myeloid leukemia (see Chap. 4, Sec. 4.3.2, and Chap. 5, Sec. 5.4.4), thus providing immediate and directly quantitative diagnostic information.

3.4.5 Comparative Genomic Hybridization

If the cytogenetic abnormalities are unknown, it is not possible to select a suitable probe for FISH detection in metaphase or interphase nuclei. Fortunately a new screening method called *comparative genomic hybridization* (CGH) has been developed that allows investigators to produce a detailed map of the differences between chromosomes in different cells. This method detects increases (amplifications) or decreases (deletions) of segments of DNA (Kallioniemi et al., 1992).

In typical CGH experiments, DNA from malignant and normal cells such as fibroblasts is labeled with two different fluorochromes and then hybridized simultaneously to *normal* chromosome metaphase spreads. Tumor DNA is labeled with biotin and detected with fluorescein (green fluorescence); the control DNA is labeled with digoxigenin and detected with rhodamine (red fluorescence). Regions of gain or loss of DNA sequences in the tumor, such as deletions, duplications, or amplifications, are seen as changes in the ratio of the intensities of the two fluorochromes along the target chromosomes (Fig. 3.16). An amplified sequence will generate increased green fluorescence, whereas a deletion will shift the red/green ratio toward red. For low-copy-number amplifications and hemizygous deletions, this change in fluorescence ratio is difficult to distinguish by eye and requires specialized image analysis software. One disadvantage of CGH is that it can detect only large blocks (>5 Mb) of over- or underrepresented chromosomal DNA; balanced rearrangements such as inversions or translocations escape detection. The CGH method has gained wide acceptance as a new and promising approach for understanding the complex cytogenetic changes in solid tumors (Bryndorf et al., 1995).

Subtle rearrangements in the karyotype that do not change the copy number can be detected by spectral karyotyping or the *"SKY" technique* (Schrock et al., 1996). It allows for the simultaneous recognition of all human chromosomes using combinations of 23 different colored probes (paints) as a "cocktail probe." Subtle differences in fluorochrome labeling profiles within the cocktail allow the computer to assign a unique color to each chromosome pair, so that extremely complex rearrangements in the karyotype can be identified by the pattern of color distribution along the abnormal chromosome. In combination, CGH and SKY will likely provide a much more detailed description of the highly abnormal karyotypes often present in advanced carcinomas.

3.4.6 Analysis of Tissue Sections and Single Cells

Tissue in situ hybridization techniques rely upon the hybridization of a specifically labeled nucleic acid probe to the cellular RNA in individual cells or tissue sections (Ausubel et al., 1996). Early studies described the localization of viral or abundant cellular messages in cultured cells or tissue sections using

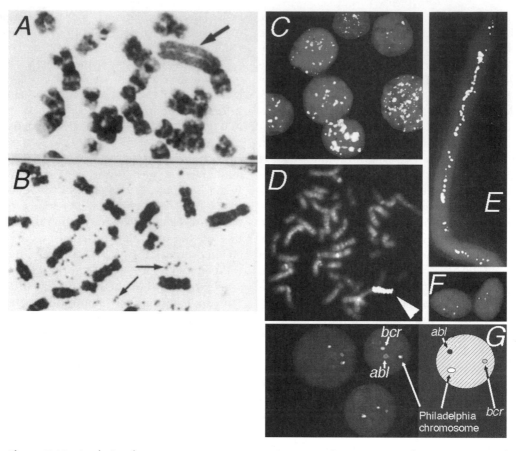

Figure 3.15. Analysis of oncogene rearrangements in tumors by conventional cytogenetics and FISH analysis. *A.* An abnormally long chromosome (*arrowed*). The extended region of this chromosome has no identifiable bands and is called a *homogeneously staining region* (HSR). *B.* Multiple paired dots of chromatic material. These chromosomal abnormalities are called *double minutes* (DM). Both HSRs and DMs are associated with gene amplification. *C.* Interphase nuclei from a neuroblastoma with DMs previously identified by metaphase analysis. The bright dots within each nucleus are the FISH signals from the N-*myc* oncogene, which is known to be amplified at 50 to 100 copies per cell in this patient's tumor. *D.* A metaphase from another neuroblastoma that has N-*myc* amplification and an HSR. In this FISH preparation, the additional N-*myc* signals can be seen to decorate the HSR (*arrowhead*). *E.* A HSR in a neuroblastoma cell line with gene amplification of N-*myc*. In this preparation, the HSR has been "stretched" so that, in the extended form, multiple N-*myc* signals can be seen as a linear array. (Courtesy of Ajay Pandita, Pathology Department, University of Toronto.) *F.* Interphase nuclei of a leukemia sample with three copies of chromosome 8. The specific centromere signal from chromosome 8 allows each nucleus to be analyzed for the presence or absence of this abnormality. *G.* Interphase cytogenetic analysis of a leukemia to identify the Philadelphia chromosome using FISH with the *bcr* and *abl* probes. The *abl* probe has been labeled with a red fluorochrome (*black dot*) and the *bcr* with a green fluorochrome (*shaded dot*). When the Philadelphia chromosome is present in a nucleus, both the red and green signals become superimposed, producing one strong yellow signal (*white dot*). If the nucleus does not have this abnormality, two red signals and two green signals will be present.

radioactively labeled probes. Nonradioactive techniques for the detection of cellular messages employ biotinylated probes, which are then detected by either a fluorescent or enzymatic system.

Successful in situ hybridization to cellular RNA relies on a number of factors. The most suitable cy-

tologic fixation procedure should retain good cellular morphology but must not be so extensive that it inhibits probe access. The most widely used fixative is paraformaldehyde, although many other fixatives have also been used successfully. The length of fixation time and type of fixative should be empiri-

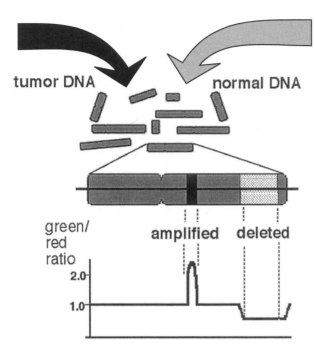

Figure 3.16. Comparative genomic hybridization (CGH). Tumor DNA is labeled with a green fluorochrome (*black arrow*), normal reference DNA is labeled with a red fluorochrome (*shaded arrow*), and an equal mixture of each is hybridized to normal human metaphase chromosomes. Unlabeled repetitive human DNA is included to suppress binding of labeled DNA to repetitive elements. Regions of DNA gain are seen as an increased green fluorescence intensity on the target chromosomes (green to red ratio >1.0); regions of DNA loss are seen as increased red fluorescence intensity (ratio <1.0). Regions on the chromosome that are stained equally for both green and red indicate equal copy number for tumor and reference DNA. It can be seen that the DNA derived from the tumor being studied has both gene amplification (*black region*) and a deletion (*pale shading*) for this particular chromosome.

cally determined for the tissue of interest. Limited proteolytic digestion with pepsin or proteinase K is commonly used to increase probe access to fixed tissues. The probe may be either DNA or RNA. DNA probes labeled by either nick translation or random primer labeling are thought to form networks on the cytologic hybrid, thus increasing the hybridization signal. Self-annealing of probe also occurs; however, this decreases the effective probe concentration. This problem has been circumvented by using *single-stranded RNA probes* transcribed by phage polymerases from plasmids containing SP6 or T7 promoters. These highly specific radioactive probes are easily synthesized in large quantities. RNA probes generally give lower backgrounds than equivalent DNA probes because nonspecifically bound probe is removed by subsequent ribonuclease treatment.

The sensitivity for detecting intracellular mRNA has been improved by performing RT-PCR directly inside the cells, without extraction of the nucleic acid. This technique, called *in-cell RT-PCR*, has been used to detect hybrid *bcr/abl* transcripts (see Chap. 5, Sec. 5.4.4) within single cells. After cellular permeabilization and fixation of single cells in suspension, the mRNA is reverse-transcribed into cDNA and the cDNA is amplified by PCR with fluorescent primers specific for *bcr/abl*. The amplified cells are observed by fluorescent microscopy and positive cells can easily be detected (Testoni et al., 1996). This technique will be of great use for the detection of minimal residual disease or when cell numbers are limited.

Another approach to providing a molecular analysis using very small numbers of cells is *random PCR* (Von Eggeling and Spielvogel, 1995). This technique allows for amplification of all DNA sequences present in microdissected cells, thereby increasing globally the amount of DNA for subsequent analysis. The method can also be adapted to generate representative amplification of the mRNA in a small number of cells. The technique has been useful in providing DNA for molecular genetic studies using microdissected DNA from paraffin blocks, cDNA from single-cell RT-PCR reactions, and chromosome band-specific probes derived for microdissected chromosomal DNA.

One problem associated with the molecular genetic analysis of small numbers of tumor cells is that often substantial numbers of normal cells will be present and can confound interpretation. This contamination is often scattered throughout a tumor section, and it is not possible to microdissect a pure population of tumor cells cleanly. This problem has recently been circumvented by the use of *laser capture microdissection,* in which tumor sections are coated with a clear ethylene vinyl acetate (EVA) polymer prior to microscopic examination (Emmert-Buck et al., 1996). Tumor cells can be captured for subsequent analysis by briefly pulsing the area of interest with an infrared laser. The EVA film becomes sticky and will selectively attach to the tumor cells directly in the laser path. When sufficient cells have been fused to the EVA film, it is placed into nucleic acid extraction buffers and used for PCR or other molecular analyses.

The most recent develpment in molecular analysis of tumors involves combining some of the principles of electronic semiconductor techniques with small-scale nucleic acid hybridization analysis. Typically *gene chip hybridization* technology involves use of a microscopic high-density microarray containing thousands of DNA probes to search for differences or characteristic patterns of gene expression (DeRisi et al., 1996). The fluorescence signals representing hybridization to each arrayed gene are used to detect mutations of specific genes. Microarray chips will be widely applicable to basic and applied cancer research studies and are likely to have an important role in the molecular diagnostic analysis of patient samples in the future.

3.5 SUMMARY

Refinements in the techniques of molecular biology have allowed a rapid increase in the understanding of all aspects of tumor cell biology and are being used routinely in the analysis of clinical samples. Recognition of chromosomal abnormalities first suggested that specific genetic lesions might be associated with some types of human tumors. Methods that allow the identification, isolation, and sequencing of genes have developed rapidly, providing a firm genetic basis for fundamental research related to the molecular changes that occur in malignancy. A number of novel technologies are providing detailed descriptions of the molecular rearrangements and functional abnormalities in tumors. As more genes are identified whose structure and/or function is modified in tumors, there are ultimately likely to be more opportunities to identify unique targets in human tumors for therapeutic intervention.

REFERENCES

Ausubel FA, Brent R, Kingston RE, et al, eds: *Current Protocols in Molecular Biology*. New York: Wiley, 1996

Bryndorf T, Kirchhoff M, Rose H, et al: Comparative genomic hybridization in clinical cytogenetics. *Am J Hum Genet*, 1995; 57:1211–1220.

Crooke ST, Lebleu B: *Antisense Research and Applications*. Boca Raton, FL: CRC Press; 1993.

DeRisi J, Penland L, Brown P O, et al: Use of a cDNA microarray to analyze gene expression patterns in human cancer. *Nature Genet.* 1996; 14:457–60

Dracopoli NC, Haines JC, Korf BR, et al., eds *Current Protocols in Molecular Genetics*. New York: Wiley; 1996.

Dunn JM, Phillips RA, Zhu X, et al: Mutations in the RB1 gene and their effects on transcription. *Mol Cell Biol* 1989; 9:4596–4604.

Emmert-Buck MR, Bonner RF, Smith PD, et al: Laser capture microdissection. *Science*, 1996; 274:998–1001.

Graham FL, van der Eb AJ: A new technique for the assay of infectivity of human adenovirus 5 DNA. *Virology* 1973; 52:456–467.

Heim S, Mitelman F: (1995) *Cancer Cytogenetics*. New York: Wiley; 1995.

Heisterkamp N, Stephenson JR, Groffen J, et al: Localization of the c-*abl* oncogene adjacent to a translocation break point in chronic myelocytic leukemia. *Nature* 1983; 306:239–242.

Kallioniemi A, Kallioniemi OP, Sudar D, et al: Comparative genomic hybridization for molecular cytogenetic analysis of solid tumors. *Science* 1992; 258:818–821.

Keen J, Lester D, Ingelhearn C, et al: Rapid detection of single base mismatches as heteroduplexes on hydrolink gels. *Trends Genet* 1991; 7:5–6.

Liang P, Pardee AB: Differential display of eukaryotic messenger RNA by means of the polymerase chain reaction. *Science* 1992; 257:967–971.

Liang P, Averboukh L, Keyomarsi K, et al: Differential display and cloning of messenger RNAs from human breast cancer versus mammary epithelial cells. *Cancer Res* 1992; 52:6966–6968.

Lichter P, Tang CC, Call K, et al: High-resolution mapping of human chromosome 11 by in situ hybridization with cosmid clones. *Science* 1990; 247:64–69.

Nowell PC, Hungerford DA: A minute chromosome in human chronic granulocytic leukemia. *Science* 1960; 132:1497.

Palmiter RD, Brinster RL: Transgenic mice. *Cell* 1985; 41:343–345.

Roest PA, Roberts, RG, Sugino S, et al: Protein truncation test (PTT) for rapid detection of translation-terminating mutations. *Hum Mol Genet* 1993; 2:1719–1721.

Rowley JD: A new consistent chromosomal abnormality in chronic myelogenous leukaemia identified by quinacrine fluorescence and Giemsa staining. *Nature* 1973; 243: 290–293.

Sanger F: Determination of nucleotide sequences in DNA. *Science* 1981; 214:1205–1210.

Schaffner W: Direct transfer of cloned genes from bacteria to mammalian cells. *Proc Natl Acad Sci USA* 1980; 77:2163–2167.

Schrock E, du Manoir S, Veldman T et al: Multicolor spectral karyotyping of human chromosomes. *Science,* 1996; 273:494–497.

Sheer D, Squire JA: Gene rearrangements and cancer. Series edition of Seminars in Cancer Biology. Academic Press. *Clinical applications of Genetic Rearrangements in Cancer* 1996; 7:25–32.

Sheffield V, Beck J, Kwitek A et al: The sensitivity of single-strand conformation polymorphism analysis for the detection of single base substitutions. *Genomics* 1993; 16:325–332.

Southern EM: Detection of specific sequences among DNA fragments separated by gel electrophoresis. *J Mol Biol* 1975; 98:503–517.

Testoni N, Martinelli G, Farabegoli P, et al: A new method of "in-cell reverse transcriptase-polymerase chain reaction" for the detection of BCR/ABL transcript in chronic myeloid leukemia patients. *Blood* 1996; 87: 3822–3827.

Verma RS and Babu A: *Human Chromosomes*. New York: McGraw-Hill; 1995.

Von Eggeling F, Spielvogel H: Applications of random PCR. *Cell Mol Biol* 1995; 41:653–70.

Walter MA, Spillet DJ, Thomas P, et al: A method for constructing radiation hybrid maps of whole genomes. *Nature Genet* 1994; 7:22–28.

Woolley AT, Mathies RA: Ultra-high-speed DNA sequencing using capillary electrophoresis chips. *Anal Chem* 1995; 67:3676–3680.

Yanagi Y, Yoshikai Y, Leggett K, et al. A human T cell specific cDNA clone encodes a protein having extensive homology to immunoglobulin. *Nature* 1984; 308: 145–149.

Zimmer A: Manipulating the genome by homologous recombination in embryonic stem cells. *Ann Rev Neurosci* 1992; 15:115–137.

BIBLIOGRAPHY

Karger S: In: Mitelman F, ed. *An International System for Human Cytogenetic Nomenclature,* (published in collaboration with Cytogenetics and Cell Genetics). Basel, Switzerland: S. Karger AG; 1992.

Lewin BM: *Genes,* 5th ed. Oxford, England: Oxford University Press; 1994.

Verma RS and Babu A: *Human Chromosomes.* New York: McGraw-Hill; 1995.

4

Genetic Basis of Cancer

Jeremy A. Squire, Gordon F. Whitmore, and Robert A. Phillips

4.1 INTRODUCTION

4.2 BASIC CONCEPTS OF CANCER GENETICS
    4.2.1 Relationship between Cancer Incidence and Age
    4.2.2 Cellular and Genetic Bases of Cancer
    4.2.3 Types of Genetic Risk Factors for Cancer
    4.2.4 Mutations Leading to Intermediate Degrees of Genetic Risk
    4.2.5 Mutations Leading to High Degrees of Genetic Risk

4.3 CHROMOSOME ABNORMALITIES IN TUMORS
    4.3.1 Molecular Genetic Consequences of Chromosome Aberrations
    4.3.2 Cytogenetics of Hematologic Malignancies
    4.3.3 Cytogenetics of Solid Tumors

4.4 DNA REPAIR
    4.4.1 Repair Deficiency Diseases
    4.4.2 Mutations leading to Deficiencies in DNA Repair

4.4.3 Damage Reversal
4.4.4 Mismatch Repair
4.4.5 Base and Nucleotide Excision
4.4.6 Sensitivity to Ionizing Radiation and Repair of Strand Breaks
4.4.7 DNA Repair, Cellular Control, and Disease

4.5 HERITABLE CANCER
    4.5.1 Retinoblastoma and Knudson's Hypothesis
    4.5.2 The Retinoblastoma Gene
    4.5.3 Tumor Suppressor Genes in Other Malignancies
    4.5.4 Colon Carcinoma
    4.5.5 Breast Cancer

4.6 SUMMARY

REFERENCES

BIBLIOGRAPHY

4.1 INTRODUCTION

There is overwhelming evidence that mutations can cause cancer. In this context, mutations are defined broadly to include any changes in the genome such as point mutations, deletions, insertions, translocations, and amplifications. Major evidence for the genetic origin of cancer (Table 4.1) includes (1) the observation of Ames (1983) that many carcinogens are also mutagens and (2) the finding that genetically determined traits associated with a deficiency in the enzymes necessary to repair lesions in DNA are associated with an increased risk of cancer. Mutations may occur in the germline of an individual and be represented in every cell in the body, or they may occur in a single somatic cell and be identified in a tumor following clonal proliferation. When mutations occur in the germline, then cancers should be inherited like other genetic traits. There are several examples of heritable human cancers. Since mutations are rare events, tumors should also be rare events, with each tumor arising from a single mutant cell; in fact, there is much evidence for the clonal origin of human malignancies (see Chap. 7, Sec. 7.6.2).

This chapter reviews information about the genetic nature of cancer deduced from epidemiologic studies. It describes some key examples of the common chromosomal abnormalities observed in hematologic and solid tumors, and discusses inherited DNA-repair defects associated with certain cancer syndromes. The way in which positional cloning can be used to clone a tumor suppressor gene is reviewed, using retinoblastoma and breast cancer as examples. The different types of genes associated with heritable cancer are discussed in the light of what is known about retinoblastoma, Wilms' tumor, colon carcinoma, and breast cancer.

Table 4.1. Evidence That Mutations Cause Cancer

- Many carcinogens are mutagens
- Susceptibility to certain carcinogens is dependent on the ability of cellular enzymes to convert them to a mutagenic form
- Defects in DNA repair increase the probability of cancer
- Chromosomal and genomic instability is observed in many types of cancer
- Some cancers are inherited
- Malignant tumors are clonal
- Some tumors contain mutated oncogenes
- Some tumors have lost or mutated tumor suppressor genes

4.2 BASIC CONCEPTS OF CANCER GENETICS

4.2.1 Relationship between Cancer Incidence and Age

The incidence of most types of cancer increases as the fourth to sixth power of age (Fig. 4-1 and Chap. 2, Sec. 2.3.3). The simplest mathematical analysis of such data suggests that five to seven mutations are necessary for malignant transformation of a normal cell. However, there are difficulties with models requiring many mutations for induction of cancer. To create the necessary age-incidence curves, multihit models assume that all of the cells are present for the lifetime of the individual, that cells with fewer than the required number of mutations have no growth advantage, that each tissue has a very large number of targets for malignant transformation, and that the presence of a putative environmental carcinogen leads to unusually high mutation frequencies. For example, Ashley (1969) had to postulate 10^9 target cells in the stomach and a mutation frequency of 10^{-3} per cell per generation to derive an incidence curve for gastric cancer that increased as the fifth power of age. It is unlikely that 10^9 progenitors remain in the lining of the stomach for the lifetime of the individual. Spontaneous mutations occur at a frequency of 10^{-6} to 10^{-7} per cell per generation. High concentrations of mutagens can increase this frequency 10- to 100-fold, but it is unlikely that tolerable doses of any known carcinogen can increase the mutation frequency to the levels required by the Ashley model.

Because of the apparent requirement for an unobtainable frequency of mutation, some investigators have proposed that cancer does not arise by mutation but that other events modify the expression of existing genes. For example, some results indicate that changes in patterns of DNA methylation can turn genes on or off, and that the frequency of these events can be as high as 10^{-3} per cell per gen-

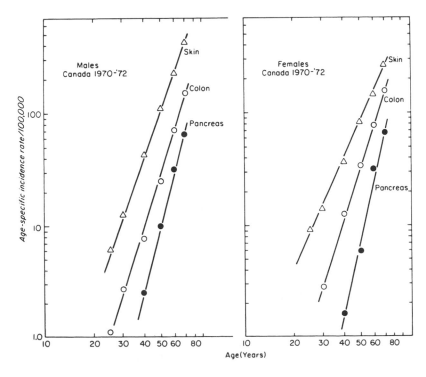

Figure 4.1. Age-specific incidence rates for cancers of the skin, colon, and pancreas in males and females in Canada for the years 1970 to 1972. All these curves are straight lines when plotted using logarithmic axes, fitting the multi-hit models for induction of cancer. According to the models, the cancers require between 5 (skin) and 7 (pancrease) mutations for induction of the malignant state. (Data from *Cancer Patterns in Canada*, 1931–1974. Published by the authority of the Minister of National Health and Welfare, Bureau of Epidemiology. Laboratory Centre for Disease Control, Health Protection Branch, 1982.)

eration. One difficulty with such epigenetic models is that the high frequency of epigenetic changes would make the malignant phenotype highly unstable. Reversion of the malignant phenotype appears to be very rare, but there is evidence that some murine teratocarcinoma cells can revert at high frequency to normal functional cells (Mintz and Illmensee, 1975). In this model, either the mutant genes initiating the tumor are turned off, or the initiating events involve inappropriate gene expression rather than mutation; this abnormal expression could then revert to give normal, tissue-specific expression.

Genomic imprinting has been shown to be an unusual and essentially epigenetic way of regulating certain genes during normal mammalian development. Imprinting is determined by a modification or "imprint" being placed on the DNA of each allele of an imprinted gene during gametogenesis. This imprint can lead to one parental allele becoming inactive and the other being expressed. For example, one particular cell type may express only the paternal copy of a particular gene, while the maternal allele will be transcriptionally silent or "imprinted." Imprinting has been shown to be accompanied by specific DNA methylation and chromatin changes. Often the genes that appear to be "imprinted" are growth factors or are involved in growth control (reviewed in Squire and Weksberg, 1996). For example, some sporadic breast, lung, and kidney tumors undergo epigenetic changes leading to re-expression of the normally silent maternal insulin-like growth factor 2 *(IGF2)* gene accompanied by characteristic alterations in patterns of methylation of the *IGF2* gene. Despite these examples of nonmutational events associated with cancer, most tumors appear to result from stable genetic changes, and the remainder of the chapter summarizes findings related to these stable events.

4.2.2 Cellular and Genetic Bases of Cancer

Evidence for the monoclonal origin of tumors has accrued from analysis of X-linked genes or gene products in cells from tumors in women who are heterozygous at these genetic loci (see Chap. 7, Sec. 7.6.2). These techniques have confirmed clonality in at least 95 percent of the wide range of tumors that have been examined.

Almost all cancers arise in renewing cell populations where a few progenitors with extensive proliferative potential produce large numbers of differentiated cells. However, most of these progenitors have a limited life span and disappear after some number of divisions. Therefore, realistic models for the induction of cancer must take into account the following properties of cell renewal systems (Chap. 7, Sec. 7.5):

1. The immature stem cells, which give rise to undifferentiated progenitor cells and which are the probable targets for transformation, make up only a small proportion of the total number of cells in that tissue or organ.
2. The limited life span of progenitor cells means that mutations that accumulate in a progenitor cell will disappear when this cell completes its life span and when it and its progeny disappear from the animal.
3. Most organs and tissues show marked variations in their proliferative rate during the lifetime of the animal. Some tissues proliferate early in childhood, others during puberty, and others (e.g., bone marrow, intestine, and skin) contain proliferating cells during the entire life span of the individual. These changes in proliferative rate can markedly influence the number of cells that are targets for malignant transformation.

Moolgavkar and Knudson (1981) have proposed a model for carcinogenesis (Fig. 4.2) that takes into account these properties of normal cells. In their model, conversion of a normal progenitor cell into a malignant cell requires only two mutations. Both normal stem cells and "initiated" stem cells, which have accumulated one of the two mutations necessary for transformation, retain normal ability to dif-

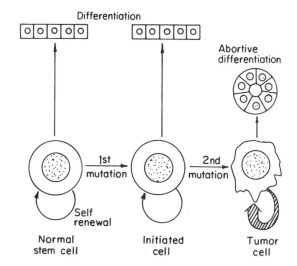

Figure 4.2. In this model of carcinogenesis, the normal stem cells and initiated cells have similar properties; both differentiate and self-renew normally. Following a second mutation, however, self-renewal potential is greatly increased and differentiation becomes grossly abnormal.

ferentiate. An important assumption in this model is that only mutations in stem cells lead to malignant disease; mutations in differentiated cells with little or no potential for self-renewal cannot give rise to tumors.

A feature of this model is that the rate of transformation is more dependent on the growth kinetics of the tissue than on the frequency of mutation. At any cell division, a stem cell has two choices: differentiation or self-renewal. If most stem cells differentiate rapidly and have limited potential for self-renewal, most mutations will be eliminated from the stem-cell pool when the stem cells differentiate. It is the difference between the probability of self-renewal and the probability of differentiation that determines the slope of age-specific incidence curves of the type shown in Fig. 4.1.

The incidence of cancer at any age is directly proportional to the number of initiated stem cells accumulated at that age. In some cancers, there are indications that the initiating event (e.g., smoking in lung cancer) alters the growth kinetics of the target tissue; these changes can be accommodated by the model. Other cancers occur in target tissues that normally change during the lifetime of the animal; examples are embryonic cells that differentiate and disappear early in life and breast tissue that changes both at puberty and at menopause. Perhaps the simplest example is in the developing retina of humans, where as few as two mutations have been shown to lead to retinoblastoma in children (see Sec. 4.5). While the model proposed by Moolgavkar and Knudson is almost certainly an oversimplification of the carcinogenic process in general, it merits consideration because it predicts the unusual age-incidence curves of childhood cancers and breast cancer.

4.2.3 Types of Genetic Risk Factors for Cancer

Occasionally mutations that can cause cancer occur in the germline, giving rise to a heritable predisposition to malignant disease. However, changes in genes other than those directly responsible for malignant disease can also lead to an increased risk of cancer. Mutations predisposing to malignant disease can be grouped into three categories depending on the level of risk involved (Peto, 1980; Table 4.2). Mutations that give a 1000-fold or greater increase in the risk of malignant disease (see Sec. 4.2.5) are easy to detect but account for a very small proportion of total cancers. In his analysis, Peto demonstrated the extreme difficulty of identifying factors that increase the risk of cancer by as much as 10- to

Table 4.2. Categories of Genetic Risk

Increase in Risk of Malignant Disease	Examples	Ease of Identifying Existence of Risk Factor
>1000	Retinoblastoma, polyposis coli, xeroderma pigmentosum	Easy
10–100	Breast cancer?	Difficult
<10	?	Almost impossible

Source: Adapted from Peto, 1980.

100-fold above that in the control population. The major difficulty is the identification of a suitable control group. Unless the genetic risk factor can be identified by its effects on normal cellular function (e.g., inhibition of DNA repair in xeroderma pigmentosum), all control groups will be a mixture of normal and high-risk individuals. The presence of the latter reduces the difference between the experimental and control groups, making identification of the high-risk group difficult. It is probable that many cancers are associated with genetic risk factors that have not yet been identified.

4.2.4 Mutations Leading to Intermediate Degrees of Genetic Risk

One approach to detecting risk factors is to study defined, partially inbred populations. In such populations, it is possible to correlate the incidence of particular malignancies with the degree of relatedness. For example, studies of the Mormon population in Utah have identified several types of human cancer with probable genetically determined risk factors (Skolnick et al., 1981). The combination of accurate genealogic data, a good cancer registry, large families, and a relatively stable, homogeneous population makes possible the identification of genetic risk factors that cannot be detected in other populations.

If genetic factors are important in a specific cancer, individuals with that malignancy will be more closely related than an age-matched control group chosen at random from the Mormon population. Thus members of the Mormon population with specific malignancies were identified, and the degree of relatedness of individuals with the malignancy was calculated. The degree of relatedness of two individuals was expressed as a kinship coefficient, which is essentially the probability that randomly selected homologous chromosomes are identical by descent from a common ancestor; the genealogical index (GI) describes the average relatedness of specific groups in the population. The larger the GI value, the more closely related is the population; the GI for the control Mormon population is 1.39×10^{-5}. Table 4.3 shows the GI obtained for groups of patients with several common malignancies. Of the malignancies listed, only lymphoma shows no familial clustering. In these studies, one cannot separate genetic risk from environmental or dietary factors that may show familial clustering because families often share the same environment and diet. Nevertheless, this method has identified malignancies that merit detailed investigation for the presence of genetic risk factors.

4.2.5 Mutations Leading to High Degrees of Genetic Risk

Mulvihill (1977) reviewed over 200 mutations that predispose to malignancy in humans. Most of these mutations cause substantial increases in risk and fall into the first category described by Peto. Some mutations cause tumors by indirect mechanisms, but at least 100 of them probably act directly to cause tissue-specific tumors. The best-characterized mutations lead to cancers inherited as autosomal dominant traits; some examples of such mutations are described in detail in Sec. 4.5. Some of these mutations have been mapped to a chromosomal location, and for several tumors, the specific genes have been identified and characterized (Table 4.4).

Table 4.3. Genealogical Index among Groups of the Mormon Population with Specified Types of Cancer

Cancer Type	Mean Genealogic Index ($\times 10^{-5}$)
Lip	3.84
Melanoma	3.36
Ovary	3.07
Prostate	2.59
Colon	2.31
Breast (<50 years)	2.23
Breast (>50 years)	2.11
Lymphoma	1.27
Control population	1.39

Source: Adapted from Skolnick et al., 1981.

As described in Chap. 5, all species have numerous genes called *cellular oncogenes* (or *proto-oncogenes*), many of which are homologous to transforming oncogenes carried by specific RNA retroviruses. Some human tumors have mutations in these oncogenes that may have led to their activation. However, there is no evidence for germline mutations in cellular oncogenes, perhaps because such mutations in the germline are lethal even in the heterozygous state. In contrast, there is good evidence (described in Sec. 4.5) for germline mutations affecting tumor suppressor genes and leading to familial clustering of cancer or transmission of predisposition to tumors as a simple Mendelian gene (Table 4.4).

Many mutations result in instability of the genome and lead indirectly to high degrees of risk for cancer, presumably because the initial germline mutation increases the likelihood of somatic mutations occurring in direct-acting genes. The best examples of this type of mutation are the well-characterized autosomal recessive diseases with known defects in their ability to repair DNA damage (see Sec. 4.4) and in some tumors in which somatic mutations of the *p53* gene result in genetic instability (see Sec. 4.5.3 and Chap. 5, Sec. 5.5.2).

Other mutations may predispose to malignant disease, but in most cases the data are only circumstantial. Since many carcinogens must be metabolized before they can cause mutations (Chap. 8, Sec. 8.2), mutations in genes that code for enzymes in the activation pathways could lead to changes in the incidence of malignant disease caused by these carcinogens. Mutations in genes that determine host resistance might also predispose to cancer. While immune suppression can accelerate the development of chemically or virally induced tumors in experimental animals, immune suppression does not always lead to marked increases in tumor incidence. For example, nude mice, which lack a thymus and are unable to reject foreign tumor grafts, do not have an increased incidence of malignant disease. In contrast, patients with immune deficiency disease of either genetic or acquired origin have an increased incidence of lymphoid tumors. However, since tumors develop within the system that is defective, it is unclear whether the malignancies occur because of immune suppression or because of the abnormality in the development of lymphocytes.

Viruses can cause malignant tumors in experimental animals, and numerous genetic factors influence susceptibility to transformation by these viruses. For example, Friend leukemia virus (FLV) induces erythroleukemia in many inbred strains of

Table 4.4. Some Examples of Cloned Tumor Suppressor Genes and Familial Human Cancer Genes

Tumor Suppressor Gene	Chromosomal Location	Malignancy
hMSH2[a]	2p22-21	Hereditary nonpolyposis colorectal cancer (HNPCC)
FHIT	3p14.2	Various tumor types
hMLH1[a]	3p21.3-p23	HNPCC
VHL	3p25-p26	Von Hippel-Lindau disease
APC	5q21	Familial polyposis
CDKN2	9p21	Familial melanoma
RET	10q11.2	Multiple endocrine neoplasia 2
PTEN/MMAC1	10q23.3	Various tumor types
WT-1	11p13	Wilms' tumor
MEN1	11q13	Multiple endocrine neoplasia 1
BRCA2	13q12-13	Familial breast cancer (early onset)
RB1	13q14	Retinoblastoma
p53	17p12-13	Li-Fraumeni syndrome, many tumor types
NF-1	17q12-22	Neurofibromatosis 1
BRCA1	17q21	Familial breast and ovarian cancer
Smad4/DPC4	18q21.1	Pancreatic cancer
MADR2	18q21	Colorectal cancer
NF-2	22q12.2	Neurofibromatosis 2

[a]Mismatch repair genes.

mice. Resistance to infection and tumorigenesis is regulated by as many as six different genetic loci in mice (Shibuya and Mak, 1982). Viruses have also been implicated in human malignancies, especially papillomaviruses in cervical cancers (see Chap. 5, Sec. 5.2.3), although there is currently little evidence for genetic predisposition to infection with these putative human tumor viruses. Many of the human DNA tumor viruses inactivate the proteins of human tumor suppressor genes early in the infection process when they transform human cells in tissue culture (see Chap. 5, Sec. 5.2), indicating the critical role that these genes play in controlling proliferation in normal cells.

4.3 CHROMOSOME ABNORMALITIES IN TUMORS

In most tumors, a variety of chromosomal abnormalities can be observed. Some of these chromosomal abnormalities have provided clues about basic genetic mechanisms and others have been found to have prognostic significance. The acquisition of these diverse chromosomal changes is thought to re-sult from chance errors during DNA replication and cell division. If the acquired change confers a selective advantage, then the cell containing the abnormality (and its progeny) will persist. If not, then the abnormality will not be a common feature of that particular type of tumor. In the following sections, those chromosome abnormalities that are reproducible and representative of a specific malignancy are discussed.

4.3.1 Molecular Genetic Consequences of Chromosome Aberrations

Progress in molecular biology and the mapping of human genes has facilitated our understanding of the significance of the acquisition of chromosome aberrations and genetic mutations in cancer. The molecular consequences of chromosome aberrations influence the functioning of two distinct classes of genes in human tumors: dominantly acting oncogenes and tumor suppressor genes.

Dominantly Acting Oncogenes   When an oncogene becomes inappropriately activated, it can stimulate cells to continue to proliferate, leading to a tumor (see Chap. 5, Sec. 5.4). There are at least three chromosomal mechanisms for activating oncogenes (Fig. 4.3):

1. Fusion of the oncogene with a second gene at a site of translocation or inversion of chromosomes generating a chimeric gene and a new protein (Figure 4.3*A*). This mechanism is found predominantly in leukemias, lymphomas, and sarcomas (reviewed in Rabbitts, 1994). The best-known example of this type of fusion is the activation of the *abl* oncogene by translocation with *bcr,* generating the Phildelphia chromosome (see Sec. 4.3.2 and Chap. 5, Sec. 5.4.4).
2. Juxtaposition of the oncogene to regulatory elements in immunoglobulin or T-cell receptor genes in B- and T-lymphocyte malignancies, respectively, leading to inappropriate expression of the oncogene (Fig. 4.3*B*). This mechanism is one of the commonest methods of oncogene activation in hematologic malignancies (see Sec. 4.3.2).
3. Increase in the amount of DNA from a specific region of a chromosome (Fig. 4.3*C*), resulting in areas on chromosomes referred to as *homogeneously staining regions* (HSR) (see Chap. 3, Fig. 3.15). Such HSRs are associated with extensive gene amplification, commonly associated with drug resistance and overexpression of onco-

genes. Another form of gene amplification leads to chromosomal abnormalities called *double minutes* (DMs), which appear as two small dots of dark-staining material in a metaphase preparation (see Chap. 3, Fig. 3.15). In some instances, the number of DMs can be very large, approaching several hundred. There is evidence that DMs represent the first stage in gene amplification and that some HSRs result from the integration of DMs into the chromosome. Various mechanisms have been proposed for the amplification process, based on molecular analysis of the regions of amplified DNA (known as *amplicons*) in different cell types (Hahn, 1993). Gene amplification occurs frequently in solid tumors but is seldom found in hematologic malignancies.

Tumor Suppressor Genes When these genes (sometimes called *recessive oncogenes*) are functioning normally, they inhibit cell proliferation. For these genes, loss or inactivation removes the normal constraints on cellular growth, resulting in a tumor (see Sec. 4.5 and Chap. 5, Sec. 5.5). The first experimental evidence of tumor suppression came from studies in which normal cells were fused with tumor cells; the resulting hybrids lost the characteristics of a tumor cell line, such as continuous growth in culture. Experiments with different combinations of

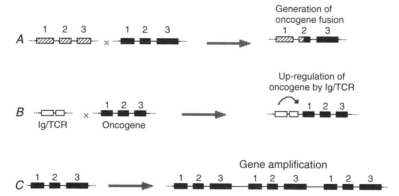

Figure 4.3. Schematic depiction of three classes of oncogene activation, with exons shown as solid, open, or hatched boxes. *A.* Fusion of the oncogene with a second gene by chromosomal translocation, generating a fusion gene with altered properties. *B.* Juxtaposition of the oncogene to regulatory elements in immunoglobulin (Ig) or T-cell receptor genes (TCR) in B- and T-lymphocyte malignancies, respectively, leading to inappropriate expression of the oncogene. *C.* Gene amplification, i.e., the generation of multiple gene copies in DMs or HSRs (also see Chap. 3, Fig. 3.15), leading to elevated expression of the oncogene in cells with amplification.

normal cells and tumor cells showed that hybrid cells were always nontumorigenic, like the normal parent cell line (Anderson and Stanbridge, 1993). This observation led to the idea that there was a class of genes in normal cells capable of reversing or suppressing the activity of growth-promoting genes.

As discussed in Sec. 4.5.1, analysis of constitutional deletions of chromosome 13 associated with the inherited form of retinoblastoma led to the development of the "two-hit" model of tumorigenesis (Knudson, 1971). This model predicted that certain genes, now called tumor suppressor genes, exert a tumorigenic effect when both alleles become inactivated by mutation or chromosomal deletion. The first allele is inactivated either in the germ cells, where it confers dominant familial susceptibility to cancer, or in the somatic cells. The second allele is inactivated in the somatic cells. The mutation or deletion that is inherited as a dominant trait is thus recessive at the cellular level. For most genetic loci, there is heterogeneity between the alleles on the maternal and paternal chromosomes. Malignant transformation requires loss of function of a tumor suppressor gene, and a common mechanism involves recombination such that the mutated or deleted allele is carried on *both* maternal and paternal chromosomes; i.e., there is *loss of heterozygosity* (LOH) at the locus of the tumor suppressor gene (see Sec. 4.5.1 and Chap. 5, Sec. 5.5.1). Molecular studies of chromosomal deletions and regions showing LOH in other hereditary and sporadic tumors have now enabled the isolation of several tumor suppressor genes (Table 4.4).

4.3.2 Cytogenetics of Hematologic Malignancies

Leukemias and lymphomas usually have few chromosome rearrangements in comparison with solid tumors. Chromosome numbers are typically in the diploid range—i.e., close to 46 chromosomes per cell—and chromosome rearrangements are therefore relatively easy to define. Consistent and in some cases highly specific chromosome aberrations have been found in hematologic malignancies (Table 4.5; Hogge, 1994; Heim and Mitelman, 1995).

Table 4.5. Common Chromosomal Abnormalities in Lymphoid and Myeloid Malignancies

Malignancy	Chromosomal Aberration[a]	Molecular Lesion
Acute myeloid leukemia (AML)		
M1, M2 subtypes	t(8;21)(q22;q22)	*AML1-MTG8* fusion
M3 subtype	t(15;17)(q22;q11.2)	*PML-RARA* fusion
M4Eo subtype	inv(16)(p13;q22) or t(16;16)(p13;q22)	*MYH11-CBFB* fusion
M2 or M4 subtypes	t(6;9)(p23;q24)	*DEK-CAN* fusion
Therapy-related AML	− 5/del(5q), − 7/del(7q)	
Chronic myeloid leukemia (CML)	t(9;22)(q34;q11) (Ph¹ chromosome)	*BCR-ABL* fusion encoding p210 protein
CML blast crisis	(9;22)(q34;q11), +8, +Ph¹, +19, or i(17q)	*BCR-ABL* fusion encoding p210 protein, *TP53* mutation
Acute lymphocytic leukemia (ALL)	t(9;22)(q34;q11)	*BCR-ABL* fusion encoding p190 protein
pre-B ALL	t(1;19)(q23;p13.3)	*E2A-PBX1* fusion
pre-B ALL	t(17;19)(q22;p13.3)	*E2A-HLF* fusion
B-ALL, Burkitt's lymphoma	t(8;14)(q24;q32) t(2;8)(p12;q24) t(8;22)(q24;q11)	Translocations between *myc* and *IgH*, *IgL*κ and *IgL*λ loci
B-Chronic lymphocytic leukemia	+12,t(14q32)	Translocations of *IgH* locus

[a]For an interpretation of the nomenclature of chromosomal rearrangements, see Chap. 3, Sec. 3.2.1.

Source: Adapted from Sheer and Squire, 1996.

Chronic myelogenous leukemia (CML) was the first malignancy in which a reproducible chromosomal abnormality was described. In almost all patients with CML, the leukemic cells contain a unique small chromosome called the *Philadelphia chromosome* (commonly abbreviated Ph[1] or simply Ph; see also Chap. 5, Sec. 5.4.4). Rowley (1973) suggested that the Ph chromosome resulted from a reciprocal translocation between chromosomes 9 and 22 (see Chap. 3, Fig. 3.1). With usual banding techniques, the tip of the long arm of chromosome 22 stains faintly, and most investigators did not detect the translocated fragment at the tip of the long arm of chromosome 9. The precise location of the break on chromosome 22 has now been identified, and there is unequivocal evidence that the rearrangement is indeed a reciprocal translocation and that it alters the structure of the *abl* oncogene (Chap. 5, Sec. 5.4.4). The Ph chromosome has also provided information about the patterns of hematopoietic differentiation. During periods of remission, when malignant cells are undetectable, all of the dividing myeloid cells (i.e., progenitors for erythrocytes, granulocytes, and megakaryocytes) contain the Ph chromosome. This finding indicates that the Ph chromosome arose in a pluripotent stem cell with high self-renewal ability, allowing this clone to dominate the entire hematopoietic system. In the chronic phase of CML, the tumor cells are diploid, with the Ph chromosome translocation being the only detectable karyotypic abnormality. When patients enter the blast crisis phase, other chromosome abnormalities frequently appear. Among the most common changes are the appearance of a second Ph chromosome, an isochromosome of the long arm of chromosome 17, or an extra copy of chromosome 8. Such changes in karyotype are a grave prognostic sign, and death usually occurs within a few months.

Another consistent chromosomal abnormality occurs in acute promyelocytic leukemia. In the majority of patients, the malignant cells have a translocation involving chromosomes 15 and 17 (Gillard and Solomon, 1993). The translocation break points occur within the retinoic acid receptor (*RARA*) gene on chromosome 17 and a gene designated *PML* (for promyelocytic leukemia) on chromosome 15, generating a chimeric *RARA-PML* gene. The RARA protein normally binds to retinoic acid and also has amino acid sequence motifs called "zinc fingers" that indicate DNA-binding properties (Chap. 6, Sec. 6.3.6). The *PML* gene also has DNA-binding motifs, including a zinc finger. The molecular consequence of this chromosome translocation is a chimeric transcription factor that retains the zinc fingers from both molecules but also keeps the ligand-binding domain of RARA. Transformation presumably results from aberrant regulation of genes involved in myeloid differentiation that are normally regulated by PML or RARA. These findings also helped to explain the molecular basis for the beneficial effects of therapy with retinoic acid in acute promyelocytic leukemia.

Burkitt's lymphoma was the first tumor where a chromosomal abnormality was demonstrated to involve the translocation of a specific gene. The common translocations involving chromosome 8 and chromosomes 2, 14, or 22 result in the relocation of the *myc* oncogene near to genes that code for immunoglobulin molecules (see also Chap. 5, Sec. 5.4.4). The most common abnormality is a reciprocal translocation between chromosomes 8 and 14. The *myc* oncogene moves from chromosome 8 to a location near the constant region of the immunoglobulin heavy-chain gene (IgH) on chromosome 14; the variable region of the immunoglobulin gene is transferred from chromosome 14 to chromosome 8 (Fig. 4.4). Similar rearrangements involv-

Figure 4.4. The common translocation between chromosomes 8 and 14 in Burkitt's lymphoma is illustrated. The arrows indicate the position of the break points in the translocated chromosomes shown on the right of each pair.

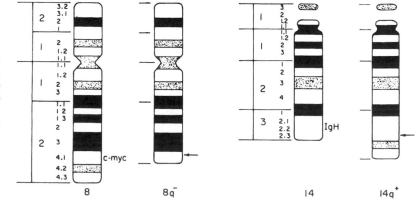

ing the light-chain loci play a role in translocations with chromosomes 2 (κ chain) and 22 (λ chain). The possible role of translocations in activating oncogenes is discussed in Chap. 5, Sec. 5.4.4.

4.3.3 Cytogenetics of Solid Tumors

It has proved difficult to obtain comprehensive information about chromosomal abnormalities in solid tumors. The major reason is the difficulty in obtaining suitable cellular preparations for chromosome analysis. In contrast to leukemias, which grow naturally as single-cell suspensions or are easily disrupted into single cells, the cells in solid tumors are held together by tight junctions. Disruption of tumors into a single-cell suspension suitable for karyotype analysis often results in cell death. When chromosomes are obtained, their morphology is usually poor. Nevertheless, data are beginning to emerge showing distinct characteristic aberrations in different categories of solid tumors (Table 4.6). Identification of these characteristic chromosomal

aberrations can enable accurate diagnoses to be made (Ilson et al., 1993; Sreekantaiah et al., 1994). Some tumors can also be assigned to good or bad prognostic categories according to their cytogenetic profiles. The following paragraphs describe examples of tumors where acquisition of a common chromosome abnormality can be observed.

Sarcomas, including soft tissue tumors, often have characteristic chromosome translocations (Table 4.6) that result in the formation of chimeric genes encoding transcription factors (Sorensen and Triche, 1996). As in leukemias and lymphomas, the chimeric transcription factor often retains the DNA binding domain from one of the translocated genes and the transcriptional transactivating domain from the other. Other sarcomas show recurrent chromosome aberrations preferentially affecting particular chromosomal regions. For example, rhabdomyosarcoma, a malignancy of striated muscle that usually occurs in children, can be diagnosed using immunohistochemical muscle markers, but classification of the two major tumor subtypes is often diffi-

Table 4.6. Common Chromosomal Abnormalities and Respective Oncogene Fusions in Solid Tumors

Tumor	Chromosomal Aberration[a]	Molecular Lesion
Lipoma	t(3;12)(q27-28;q13-14)[b]	
Ewing's sarcoma and pPNET[c]	t(11;22)(q24;q12)	*EWS-FLI-1* fusion
pPNET[c]	t(7;22)(p22;q12) t(21;22)(q22;q12)	*EWS-ETV1* fusion *EWS-ERG* fusion
Clear cell sarcoma	t(12;22)(q13;q12)	*EWS-ATF1* fusion
Extraskeletal myxoid chondrosarcoma	t(9;22)(q22;q12)	*EWS* translocation
Alveolar rhabdomyo-sarcoma	t(2;13)(q35-37;q14) t(1;13)(p36;q14)	*PAX3-FKHR* fusion *PAX7-FKHR* fusion
Synovial sarcoma	t(X;18)(p11.2;q11.2)	*SYT-SSX1* *SYT-SSX2*
Myxoid liposarcoma	t(12;16)(q13;p11)	*FUS-CHOP* fusion
Germ cell tumor	i(12p)	
Small cell lung carcinoma	del(3)(p14-23)	
Renal cell carcinoma	t/del(3)(p11-21)	
Neuroblastoma	del(1)(p32), DMs	N-*myc* amplification
Meningioma	− 22	
Glioblastoma multiforme	− 10/del(10)p/q	

[a]For an interpretation of the nomenclature of chromosomal rearrangements, see Chap. 3, Sec. 3.2.1.

[b]A hyphen in between chromosome band numbers indicates that the exact position of the translocation breakpoint is uncertain.

[c]pPNET = peripheral primitive neuroectodermal tumor.

Source: Adapted from Sheer and Squire, 1996.

cult. Accurate recognition of rhabdomyosarcoma subtype is vital because alveolar tumors require more aggressive treatment than embryonal tumors. A combination of tumor cytogenetics and molecular biology has helped to distinguish the subtypes. The majority of alveolar rhabdomyosarcoma tumors have a unique translocation between chromosome bands 2q35-7 and 13q14. In these translocations, the *FKHR* gene at 13q14, encoding a transcription factor protein, becomes juxtaposed with the *PAX3* (also a transcription factor) gene at 2q35-37. The resulting chimeric gene combines the transcriptional transactivating domain of *FKHR* and the DNA-binding domains of the *PAX* gene, presumably encoding a fusion protein that inappropriately activates the *PAX* target genes (Fredericks et al., 1995). In contrast, embryonal tumors do not have this chromosomal rearrangement but often have lost heterozygous restriction fragment length polymorphisms (RFLPs) at band 11p15, indicating a deletion or other molecular genetic change at this locus.

In addition to translocations and deletions, cells in solid tumors often show increases in genetic material associated with overexpression of oncogenes. Solid tumors frequently have large numbers of chromosomes, often approaching a tetraploid number, and increases in specific chromosomes or in portions of a chromosome are also detected. Cells from many tumors show double minutes (DMs), which are diagnostic of gene amplification. Some of the gene amplifications studied in detail include the oncogenes N-*myc*, *erb*B-2/*neu*, *gli*, *erb*B-1, *HST1*, *INT2*, and *MDM2;* some of the cell-cycle control genes; and those genes involved in drug resistance such as *mdr1* (Stein et al., 1996). For example, in neuroblastoma, the N-*myc* oncogene is frequently amplified, presenting cytologically as DMs or homogeneously staining regions (see Chap. 3, Fig. 3.15). The presence of this amplification is recognized as one of the primary determinants of aggressive disease (reviewed in Sheer and Squire, 1996). Newer molecular cytogenetic technologies, including fluorescence in situ hybridization (FISH) (see Chap. 3, Sec. 3.4.4) and comparative genomic hybridization (CGH) (see Chap. 3, Sec. 3.4.5), have shown that gene amplification is common in solid tumors. The acquisition of additional chromosomal regions and increased gene copy number is likely to confer a strong selective advantage to some tumors, and the further characterization of amplified genes may give useful prognostic information about various solid tumors.

Despite the technical difficulties in obtaining good-quality karyotypes from *carcinomas,* data are now available indicating the presence of some consistent genetic aberrations, including chromosome deletions/LOH, chromosome gains, mutations, and gene amplification (Table 4.6; Rodriguez et al., 1994). Consistent translocations have been described in only a few carcinomas and adenomas (Bongarzone et al, 1994). The presence of consistent chromosomal deletions and regions showing LOH indicates the involvement of multiple tumor suppressor genes in carcinomas. In fact, all the cloned tumor suppressor genes that play a role in hereditary cancer (see Chap. 5, Sec. 5.5) have been found to be mutated in sporadic carcinomas as well, and the locations of these mutations coincide with many of the mutations that occur in the hereditary forms of the disease. Genetic changes have been studied in detail in colon carcinomas, with a well-defined progression from premalignant adenomas to metastatic carcinomas (see Sec. 4.5.4).

4.4 DNA REPAIR

The interactions of cells with ionizing radiation, ultraviolet light, and endogenous and exogenous chemical agents produce a variety of lesions in DNA. These lesions include single- and double-strand breaks, base alterations, and cross-links, both inter- and intrastrand as well as between DNA and proteins. Also, errors during DNA synthesis can lead to the insertion of incorrect bases or the addition or deletion of base sequences. To maintain genetic integrity, cells have developed multiple repair processes that alleviate or eliminate the effects of these various lesions. Many of the proteins involved in DNA repair have been highly conserved throughout evolution, attesting to the importance of these processes. Repair of DNA plays an important role in determining cancer predisposition, thus providing further evidence that genetic change is a primary event in malignant transformation. DNA repair proteins are also involved in cell-cycle control and the generation of immune diversity; defects in these proteins are manifest in disease symptoms in addition to malignancy.

4.4.1 Repair Deficiency Diseases

At least seven human disease syndromes are associated with pronounced cellular sensitivity to DNA-damaging agents and are either known or assumed to arise from hereditary deficiencies in DNA repair or cell signaling pathways responsive to DNA damage (Table 4.7). Xeroderma pigmentosum (XP), ataxia telangiectasia (AT), Bloom's syndrome (BS), and Fanconi's anemia (FA) are autosomal recessive diseases. In addition to the clinical symptoms indicated

Table 4.7. Clinical and Cellular Characteristics of Human Hereditary Diseases with Defective DNA Repair

Human Genetic Disease	Clinical Characteristics	Cellular Characteristics
Xeroderma pigmentosum (XP)	Photosensitivity Parchment skin Skin pigmentation Neurologic abnormalities Physical impairment Skin tumors Autosomal recessive	UV sensitive Sensitive to alkylating and cross-linking agents Defective excision repair Seven complementation groups
Ataxia telangiectasia (AT)	Ataxia Telangiectasia Reduced immune competence Lymphoreticular tumors Sensitive to radiotherapy Autosomal recessive	Frequent chromosome abnormalities X-ray sensitive Sensitive to DNA-breaking agents DNA synthesis is resistant to radiation Four complementation groups
Bloom's syndrome (BS)	Low birth weight Stunted development Light-induced telangiectasia Increased malignancy Autosomal recessive	Reduced DNA ligase I activity Defective DNA synthesis Increased sister chromatid exchanges Slow growth rate
Fanconi's anemia (FA)	Growth retardation Hyperpigmentation Skeletal abnormalities Pancytopenia Increased leukemias and solid tumors Autosomal recessive	Chromosome aberrations Sensitive to cross-linking agents No UV or x-ray sensitivity Five complementation groups
Cockayne's syndrome (CS)	Dwarfism Photosensitivity Mental deficiency Optic and aural defects Mean age at death approx. 12 years No increased malignancy Autosomal recessive	Deoxyguanosine sensitive Camptothecin sensitive Defective repair of UV-induced dimers Defective recovery of RNA synthesis Two complementation groups
Trichothiodystrophy (TTD)	Brittle hair with reduced sulfur content Impaired mental and physical development Icthyosis Variable sun sensitivity No increased malignancy Autosomal recessive	Variable excision repair deficiency Three complementation groups
Hereditary nonpolyposis colon cancer (HNPCC)	Increased colon, ovarian, and endometrial cancer Autosomal dominant	Hypermutability Microsatellite instability

in Table 4.7, patients with several of these syndromes show marked predisposition to malignancy. Patients suffering from XP are sun-sensitive and have an extreme predisposition to skin cancer—an increase in incidence of perhaps 1000-fold. Patients with AT have a very high incidence of lymphomas, often before the age of 20. The incidence of lymphomas is also increased markedly in FA and BS patients.

The above diseases are rare. Ataxia telangiectasia occurs in approximately 1 of 40,000 births; BS appears in 1 of 58,000 Ashkenazi Jews but much less frequently in the general population. However, heterozygous individuals probably occur at frequencies of 1:100 to 1:400 in the general population. The frequency of malignancies in heterozygotes is unknown, but it has been estimated that AT heterozygotes may account for 5 percent of all patients who die of cancer before age 45 and 8 percent of all breast cancer patients (Swift et al., 1987; Easton, 1994). These individuals may also be at increased risk for treatment-related complications because of the increased sensitivity of their cells to ionizing radiation and certain chemical agents (Weeks et al., 1991; Deschavanne and Fertil, 1996). Human non-polyposis colon cancer (HNPCC), which is hereditary and diagnosed on the basis of a familial predisposition to colon cancer in the absence of premalignant polyps, is now known to be caused by a deficiency in DNA mismatch repair (Rhyu, 1996). Finally, there are at least two diseases, Cockayne's syndrome (CS) and trichothiodystrophy (TTD), that involve deficiencies in DNA repair but do not appear to exhibit an increase in malignancy (Table 4.7).

Cells derived from XP patients are extremely sensitive to killing by ultraviolet light and are also defective in unscheduled DNA synthesis, an indicator of nucleotide excision repair (see Sec. 4.4.5). Cells from AT patients show increased chromosomal aberrations and are very sensitive to ionizing radiation and chemicals known to produce double-strand breaks in DNA (Paterson, 1979). Cells from AT heterozygotes show a range of sensitivities to ionizing radiation intermediate between that of cells from AT patients and those from normal controls (Weeks et al., 1991). Cells from FA patients are extremely sensitive to DNA cross-linking agents, and cells from patients with BS show an increased frequency of sister chromatid exchanges, assumed to arise from a reduced ability to repair DNA single-strand breaks. However, the defects in DNA repair have not yet been defined precisely in AT, FA, or BS cells.

4.4.2 Mutations Leading to Deficiencies in DNA Repair

Characterization of genetic abnormalities in cells derived from patients or heterozygotes with one of the syndromes listed in Table 4.7 is providing information about some of the processes involved in DNA repair. However improved understanding of repair processes in mammalian cells has come largely from the isolation of repair-deficient mutant cells from established cell lines, predominantly rodent cells. A variety of techniques has been used to isolate cells with unusual sensitivity to ultraviolet (UV) light, ionizing radiation, and various chemical agents (for reviews, see Collins, 1993; Weeda et al., 1993). The use of such cell lines has several advan-

tages. Studies based on cells derived from patients will be limited to those defects that are compatible with life, but the introduction of defective repair genes into transgenic mice (Chap. 3, Sec. 3.3.12) suggests that not all repair defects fall into this category. Mutants can also be selected for sensitivity to a particular agent or class of agents. In addition to their immortality, rodent cell lines accept transfected DNA from both rodent or human donors with much greater efficiency than human cells— both major advantages for gene cloning approaches.

Studies of the sensitivity of both human cells and rodent cell lines to various agents have revealed a variety of phenotypes (see Fig. 4.5). Some cells exhibit extreme sensitivity to ultraviolet light and cross-linking agents such as mitomycin C but little or no sensitivity to x-rays. Other cells exhibit sensitivity to x-rays and chemical agents known to cause DNA breakage but little or no sensitivity to UV light or cross-linking agents. These various phenotypes, which are similar to those characterized previously in bacteria and yeast mutants, indicate the involvement of several repair pathways and gene products.

Determination of whether mutants sensitive to the same agent are defective in the same gene involves complementation analysis using cell-cell hybridization (see Chap. 3, Sec. 3.4.2). In this process, two mutant cells are fused to form a single viable cell. If the offspring of this hybrid cell remain sensitive, the two mutants are considered noncomplementing and are probably defective in the same gene. If the hybrid cells are resistant, the two mutants are considered complementing and assumed to be defective in two different genes. Selective results from complementation analyses carried out with cell lines derived from patients, with mutant rodent cells, and with mixed human-rodent hybrids are summarized in Tables 4.7, 4.8, and 4.9. Table 4.7 indicates that several of the human diseases comprise multiple complementation groups, with xeroderma pigmentosum having a total of seven, XPA to XPG, all of which are defective in nucleotide excision repair. Table 4.8 lists 11 complementation groups for rodent cells defective in excision repair processes (see Sec. 4.4.5). Six of these groups correspond to genes that have been located to human chromosomes and are responsible for some of the complementation groups associated with the repair-deficiency syndromes XP, CS, and TTD. A total of thirty or more gene products might be involved in excision repair pathways (Lehmann, 1995a; Sec. 4.4.5). Table 4.9 lists mutant cells from rodents in

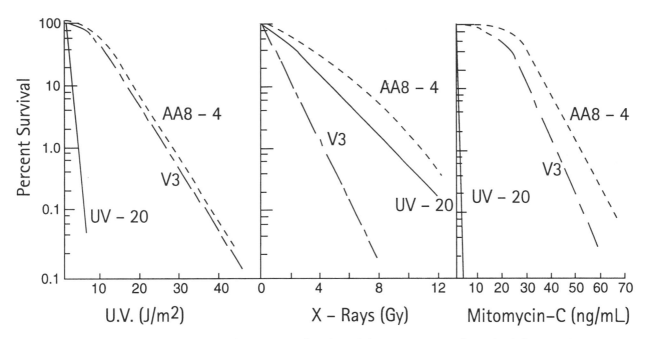

Figure 4.5. Survival curves for mutant cells selected for sensitivity to ultraviolet light (UV-20), x-rays (V3), and the parental line (AA8-4) following exposure to ultraviolet light, x-rays, and mitomycin C. Note the differing patterns of sensitivity to these treatment modalities.

eight complementation groups that have been isolated and exhibit sensitivity to ionizing radiation; these groups, plus AT, imply the involvement of multiple gene products in the repair of damage induced by ionizing radiation and by certain classes of chemical agents (Jeggo et al., 1994).

Complementation analysis provides information about the number of gene products likely to be involved but little or no insight into their nature and function. Such insights have resulted largely from the cloning of complete genes or appropriate cDNAs. A typical cloning strategy involves cotransfecting a recipient rodent mutant cell with plasmid DNA containing a dominant selectable marker (e.g., the neo gene, which confers resistance to the antibiotic G418) together with genomic or cDNA derived from a repair-proficient cell line (often human). Following transfection, cells are selected for the presence of the dominant selectable marker and for resistance to the appropriate DNA-damaging agent. DNA from cells exhibiting resistance is used to construct a DNA library in either λ-phage or cosmids (see Chap. 3, Sec. 3.3.3). The library is screened for the presence of either human repetitive sequences or sequences associated with the dominant selectable marker. DNA from selected phage or cosmids is then tested for its ability to confer resistance following transfection into sensitive re-cipient mutants. Once isolated, appropriate sequences can be used to isolate entire genes or cDNAs from appropriate libraries or as probes to determine the chromosomal location of the gene in either humans or rodents. The existence of complementation groups usually indicates the involvement of several genes, but the recent cloning of the ATM (AT mutated) gene indicates that all four of the AT complementation groups involve mutations in a single large gene located on human chromosome 11q22-23 (Savitsky et al., 1995).

Assignment of chromosomal locations for the human counterparts of the rodent genes involved in repair of damage induced by UV light and x-rays has been made possible because either the gene or its cDNA counterpart has been sufficiently cloned to be used as a probe for chromosome mapping. Sequencing of cloned genes has also made it possible to assign putative functions to some of their protein products; this is often done on the basis of homology of the human genes with genes of known function in yeasts or bacteria.

There are a variety of repair processes that can lead to repair of diverse lesions produced in DNA. These processes are described in subsequent sections and can be divided into four general classes: (1) damage reversal, (2) mismatch repair, (3) base and nucleotide excision, and (4) repair of strand

Table 4.8. Rodent and Human Genes Involved in Nucleotide Excision Repair

Complementation Group	Typical Rodent Mutants	Human Counterpart[a]	Human Chromosome	Putative Protein Properties
RCG1	UV20, 43-3B	ERCC-1	19q13.2	Nuclease Complex with RCG4 and XPA
RCG2	UV5, VH-1	XPD, XP/CS, TTD	19q13.2	5'-3' helicase TF11H subunit Essential gene
RCG3	UV24, 27-1	XPB, XP/CS, TTD	2q21	3'-5' helicase TF11H subunit Essential gene
RCG4	UV41	XPF	16p13	Nuclease Complex with RCG1 and XPA
RCG5	UV135	XPG, XP/CS	13q32-33	Nuclease
RCG6	UV61	CSB	10q11-21	Helicase
RCG7	VB11			
RCG8	US31			
RCG9	CHO4PV			
RCG10	CHO7PV			
RCG11	UV51			
XPA			9q34	DNA binding Recognizes 6-4 photoproduct Complex with RCG1 and RCG4
XPC			3p25	Defective repair of transcribed strands
XPE				Inducible DNA binding
CSA				
TTDA				TF11H subunit

[a]Based on complementation analysis or DNA transfection.

breaks (see also Friedberg et al., 1995). Some gene products may be components of more than one process. The processes differ in the fidelity of the repair achieved, leading to the concepts of error-prone and error-free repair. Error-prone processes may increase cell survival following exposure to DNA-damaging agents, but increased survival may be achieved at the cost of increased mutagenic frequency.

4.4.3 Damage Reversal

Damage reversal processes revert damaged DNA to its original state without replacement of constituents. Exposure of DNA to UV light results in the formation of pyrimidine-pyrimidine cyclobutane dimers and (6-4) photoproducts (i.e., production of a linkage between positions 6 and 4 of adjacent pyrimidine rings; Fig. 4.6). In bacterial cells, such dimers can be returned to their initial state by light-activated or photolyase enzymes in a process known as *photoreactivation* (Sancar, 1996). Photolyases have been identified in bacteria, yeast, and *Drosophila melanogaster;* a human protein with a high degree of homology to the *Drosophila* (6-4) photolyase has been identified, but a definitive role for photolyases has not been determined for human cells (Sancar, 1996; Todo et al., 1996). In mammalian cells, photoproducts are repaired primarily by nucleotide excision (Sec. 4.4.5).

A variety of alkylating agents, many of which are known or suspected carcinogens, are capable of reaction with nucleophilic sites in the bases and phosphotriester bonds of DNA. Alkylation, especially at the O^6 position of guanine and the O^4 position of thymine, may lead to mispairing during later DNA

Table 4.9. X-ray Sensitive Mutants

Complementation Group	Typical Rodent Mutants	Human Chromosome	Cell Phenotype; Putative Protein Properties
IR1	EM9	19p13.2-13.3	High sensitivity to mutagens Hypermutable Delayed SSB repair Protein complexes with ligase III
IR2	irs1	7q36.1	Defective DSB rejoining Radioresistant DNA synthesis
IR3	irs1SF	14q32.3	Collateral sensitivity to UV Normal DSB rejoining Hypermutable Defective SSB rejoining
IR4	XR-1	5q13-14	Defective DSB rejoining Defective V(D)J recombination
IR5	xrs1-7 XR-V15B XR-V9B sxi-2,3	2q34-36	Defective DSB rejoining Defective V(D)J recombination Complemented by Ku80 cDNA
IR6		22q13	Complemented by Ku80 cDNA
IR7	V3 SCID irs-20	8p11.1-q11.1	Defective DSB rejoining Defective V(D)J recombination Radioresistant DNA synthesis Defective DNA-PK$_{CS}$
IR8	irs-2 V-C4		Normal DSB rejoining Radioresistant DNA synthesis Not complemented by ATM
Ataxia telangiectasia		11q22-23	Normal DSB rejoining Radioresistant DNA synthesis Normal V(D)J recombination Defective/delayed G_1S, S, and G_2 cell cycle checkpoints Phosphatidylinositol (PI-3) kinase

synthesis and to the potential for mutagenesis and carcinogenesis. Both bacteria and higher animals including humans possess alkyl transferase enzymes capable of removing methyl and larger alkylating groups from the O^6 position of guanine and to a lesser extent from the O^4 position of thymine. Reaction with the transferase results in the transfer of the alkyl group to the cysteine residue in the transferase enzyme (Fig. 4.7). Each transferase molecule is capable of only one abstraction, leading to the designation of these molecules as "suicide enzymes." Intertissue variations in the levels of alkyl transferase enzymes may account for the highly variable organ responses to various carcinogens.

A final example of damage reversal is the rejoining, by a ligase, of a single-strand break. If the ligase is to function, the break must contain a 3'-OH and a 5'-PO$_4$ group (Fig. 4.8). Any other type of break will require additional processing, possibly including

nucleotide or polynucleotide removal and replacement, prior to ligation (see Sec. 4.4.5).

4.4.4 Mismatch Repair

In *Escherichia coli* bacteria, the mismatch repair (MMR) system is capable of repairing single-base mispairs and small insertion/deletion mispairs leading to loops of up to four or more bases (Kolodner, 1995). Bacteria incapable of mismatch repair (also known as replication error repair; RER) have a high frequency of mutations. In bacteria, the repair reaction involves mismatch recognition by the MutS protein, recruitment of MutL by MutS, and incision of the DNA by the endonuclease MutH. Incision is then followed by the excision, resynthesis, and ligation steps of RER. These latter steps require an exonuclease, polymerase, single-strand binding protein, and DNA ligase. Currently no function is

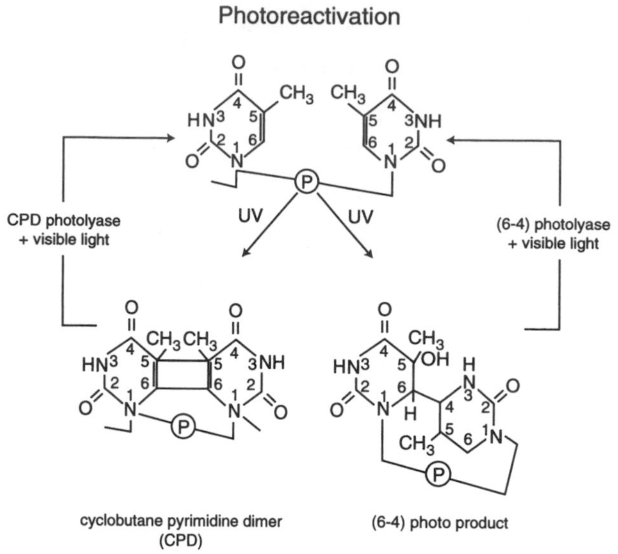

Photoreactivation

Figure 4.6. Ultraviolet-induced formation of a thymine-thymine cyclobutane dimer and a thymine-thymine (6-4) photoproduct and their reversal by CPD (cyclobutane pyrimidine dimer) photolyase, and (6-4) photolyase, respectively. In each case photoreactivation requires exposure to visible light. (Adapted from Sancar, 1996.)

known for MutL, but it may stabilize the binding of MutS and is required for MutH incision (Modrich and Lahue, 1996).

Human cells express related mismatch repair genes: *hMSH2* is a homologue of the *E. coli MutS* gene and *hMLH1* is a homologue of *MutL*. Two other human homologues of *MutL*, *hPMS1* and *hPMS2*, and another human *MutS* homologue, *GTBP/P160*, have been identified. A model for the involvement of the protein products of these genes in human mismatch repair is presented in Fig. 4.9. All mismatches require hMSH2 for repair. Some lesions in DNA, including single-base mispairs, require a heterodimer comprising hMSH2 and GTBP/P160. Other lesions may be recognized by hMSH2 alone or in combination with an unknown protein (Karran, 1995). All mismatches also require hMLH1, which exists as a heterodimer with hPMS2 and is recruited by the hMSH2 complex. Removal of the mismatch followed by resynthesis and ligation completes the repair process.

Human nonpolyposis colon cancer (HNPCC) is one of the most common inherited cancer syn-

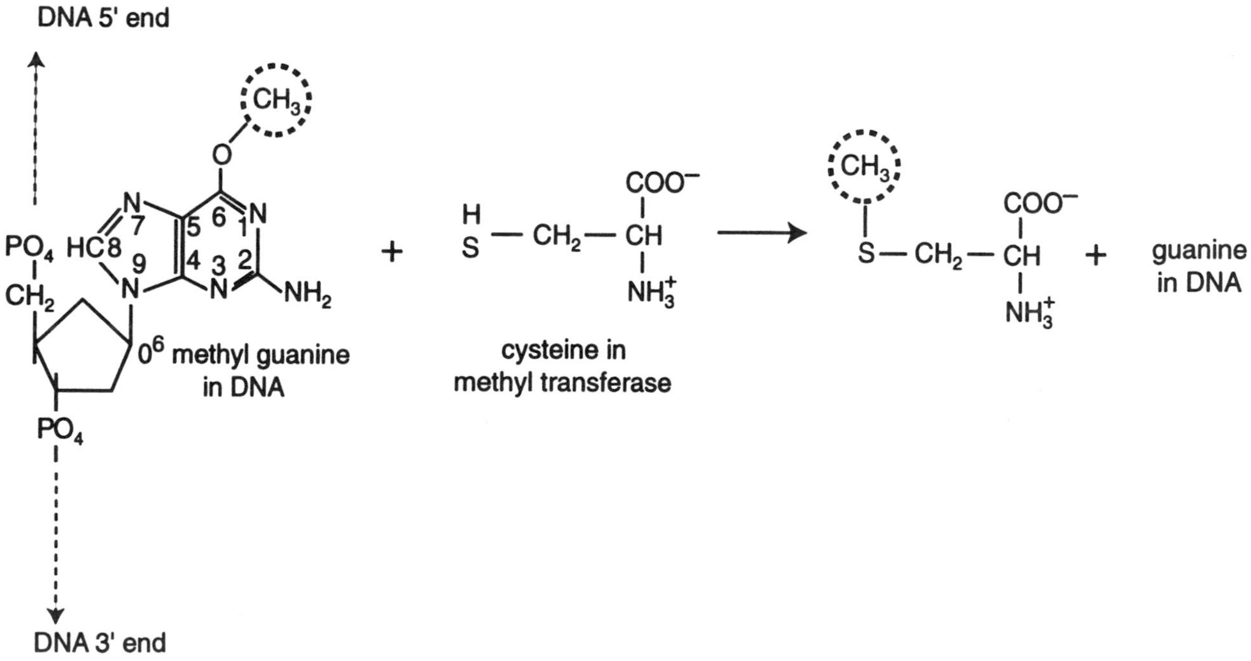

Figure 4.7. Alkyl transferase repair of O^6 methyl guanine. In the example, the methyl group is transferred to a cysteine group in the methyl transferase, resulting in the restitution of guanine and causing inactivation of the methyl transferase protein. (Adapted from Friedberg et al., 1995.)

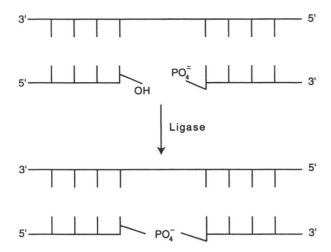

Figure 4.8, Simplest form of DNA single-strand break repair. Because the break is bounded by a 3'-OH and a 5'-PO$_4$, rejoining requires only the action of a ligase. (Adapted from Friedberg et al., 1995.)

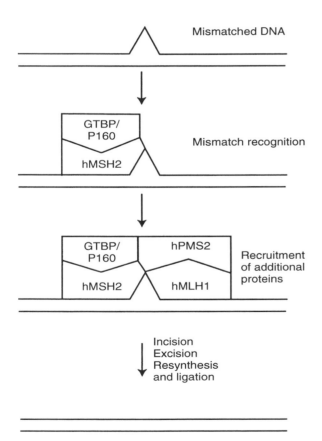

Figure 4.9. Proteins involved in human mismatch repair. The mismatch may occur by mispairing or by addition or deletion of base(s). The mismatched lesion is recognized by the hMSH2 protein or the hMSH2:GTBP/P160 heterodimer. Recognition is followed by the recruitment of hPMS2 and hMLH1. Completion of repair requires incision, excision, resynthesis, and ligation by proteins as yet unidentified.

dromes; it may account for approximately 5 percent of all colorectal cancers (Kolodner, 1995). Members of HNPCC families also show marked increases in the incidence of other cancers, especially of the ovary, stomach, and endometrium. The following evidence suggests that the HNPCC syndrome may be related to a defect in mismatch repair. Cells from HNPCC tumors exhibit a high degree of instability in microsatellite DNA: runs of approximately four to forty repeated mononucleotides or dinucleotides such as TTTT... or CACACA... occur at multiple sites in the genome and alterations in base sequence are easily detected within them. Microsatellite instability is a characteristic of mismatch repair-defective mutants in *E. coli* and yeast. Second, kindred analysis indicates that two HNPCC loci are located on chromosomes 2p and 3p, the locations of the human mismatch repair genes *hMSH2* (2p21-23) and *hMLH1* (3p21), respectively. Other HNPCC loci correspond to those of *hPMS1* and *hPMS2*. The absolute requirement for the hMSH2 and hMLH1 products and the lesser role played by GTBP/P160, hPMS1, and hMPS2 may account for the different phenotypes exhibited by cells from HNPCC tumors.

4.4.5 Base and Nucleotide Excision

The mismatch repair processes described above involve excision of mispaired nucleotides arising primarily as a result of erroneous DNA synthesis. The repair of damaged bases can also be achieved by excision of a single base in base-excision repair or of polynucleotide fragments in nucleotide excision repair.

Base-excision repair involves the enzymatic removal of one damaged base by a DNA glycosylase, specific to the altered base, leaving an apurinic or apyrimidinic site (Fig. 4.10). This site can be restored by the nicking action of an endonuclease and an exonucleolytic removal of the sugar residue and perhaps a neighboring nucleotide, followed by DNA synthesis using the opposite strand as a template and ligation. Base-excision repair tends to be limited to small lesions such as deaminated cytosines and the repair patches consist usually of only one or two nucleotides (short patch repair). Base-excision repair may also be one category of mismatch repair.

Three major features distinguish base-excision repair from nucleotide excision repair (NER): (1) base-excision repair operates primarily on small base adducts, whereas NER operates on bulky lesions such as pyrimidine dimers, other photoproducts, larger chemical adducts, and cross-links produced by agents such as mitomycin C;

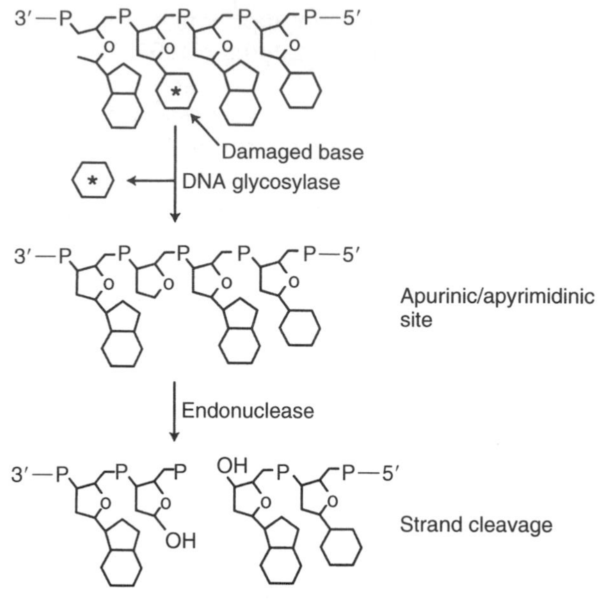

6

CHAPTER 4

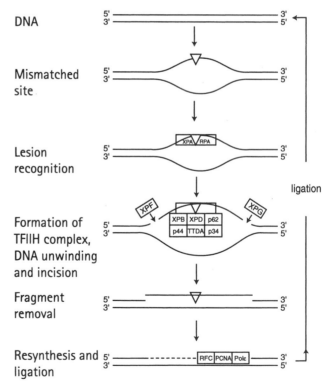

model, damaged sites are recognized by the protein product of the XPA and possibly XPE genes. Binding of XPA to RPA, a single-stranded binding protein, improves the attachment of XPA to damaged DNA. XPA recruits the TF11H transcription factor, three subunits of which are the XPB, XPD, and TTDA gene products. Once attached to the DNA, the helicase activities of XPB and XPD unwind the DNA in opposite directions and incisions leading to oligonucleotide removal are made at the opposite Y junctions by products of the XPF and XPG genes. Incision may also require the XPC product and is stimulated by the XPE product. Following removal of the oligonucleotide fragment, repair synthesis then involves DNA polymerase ε and accessory factors such as replication factor C (RFC) and proliferating cell nuclear antigen (PCNA). Ligation completes the repair process.

TF11H is involved in both transcription and repair but may interact with one group of proteins to

Figure 4.10. Base-excision repair utilizes a damage-specific glycosylase to remove the damaged base, leaving an apurinic or apyrimidinic site, which becomes a point of attack for endonuclease followed by exonuclease (or phosphodiesterase) removal of the sugar residue. Completion of repair requires nucleotide replacement using the complementary strand as a template followed by ligation. (Adapted from Friedberg et al., 1995.)

(2) base-excision results ultimately in the replacement of one or two nucleotides (short patch repair), whereas NER results in replacement patches of the order of thirty nucleotides (long patch repair); and (3) during base-excision repair, the damaged base is released as a free base, whereas in NER, the damaged site is excised as part of a long single-strand fragment. Since both types of excision repair utilize the complementary strand of DNA for repair synthesis, both are considered error-free processes.

Nucleotide excision repair is the most studied and perhaps the most complex of the DNA repair processes, involving as many as twenty to thirty genes. Lehmann (1995b) has suggested a possible model for NER (Fig. 4.11) and its relation to both transcription and cell-cycle control. The model has developed as a result of (1) the cloning of a number of genes involved in NER and the transcription factor TF11H; (2) comparison of nucleotide and derived amino acid sequences with proteins with known repair functions in bacteria and yeasts; (3) purification and biochemical testing of gene products; and (4) introduction of cloned genes and purified proteins into repair-deficient cells and use of in vitro systems to assay for their function. In the

Figure 4.11. Nucleotide excision repair in humans involves lesion recognition by XPA and RPA proteins. The XPA/RPA complex recruits the TF11H complex, leading to DNA unwinding by the XPB and XPD helicases. Endonuclease attack by XPF and XPG removes an oligonucleotide containing the lesion. Resynthesis involves RFC, PCNA, and Polε, followed by ligation. (Adapted from Lehmann, 1995a.)

control repair and another group to control transcription (Lehmann, 1995a). In addition to the gene products mentioned above, there is increasing evidence that the tumor suppressor gene p53 plays a major role in cellular response to genotoxic agents (see Sec. 4.5.3). Smith et al. (1995) have shown that cells with functional as opposed to nonfunctional p53 show greater repair activity following exposure to both ionizing radiation and UV light. They provide evidence that the effect seen with UV light is a result of enhanced NER, perhaps mediated by the interaction of the p53-regulated protein Gadd45 with proliferating cell nuclear antigen (PCNA; Smith et al., 1994).

Synthesis of both DNA and RNA is inhibited temporarily following exposure to UV light. RNA synthesis normally recovers rapidly, but this recovery is markedly slower in cells from CS patients. This led to the finding that NER is more rapid in transcribed regions of DNA than in untranscribed regions (Mellon et al., 1987). In CS cells, this transcription-coupled preferential repair is markedly inhibited and repair of transcribed strands proceeds at the same rate as that of untranscribed strands.

4.4.6 Sensitivity to Ionizing Radiation and Repair of Strand Breaks

Ionizing radiation is capable of producing both single- (SSB) and double-strand breaks (DSB) in DNA. Single-strand breaks are produced at high frequency and in general are repaired rapidly. Because radiation-induced single strand breaks are unlikely to be suitable substrates for direct ligation, as shown in Fig. 4.8, some degree of processing, perhaps requiring nucleotide removal and resynthesis using the complementary strand as a template, will be required before ligation can complete the repair process. Some single-strand breaks may also be repaired by recombinational events similar to those shown in Fig. 4.12, but overall the repair of radiation-induced single-strand breaks is poorly understood.

While DSB are induced far less frequently than SSB, unrepaired or misrepaired DSB are probably responsible for most of the cellular effects of ionizing radiation. In bacteria and yeast, repair of DSB is often accomplished by recombinational processes: In the yeast *Saccharomyces cerevisiae*, the RAD51,

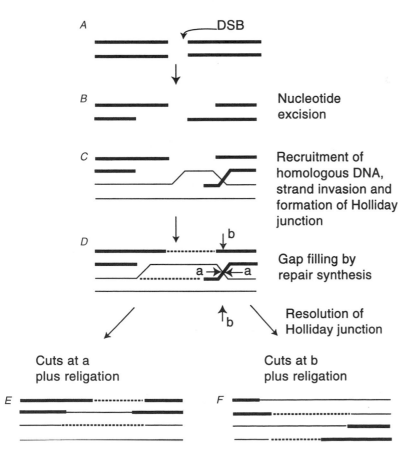

Figure 4.12. Repair of double-strand breaks (*A*) begins with nucleotide removal from both strands (*B*), followed by recruitment of complementary DNA double strands (*C*), which, in bacteria, are present in multiple copies. This allows synthesis to close the gaps using the opposite strand as a template (*D*). Endonucleases then cut the strands at either (*a*) or (*b*), and ligation of the cut ends allows repair of the lesion (*E* or *F*). (Adapted from Shinohaia and Ogawa, 1995.)

RAD52, and RAD54 gene products are involved in recombination repair. Homologues of these yeast genes have been isolated from human cells, suggesting the involvement of recombination in the repair of DSB in mammalian cells.

Figure 4.12 illustrates a possible recombination model for repair of DSB. This model requires recruitment of homologous strands that, after a process of interaction known as *strand invasion,* provide templates for synthesis to fill the two single-strand gaps. Such homologous strands are available in multiple copies in bacterial cells. How homologous strands are recruited in mammalian cells is not clear, nor is the length of homology required. The use of nonhomologous strands is, however, likely to lead to errors in repair. Panels *C* and *D* of Fig. 4.12 show the formation of a Holliday junction caused by the crossing over of single strands from two adjacent DNA duplexes. This junction requires resolution before repair and duplex separation are complete. The pairs of arrows, *a* and *b* in panel *D* of Fig. 4.12, show the positions at which specific endonucleases

(resolvases) can cut DNA strands to resolve the Holliday junction, resulting in two possible types of recombinant molecules, (*E*) or (*F*), with each molecule also containing a repair patch.

Another type of repair process, known as *daughter strand gap repair* (Fig. 4.13), involves aspects of both recombination and excision repair. DNA synthesized on unrepaired templates may contain gaps in the newly synthesized DNA. It is postulated that the existence of these gaps leads to strand invasion, the formation of a Holliday junction, and synthesis of a repair patch using a newly synthesized DNA strand as a template. Once again, resolution of the Holliday junction leads to two possible outcomes, with the original lesion contained either in its original parental strand or, alternatively, transferred to a newly synthesized strand. In either case, complete repair requires the removal of the original lesion by an excision repair process. Because repair is not complete prior to DNA synthesis, this is sometimes referred to as damage-tolerance repair or postsynthesis repair.

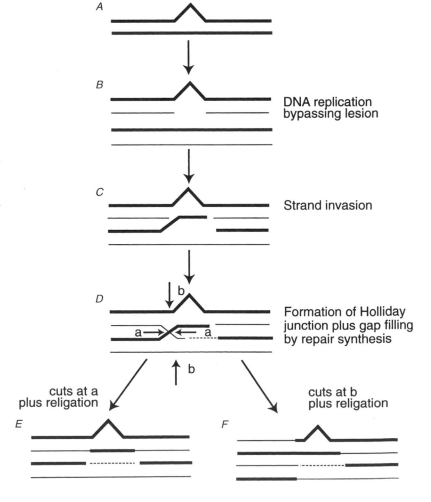

Figure 4.13. A lesion in one strand of parental DNA (*A, heavy line*) leads to a gap when used as a template for synthesis of a daughter strand (*B, light line*). Recombination (*C*) is followed by synthesis using the opposite strand as a template to close the gap (*D*). Cuts in the strands and religation can lead to complete strands as shown in *E* or *F*. Completion of repair requires repair of the initial lesion by base, nucleotide, or mismatch repair.

DNA replication bypassing lesion

Strand invasion

Formation of Holliday junction plus gap filling by repair synthesis

cuts at a plus religation

cuts at b plus religation

As shown in Table 4.9, at least eight complementation groups that confer sensitivity to ionizing radiation have been identified in rodent cells. Mutants of groups 2, 4, 5, and 7 exhibit defective rejoining of DSB and are highly sensitive to x-ray killing; cells from groups 4, 5, and 7 also exhibit pronounced defects in a plasmid assay for V(D)J recombination (Taccioli et al., 1993, 1994a; see also Chap. 11 Secs. 11.2.6 and 11.3.4)—a process responsible for the generation of immunologic diversity that involves site-specific rearrangements in DNA. Subsequent studies indicated that mutant cells of group 5 are deficient in Ku80, an end-binding protein which may protect DNA ends from degradation (Taccioli et al., 1994b). Ku80 forms a dimeric complex with another protein (Ku70), which serves as the DNA binding component of a DNA-dependent protein kinase (DNA-PK) complex. Reduced activity of the DNA-PK is responsible for the radiation sensitivity seen in mutant cells of group 7 and also for the immune defect seen in severe combined immunodeficiency (SCID) mice (Blunt et al., 1996). Cells from AT and BS patients do not appear to be defective in the plasmid assay for V(D)J recombination, so the reasons for the immunologic deficiencies seen in AT and BS patients are not yet apparent.

Cells from AT patients exhibit sensitivity to x-ray killing, a propensity to apoptotic death, but normal rejoining of double-strand breaks. The recent cloning of the AT gene, designated ATM, provided evidence that a portion of the AT gene product bears striking homology to phosphatidylinositol-3-kinases (PI-3 kinases; Lavin et al., 1995; Savitsky et al., 1995). PI-3 kinases are involved in a variety of cell signaling pathways (see Chap. 6, Sec. 6.3.3), suggesting that the AT gene product may be involved in recognition of damage and control of the cell cycle. This conclusion is strengthened by the observation that DNA synthesis in AT cells is more resistant to radiation than in normal cells and by similarities between the AT gene and a variety of yeast and *Drosophila* genes, all of which are involved in processing of DNA damage, control of the cell cycle, and maintenance of genetic stability. The use of antisera against the ATM gene product has demonstrated that the product is localized primarily in the nucleus, is not regulated by exposure to either ionizing radiation or UV, and is expressed in a wide variety of normal cells and tissues, but that expression is drastically reduced in all AT patients (Lakin et al., 1996).

Ionizing radiation is capable of producing a wide variety of lesions in DNA, including base damage and single- and double-strand breaks. It is probable that several repair processes are involved, including excision repair, single-strand break repair, recombination repair, and possibly a process of end-joining repair that is not yet defined. The observation that the products of the ATM and DNA-PK genes are involved in cell signaling and cell-cycle control processes suggests that not all gene products involved in determining cell sensitivity are involved directly in the mechanics of repair (Lavin et al., 1995; Meyn, 1995; Savitsky et al., 1995). Rather, these products may provide for cell-cycle checkpoints that allow time for DNA repair prior to crucial functions such as DNA synthesis and mitosis. These concepts are discussed briefly in the following section.

4.4.7 DNA Repair, Cellular Control, and Disease

Several of the proteins known to be defective in XP, CS, and TTD are related to the TF11H transcription complex. This observation suggests that, in addition to their roles in nucleotide excision repair, these proteins participate in the regulation of normal transcription and may act as transcription-coupled repair factors. The central role played by TF11H in both the regulation of transcription and in DNA repair may provide clues to the variety and variability of symptoms seen with XP, CS, and TTD (Lehmann, 1995a). If TF11H combines with different proteins to regulate transcription and to effect nucleotide excision repair, then certain mutations in the XP, CS, and TTD genes might lead to effects on repair whereas others might lead to effects related to transcription or to both transcription and repair. Some mutations might be of sufficient severity to prevent transcription and be incompatible with life. Others might lead to impaired transcription of certain genes and to some of the symptoms listed in Table 4.7 for XP, CS, and TTD patients. Other symptoms may arise because of inability to repair endogenously induced oxidative damage, especially in neuronal cells.

The observation that AT cells are highly sensitive to ionizing radiation led initially to the assumption that AT cells were defective in the repair of DNA strand breaks. However, most studies have suggested that AT cells are essentially normal with respect to the mechanical rejoining of DNA strand breaks, although plasmid assays have provided some evidence for reduced fidelity of DNA repair. In contrast to normal cells, AT cells treated with ionizing radiation exhibit delayed or defective induction of p53, p21 (WAFI/CIPI; see Chap. 7, Sec. 7.2.3), Gadd45, and other proteins that function in the p53 signaling pathway. Induction of p53 does, however, appear normal in AT cells exposed to UV radiation (Canman et al., 1994). The suboptimal induction of p53 in AT cells, leading to lack of cell-cycle inhibition at the G1/S boundary, could explain the radiation-resistant DNA synthesis.

Because the catalytic domain of the DNA-PK protein shows structural similarity to the AT gene, DNA-PK might play a role in the p53-mediated signaling pathway that controls cellular response to DNA damage induced by ionizing radiation. Jongmans et al. (1996) have, however, provided evidence that DNA-PK does not play a major role in the activation of p53, nor can it substitute for the ATM gene product in the control of cellular response to ionizing radiation. Rather, the two proteins appear to operate in separate signal transduction pathways, with DNA-PK activating strand break repair whereas the ATM protein serves to upregulate p53 and inhibit cell-cycle progression. DNA-PK and the ATM product cooperate to achieve repair and prevent cell cycle progression until repair is complete (Meyn, 1995; Jongmans et al., 1996).

Patients with AT show reduced immunocompetence and an increased frequency of lymphoid tumors. The generation of immunologic diversity requires site-specific DNA rearrangements (see Chap. 11, Secs. 11.2.6 and 11.3.4), and the ATM gene product may detect these breaks and lead to cell cycle delay until the breaks are rejoined (Meyn, 1995). Cells lacking the ATM gene product would progress through the cell cycle before the breaks were rejoined, leading to accumulation of chromosome translocations due to misjoining of unrepaired breaks and loss of immune competence due to improper rejoining. Such translocations would be especially frequent in regions involving the immunoglobin genes—an observation seen in B and T lymphocytes from AT patients (Kojis et al., 1991). DNA breaks arising spontaneously in non-immune-related regions of the genome would lead to the high frequency of chromosome rearrangements seen in fibroblasts from AT patients. Inappropriate activation of apoptosis in cells containing DNA damage might lead also to preferential loss of neuronal and other cell types prone to apoptosis, leading to ataxia and other neurologic defects present in AT patients (Meyn, 1995). Further interrelationships between cell-cycle control, apoptosis, and DNA repair are likely to be defined in the next few years.

4.5 HERITABLE CANCER

In the preceding section, some inherited syndromes with a deficiency in DNA repair and a high incidence of cancer were described. Studies of some of the other rare examples of predisposition to cancer that are inherited as a simple Mendelian trait have provided important insights into the concept of tumor suppressor genes. In this section, retinoblastoma and Knudson's hypothesis will be used to show how inheritance of inactivating mutations in a single gene can lead to cancer. More complex inherited cancers, such as familial breast and colon carcinoma, are based on the same genetic principles but with more complex etiology that may involve multiple genetic pathways and confounding factors such as incomplete penetrance of the predisposing mutation.

4.5.1 Retinoblastoma and Knudson's Hypothesis

Retinoblastoma is a tumor of the eye found exclusively in young children. It occurs in both hereditary and nonhereditary forms. The nonhereditary form, found in 60 percent of patients, is always unilateral. The remaining 40 percent of patients have a germline mutation that predisposes to retinoblastoma. About 80 percent of people with the germline mutation have bilateral disease (i.e., tumors arise independently in both eyes), about 15 percent have unilateral tumors, and 5 percent of individuals are asymptomatic carriers of the retinoblastoma mutation. The high cure rate in this malignancy has allowed analysis of its inheritance. In most families, the penetrance of the mutation is 90 to 95 percent, and it is inherited as an autosomal dominant trait. Linkage analysis, and characterization of the small percentage of retinoblastoma patients with a constitutional chromosome 13 deletion, has placed the retinoblastoma locus at the center of the 13q14 band.

The normal cells that are able to transform into retinoblastoma tumor cells probably disappear with age. The most likely explanation for the disappearance of these cells is that they are embryonic cells that differentiate into mature photoreceptors. Once the cells are terminally differentiated, they are no longer at risk for transformation by mutations. Knudson (1971) presented convincing evidence that the transformation of these embryonic target cells into tumor cells requires two mutations. For nonhereditary unilateral retinoblastoma, both mutations are somatic and must occur in the same cell. Because mutation frequencies are low and the putative target cells gradually disappear from the eye, it is not surprising that retinoblastoma is a very rare malignancy and occurs unilaterally. However, when the first mutation occurs in the germline, every potential target cell in the retina has undergone the first mutation and is an "initiated cell" in terms of the model shown in Fig. 4.2. A second mutation in any of the target cells will lead to malignancy. The large number of target cells in the retina almost guarantees that one or more will undergo the second mutation and develop into a tumor cell; in fact, most patients develop more than two tumors.

On the basis of the two-hit model and the occurrence of retinoblastoma in some patients with deletion of large portions of the long arm of chromosome 13, the first mutation in both hereditary and nonhereditary tumors occurs on this chromosome and involves loss of gene function. Cells carrying this mutation are therefore heterozygous at the RB locus, with one normal and one mutant allele (Fig. 4.14). Molecular studies indicate that the second mutation occurs in the remaining normal allele at the *RB* locus. Although most tumors retain two apparently normal copies of chromosome 13, a detailed genetic analysis of chromosome 13 restriction fragment length polymorphism (RFLP; Chap. 3, Sec. 3.3.5) shows that for 70 percent of tumors, the long arm of chromosome 13 becomes homozygous (i.e., there is loss of heterozygosity) at almost all loci (Figs. 4.14 and 4.15). Cavenee et al. (1985) showed that many tumors have two duplicate copies of the chromosome carrying the *RB1* mutation and have lost the chromosome carrying the normal allele (Fig. 4.15A). Sometimes tumors have only a single copy of chromosome 13 (Fig. 4.15B) or have a deleted chromosome 13 (Fig. 4.15C); they have presumably retained the chromosome carrying the mutant allele at the *RB1* locus and lost the one with the normal allele. A few tumors remain heterozygous at loci near the centromere and become homozygous for all distal loci; in these tumors, mitotic recombination probably creates the observed pattern of homozygosity (Fig. 4.15D). Thirty percent of retinoblastoma tumors remain heterozygous at all loci tested on chromosome 13; subsequent work has shown that in these tumors, a second independent mutation has inactivated the normal allele (Fig. 4.15E).

The loss of heterozygosity on chromosome 13 occurs in both heritable and sporadic forms of retinoblastoma, indicating that the same mutations are involved in both forms of the disease. Other chromosomes retain the same heterozygous state detected in normal cells from the same individuals. Interestingly, osteosarcomas arising in patients with a germline mutation at the retinoblastoma locus are also homozygous for chromosome 13, and there is an increased incidence of a similar homozygosity in osteosarcoma patients who do not have the germline mutation. Thus, mutations of the *RB* gene appear to be responsible for at least two different tumors, retinoblastoma and osteosarcoma; for both tumors, identical genetic mechanisms appear responsible for tumor formation. The mutation is recessive at the cellular level and only appears dominant in the individual because of the large number of target cells at risk for a second somatic event.

4.5.2 The Retinoblastoma Gene

The retinoblastoma or *RB* gene (locus name is *RB1*) was cloned by isolating and sequencing genomic DNA fragments derived from band 13q14 on chromosome 13. Friend et al. (1986) identified the *RB* gene and several different investigators confirmed that the *RB* gene was subject to unique inactivating mutations in retinoblastomas and osteosarcomas and

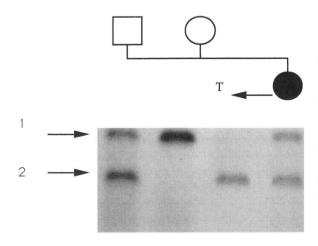

Figure 4.14. The usefulness of restriction fragment length polymorphisms (RFLPs) to identify the loss of genetic information in a retinoblastoma tumor is illustrated. In this particular example, DNA probe p88 detects an RFLP (with the restriction enzyme Xba1) in the RB1 gene. As shown in the figure, the mother is homozygous for this marker (*lane 2*), having only allele 1, and the father heterozygous, having both alleles 1 and 2 (*lane 1*). The daughter inherited one allele from each parent and is also heterozygous in the majority of her cells (*lane 4*). However, the retinoblastoma that arose in the child (*lane 3*) shows a loss of the allele (*upper band 1*) inherited from the mother and retains only the RB1 allele inherited from the father. (Figure courtesy of Xiaoping Zhu, Hospital for Sick Children, Canada.)

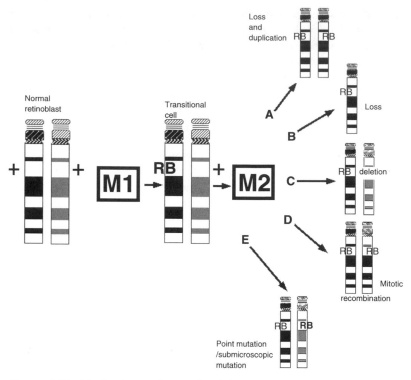

Figure 4.15. Mechanisms of mutational inactivation of a tumor suppressor gene illustrated using the retinoblastoma gene *(RB1)*. Retinoblastoma tumors appear to occur when two independent mutations, M1 and M2, inactivate both normal alleles at the *RB1* (RB) locus on chromosome 13 at band 13q14. In most cases the first mutation, M1, is localized to the *RB1* locus. One of several different mechanisms generate the second mutation, M2, in the remaining normal allele at the RB1 locus. The most frequently observed mechanism results in the chromosome carrying the normal allele being lost entirely and the chromosome bearing the mutant RB1 allele being duplicated (*A*). Sometimes the normal chromosome is lost and the mutant chromosome remains as an apparent monosomic chromosome (*B*). Occasionally it is possible to detect a small cytogenetic deletion at band 13q14 (*C*); this loss will have the same genetic effect as mechanisms *A* and *B*. Mitotic recombination is another mechanism, such that the proximal part of chromosome 13 retains paternal and maternal markers but the distal portions of chromosome 13 contain only the RFLP markers characteristic of the chromosome carrying the retinoblastoma mutation (*D*). In about 30 percent of cases, there is no gross chromosomal mechanism involved; rather, these patients have two independent mutations in each RB1 allele (*E*). Molecular methods such as sequencing, single-stranded conformational polymorphism analysis, or RNase protection are required to detect this type of mutation (see Chap. 3).

in the germline of patients with heritable retinoblastoma (reviewed in Gallie et al., 1990). These data provided unequivocal evidence that the first gene responsible for a human malignancy had been cloned.

The *RB* gene appears to be transcribed in all cells, and it is not clear why the mutant allele predisposes retinal or osteoid cells, in particular, to malignancy. In fact, mutations in the *RB* gene may predispose other types of cell to malignant transformation. Some individuals who develop breast, bladder, or lung cancer have structural abnormalities of the retinoblastoma gene (Harbour et al., 1988; Lee et al., 1988), suggesting that the *RB* gene may play a role in carcinogenesis in several different types of cancer. Characterization of *RB* gene mutations and of their gene products supports the proposal that it is loss of normal *RB* function which leads to malignancy. Thus *RB* is a tumor suppressor gene.

The *RB* gene product, pRB, which is 928 amino acids long and has a molecular weight of 110 kDa, is found in cell nuclei. The RB protein probably has a fundamental role in regulating normal cell proliferation (see Chap. 7, Sec. 7.2). The RB protein exists in both phosphorylated and dephosphorylated forms. Phosphorylation of pRB is at a low level at the beginning of the cell cycle (G_1) and increases as the cycle progresses (S and G_2). Recent work has shown that pRB binds to and potentially inactivates the E2F transcription complex, which is involved in cell cycle regulation (Weinberg, 1995). This binding is inhibited by phosphorylation of pRB protein just before S phase in the cell cycle. The release of the E2F transcription complex from pRB control allows the cell cycle to proceed. Because of the pivotal role played by pRB in cell-cycle regulation, loss of the *RB* gene by mutation may contribute to a deregulated cell cycle, to uncontrolled cell division, and thus to tumor development.

The RB protein may be important for transformation of a variety of cell types by DNA tumor viruses of the adeno-, polyoma-, and papillomavirus classes (see Chap. 5, Sec. 5.2). Each of these viruses encodes one or more transforming proteins able to bind pRB (Weinberg, 1995). For example, pRB binds to the E1A-encoded transformation protein of adenovirus, which activates transcription of both viral and cellular genes. In fact, malignant transformation of cells by DNA tumor viruses requires that the viruses be able to inactivate both pRB and p53. Intriguingly, all three classes of unrelated DNA tumor viruses have evolved an identical mechanism for activating host-cell proliferation.

4.5.3 Tumor Suppressor Genes in Other Malignancies

As described in Secs. 4.5.1 and 4.5.2, mutations in a tumor suppressor gene contribute to the malignant process when both normal alleles have inactivating mutations. Based on observations in retinoblastoma (Fig. 4.15) and in Wilms' tumor (another inherited form of cancer occurring in children), the most common sequence for acquiring mutations in both alleles is for an initial mutation to occur in one allele and for a mitotic recombination to occur between the chromosome carrying the mutant allele and the chromosome carrying the normal allele. After mitosis, one daughter cell will have two mutant alleles and one daughter cell two normal alleles. In addition, the mitotic recombination leads to the daughter cells having two copies of the paternal chromosome or two copies of the maternal chromosome. The easiest way to identify mitotic recombi-

natin is offered by RFLPs that distinguish the maternal and paternal chromosomes. If mitotic recombination has occurred in a tumor, RFLPs that distinguish the maternal and paternal chromosomes in normal cells of a patient will show only one allele in the tumor (Fig. 4.14). Regions of the genome in a tumor frequently showing *loss of heterozygosity* (LOH) for informative RFLP may contain tumor suppressor genes. Thus, a common analysis of tumors now involves RFLP analysis of regions subject to recurrent LOH, followed by a detailed investigation of the region commonly deleted to isolate the tumor suppressor gene involved.

Wilms' tumor is a kidney tumor of childhood, which has many characteristics in common with retinoblastoma. It occurs in both heritable and nonheritable forms, and the heritable form is frequently bilateral. In Wilms' tumor, deletions or mutations are found in a gene on the short arm of chromosome 11 in the 11p13 region. Utilizing a similar strategy to that described for the *RB* gene, the *WT1* gene was isolated by positional cloning (Rose et al., 1990). However, linkage studies in some families with Wilms' tumor have now shown an absence of linkage to chromosome 11, suggesting that mutations in another as yet unidentified genetic locus can also predispose to this tumor. These results indicate that the genetic events leading to Wilms' tumor are more complex than those leading to retinoblastoma.

Many investigators have observed LOH in a variety of cancers and have proposed the identified region to be etiologically involved: genetic analysis of some of these loci has led to characterization of tumor suppressor genes (see Table 4.4). Other loci that commonly show LOH include chromosome 3p in small-cell carcinoma of the lung and renal cell carcinoma, chromosome 2 in bladder carcinoma, chromosome 22 in acoustic neuroma and meningioma, and chromosome 1 in neuroblastoma (reviewed in Strachan and Read, 1996). It remains to be established whether recurrent chromosome deletions, LOH, or monosomies involving a large number of other genomic regions in sporadic malignancies indicate the presence of many more tumor suppressor genes present in the human genome.

The *p53* tumor suppressor gene is located on the short arm of chromosome 17 and encodes a 393–amino acid nuclear phosphoprotein. Mutations of this gene are among the commonest somatic genetic changes found in human cancer (Holstein et al., 1991; see also Chap. 5, Sec. 5.5.2). The *p53* gene is not required for normal development, but lack of p53 function confers a greatly elevated risk of malignancy. Germline mutations of *p53* have been identified as the cause of Li-Fraumeni syndrome as well as a predisposition to a spectrum of tumors of which breast and brain tumors are the most common (reviewed in Knudson, 1993). A better understanding of the role of p53 as a tumor suppressor, functioning as "the guardian of the genome," has emerged in recent years (Lane, 1993). Loss of normal p53 protein is associated with genetic instability. The p53 protein is usually present in minute amounts, but when cells are exposed to agents that could potentially damage DNA, p53 levels rise to initiate a protective response by blocking the cell cycle or by inducing apoptosis (see Chap. 7, Sec. 7.3). Loss of p53 function allows cells that sustain genetic damage to survive and propagate, leading to the development of neoplasia.

4.5.4 Colon Carcinoma

Colon carcinoma is particularly suitable for the study of tumor progression because it develops slowly over several years and progresses through cytologically distinct benign and malignant stages of growth. In colon carcinoma, one of the chromosomal regions showing cytogenetic changes, 5p, also shows linkage to colon carcinoma in rare familial cases. Vogelstein et al. (1989) analyzed genetic regions showing deletion or mutation in colon cancer and proposed an etiologic combination of genetic events for the development of colon cancer (Fig. 4.16). They proposed that a mutation that involves a predisposing gene called *APC* (adenomatous polyposis coli) on chromosome 5p transforms normal epithelial tissue lining the gut to hyperproliferating tissue. Hypomethylation of DNA, activation of the Kirsten *ras* (*K-ras*) proto-oncogene, and loss of the *DCC* (deleted in colon carcinoma) gene are involved in the progression to a benign adenoma. Loss of the *p53* gene and other chromosomal losses

are involved in the progression to malignant carcinoma and metastasis. This sequence of events is not invariable, however, and may differ in some colon cancers.

Mutations of K-*ras* and DCC appear to be associated with the intermediate stage of colorectal tumorigenesis. Activating mutations in codons 12 or 13 of the *K-ras* gene occur in 50 percent of colorectal carcinomas and adenomas (Fearon and Vogelstein, 1990). The *ras* gene family are cytoplasmic proto-oncogenes with signal transduction functions (see Chap. 6, Sec. 6.3.4) that, when defective, send inappropriate growth signals to downstream proteins. DCC is expressed at a low level in many tissues, including normal colonic mucosa, but expression is reduced or absent in colorectal cancer tissue. This finding is consistent with DCC being a tumor suppressor gene in colon carcinoma, since both copies of the gene are inactivated in large adenomas as well as carcinomas. Some types of colon carcinoma families have an hereditary form involving defective DNA repair (see Sec. 4.4.4). In these patients, loss of mismatch repair function leads to accumulated mutations that arise because of uncorrected misalignments or DNA slippage between template and daughter DNA strands during replication (Karran, 1996; Stratton, 1996). As the malignancy develops, this defect confers a general mutator phenotype that accelerates the accumulation of mutations in critical target genes as the tumor progresses.

The different genetic changes discovered in colon carcinoma illustrate that most cancers arise from a progressive series of events that incrementally increase the extent of transformation of a cell; eventually a cell emerges whose descendants multiply without appropriate restraints. Further changes give these cells the capacity to invade and metastasize to adjacent tissues. The requirement for several mutations to produce a cancer has been called the *multi-hit concept of carcinogenesis* (reviewed in Vogelstein and Kinzler, 1993). Some cancers may arise follow-

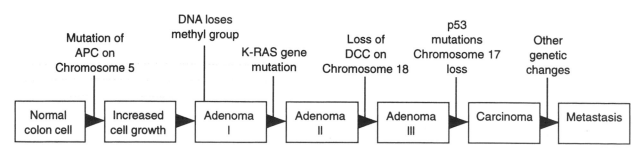

Figure 4.16. Genetic changes and progression in colon cancer. (Modified from Fearon and Vogelstein, 1990.)

ing an orderly sequence of specific genetic changes, in many cancers, however, the transition from normal to malignant cell can likely occur by several pathways involving different genes. In many instances, initial genetic changes may not alter normal cellular function. Multistep schemes of tumor progression have also been proposed for malignancies of the bladder, prostate, brain, cervix, and breast.

4.5.5 Breast Cancer

Familial breast cancer occurs in about 5 percent of patients; it is characterized by early onset and by bilateral disease. Segregation studies suggest an autosomal dominant inheritance of susceptibility genes with incomplete penetrance predisposing to breast cancer. Analysis of breast cancer families by Hall et al. (1990) demonstrated the existence of a breast cancer susceptibility gene on the long arm of human chromosome 17. This gene was subsequently named *BRCA1*. Constitutional mutations of the *BRCA1* gene are estimated to account for 45 percent of families with a high incidence of breast cancer and at least 80 percent of families with an increased incidence of both breast and ovarian cancer. The *BRCA1* gene has been cloned and found to be a large gene that shows only limited homology to other known genes (Miki et al., 1994). Near the amino terminus of the predicted protein is a RING-finger motif associated with DNA-binding proteins and gene regulation. Virtually all inherited mutations cause the BRCA1 protein to be prematurely truncated, in keeping with its predicted role as a tumor suppressor gene (reviewed in Cannon-Albright and Skolnick, 1996). SSCP analysis (Sec. 3.3.8) and DNA sequencing (Sec. 3.3.6) have been used to identify mutations within the *BRCA1* gene. Using these techniques, mutations were identified in 16 percent of women with a family history of breast cancer. However, the rates were found to be higher among women from families with a history of both breast cancer and ovarian cancer (Couch et al., 1997). A large number of distinct mutations have been reported, although some families have identical mutations, probably due to a founder effect. There is some evidence to suggest that mutations at the 5' end of the gene carry a higher risk of ovarian cancer than those at the 3' end. *BRCA1* is infrequently mutated in sporadic breast or ovarian cancer (Stratton, 1996), although LOH in regions adjacent to *BRCA1* is common, suggesting that other genes close to *BRCA1* may be important in sporadic forms of both types of tumor.

Genetic linkage analysis has mapped another breast cancer susceptibility gene, *BRCA2*, to chromosome 13q12-13. This gene has recently been cloned and germline mutations of *BRCA2* in breast cancer families have been identified (Wooster et al., 1995). Mutations of *BRCA2* invariably cause disruption to the open reading frame of the transcriptional unit of the gene, again suggestive of a tumor suppressor function. Mutations in *BRCA2* appear to account for an additional 45 percent of familial breast cancers. *BRCA2* carries a risk of breast cancer similar to that of *BRCA1*, but it is associated with a lower risk of ovarian cancer and a higher risk of male breast cancer. Somatic mutations of *BRCA2* in sporadic breast and ovarian cancer are very rare. Between them, *BRCA1* and *BRCA2* may be responsible for about 90 percent of hereditary breast cancers. Defects in other genes, such as *p53*, the ataxia telangiectasia gene, and other as yet unidentified breast cancer susceptibility genes are likely to explain the predisposition to breast cancer in other familial cases.

As the complex genetic nature of common malignancies such as breast cancer becomes elucidated, there are increasing concerns about the potential impact of laboratory-based predictive genetic testing. These concerns include the development of recommendations for women with mutations in breast cancer susceptibility genes (bilateral mastectomy with or without oophorectomy versus observation), advice about family planning, access to insurance for life and health care, and management of anxiety and psychosocial issues (Malkin and Knoppers, 1996).

4.6 SUMMARY

Strong evidence supports the conclusion that cancer is a genetic disease. Cancer onset probably requires two or more mutations in the stem cells of the tissue, but development of a tumor likely depends on the kinetics of cellular proliferation and numerous host factors, such as availability of growth factors and presence of host resistance. Certain cancers, such as retinoblastoma and Wilms' tumor, appear to arise primarily through the acquisition of inherited and somatic genetic alterations at a single genetic locus, while others, including sporadic carcinomas of the lung, bladder, and colon, result from acquired genetic abnormalities in multiple genes, perhaps as a result of exposure to environmental factors. Most cancers probably have a heritable subgroup. Studies of partially inbred populations, such as the Mormon population in Utah, suggest that the risk of developing most of the common cancers is associated with genetic factors. However, mutations associated with this increase in risk have not been identified, and some of the observations might be explained by environmental factors.

Individuals suffering from genetic defects resulting in deficiency of DNA repair may exhibit increased malignancy and/or other clinical symptoms. Some individuals will also exhibit extreme sensitivity to radiation and/or chemotherapy. Cells obtained from these individuals as well as repair-deficient mutants of rodent cell lines have demonstrated the existence of a variety of pathways for DNA repair, each relatively specialized for certain types of spontaneous or induced lesions. Each pathway involves several gene products. Some of these gene products are involved in other cellular processes, including control of transcription, control of the cell cycle, and the generation of immune diversity. Improved understanding of these properties should lead to further elucidation of the mechanisms of DNA repair in mammalian cells and of the mechanisms and diversity of oncogenic processes, including disease-site specificity.

Chromosomal abnormalities are associated with many types of tumors. Some of these, such as the rearrangements of Burkitt's lymphoma and the Philadelphia chromosome in CML, involve the breakage of chromosomes close to known oncogenes. Many of these chromosomal abnormalities may be early or initiating events. The progression of genetic changes leading to cancer is best understood for colon carcinoma. Other mutations involve amplification of genes or the addition or deletion of chromosomal material. Analyses of common abnormalities have provided important clues to the sites of genes involved in cancer causation and progression. There has been rapid progress in the isolation and characterization of genes involved in human cancer.

REFERENCES

Ames BN: Dietary carcinogens and anticarcinogens. *Science* 1983; 221:1256–1264.

Anderson MJ, Stanbridge EJ: Tumor suppressor genes studied by cell hybridization and chromosome transfer. *FASEB J* 1993; 7:826–833.

Ashley DJB: The two "hit" and multiple "hit" theories of carcinogenesis. *Br J Cancer* 1969; 23:313–328.

Blunt T, Gell D, Fox M, et al: Identification of a nonsense mutation in the carboxyl-terminal region of DNA-dependent protein kinase catalytic subunit in the SCID mouse. *Proc Natl Acad Sci USA* 1996; 93:10285–10290.

Bongarzone I, Butti MG, Coronelli S et al. Frequent activation of ret protooncogene by fusion with a new activating gene in papillary thyroid carcinomas. *Cancer Res* 1994; 54: 2979–2985.

Canman CE, Wolff AC, Chen CY, et al: The p53-dependent G_1 cell cycle checkpoint pathway and ataxia telangiectasia. *Cancer Res* 1994; 54:5054–5058.

Cannon-Albright LA, Skolnick MH: The genetics of familial breast cancer. *Semin Oncol* 1996; 23:1–5.

Cavenee WK, Hansen MF, Nordenskjold M, et al: Genetic origin of mutations predisposing to retinoblastoma. *Science* 1985; 228:501–503.

Collins ARS: Mutant rodent cell lines sensitive to ultraviolet light, ionizing radiation and cross-linking agents; A comprehensive survey of genetic and biochemical characteristics. *Mutat Res* 1993; 293:99–118.

Couch FJ, DeShano ML, Blackwood MA: *BRCA1* mutations in women attending clinics that evaluate the risk of breast cancer. *N Eng J Med* 1997; 336:1409–1415.

Deschavanne PJ, Fertil B: A review of human cell radiosensitivity in vitro. *Int J Radiat Oncol Biol Phys* 1996; 34:251–266.

Easton DF: Cancer risks in A-T heterozygotes (review). *Int J Radiat Biol* 1994; 66(supp 6):5177–5182.

Fearon ER, Vogelstein B: A genetic model of colorectal tumorigenesis. *Cell* 1990; 61:759–767.

Fredericks WJ, Galili N, Mukhopadhyay S, et al: The pax3-fkhr fusion protein created by the t(2/13) translocation in alveolar rhabdomyosarcoma is a more potent transcriptional activator than pax3. *Mol Cell Biol* 1995; 15:1522–1535.

Friedberg EC, Walker GC, Siede W: *DNA Repair and Mutagenesis.* Washington DC: ASM Press; 1995.

Friend SH, Bernards R, Rogelj S, et al: A human DNA segment with properties of the gene that predisposes to retinoblastoma and osteosarcoma. *Nature* 1986; 323: 643–646.

Gallie BL, Squire JA, Goddard A, et al: Mechanism of oncogenesis in retinoblastoma. *Lab Invest* 1990; 62: 394–408.

Gillard EF, Solomon E: Acute promyelocytic leukaemia and the t(15;17) translocation. *Semin Can Biol* 1993; 4:359–368.

Hahn PJ: Molecular biology of double minute chromosomes. *Bioessays* 1993; 15:477–484.

Hall JM, Lee MK, Newman B, et al. Linkage of early-onset familial breast cancer to chromosome 17q21. *Science* 1990; 250:1684-1689.

Harbour JW, Lai SL, Whang PJ, et al: Abnormalities in structure and expression of the human retinoblastoma gene in SCLC. *Science* 1988; 241:353–357.

Hogge DE: Cytogenetics and oncogenes in leukemia. *Curr Opin Oncol* 1994; 6:3–13.

Holstein M, Sidransky D, Vogelstein B, et al: p53 in human cancer. *Science* 1991; 253:49–53.

Ilson DH, Motzer RJ, Rodriguez E, et al: Genetic analysis in the diagnosis of neoplasms of unknown primary tumor site. *Semin Oncol* 1993; 20: 229–37.

Jeggo PA, Carr AM, Lehmann AR: Cloning human DNA

repair genes involved in ionizing radiation sensitivity. *Int J Radiat Biol* 1994; 66:573–577.

Jongmans W, Artuso M, Vuillaume M, et al: The role of ataxia telangiectasia and the DNA-dependent protein kinase in the p-53-mediated cellular response to ionizing radiation. *Oncogene* 1996; 13:1133–1138.

Karran P: Appropriate partners make good matches. *Science* 1995; 268:1857–1858.

Karran P: Microsatellite instability and DNA mismatch repair in human cancer. *Semin Cancer Biol* 1996; 7: 15–24.

Knudson AG: Antioncogenes and human cancer. *Proc Natl Acad Sci USA* 1993; 90:10914–10921.

Kojis TL, Gatti RA, Sparkes RS: The cytogenetics of ataxia telangiectasia. *Cancer Genet Cytogenet* 1991; 56:143–156.

Kolodner RD: Mismatch repair: mechanisms and relationship to cancer susceptibility. *Trends Biochem Sci* 1995; 20:397–401.

Lakin ND, Weber P, Stankovic T: Analysis of the ATM protein in wild-type and ataxia telangiectasia cells. *Oncogene* 1996; 13:2707–2716.

Lane DP: Cancer: A death in the life of p53. *Nature* 1993; 362:786–787.

Lavin MF, Khanna KK, Beamish H: Relationship of the ataxia telangiectasia protein to phosphoinositide 3-kinase. *Trends Biochem Sci* 1995; 20:382–383.

Lee EY, To H, Shew JY, et al: Inactivation of the retinoblastoma susceptibility gene in human breast cancers. *Science* 1988; 241:218–221.

Lehmann AR: Workshop on eukaryotic DNA repair genes and gene products. *Cancer Res* 1995a; 55:968–970.

Lehmann AR: Nucleotide excision repair and the link with transcription. *Trends Biochem Sci* 1995b; 20: 402–405.

Malkin D, Knoppers BM: Genetic predisposition to cancer—Issues to consider. *Semin Cancer Biol* 1996; 7:49–53.

Mellon I, Spivak G, Hanawalt PC: Selective removal of transcription-blocking DNA damage from the transcribed strand of the mammalian DHFR gene. *Cell* 1987; 51:241–249.

Meyn MS: Ataxia telangiectasia and cellular responses to DNA damage. *Cancer Res* 1995; 55:5991–6001.

Miki Y, Swensen J, Shattuck-Eidens D, et al. A strong candidate for the breast and ovarian cancer susceptibility gene BRCA1. *Science* 1994; 266:66–71.

Mintz B, Illmensee K: Normal genetically mosaic mice produced from malignant teratocarcinoma cells. *Proc Natl Acad Sci USA* 1975; 72:3585–3589.

Modrich P, Lahue L: Mismatch repair in replication fidelity, genetic recombination and cancer biology. *Annu Rev Biochem* 1996; 65:101–133.

Moolgavkar SH, Knudson AG Jr: Mutation and cancer: a model for human carcinogenesis. *J Natl Cancer Inst* 1981; 66:1037–1052.

Mulvihill JJ: Genetic repertory of human neoplasia. In: Mulvihill JJ, Miller RW, Fraumeni JF Jr, eds. *Genetics of Human Cancer*. New York: Raven Press; 1977:137–143.

Paterson MC: Ataxia telangiectasia: An inherited human disorder involving hypersensitivity to ionizing radiation

and related DNA-damaging chemicals. *Annu Rev Genet* 1979; 13:291–318.

Peto J: Genetic predisposition to cancer. In: Cairns J, Lyon JL, Skolnick M, eds. *Banbury Report 4: Cancer Incidence in Defined Populations*. Cold Spring Harbor, NY: Cold Spring Harbor Laboratory; 1980:203–213.

Rabbitts TH: Chromosomal translocations in human cancer. *Nature* 1994; 372:143–149.

Rhyu MS: Molecular mechanisms underlying hereditary nonpolyposis colorectal carcinoma. *J Natl Cancer Inst* 1996; 88:240–251.

Rodriguez E, Sreekantaiah C, Chaganti RSK: Genetic changes in epithelial solid neoplasia. *Cancer Res* 1994; 54:3398–3406.

Rose EA, Glaser T, Jones C, et al: Complete physical map of the WAGR region of 11p13 localizes a candidate Wilms' tumor gene. *Cell* 1990; 60:495–508.

Rowley JD: A new consistent chromosomal abnormality in chronic myelogenous leukemia identified by quinacrine fluorescence and Giemsa staining. *Nature* 1973; 243: 290–293.

Sancar A: No "end of history" for photolyases. *Science* 1996; 272:48–49.

Savitsky K, Bar-Shiva A, Gilad S, et al: A single ataxia telangiectasia gene with a product similar to PI-3 kinase. *Science* 1995; 268:1749–1753.

Sheer D, Squire JA: Clinical applications of genetic rearrangements in cancer *Semin Cancer Biol* 1996; 7: 25–32.

Shibuya T, Mak TW: Host control of susceptibility to erythroleukemia and to types of leukemia induced by Friend murine leukemia virus: Initial and late stages. *Cell* 1982; 31:483–493.

Shinohaia R, Ogawa T: Homologous recombination and the roles of double strand breaks. *Trends Biochem Sci* 1995; 20:387–391.

Skolnick M, Bishop DT, Carmelli D, et al: A population-based assessment of familial cancer risk in Utah Mormon genealogies. In: Arrighi FE, Rao PN, Subblefield E, eds. *Genes, Chromosomes and Neoplasia*. New York: Raven Press, 1981:477–500.

Smith ML, Chen IT, Zhan Q, et al: Interaction of the p53-regulated protein Gadd45 with proliferating cell nuclear antigen. *Science* 1994; 266:1376–1380.

Smith ML, Chen IT, Zhan Q, et al: Involvement of the p53 tumour suppressor in repair of UV-type DNA damage. *Oncogene* 1995; 10:1053–1059.

Sorensen PHB, Triche TJ: Gene fusions encoding chimeric transcription factors in solid tumors. *Semin Cancer Biol* 1996; 7:3–14.

Squire JA, Weksberg R: Genomic imprinting in tumours. *Semin Cancer Biol* 1996; 7:41–47.

Sreekantaiah C, Ladanyi M, Rodriguez E, Chaganti RSK: Chromosomal aberrations in soft tissue tumors: Relevance to diagnosis, classification, and molecular mechanism. *Am J Pathol* 1994; 144:1121–1134.

Stein U, Shoemaker RH, Schlag PM: MDR1 gene expression: evaluation of its use as a molecular marker for prognosis and chemotherapy of bone and soft tissue sarcomas. *Eur J Cancer* 1996; 32A:86–92.

Stratton MR: Recent advances in understanding of genetic susceptibility to breast cancer. *Hum Molec Genet* 1996; 5:1515–1519.

Swift M, Reitnauer PJ, Morrell D, et al: Breast and other cancers in families with ataxia telangiectasia. *N Engl J Med* 1987; 316:1289–1294.

Taccioli GE, Rathbun G, Oltz E, et al: Impairment of V(D)J recombination in double strand break repair mutants. *Science* 1993; 260:207–210.

Taccioli GE, Cheng HL, Varghese AJ, et al: A DNA repair defect in Chinese hamster ovary cells affects V(D)J recombination similarly to the murine SCID mutation. *J Biol Chem* 1994a; 269:7439–7442.

Taccioli GE, Gottlieb TM, Blunt T, et al: Ku80: product of the XRCC5 gene and its role in DNA repair. *Science* 1994b; 265:1442–1445.

Todo T, Ryo H, Yamamoto K, et al: Similarity among the drosophila (6-4) photolyase, a human photolyase homolog and the DNA photolyase-blue-light photoreceptor family. *Science* 1996; 272:109–112.

Vogelstein B, Fearon ER, Kern SE, et al: Allelotype of colorectal carcinomas. *Science* 1989; 244:207–211.

Vogelstein B, Kinzler KW: The multistep nature of cancer. *Trends Genet* 1993; 9:138–141.

Weeda G, Hoeijmakers JHJ, Bootsma D: Genes controlling nucleotide excision repair in eukaryotic cells. *Bioessays* 1993; 15:249–258.

Weeks DE, Paterson MC, Lange K, et al: Assessment of chronic γ radiosensitivity as an in vitro assay for heterozygote identification of ataxia telangiectasia. *Radiat Res* 1991; 128:90–99.

Weinberg RA: The retinoblastoma protein and cell cycle control. *Cell* 1995; 81:323–330.

Wooster R, Bignell G, Lancaster J, et al: Identification of the breast cancer susceptibility gene BRCA2. *Nature* 1995; 378:789–792.

BIBLIOGRAPHY

Heim S, Mitelman F: Cancer Cytogenetics. New York: Wiley; 1995.

Knudson AG Jr: Mutation and cancer: Statistical study of retinoblastoma. Proc Natl Acad Sci USA 1971; 68: 20–823.

Strachan T, Read A: Human Molecular Genetics. Oxford, England: Bios Scientific Publishers; 1996.

5

Viruses, Oncogenes, and Tumor Suppressor Genes

Sam Benchimol and Mark D. Minden

5.1 INTRODUCTION

5.2 DNA TUMOR VIRUSES
    5.2.1 Simian Virus 40 and Polyomavirus
    5.2.2 Human Adenoviruses
    5.2.3 Human Papillomaviruses
    5.2.4 Epstein-Barr Virus
    5.2.5 Hepatitis B Virus

5.3 RETROVIRUSES
    5.3.1 Life Cycle
    5.3.2 Acute Transforming Viruses
    5.3.3 Chronic Tumor Viruses
    5.3.4 Human T-Cell Leukemia Virus
    5.3.5 HTLV-2 and HIV

5.4 ONCOGENES IN HUMAN CANCER
    5.4.1 Identification of Oncogenes by Transfer of DNA
    5.4.2 Activation of Oncogenes by Mutation
    5.4.3 Amplification of Oncogenes
    5.4.4 Chromosome Translocation and Gene Rearrangement
    5.4.5 Multiple Oncogenes
    5.4.6 Protein Products of Oncogenes

5.5 TUMOR SUPPRESSOR GENES
    5.5.1 Tumor Suppressor Genes and Loss of Heterozygosity
    5.5.2 The p53 Gene
    5.5.3 Other Tumor Suppressor Genes

5.6 SUMMARY

REFERENCES

5.1 INTRODUCTION

Cancer is a complex disease, and a large number of cellular genes have now been implicated in the development of malignancy (see Chap. 4). These genes can be divided into two distinct groups, known as the oncogenes and the tumor suppressor genes.

Oncogenes were identified initially in cancer-causing viruses. These viruses fall into two groups: the DNA tumor viruses that contain either linear or circular double-stranded DNA and the RNA-containing tumor viruses (also called *retroviruses*). Stehelin et al. (1976) demonstrated that Rous sarcoma virus (a retrovirus that causes sarcomas in chickens) contained nucleotide sequences that were not found in related but nontransforming retroviruses. These novel retroviral sequences, however, were closely related to nucleotide sequences present in the DNA of normal chickens. This important discovery indicated that a viral transforming gene (in this case v-*src*) was derived from a normal cellular gene. Many other retroviruses have been studied since and have been shown to contain different oncogenes derived from and closely related to their cellular counterparts (Bishop, 1985). DNA tumor viruses also contain transforming genes; however, the derivation of these genes is not as well understood as it is for the transforming retroviruses.

The normal cellular genes from which the viral oncogenes (v-*onc*) are derived are referred to as *proto-oncogenes* (or c-*onc*). The process by which proto-oncogenes become integrated into the viral genome and are converted to viral oncogenes with overt transforming activity is complex; it involves recombination between the retroviral and cellular genomes following integration of a retrovirus adjacent to a cellular proto-oncogene. This process, known as *transduction,* is accompanied by alterations in the structure and regulation of oncogene sequences (Varmus, 1988).

Many of the oncogenes found in transforming retroviruses have also been identified independently in spontaneously arising tumors of nonviral origin, where they appear to be activated by other mechanisms, including point mutation, gene amplification, and chromosomal translocation. Activation of proto-oncogenes is associated with genetic alterations that result in either deregulation of (and increase in) expression of the normal gene or alteration in the structure (and function) of the encoded protein. The startling implication of these studies is that every cell in the human body contains a set of genes that can participate in malignancy following appropriate activation or deregulation. Proto-oncogenes encode a wide range of protein products involved in the control of cell proliferation and differentiation, including growth factors, growth factor receptors, components of signal transduction pathways, and transcription factors that regulate the transcription of mRNA and hence the expression of other genes (see Chap. 6).

Tumor suppressor genes, in contrast, represent genes that are likely to play a role in negatively regulating cell growth. Loss or inactivation of tumor suppressor genes is associated with malignancy (Weinberg, 1991; Knudson, 1993). The cellular *p53* gene, for example, undergoes a variety of rearrangements, deletions, and point mutations that abrogate its function in a wide range of human malignancies (Lane and Benchimol, 1990; Greenblatt et al., 1994). Another tumor suppressor gene, the retinoblastoma susceptibility (*RBI*) gene, undergoes deletion or mutation of both alleles in human retinoblastoma and other cancers (Weinberg, 1992). In the present chapter, the mechanisms of cellular transformation by oncogenic viruses are described first; these mechanisms provide clues to more general mechanisms of transformation due to changes in dominantly acting oncogenes or tumor suppressor genes. Studies of DNA tumor viruses suggest that some of them may cause malignant transformation by inhibiting the normal function (growth control) of tumor suppressor genes.

5.2 DNA TUMOR VIRUSES

5.2.1 Simian Virus 40 and Polyomavirus

The papovaviruses—Simian virus 40 (SV40) and polyomavirus—have given valuable information about the process of cellular transformation by DNA

viruses. Both viruses may cause tumors in newborn hamsters but have not been associated directly with human cancer. Widespread interest in SV40 virus began in 1960 when it was discovered as a contaminant in poliomyelitis virus vaccines prepared in rhesus monkey cells. The virus was injected unwittingly into millions of people. Epidemiologic studies of people who received the vaccine have given no evidence that it can cause cancer in humans. However, SV40 gene sequences were recently identified in a small number of human tumors (reviewed by Pennisi, 1997). The significance of these findings is uncertain.

The papovaviruses interact with susceptible cells in two different ways. In permissive cells that support productive infection, the lytic cycle proceeds in two phases: an early phase in which nonstructural, regulatory proteins are synthesized and a late phase during which viral DNA is replicated, coat protein is made, and progeny virions are assembled. Viral DNA is not integrated in the cellular genome during the lytic cycle. Release of mature virus particles results in lysis and cell death. Monkey cells are permissive for SV40 infection, whereas mouse cells are permissive for polyoma infection. A second type of interaction leads to a small proportion of surviving transformed cells that contain viral DNA integrated randomly into host chromosomes. Transformation occurs more commonly in cells that are unable to support viral replication well. In contrast to normal cells, virus-transformed cells show little or no contact inhibition and therefore grow to high cell density in culture; they give rise to multilayered and disorganized cell colonies, show anchorage-independent growth in a semisolid medium containing agar or methylcellulose, and exhibit a decreased requirement for serum. Moreover, the cells transformed in culture after infection give rise to tumors when inoculated into susceptible animals (see Sec. 5.4.1).

Molecular characterization of SV40-transformed cells showed that the only common feature was the presence of integrated viral DNA sequences that encode two proteins called large-T and small-t antigens (Fig. 5.1). Transfection of the gene encoding large-T antigen may alone cause the malignant transformation of normal rodent cells, although the presence of the small-t antigen contributes to the full expression of an SV40-transformed phenotype. The functions of the large T-antigen have been identified through the use of naturally occurring and genetically engineered mutants: these functions include the ability to bind to (and inactivate) the protein products of the tumor suppressor genes *p53*

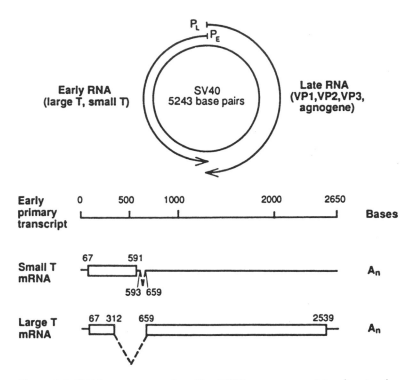

Figure 5.1 SV40 gene expression. The SV40 genome consists of a circular duplex DNA molecule containing 5243 base pairs. Two primary transcripts are expressed from opposite strands that are further processed to produce early and late viral mRNA. These transcripts initiate from the early (P_E) and late (P_L) SV40 promoters. The early region of SV40 is expressed as one primary RNA transcript of about 2650 nucleotides that can be alternatively spliced. Two discrete donor 5' splice sites and one common acceptor 3' splice site are used to form two different mRNA molecules. The smaller of the two early mRNAs encodes large-T antigen. In the other mRNA, fewer nucleotides are removed by splicing and the additional mRNA sequences contain an in-phase translation termination codon. This mRNA encodes small-t antigen. The amino-terminal 82 residues of these proteins are identical. The open boxes denote protein coding regions; the lines, noncoding regions; the intron sequences that are removed by splicing are indicated by dashed lines. A_n is the stretch of adenylic acid residues present on the 3' end of the mRNA also known as the poly-A tail. The nucleotide numbering is approximate because of heterogeneity in the start sites for transcription and for termination. For this purpose, nucleotide number 1 for early transcription is defined as position 5231 on the SV40 genome. The late mRNA encodes the structural proteins indicated.

and *RB* (Fig. 5.2*A*; see also Sec. 5.5). Transgenic mice that contain the SV40 *large-T antigen* gene develop a high incidence of tumors in organs in which the gene is expressed.

Large-T antigen contains three domains involved in the transformation and immortalization of rodent cells (Conzen and Cole, 1995). One is localized at the N-terminus and includes amino acids 1 to 82. The second domain of large-T antigen required for transformation includes residues 102 to 114 (including the LXCXE motif; see Fig. 5.2*D*). This region is required for binding to pRB as well as two other cellular proteins, p107 and p130, closely related to pRB on the basis of amino acid sequence similarity. The RB protein and related proteins p107 and p130 function in part by binding to and inactivating the transcription factor designated E2F (Sec. 5.5). The binding of large-T antigen to pRB and related proteins disrupts the pRB-E2F interaction, resulting in the release of E2F and the activation of

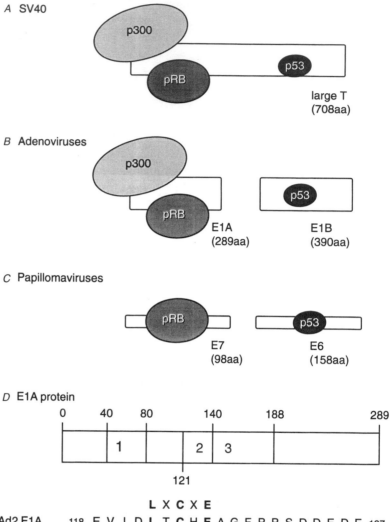

A SV40

B Adenoviruses

C Papillomaviruses

D E1A protein

Figure 5.2 Schematic representation of protein interactions involving viral oncoproteins and cellular proteins. Both p53 and pRB, the products of two cellular tumor suppressor genes, bind to the SV40 large-T antigen (*A*), whereas each binds to separate adenovirus (*B*) and HPV-encoded proteins (*C*). E1A and E1B are required for complete transformation of primary cells by adenoviruses as are E6 and E7 for HPV-mediated transformation. Not shown in the figure are the pRB-related proteins, p107 and p130, which also bind SV40 large-T antigen, Ad E1A protein, and HPV E7 protein. The p300 transcriptional adaptor protein has been shown to bind large-T antigen and E1A protein. The three regions of the 289–amino acid adenovirus E1A protein that are conserved among the different adenovirus serotypes are shown in *D*. The amino acid sequence of conserved region 2 of the Ad E1A protein is compared with functionally related regions of SV40 large-T antigen and HPV16 E7 protein. The LXCXE sequence motif present in the proteins that is necessary for binding to pRB, p107 and p130 is indicated.

```
                        L X C X E
Ad2 E1A      118  E V I D L T C H E A G F P P S D D E D E  137
HPV16 E7      18  E T T D L Y C Y E Q L N D S S E E E D E  37
SV40 large T  99  N E E N L F C S E E M - P S S D D E A T  117
```

E2F-responsive genes, which are associated with cell-cycle progression. The third domain is localized between amino acid residues 350 to 560, a region required for p53 binding. While the p53 binding region of large-T antigen is crucial for extending the life span of primary mouse fibroblasts, the extreme N terminal and the pRB binding region are also necessary for efficient immortalization of primary rodent cells.

Large-T antigen also interacts with p300, a transcriptional coactivator protein (coactivators physically connect many DNA binding/transcription factors to the basal transcription machinery) that shows considerable similarity to the transcriptional coactivator CBP, a protein that binds specifically to the DNA-binding protein CREB (cAMP response

element–binding protein). p300 and CBP define a family of transcriptional coactivator proteins targeted not only by SV40 large-T antigen but also by the adenovirus E1A protein (see below; Eckner et al., 1994). The region of large-T encompassing amino acid residues 251–708 is required for binding to p300. Interestingly, T-antigen mutants defective in p53 binding do not bind to p300 (Lill et al., 1997). The recent demonstration that p300 binds to p53 in the absence of viral oncoproteins raises the possibility that p300 may bind to T-antigen indirectly through its association with p53.

Expression of large-T antigen in human diploid fibroblast strains extends cellular life span in culture. This is associated with inactivation of pRB (and pRB-related proteins) and p53 (reviewed in

Bryan and Reddel, 1994). These cells, however, inevitably cease dividing and enter a crisis period in culture where there is a balance between cell growth and cell death. Rare immortal clones arise from such cultures presumably as a result of one or more genetic changes.

5.2.2 Human Adenoviruses

Adenoviral infections of the upper respiratory and intestinal tracts are very common and most people have antibodies directed against one or more of these viruses. A few types (12, 18, and 31) are highly oncogenic in newborn rodents, whereas others are weakly oncogenic or nononcogenic. In addition, many adenoviruses transform rodent cells in culture. Cells transformed with adenoviruses contain an incomplete viral genome that always includes the viral *E1A* (early region 1A) and *E1B* genes integrated into host DNA (for review, see Pettersson and Roberts, 1986). This minimal region of adenovirus DNA was shown to be capable of transforming rat embryo cells following DNA-mediated gene transfer. These viruses are not known to cause human cancer.

Two mRNA species, 12S and 13S, are produced by differential splicing from the *E1A* gene and encode similar proteins of 243 and 289 amino acids, respectively. These two proteins differ internally by an additional 46 amino acids that are unique to the 13S product. Multiple transcripts also originate from the *E1B* gene, giving rise to two major proteins of 19 and 58 kDa. In gene-transfer experiments, both E1A gene products immortalize primary rodent cells and complement an activated *ras* gene to transform these cells. *E1B* can replace *ras* in this type of assay. Additional functions attributed to E1A protein include its ability to either activate or repress transcription from cellular and viral genes dependent on enhancer sequences.

Comparison of the E1A amino acid sequence among several adenovirus serotypes shows the presence of three conserved regions (CR1, CR2, and CR3). Mutational analysis of the E1A region has revealed that CR1 (amino acids 40 to 80) and CR2 (amino acids 121 to 139) are necessary for transformation, whereas CR3 (amino acids 140 to 188) is dispensable (Moran and Mathews, 1987). Since CR3 is solely responsible for transactivation and is missing in the transformation competent 243 amino acid E1A protein, it is unlikely that the transactivation (i.e., activating the transcription of genes) function of E1A is required for immortalization and *ras* complementation. The E1A regions required for

control of cell growth, blockade of differentiation, and transformation comprise the nonconserved amino terminus together with CR1 and CR2. CR2 contains the LXCXE motif that is present in SV40 large-T antigen and in the E7 protein of human papillomaviruses (Fig. 5.2D).

Two noncontiguous regions of E1A, the N-terminus of CR1 and CR2, are required for binding to pRB and the related proteins, p107 and p130. The N-terminus of the E1A protein and the carboxy-terminal half of CR1 are involved in binding to p300. Genetic studies have revealed a correlation between the repressive activity of E1A on enhancer elements and the ability of E1A to bind and repress the coactivator function of p300. It is likely that transcriptional repression of a certain class of genes plays a role in E1A-mediated transformation. The E1B 55-kDa protein has been shown to bind to the N-terminus of p53 and to inhibit its transactivation function (Fig. 5.2B).

5.2.3 Human Papillomaviruses

Human papillomaviruses (HPV) make up a large family with the same overall genome organization of at least seven "early" genes (*E1* to *E7*) and two "late" genes (*L1* and *L2*) (Fig. 5.3). Different types of HPV are identified on the basis of DNA homology following hybridization under conditions of low stringency with established prototypes (de Villiers, 1989; Sousa et al., 1990) or by the use of sensitive and specific polymerase chain reaction assays. These viruses infect only epithelial cells and are associated mostly with benign mucosal and cutaneous lesions. The low-risk types—including HPV6, 10, and 11—infect the genital tract and are associated with benign genital warts and low grades of cervical intraepithelial neoplasia that regress spontaneously; they are rarely found in malignant tumors. In contrast, viral DNAs from the high-risk types—including HPV16, 18, 31, 33, and 45—are found in about 90 percent of all cervical cancers (Vousden, 1989; Lowy et al., 1994). However, these types have also been detected in nonmalignant cervical tissue, and only a small proportion of women with clinically apparent high-risk HPV infection eventually develop cervical carcinoma, possibly because many of these infections may be transient. When the epidemiologic and clinical evidence is viewed jointly with laboratory studies demonstrating the transforming potential of HPV DNA in cell-culture systems, it seems likely that persistent infection with certain strains of HPV contributes to the development of cervical cancer. There is widespread agreement that HPV infection

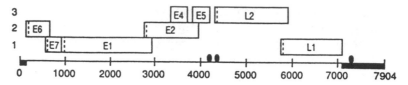

Figure 5.3 Organization of the HPV-16 genome. The papillomavirus DNA molecule is circular, but the genome is represented conventionally as a linear molecule opened at the regulatory region. The open reading frames (ORFs) in all three possible translation phases are indicated by the open boxes and are based on the complete DNA sequence. E and L stand for early and late region ORFs, respectively. The vertical dotted line represents the first ATG initiation codon of each ORF. Black circles show polyadenylation sites. The bold black lines indicate the regulatory region.

is not sufficient for tumor development and that other factors—such as smoking, use of oral contraceptives, recurrent infection, early pregnancy, and the immunologic and hormonal status—may play a role in progression to malignancy. Herpes simplex virus type 2 (HSV-2) was thought previously to be involved in cervical cancer on the basis of epidemiologic studies, but HSV-2 DNA is not found in most tumors and does not appear to contribute to the generation of cervical cancer.

Although present in benign warts, the HPV genome is maintained as an episome (nonintegrated, circular form). In malignant cells, HPV DNA is randomly integrated into various chromosomes, resulting in substantial deletions or disruption of the viral genome, particularly the *E2* gene, which has a negative regulatory effect on the expression of the HPV proteins E6 and E7. These latter two proteins are always retained and consistently expressed in cervical tumor tissue and cervical tumor cell lines, suggesting that one or both of these proteins may be required for transformation by HPV.

Gene transfer experiments demonstrate that either the *E6* or *E7* genes from the high-risk HPV types but not from the low-risk HPV types extend the life span of human epithelial cells in culture. These cells, however, will not form tumors when injected into nude mice and enter a crisis period in culture. Thus, HPV alone is not carcinogenic—a finding that is consistent with epidemiologic and clinical data. This has led to the idea that malignant transformation of HPV-infected cells requires additional genetic alterations. The transforming ability of the E6 and E7 proteins depends on their binding to p53 and pRB tumor suppressor proteins, respectively. E6 binds to p53, resulting in rapid degradation of p53 protein via the ubiquitin-dependent proteolytic pathway. E7 binds to several cellular

proteins (Fig. 5.2*C*) including pRB, p107, p130, and cyclin A. Binding of E7 to pRB results in the release of the bound E2F1 transcription factor from pRB. Thus, related mechanisms of transformation are evident for papovaviruses, adenoviruses, and papillomaviruses (Fig. 5.2).

5.2.4 Epstein-Barr Virus

Cultured tumor cells from Burkitt's lymphoma in African children release a herpesvirus named *Epstein-Barr virus* (EBV). EBV is transmitted horizontally, infecting more than 90 percent of the human population by the age of 20, usually without any manifestation of disease. EBV strains can be classified into two main types, type 1 and type 2, based on polymorphisms (genetic differences) within certain viral genes. Type 1 strains are more common in western countries, whereas type 2 strains are prevalent in central Africa and New Guinea. Strong epidemiologic and clinical data have associated EBV infection with three lymphoproliferative diseases of B-cell origin, namely infectious mononucleosis, Burkitt's lymphoma, and lymphoma of the immunocompromised host, particularly in the setting of organ transplantation and HIV infection.

There is also a very strong association between EBV infection and undifferentiated nasopharyngeal carcinoma (NPC), and recent evidence has implicated EBV in the pathogenesis of another lymphoid tumor, Hodgkin's disease (Weinreb et al., 1996). However, geographic and ethnic variation have been recognized in the incidence of these EBV-associated malignancies, indicating involvement of genetic and environmental factors. EBV can infect B lymphocytes and epithelial cells, both of which express the CR2 cell surface receptor molecule for

C3d serum complement (also known as CD21), which also serves as the receptor for EBV.

In the cell culture, the virus infects preferentially B cells and immortalizes these cells with high efficiency (Sugden, 1989). Upon infection of human B lymphocytes, the 172-kbp EBV genome forms a covalently closed circle via its terminal repeats. EBV encodes about 100 genes, of which about 10 are expressed in B lymphocytes that are immortalized after infection. Four of these genes are considered most likely to play a role in cellular transformation, *EBNA-1* (Epstein-Barr virus nuclear antigen 1), *EBNA-2*, and *LMP1* (latent membrane protein 1) and *LMP2*. EBNA-1 protein is required for DNA replication of the extrachromosomal viral plasmids in EBV-infected cells. It binds to the viral origin of replication and is essential for maintenance of multiple viral genomes in an episomal form. The gene *EBNA-2* encodes a 90-kDa transcriptional activator protein that is localized in the nucleus of infected cells. The EBNA-2 protein transactivates expression of cellular and viral genes through interaction with at least two sequence-specific DNA-binding proteins, J kappa and PU.1. The amino acid sequence of LMP1 and LMP2 predicts proteins with multiple membrane-spanning segments, reminiscent of an ion channel or of a growth factor receptor. In gene transfer experiments, LMP1 expression results in transformation of established rodent cell lines. In human keratinocytes, LMP1 expression results in morphologic transformation and inhibition of terminal differentiation. LMP2 protein associates with src family tyrosine kinases, LMP1, and several other unidentified cell proteins.

A chromosomal translocation is present in approximately 80 percent of Burkitt's lymphomas involving the immunoglobulin (Ig) heavy-chain locus on chromosome 14 and the c-*myc* oncogene on chromosome 8. In the remaining tumors, translocations involving chromosome 8 with chromosome 2 (Ig κ light chain) or with chromosome 22 (Ig λ light chain) are detected. These translocations are believed to result in deregulation of c-*myc* expression as a result of proximity to the Ig enhancer sequences, thus preventing the normal downregulation of c-*myc* expression in maturing B lymphocytes.

The importance of EBV infection in the development of Burkitt's lymphoma has been described by Klein and Klein (1986) in the following way:

> The risk of all genetic accidents increases in direct relation to the number of cell divisions. The tumorigenic myc/Ig translocation is probably a very rare accident, but with a high selective value. In the African

endemic form of Burkitt's lymphoma, EBV and chronic malaria may act as the main predisposing combination. EBV extends the life of the short-lived B cell toward potential immortality. The heavy parasite load associated with the hyperendemic form of tropical malaria may increase the likelihood of the translocation event by a continuously ongoing process of B-cell activation and may facilitate the outgrowth of the highly immunogenic EBV-carrying cells by a relative T-cell suppression.

The role of EBV in nasopharyngeal cancer (NPC) is poorly understood, although racial, genetic, and environmental cofactors appear to be important (Liebowitz, 1994). Four EBV proteins have been detected in NPC cells, namely the nuclear antigen EBNA-1, LMP1, LMP2A, and LMP2B. LMP2A and LMP2B are generated by alternative splicing of the *LMP2* transcript, each species having a distinct first exon. LMP1 is detected in about 65 percent of tumors. The profound growth-stimulating effect of LMP1 on keratinocyte cultures suggests that LMP1 expression may exert similar effects in the nasopharyngeal epithelium. It has been suggested that EBV infection of nasopharyngeal epithelial cells could provide an expanded pool of target cells susceptible to the further genetic changes (in oncogenes and tumor suppressor genes) necessary for malignant transformation of these cells and development of NPC. EBV is likely to be acting as a major cofactor in the etiology of NPC.

An association between EBV and Hodgkin's disease (HD) is now supported by a variety of evidence. EBV DNA sequences and transcripts have been detected in malignant Reed-Sternberg cells and their mononuclear variants, Hodgkin cells, by in situ hybridization and polymerase chain reaction (PCR)–based assays (see Chap. 3, Secs. 3.3.7 and 3.4.4). LMP1 protein has also been detected by immunohistochemical staining of lymph nodes from patients with HD. The association of EBV with this disease varies greatly from country to country, and HD in developing countries differs from HD in western countries in terms of epidemiologic, pathologic, and clinical characteristics. In recent reports, 100 percent of Kenyan children with HD were found to be EBV positive (53 of 53 cases), while 51 percent of children from the United States and the United Kingdom (46 of 90 cases) showed evidence of EBV in their malignant cells (Weinreb et al., 1996).

5.2.5 Hepatitis B Virus

Most individuals infected with the hepatitis B virus (HBV) develop either an acute transient illness or an asymptomatic infection that leaves them immune. About 10 percent of infected individuals, however, develop chronic hepatitis, which can progress to more severe conditions such as chronic active hepatitis, cirrhosis, and liver cancer. There are estimated to be 200 million chronic carriers of HBV worldwide. There is strong epidemiologic evidence indicating the importance of chronic HBV infection in the development of human hepatocellular carcinoma (HCC). More than 80 percent of individuals with HCC are chronically infected by HBV.

HBV is an enveloped DNA-containing virus. The envelope carries a surface-exposed glycoprotein that acts as the major surface antigenic determinant (HBsAg). This molecule interacts with a specific HBV receptor on the plasma membrane of susceptible hepatocytes in the first step of infection. The viral DNA genome as found in viral particles is composed of one 3.2-kb strand (minus strand) base-paired with a shorter "plus" strand of variable length. Because the 5' ends of both strands invariably overlap by about 300 bases, the DNA retains a circular configuration, although neither strand is itself a closed circle. Replication is complex and proceeds through an RNA intermediate that is made in an early step in the infection cycle and used as a template for reverse transcription into DNA.

Integrated HBV DNA is found frequently in the cellular DNA of hepatocellular carcinoma. The implications of viral DNA integration are controversial. An animal model for studying transformation by HBV is provided by the woodchuck. In the woodchuck, HBV DNA is commonly integrated adjacent to c-*myc*, N-*myc*, and the woodchuck N-*myc* retroposon (intronless complementary DNA gene), resulting in insertional activation of these genes. However, HBV is not believed to act as an insertional mutagen in humans. HBV integration in human cells frequently induces deletions and translocations in a seemingly random way. HBV insertion and disruption of the cellular genes encoding the β-retinoic acid receptor and cyclin A have been reported, but the importance of these events for the development of liver cancer is not known.

Only two viral genes, *HBx* and *preS2/S*, are usually retained intact after viral DNA integration. Both of these genes encode proteins with transcriptional activity. The HBx protein plays an essential role during viral infection by regulating viral gene expression. Moreover, the *HBx* gene has oncogenic potential; its expression transforms immortalized mouse hepatocytes in culture and induces liver can-

cer in mice that carry it as a transgene (see Chap. 3, Sec. 3.3.12; Kim et al., 1991). Expression of the *HBx* gene in cultured cells stimulates DNA synthesis and cell proliferation and activates the Ras-Raf-mitogen activated protein (MAP) kinase pathway, which is required for activation of the transcription factor AP-1 and cell division (see Chap. 6, Sec. 6.3). Recently, the HBx protein was reported to form a complex with p53 protein and to inhibit its sequence-specific DNA binding and transcriptional transactivator activity (Wang et al., 1994), but the significance of this interaction in HCC is unknown.

5.3 RETROVIRUSES

5.3.1 Life Cycle

The retroviruses are enveloped viruses about 120 nm in diameter. The outer envelope is a lipid bilayer derived from the plasma membrane of the previous host cell. It is enriched by viral glycoproteins encoded by the viral *env* gene. The envelope surrounds a core that consists of capsid proteins encoded by the viral *gag* gene. The core includes two identical single strands of viral RNA that are linked together near their 5' termini. The RNA comprises the genetic information that is necessary for the virus to synthesize its components and thereby reproduce itself. Bound to the RNA are several copies of the enzyme reverse transcriptase (RT) encoded by the viral *pol* gene.

The life cycle of a retrovirus occurs in discrete steps, illustrated in Fig. 5.4. Absorption of the virus to a cell is mediated by interaction between the envelope proteins of the virus and specific receptor molecules on the cell surface. Entry of the virus into a cell occurs by receptor-mediated endocytosis, a process that mimics the normal role of these receptors to recognize and internalize substances that are beneficial to the cell. Specificity at the level of virus absorption accounts in large part for the restricted host and cell range of many types of viruses. Human immunodeficiency virus (HIV), for example, attaches to and enters a cell through the CD4 cell surface antigen. As a result, only CD4-positive cells (primarily helper T lymphocytes, see Chap. 11, Sec. 11.3.3) are susceptible to infection by HIV.

Once the virus is inside the cell, loss of the viral envelope and core proteins results in release of the viral RNA into the cytoplasm. The RNA is then converted to double-stranded DNA through the activity of the virus-encoded reverse transcriptase. During this process of reverse transcription (RNA to DNA), a small nucleotide repeat sequence at both ends of

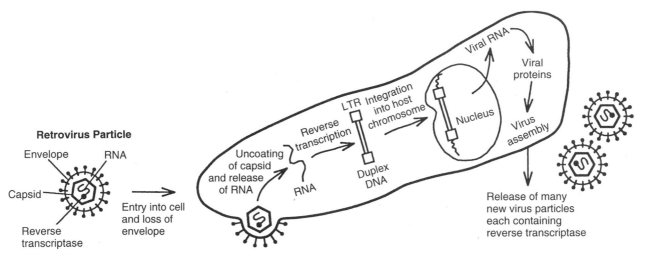

Figure 5.4 The life cycle of a retrovirus. The virus contains two identical RNA strands, only one of which is shown for clarity. After penetrating the plasma membrane, the single-stranded viral RNA genome is reverse-transcribed to a double-stranded DNA form, which has at its ends a duplication called the long-terminal repeat (LTR). The viral DNA migrates to the nucleus and integrates into the chromosomal DNA. The single viral transcript can form the genome for progeny viruses or can be processed and translated to generate viral structural proteins.

the viral RNA is extended to form a long terminal repeat (LTR) on the double-stranded DNA. These linear DNA molecules then proceed to the nucleus, where one or a few molecules integrate randomly into the host chromosomes. The integrated form of the virus is called the *provirus* (Fig. 5.5).

Once integrated, the proviral DNA acts as a template for transcription. Although both LTRs are identical and contain promoter and enhancer sequences as well as polyadenylation sequences necessary for synthesis of viral RNA, the upstream LTR acts to promote transcription whereas the down-

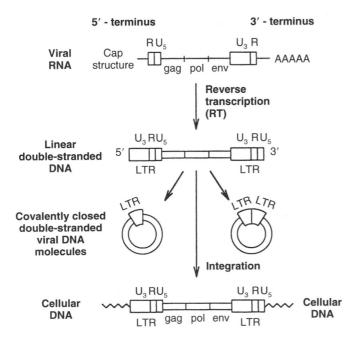

Figure 5.5 Replication and integration of the retroviral genome. The retroviral genome contains three coding regions and two terminal sequences consisting of R, a repeated sequence of 20–80 nucleotides that is present at both ends of the genome, and U5 or U3, unique segments found at the 5' or 3' end of the viral RNA, respectively. The *pol* sequence encodes the enzyme reverse transcriptase that first makes an initial DNA copy of the viral RNA molecule and then a second DNA strand, generating a double-stranded DNA copy of the viral genome. During the process of reverse transcription, each terminus is extended by the addition of the U segment of the opposite end resulting in the creation of the long-terminal repeats (LTRs). The linear double-stranded molecule is transported to the nucleus and a small proportion is circularized to generate secondary forms that have a single or tandem LTR. The linear form integrates into cellular DNA, where it is referred to as a provirus. (The relative lengths of the genes and LTRs are not drawn to scale.)

stream LTR specifies termination. Between the LTRs are coding sequences for the *gag, pol,* and *env* genes. Two transcripts are synthesized from the proviral DNA. A full-length genomic transcript serves as the mRNA for the synthesis of both gag and gag-pol fusion proteins. This transcript can also be packaged into virus particles and therefore acts as the genome of the virus. A spliced transcript, which is not packaged, serves as the mRNA for the env protein. The viral RNA, the proteins, and their mature products after cleavage—and, in some cases, after glycosylation and phosphorylation—assemble into virions that are released from the cell. This is accomplished by a budding process that encloses the virion within a membrane envelope and gives rise to mature virus particles. Infected cells may continue to assemble and release virus particles over long periods of time without affecting their survival.

5.3.2 Acute Transforming Viruses

Transforming retroviruses can be separated into two major groups based on their different mechanisms of transformation (Varmus, 1988). The more intensely studied group consists of viruses that contain a viral oncogene, and these have been termed *acute* or *rapidly transforming viruses.* More than 20 viral oncogenes have been identified; each of these has been found to have a counterpart in normal cells. Viruses in the second group do not contain an oncogene and are referred to as the *chronic tumor* or *slowly transforming viruses.*

Acute transforming viruses are almost always replication-defective due to replacement of viral sequences required for replication with host-derived oncogene sequences. As a result, these transforming viruses require the presence of replication-competent helper viruses that assist in virus replication and assembly by supplying the necessary viral gene products. Because viral oncogenes come under the control of the efficient retroviral promoter present on the LTRs and are no longer tightly regulated by cellular mechanisms that normally act on the natural promoter, these genes can be expressed at inappropriately high levels. The viral oncogenes are frequently mutated because of the poor fidelity of retroviral replication, with point mutations, deletions, substitutions, and insertions compared with the proto-oncogenes from which they are derived. In addition, viral oncogenes differ from proto-oncogenes in not containing intron (i.e., noncoding) sequences. Retroviruses containing oncogenes can transform cells in culture after several days and can induce leukemias and sarcomas in infected animals relatively quickly. Expression of the v-*onc* gene transforms every infected cell. Consequently, polyclonal tumors develop from many different infected progenitor cells. Figure 5.6 provides an example of an acute transforming retrovirus, the avian myelocytomatosis-29 virus (MC29), which contains an oncogene called v-*myc*, and compares it with its normal cellular counterpart, the proto-oncogene c-*myc*. MC29 is a defective virus missing all of the *pol* gene and parts of *gag* and *env.*

5.3.3 Chronic Tumor Viruses

The replication-competent chronic tumor viruses do not contain viral oncogenes but transform infected cells through a mechanism known as *insertional mutagenesis,* in which proviral integration leads to the aberrant activation of adjacent cellular genes. Several of the proto-oncogenes identified initially as

Figure 5.6 Structure of the normal c-*myc* gene, the MC29 proviral genome, and the transforming protein encoded from it. The Δ*gag-myc* transforming gene of MC29 is a genetic hybrid that consists of 1.5 kb derived from the *gag* gene of the avian leukemia virus and 1.6 kb derived from the avian c-*myc* gene. All of the exon 2 and exon 3 sequences of c-*myc* are present in MC29. The c-*myc* and v-*myc* genes also differ by a number of missense mutations.

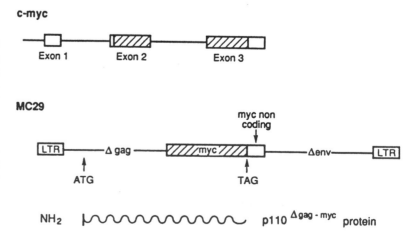

progenitors to retroviral oncogenes (c-*erb*B, c-*mos*, c-*myb*, c-*myc*, c-H-*ras*, c-K-*ras*, c-*fms*), as well as genes known to be important in regulating cell growth (*IL-2*, *IL-3*), have been identified as targets for insertional mutagenesis in animal species.

Avian leukemia virus (ALV) is typical of slow-acting retroviruses. In ALV-induced B-cell lymphomas, malignant clones independently transformed by these viruses contain proviruses integrated in the vicinity of the c-*myc* gene (Hayward et al., 1981). In most tumors, the provirus is integrated upstream of c-*myc* and in the same transcriptional orientation (Fig. 5.7A). In such cases the 3′ LTR, which normally acts to terminate viral transcription, promotes transcription of c-*myc* sequences. The resulting hybrid RNA transcripts contain both viral and c-*myc* sequences and are present at levels 30- to 100-fold higher than that of c-*myc* RNA in normal tissues. Such c-*myc* transcripts appear to encode a normal c-myc protein. This mechanism is called *promoter insertion*. In other tumors, the provirus is integrated upstream of c-*myc* but oriented in the transcriptional direction opposite to that of the gene, or it is integrated downstream of the gene (Fig. 5.7B through D). The strong enhancer properties of the LTRs are then believed to be responsible for activation of c-*myc* transcription, and this mechanism of transformation is known as *enhancer insertion*.

The majority of B-cell lymphomas induced by ALV contain proviral sequences adjacent to c-*myc*. However, in transformation assays of normal cells in culture, the *myc* oncogene requires the cooperative function of a second oncogene (see Sec. 5.4), an analysis of DNA from B-cell lymphomas indicates that other cellular genes may be activated during oncogenesis. Because integration adjacent to c-*myc* is a random, rare event and secondary genetic events are required for tumor progression, ALV-induced leukemia may arise slowly and is clonal in origin.

In other tumors, proviral insertion may disrupt or alter the protein-coding sequence of resident cellular genes. For example, in ALV-induced erythroblastosis, proviral insertions commonly map to a small region in the middle of the epidermal growth-factor (EGFR) receptor gene (c-*erb*B). The resulting transcripts contain viral *gag* and *env* sequences fused to c-*erb*B sequences. The amino acid sequence predicted from this hybrid transcript would contain amino acids encoded by *gag* and *env* fused to carboxy-terminal amino acid sequences encoded by c-*erb*B. Thus, expression of an altered, truncated EGFR molecule appears necessary for the development of ALV-induced erythroblastosis.

5.3.4 Human T-Cell Leukemia Virus

Adult T-cell leukemia (ATL) is a rare but virulent leukemia that is endemic in southern Japan, the Caribbean, northern South America, parts of Africa, and the southeastern United States. Transmission of this disease may occur through blood transfusion, breast feeding, and sexual intercourse. In 1980, the first viral isolates from patients with ATL were ob-

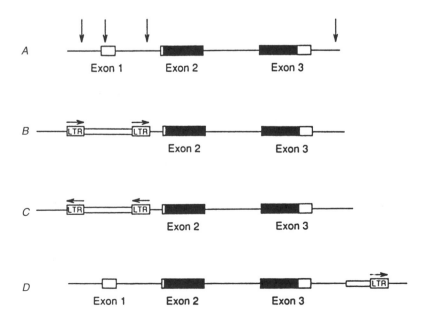

Figure 5.7 Insertional mutagenesis of c-*myc* by the avian leukemia virus. Structure of the normal c-*myc* gene showing regions (*indicated by arrows*) where activation by retroviral promoter and enhancer insertions can occur (*A*). The coding sequences are shown in black. Promoter insertion can occur when the retrovirus integrates upstream of the *myc* coding sequences either in intron 1, exon 1, or 5′ of exon 1. The retroviral long-terminal repeat (LTR) can then act to increase the transcription of c-*myc* (*B*). Enhancer insertion occurs when the retrovirus integrates upstream of c-*myc* but in the opposite transcription direction (*C*) or downstream of c-*myc* (*D*). In both cases the viral LTR increases transcription indirectly as a result of its enhancing properties. As indicated in *D*, truncation of the provirus resulting in loss of the 5′ LTR can occur during enhancer insertion.

tained in the United States and later, independently, in Japan. Nucleotide sequence determination of the viral genomes (Table 5.1) revealed subsequently that the Japanese and American isolates were very closely related strains of a single retrovirus now called human T-cell leukemia virus (HTLV-1) (Wong-Staal and Gallo, 1985; Yoshida, 1987). The data that support HTLV-1 as being the causative agent of ATL are summarized in Table 5.1. Adult T-cell leukemia is the only human malignancy that is clearly associated with a retrovirus as the causative agent.

Unlike the common oncogenic retroviruses of animals, HTLV-1 does not carry a host-derived oncogene and does not activate cellular proto-oncogenes by insertional mutation. HTLV-1 is believed to initiate a multistep process leading to ATL. Following infection of CD4-positive lymphocytes by HTLV-1, all the cells develop IL-2 receptors, and the provirus is found randomly integrated into the cellular genome. The infected cell population undergoes a transient polyclonal expansion followed by a latency period that is variable in duration; it can be as short as a few years if infection occurs in adulthood or as long as 40 years if infection occurs in infancy. Not all individuals infected by the virus develop ATL, and the latent state may be maintained by immunologic clearance of the infected cells. When ATL is clinically evident, however, all the leukemic cells in a patient have a common proviral integration site in the host DNA, but no two patients have the same integration site. These observations suggest that

Table 5.1. Evidence That Supports HTLV-1 as the Causative Agent of Adult T-Cell Leukemia (ATL)

- Isolation of HTLV-1 from the leukemic T cells of patients with ATL.

- HTLV-1 virus particles isolated from ATL cells can infect and immortalize normal, human CD4-positive T cells. These infected cells continue to proliferate in the absence of exogenous interleukin 2.

- HTLV-1 proviral DNA is found integrated into the cellular genome of leukemic T cells from ATL patients.

- Although HTLV-1 proviral DNA integrates randomly into host DNA, the malignant cells in ATL constitute a clone in which all the leukemic cells of a patient contain a common site of proviral integration. This suggest that infection probably preceded the growth of the tumor.

- Serum from all ATL patients contains antibodies that react with HTLV-1.

- Monoclonal antibodies made to HTLV-1 proteins react with ATL cells but not with normal cells.

HTLV-1 is derived from a single infected progenitor cell but that subsequent genetic events are required to induce ATL (Fig. 5.8).

The genome of HTLV-1 is shown in Figure 5.9A. In addition to *gag, pol*, and *env* genes, HTLV-1 encodes two other proteins, Tax and Rex. From the numerous experiments using T cells from infected patients, transgenic mice, and tissue culture transformation assays, the Tax protein has been shown to be the transforming component of HTLV-1. Tax protein is critical for viral replication and functions as a transcriptional coactivator of viral and cellular gene expression (Yoshida et al., 1995). Tax protein does not bind directly to promoter sequences; its mode of action is through the modification of host transcription factors, including CREB and NF-κB. Cellular genes that are responsive to transcriptional activation by Tax include *IL-2*, the α subunit of the interleukin-2 (IL-2) receptor, granulocyte-macrophage colony-stimulating factor, and the proto-oncogenes c-*sis* and c-*fos*. Tumor cells from ATL patients as well as T lymphocytes transformed in culture with HTLV-1 display an activated T-cell phenotype characterized by expression of IL-2 cell surface receptors. Expression of the HTLV-1 *tax* gene in transgenic mice leads to various abnormalities, including the development of fibroblastic tumors and leukemia (Nerenberg et al., 1987). Thus, expression of the *tax* gene has the potential to perturb normal cellular functions leading to malignancy.

The HTLV-1 Rex protein is essential for viral replication and acts posttranscriptionally to enhance the expression of incompletely spliced viral transcripts that encode the viral structural proteins. The Rex protein interacts with a complex stem-loop structure termed the *Rex RNA response element* present at the 3' end of viral transcripts. It is unclear whether Rex directly affects splicing or only the nuclear-to-cytoplasmic transport of viral mRNA.

5.3.5 HTLV-2 and HIV

Two other human retroviruses, related to HTLV-1 on the basis of their complex genomic structure and common tropism for CD4-positive helper T lymphocytes, are HTLV-2 and HIV (human immunodeficiency virus). The genomic structure of HIV is shown in Fig. 5.9B. All three viruses encode proteins with trans-activation activity. HTLV-2 is most closely related to HTLV-1 and has been detected only rarely in humans. Although it was first isolated from a patient with hairy cell leukemia, it has not been linked to any human disease.

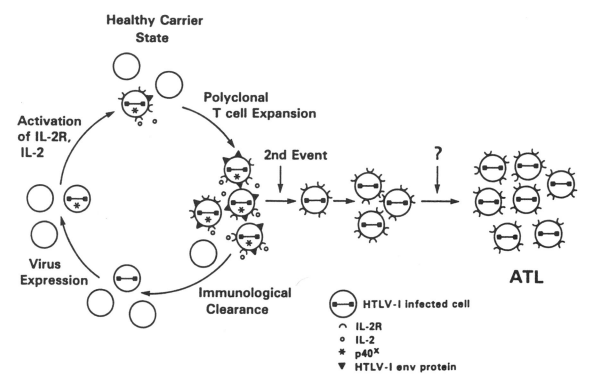

Figure 5.8 Development of adult T-cell leukemia (ATL). The multistep process through which HTLV-1 induces ATL is shown in the diagram and described in the text. p40^x refers to the 40-kDa protein encoded by the HTLV-1 *tax* gene; IL-2R refers to the interleukin-2 receptor. (Diagram was kindly provided by Dr. R. C. Gallo and is based on a diagram by Dr. Yoshida.)

HIV is recognized widely as the causative agent of acquired immunodeficiency syndrome (AIDS), in which the primary consequence of infection is depletion of the target-cell population, leading to immunosuppression and opportunistic infections. HIV subtypes have distinct geographic distributions, with A, C, D, and E predominant in sub-Saharan Africa and Asia and B predominant in the United States, the Caribbean, South America, and western Europe (Royce et al., 1997). HIV infection predisposes to several neoplastic conditions, especially non-Hodgkin's lymphoma, Kaposi's sarcoma, intraepithelial cervical neoplasia, and anal tumors. The role of HIV in malignancy is probably linked to its immunosuppressive effect and interference with immune-mediated tumor surveillance (Schulz et al., 1996; see also Chap. 11, Sec. 11.4.2), although additional mechanisms are involved in the induction of Kaposi's sarcoma.

Kaposi's sarcoma (KS) is frequently associated with HIV infection. Until recently, Kaposi's sarcoma was thought to arise as a consequence of the immunosuppressed state induced in patients by HIV infection. Compelling evidence, however, indicates that the trans-activating protein encoded by HIV, known as the Tat protein, can be released from infected CD4-positive cells as a biologically active protein and that it can act extracellularly as a growth stimulator for cells derived from KS tumors of AIDS patients (Ensoli et al., 1990). This, together with the observations that HIV nucleotide sequences are absent in the DNA from KS lesions and that transgenic mice carrying the HIV *tat* gene develop KS-like lesions and express *tat* in the skin but not in the tumor cells (Vogel et al., 1988), indicates that the role of HIV in KS is indirect and that Tat may contribute to the development of KS in HIV-infected patients through its growth-promoting properties on appropriate target cells. The ability of Tat to induce angiogenesis from normal vascular endothelial cells may be important in this regard.

Tat is also required for high-level expression of HIV genes in infected cells. The mechanism of HIV Tat trans-activation appears to be different from that of the HTLV-1 Tax protein. Transcriptional regulation by Tat requires binding to nascent viral RNA. The target sequence for Tat has been mapped to an RNA stem-loop structure (TAR, or transactivation

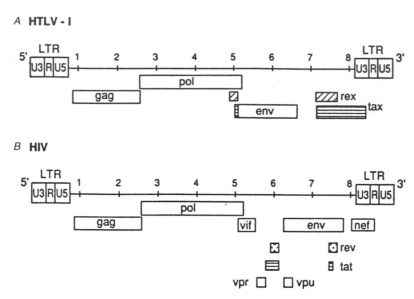

Figure 5.9 Genome organization of HTLV-1 and HIV. *A.* In addition to the long-terminal repeats (LTRs) and the typical *gag, pol,* and *env* genes found in other replication-competent retroviruses, a novel region exists at the 3' end of the HTLV-1 genome encoding two regulatory proteins, Tax (transactivator) and Rex (regulator of expression). Three different mRNA species have been identified for HTLV-1. The full-length genomic mRNA encodes the gag and pol proteins and is also packaged into virions. A singly spliced mRNA encodes the env protein and the doubly spliced mRNA encodes Tax and Rex. Numbers indicate kilobases. *B.* HIV encodes nine genes. In addition to *gag, pol,* and *env* genes, HIV encodes six genes important for regulating viral gene expression and replication. These are *rev, tat, vif, nef, vpr,* and *vpu.*

response element) located immediately downstream of the transcriptional start site on the HIV LTR. Various studies suggest that Tat can activate initiation of transcription and facilitate the elongation of nascent transcripts (Cullen, 1993).

The recent discovery of human herpesvirus-8 in over 90 percent of KS tissues obtained from patients with AIDS indicates that HHV-8 (also referred to as *Kaposi's sarcoma–associated herpesvirus,* KSHV) may play a role in the development of this disease, but a casual relation between disease and HHV-8 infection has not been established (Chang et al., 1994). Since the initial finding, HHV-8 viral DNA sequences have been found in KS lesions of all types, including AIDS-related, classical (in HIV-negative individuals), and the endemic form found in Africa. HHV-8 has also been detected in the rare condition known as pleural effusion lymphoma and in AIDS-related Castleman's disease. The possible mechanistic basis for pathogenesis mediated by HHV-8 is not known. The identification of HHV-8 genes encoding functional homologues of IL-6 and macrophage inflammatory protein could be important for HHV-8 associated malignancies (Nicholas et al., 1997). It has been suggested that

the growth-promoting properties of Tat might be responsible for the more aggressive nature of AIDS-associated KS compared with classical KS.

5.4 ONCOGENES IN HUMAN CANCER

The studies of RNA tumor viruses described in Sec. 5.3 have identified a variety of genetic events important in the development of malignancy in animal models. These include activation of specific genes carried by the virus or activation of cellular genes by insertional mutagenesis; these genes are referred to as *viral* or *cellular oncogenes* (Table 5.2). In the following section, experimental strategies that led to the discovery of these and other dominantly acting oncogenes in human tumors are discussed. The protein products of these genes are involved in a variety of cellular processes linked to intracellular signaling and cell-cycle control (see Chaps. 4, 6, and 7).

5.4.1 Identification of Oncogenes by Transfer of DNA

Dominantly acting transforming genes have been identified by extracting DNA from chemically trans-

Table 5.2. Oncogene Groups

Oncogene	Function
Growth Factors	
int-1	Matrix protein
int-2	Fibroblast growth factor–related protein
sis	Platelet-derived growth factor
Growth-factor receptors	
erbB-1	Epidermal growth factor receptor
fms	CSF-1 receptor
kit	Stem-cell growth factor receptor
met	Hepatic growth factor receptor
neu/erbB-2	Heregulin receptor
ret	Glial cell derived neurotrophic factor receptor
ros	Unknown ligand
trkA	Nerve growth factor receptor
G proteins	
H-ras	GTPase
K-ras	GTPase
N-ras	GTPase
Cytoplasmic kinases	
bcr-abl	Tyrosine kinase
fes/fps	Tyrosine kinase
fgr	Tyrosine kinase
hck	Tyrosine kinase
lck	Tyrosine kinase
pim	Tyrosine kinase
src	Tyrosine kinase
yes	Tyrosine kinase
raf/mil	Serine-threonine kinase
mos	Serine-threonine kinase
Other cytoplasmic proteins	
bcl-2	Anti-apoptosis
Nuclear proteins	
erbA	Thyroid hormone receptor
ets	Transcription factor
fos	Transcription factor
jun	Transcription factor
L-myc	Transcription factor
lyl-1	Transcription factor
myc	Transcription factor
N-myc	Transcription factor
rel	Transcription factor
ski	Transcription factor
tal-1	Transcription factor

formed rodent cells or human tumor cell lines and transferring the DNA to nonmalignant mouse or rat cells. A cell line designated NIH/3T3, derived from mouse embryo fibroblasts, was used as the recipient in many of these experiments. Although this cell line has a normal phenotype in culture, it was selected for its ability to propagate indefinitely (i.e., it is immortal). Following transfection, the cells were assayed for the development of a transformed phenotype using one or more of the following assays (Fig. 5.10).

1. *The focus formation assay.* Normal fibroblasts are contact-inhibited and will stop growing when they become confluent. Transformed cells are not contact-inhibited and continue to grow. This results in the development of a focus of cells on a background of contact-inhibited fibroblasts (see Chap. 8, Sec. 8.5.1).

2. *Anchorage-independent growth.* Normal fibroblasts will not grow unless they are adherent to a supporting matrix such as glass or plastic. In contrast, transformed cells do not need such attachment and are capable of growing when suspended in a semisolid medium such as agar that prevents adherence to the bottom of the culture vessel.

3. *Tumor formation.* Normal fibroblasts will not form tumors when inoculated into syngeneic or immunologically deficient animals, whereas transformed fibroblasts can do so.

Initial experiments that sought the presence of transforming activity in DNA from human tumor cells were mostly unsuccessful, but a few positive results were obtained. For example, DNA obtained from the EJ cell line, derived from a human bladder cancer, was able to transform NIH/3T3 cells. If the

(1) Focus formation

Normal growth of fibroblasts in monolayer

Formation of focus

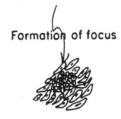

(2) Anchorage independence

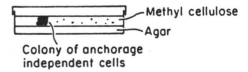

Colony of anchorage independent cells — Methyl cellulose — Agar

(3) Tumor formation

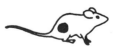

Figure 5.10 Assays of the malignant phenotype. Malignant transformation of a cell may be recognized in tissue culture (1) by cells piling up on the bottom of the culture dish to form a focus; (2) by growth under anchorage-independent conditions in semisolid media such as methylcellulose or agar; or (3) by tumor formation in syngeneic or immune-deprived animals.

DNA from the transformed cells was used in a further transfection assay, it was able to generate further transformants (Shih and Weinberg, 1982).

The transformants obtained after transfer of DNA from human malignant cells to murine fibroblasts were studied with the Southern blotting technique (see Chap. 3, Sec. 3.3.4) using either radioactively labeled total human DNA or a cloned Alu probe, which recognizes characteristic repetitive sequences in human DNA. Primary transformants were found to have varying amounts of human DNA, and some samples showed extensive hybridization, indicating the presence of a large amount of human DNA. The complex pattern seen in primary transformants was simplified in secondary and tertiary transformants. Independent transformants derived from the same source of DNA then contained the same pattern of discrete bands when studied by Southern blotting, indicating that in each case the same gene had been transferred. Transformants derived from different sources of tumor DNA revealed a few different patterns of bands; this suggested that the same gene was being transferred from different sources of DNA and that a limited number of genes were being detected as active in the transfection assay.

To determine which gene or genes were being transferred, the DNA of a secondary transformant was cloned into a bacteriophage (see Chap. 3, Sec. 3.3.3) and individual bacteriophage plaques (resulting from multiple rounds of lytic infection of bacterial cells by a single bacteriophage) containing human DNA were detected by hybridization analysis and isolated (Fig. 5.11). DNA from some of the clones isolated in this manner was found to be extremely efficient in inducing malignant transformation of a murine fibroblast cell line (NIH/3T3 cells). Thus, a gene (oncogene) had been isolated from a malignant human cell that was capable of inducing a transformed phenotype in nonmalignant cells.

The transfected DNA in the transformed cells was examined by Southern blot analysis using labeled DNA probes derived from RNA tumor viruses. Surprisingly, the transfected DNA in many of the transformants, including that from the EJ bladder cancer cell line, was found to be homologous to the viral oncogenes of the Harvey and Kirsten sarcoma viruses (Parada et al., 1982; Santos et al., 1984). These two genes, known as H-*ras* and K-*ras*, both encode proteins of 21,000 Da molecular weight that are similar in amino acid sequence. These proteins are referred to as p21 ras proteins, or p21^{ras}, and are located in the cytoplasm adjacent to the cell membrane; it has been determined that they bind to GTP, have GTPase activity, and are involved in signal

A

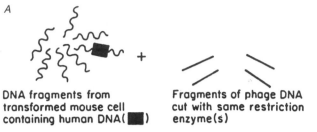

DNA fragments from
transformed mouse cell
containing human DNA(■)

Fragments of phage DNA
cut with same restriction
enzyme(s)

B **Ligation of DNA fragments**

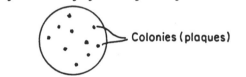

C **Phage containing ligated fragments grown in bacteria**

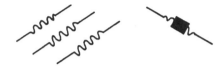

Colonies (plaques)

D **Plaque screened with a radioactive probe to human DNA**

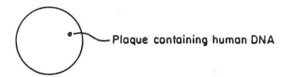

Plaque containing human DNA

Figure 5.11 Cloning of transforming sequences. *A.* DNA from a murine cell that contains human DNA is mixed with DNA from a bacteriophage. When the same restriction enzymes are used to cut the DNA, spontaneous ligation between the different types of DNA may occur, as shown in (*B*). The ligated DNA (*C*) is then packaged into mature bacteriophages that form plaques on a plate containing bacteria. *D.* The plaques are then screened with a radioactive probe that recognizes the specific human DNA of interest.

transduction (Barbacid, 1987; see also Chap. 6, Sec. 6.3.4).

A majority of cells transformed by DNA from human tumor cells have been found to contain human DNA that will hybridize to either the H-*ras* or K-*ras* genes. A transformant that did not contain such DNA was derived following transfection with DNA from a neuroblastoma. The gene responsible for this transforming activity was found to have weak homology with K-*ras* or H-*ras* and also encoded a protein with a molecular weight of 21,000, which cross-reacted with antibodies against the H-ras and K-ras proteins. This new gene, therefore, was named N-*ras*. N-*ras* has since been found in other transformants, especially those derived by transfection of

DNA from leukemias and lymphomas. Cells from up to 70 percent of acute leukemias have an activated N-*ras* gene (Eva et al., 1983).

Other cells that have been transformed by DNA from human tumors yet do not contain a transfected *Ras* gene have been found to contain the *neu*/c-*erb*B-2/*HER*-2, *Ret*, or *Trk* oncogenes (see Secs. 5.4.3 and 5.4.4). These genes encode transmembrane receptors with tyrosine kinase activity (see Chap. 6, Sec. 6.7.2).

DNA from almost all histologic types of human tumors has been able to transform NIH/3T3 cells to a malignant phenotype; however, only a small percentage (in general less than 10 percent) of tumors of a particular type score as positive in the focus formation assay. Exceptions are the leukemias and lymphomas, in which up to 70 percent of tumors score as positive. It is likely that the transfection assay does not detect activated oncogenes in many tumors for purely technical reasons, such as (1) the assay system is insensitive, (2) the activated oncogenes may be sufficiently large that they are broken during the extraction and transfer of tumor cell DNA, (3) the subjectivity of deciding what is to be called a transformed cell, and (4) the oncogene is not transforming in the target cell. For example, mutated forms of oncogenes found in pituitary tumors do not cause malignant transformation of NIH/3T3 cells (Clementi et al., 1990).

Transfection assays have identified genes that have the potential for malignant transformation, but such assays are slow and difficult to reproduce. For this reason, once an activating mutation has been identified in an oncogene, it is simpler to determine if other tumors carry the same or a similar abnormality either by Southern blot analysis, probing with allele-specific oligonucleotides, or by combining gene amplification by PCR with DNA sequencing (see Chap. 3, Sec. 3.3).

5.4.2 Activation of Oncogenes by Mutation

The H-*ras* gene from the EJ bladder tumor cell line was active in transfection/transformation assays while a *ras* gene cloned from a normal cell was inactive. When the normal and tumor-derived genes were sequenced, it was found that there was a change in a single base pair in the 12th codon that resulted in substitution of valine (Val) for glycine (Gly) in the corresponding p21 ras protein. The significance of this point mutation was confirmed in a number of ways. First, a mutation at the same position was found in *ras* genes derived from other tumors. Second, when genes that were specifically mu-

tated at this point were synthesized, they were found to have transforming activity. Thus a single point mutation can significantly alter the biologic behavior of a normal gene.

The K-*ras* and N-*ras* genes that are active in the transfection assay have also been cloned and sequenced. In addition to changes in the 12th amino acid, changes in the 13th and 61st amino acids have also been found to convey the ability to transform fibroblasts to a malignant phenotype. The proteins produced by the mutated genes have decreased GTPase activity as compared with the p21 protein derived from the normal *Ras* gene. The GTP-bound form of p21 ras protein is the active form of the protein. The p21 ras protein is activated in response to extracellular stimuli and initiates a signaling pathway (mitogen-activated protein kinase pathway) that results in gene expression leading to cell proliferation (see Chap. 6, Secs. 6.3.4 and 6.3.5).

Point mutations implicated in the development of transforming ability have been observed in a number of other genes. In the transmembrane region of the *neu* gene, the activating mutation changes the protein from a ligand-regulated tyrosine kinase receptor to a constitutively active tyrosine kinase protein (Bargmann et al., 1986). In the fms protein (a receptor for the growth factor CSF-1) involved in malignant transformation, mutations of amino acid 301 have been shown to result in constitutive activation of the receptor in the absence of ligand, while mutations of amino acid 969 result in enhanced activity of the gene once ligand has been bound (Roussel et al., 1988). Point mutations of amino acids 301 and 969 have also been found in the *fms* gene in acute myeloblastic leukemia (AML) and myelodysplastic syndromes (Ridge et al., 1990).

Many chemical carcinogens are mutagenic (see Chap. 8, Sec. 8.2.2), and the DNA from chemically induced tumors in rodents often contains mutated oncogenes. For example, DNA from rat mammary tumors induced by the carcinogen nitrosomethylurea (NMU) was found to contain an activated H-*ras* gene that led to malignant transformation of fibroblasts in transfection experiments. A majority of these tumors contained an activated H-*ras* gene in which a G-to-A transition occurred at the second nucleotide of codon 12. Over 90 percent of skin tumors initiated with dimethylbenzanthracene (DMBA) in mice have a specific A-to-T transversion at the second nucleotide of codon 61 of the H-*ras* gene. Mutation and consequent activation of oncogenes has also been reported following ionizing radiation (see Chap. 8, Sec. 8.5.3).

5.4.3 Amplification of Oncogenes

A number of mechanisms other than point mutation of an endogenous gene have been implicated in the development of malignancy. Cytogeneticists have recognized a large number of chromosomal abnormalities in malignant cells (see Chap. 4, Sec. 4.3); they include breaks and translocations, deletions, duplications, homogeneously staining regions (HSRs), and double minute chromosomes (DMs). Schimke et al. (1980) have demonstrated that HSRs and DMs are the result of amplification of genes.

Gene amplification results from several rounds of unscheduled DNA synthesis occurring during a single cell cycle. Such abnormal DNA replication has been shown to occur in cells exposed to transient hypoxia or cells that have been treated with cytotoxic agents, such as methotrexate, that inhibit DNA synthesis (Schwab, 1990). The region of amplification is usually several hundred kilobases in size, so that not one but a number of genes are increased in copy number. Amplified genes may be located at the site at which the normal gene is located, as small extrachromosomal fragments (DMs), as part of "marker chromosomes," or as HSRs in chromosomes that do not normally contain the gene (Schwab, 1990).

Malignant cells are sometimes found to contain HSRs and/or DMs. The genes contained in these HSRs and DMs have been studied using Southern blots and/or in situ hybridization (Chap. 3, Secs. 3.3.4 and 3.4.4). Amplification of a proto-oncogene (c-*myc*) was first reported for the HL-60 cell line derived from a patient with acute myelocytic leukemia (AML) (Collins and Groudine, 1982). Cells from neuroblastomas often contain HSRs that include amplified copies of the N-*myc* gene, and the presence of amplified N-*myc* is associated with poor prognosis (Schwab et al., 1983). N-*myc* is located on chromosome 2 and is one of a number of genes that bears homology to c-*myc* on chromosome 8. Another member of the *myc* gene family is L-*myc*, which, along with c-*myc*, has been found to be amplified in cell lines derived from small-cell cancer of the lung, where they seem to correlate with biologic subtypes showing aggressive clinical behavior (Little et al., 1983).

The *neu* gene was obtained in transfections using DNA from a rat neurogenic tumor; a mutation in the transmembrane region was responsible for activating the tyrosine kinase potential of the protein. The human homologue of the rat *neu* gene, called c-*erb*B-2 or *HER*-2, shows extensive homology to the epidermal growth factor receptor (c-*erb*B-1) and was shown to be amplified in nonneurogenic human tumors, primarily in a high proportion of breast and ovarian cancers (Slamon et al., 1989). Mutation of the c-*erb*B-2 gene was not found in these tumors; instead, the amplification resulted in overexpression of the normal gene product. Recently the product of the c-*erb*B-2 gene together with the products of related genes, c-*erb*B-3 and c-*erb*B-4, were shown to act as receptors for the ligand heregulin (Lupu et al., 1995). It is likely that heregulin-mediated activation of these receptors plays an important role in breast cancer. Thus, increased production of the normal protein products of amplified proto-oncogenes contribute to the development of the malignant phenotype.

5.4.4 Chromosome Translocation and Gene Rearrangement

Chromosome translocations occur at a high frequency in some types of tumors, suggesting that they may play a role in the development (or progression) of these tumors. Examples of recurring translocations are the Philadelphia (Ph) chromosome (a 9;22 translocation) in chronic myelogenous leukemia (CML) and in a subset of acute lymphoblastic leukemia (ALL), the 15;17 translocation in promyelocytic leukemia, and the several translocations involving chromosome 8 that occur in lymphoid malignancies (see Chap. 4, Sec. 4.3.2). Common sites of chromosome translocations in malignant cells have breakpoints that are frequently found to be near an oncogene (Rowley, 1989), suggesting that chromosomal breaks might lead to activation of oncogenes.

A number of investigators have cloned genes from the sites of chromosomal translocations (Groffen et al., 1984; de The et al., 1990). This can be illustrated by analysis of genes at the site of the translocation between chromosomes 9 and 22 in the Ph chromosome of CML patients (Fig. 5.12). The translocation leads to an aberrant juxtaposition of the *bcr* gene (breakpoint cluster region) present on chromosome 22 with c-*abl* sequences from chromosome 9. This results in the expression of a chimeric 8.5-kb *bcr-abl* hybrid mRNA transcript that encodes the p210 bcr-abl fusion protein, in which amino-terminal *abl* sequences are replaced by sequences from the *bcr* gene (Shtivelman et al., 1985). In normal cells, the *abl* mRNA is 5000 base pairs long and encodes a tyrosine kinase protein of about 145 kDa. While the break points in the *bcr* gene occur over a limited region, they are spread out over a relatively large region of approximately 100 kb in the *abl* gene. The p210 bcr-abl fusion protein exhibits elevated tyrosine-specific protein kinase activity.

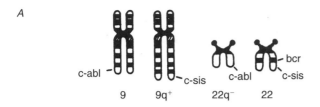

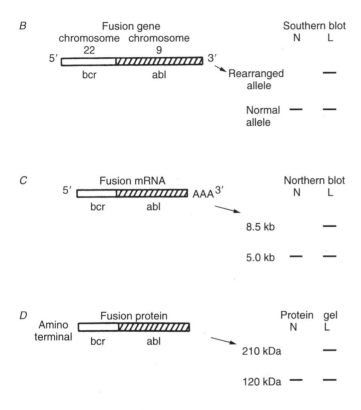

Figure 5.12 Cloning of genes from the Ph translocation. *A.* A schematic presentation of the normal chromosomes 9 and 22 and of the chromosomes 9q⁺ and 22q⁻ following translocation in CML. The Ph chromosome is 22q⁻. *B.* Rearrangement of the c-*abl* oncogene was found in a patient. A probe derived from this rearranged region (see text) was used to probe Southern blots from normal cells (*N*) and those from patients with CML (*L*). Rearrangement was found in almost all patients with CML. *C.* Schematic diagram of the mRNA from the fused region, and of a Northern blot demonstrating an increase in size of the mRNA from the *abl* oncogene in Ph-positive cells. *D.* Schematic diagram of the protein product of the fused gene and of a polyacrilamide gel electrophoresis demonstrating the increased size of the c-*abl* protein in Ph-positive CML cells. Note that CML cells contain both the abnormal enlarged (210-kDa) protein and the normal (120-kDa) protein.

In some forms of acute lymphoblastic leukemia (ALL) and acute myeloblastic leukemia (AML), a Ph chromosome may be identified. The *bcr* gene on chromosome 22 and the *abl* gene on chromosome 9 are both involved in the translocation, but the break point of the *bcr* gene occurs between the first and second exons of *bcr* (Heisterkamp et al., 1988; Fig. 5.13). The resulting fusion protein has a molecular mass of 190 kDa. Like the 210-kDa bcr-abl fusion protein, this protein is localized in the cytoplasm and has enhanced tyrosine kinase activity. In vivo experiments comparing the transforming efficiency of the 190-kDa protein with that of the 210-kDa protein demonstrate that the 190-kDa protein has greater transforming ability. This difference in activity of the two genes may account for the association of the 190-kDa protein with acute leukemias and the 210-kDa protein with chronic leukemia.

A number of groups have infected normal mouse bone marrow cells with retroviruses carrying the gene encoding the 210-kDa form of the bcr-abl fusion protein. After several weeks, a condition similar to CML develops in some of the animals. In some mice, acute lymphoid leukemias develop. These studies indicate that the *bcr-abl* gene is causative in the development of CML, but the long latency period and the fact that not all animals develop tumors suggests that other genetic changes occur in the infected cells before disease becomes evident (Daley et al., 1990).

Other chromosome translocations also give rise to fusion proteins. About 25 percent of children with pre-B-cell acute lymphoblastic leukemia (ALL) have a chromosomal translocation involving chromosomes 1 and 19, t(1;19)(q23;p13). This translocation juxtaposes the *E2A* gene on chromosome 19 to the *PBX1* gene on chromosome 1, leading to production

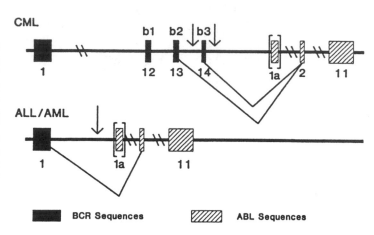

Figure 5.13 A schematic diagram illustrating the different forms of chromosome translocation that can result in the Ph chromosome. In the upper part of the diagram is shown the translocation found in CML. The *bcr* exons of the major breakpoint cluster are numbered b1, b2, and b3. The vertical arrows demonstrate the usual sites of translocation. In the bottom panel is shown the translocation that is often found in de novo acute leukemias. In this case the translocation occurs in the first intron of the *bcr* gene, as illustrated by the vertical arrow.

of a fusion transcript. As a result of this translocation, two proteins involved in transcription are fused (Nourse and Cleary, 1990). This translocation has been shown to have important prognostic and therapeutic implications in ALL patients. A characteristic chromosome translocation involving chromosomes 15 and 17 occurs in acute promyelocytic leukemia. As a result of the translocation, a fusion protein between the *PML* gene from chromosome 15 (of unknown function) is fused to the retinoic acid receptor α (*RAR*α) gene on chromosome 17. The fusion alters the DNA binding and transcriptional properties of the receptor. The fusion protein may bring about the malignant phenotype in several ways. First, the removal of the trans-activation domain of RARα may block the normal function of this protein. Second, the fusion may interfere with the normal function of PML, probably by the ability of RARα to form homo- and heterodimers with a variety of proteins through sequences retained in the PML-RAR fusion protein. The protein product of the PML gene in normal hematopoietic cells is localized in discrete nuclear structures composed of multiprotein complexes referred to as PODs (PML oncogenic domains); there are several in each cell. In acute promyelocytic leukemia, these structures are disrupted, but treatment of acute promyelocytic cells with retinoic acid allows the reappearance of the PODs. The exact function of PML is not known, but PML protein appears to block cell growth. One hypothesis is that the PML-RAR fusion protein is acting in a dominant manner to inhibit the function of the PML protein by sequestering it away from the POD structure. The inhibition of the normal function of RAR and PML by the fusion protein leads to a block in the differentiation capacity and possibly increased cell growth of hematopoietic stem cells (Dyck et al., 1994). The addition of retinoic acid may restore some degree of growth control and transient remission, but only in patients whose leukemic cells carry the 15;17 translocation (de The et al., 1990).

The nerve growth factor receptor trkA was initially isolated as a transforming oncogene, *trk*, in which most of the extracellular receptor part is replaced by the coding sequence for a tropomyosin-encoding gene. Two closely related genes, *trkB* (receptor for brain-derived neurotrophic factor) and *trkC* (receptor for neurotrophin 3), have been isolated and, together with *trkA*, form the neurotrophin family of receptor tyrosine kinases. Neurotrophins regulate the survival and differentiation of specific populations of neurons.

The *RET* oncogene was obtained from transfections with DNA from a thyroid carcinoma. The *RET* proto-oncogene encodes a receptor for GDNF (glial cell–derived neurotrophic factor). Oncogenic activation of this gene occurs by a rearrangement in which the tyrosine kinase domain is truncated and fused to heterologous genes resulting in novel fusion proteins with constitutive tyrosine kinase activity. Recently, oncogenic activation of the *RET* gene was detected in thyroid carcinomas from children exposed to the Chernobyl nuclear accident (Fugazzola et al., 1995). In addition, missense germline mutations of the *RET* proto-oncogene have been identified in the hereditary cancer syndromes multiple endocrine neoplasia types 2A and 2B (MEN2A and MEN2B) and familial medullary thyroid carcinoma (FMTC), all characterized by medullary carcinoma. Inherited cancer syndromes predispose an individual to development of specific tumors. Germline mutations of *RET* have also been associated with a nonneoplastic congenital disease, Hirschsprung disease, a disorder of gut development (Mak and Ponder, 1996).

In the above examples, translocation results in the production of a new protein. In other translocations, such as those involving immunoglobulin genes and the *myc* gene (2;14, 8;14, and 22;14 translocations) observed in lymphomas, the regulation of the *myc* gene is altered (Feo et al., 1985). The *myc* gene appears to be involved in the control of differentiation and proliferation. Normally the expression of this gene is tightly regulated, but in cells in which a translocation has occurred, the gene is constitutively expressed; that is, rather than being regulated, the gene product is always being produced. It seems possible that this alteration in the expression of the gene contributes to development of the malignant phenotype. A majority of follicular lymphomas display a t(14;18) translocation that places the *bcl-2* gene into juxtaposition with the Ig heavy-chain (H) gene locus, resulting in overexpression of *bcl-2* (Cotter, 1990)). The *tal-1* gene on chromosome 1 is another gene whose regulation is altered by translocation with a gene on chromosome 14 (1:14 translocation). The *tal-1* gene is rearranged in approximately 20 percent of cases of T-cell ALL (Chen et al., 1990).

5.4.5 Multiple Oncogenes

The previous discussion of the ways in which the various oncogenes might become activated has not addressed whether any one of these changes is sufficient to produce the malignant phenotype. Evidence reviewed in Chap. 4, Secs. 4.2 and 4.5.1, suggests that at least two genetic changes are needed to produce a cancer cell, and studies of oncogenes support this view. Some cell lines contain at least two activated oncogenes. For example, the cell line HL-60 contains an amplified *myc* gene as well as an activated N-*ras* gene, while some cell lines derived from Burkitt's lymphoma contain a rearranged *myc* gene and an activated N-*ras* gene (Murray et al., 1983). In colon cancer, at least six different genetic alterations have been observed (Fearon and Vogelstein, 1990; Chap. 4, Sec. 4.5.4).

Experimental support for the involvement of two or more oncogenes in malignant transformation has been obtained using gene transfer. The DNA transfection experiments described in Sec. 5.4.1 all used NIH/3T3 cells as recipients; this cell line has a normal phenotype but has been selected for its ability to be propagated indefinitely in tissue culture. Normal fibroblasts obtained fresh from an individual or an animal, referred to as *primary fibroblasts,* do not have this property and will die after approximately 20–60 generations in culture. When primary rat embryo fibroblasts are transfected with a rearranged *myc* gene, it is possible to obtain permanent (immortalized) cell lines; however, they are phenotypically normal. If an activated *ras* gene is used instead, morphologic transformation may occur, but these cells are unable to grow indefinitely and will not form tumors in animals. Transfection with both an activated *ras* gene and a rearranged *myc* gene leads to morphologic transformation, the development of permanent cell lines, and the development of tumors on injection into animals (Land et al., 1983). However, these tumors grow to a limited size and then stop growing; this suggests that further events may be needed to produce a tumor that can grow to kill the animal.

There are contradictory observations about the sequence of genetic changes occurring during malignant transformation. In the development of carcinogen-induced skin tumors, *ras* mutations have been found to precede the development of tumors (Kumar et al., 1990). In contrast, mutations of *ras* are rare in CML; if present, they occur late in the course of the disease (Collins et al., 1989). In some diseases such as follicular lymphoma, the biologic behavior of the disease changes from a slow-growing, relatively benign malignancy to a rapidly growing, aggressive tumor. In the early phase of the disease, a characteristic t(14;18) chromosome translocation involving the immunoglobulin heavy-chain locus on chromosome 14 and the *bcl-2* gene on chromosome 18 is often observed. In more aggressive tumors, in addition to the t(14;18) translocation, it is common to observe a t(8;14) translocation that involves the *myc* gene on chromosome 8 and the immunoglobulin gene on chromosome 14 (De Jong et al., 1988); the reverse sequence of translocations has not been reported. In the development of colon carcinoma, a number of characteristic changes appear to occur in a steplike manner (Fearon and Vogelstein, 1990). The evidence suggests that the development of some tumors may be dependent on the activation of oncogenes in a preferred sequence, while in others the development of a tumor is governed by the accumulation of specific genetic changes and not the order in which the changes arise.

5.4.6 Protein Products of Oncogenes

Proto-oncogenes encode proteins whose normal function is to regulate cellular responses to external signals that elicit cell growth and differentiation. These proteins form a biochemical network by which information from the outside of the cell is interpreted, resulting in changes in gene expression, DNA synthesis, cytoskeletal architecture, cell-cell contacts, and cellular metabolism. Structural alteration or overexpression of these proteins, which occurs frequently as a consequence of oncogenic mutations, can induce the constitutive activation of intracellular biochemical pathways that stimulate cell proliferation in the absence of a bona fide signal. Hence, a cell carrying an activated oncogene is no longer dependent for its own growth on factors produced by other cells.

The protein products of proto-oncogenes and their transforming variants can be grouped into distinct classes based on their subcellular localization and biochemical activity. These include (1) growth factors; (2) growth-factor receptors with tyrosine kinase activity; (3) cytoplasmic protein tyrosine kinases; (4) membrane-associated guanine nucleotide–binding proteins; (5) soluble cytoplasmic serine-threonine–specific protein kinases; (6) nuclear proteins, and (7) cytoplasmic proteins that affect cell survival. Examples of proteins that fall into each class have been presented in Table 5.2. The functions of the gene products in these various classes are discussed in Chaps. 6 and 7.

5.5 TUMOR SUPPRESSOR GENES

Tumor Suppressor Genes and Loss of Heterozygosity

In contrast to the oncogenes described above, a variety of genes referred to as *tumor suppressor genes* have been identified (see Chap. 4, Table 4.4). As their name suggests, these genes are involved in preventing the development of malignancy. Tumor suppressor genes differ from activated oncogenes in a number of important ways. First, activated oncogenes act in a dominant manner and the activating event is usually acquired. In contrast, tumor suppressor genes act in a recessive manner. Mutations represent inactivating events and mutated forms of the gene may be inherited. Thus, tumor suppressor genes figure prominently in the development of familial cancers, but mutations of tumor suppressor genes also occur commonly in sporadic forms of cancer.

Tumor suppressor genes were identified initially through the study of somatic cell hybrids and hereditary cancers. When tumor cells were fused with normal cells, the resulting hybrids were suppressed in their ability to form tumors. Tumor-forming cells arose from the hybrid cell populations, with reexpression of tumorigenicity often associated with loss of a specific chromosome. These findings suggested that malignancy behaves as a recessive trait in hybrid cells and that genes responsible for suppression of malignancy must be lost or inactivated for the hybrid cells to regain the capacity to form tumors.

Cytogenetic analysis of tumor cells in patients with hereditary cancers, such as retinoblastoma and Wilms' tumor, revealed the presence of chromosome deletions associated with these diseases. In particular, deletions of chromosome 13q14 are associated with retinoblastoma, and deletions of chromosome 11p13 are associated with Wilms' tumor. These findings suggested that loss of chromosomal DNA was required for the development of specific cancers. These chromosomal sites are now known to be the location of the retinoblastoma (*RB1*) and Wilms' (*WT-1*) tumor suppressor genes.

Knudson's analysis of the age-specific incidence of familial and sporadic forms of retinoblastoma and other childhood cancers led him to suggest that development of these cancers requires two events (or mutations). He proposed that, in familial cancers, one mutation is transmitted through the germline and that the second mutation occurs somatically. In noninherited (sporadic) cancers, both mutations have to occur within the same somatic cell. In nearly all the hereditary cancers, the two mutations occur on both copies (alleles) of the same tumor suppressor gene and the mutations result in complete loss of tumor suppressor function. The germline loss of the first copy of the gene in familial retinoblastoma is visible at the cytogenetic level in a few cases. Usually, there is no cytogenetic abnormality, and the inherited mutation is either a small deletion or a point mutation. In contrast, the loss of the second allele in the tumor cells often involves loss of a larger chromosome segment (see Chap. 4, Sec. 4.5.2). The presence of DNA sequence polymorphisms throughout the human genome has provided a means to search for allele loss in tumors (Knudson, 1993). At most genetic loci, there are differences in sequence between the alleles on the maternal and paternal chromosomes (i.e., heterozygosity). Mechanisms such as chromosomal nondisjunction, mitotic recombination, or gene conversion, in which the wild-type allele is replaced by a duplicated copy of the homologous chromosome region that carries the mutant allele, lead to loss of heterozygosity (LOH): the tumor would then contain two identically mutated alleles. Alternatively, LOH may occur by deletion of the normal allele or by complete or partial chromosome loss, in which case the tumor would contain one copy of the mutated allele and no wild-type allele (see Chap. 4, Fig. 4.15). The repeated observation of LOH of a specific, polymorphic, chromosomal marker in cells from a particular tumor type (familial or sporadic) suggests the presence of a tumor suppressor gene located close by.

5.5.2 The p53 Gene

The *p53* tumor suppressor gene is a frequent target for recessive mutations in many human and rodent malignancies (Greenblatt et al., 1994). The loss of wild-type p53 expression in tumor cells provides these cells with a selective growth advantage, and much effort is currently directed at understanding the role of p53 in growth regulation and tumor suppression. Studies with genetically engineered p53-null (p53-knockout) mice (see Chap. 3, Sec. 3.3.12) indicate that p53 protein function is required neither for normal cell proliferation nor for development. However, the increased incidence of spontaneous tumors in p53-null mice and the enhanced susceptibility of p53-null mice to carcinogen- and radiation-induced tumorigenesis indicate a role for p53 in tumor suppression (Donehower et al., 1992). The Li-Fraumeni syndrome provides another example illustrating the role of p53 in cancer susceptibility and tumor development. This rare autosomal dominant syndrome in humans is characterized by the occurrence, at an early age, of diverse mesenchymal and epithelial tumors at multiple sites. Affected individuals from certain families with this syndrome carry a heterozygous *p53* mutation in the germline, and the occurrence of tumors is associated with loss of the remaining wild-type *p53* allele in the tumor cells (Malkin et al., 1990).

Despite intensive study of the properties of the p53 protein, the mechanisms by which p53 functions as a tumor suppressor gene are unknown. There is widespread agreement that p53 plays a critical role in the cellular response to DNA damage leading to cell cycle arrest in G1 or apoptosis. Transient arrest in G1 is postulated to allow time for repair of damaged DNA, which might otherwise interfere with accurate DNA replication, and for repair of lesions that might be perpetuated as mutations in cells entering S phase. Cells that lack p53 expression may enter S phase inappropriately after treatment with metabolic inhibitors that normally arrest cells in G1 and have a higher incidence of genetic instability and gene amplification (Kastan et al., 1991; Lu and Lane, 1993).

p53 has been shown to initiate apoptosis in cells exposed to agents that cause DNA strand breakage, including γ-irradiation and various chemotherapeutic drugs. For example, normal murine thymocytes and quiescent lymphocytes exposed to ionizing radiation in culture undergo apoptosis, whereas thymocytes and lymphocytes obtained from p53-null mice remain viable after irradiation (Clarke et al., 1993;

Lowe et al., 1993). Oncogenes such as c-*myc* and *E1A* can induce apoptosis, particularly after serum depletion, and this form of apoptosis has also been shown to be p53-dependent. Loss of p53-mediated apoptosis could result in the survival of oncogene-expressing cells undergoing inappropriate cell growth and in the survival of cells carrying mutations and carcinogenic lesions. Failure to eliminate such cells could contribute to tumorigenesis (Lowe et al., 1994).

The p53 protein has also been implicated in DNA repair (see Chap. 4, Sec. 4.4.7). The ability of p53 protein to interact with the DNA helicases encoded by the xeroderma pigmentosa XPB and XPD genes supports this possibility; cells lacking either one of these proteins are defective in nucleotide excision repair. Loss of p53 may lead to genomic instability by reducing the efficiency of DNA repair.

The finding that wild-type p53 protein has site-specific double-stranded DNA binding activity and that it possesses transcription regulatory activities suggests that the p53-mediated G1 arrest and the p53-dependent apoptosis pathway might involve downstream effector genes. The p53 protein has been shown to promote transcription of genes containing a p53-responsive element and to repress transcription of numerous other genes that lack a p53 consensus binding sequence. Almost all of the mutant p53 proteins associated with malignancies lose the ability to regulate transcription. Furthermore, transcriptional activation by p53 has been shown to be intimately associated with its ability to act as a tumor suppressor and as a growth suppressor (Pietenpol et al., 1994).

Two of several genes that are transcriptionally activated by p53 are *GADD45* and *p21/WAF1*. *GADD45* belongs to the gadd (growth arrest and DNA damage inducible) family of genes and contains a conserved p53-binding motif in its third intron (Kastan et al., 1992). Induction of *GADD45* by γ-irradiation is strictly dependent on p53 function. In gene transfer experiments, *GADD45* expression results in growth inhibition as measured by reduced ability of recipient cells to generate colonies in culture. GADD45 protein can bind to the proliferating cell nuclear antigen (PCNA), a normal component of cyclin-dependent kinase (CDK) complexes and a protein involved in DNA replication and repair. This interaction between GADD45 protein and PCNA may be involved in the inhibitory effect of *GADD45* expression on cell growth. The *p21/WAF1* gene contains a p53-binding motif in its promoter (El-Deiry et al., 1993) and encodes a 21000-Da protein (p21) that inhibits the activity of cyclin-dependent kinases necessary for the G1-S transition (Chap. 7, Sec. 7.2.3). Gene transfer experiments indicate that *p21* expression in recipient cells inhibits cell growth. Like GADD45, p21 protein also binds to PCNA and inhibits its DNA replication function. The presence of CDK and PCNA inhibitory activities in p21 suggests that this protein may prevent S-phase entry in two ways: by inhibiting CDKs required for the G1-S transition, and by inhibiting PCNA, which would interfere directly with DNA replication. The *p21/WAF1* gene is considered to be a critical downstream effector in the p53-specific pathway of G1 cell-cycle control (Dulic et al., 1994; El-Deiry et al., 1994).

5.5.3 Other Tumor Suppressor Genes

Studies of loss of heterozygosity (LOH) have led to the identification and isolation of numerous tumor suppressor genes. A listing of these can be found in Chap. 4, Table 4.4. Functional studies of these genes indicate that tumor suppressor proteins are involved in a wide array of cellular functions. *WT-1*, like the *p53* gene, encodes a transcription factor; *VHL* encodes a protein that associates with the elongin/sIII transcription elongation complex; *DPC4* encodes a component of the TGFβ signaling pathway; *CDKN2/INK4A* encodes p16, a protein that acts as an inhibitor of cyclin-dependent kinases; *MSH2, MLH1,* and *PMS2* each encode proteins involved in DNA mismatch repair. Tumor suppressor genes may regulate the growth of tumors directly by inhibiting growth or promoting death. Alternatively, genes such as *MSH2* may promote tumorigenesis indirectly. Genes involved in DNA repair may be required to maintain genomic stability, and their inactivation may lead to an accelerated rate of mutation in other genes that directly control cell growth and death.

5.6 SUMMARY

Some DNA- and RNA-containing viruses are known to induce tumors in animals. An essential step in malignant transformation of normal cells by most tumor viruses is integration of all or part of the viral DNA (or DNA copy of retroviral RNA) into the host-cell genome. For certain viruses, specific viral genes (oncogenes) have been identified that, when expressed in normal cells, lead to malignant transformation. Other viruses, through the process of integration, activate the expression of normal cellular genes. When these genes encode proteins normally involved in the regulation of cell proliferation, their overexpression can lead to cellular transformation. Viral integration can also result in disruption of cellular genes. If these genes encode proteins that negatively regulate cell growth, their inactivation can lead to uncontrolled cell growth.

Links between human viruses and certain cancers have been established on the basis of epidemiologic, clinical, and molecular biologic studies. The links are strongest for HTLV-1 and adult T-cell leukemia. Compelling evidence also exists for a role of human papillomaviruses in the development of cervical cancer, Epstein-Barr virus in the development of Burkitt's lymphoma and nasopharyngeal carcinoma, human hepatitis B virus in the pathogenesis of hepatocellular carcinoma, and HIV and herpesvirus-8 in Kaposi's sarcoma. In each of the human malignancies where viruses are suspected of playing an important role, other genetic changes are required in the infected cell.

The identification of cellular genes related to the oncogenes present in RNA tumor viruses provided the first demonstration that deregulated and/or altered cellular proto-oncogenes could lead to cancer. Subsequently, gene transfer experiments led to the discovery of novel oncogenes. Other oncogenes have been identified at the sites of recurring chromosomal translocations in human cancer and on regions of the genome that become amplified in tumors. Proto-oncogenes encode proteins that are normally involved in the promotion of cell growth; their activation—by a variety of mechanisms including mutation, amplification, and translocation—can lead to the development of malignancy.

Tumor suppressor genes encode proteins involved in regulating cell proliferation, in cell death, and in maintaining genomic integrity. Tumor suppressor genes become inactivated in human cancer. Generally, inactivation occurs through genetic mechanisms that disrupt gene expression or gene function. Occasionally, tumor suppressors are inactivated through protein interactions involving other cellular or viral proteins. Cancer susceptibility genes may be considered as a subset of the tumor suppressor genes. A single defective copy of a cancer susceptibility gene may be inherited and can predispose a person to neoplasia. However, additional genetic changes are required to convert a predisposed cell to a tumor cell, including the inactivation of the homologous copy of the cancer susceptibility gene.

REFERENCES

Barbacid M: Ras genes. *Annu Rev Biochem* 1987; 56:779–827.

Bargmann CI, Hung M-C, Weinberg RA: The neu oncogene encodes an epidermal growth factor receptor related protein. *Nature* 1986; 319:226–230.

Bishop JM: Viral oncogenes. *Cell* 1985; 42:23–38.

Bryan TM, Reddel RR: SV40-induced immortalization of human cells. *Crit Rev Oncol* 1994; 5:331–357.

Chang Y, Cesarman E, Pessin MS, et al: Identification of herpesvirus-like DNA sequences in AIDS-associated Kaposi's sarcoma. *Science* 1994; 266:1865–1869.

Chen Q, Cheng J-T, Tsai L-H, et al: The tal gene undergoes chromosome translocation in T-cell leukemia and potentially encodes a helix-loop-helix protein. *EMBO J* 1990; 9:415–424.

Clarke AR, Purdie CA, Harrison DJ, et al: Thymocyte apoptosis induced by p53-dependent and independent pathways. *Nature* 1993; 362:849–852.

Clementi E, Malgaretti N, Meldolesi J, et al: A new constitutively activating mutation of the Gs protein alpha subunit-gsp oncogene is found in human pituitary tumors. *Oncogene* 1990; 5:1059–1061.

Collins S, Groudine M: Amplification of endogenous myc-related DNA sequences in a human myeloid leukaemia cell line. *Nature* 1982; 298:679–681.

Collins SJ, Howard M, Andrews DF, et al: Rare occurrence of N-ras point mutations in Philadelphia chromosome positive chronic myeloid leukemia. *Blood* 1989; 73:1028–1032.

Conzen SD, Cole CN: The three transforming regions of SV40 T antigen are required for immortalization of primary mouse embryo fibroblasts. *Oncogene* 1995; 11:2295–2302.

Cotter FE: The role of the bcl-2 gene in lymphoma. *Br J Haematol* 1990; 75:449–453.

Cullen BR: Does HIV-1 Tat induce a change in viral initiation rights? *Cell* 1993; 73:417–420.

Daley GQ, van Etten RA, Baltimore D: Induction of chronic myelogenous leukemia in mice by the p210 bcr/abl gene of the Philadelphia chromosome. *Science* 1990; 247:824–830.

De Jong D, Voetdijk MB, Beverstock GC, et al: Activation of the c-myc oncogene in a precursor-B-cell blast crisis of follicular lymphoma, presenting as composite lymphoma. *N Engl J Med* 1988; 318:1373–1378.

de The H, Chomienne C, Lanotte M, et al: The t(15;17) translocation of acute promyelocytic leukemia fuses the retinoic acid receptor alpha gene to a novel transcribed locus. *Nature* 1990; 347:558–561.

de Villiers EM: Heterogeneity of the human papillomavirus group. *J Virol* 1989; 63:4898–4903.

Donehower LA, Harvey M, Slagle BL, et al: Mice deficient for p53 are developmentally normal but susceptible to spontaneous tumours. *Nature* 1992; 356:215–221.

Dulic V, Kaufmann WK, Wilson SJ, et al: p53-dependent inhibition of cyclin-dependent kinase activities in human fibroblasts during radiation-induced G1 arrest. *Cell* 1994; 76:1013–1023.

Dyck JA, Maul GG, Miller WH Jr, et al: A novel macromolecular structure is a target of the promyelocyte-retinoic acid receptor oncoprotein. *Cell* 1994; 76:333–343.

Dyson N, Harlow E: Adenovirus E1A targets key regulators of cell proliferation. In: Levine AJ, ed: *Cancer Surveys 12: Tumor Suppressor Genes, The Cell Cycle and Cancer.* Cold Spring Harbor, NY: Cold Spring Harbor Laboratory; 1992:161–195.

Eckner R, Ewen ME, Newsome D, et al: Molecular cloning and functional analysis of the adenovirus E1A-associated 300 kD protein (p300) reveals a protein with properties of a transcriptional adaptor. *Genes Dev* 1994; 8:869–884.

El-Deiry WS, Harper JW, O'Connor PM, et al: WAF1/CIP1 is induced in p53-mediated G1 arrest and apoptosis. *Cancer Res* 1994; 54:1169–1174.

El-Deiry WS, Tokino T, Velculescu VE, et al: WAF1, a potential mediator of p53 tumor suppression. *Cell* 1993; 75:817–825.

Ensoli B, Barillari G, Salahuddin SZ, et al: Tat protein of HIV-1 stimulates growth of cells derived from Kaposi's sarcoma lesions of AIDS patients. *Nature* 1990; 345:84–86.

Eva A, Tronick SR, Gol RA, et al: Transforming genes of human hematopoietic tumors: frequent detection of ras related oncogenes whose activation appears to be independent of tumor phenotype. *Proc Natl Acad Sci USA* 1983; 80:4926–4930.

Fearon ER, Vogelstein B: A genetic model of colorectal tumorigenesis. *Cell* 1990; 61:759–767.

Feo S, ar-Rushdi A, Huebner K, et al: Suppression of the normal mouse c-myc oncogene in human lymphoma cells. *Nature* 1985; 313:493–495.

Fried M, Prives C: The biology of simian virus 40 and polyomavirus. In: Botchan M, Grodzicker T, Sharp PA, eds. *Cancer Cells 4: DNA Tumor Viruses.* Cold Spring Harbor, NY: Cold Spring Harbor Laboratory; 1986:1–16.

Fugazzola L, Pilotti S, Pinchera A, et al: Oncogenic rearrangements of the RET proto-oncogene in papillary thyroid carcinomas from children exposed to the Chernobyl nuclear accident. *Cancer Res* 1995; 55:5617–5620.

Greenblatt MS, Bennett WP, Hollstein M, Harris CC: Mutations in the p53 tumor suppressor gene: Clues to cancer etiology and molecular pathogenesis. *Cancer Res* 1994; 54:4855–4878.

Groffen J, Stephenson JR, Heisterkamp N, et al: Philadelphia chromosomal breakpoints are clustered within a limited region bcr on chromosome 22. *Cell* 1984; 36:93–99.

Hayward WS, Neel BG, Astrin SM: Activation of a cellular onc gene by promoter insertion in ALV-induced lymphoid leukosis. *Nature* 1981; 290:475–480.

Heisterkamp N, Knoppel E, Groffen J: The first BCR gene intron contains breakpoints in Philadelphia chromosome positive leukemia. *Nucleic Acids Res* 1988; 16:10069–10081.

Kastan MB, Onyekwere O, Sidransky D, et al: Participation of p53 protein in the cellular response to DNA damage. *Cancer Res* 1991; 51:6304–6311.

Kastan MB, Zhan Q, El-Deiry WS, et al: A mammalian cell cycle checkpoint pathway utilizing p53 and GADD45 is defective in ataxia-telangiectasia. *Cell* 1992; 71:587–597.

Kim CM, Koike K, Saito I, et al: *HBx* gene of hepatitis B virus induces liver cancer in transgenic mice. *Nature* 1991; 351:317–320.

Klein G, Klein E: Conditioned tumorigenicity of activated oncogenes. *Cancer Res* 1986; 46:3211–3224.

Knudson AG: Antioncogenes and human cancer. *Proc Natl Acad Sci USA* 1993; 90:10914–10921.

Kumar R, Sukumar S, Barbacid M: Activation of ras oncogenes preceding the onset of neoplasia. *Science* 1990; 248:1101–1102.

Land H, Parada LF, Weinberg RA: Tumorigenic conversion of primary embryo fibroblasts requires at least two cooperating oncogenes. *Nature* 1983; 304:596–602.

Lane DP, Benchimol S: p53: Oncogene or anti-oncogene? *Genes Dev* 1990; 4:1–8.

Levine AJ, Momand J: Tumor suppressor genes: the p53 and retinoblastoma sensitivity genes and gene products. *Biochim Biophys Acta* 1990; 1032:119–136.

Liebowitz D: Nasopharyngeal carcinoma: the Epstein-Barr virus association. *Semin Oncol* 1994; 21:376–381.

Lill NL, Tevethia MJ, Eckner R, et al: p300 family members associate with the carboxyl terminus of simian virus 40 large tumor antigen. *J Virol* 1997; 71:129–137.

Little CD, Nau MM, Carney DN, et al: Amplification and expression of the c-myc oncogene in human lung cancer cell lines. *Nature* 1983; 306:194–196.

Livingston DM: Functional analysis of the retinoblastoma gene product and of RB-SV40 T antigen complexes. In: Levine AJ, ed: *Cancer Surveys 12: Tumor Suppressor Genes, The Cell Cycle and Cancer.* Cold Spring Harbor, NY: Cold Spring Harbor Laboratory; 1992:153–160.

Lowe SW, Bodis S, McClatchy A, et al: p53 status and the efficacy of cancer therapy in vivo. *Science* 1994; 266:807–810.

Lowe SW, Schmitt EM, Smith SW, et al: p53 is required for radiation-induced apoptosis in mouse thymocytes. *Nature* 1993; 362:847–849.

Lowy DR, Kirnbauer R, Schiller JT: Genital human papillomavirus infection. *Proc Natl Acad Sci USA* 1994; 91:2436–2440.

Lu X, Lane DP: Differential induction of transcriptionally active p53 following UV or ionizing radiation: Defects in chromosome instability syndromes? *Cell* 1993; 75: 765–778.

Lupu R, Cardillo M, Harris L, et al: Interaction between erbB-receptors and heregulin in breast cancer tumor progression and drug resistance. *Semin Cancer Biol* 1995; 6:135–145.

Mak YF, Ponder BA: RET oncogene. *Curr Opin Genet Dev* 1996; 6:82–86.

Malkin D, Li FP, Strong LC, et al: Germ line p53 mutations in a familial syndrome of breast cancer, sarcomas and other neoplasms. *Science* 1990; 250:1233–1238.

Moran E, Mathews MB: Multiple functional domains in the adenovirus E1A gene. *Cell* 1987; 48:177–178.

Munger K, Scheffner M, Huibregtse JM, Howley PM: Interactions of HPV E6 and E7 oncoproteins with tumor suppressor gene products. In: Levine AJ, ed: *Cancer Surveys 12: Tumor Suppressor Genes, The Cell Cycle and Cancer.* Cold Spring Harbor, NY: Cold Spring Harbor Laboratory; 1992:197–217.

Murray MJ, Cunningham JM, Parada LF, et al: A ras oncogene coexisting with altered myc genes in hematopoietic tumors. *Cell* 1983; 33:749–757.

Nerenberg M, Hinrichs SH, Reynolds RK, et al: The tax gene of human T-lymphotropic virus type I induces mesenchymal tumors in transgenic mice. *Science* 1987; 237:1324–1329.

Nicholas J, Ruvolo VR, Burns WH, et al: Kaposi's sarcoma-associated human herpesvirus-8 encodes homologues of macrophage inflammatory protein-1 and interleukin-6. *Nature Med* 1997; 3:287–292.

Nourse J, Cleary ML: Chromosomal translocation t(1;19) results in synthesis of a homeobox fusion mRNA that codes for a potential chimeric transcription factor. *Cell* 1990; 60:535–545.

Parada LF, Tabin CJ, Shih C, et al: Human EJ bladder carcinoma oncogene is homologue of Harvey sarcoma virus ras gene. *Nature* 1982; 297:474–478.

Pennisi E: Monkey virus DNA found in rare human cancers (editorial). *Science* 1997; 275:748–749.

Pettersson U, Roberts RJ: Adenovirus gene expression and replication: A historical review. In: Botchan M, Grodzicker T, Sharp PA, eds. *Cancer Cells 4: DNA Tumor Viruses.* Cold Spring Harbor, NY: Cold Spring Harbor Laboratory; 1986:37–57.

Pietenpol JA, Tokino T, Thiagalingam S, et al: Sequence-specific transcriptional activation is essential for growth suppression by p53. *Proc Natl Acad Sci USA* 1994; 91:1998–2002.

Ridge SA, Worwood M, Oscier D, et al: FMS mutations in myelodysplastic, leukemic and normal subjects. *Proc Natl Sci USA* 1990; 87:1377–1380.

Roussel MF, Downing JR, Rettenmier CW, et al: A point mutation in the extracellular domain of the human CSF-1 receptor (c-fms proto-oncogene product) activates its transforming potential. *Cell* 1988; 55: 979–988.

Rowley JD: Finding order in chaos. *Perspect Biol Med* 1989; 32:371–384.

Royce RA, Sena A, Cates W Jr, Cohen MS: Sexual transmission of HIV. *N Engl J Med* 1997; 336:1072–1078.

Santos E, Martin-Zanca D, Reddy EP, et al: Malignant activation of a K-ras oncogene in lung carcinoma but not in normal tissue of the same patient. *Science* 1984; 223:661–664.

Schimke RT, Brown PC, Kaufman RJ, et al: Chromosomal and extrachromosomal localization of amplified dihydrofolate reductase genes in cultured mammalian cells. *Cold Spring Harb Symp Quant Biol* 1980; 45:785–797.

Schulz TF, Boshoff CH, Weiss RA: HIV infection and neoplasia. *Lancet* 1996; 348:587–591.

Schwab M: Oncogene amplification in neoplastic development and progression of human cancers. *Crit Rev Oncogen* 1990; 2:35–52.

Schwab M, Alitalo K, Klempnauer K-H, et al: Amplified DNA with limited homology to myc cellular oncogene is shared by human neuroblastoma cell lines and a neuroblastoma tumour. *Nature* 1983; 305:245–248.

Shih C, Weinberg RA: Isolation of a transforming sequence from a human bladder carcinoma cell line. *Cell* 1982; 29:161–169.

Shtivelman E, Lifshitz B, Gale RP, et al: Fused transcript of abl and bcr genes in chronic myelogenous leukemia. *Nature* 1985; 315:550–554.

Slamon DJ, Godolphin W, Jones LA, et al: Studies of the HER-2/neu proto-oncogene in human breast and ovarian cancer. *Science* 1989; 244:707–712.

Sousa R, Dostatni N, Yaniv M: Control of papillomavirus gene expression. *Biochim Biophys Acta* 1990; 1032:19–37.

Stehelin D, Varmus HE, Bishop JM, Vogt PK: DNA related to the transforming gene(s) of avian sarcoma viruses is present in normal avian DNA. *Nature* 1976; 260:170–173.

Sugden B: An intricate route of immortality. *Cell* 1989; 57:5–7.

Varmus H: Retroviruses. *Science* 1988; 240:1427–1435.

Vogel J, Hinrichs SH, Reynolds RK, et al: The HIV tat gene induces dermal lesions resembling Kaposi's sarcoma in transgenic mice. *Nature* 1988; 335:606–611.

Vousden KH: Human papillomaviruses and cervical carcinoma. *Cancer Cells* 1989; 1:43–50.

Wang XW, Forrester K, Yeh H, Feitelson MA, et al: Hepatitis B virus X protein inhibits p53 sequence-specific DNA binding transcriptional activity, and association with transcription factor ERCC3. *Proc Natl Acad Sci USA* 1994; 91:2230–2234.

Weinberg R: The retinoblastoma gene and gene product. In: Levine AJ, (ed): *Cancer Surveys 12: Tumor Suppressor Genes, The Cell Cycle and Cancer.* Cold Spring Harbor, NY: Cold Spring Harbor Laboratory; 1992:43–57.

Weinberg R: Tumor suppressor genes. *Science* 1991; 254:1138–1146.

Weinreb M, Day PJR, Niggli F, et al: The consistent association between Epstein-Barr virus and Hodgkin's disease in children in Kenya. *Blood* 1996; 87:3828–3836.

Weiss R, Teich N, Varmus H, Coffin J, eds. *RNA Tumor Viruses.* Cold Spring Harbor, NY: Cold Spring Harbor Laboratory; 1985.

Wong-Staal F, Gallo RC: Human T-lymphotropic retroviruses. *Nature* 1985; 317:395–403.

Yoshida M: Expression of the HTLV-1 genome and its association with a unique T-cell malignancy. *Biochim Biophys Acta* 1987; 907:145–161.

Yoshida M, Suzuki T, Fujisawa J, Hirai H: HTLV-1 oncoprotein tax and cellular transcription factors. *Curr Top Microbiol Immunol* 1995; 193:79–89.

6

Growth Factors and Intracellular Signaling

Brent W. Zanke

6.1 INTRODUCTION

6.2 EXTRACELLULAR GROWTH FACTORS

6.3 SIGNALING PATHWAYS TRIGGERED
BY GROWTH FACTORS
6.3.1 Growth-Factor Receptors
6.3.2 Binding of Receptors to Cytoplasmic Proteins
6.3.3 Receptor-Substrate Complexes: Propagation
of the Signal
6.3.4 Activation of Ras Proteins
6.3.5 Mitogen-Activated Protein Kinase Signaling Pathways
6.3.6 Activation of Transcription Factors
6.3.7 Function of Growth Factor–Stimulated Signaling Pathways

6.4 STRESS-ACTIVATED SIGNALING PATHWAYS
6.4.1 Stress-Activated Protein Kinases
6.4.2 Physiologic Consequences of SAPK/p38 Signaling
6.4.3 Interpathway Control of Signaling

6.5 SIGNALING THROUGH CYTOKINE RECEPTORS
6.5.1 Structure of Cytokine Receptors
6.5.2 Cytokine-Induced Signaling Pathways

6.6 SIGNALING THROUGH ANTIGEN RECEPTORS
6.6.1 Lymphocyte Antigen Receptors
6.6.2 Cytoplasmic Signaling

6.7 SIGNAL TRANSDUCTION IN CANCER
6.7.1 Abnormalities of Extracellular Signaling Molecules
6.7.2 Abnormalities of Growth Factor Receptors
6.7.3 Abnormalities in Cytoplasmic Signaling Transducers
6.7.4 Abnormalities in Nuclear Transcription Factors

6.8 SUMMARY

REFERENCES

6.1 INTRODUCTION

Cell growth and differentiation is triggered by the recognition of extracellular signals at the cell surface, resulting in the activation of linked cytoplasmic and nuclear biochemical cascades. Perhaps the greatest advance in our understanding of the molecular cell biology of cancer has been the recognition that, when dysregulated, normal growth-signaling pathways can cause malignant transformation in human cells. What normally is a coordinated and measured process becomes unbridled and destructive. This chapter reviews what is known about these signaling pathways and highlights identified abnormalities relevant to the understanding and management of human cancer.

6.2 EXTRACELLULAR GROWTH FACTORS

As multicellular organisms became more complex with evolution, sensitivity to the pericellular environment evolved to allow coordinated cell growth and differentiation. Much cell regulation in higher organisms is controlled by secreted polypeptide molecules called *growth factors* or *cytokines* or by antigen stimulation in immune cells. Our understanding of how these molecules interact with complementary receptors on the cell surface and modify intracellular biochemical signaling pathways has developed rapidly and provides new insights into the control of cellular responses, especially cell proliferation. This understanding will probably translate into effective patient care as new and specific anticancer therapeutic agents are designed.

Much of this information has derived from studies of tissue culture cells, which are dependent for their survival on the addition of serum or tissue extracts to their growth medium. Growth factors were first identified following their isolation from such a medium, with the subsequent demonstration that they could independently support cell growth. That malignant transformation might involve independence from the action of external growth factors was suggested by experiments on virally transformed cells: such cells displayed lower requirements for exogenous sources of growth factors than did normal cells. Growth factors include a large number of molecules, although surprisingly few have been associated with the process of malignant transformation (described in Sec. 6.7.2). Most growth factors bind to receptor proteins that have tyrosine kinase activity; but one, TGF-ß, which stimulates the proliferation of various mesenchymal cells and inhibits the proliferation of many epithelial cells, binds to a receptor that has serine/threonine kinase activity (Derynck, 1994). The characteristics of selected growth factors are summarized in Table 6.1.

While specific growth factor molecules (ligands) share the ability to stimulate receptor kinases, their structures are quite diverse. Most are small monomeric (i.e., single chain) polypeptides, such as the epidermal growth factor (EGF) and the members of the fibroblast growth factor (FGF) family. Dimeric polypeptides (i.e., those containing two chains of amino acids), such as platelet-derived growth factor (PDGF), also exist.

6.3 SIGNALING PATHWAYS TRIGGERED BY GROWTH FACTORS

6.3.1 Growth-Factor Receptors

Receptors for growth factors share the ability to phosphorylate cytoplasmic proteins on tyrosine residues, thereby activating a signaling cascade. These molecules, referred to as *receptor protein tyrosine kinases* (RPTKs), are transmembrane proteins, having a protruding growth factor–binding amino terminus several hundred amino acids in length (van der Geer et al., 1994). These extracellular domains are grouped by sequence homology, by the position of conserved cysteine amino acids, or by similarity to other signaling molecules such as the immunoglobulins. The extracellular domain is attached to a short single hydrophobic α helix transmembrane component, which, in turn, is attached

to the intracellular catalytic tyrosine kinase domain. This catalytic site is typically about 260 residues in length and is as much as 90 percent identical from molecule to molecule (Hanks and Quinn, 1989; Zhang et al., 1994). The degree of divergence and conservation of amino acid sequence within this general structure has allowed the subgrouping of over 50 tyrosine kinase receptors (van der Geer et al., 1994; Table 6.2; Fig. 6.1).

After binding of the growth factor ligand, a conformational alteration in the extracellular domain results in dimerization (i.e., joining together) of receptor tyrosine kinases (Kashles et al., 1991; Fig. 6.2). Some ligands, such as PDGF, are themselves dimeric forms of a single subunit and naturally induce a symmetric ligand/receptor dimer. Other ligands that exist as monomers, such as EGF, likely have two distinct receptor binding sites. Receptor dimerization brings together their two catalytic domains, which then phosphorylate each other (transphosphorylation), resulting in propagation of the signal. The importance of transphosphorylation to growth factor signaling is illustrated by experiments in which mutant growth-factor receptors that lack kinase activity are expressed in cells with their normal counterparts. Dimers of one catalytically competent receptor with the kinase-inactive mutant are unable to signal. The expression of the mutant thereby neutralizes the wild-type receptor (Ueno et al., 1991). Conversely, abnormal RPTKs that can dimerize in the absence of growth factor stimulation may be active in the absence of ligand. For example, the *HER2/neu* oncogene encodes an RPTK that has a mutation in its transmembrane region, which allows the association of multiple receptor proteins in the absence of ligand, generating continuous activation and inappropriate cellular signaling (Peles and Yarden, 1993; see Sec. 6.7.2). These observations suggest that receptor dimerization is the primary conformational change induced by ligand and is central to distal signaling events. This important principle helps explain how many oncogenic mutations induce abnormal cell division.

6.3.2 Binding of Receptors to Cytoplasmic Proteins

Signaling molecules at the cell surface, such as the RPTKs, communicate with cytoplasmic molecules that propagate the signal (Pawson, 1995). Multiple molecules, active in cell signaling, complex at the cell surface in association with each other and with

Table 6.1. Properties of Some Selected Polypeptide Growth Factors

Growth Factor	Description	Sources	Receptors
Platelet-derived growth factor	Dimers of A (17 kDa) and B (16 kDa) chains	Platelets, placenta, endothelial cells	Transmembrane tyrosine kinases α (170 kDa) and β (180 kDa)
Epidermal growth factor (EGF)	6 kDa, released by proteolysis of membrane bound precursors	Submaxillary gland, Brunner's gland	Transmembrane tyrosine kinase (175 kDa)
Transforming growth factor-α (TGF-α)	Similar to EGF	Embryos, placenta, transformed cells	Intracellular domain homologous with product of c-*erbB* proto-oncogene
Fibroblast growth factors:			
FGF1,2	"Acidic" and "basic" FGF, respectively; 16–17 kDa; 55% identical	Many normal and transformed cells and proteins associated with extracellular matrix	FGFR1 FGFR2
FGF3	Translation product of int-2 oncogene	Many embryonic and tumor tissues	
FGF4,5	19 kDa and 26 kDa, respectively; identified as dominant-acting oncogenes	Skeletal muscle	Unknown
FGF 6-9	Small polypeptides	Mesodermal tissue	FGFR2 (FGF 9) FGFR3 (FGF 9)
Transforming growth factor-β family			
TGF-β1 TGF-β2 TGF-β3 TGF-β4 TGF-β5	25-kDa homodimers, secreted in latent form	Widespread, embryonic and adult tissues	Three receptors: 60 kDa, 90 kDa, 250 kDa; specificity for TGF-β forms is unknown
Insulin-like growth factors			
IGF-1 IGF-2	7-kDa peptides	IGF-1: liver IGF-2: many cell types	IGF-1 receptor is a dimer (130 kDa and 90 kDa) protein tyrosine kinase; IGF-2 receptor is a distinct 250-kDa protein
Neurotrophins			
NGF BDNF HGF	Polypeptides Glycosylated heterodimer, disulfide	Many endocrine and immune tissues, stromal tissues	TRK A TRK B c-MET
GAS6	Globular (G) domain containing protein with EGF-like repeats		AXL Tse/Tyro3/SKY/RSE/BRT
LERK 1-7 ELK-L3 ELF-1 Many others	Glycosyl phosphatidyl inositol (GPI) linked or transmembrane members		EPH family members
Melatonin		Pineal gland	ROR family members

Table 6.2. Receptor Protein Tyrosine Kinases

Subfamily	Members
PDGFR	PDGFRα, PDGFRβ, SCF, c-KIT, CSF-1R, cFMS, FLK2, FLK3
FGFR	FGFR (1-4)
INSR	Insulin R, IGF-1R, ROS
EGFR	EGFR, c-erbB, Neu, HER2,
NGFR	NGFR, TRK(A-C)
HGFR	HGF, c-MET, c-SEA
EPH	EPH, HEK2, HEK11, EL, CEK (4-10), EEK
AXL	AXL, EYK, SKY, TIF
DDR	TKT, DDR, NEP, TRK E, CAK
TIE	TEK, TIE
ROR	ROR (1-2), RET

^aThe receptors are grouped by similarity of structure and catalytic sites. Members of each family likely evolved from a common precursor kinase.

the growth-factor receptor through specific binding sites. While this type of protein-protein interaction is not specific to growth factor signaling, it was first identified through the study of these pathways. It

appears to be conserved throughout evolution, defining molecules that are able to bind to one another. Although many binding modules have been defined, the *Src homology-2* (SH2), and *Src homology-3* (SH3) binding domains are representative and are discussed here (Pawson, 1994). Individual signaling molecules may contain various combinations of these and other domains, leading to a complex series of potential interactions.

The SH2 domains were first identified as regions of similarity of amino acid sequences found among the src family protein tyrosine kinases (*Src* is the mammalian homologue of the Rous sarcoma virus oncogene. The SH2 domains, which are critical mediators of the association of many molecules, lie outside the actual kinase site. They bind other signaling molecules specifically to phosphotyrosine, adjacent to specific flanking amino acids. X-ray crystallographic data of SH2 domains shows that bound phosphotyrosine is found in a depression lined by conserved basic residues that associate with both the negatively charged phosphate residue and the large aromatic ring of tyrosine (Fig. 6.3A; Marengere and Pawson, 1994). The amino acid that is three residues downstream of the phosphotyrosine interacts with a sepa-

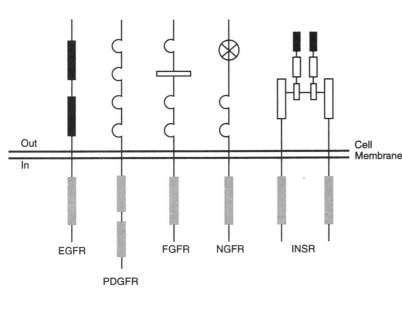

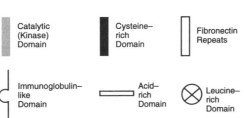

Figure 6.1. The receptor tyrosine kinases. Representative molecules from selected classes of receptor tyrosine kinases are shown. Each has a conserved intracellular kinase domain. Shared structural elements are found within the extracellular ligand-binding domains of each receptor. These include cysteine- or leucine-rich domains, sequences resembling the protein fibronectin, domains rich in acidic amino acids, or areas showing similarity to the immunoglobulins. Each of these extracellular domains has a specialized ligand-binding function. EGFR = epidermal growth-factor receptor; PDGFR = platelet-derived growth-factor receptor; FGFR = fibroblast growth-factor receptor; NGFR = nerve cell growth-factor receptor; INSR = insulin receptor.

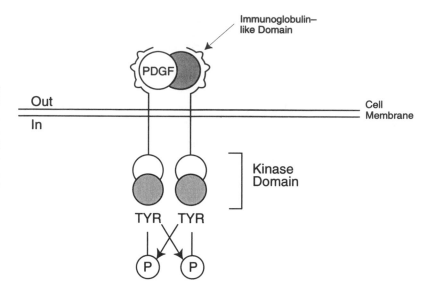

Figure 6.2. Functional significance of PDGF binding to its receptor. PDGF binds two receptor molecules, facilitating phosphorylation of their intracellular components. This allows recruitment of additional intracellular signaling molecules, which bind to phosphotyrosine, thus propagating the signal. TYR = tyrosine, P = phosphate.

rate pocket in many SH2 domains and provides binding specificity (Fig. 6.3*A*; Songyang et al., 1993). Binding of SH2-containing molecules to activated receptor tyrosine kinases facilitates their phosphorylation on tyrosine, resulting in alteration of their enzymatic activities and propagation of the signal (see Sec. 6.3.3). Binding may also result in conformational changes that are independent of phosphorylation yet may also lead to activation of the target molecule; this has been described for the SH2-containing phosphoinositol-3-kinase, where binding to RPTKs may increase its activity by as much as an order of magnitude (Shoelson et al., 1993). Finally, binding of SH2-containing proteins to RPTKs may serve to bring these proteins closer to

their own substrates, increasing the efficiency of signal propagation.

The SH3 domains are found in both signaling molecules and cytoskeletal structural proteins, providing a potential link between cell signals and alteration in cellular architecture. Sites on target molecules that bind to SH3 domains are defined by proline-rich segments containing the somewhat symmetrical consensus sequence X-P-p-X-P, where X is often a hydrophobic amino acid, P is proline necessary for binding affinity, and p also tends to be proline (Pawson, 1994). Each X-P unit fits into hydrophobic pockets formed by aromatic amino acid residues on SH3 domains (Musacchio et al., 1992; Fig. 6.3*B*). Specificity

Figure 6.3. *A*. Schematic diagram of the SH2 domain peptide binding site. A pocket of basic amino acids binds the phosphotyrosine of a ligand while a distinct pocket binding the third downstream amino acid residue provides relative specificity for individual peptides. *B*. Schematic diagram of the SH3 domain peptide-binding site. The SH3 peptide ligand is a seven-residue core forming a helix with the consensus X-P-p-X-P-X-X, (where X is a nonconserved amino acid, P is a proline, and p also tends to be proline). Each X-P forms a binding site for hydrophobic SH3 binding pockets. A third binding site stabilizes the interaction and is composed of variable residues.

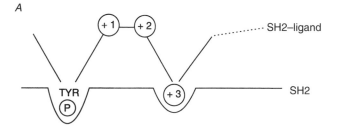

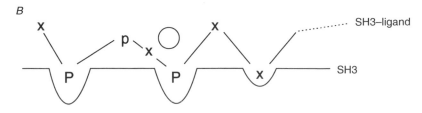

of particular ligands for individual SH3 domains is provided by two variable conserved loops surrounding the proline-rich binding region. Binding by other signaling molecules to either of these loops may affect the strength of association between SH3 domains and SH3 ligand–containing binding partners. Through these mechanisms, SH3 domains induce the formation of signaling complexes as part of an activated signaling pathway.

6.3.3 Receptor-Substrate Complexes: Propagation of the Signal

As described above, auto- or trans-phosphorylation of the receptor tyrosine kinases allows binding of SH2-containing cytoplasmic proteins. These cytoplasmic proteins are often enzymes, which include phospholipases, phosphatidylinositol-3-kinase, protein tyrosine phosphatases, and Src kinases (Fig. 6.4). These binding molecules may also be adaptor molecules without obvious catalytic activities but which provide links to signaling pathways. Targets also include structural proteins whose phosphorylation results in cytoskeletal modification that is associated with cellular activation. The properties of each of these types of target molecules are described below.

Phospholipases Turnover of membrane phospholipid results from the regulated activities of phospholipase C (PLC), phospholipase A2 (PLA2), and phospholipase D (PLD). PLA2 appears to mediate the generation of inflammatory prostaglandins and leukotrienes from membrane phospholipids (Axelrod et al., 1988), while PLC and PLD lead to activation of protein kinase C (PKC), which is a known mediator of cell proliferation and tumor growth, and is considered here in more detail.

All PLC isoforms hydrolyze phosphatidylinositol 4,5-diphosphate (PIP_2) to diacylglycerol (DAG) and inositol-1,4,5-triphosphate (ITP). Diacylglycerol, like tumor-promoting phorbol esters, activates protein kinase C, which induces cell proliferation and malignant transformation through mechanisms that remain to be elucidated, while inositol triphosphate increases cytoplasmic calcium. One isoform of PLC, PLC-γ, contains two SH2 domains, which interact directly with most activated RPTKs, and one SH3 domain that anchors this molecule to the cytoskeleton. After stimulation of the tyrosine kinase receptors (e.g., by binding to a growth factor), PLC-γ binds to them at specific phosphorylated tyrosine residues. It then becomes activated by phosphorylation on three

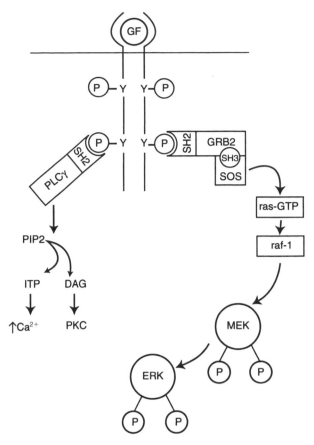

Figure 6.4. Cytoplasmic signaling molecules recruited by receptor protein tyrosine kinases. Binding of a receptor to its ligand (e.g., a growth factor) results in phosphorylation of the intracellular components on tyrosine (Y); this allows the SH2-mediated association of enzymes such as phospholipase C γ (PLC-γ). PLC-γ catalyses the lysis of phosphatidyl inositol (PIP2) into inositol triphosphate (ITP), which increases cytoplasmic calcium concentration and diacylglycerol (DAG), which activates the mitogenic protein kinase C (PKC). Linker molecules such as growth factor receptor binding protein 2 (GRB2) also bind activated growth factor receptor molecules via an SH2 linkage. Association of son-of-sevenless (SOS) to GRB2 occurs via an SH3 linkage. SOS then catalyzes the exchange of *ras*-GDP for *ras*-GTP, which then activates the serine/threonine kinase *raf*-1. *Raf*-1 phosphorylates and activates the dual specificity (serine/threonine and tyrosine) kinase MEK, which, in turn, phosphorylates and activates ERK on threonine and tyrosine. (For abbreviations, see legend to Fig. 6.6).

defined tyrosine residues, although the precise conformational change that produces enzymatic activation is unknown (Rottapel et al., 1991).

Phosphatidylinositol 3 (PI-3) Kinase The PI-3 kinase exists as a heterodimer of an 85-kDa regulatory subunit and a 110-kDa catalytic subunit that phosphorylates phosphatidylinositol, a membrane-derived phospholipid, on the inositol sugar ring. This enzyme is coupled to mitogenic signaling pathways and is necessary for transformation of animal cells by the polyoma middle T antigen and by a number of retroviral transforming oncogenes (Whitman et al., 1987; see Chap. 5, Sec. 5.3).

The 85-kDa regulatory subunit of PI-3 kinase contains an N-terminal SH3 domain and two SH2 domains. Binding of the regulatory subunit to the 110-kDa catalytic subunit occurs through the region found between the two SH2 domains (Klippel et al., 1993), while its binding to tyrosine-phosphorylated receptors occurs within the two SH2 domains (Songyang et al., 1993). Phosphorylation of the catalytic p110 subunit has not been described, suggesting that its activity may be regulated by p85 mediated-binding to the receptors (Hayashi et al., 1992). Despite the known association of PI-3 kinase activation with the appearance of 3′ phosphoinositides and mitogenesis, subsequent molecular events remain largely unknown.

Protein Tyrosine Phosphatases (PTP): Tyrosine phosphatases (which remove phosphate groups) in addition to tyrosine kinases (which add phosphate groups) have been recognized recently as mediators of cellular transformation. Since tyrosine phosphorylation of individual signaling molecules may result in either activation of a pathway or its repression, the influence of phosphatases or kinases may be difficult to predict (Fischer et al., 1992). Just as the tyrosine kinases contain structural similarities, the tyrosine phosphatases share sequence motifs that define regions catalyzing tyrosine dephosphorylation. Molecular techniques exploiting these areas of structural similarity have identified over 50 distinct tyrosine phosphatase genes. Although the signaling role of most tyrosine phosphatases has not yet been elucidated, several members have been identified that contain SH2 domains and have been implicated in mitogenic signaling pathways (Shen et al., 1991).

The protein tyrosine phosphatase SH-PTP1 (for Src homology 2–protein tyrosine phosphatase 1), which is expressed exclusively in hematopoietic cells, can bind to a variety of receptor tyrosine kinases through two SH2 domains and can dephosphorylate colony stimulating factor (CSF-1) and stem cell factor (SCF) receptors in vitro (Zhao et al., 1993). Mice with the "moth-eaten" mutation lack SH-PTP1 and demonstrate CSF-1 independent proliferation of macrophages as well as other developmental abnormalities. Other substrates of SH-PTP1 are unknown.

Another tyrosine phosphatase SH-PTP2 (for Src homology 2–protein tyrosine phosphatase 2) is expressed ubiquitously and associates via an amino-terminal SH2 domain with receptor protein tyrosine kinases including the PDGF and the EGF receptors, although it is unable to dephosphorylate them. This phosphatase itself becomes phosphorylated through these associations and mediates the binding of a linker sequence, GRB2, to the PDGF receptor (Li et al., 1994). This, in turn, may influence mitogenic signaling through the ras GTP-binding proteins, as described in Sec. 6.3.4.

Src Kinases   Nine structurally similar cytoplasmic tyrosine kinases containing SH2, SH3, and catalytic domains have been identified, many of which participate in the transmission of mitogenic signals from receptor kinases. *Src,* the mammalian homologue of the Rous sarcoma virus oncogene v-*src*, encodes the prototype of these kinases. It is through the comparison of member kinases that src homology domains were defined. These molecules are regulated through phosphorylation of a carboxy-terminal tyrosine. This residue inhibits enzymatic activity by internal binding to the amino-terminal SH2 domain, which imposes a conformational shift, causing inhibition of the catalytic site. For two Src family kinases, Src itself and leukocyte kinase (Lck), this carboxy-terminal phosphorylation is mediated by the cytoplasmic kinase Csk, which efficiently inhibits catalytic activity (Murphy et al., 1993). Src family kinases have been implicated in signaling through the T-cell antigen receptor, through numerous cytokines, and through growth factor receptor tyrosine kinases such as those for PDGF and CSF-1 (Twamley-Stein et al., 1993).

Adaptor Proteins   Increased activation of substrate molecules by enzymes involved in signaling may occur either through enhanced catalytic activity or through their improved association with substrates. Small oncogenic molecules containing only protein association modules have been identified that probably transform cells by effecting the association of activated signaling kinases and their substrates. These adaptor molecules commonly contain both SH2 and SH3 domains or, alternatively, just have sites of multiple tyrosine phosphorylation. Intermolecular associations are effected because enzyme and substrate each bind to either the SH2 and SH3 domains of linkers. Alternatively, SH2-containing enzymes and substrates may each bind to different sites of multiply tyrosine-phosphorylated linker molecules, as occurs on insulin-receptor substrate-1 (IRS-1) and IRS-2, which are linker substrates of the insulin receptor (White, 1994).

The GRB2 linker molecule contains two SH3 domains separated by one SH2 domain and links receptor tyrosine kinases directly with ras-mediated mitogenic signaling pathways. GRB2, through its SH2 domain, directly binds to tyrosine-phosphorylated receptors (Suen et al., 1993), to other linkers such as IRS–1 and, through the SH2 domains of the SH-PTP2 tyrosine phosphatase, to the PDGF receptor. Despite these associations, it does not itself become phosphorylated. While bound to a receptor kinase, GRB2 SH3 domains mediate binding to proline-rich sequences in the guanine nucleotide exchange factor son of sevenless (SOS) (see Fig. 6.4; Olivier et al., 1993). SOS, as described below, then catalyzes the exchange of guanosine diphosphate (GDP) bound to the ras protein for guanosine triphosphate (GTP), thus causing activation of the ras protein (see below). This illustrates the role of a linker molecule in inducing activation of a cytoplasmic cascade, although it has no catalytic activity itself. Linker molecules may induce transformation when overexpressed, as described below.

6.3.4   Activation of Ras Proteins

Abnormalities in ras proteins have been identified in many human malignancies. Three normal mammalian ras proteins—H-ras, K-ras, and N-ras—have been identified, which differ only at their carboxy termini (see also Chap. 5, Sec. 5.4.1). They have a molecular weight of 21 (hence the designation p21ras) and have few, if any, functional differences. The p21^{ras} protein cycles as a molecular binary switch between the GTP-bound "on" and the GDP-bound "off" configurations in response to extracellular signals (Fig. 6.5). The ras protein itself has intrinsic GTPase activity, which converts ras-bound GTP to GDP, causing its autoinactivation. This activity can be enhanced by a family of GTPase-activating proteins (GAPs), represented by p120^{GAP}, which may themselves be regulated by signaling cascades (Schlessinger, 1994). Balancing this are the effects of guanine nucleotide exchange proteins, such as SOS, described above, which can exchange free GTP for ras-bound GDP (Fig. 6.5). Several oncogenic mutations of ras have been identified that inhibit its intrinsic GTPase activity, trapping proportionately more in the activated GTP-bound state. Conversely, dominant inhibiting forms have been

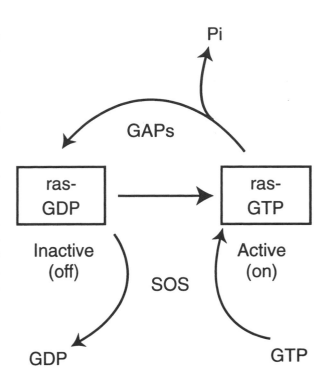

Figure 6.5. GDP-bound *ras* becomes active only when transformed into the GTP-bound state. This reflects a balance between the activities of guanine nucleotide exchangers, such as SOS (sons of sevenless), and the intrinsic GTPase activity of ras itself, which is enhanced by the GTPase activating proteins (GAPs).

developed that demonstrate enhanced ability to hydrolyze GTP (see Sec. 6.7). Constitutively active mutations of *ras* lead to cell transformation, while the dominant inhibiting forms can prevent experimental transformation by other oncogenes.

Considerable evidence links the ras protein to receptor tyrosine kinase signaling. Early experiments utilized the injection of neutralizing ras antibody into cells, which prevented growth factor–induced mitogenesis (Smith et al., 1986). Later studies involved the introduction of a dominant inhibiting mutant version of ras in which asparagine was substituted for tyrosine at amino acid position 12. Cells transfected with this dominant negative mutant of ras could not become stimulated after treatment with epidermal or neuronal growth factor (Hallek et al., 1992). In contrast, cells expressing the dominantly active mutant of ras, which contains valine at this critical residue, behave as if they were perpetually stimulated by growth factor (Burgering and Bos, 1995). A complex signaling web probably links tyrosine kinase receptors and this central growth regulating molecule.

Experiments described above suggest that activation of the ras protein is crucial for the transmission of mitogenic stimuli. Activated ras causes the activation of the raf-1 serine/threonine protein kinase, to which it physically binds (Vojtek et al., 1993). This association provides a critical link from activated growth factor receptors to distal activational pathways. Protein kinase C, which is activated through PLC-γ, as described in Sec. 6.3.3, can phosphorylate raf-1 (Kolch et al., 1993), and together with other kinases may participate in its activation (Fabian et al., 1993).

6.3.5 Mitogen-Activated Protein Kinase Signaling Pathways

A mutant form of the *raf*1 gene, which is truncated at its amino-terminal end, is constitutively active, presumably freed from negative regulators that would otherwise bind this region. This mutant, and the ras-stimulated naturally occurring form, causes the activation of a well-described signaling pathway leading to the activation of the *extracellular regulated kinases* (ERKs), which are members of the *mitogen-activated protein kinase* (MAPK) family (Howe et al., 1992; Fig. 6.6). Multiple forms of the ERK protein have been isolated. These forms are thought to be functionally redundant and are considered together. ERK kinase activation appears to be part of the final common pathway used by diverse proliferative stimuli; this is accomplished through the sequential activation of linked serine/threonine kinases, which are described below.

Raf-1 directly activates a family of closely related ERK kinase isoforms, referred to as the *MAPK or ERK kinases* (MEK; Kyriakis et al., 1992). MEK activation is induced by phosphorylation on serine residues (Alessi et al., 1994), which enhances the availability of the catalytic site to potential substrates. Other sites of regulatory phosphorylation may exist on MEK, although their physiologic role remains under investigation. Activated MEK is rare among known protein kinases in being able to phosphorylate both tyrosine and serine/threonine residues (Seger and Krebs, 1995). It is one of the only kinases identified thus far where this ability is important for the efficient activation of a target molecule, in this case the ERK kinases.

MEK-induced phosphorylation of ERK occurs on threonine and tyrosine at the TEY [single-letter amino acid abbreviation for threonine (T), glutamic acid (E), tyrosine (Y)] motif, which induces both catalytic activation of ERK and its translocation to the nucleus. Nuclear ERK regulates transcription, thereby completing the transmission of the signal from the cytoplasmic membrane to DNA in the nuclei of cells.

Figure 6.6. Three parallel signaling pathways. The mammalian "MAPK" signaling pathways involve structurally related molecules derived through evolution from common precursors. The outcome of stimulation of each is quite different: ERK stimulation causes cell division, while SAPK and p38^HOG stimulation results in growth arrest. MAPK = mitogen activated protein kinase; MKK = MAPK kinase; MAPKKK = MAPKK kinase, TF = transcription factors; HSPs = heat-shock proteins, ERK = extracellular stimulus regulated kinase, SAPK = stress-activated protein kinase; p38^HOG = the mammalian equivalent of the yeast hyperosmolarity glycerol gene; SEK is inappropriately named as SAPK and ERK kinase; MEKK is inappropriately named as MEK kinase; MEK = MAPK or ERK kinase.

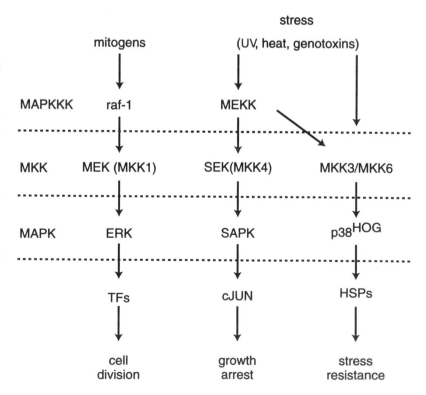

ERK kinases recognize proline-containing sequences that target them to their substrates. The most stringent consensus sequence for substrate recognition is PL(S or T)P, where P is proline, L is leucine, S is serine, and T is threonine, although there are known targets without this consensus motif (Alzarez et al., 1991). Numerous ERK targets, which are often regulatory molecules, are found in both the cytoplasm and the nucleus. They include many transcription factors (i.e., molecules that bind to DNA and influence the transcription of genes; see Sec. 6.3.6). In vitro targets for activated ERKs also include proteins that initiate or propagate signals leading to their own activation, including the neuronal growth factor receptor, the epidermal growth factor (EGF) receptor, SH-PTP2, SOS, raf-1, and MEK. The physiologic significance of this potential positive feedback loop remains to be demonstrated. Activated ERKs may also target cytoskeletal proteins (Minshull et al., 1994). With such a broad range of potential targets, the ERKs could coordinate a complex act such as regulation of cell-cycle progression (see Chap. 7, Sec. 7.2). Such a commanding role would demand the ability to integrate DNA replication, cell morphology, cell adhesion, and nuclear membrane disruption and would explain the prominent role of ERK activators in malignant transformation (see Sec. 6.7).

6.3.6 Activation of Transcription Factors

Activation of mitogenic signaling pathways leads to transcription of new genes that coordinate cell growth. Transcription of genes is catalyzed by the enzyme RNA polymerase II and other supporting molecules collectively termed *transcription factors.* Transcription factors influence the regulation of genes by binding to specific DNA recognition sequences, typically 6 to 8 base pairs in length, found in the promoter regions at the start of genes. The formation of RNA transcripts is influenced by the interaction of these gene-specific factors with elements of a common core of molecules regulating the activity of RNA polymerase II. The activity of transcription factors can be modified, most often by phosphorylation, through the activity of many of the signaling pathways described previously. They may also be enhanced through interaction with small molecules (e.g., steroid hormones) (see Chap. 12, Sec. 12.2.5). Mutation of transcription factors, which may cause unregulated activation and expression of genes, can lead to transformation and has been implicated in human cancers (Cleary, 1992; see Sec. 6.7.4). Based on the structure of their DNA-

binding domains, transcription factors can be placed into helix-turn-helix (HTH), helix-loop-helix (HLH), zinc-finger, or leucine-zipper groupings (Papavassiliou, 1995; Fig. 6.7).

The HTH transcription factors are made up structurally of three α helices. Two helices mediate interaction with signaling molecules or other transcription elements, while the third interacts with specific sequences in target DNA. HLH transcription factors, such as the product of the c-*myc* proto-oncogene, contain two α helices separated by a short DNA-binding peptide loop and become activated after heterodimerization. Both structural classes often regulate genes that control development in humans.

Zinc-finger transcription factors contain a sequence of 20 to 30 amino acids having two paired cysteine or histidine residues that are coordinated by a zinc ion. The sequence between the paired cysteines protrudes as a finger, giving these transcription factors their name (Fig. 6.7). DNA-binding specificity is provided by the sequence at the base of the loop. Members of this group of transcription factors mediate differentiation and growth signals, including those due to binding of steroid hormones to receptors; they have been implicated in malignancy (see Sec. 6.7.4).

Leucine-zipper transcription factors contain helical regions with leucine residues occurring at every seventh amino acid, which all protrude from the same side of the α-helix. These leucines interact hydrophobically with leucines of similar proteins in an antiparallel fashion. These factors, which exist as homo- or heterodimers, include the fos/jun pair (called the AP1 transcription factor), which becomes activated by cellular stress, as described in Sec. 6.4.1. Members of this group also tend to become activated by proliferative and developmental stimuli.

6.3.7 Function of Growth Factor–Stimulated Signaling Pathways

Cell Proliferation There is correlative evidence that agents causing cellular proliferation also lead to activation of the signaling pathways described above. The most convincing evidence linking the ERK activational cascade to growth factors and cell division has come from mutational studies. Inhibition of *raf*-1 by antisense oligonucleotides (see Chap. 3, Sec. 3.3.11) interferes with proliferation of NIH-3T3 cells, while constitutively activated *raf*-1 enhances proliferation (Miltenberger et al., 1993). Overex-

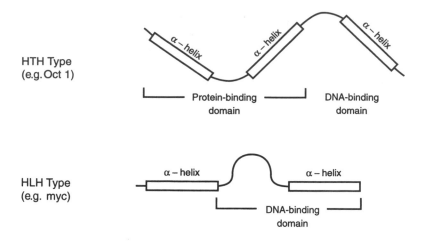

HTH Type
(e.g. Oct 1)

HLH Type
(e.g. myc)

Figure 6.7. The transcription factors. The general structure of each of the major classes of transcription factors is shown. Each structure is illustrated with an example (indicated in brackets). HTH = helix-turn-helix; HLH = helix-loop-helix.

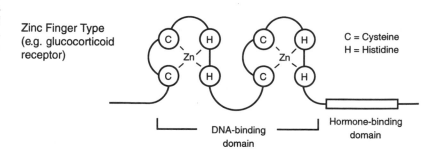

Zinc Finger Type
(e.g. glucocorticoid receptor)

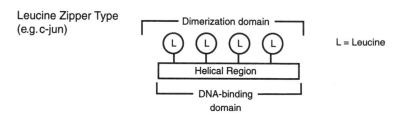

Leucine Zipper Type
(e.g. c-jun)

pression of nonactivatable forms of *MEK* and dominant negative mutations of *ERK* in NIH-3T3 cells reduces the rate of proliferation, while activated forms of *MEK* accelerate cell growth (Pages et al., 1993). Not all cell proliferation, however, is associated with activation of ERK. For example, the cytokine interleukin 4 (IL-4) stimulates hematopoietic cell proliferation independent of ERK (Wang et al., 1992; see Sec. 6.5).

Malignant Transformation Activation of signaling pathways occurs normally in response to growth factor stimulation and occurs in a coordinated and controlled fashion. Through mutation, which liberates signaling molecules from regulation, or through

deletion of negative regulators, these pathways may be activated constitutively, resulting in an inappropriate, sustained growth signal. Overexpression or deletions in the EGF receptor and point mutations in *ras* are examples of naturally occurring mutations associated with human cancer (see Sec. 6.7).

Differentiation Growth factor stimulation with resulting activation of ERK protein kinases usually causes cell division, but in some cellular contexts the same signals result in cell differentiation with reduced growth potential. For example, ERK stimulation has been implicated in monocytic differentiation of prolymphocytes (Han et al., 1993), axonal differentiation of the primitive neuroectodermal cell line PC12 (Qui and Green, 1996), T-cell maturation (Alberola-Ila et al., 1995), and hematopoietic mast cell development (Tsai et al., 1993). Since proliferation and differentiation are opposite outcomes of growth factor stimulation, the use of an identical signaling pathway to control these two cell outcomes seems paradoxical. The duration and/or extent of ERK activation may in part determine the cellular outcome. PC-12 cells can be induced to proliferate by EGF, while stimulation with NGF causes their differentiation (Qui and Green, 1996). EGF stimulation of ERK is transient, whereas NGF-stimulated ERK activity is sustained, suggesting a basis for the differences observed after stimulation by these two agents (Traverse et al., 1992). Also, experimental augmentation of the number of EGF receptors on PC12 cells causes them to differentiate rather than divide after EGF stimulation (Traverse et al., 1994). Other unidentified signaling pathways, exclusively stimulated by one agent or the other, may also contribute to this difference.

6.4 STRESS-ACTIVATED SIGNALING PATHWAYS

6.4.1 Stress-Activated Protein Kinases

As described in Sec. 6.3, mitogenic extracellular signals such as growth factors trigger signaling pathways, which cause activation of the ERK protein kinases. Related pathways have been described that are stimulated by cellular stress rather than by mitogens (Fig. 6.6). These signaling pathways may coordinate attempts by a cell to repair damage caused by stress or may coordinate programmed cell death, or apoptosis, if damage is too extensive (see Chap. 7, Sec. 7.3). The pathways may have evolved from a common primitive signaling complex.

The environment of cells provides a variety of physical stresses such as extremes of heat, exposure to ultraviolet and ionizing radiation, and exposure to potentially damaging biologic agents such as the cytokines IL-1 and tumor necrosis factor α (TNF-α). Each of these stresses results in phosphorylation of two serine residues of c-jun, a component of the AP-1 transcription factor complex. These sites, serine 63 and 73, are found within a part of the c-jun molecule that influences its binding to other molecules involved in DNA transcription (known as a transactivating domain). This domain is deleted in the corresponding viral oncogene v-*jun* (Vogt and Bos, 1990), implying their importance in negative growth regulation. These serine residues are each adjacent to a proline, suggesting that the responsible kinases may bind to proline-containing sequences, as described for the mitogen-activated protein (MAP) kinases (Sec. 6.3.5; Davis, 1993). While the ERK family of MAP kinases activate c-jun poorly, a structurally related family of stress-activated protein kinases (SAPKs) binds to and phosphorylates c-jun on these two serine residues in response to cell stress (Fig. 6.8).

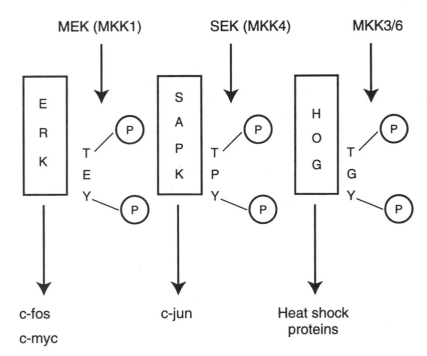

Figure 6.8. The MAPKs are activated by dual phosphorylation on threonine (T) and on tyrosine (Y). The primary sequence surrounding these sites of activation differs (E = glutamic acid, P = proline, G = glycine), producing, in each, unique conformations that can only be recognized by their activators. This feature "insulates" these three pathways. Once activated, ERK causes activation of specific mitogenic transcription factors such as c-fos and c-myc. Activation of SAPK results in the activation of the c-jun transcription factor, resulting in growth arrest or apoptosis. The targets of p38^{HOG} kinase cause the activation of low-molecular-weight heat-shock proteins, conferring resistance to heat-induced cell injury. (For abbreviations, see legend to Fig. 6.6.)

SAPK and ERK are components of parallel but different activation pathways, insulated from each other by virtue of highly specific intermolecular interactions (Fig. 6.8). A serine/threonine kinase called *SAPK and ERK kinase* (SEK), which is homologous to MEK (Sec. 6.3.5), phosphorylates SAPK in vivo; SEK, in turn, is activated through phosphorylation by the inappropriately named MEK kinase (MEKK), the functional homologue of the MEK activator raf (Davis, 1994; Yan et al., 1994; Fig. 6.6). MEKK, which was identified initially as a potential MEK kinase by in vitro experiments (hence its name), is actually a very poor phosphorylator of MEK and prefers SEK as a substrate under physiologic conditions. Since these structurally related pathways are controlled by stimuli having very different physiologic consequences (i.e., mitogenesis or the stress response) the pathways and effector molecules, although related through evolution, have become functionally distinct.

p38^{HOG} Signaling Lower eukaryotic cells such as the yeast *Saccharomyces cerevisiae* have additional MAPK structural homologues that control cellular response to diverse extracellular stimuli. One yeast homologue becomes activated after exposure to hyperosmolarity, participating in the generation of intracellular glycerol, which is protective (Brewster et al., 1993); it has been named high osmolarity glycerol (HOG). Through techniques based on molecular similarity, a mammalian homologue, $p38^{HOG}$, has been identified, which is most closely related to the SAPK family of enzymes (Han et al., 1994).

$p38^{HOG}$ is similar to the ERKs and to SAPKs, containing the characteristic amino acid motif TXY (where X is any amino acid), in this case TGY, at the site of activation (Raingeaud et al., 1995). The threonine and tyrosine residues, which are separated by glycine, become phosphorylated in response to a wide variety of stress stimuli including hyperosmolarity, heat shock, ultraviolet (UV) irradiation, oxidative stress, and inhibitors of protein synthesis. The TGY activation site appears to be characteristic for $p38^{HOG}$ and suggests a distinct signaling pathway, despite the similarity of agents that stimulate SAPK and $p38^{HOG}$ (Fig. 6.8). While SEK, the SAPK activator, can phosphorylate $p38^{HOG}$ in vitro, a related pair of mammalian serine/threonine kinases, MAP kinase kinase 3 (MKK3) and MAP kinase kinase 6 (MKK6), appear to activate $p38^{HOG}$ in vivo (Han et al, 1996; Figs. 6.6 and 6.8). Both MKK3 and MKK6 have structural similarity to SEK (also known as MKK4) and MEK (also known as MKK1), suggesting evolution from a common precursor molecule.

Both the SAPK and $p38^{HOG}$ kinase pathways are triggered by serine/threonine kinases, which are themselves activated by kinases associated with GTP-binding proteins. Family members of these GTP-binding proteins (known as rho) act in a similar way to the ras proteins described in Sec. 6.3.4. These proteins respond to stress, such as that induced by IL-1 and result in the ultimate activation of $p38^{HOG}$ and SAPK (Zhang et al., 1996). Dominant inhibiting forms of the rho family of GTP-binding proteins prevent IL-1–induced activation of both SAPK and $p38^{HOG}$, suggesting that this form of biologic stress mediates signals through this class of GTP-binding proteins.

6.4.2 Physiologic Consequences of SAPK/p38 Signaling

Activation of the ERK pathway occurs after extracellular growth-promoting stimuli result in mitogenesis; this helps to explain the transforming abilities of dominantly acting mutant members of this pathway. Conceptually, cell stress, which results in macromolecular damage, induces either the activation of repair mechanisms or cell death if the damage is too extensive. This binary outcome of stress reflects a balance between the requirements of an organism to preserve cell mass after minor stress and the need to eliminate critically damaged or mutated transformed cells after major insult.

The outcome of SAPK activation may be apoptosis. Cell lines have been identified that are constitutively resistant to the toxic effects of diverse stresses and coincidentally are resistant to SAPK activation (Zanke et al., 1996). This observation suggests that SAPK activation may cause cell death after some forms of stress. This hypothesis has been tested formally in several unrelated cell systems. Thermosensitive cells can be made resistant to the lethal effects of heat shock by inhibiting SAPK activation through the expression of a dominantly inhibiting mutant form of SEK. This mutant competes for SAPK binding with wild-type SEK, resulting in the complete biochemical inhibition of SAPK. Such cells are markedly resistant to the lethal consequences of a variety of cell stresses, including heat shock and many forms of chemotherapy. These observations indicate that the selection of cells that have deficient activation of SAPK might convey therapeutic resistance to multiple agents and is a possible cause of pleiotropic drug resistance (see Chap. 17, Sec. 17.2.8).

Inhibition of stress-activated protein kinases may also prevent apoptosis following withdrawal of growth factor. The primitive neuroepithelial cell line PC12 can be made to differentiate into axon-like cells in tissue culture by exposure to neuronal growth factor (NGF). Once differentiated, these cells die by apoptosis if NGF is withdrawn. Apoptotic cell death can be prevented by inhibition of either SAPK or p38^{HOG} through the expression of dominantly inhibiting forms of SEK or dominant negative inhibitors of the p38^{HOG} activator MKK3 (Xia et al., 1995). These data suggest that death after the withdrawal of trophic influences occurs not simply by silencing of ERK activated effector molecules but is an active process, coordinated by the stimulation of these related stress-stimulated signaling pathways.

Activation of p38^{HOG} does not always result in cell death. Cells of the monocytic lineage stimulate p38^{HOG} after exposure to lipopolysaccharide (LPS), a bacterial cell wall component critical for the development of septic shock, through the secretion of inflammatory cytokines such as tumor necrosis factor (TNF). Pyridinyl-imidazole compounds have been discovered that prevent the elaboration of inflammatory cytokines from LPS-stimulated cultured monocytes (Lee et al., 1994). These molecules, termed *cytokine suppressive anti-inflammatory drugs* (CSAIDS), bind to p38^{HOG} and prevent its activation. In this context, p38^{HOG} seems to be functioning as a mediator of cytokine synthesis and release, which can be pharmacologically inhibited by these drugs. Other data suggest that p38^{HOG} may result in the activation of low-molecular-weight heat-shock proteins and can confer cell resistance to heat-induced cell death. These data imply that activation of p38^{HOG}, unlike activation of SAPK, may in some cells ameliorate the toxic effects of cellular stress.

6.4.3 Inter-Pathway Control of Signaling

Since activation of the three known mammalian MAPK signaling pathways (ERK, SAPK, and p38^{HOG}; see Fig. 6.6) results in differing cellular outcomes, mechanisms for controlling the relative activities of each pathway within a single cell are necessary. Some measure of control is inherent in that different extracellular factors activate each pathway. Mitogenic effectors such as growth factors are generally poor activators of SAPK and p38^{HOG}, while stressful stimuli such as cytotoxic drugs, inhibitors of protein synthesis, and toxic physical stimuli do not stimulate the ERKs. Additional mechanisms of control have evolved, as exemplified by the ability of activated SAPK to inhibit ERK kinase activity in cells. This inhibition is accomplished through increased translation of a protein phosphatase, MAP kinase phosphatase-1 (MKP-1), which is capable of specifically removing phosphate from both the threonine and tyrosine found in the activating loop of the ERKs (Keyse and Ginsburg, 1993; Emslie et al., 1994).

The phosphatase MKP-1 turns off mitogenic signaling pathways that are stimulated by growth factors through the inhibition of ERK (Bokemeyer et al., 1996). This mechanism of control allows coordination of the cellular response to mixed stimuli. Although not yet identified, it is probable that activated ERKs are able to inhibit SAPK and p38^{HOG} pathways, thus allowing reciprocal modulation of mitogenic and stress stimuli. In this way relative activities of these pathways can be coordinated, resulting in an inhibition of ERK-induced cell division while SAPK-induced cell death or p38^{HOG}-mediated repair may occur. Such coordination is important to prevent the replication of mutated DNA, which would result in enhanced malignant transformation after mutagenic exposures.

6.5 SIGNALING THROUGH CYTOKINE RECEPTORS

Stimulation of cell proliferation or differentiation may be transmitted through receptors that do not appear to be enzymes but which stimulate phosphorylation of tyrosine in cytoplasmic proteins. These receptors, collectively called the *cytokine-receptor superfamily*, mediate hematopoietic, neural, and embryonal development by interleukins, interferons, and colony-stimulating factors. Malignant transformation through cytokine deregulation has not been reported. Cytokines are used clinically, both therapeutically and as agents of supportive care (see Chap. 7, Sec. 7.5.1, and Chap. 18, Sec. 18.3.1).

6.5.1 Structure of Cytokine Receptors

Cytokine receptors have been identified that transmit intracellular signals after binding to their ligand (Taniguchi, 1995). While receptors for G-CSF and erythropoietin are single chains, most cytokine receptors exist as multisubunit structures. These receptors contain unique extracellular ligand-binding segments coupled to intracellular components that are linked to signaling pathways. Many cytokine receptors share intracellular components and are presumably linked to the same signal transducing pathways.

The functional redundancy seen in the effects of different cytokines is probably explained by the common use of intracellular signaling components. Four distinct signaling molecules have been identified that are used by most multisubunit cytokine receptors (Fig. 6.9). The gp130 molecule (IL-6Rβc, where "c" denotes that these chains are common to other cytokine receptors) is shared by the receptors for IL-6, ciliary neurotrophic factor (CNTF), leukemia inhibitory factor (LIF), oncostatin M (OM), and IL-11 (Miyajima et al., 1992). These cytokines have overlapping effects on cells that have these receptors. Similarly, the response to IL-3, IL-5, and granulocyte-macrophage colony stimulating factor (GM-CSF) overlaps in various hematopoietic cells, which is explained by the common use of the IL-3Rβc signal-transducing chain (also known as the KH97 chain) in the receptors for these cytokines (Miyajima et al., 1992). The IL-2 receptor is composed of three subunits: the α, β, and γ chains, formally designated as IL-2Rα, IL-2Rβc and IL-2Rγc (Davies and Wlodawer, 1995). The β subunit is used by the IL-15 receptor, while the γ subunit is used as part of the receptors for IL-4, IL-7, and IL-9 (Kondo et al., 1993; Giri et al., 1994; Fig. 6.9).

6.5.2 Cytokine-Induced Signaling Pathways

Although the common cytokine receptor chains do not have intrinsic tyrosine kinase activity, they associate with specific cytoplasmic Janus family tyrosine kinases (JAKs, for janus kinase or "just another kinase") (Darnell et al., 1994). These SH2-containing proteins have two tandem kinase-like domains and thus were named for the Roman god with two faces. Binding of JAKs to cytokine receptor subunits occurs in a sequence-specific manner and is dependent on a short conserved juxtamembrane region. Some receptors such as the erythropoietin receptor bind only one type of JAK (Witthuhn, 1993), while others, such as the gp130 molecule, may bind as many as three distinct JAK subtypes (Lutticken et al., 1994). Other tyrosine kinases, such as src family members, associate with some receptor subunits at the C-terminal tail of the IL-2βc chain and to the gp130 chain distal to the JAK binding sites. These kinases probably transmit a distinct second signal after cytokine binding, thereby recruiting additional signaling pathways (Minami et al., 1995).

In common with signaling initiated by ligands of protein tyrosine kinase receptors, cytokines induce dimerization of receptor components as one step to-

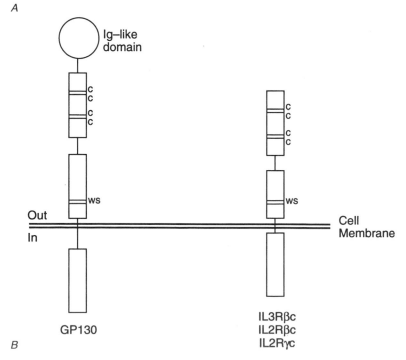

Cytokine Receptor Chains

GP130	IL3Rβc	IL2Rβc	IL2Rγc
Component of receptors for:			
IL6	IL3	IL2	IL4
CNTF	IL5	IL15	IL7
LIF	GM–CSF		IL9
OM			IL13
IL11			

A

Figure 6.9. *A.* Common cytokine receptor chains. Four receptor chains are shared among many cytokine receptors. This commonality partially explains the similar effects seen after ligand binding. These common chains function as connectors to cytoplasmic signaling cascades rather than as ligand binders. CNTF = ciliary neurotropic factor; LIF = leukemia inhibitory factor; OM = oncostatin M; GM-CSF = granulocyte-macrophage colony-stimulating factor. *B.* While the structures of these common chains are similar, the GP 130 molecule contains an additional proximal immunoglobulin-like domain. Both types of shared receptors contain cysteine-rich domains and "WS" motifs (WSXWS: W is tryptophan, S is serine, and X is a nonconserved residue), which are thought to function as a ligand interaction site.

B

ward the initiation of cytoplasmic signaling pathways. The single subunit receptors for G-CSF and erythropoietin accomplish this by forming homodimers that bring two receptors together. Dimerization-induced tyrosine phosphorylation of each binding partner then occurs, an event mediated by activated JAK- or src-family kinases. This critical step generates binding sites for SH2-containing signaling proteins, resulting in signal propagation (Hatakeyama et al., 1991; Schieven et al., 1992). One group of SH2-proteins that associates with activated cytokine receptors is the STAT (signal transducers and activators of transcription) family of transcription factors. Remarkably, stimulation of specific cytokine receptors results in the specific activation of individual STAT molecules. This occurs by the interaction of STAT SH2 domains with phosphotyrosine residues found in a particular

sequence on individual cytokine receptor molecules (Taniguchi, 1995; Fig. 6.10A and B).

STATs were first identified as specific mammalian transcription factors that mediated interferon-regulated gene expression, but they have since been implicated in several cytokine signaling pathways. Many STAT proteins have been identified and the genes encoding them co-localize to three chromosomal locations. This suggests duplication of an ancestral gene, a process necessary to permit the complex signaling patterns seen in higher mammals (Ihle and Kerr, 1995). Stimulation of various cytokine receptors results in an overlapping pattern of STAT activation (Fig. 6.10C). This further explains the similarity of cellular responses to individual cytokines. STATs share conserved functional domains: all have phosphotyrosine-binding SH2 domains and

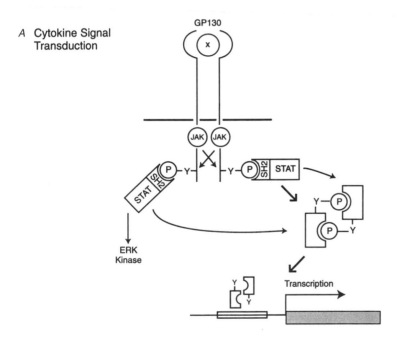

A **Cytokine Signal Transduction**

ERK Kinase

Transcription

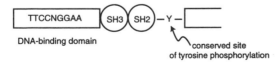

B **STAT Structure**

TTCCNGGAA — SH3 SH2 — Y —

DNA-binding domain

conserved site of tyrosine phosphorylation

C **Binding of receptors to STATs**

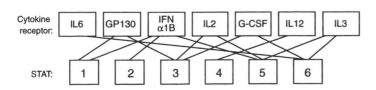

Cytokine receptor: IL6 | GP130 | IFN α1B | IL2 | G-CSF | IL12 | IL3

STAT: 1 | 2 | 3 | 4 | 5 | 6

Figure 6.10. Cytokine signal transduction. *A.* Ligands induce dimerization of specific receptor chains, resulting in receptor transphosphorylation through the action of the JAK kinases. Receptor phosphotyrosine attracts signaling molecules such as the STAT molecules through SH2 domains. STATs also become phosphorylated on tyrosine, dissociating from the receptor by autodimerization, and travel to the nucleus where they activate transcription. *B.* General structure of the STATs. A conserved DNA binding domain induces transcription of target genes. SH3 and SH2 domains mediate binding of molecules involved in specific signaling pathways. The conserved tyrosine (Y), when phosphorylated, also mediates intermolecular binding. *C.* Cytokine receptors utilize multiple STAT molecules that are not exclusive to particular receptors. This partially explains the similarity of cellular response after stimulation of different cytokines.

conserved sites of tyrosine phosphorylation, which allows homo- or heterodimerization after activation of the cytokine receptor complex. Binding of STATs to DNA occurs through a conserved amino terminal domain that is specific to these molecules, which recognizes specific sequences found in the promoter regions of cytokine-stimulated genes (Kishimoto et al., 1994; Schindler, 1995).

Although the sequence of JAK activation followed by STAT phosphorylation after ligation of cytokines to their receptors has been well defined, stimulation of cytokine receptors may also activate ERK kinases in a signaling pathway that involves the ras protein. Phosphorylation of cytokine receptors, such as that for erythropoietin, introduces SH2 binding sites for linker molecules of the ras signaling pathway (see Sec. 6.3.4). Moreover, a number of cytokines induce the phosphorylation of the p85 subunit of phosphatidylinositol-3 kinase, thus linking cytokine and lipid kinase signaling pathways (Ihle and Kerr, 1995). These observations suggest that stimulation of cytokine receptors can induce diverse cell-signaling pathways, which are presumably necessary to produce an optimal cellular response. Activation of STATs may also occur after stimulation through receptors other than those of the cytokine superfamily. STAT1 and STAT3 can be activated by the epidermal growth factor (EGF) receptor in vivo and are directly phosphorylated by this receptor tyrosine kinase in vitro. CSF-1 and the PDGF receptors may also phosphorylate STATs suggesting that some overlap occurs between growth-factor- and cytokine-mediated signaling pathways (Kishimoto et al., 1994).

6.6 SIGNALING THROUGH ANTIGEN RECEPTORS

Unlike cell stimulation by growth factors or cytokines, signaling through cell-surface antigen receptors occurs after interaction with one of a huge number of potential stimulants. B and T lymphocytes, which are stimulated by foreign antigens, utilize signaling pathways that share characteristics with those described previously (see also Chap. 11, Sec. 11.3.5). The process of antigen-driven proliferation of lymphocytes can be subverted during malignant transformation through mutation of signaling components or through overexpression of signaling proteins, which results in constitutive activation of the signaling pathways.

6.6.1 Lymphocyte Antigen Receptors

Antigen recognition by T cells is provided by the T-cell receptor, which has two subunits, the α and β

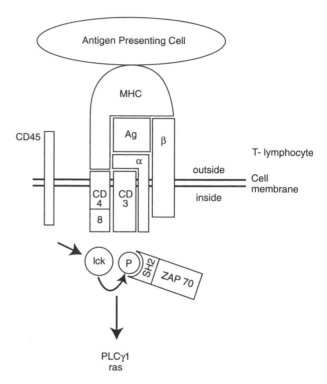

Figure 6.11. The T-cell receptor signaling complex. Antigen bound to major histocompatibility complex (MHC) molecules on antigen-presenting cells is recognized by the T-cell receptor (TCR) of T lymphocytes. The α and β chains of the TCR recognize antigen and CD4 or CD8, which is bound to MHC molecules of class 2 or 1, respectively. The protein tyrosine kinase lck, which is bound to the tail of the CD4 or CD8 molecules, is activated by the protein tyrosine phosphatase CD45 and then phosphorylates the zeta chain of the CD3 molecule (shown here as a single chain for simplicity). This allows binding of the SH2 containing 70-kDa, zeta-associated protein kinase (ZAP 70). ZAP 70 is connected to downstream signaling cascades.

chains, that are structurally similar to the antigen-binding immunoglobulin molecules found in B lymphocytes (Fig. 6.11; see also Chap. 11, Sec. 11.3.4). As a rule, all of these antigen-binding molecules have very short cytoplasmic portions and are coupled to cytoplasmic signaling pathways through the multisubunit CD3 and CD4 or CD8 molecules in T cells and through heterodimers of the immunoglobulin α and β chains in B cells. These components of the T- and B-cell receptors are coupled to intracellular kinase signaling cascades through conserved motifs consisting of paired tyrosines (Y) and leucines (L) having the consensus sequence $(D/E)XXYXXL(X)_{6-8}YXXL$ (where D is aspartic acid, E is glutamic acid, Y is tyrosine, L is leucine, and X is any amino acid), termed the *antigen recognition activation motif* (ARAM) (Romeo et al., 1992). ARAM sequences are phosphorylated on tyrosine by cytoplasmic kinases and become bound by SH2 containing cytoplasmic signaling molecules.

T lymphocytes will not respond to antigens except in association with molecules of the major histocompatability complex (MHC; see Chap. 11, Sec. 11.3.2); molecules which are recognized by CD8 or CD4 on the surface of T lymphocytes (Cammarota et al., 1992; Konig et al., 1992). The src family protein tyrosine kinase, known as lck, associates with the cytoplasmic tail of these accessory molecules through N-terminal glycine residues. It couples to cytoplasmic signaling pathways by providing its own SH2 domain as a binding site for tyrosine phosphorylated signaling molecules (Rudd, 1990; Veillette et al, 1991). In addition, Lck, when activated, phosphorylates tyrosine residues on the ARAM sequences of CD3, allowing the binding of an additional kinase with an SH2 domain, p70 zeta-associated protein kinase (ZAP-70; Chan et al., 1992). ZAP-70 becomes activated upon association with CD3 either through its phosphorylation by src kinases or through allosteric structural changes induced by this binding with CD3. A ZAP-70 homologue becomes activated in a similar way after stimulation of B lymphocytes and associates with the invariant chains of antigen receptors of B cells through SH2/ARAM mediated binding (Taniguchi et al., 1991). The molecules CD19, and possibly CD21, may act in B lymphocytes as the functional equivalents of the T-cell accessory molecules CD4 and CD8, binding src family kinases and mediating phosphorylation of a ZAP-70 homologue (Law et al., 1993).

A central role in lymphocyte signal transduction is played by the transmembrane protein tyrosine phosphatase CD45. Phosphatases can be expected to counter the effects of protein tyrosine kinases if they both act on the same tyrosine. Alternatively, phosphatases that target inhibitory phosphotyrosine residues on kinases may increase the activities of these kinases (Cooper et al., 1986). Mice lacking CD45, generated by gene-targeted disruption (see Chap. 3, Sec. 3.3.11), show impaired responses following antigenic stimulation of T and B cells (Kishihara et al., 1993). This is probably related to impaired activation of critical src kinases, which require removal of inhibitory carboxy-terminal phosphotyrosine residues by the CD45 phosphatase (Sieh et al., 1993).

6.6.2 Cytoplasmic Signaling

Ligation of antigens to their receptors on T and B cells activates the signaling complex described above and leads to the activation of phospholipase C γ-1 through phosphorylation of tyrosine. This leads, in turn, to the generation of inositol-triphosphate and diacylglycerol as described in Sec. 6.3.3 (Secrist et al., 1991; Weiss 1991). Activation of inositol-triphosphate results in a rapid and sustained elevation in cytoplasmic calcium due to liberation from intracellular stores. Enhanced cytoplasmic calcium increases the activity of the serine phosphatase known as calcinurin and leads to activation of transcription factors that regulate expression of cytokine genes (Liu et al., 1993). The immunosuppressive drugs cyclosporin A and FK506 inhibit calcinurin function and hence this calcium-dependent part of T-lymphocyte signaling (Clipstone and Crabtree, 1992).

Stimulation of both T and B lymphocytes also leads to the rapid activation of $p21^{ras}$ (Downward et al., 1992), possibly through the inhibition of ras-GTPase activating protein and activation of guanine nucleotide exchange activities (see Sec. 6.3.4). As is seen with growth factor stimulation, ras activation is coupled to sequential activation of raf-1 and ERK protein kinases and leads to regulation of gene transcription (Nel et al., 1990). As is detailed in Sec. 11.3.5, optimal T-cell signaling depends both on TCR stimulation and on a "second signal." This second signal, provided by ligation of the CD28 surface molecule, results in lymphocyte secretion of IL-2. The molecular interaction of TCR and second signal pathways remains unknown.

Although human hematopoietic malignancies that are caused by disruption of these lymphocyte signaling molecules have not yet been identified, overexpression in experimental settings results in clonal proliferation of cells. Future studies of human lymphoma or myeloma could identify abnormalities of these molecules and suggest specific molecular therapeutic strategies.

6.7 SIGNAL TRANSDUCTION IN CANCER

Signal transducing molecules form a biochemical network through which extracellular information results in changes to gene expression, DNA synthesis, cytoskeletal architecture, and cellular metabolism. Structural alteration or overexpression of these proteins can induce the constitutive activation of intracellular biochemical pathways that stimulate cell proliferation in the absence of a bona fide signal and thereby lead to malignant transformation. Hence, a cell carrying an activated oncogene is no longer dependent on factors produced by other cells for its own growth. Genes that encode normal signaling components homologous to oncogenes have been termed *proto-oncogenes* in recognition of their potential to become mediators of oncogenesis when dysregulated.

Although numerous growth-mediating signal transducers have been described in this chapter, in few cases have they been linked to cancer in humans or animals. Indeed, for most types of human cancer the genetic basis of unregulated growth is yet to be elucidated. Some molecular abnormalities have been identified and serve as markers of disease; in the future, they may form the basis for rationally designed specific therapies. These abnormalities are described in the organizational context of growth factor–and cytokine-mediated signaling pathways (Table 6.3).

6.7.1 Abnormalities of Extracellular Signaling Molecules

Platelet-derived growth factor (PDGF) appears to function as a normal regulator of connective tissue growth (Westermark et al., 1989) and exists as a dimer of two polypeptide chains, A and B. All combinations of subchains (AA, AB, BB) have been identified and bind to PDGF receptors. The product of the *sis* oncogene, identified originally as the transforming oncogene of simian sarcoma virus (SSV), is homologous to the PDGF receptor β-chain (Waterfield et al., 1983). Studies of SSV-transformed monkey cells suggest that overexpression of *sis* is involved in their malignant transformation, since (1) the transformed cells produce a growth factor that interacts with PDGF receptors, (2) only cell types that express PDGF receptors are transformed by the SSV, and (3) transformation is inhibited by anti-PDGF antibodies (Westermark et al., 1989). Cellular transformation cannot be achieved in the absence of virus just by supplying large amounts of exogenous PDGF, suggesting that additional SSV-mediated events are necessary for malignant transformation.

Table 6.3. Signaling Molecule Abnormalities in Cancer

Molecule	Abnormality	Cancer Type	Organism
PDGF	Overexpression (sis)	Sarcoma	Monkey
VEGF	Overexpression	? Kaposi's sarcoma	Human
FGF	Overexpression	Mammary cancer	Mouse
Neu	Gene amplification or mutation-causing dimerization	Breast Neuroblastoma	Human Rat
RET	Mutation	MEN 1 or MEN 2	Human
KIT	Overexpression	? Leukemia	Human
FMS	Mutation	? Leukemia	Human
FLT-3	Overexpression	? Leukemia	Human
ALK	Translocation-induced overexpression	Lymphoma	Human
Ras	Mutation	Lymphoma Leukemia Oral cancer Pancreas	Human
bcr/abl	Fusion protein by chromosomal translocation	Chronic myelogenous leukemia	Human
PBX-1/E2A	Fusion protein by chromosomal translocation	Leukemia	Human
Myc	Fusion protein by chromosomal translocation; amplification	Burkitt's lymphoma; neuroblastoma	Human
RARα	Fusion protein making dominant inhibitor	Acute promyelocytic leukemia	Human
WT1	Inactivation	Wilm's tumor	Human

Cell lines derived from several types of human tumors produce PDGF. Best characterized are cell lines derived from human brain tumors (gliomas), where there is often both secretion of PDGF-like molecules and expression of PDGF receptors. Autocrine stimulation of these cell lines by PDGF has been demonstrated in vitro and may play a role in the growth of human brain tumors (Hammacher et al., 1988; Nister et al., 1991).

Vascular endothelial growth factor (VEGF) is a specific mitogen for vascular endothelial cells and is structurally related to PDGF. VEGF expression is important for tumor angiogenesis (Chap. 9, Sec. 9.3.2), a process necessary for the growth of solid tumors (Folkman, 1990). Neutralizing antibodies to VEGF inhibit vascularization and the growth of VEGF-producing tumors such as glioblastomas (Kim et al., 1993). A possible direct role for VEGF as a mitogen for malignant cells has been proposed in the growth of Kaposi's sarcoma, a vascular tumor associated with the acquired immunodeficiency syndrome (AIDS). These cells respond to VEGF, which might act, in this special case, as a conventional growth factor (Weindel et al., 1992).

Members of the *fibroblast growth factor (FGF)* gene family have been identified through their involvement in malignant transformation. The *INT-2* gene was identified as a frequent site of viral integration during mouse mammary tumor virus carcinogenesis. The *INT-2* gene encodes an FGF-related peptide. Two other FGF-related peptides have been identified as oncogenes by their ability to transform NIH/3T3 cells in transfection experiments (see Chap. 5, Sec. 5.4.1). FGF isoforms have been isolated from human gastric carcinoma, Kaposi's sarcoma, and others (Burgess and Maciag, 1989). The FGF family may be involved in cell transformation in a similar manner to the v-*sis* (PDGF B chain) oncogene by activating a receptor tyrosine kinase through an autocrine mechanism.

6.7.2 Abnormalities of Growth Factor Receptors

The Epidermal Growth Factor Receptor (EGFR) Several viral and cellular oncogenes encode aberrant growth factor receptors that are not dependent on ligand for activation. The structure of these naturally occurring mutants has provided insight into normal receptor function and regulation. Molecular cloning and characterization of the human homologue of the avian erythroblastosis virus (AEV) transforming protein (v-erbB) has defined a new family of human receptor tyrosine kinases. These new receptors are called ErbB types 1 to 4 (Peles and Yarden, 1993; Carraway and Cantley, 1994). ErbB-1 binds EGF, while ErbB-3 and ErbB-4 bind a related factor called *neu differentiation factor* (NDF). ErbB-2(neu), which is most closely related to the AEV transforming protein, binds no known ligand (Dougall et al., 1994) but can dimerize with ErbB-1 to bind EGF and with ErbB-3 or ErbB-4, increasing their affinity for NDF (Karunagaran et al., 1996). Overexpression of ErbB-2, usually due to gene amplification, is associated with certain human malignancies such as glioblastoma, breast carcinoma, and bladder carcinoma.

The human *neu* oncogene has sequence similarity to the EGFR and was identified originally through transfection of DNA from rat neuroblastomas induced by the mutagen ethylnitrosourea (Bargmann et al., 1986). The activated *neu* gene in rat neuroblastomas had sustained a single T⇒A base change, presumably induced by the carcinogen, which resulted in a substitution of glutamic acid for valine in the transmembrane region of this receptor tyrosine kinase. This single mutation induces constitutive dimerization, and, as described in Sec. 6.3.3, dimerization allows mutual receptor phosphorylation with subsequent binding of signaling molecules. Gene amplification and overexpression of the mutated *neu* gene (also called *HER-2*) is common in some human malignancies, notably breast and ovarian carcinoma, and the degree of overexpression has been linked to poor prognosis in breast carcinoma.

Ret Germline mutations in the *ret* gene, which encodes a receptor protein tyrosine kinase, are associated with multiple endocrine neoplasia type 2A (MEN 2A) and type 2B (MEN 2B) and with familial medullary thyroid carcinoma (Ponder, 1994; Goodfellow and Wells, 1995). MEN 2A consists of medullary thyroid carcinoma, benign pheochromocytomas, and benign parathyroid tumors. In addition to endocrine malignancies, patients with MEN 2B have a characteristic facial appearance (Schimke, 1984) but have a reduced incidence of parathyroid abnormalities. In MEN 2A, mutations of multiple extracellular cysteine amino acids in *ret* have been documented (Mulligan et al., 1993). In familial medullary thyroid cancer, substitution of aspartic acid for glutamic acid and replacement of valine for leucine in the intracellular tyrosine kinase domain of *ret* has been described (Donis-Keller et al., 1993). MEN 2B results from substitution of threonine for methionine in the same region (Hofstra et al, 1994). As many as one-third of spontaneous medullary thyroid carcinomas have these same mutations (Goodfellow and Wells, 1995).

All identified mutations of *ret* appear to be dominant. The extracellular cysteine mutations in MEN 2A may affect ligand binding, although this has not yet been characterized. Alternatively, these extracellular mutations may cause receptor dimerization resulting in transphosphorylation, as seen in mutation of the *neu* gene. Mutations in the catalytic core of the receptor are seen in MEN 2B and may result in the activation of inappropriate signaling molecules (Songyang et al., 1995).

With the identification of specific mutations in a single gene that give rise to these familial cancer syndromes, it has become possible to screen unaffected family members by direct DNA sequencing for the presence of such germline mutations (Lips et al., 1994). Detection of germline mutations makes prophylactic ablative surgery of the thyroid a possibility, thus avoiding the development of potentially fatal medullary carcinoma in later life. For few malignancies is such screening possible or beneficial.

Kit, Fms and Flt-3 These receptor tyrosine kinases, which share significant structural similarity, are stimulated normally by their respective ligands, stem-cell factor (SCF), macrophage colony-stimulating factor (M-CSF) and flt-3 ligand (Meierhoff et al., 1995). Each receptor is overexpressed or mutated in various hematologic malignancies and may contribute to their etiology.

The c-kit protein plays an important role in the early development of myeloid and lymphoid precursors (Brandt et al., 1992; Broudy et al., 1992) potentiating the effect of lineage-specific growth factors such as erythropoietin, IL-3, GM-CSF, and G-CSF (Broxmeyer et al., 1991). The c-kit protein is coexpressed with the hematopoietic stem cell marker CD34 on normal cells and on immature acute leukemic cells (Kubota et al., 1994). The c-kit protein is functional in a large proportion of leukemic cells, which also express functional c-kit ligand, raising the possibility of growth potentiation through an autocrine growth loop (Broudy et al., 1992). Specific mutations of the c-*kit* gene in human malignancies have not yet been identified.

The protein product of the retroviral transforming oncogene v-*fms* (Chap. 5, Sec. 5.4.2) escapes dependence on its ligand through deletion of its carboxy terminus (Coussens et al., 1986) and can transform murine myeloid cells (Sherr et al., 1985). In contrast to c-*kit*, in which mutant sequences have not yet been isolated, miscellaneous point mutations of c-*fms* have been found in the affected cells

of approximately 25 percent of patients with acute myelogenous leukemia or myelodysplastic syndromes (Ridge et al., 1990). These data suggest that mutations of c-*fms* may be an important feature of the malignant transformation of myeloid cells.

Fms-like Tyrosine kinase 3 (FLT-3) is expressed with its ligand by diverse hematopoietic malignant cells, suggesting the presence of autocrine stimulation, as has been postulated for c-*kit* (Meierhoff et al., 1995). FLT-3 can function as a proliferation factor on primitive hematopoietic cells (Lyman et al., 1993; Hannum et al., 1994) and may participate in malignant hematopoiesis.

The chromosomal translocation t(2;5) occurs in T-lymphocyte anaplastic large-cell lymphomas and fuses the NPM nucleolar phosphoprotein on chromosome 5q35 to the receptor tyrosine kinase ALK (anaplastic large-cell kinase) on chromosome 2 (Morris et al., 1994). ALK is normally expressed in intestines, testis, and brain, suggesting that its abnormal expression as a mutated form in lymphoid tissue may contribute to transformation. NPM, a nonribosomal nucleolar phosphoprotein, contributes its promoter and replaces a potential regulating sequence in the carboxy terminus of this tyrosine kinase.

6.7.3 Abnormalities in Cytoplasmic Signaling Transducers

Ras Transforming alleles of one of the three closely related *ras* genes have been identified in a variety of human tumors (Bos, 1989). These *ras* genes differ from their normal counterparts in carrying mutations in the phosphate-binding region of the nucleotide-binding site. As a result, the GTPase activity is lost, resulting in accumulation of ras protein in the GTP-bound state. These oncogenic mutants can still bind GTPase activating protein but are insensitive to its GTPase stimulating activity. In humans, activation of K-*ras* is observed in lung cancer (Mitsudomi et al., 1991) and colorectal carcinoma (Burner et al., 1991; Sasaki et al., 1990). N-*ras* is often mutated in leukemia and lymphoma (Farr et al., 1988; Janssen et al., 1987) and H-*ras* is often mutated in oral and other cancers (Saranath et al., 1991). Either N or H-*ras* mutations have been detected in thyroid and skin cancers (Corominas et al., 1989; Shi et al., 1991)

Bcr/abl Chronic myelogenous leukemia is characterized by a unique chromosomal translocation that generates the Philadelphia chromosome, t(9;22) (see Chap. 4, Sec. 4.3.2, and Chap. 5, Sec. 5.4.4). This translocation produces a fusion protein involving bcr, an SH2 domain–containing serine/threonine kinase (Pendergast et al., 1991), and the cellular homologue of the v-*abl* oncogene (Kurzrock et al., 1988). Two fusion products can be formed, 210 or 190 kDa in size, which can both cause leukemia when expressed in transgenic mice (Daley et al., 1990; Kelliher et al., 1990). The bcr/abl fusion protein has constitutive tyrosine kinase activity. In vitro, the SH2 domain of the GRB2 linker molecule (Sec. 6.3.3) binds the bcr-abl protein at a phosphotyrosine, suggesting a direct link between bcr-abl and ras activation (Puil et al., 1994). Bcr-abl has also been linked to SAPK activation (Raitano et al, 1995). It remains to be defined how bcr-abl integrates these two signaling pathways and what the critical determinants of transformation are.

The detection of the bcr/abl fusion protein from clinical samples has utility as a marker of malignant cells among normal marrow elements. The gene encoding this fusion protein is found only in cells derived through the transforming process and can be detected in DNA of bone marrow by using the polymerase chain reaction (PCR) to amplify a segment across the break point (see Chap. 3, Sec. 3.3.7). Alternatively, Southern blot analysis can be used to demonstrate unique restriction fragments indicative of the presence of the malignant clone (see Chap. 3, Secs. 3.3.4 and 3.3.5). While Southern blot analysis can detect malignant cells comprising 1 percent or more of the total cell population, PCR can theoretically detect as little as one malignant cell within a particular marrow sample. These tests are used clinically to detect residual disease in patients as a measure of treatment efficacy (Howe and Weiss, 1995).

ARAM Sequences The ability of two viruses to transform hematopoietic cells may be explained by their ability to mimic normal signaling mechanisms. The bovine leukemia virus (BLV), in the cytoplasmic portion of its envelope glycoprotein, and the Epstein-Barr virus (EBV), in the latent membrane protein 2 (LMP2), contain functional ARAM sequences (Sec. 6.6.1). These two transforming viruses induce lymphocyte proliferation by coupling directly to cytoplasmic tyrosine kinases (Alber et al., 1993).

6.7.4 Abnormalities in Nuclear Transcription Factors

Transcription factors control the expression of genes and are often regulated by extracellular stimuli such as growth factors or cytokines. When their activities become dysregulated through gene amplification or mutation, abnormalities of cell growth or cellular differentiation can occur, leading to malignant transformation. Each of the structural classes of transcription factors has been implicated in human malignancy (see Sec. 6.3.6).

Helix turn helix (HTH) transcription factors may be dysregulated in childhood leukemias, with the fusion of the PBX-1 and E2A transcription factors being the best studied example. The fusion of these two HTH transcription factors is produced by the t(1;19) translocation, found in 25 percent of childhood pre–B cell acute lymphocytic leukemias (Crist et al., 1990; Hunger et al., 1991). The product contains the DNA binding domain of PBX-1, which is probably regulated in a novel way and contributes to the expression of lymphocytic transforming genes.

Helix loop helix (HLH) transcription factors, when dysregulated, may cause primitive tumors such as acute leukemias or undifferentiated lymphomas in both children and adults. Typically, overexpression occurs after a chromosomal translocation brings these transcription factor genes under the spurious control of some other actively transcribed gene (Cleary, 1992). The prototypic HLH transcription factor is the myc protein, which becomes dysregulated in Burkitt's lymphoma by the t(8;14) translocation, bringing it under the control of the immunoglobulin heavy chain promoter (Kluin and van Krieken, 1996; Chap. 4, Sec. 4.3.2). Other HLH transcription factors implicated in hematologic malignancies include lyl-1, tal-1/scl, and tal-2, all of which may be activated by translocation into the T-cell receptor locus in acute T-cell leukemias (Xia et al., 1991). Amplification of the N-*myc* gene has also been observed in solid tumors such as pediatric neuroblastoma, where it portends a poor prognosis (Seeger et al., 1985).

The receptor for thyroid hormone is a zinc finger–containing transcription factor. A form lacking the hormone-binding region, the avian erythroblastosis virus oncogene v-*erb*A is able to transform susceptible cells. v-*erb*A may act in concert with v-*erb*B, described above, as a dominant inhibitor to eliminate the differentiating effects of the normal hormone (Wong and Privalsky, 1995). Other dysregulated members of the zinc-finger family of transcription factors include mutated estrogen-binding proteins, which may play a role in establishing growth independence from estrogen in human breast carcinoma (Catherino and Jordan, 1995;

Tonetti and Jordan, 1995); the *bcl*-6 oncogene, which becomes overexpressed in large-cell lymphoma (Dalla-Favera et al., 1994); and the tumor suppressor protein WT-1 which is inactivated in children with Wilms' tumor (Schneider et al., 1993; see Chap. 4, Sec. 4.5.3). Acute promyelocytic leukemia is characterized by the t(15;17) translocation, which produces a chimeric transcription factor through fusion of the retinoic acid receptor α (RAR-α) to a previously undescribed gene named *pml* (Mu et al., 1994). This hybrid protein may target genes responsive to either RAR-α or *pml*, since it contains the DNA-binding domains of each factor. Since the RAR-α/*pml* fusion can compete with endogenous RAR-α, it may, like v-*erb*A, act as a dominant inhibitor, suppressing the expression of differentiating genes induced by RAR-α.

Leucine-zipper transcription factors include v-*jun*, which was found initially in the transforming avian sarcoma virus and v-*fos*, which was characterized in the FBJ murine osteosarcoma virus. Human tumors have not, however, been shown to contain mutations of these genes.

6.8 SUMMARY

Proliferation of mammalian cells and their responses to stressful stimuli are carefully controlled. This control derives from complex evolutionary pressure, which has resulted in the ability to initiate cell division during normal development and to maintain static the mass of mature tissues. All mammalian cells contain genes, known as proto-oncogenes, that control these processes but when dysregulated contribute to the development of malignancy. The proto-oncogenes encode proteins involved with all aspects of cell signaling that result in cell proliferation, cell differentiation, or cell death. These proteins include growth factors, growth-factor receptors, cytoplasmic kinases involved in signal transduction, and nuclear proteins involved in the control of gene expression.

The binding of a growth factor to its receptor can result in the proliferation or differentiation of a cell. Activated growth factor receptors induce a variety of biochemically distinct signal-transduction pathways that carry information from the membrane to the nucleus. These pathways generally involve a cascade of signaling proteins that act to phosphorylate the next protein in the signaling cascade. These pathways eventually influence the activity of transcription factors, which bind to DNA and control the expression of specific genes. Related signaling pathways are induced by stressful stimuli,

such as exposure to heat, radiation, or cytotoxic drugs. Other pathways, with both specific and common elements, are initiated by binding of cytokines to their receptors or by interaction of antigens with receptors on lymphocytes. As the molecules involved in signal transduction and the genes involved in the regulation of cell proliferation and differentiation are identified, novel opportunities for controlling malignancy are likely to follow.

REFERENCES

Alber G, Kim K-M, Weiser P, et al: Molecular mimicry of the antigen receptor signaling motif by transmembrane proteins of the Epstein-Barr virus and the bovine leukemia virus. *Curr Biol* 1993; 3:333–339.

Alberola-Ila J, Forbush KA, Seger R, et al: Selective requirement for MAP kinase activation in thymocyte differentiation. *Nature* 1995; 373:620–623.

Alessi DR, Saito Y, Campbell DG, et al: Identification of the sites in MAP kinase kinase-1 phosphorylated by p74raf-1. *EMBO J* 1994; 13:1610–1619.

Alzarez E, Northwood IC, Gonzalez FA, et al: Pro-Leu-Ser/Thr-Pro is a consensus primary sequence for substrate protein phosphorylation. Characterization of the phosphorylation of c-myc and c-jun proteins by an epidermal growth factor receptor threonine 669 protein kinase. *J Biol Chem* 1991; 266:15277-15288.

Axelrod J, Burch RM, Jelsema CL: Receptor mediated activation of phospholipase A2 via GTP binding proteins: arachidonic acid and its metabolites as second messengers. *Trends Neurosci* 1988; 11:117-123.

Bargmann CI, Hung MC, Weinberg RA: Multiple independent activations of the neu oncogene by a point mutation altering the transmembrane domain of p185. *Cell* 1986; 45:649–657.

Bokemeyer D, Sorokin A, Yan M, et al: Induction of mitogen activated protein kinase phosphatase 1 by the stress activated protein kinase signaling pathway but not by extracellular signal regulated kinase in fibroblasts. *J Biol Chem* 1996; 271:639–642.

Bos JL: Ras oncogene in human cancer: a review. *Cancer Res* 1989; 49:4682–4689.

Brandt J, Briddell RA, Srour EF, et al: Role of c-kit ligand in the expansion of human hematopoietic progenitor cells. *Blood* 1992; 79:634–641.

Brewster JL, De Valoir T, Dwyer ND, et al: An osmosensing signal transduction pathway in yeast. *Science* 1993; 259:1760–1763.

Broudy VC, Smith FO, Lin N, et al: Blasts from patients with acute myelogenous leukemia express functional receptors for stem cell factor. *Blood* 1992; 80:60–67.

Broxmeyer HE, Cooper S, Lu L, et al: Effect of murine mast cell growth factor (c-kit proto oncogene ligand) on colony formation by human marrow hematopoietic progenitor cells. *Blood* 1991; 77:2142–2149.

Burgering BM Bos JL: Regulation of Ras-mediated signaling: More than one way to skin a cat (review). *Trends Biochem Sci* 1995; 20;18–22.

Burgess WH Maciag T: The heparin binding (fibroblast) growth factor family of proteins. *Annu Rev Biochem* 1989; 58:575–606.

Burner G, Rabinovitch P, Loeb L: Frequency and spectrum of c-Ki-ras mutations in human sporadic colon carcinoma, carcinomas arising in ulcerative colitis and pancreatic adenocarcinoma. *Environ Health Perspect* 1991; 93:27–31.

Cammarota G, Schierle A, Takacs B, et al: Identification of a CD4 binding site on the β-2 domain of HLA-DR molecules. *Nature* 1992; 356:799–801.

Carraway KL, Cantley LC: A neu acquaintance for erbB3 and erbB4: A role for receptor heterodimerization in growth signaling (review). *Cell* 1994; 78:5–8.

Catherino WH, Jordan VC: The biological action of cDNAs from mutated estrogen receptors transfected into breast cancer cells. *Cancer Lett* 1995; 90:35–42.

Chan AC, Iwashima M, Turch CW, Weiss A: A 70 KDa protein tyrosine kinase that associates with the TCR zeta chain. *Cell* 1992; 71:649–662.

Cleary ML: Transcription factors in human leukemias. *Cancer Surv* 1992; 15:89–104.

Clipstone NA, Crabtree GR: Identification of calcineurin as a key signaling enzyme in T lymphocyte activation. *Nature* 1992; 357:695–697.

Cooper JA, Gould KA, Cartwright CA, Hunter T: Tyr 527 is phosphorylated in pp60c-src: Implication for regulation. *Science* 1986; 231:1431–1434.

Corominas M, Kamino H, Leon J, et al: Oncogene activations in human benign tumors of the skin (keratoacanthomas): Is H-ras involved in differentiation as well as proliferation? *Proc Natl Acad Sci USA* 1989; 86: 6372–6376.

Coussens L, Van Beveren C, Smith D, et al: Structural alteration of viral homolog of receptor proto-oncogene fms at carboxyl terminus. *Nature* 1986; 320:277–280.

Crist WM, Carrol AJ, Shuster JJ, et al: Poor prognosis of children with pre-B lymphoblastic leukemia is associated with the t(1;19)(q23;p13): A pediatric oncology group study. *Blood* 1990; 76:117–127.

Daley GQ, van Etten RA, Baltimore D: Induction of chronic myelogenous leukemia in mice by the p210 bcr/abl gene of the Philadelphia chromosome. *Science* 1990; 247:824–830.

Dalla-Favera R, Ye BH, Lo Coco F: BCL-6 and the molecular pathogenesis of B-cell lymphoma (review). *Cold Spring Harbor Symp Quant Biol* 1994; 59:117–123.

Darnell JE, Kerr IM, Stark GR: JAK-STAT pathways and transcriptional activation in response to IFNs and other extracellular signaling proteins. *Science* 1994; 264:1415–1421.

Davies DR, Wlodawer A: Cytokines and their receptor complexes (review). *FASEB* 1995; 9:50–56.

Davis RJ: The mitogen-activated protein kinase signal transduction pathway (review). *J Biol Chem* 1993; 268:14553–14556.

Davis RJ: MAPKs: new JNK expands the group (review). *Trends Biochem Sci* 1994; 19:470–473.

Derynck R: TGF-beta-receptor-mediated signaling (review). *Trends Biochem Sci* 1994; 19:548–553.

Donis-Keller H, Dou S, Chi D, et al: Mutations in the RET proto-oncogene are associated with MEN 2A and FMTC. *Hum Mol Genet* 1993; 2:851–856.

Dougall WC, Qian X, Peterson NC, et al: The neu-oncogene: Signal transduction pathways, transformation mechanisms and evolving therapies (review). *Oncogene* 1994; 9:2109–2123.

Downward J, Graves J, Cantrell D: The regulation and function of p21RAS in T cells. *Immunol Today* 1992; 13:89–92.

Emslie EA, Jones TA, Sheer D, et al: The CL100 gene, which encodes a dual specificity (Tyr/Thr) MAP kinase phosphatase, is highly conserved and maps to human chromosome 5q34. *Hum Genet* 1994; 93:513–516.

Fabian JR, Daar IO, Morrison DK: Critical tyrosine residues regulate the enzymatic and biological activity of Raf-1 kinase. *Mol Cell Biol* 1993; 13:7170–7179.

Farr C, Saiki R, Ehrlich H: Analysis of ras gene mutations in acute myeloid leukemia using the polymerase chain reaction and oligonucleotide probes. *Proc Natl Acad Sci USA* 1988; 85:1629–1633.

Fischer EH, Charbonneau H, Cool DE, et al: Tyrosine phosphatases and their possible interplay with tyrosine kinases. *Ciba Found Symp* 1992; 164:132–40; discussion, 140–144.

Folkman J: What is the evidence that tumors are angiogenesis dependent? *J Natl Cancer Inst* 1990; 82:4–7.

Giri JG, Ahdieh M, Eisenman J, et al: Utilization of the beta and gamma chains of the IL-2 receptor by the novel cytokine IL-15. *EMBO J* 1994; 13:2822–2830.

Goodfellow PJ, Wells SA Jr: RET gene and its implications for cancer. (review). *J Natl Cancer Inst* 1995; 87: 515–1523.

Hallek M, Druker B, Lepisto EM, et al: Granulocyte macrophage colony stimulating factor and Steel factor induce phosphorylation of both unique and overlapping signal transduction intermediates in a human factor dependent hematopoietic cell line. *J Cell Physiol* 1992; 153:176–186.

Hammacher A, Nister M, Westermark B, et al: A human glioma cell line secretes three structurally and functionally different dimeric forms of platelet-derived growth factor. *Eur J Biochem* 1988; 176:179–186.

Han J, Lee JD, Bibbs L, et al: A MAP kinase targeted by endotoxin and hyperosmolarity in mammalian cells. *Science* 1994; 265:808–811.

Han J, Lee JD, Jiang Y, et al: Characterization of the structure and function of a novel MAP kinase kinase (MKK6). *J Biol Chem* 1996; 271:2886–2892.

Han J, Lee JD, Tobias PS, et al: Endotoxin induces rapid protein tyrosine phosphorylation in 70Z/3 cells expressing CD14. *J Biol Chem* 1993; 268:25009–25014.

Hanks SK, Quinn AM: The protein kinase family: Conserved features and deduced phylogeny of the catalytic domains. *Science* 1989; 241:42–52.

Hannum C, Culpepper J, Campbell D, et al: Ligand for FLT3/FLK2 receptor tyrosine kinase regulates growth of hematopoietic stem cells and is encoded by variant RNAs. *Nature* 1994; 368:643–648.

Hatakeyama M, Kono T, Kobayashi N, et al: Interaction of the IL-2 receptor with the src family kinase p56lck: Identification of novel intermolecular association. *Science* 1991; 252:1523–1528.

Hayashi H, Kamohara S, Nishioka Y, et al: Insulin treatment stimulates the tyrosine phosphorylation of the alpha-type 85 kDa subunit of phosphatidylinositol 3-kinase in vivo. *J Biol Chem* 1992; 26:22575–22580.

Hofstra RM, Landsvater RM, Ceccherini I, et al: A mutation in the RET proto-oncogene associated with multiple endocrine neoplasia type 2B and sporadic medullary thyroid carcinoma. *Nature* 1994; 367:375–376.

Howe LR, Weiss A: Multiple kinases mediate T-cell-receptor signaling (review). *Trends Biochem Sci* 1995; 20:59–64.

Howe LR, Leevers SJ, Gomez N, et al: Activation of the MAP kinase pathway by the protein kinase raf. *Cell* 1992; 71:335–342.

Hunger SP, Galili N, Carroll AJ, et al: The t(1;19)(q23;p13) results in consistent fusion of E2A and PBX1 coding sequences in acute lymphoblastic leukemias. *Blood* 1991; 77: 687–693.

Ihle JN, Kerr IM: Jaks and Stats in signaling by the cytokine receptor superfamily (review). *Trends Genet* 1995; 11:69–74.

Janssen J, Steenvoorden A, Lyons J: Ras gene mutations in acute and chronic myelocytic leukemias, chronic myeloproliferative disorders and myelodysplastic syndromes. *Proc Natl Acad Sci USA* 1987; 85:1629–1633.

Karunagaran D, Tzahar E, Beerli RR, et al: ErbB-2 is a common auxiliary subunit of NDF and EGF receptors: Implications for breast cancer. *EMBO J* 1996; 15: 254–264.

Kashles O, Yarden Y, Fischer R, et al: A dominant negative mutation suppresses the function of normal epidermal growth factor receptors by heterodimerization. *Mol Cell Biol* 1991; 11:1454–1463.

Kelliher MA, McLaughlin J, Witte ON, et al: Induction of a chronic myelogenous leukemia-like syndrome in mice with v-abl and bcr/abl. *Proc Natl Acad Sci USA* 1990; 87:6649–6653.

Keyse SM, Ginsburg M: Amino acid sequence similarity between CL100, a dual-specificity MAP kinase phosphatase and cdc25. *Trends Biochem Sci* 1990; 18: 377–378.

Kim KJ, Li B, Winer J, et al: Inhibition of vascular endothelial growth factor induced angiogenesis suppresses tumor growth in vivo. *Nature* 1993; 362: 841–844.

Kishihara K, Penninger J, Wallace VA, et al: Normal B lymphocyte development but impaired T cell maturation in CD45 exon 6 protein tyrosine phosphatase deficient mice. *Cell* 1993; 74:143–156.

Kishimoto T, Taga T, Akira S: Cytokine signal transduction (review). *Cell* 1994; 76:253–262.

Klippel A, Escobendo JA, Hu Q, et al: A region of the 85 kilodalton (kDa) subunit of phosphatidylinositol 3 kinase binds the 110 kDa catalytic subunit in vivo. *Mol Cell Biol* 1993; 13:5560–5566.

Kluin PM, van Krieken JH: The molecular biology of B cell lymphoma: clinicopathologic implications. *Ann Hematol* 1996; 62:95–102.

Kolch W, Heidecker G, Kochs G, et al: Protein kinase C alpha activates RAF-1 by direct phosphorylation. *Nature* 1993; 364:249–252.

Kondo M, Takeshita T, Ishii N, et al: Sharing of the interleukin-2 (IL-2) receptor gamma chain between receptors for IL-2 and IL-4. *Science* 1993; 262:1874–1877.

Konig R, Huang L-Y, Germain RN: MHC class II interaction with CD4 mediated by a region analogous to the MHC class I binding site for CD8. *Nature* 1992; 356:796–798.

Kubota A, Okamura S, Shimoda K, et al: The c-kit molecule and the surface immunophenotype of human acute leukemia. *Leuk Lymph* 1994; 14:421–428.

Kurzrock R, Gutterman JU, Talpaz M: The molecular genetics of Philadelphia chromosome–positive leukemias (review). *N Engl J Med* 1988; 319:990–998.

Kyriakis JM, App H, Zhang XF, et al: Raf-1 activates MAP kinase-kinase. *Nature* 1992; 358:417–421.

Law DA, Chan VWF, Datta SK, et al: B cell antigen receptor motifs have redundant signaling capabilities and bind the tyrosine kinases PTK72, Lyn and Fyn. *Curr Biol* 1993; 3:645–657.

Lee JC, Laydon JT, McDonnell PC, et al: A protein kinase involved in the regulation of inflammatory cytokine biosynthesis. *Nature* 1994; 372:739–746.

Li W, Nishimura R, Kashishian A, et al: A new function for a phosphotyrosine phosphatase: Linking GRB2-SOS to a receptor tyrosine kinase. *Mol Cell Biol* 1994; 14: 509–517.

Lips CJ, Landsvater RM, Hoppener JW, et al: Clinical screening as compared with DNA analysis in families with multiple endocrine neoplasia type 2A. *N Engl J Med* 1994; 331:828–835.

Liu X, Marengere LEM, Koch CA, et al: The v-Src SH3 domain binds phosphatidylinositol 3′ kinase. *Mol Cell Biol* 1993; 13:5225–5232.

Lutticken C, Wegenka UM, Yuan J, et al: Association of transcription factor APRF and protein kinase Jak1 with the interleukin-6 signal transducer gp130. *Science* 1994; 263:89–92.

Lyman SD, James L, Vanden Bos T, et al. Molecular cloning of a ligand for the flt3/flk-2 tyrosine kinase receptor: A prolifererative factor for primitive hematopoietic cells. *Cell* 1993; 75:1157–1167.

Marengere LE, Pawson T: Structure and function of SH2 domains (review). *J Cell Sci* 1994; 18:97–104.

Meierhoff G, Dehmel U, Gruss H-J, et al: Expression of FLT3 receptor and FLT3-ligand in human leukemia-lymphoma cell lines. *Leukemia* 1995; 9:1368–1372.

Miltenberger RJ, Cortner J, Farnham PJ: An inhibitory Raf-1 mutant suppresses expression of a subset of v-raf activated genes. *J Biol Chem* 1993; 268: 15674–15680.

Minami Y, Nakagawa Y, Kawahara A, et al: Protein tyrosine kinase Syk is associated with and activated by the IL-2 receptor. Possible link with the c-myc induction pathway. *Immunity* 1995; 2:89–100.

Minshull J, Sun H, Tonks NK, et al: A MAP kinase-dependent spindle assembly checkpoint in Xenopus egg extracts. *Cell* 1994; 79:475–486.

Mitsudomi T, Viallet J, Mulshine J, et al: Mutations of ras genes distinguish a subset of non small cell lung cancer lines from small cell lung cancer lines. *Oncogene* 1991; 6:1353–1362.

Miyajima A, Kitamura T, Harada N, et al: Cytokine receptors and signal transduction. *Ann Rev Immunol* 1992; 10:295–331.

Morris SW, Kirstein MN, Valentine MB, et al: Fusion of a kinase gene, ALK to a nucleolar protein gene, NPM, in non-Hodgkin's lymphoma. *Nature* 1994; 263:1281–1284.

Mu ZM, Chin KV, Liu JH: PML, a growth suppressor disrupted in acute promyelocytic leukemia. *Mol Cell Biol* 1994; 14:6858–6867.

Mulligan LM, Kwok JB, Healey CS, et al: Germline mutations of the RET proto-oncogene in multiple endocrine neoplasia type 2A. *Nature* 1993; 363:458–460.

Murphy SM, Bergman M, Morgan DO: Suppression of c-Src activity by C-terminal Src kinase involves the c-Src SH2 and SH3 domains: Analysis with Saccharomyces cerevisiae. *Mol Cell Biol* 1993; 13:5290–5300.

Musacchio A, Noble M, Paupitit R, et al: Crystal structure of a Src-homology 3 (SH3) domain. *Nature* 1992; 359:851–854.

Nel AE, Hanekom C, Rheeder A, et al: Stimulation of MAP-2 kinase activity in T lymphocytes by anti-CD3 or anti-Ti monoclonal antibody is partially dependent on protein kinase C. *J Immunol* 1990; 144:2683–2689.

Nister M, Claesson-Welsh L, Eriksson A, et al: Differential expression of platelet-derived growth factor receptors in human malignant glioma cell lines. *J Biol Chem* 1991; 266:16755–16763.

Olivier JP, Raabe T, Henkemeyer M, et al: A drosophila SH2-SH3 adaptor protein implicated in coupling the sevenless tyrosine kinase to an activator of Ras guanine nucleotide exchange. *Cell* 1993; 73:179–191.

Pages G, Lenormand P, L'Allemain G, et al: Mitogen activated protein kinases p42MAPK and p44MAPK are required for fibroblast proliferation. *Proc Natl Acad Sci USA* 1993; 90:8319–8323.

Papavassiliou A: Transcription factors: structure, function, and implication in malignant growth. *Anticancer Res* 1995; 15:891–894.

Pawson T: SH2 and SH3 domains in signal transduction. *Adv Cancer Res* 1994; 64: 87–110.

Pawson T: Protein modules and signaling networks. *Nature* 1995; 373:573–580.

Peles E, Yarden Y: Neu and its ligands: from an oncogene to neural factors. *Bioessays* 1993; 15:815–824.

Pendergast AM, Muller AJ, Havlik MH, et al: BCR sequences essential for transformation by the BCR-ABL oncogene bind to the ABL SH2 regulatory domain in a non-phosphotyrosine-dependent manner. *Cell* 1991; 66:161–171.

Ponder BA: The gene causing multiple endocrine neoplasia type 2 (MEN 2). *Ann Med* 1994; 26:199–203.

Puil L, Liu J, Gish G, et al: Bcr-Abl oncoproteins bind directly to activators of the Ras signaling pathway. *EMBO J* 1994; 13:764–773.

Qui MS, Green SH: PC12 cell neuronal differentiation is associated with prolonged p21RAS activity and consequent prolonged ERK activity. *Neuron* 1992; 9:705–717.

Raingeaud J, Gupto S, Rogers JS, et al: Pro-inflammatory cytokines and environmental stress cause p38 mitogen-activated protein kinase activation by dual phosphorylation on tyrosine and threonine. *J Biol Chem* 1995; 270:7420–7426.

Raitano AB, Halpern JR, Hambuch TM, et al: The Bcr-Abl leukemia oncogene activates Jun kinase and requires Jun for transformation. *Proc Natl Acad Sci USA* 1995; 92:11746–11750.

Ridge SA, Worwood M, Oscier D, et al: FMS mutations in myelodysplastic, leukemic and normal subjects. *Proc Natl Acad Sci USA* 1990; 87:1377–1380.

Romeo C, Amiot M, Seed B: Sequence requirements for induction of cytolysis by the T cell antigen/Fc receptor zeta chain. *Cell* 1992; 68:889–897.

Rottapel R, Reedijk M, Williams DE, et al: The Steel/W transduction pathway: Kit autophosphorylation and its association with a unique subset of cytoplasmic signaling proteins is induced by the Steel factor. *Mol Cell Biol* 1991; 11:3043–3051.

Rudd CE: CD4, CD8 and the TCR-CD3 complex: A novel class of protein tyrosine kinase receptor. *Immunol Today* 1990; 11:400-406.

Saranath D, Chang S, Bhoite L, et al: High frequency mutation in codons 12 and 61 of H-ras oncogene in chewing tobacco related human carcinoma in India. *Br J Cancer* 1991; 63:573–578.

Sasaki M, Sugio K, Sasazuki T: K-ras activation in colorectal tumors from patients with familial polyposis coli. *Cancer* 1990; 65:2576–2579.

Schieven GL, Kallestad JC, Brown TJ, et al: Oncostatin M induces tyrosine phosphorylation in endothelial cells and activation of p62YES tyrosine kinase. *J Immunol* 1992; 149:1676–1682.

Schimke RN: Genetic aspects of multiple endocrine neoplasia. *Annu Rev Med* 1984; 35:25–31.

Schindler C: Cytokine signal transduction. *Receptor* 1995; 5:51–62.

Schlessinger J: SH2/SH3 signaling proteins. *Curr Opin Genet Dev* 1994; 4:25–30.

Schneider S, Wildhardt G, Ludwig R, et al: Exon skipping due to a mutation in a donor splice site in the WT-1 gene is associated with Wilms' tumor and severe genital malformations. *Hum Genet* 1993; 91:599–604.

Secrist JP, Karnitz L, Abraham RT: T cell antigen receptor ligation induces tyrosine phosphorylation of phospholipase C gamma-1. *J Biol Chem* 1991; 266:12135-12139.

Seeger RC, Brodeur GM, Sather H, et al: Association of multiple copies of the N-myc oncogene with rapid progression of neuroblastomas. *N Engl J Med* 1985; 313: 1111–1116.

Seger R, Krebs EG: The MAPK signaling cascade. *FASEB J* 1995; 9:726–735.

Shen SH, Bastien L, Posner BI, et al: A protein tyrosine phosphatase with sequence similarity to the SH2 domain of the protein tyrosine kinases. *Nature* 1991; 352:736–739.

Sherr CJ, Rettenmier CW, Saaca R, et al: The c-FMS proto-oncogene product is related to the receptor for the mononuclear phagocyte growth factor, CSF-1. *Cell* 1985; 41:665–676.

Shi Y, Zou M, Schmidt H, et al: High rates of ras codon 61 mutations in thyroid tumors in iodide deficient areas. *Cancer Res* 1991; 51:2690–2693.

Shoelson SE, Sivaraja M, Williams KP, et al: Specific phosphopeptide binding regulates a conformational change in the PI 3-kinase SH2 domain associated with enzyme activation. *EMBO J* 1993; 12:795–802.

Sieh M, Bolen JB, Weiss A: CD45 specifically modulates binding of LCK to a phosphopeptide encompassing the negative regulatory tyrosine of LCK. *EMBO J* 1993; 12:315–322.

Smith MR, DeGudicibus SJ, Stacey DW: Requirement for c-ras proteins during viral oncogene transformation. Nature 1986; 320:540-543.

Songyang Z, Shoelson SE, Chaudhuri M et al: SH2 domains recognize specific phosphopeptide sequences. *Cell* 1993; 72:767–778.

Songyang Z, Carraway KL, Eck MJ, et al: Catalytic specificity of protein tyrosine kinases is critical for selective signaling. *Nature* 1995; 373:536–539.

Suen KL, Bustelo XR, Pawson T, et al: Molecular cloning of the mouse GRB2 gene: Differential interaction of the GRB2 adaptor protein with epidermal growth factor and nerve growth factor receptors. *Mol Cell Biol* 1993; 13:5500–5512.

Taniguchi T: Cytokine signaling through nonreceptor protein tyrosine kinases. *Science* 1995; 268: 251–255.

Taniguchi T, Kobayashi T, Kondo J, et al: Molecular cloning of a porcine gene syk that encodes a 72 kDa protein tyrosine kinase showing high susceptibility to proteolysis. *J Biol Chem* 1991; 266:15790–15796.

Tonetti DA, Jordan VC: Possible mechanisms in the emergence of tamoxifen-resistant breast cancer. *Anticancer Drugs* 1995; 6:498–507.

Traverse S, Gomez N, Paterson H, et al: Sustained activation of the mitogen activated protein (MAP) kinase cascade may be required for differentiation of PC12 cells: Comparison of the effects of nerve growth factor and epidermal growth factor. *Biochem J* 1992; 288: 351–355.

Traverse S, Seedorf K, Paterson H, et al: EGF triggers neuronal differentiation of PC12 cells that overexpress the EGF receptor. *Curr Biol* 1994; 4:694–701.

Tsai M, Chen RH, Tam SY, et al: Activation of MAP kinases, pp90RSK and pp70-S6 kinases in mouse mast cells by signaling through the c-kit receptor tyrosine ki-

nase of Fc epsilon RI: rapamycin inhibits activation of pp70-S6 kinase and proliferation in mouse mast cells. *Eur J Immunol* 1993; 23:3286–3291.

Twamley-Stein GM, Pepperkok R, Ansorge W, et al: The Src family tyrosine kinases are required for platelet derived growth factor mediated signal transduction in NIH 3T3 cells. *Proc Natl Acad Sci USA* 1993; 90: 7696–7700.

Ueno H, Colbert H, Escobendo JA, et al: Inhibition of PDGF beta receptor signal transduction by coexpression of a truncated receptor. *Science* 1991; 252: 844–848.

van der Geer P, Hunter T, Lindberg RA: Receptor protein-tyrosine kinases and their signal transduction pathways. *Annu Rev Cell Biol* 1994; 10:251–337.

Veillette A, Abraham N, Caron L et al: The lymphocyte specific tyrosine kinase p56LCK. *Semin Immunol* 1991; 3:143–152.

Vogt P, Bos JL: Jun: Oncogene and transcription factor. *Adv Cancer Res* 1990; 55:1–34.

Vojtek AB, Hollenberg SM, Cooper JA: Mammalian Ras interacts directly with the serine/threonine kinase Raf. *Cell* 1993; 74:205–214.

Wang LM, Keegan AD, Paul WE, et al: IL-4 activates a distinct signal transduction cascade from IL-3 in factor dependent myeloid cells. *EMBO J* 1992; 11:4899–4908.

Waterfield MD, Scrace GT, Whittle N, et al: Platelet derived growth factor is structurally related to putative transforming protein p28sis of simian sarcoma virus. Nature 1983; 304:35–39.

Weindel K, Marme D, Weich HA: AIDS-associated Kaposi's sarcoma cells in culture express vascular endothelial growth factor. *Biochem Biophys Res Commun* 1992; 83:1167–1174.

Weiss A: Molecular and genetic insights into T cell antigen receptor structure and function. *Annu Rev Genet* 1991; 25:487–510.

Westermark B, Claesson-Welsh L, Heldin CH: Structural and functional aspects of the receptors for platelet- derived growth factor (review). *Prog Growth Factor Res* 1989; 1:253–266.

White MF: The IRS-1 signaling system. *Curr Opin Genet Dev* 1994; 4:47–54.

Whitman M, Kaplan D, Roberts T, et al: Evidence for two distinct phosphatidylinositol kinases in fibroblasts. *Biochem J* 1987; 247:165–174.

Witthuhn BA, Quelle FW, Silvennoinen O, et al: JAK2 associates with the erythropoietin receptor and is tyrosine phosphorylated and activated following stimulation with erythropoietin. *Cell* 1993; 74:227–236.

Wong CW, Privalsky ML: Role of the N terminus in DNA recognition by the v-erb A protein, an oncogenic derivative of a thyroid hormone receptor. *Mol Endocrin* 1995; 9:551-562.

Xia Y, Brown L, Yang C-C, et al: Tal-2, a novel helix-loop-helix gene activated by the t(7;9)(q34;q32) translocation in human T cell leukemia. *Proc Natl Acad Sci USA* 1991; 88: 11416–11420.

Xia Z, Dickensons M, Raingeaud J: Opposing effects of ERK and JNK-p38 MAP kinases on apoptosis. *Science* 1995; 270:1326–1331.

Yan M, Dai T, Deak JC, et al: Activation of stress-activated protein kinase by MEKK1 phosphorylation of its activator SEK1. *Nature* 1994; 372:798–800.

Zanke BW, Boudreau K, Rubie E, et al: The stress-activated protein kinase pathway mediates cell death following injury induced by cis-platinum, UV irradiation or heat. *Curr Biol* 1996; 6:606–613.

Zhang F, Strand A, Robbins D, et al: Atomic structure of the MAP kinase ERK2 at 2.3 A resolution. *Nature* 1994; 367:704–711.

Zhang S, Han J, Sells MA, et al: Rho family GTPases regulate p38 mitogen activated protein kinase through the downstream mediator Pak1. *J Biol Chem* 1996; 270: 23934–23936.

Zhao Z, Bouchard P, Diltz, CD: Purification and characterization of a protein tyrosine phosphatase containing SH2 domains. *J Biol Chem* 1996; 68:2816–2820.

7

Cell Proliferation and Cell Death

Joyce M. Slingerland and Ian F. Tannock

7.1 INTRODUCTION

7.2 THE CELL CYCLE AND ITS REGULATION
    7.2.1 The Cell Cycle
    7.2.2 Cyclins and Cyclin-Dependent Kinases
    7.2.3 Inhibitors of Cell Cycle Progression
    7.2.4 The Cell Cycle and Cancer

7.3 APOPTOSIS AND CELLULAR SENESCENCE
    7.3.1 Apoptosis
    7.3.2 Induction of Apoptosis
    7.3.3 Regulation of Apoptosis
    7.3.4 Apoptosis and Cancer
    7.3.5 Cellular Senescence

7.4 ASSESSMENT OF CELL KINETICS
    7.4.1 Tritiated Thymidine and Autoradiography

7.4.2 Principles of Flow Cytometry
7.4.3 Analysis of Cell Kinetics by Flow Cytometry
7.4.4 Other Applications of Flow Cytometry

7.5 CELL PROLIFERATION IN NORMAL TISSUES
    7.5.1 Hemopoietic Cells and Growth Factors
    7.5.2 Intestine

7.6 TUMOR GROWTH AND CELL KINETICS
    7.6.1 Growth of Tumors
    7.6.2 Stem Cells and Clonality
    7.6.3 Cell Proliferation in Tumors
    7.6.4 Cell Proliferation, Prognosis, and Therapy

7.7 SUMMARY

REFERENCES

7.1 INTRODUCTION

In normal tissues that undergo cell renewal, there is a balance between cell proliferation, growth arrest and differentiation, and loss of mature cells by programmed cell death, or apoptosis. Tumors grow because the homeostatic control mechanisms that maintain the appropriate number of cells in normal tissues are defective, leading to an imbalance between cell proliferation and cell death, and there is expansion of the cell population. The development of autoradiography and its use with tritiated thymidine in the 1950s and 1960s, and the more recent application of flow cytometry, have allowed a detailed analysis of tumor growth in terms of the kinetics of proliferation of their constituent cells. The proliferative rate of tumor cells varies widely between tumors; nonproliferating cells are common, and there is often a high rate of cell death. The rate of cell proliferation in tumors may be an important factor in determining prognosis, or response to radiation or chemotherapy. Several

normal tissues, including bone marrow and intestine, contain cells with high rates of proliferation, and damage to these cells may be dose-limiting for chemotherapy. An understanding of the molecular events that regulate the cell proliferation cycle and the mechanisms whereby malignant cells escape from cell cycle controls, from apoptotic cell death, and from the limitations of a finite life span are key to an understanding of the differences between growth of the normal cells and that of their malignant counterparts. These concepts are also important for understanding the interaction of drugs and radiation with tissues and are likely to provide leads for the development of new therapeutic strategies.

7.2 THE CELL CYCLE AND ITS REGULATION

7.2.1 The Cell Cycle

The demonstration that a radiolabeled precursor of DNA is incorporated into a discrete population of cells (Howard and Pelc, 1951) indicated that DNA synthesis is not continuous from one mitosis to the next but takes place only in a specific period of the cell cycle, the S phase. This and subsequent experiments using ^{3}H-thymidine have led to an appreciation that the cell cycle is comprised of four phases (see Fig. 7.1). The gaps between mitosis (M) and S phase, and between the S phase and mitosis, are respectively called the G1 and G2 phases; the duration of individual phases of the cell cycle may vary among cells of a population. Nonproliferating cells that retain the capacity to divide following an appropriate stimulus are usually arrested between the M and S phases and are referred to as G0 cells. Most cells in normal tissues of adults are in a quiescent or G0 state.

When nontransformed cells are grown in tissue culture, they will stop proliferating and enter a quiescent or G0 state if they become confluent or are deprived of serum. Subsequent replating of cells at low density, or stimulation with serum or growth factors, leads to a resumption of cell proliferation, but there is a delay prior to initiation of DNA synthesis, followed by a partially synchronized entry of cells into S phase (Pardee, 1989). A similar delay in onset of DNA synthesis is observed when proliferative stimuli are applied to resting tissues *in vivo*—e.g., partial hepatectomy that stimulates proliferation of the remaining liver cells. Cells are receptive to signals to initiate proliferation in both the G0 and G1 phases of the cell cycle. A "restriction point," or R point, has been defined in cultured cells as the point in G1 phase beyond which a cell is committed to enter DNA synthesis (Fig. 7.1). While the R point

has been operationally defined in tissue culture, the molecular events that regulate irreversible commitment to DNA synthesis, or the R point, have not been defined. In vivo, mammalian cells may respond to different growth inhibitory signals with arrest at different points in G1. Thus there may actually be several different physiologic R points in different cell types that "restrict" cell cycle progression through G1 during differentiation and development.

7.2.2 Cyclins and Cyclin-Dependent Kinases

The cell cycle is governed by a family of cyclin-dependent kinases (cdks) whose activity is regulated by the binding of positive effectors, the cyclins (Sherr, 1994; Morgan, 1995), and by both activating and inactivating phosphorylation events. Cyclin binding to its cdk is required for kinase activation, but an additional level of control is provided by two different families of cdk inhibitory molecules (see below). The cyclin-dependent kinases regulate a series of biochemical pathways, or checkpoints, that integrate mitogenic and growth-inhibitory signals, monitor chromosome integrity, and coordinate the orderly sequence of cell cycle transitions (Hartwell, 1992). In mammalian cells, the family of cdks, designated cdk1 to 7, are conserved in size, ranging from 32 to 40 kDa, and share sequence homology (>40 percent identity). They are small serine/threonine kinases that are expressed at constant levels throughout the cell cycle and are catalytically inactive unless they are bound to cyclins. Phosphorylation of a conserved threonine, located in the catalytic cleft of the kinase (e.g., Thr161 for cdk1 and Thr160 for cdk2) is required for full activation, and this is catalyzed by the cdk-activating kinase, or CAK (see Solomon, 1993, and Morgan, 1995, for reviews). Cdk activation can be inhibited by phosphorylation of conserved inhibitory sites at Thr14 and Tyr15 by wee-1 kinases. Full cdk activation requires dephosphorylation of these inhibitory sites by phosphatases of the cdc25 family (Fig. 7.2).

In general, cyclin levels oscillate during the cell cycle and cyclin mRNA and protein expression peak at the time of maximum kinase activation, contributing to discrete bursts of kinase activity at specific cell cycle transitions. Degradation of cyclin proteins is also tightly regulated and contributes to the tight temporal regulation of cdk activities (see King et al., 1996, for review). The family of mammalian cyclins includes cyclins A to H, which all share a conserved sequence of about 100 amino acids, whose mutation disrupts both kinase binding and

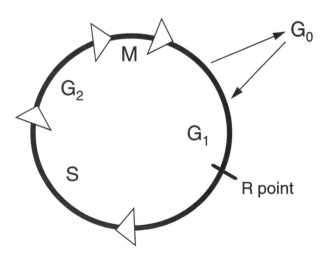

Fig. 7.1. The cell-cycle. The R (restriction) point represents the time in G_1 phase beyond which cells are committed to proceed to S phase.

**Cyclin binding
required for activation**

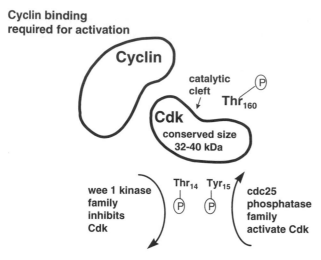

Fig. 7.2. Schematic diagram of cyclin-cdk interaction. Phosphorylation of a conserved threonine (Thr) in the catalytic cleft is required for full activity. Cdk activity is inhibited by phosphorylation of threonine and tyrosine (Tyr) at positions 14 and 15, as shown.

activation. Different cyclins have subfamilies. For example, there are two B-type cyclins, cyclin B1 and B2, and three D-type cyclins, cyclins D1, D2, and D3. Usually more than one D-type cyclin is expressed in any mammalian cell, but the combinations differ in different cell types.

Passage through G1 into S phase is regulated by the activities of cyclin D-, cyclin E-, and cyclin A-associated kinases (see Fig. 7.3, also Sherr, 1994, and Morgan, 1995, for reviews). D-type cyclins (cyclins

D1, D2, and D3) associate with cdks 2, 4, 5, and 6 and play an important role in reentry of cells into the proliferative cycle from quiescence. In cycling cells, they also effect essential steps during G1 phase. A primary role for cyclin D-associated kinases in vivo appears to be the phosphorylation of the retinoblastoma protein, pRb (see Chap. 4, Sec. 4.5.2). Phosphorylation of pRb in G1 phase is required to allow progression from G1 to S phase. Cyclin E is associated with cdk2 and, in most cells, cyclin E/cdk2 activity peaks after the peak of cyclin D/cdk activation. Overexpression of both D-type cyclins and cyclin E can accelerate the transition from G1 to S phase. That these kinases regulate independent pathways is shown by the fact that overexpression of cyclin D1 but not cyclin E causes premature phosphorylation of pRb. In addition, concurrent overexpression of both cyclins D1 and E accelerates the transistion from G1 to S to a greater extent than does either alone. Cyclin E/cdk2 activity is essential for passage from G1 into S phase: microinjection of antibodies to either cdk2 or cyclin E can prevent the transition from G1 to S phase. Cyclin A/cdk2 activation follows that of cyclin E/cdk2 and is essential for the initiation of and progression through S phase. Cyclin A may also play a role in mitosis.

In its hypophosphorylated state in early G1 phase, pRb binds the transcription factor E2F, and the pRb/E2F complex inhibits transcription of genes whose products are essential for S phase entrance (see Adams and Kaelin, 1995, and Kouzarides, 1995, for reviews). Upon phosphorylation of pRb late in

Fig. 7.3. Progression through the cell cycle is governed by a series of cyclin dependent kinases (cdks and cdc2, also known as cdk1) whose activities are positively regulated by cyclins and negatively regulated by cdk inhibitors (indicated by p15...p57). The phosphorylation and dephosphorylation of the retinoblastoma protein (pRB) in late G1 and in M phase is also necessary for cell cycle progression.

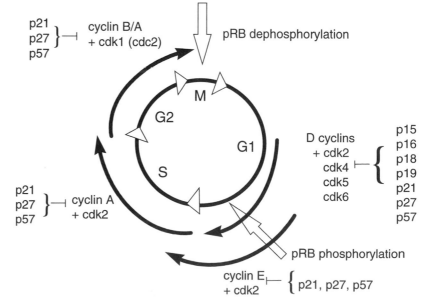

G1, E2F is released from this complex and transcription is activated. Both cyclin E- and cyclin A-associated kinases appear to play a role in modulating E2F transcriptional activity. These cyclin/cdks are found in complexes containing E2F and the pRb-related protein p107 in late G1 and early S phase respectively.

Mitotic or B-type cyclins, in association with cdk1 (also called cdc2, the name of the fission yeast homologue), control entry into and exit from mitosis. B-type cyclin levels increase during S phase. Phosphorylation of the inhibitory Thr14 and Tyr15 sites on cdk1 keeps the kinase inactive until the G2/M transition (Fig. 7.2). Dephosphorylation of these moieties by cdc25 phosphatase, and CAK activation, triggers cdk1 activation which is essential for mitosis to occur. The abrupt, controlled degradation of cyclin B by a particular protein degradation pathway called the *ubiquitin-proteasome pathway* allows exit from mitosis (see King et al., 1996, for review). The retinoblastoma protein, pRb, is also dephosphorylated at this time.

7.2.3 Inhibitors of Cell Cycle Progression

Recent work has identified two families of cdk inhibitory proteins (see Reed et al., 1994, and Sherr and Roberts, 1995, for reviews). The kinase inhibitory protein (KIP) family members include p21 (Cip1, WAF1, Sdi1), p27 (Kip1), and p57 (Kip2). p21 was identified both as a novel protein bound to cdk2 and as the product of a gene whose transcrip-

tion is activated by the negative growth regulator p53 (see Chap. 4, Sec. 4.5.3, and Chap. 5, Sec. 5.5.2); its expression is upregulated in senescent fibroblasts. p27 was identified as an inhibitory activity induced by TGF-β (see below). p57 is the most recent member of this family to be discovered. Its role in growth regulation is not yet known.

All KIP family members can bind to and inhibit a wide range of cdks, including cdks1 to 6. KIP molecules bind more efficiently to cyclin/cdk complexes than to either cyclin or cdk alone (Hall et al., 1995). Kinase inhibition is regulated by the number of KIP molecules available to bind cdk proteins. When the ratio of KIP:cdk molecules is low, the KIPs may facilitate cdk/cyclin assembly and kinase activation (LaBaer et al., 1977). However, at a certain critical point, an excess of KIP is reached and/or there are conformational changes so that the effect of the KIP binding becomes inhibitory. Thus small variations in the KIP/cdk ratios are required for cdk inactivation at critical points in the cell cycle (Fig. 7.4). All KIPs can inhibit the mitotic cyclin B/cdk1 complexes in cell-free systems, but introduction of KIP genes and overexpression of KIPs in cells induces G1 arrest. All three KIP family members—p21, p27 and p57—play important roles in differentiation, senescence, and cellular responses to negative growth-regulatory cytokines and to DNA damage (see below). Because they play important roles in restraining cell growth, some redundancy or functional overlap between the KIPs would, in theory, be beneficial in multicellular organisms. The cellular

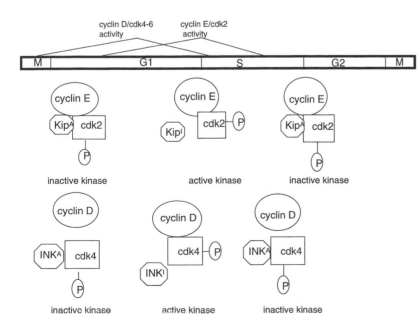

Fig. 7.4. A schematic diagram showing mechanisms of inhibition of cdks by the KIP and INK4 families of cdk inhibitors. Putative active and inactive forms of these molecules are indicated by the superscripts A and I. The KIP molecules inhibit cdks when they bind the cyclin/cdk complex. The INK4 family of inhibitors act to destabilize cyclin-cdk association and prevent reassociation of the displaced cyclin.

and tissue specificities of the three different KIP family members and which cdks they target are incompletely understood.

A second group of cdk inhibitors is the INK4 (inhibitor of cdk4) family (see Reed et al., 1994, and Sherr and Roberts, 1995, for reviews). They share a highly conserved motif that plays a role in protein/protein interactions. The INK4 proteins can inhibit specifically the cyclin D–dependent kinases, cdk4 and cdk6. The first of the INK4 genes to be cloned encodes p16 (INK4A; Serrano et al., 1993). This protein was first identified because its binding to cdk4 differed between transformed or tumor-derived cells and their normal counterparts (Xiong et al., 1993). Its gene is located on chromosome 9p13, and close to this locus lies the related p15 (INK4B/MTS2) gene (Hannon and Beach, 1994). Two other INK4 family members, p18 and p19, have been cloned recently. In contrast to the mode of action of the KIP proteins, the INK4 proteins appear to destabilize the association of the D-type cyclins with cdk4 or cdk6 (Parry et al., 1996; Sandhu et al., 1997). The INK4 proteins can displace cyclin D1 from cdk4 complexes (Fig. 7.4). The levels of p19 increase in S phase, and this inhibitor may limit cyclin D/cdk4 or cdk6 activity as cells leave G1 phase. As for the KIP family, the tissue specificities of the INK4 proteins are not fully understood. p16 appears to be important in fibroblasts and melanocytes, while p15 plays an important role in human mammary epithelial cells.

The cdk inhibitors play a role in the proliferative arrest that accompanies *differentiation*. In developing mouse embryos, p21 is localized in nonproliferating differentiated cells and its expression is prominent in skeletal muscle (Parker et al., 1995; Skapek et al., 1995). p21 is regulated in differentiating cells in both p53-dependent and independent pathways and is implicated in retinoic acid and vitamin D_3–induced differentiation of HL-60 leukemia cells (Jiang et al., 1994, Steinman et al., 1994). p27 is also induced during differentiation of HL-60 cells by vitamin D_3 (Hengst and Reed, 1996; Wang et al., 1996). The localization of p57 in mouse embryos differs somewhat from that of p21: it colocalizes with p21 in the lens epithelium and skeletal muscle but is found also in brain and cartilage (Matsuoka et al., 1995). While the KIP proteins may play a role in development, their individual function is not essential, since both p21 knockout mice (Brugarolas et al., 1995; Deng et al., 1995) and p27 knockout mice (see Chap. 3, Sec. 3.3.12) are viable. However, p27 knockout mice have multiorgan hyperplasia, indi-

cating an important antiproliferative role for this protein (Fero et al., 1996; Kiyokawa et al., 1996; Nakayama et al., 1996). There appears to be some functional redundancy among the cdk inhibitors in development.

An example of cell cycle regulators affecting differentiation is evident in muscle cell differentiation. Cyclin D1 (but not cyclins E, A, or B) can inhibit the activation of a muscle-specific gene, MyoD, and p21 and p16 overexpression can induce muscle-specific gene expression in cultured muscle cells (Skapek et al., 1995). Equally, cdk4 may regulate hemopoietic cell differentiation, as suggested by the observation that this cdk is downregulated during induced differentiation of murine erythroleukemia cells. Which combinations of KIPs and INKs play roles in the differentiation of different cell and tissue types has not yet been ascertained.

The cdk inhibitors are implicated in the G1 arrest that occurs when cultured normal cells reach the end of their finite life span in culture and undergo *senescence*. The cdk inhibitor p21 is encoded by a gene whose expression is induced as cultured fibroblasts approach the end of their finite life span (Noda et al., 1994). p16 has also been shown to increase in senescent fibroblasts (Hara et al., 1996) and different inhibitor family members may be of greater relative importance in senescence in different cell types (see Sec. 7.3.5, below).

The effects of growth factors and growth-factor receptor signal-transduction pathways on cell proliferation was discussed in Chap. 6. *Growth inhibitory cytokine* signaling pathways are less well understood. Growth-inhibitory factors mediate G1 arrest by increasing or activating the cdk inhibitors with resulting inhibition of cyclin-dependent kinases. While a number of cytokines are known to bring about G1 arrest in different cell types, the effects of transforming growth factor β (TGF-β) on cell cycle regulators are the best characterized. TGF-β is a potent growth inhibitor of many different cell types and plays important roles in growth control during development and differentiation (Massague, 1990; Moses, 1992). Loss of sensitivity to growth inhibition by TGF-β is seen in cell lines derived from many common human tumors—including adenocarcinomas, gliomas, and melanomas—and this is thought to confer a growth advantage during tumor progression (Fynan and Reiss, 1993).

TGF-β modulates cell cycle regulators to bring about cell cycle delay or arrest at the G1-to S-phase transition through a number of mechanisms (see Table 7.1; Sherr and Roberts, 1995, and references

Table 7.1. Mechanisms by Which TGF-β May Inhibit Cell Cycle Progression

Inhibits pRb phosphorylation

↓ cyclin E and cyclin A mRNAs

↑ p15^{INK4B} mRNA and protein

↑ p21^{Cip1} and p27^{Kip1} (in some cells)

↓ cdk4 and cyclin D$_1$ proteins (in some cells)

Inhibits cyclin D$_1$/cdk4, cyclin E/cdk2, and cyclin A/cdk2 activities

Increases cdk4 and cdk6 bound p15^{INK4B}

Increases cyclin E/cdk2 bound p27^{Kip1}

therein). These include inhibition of pRb phosphorylation, reduction of cyclin A and cyclin E mRNA levels and of cyclin A protein, and inhibition of cyclin E– and A–dependent kinases (Koff et al., 1993; Polyak et al., 1994; Slingerland et al., 1994). In certain cell types, TGF-β–mediated arrest involves the downregulation of cyclin D1 and cdk4 proteins, although the latter may reflect the quiescent state that follows initial arrest by TGF-β (Reynisdottir et al., 1995). The INK4 family member p15 is induced in TGF-β–sensitive cells and inhibits cdk4 and cdk6 (Hannon and Beach, 1994).

It has been proposed that the cdk inhibitors p15 and p27 cooperate to induce G1 arrest following TGF-β treatment (Reynisdottir et al., 1995). Indeed, in epithelial cells, upregulation of p15 protein and increased binding of p15 to its targets, cdk4 and cdk6, occurs concomitantly with displacement of cyclin D1 and p27 from cdk4 and an increase or stabilization of the association of p27 with cyclin E/cdk2 complexes (Reynisdottir et al., 1995; Sandhu et al., 1997). While p15 and p27 may act in concert to bring about cdk inhibition and G1 arrest in epithelial cells, this is not a universal mechanism for G1 arrest by TGF-β, since in cell lines of different tissue origin, such as melanoma cells which lack p15, p21, and p27 can cooperate to bring about G1 arrest by TGF-β (Florenes et al., 1996).

The cdk inhibitors also act to arrest the cell cycle when cells undergo DNA damage. Recent studies have demonstrated induction of the KIP protein p21, mediated by p53, in the cellular response to DNA damage by both gamma and ultraviolet (UV) irradiation (see Petrocelli et al., 1996, and references therein). The p53 protein levels increase dramatically following genomic insults and activate transcription of p21. The rise in p21 results in in-

creased binding of this inhibitor to target cdks and in kinase inhibition. Increases in p21 have been shown to result in abrupt cessation of DNA replication both in vitro and in vivo. This results from an increase in the binding of p21 to proliferating cell nuclear antigen (PCNA). PCNA acts to keep the DNA polymerase associated with the DNA template during leading strand replication. In vitro, the binding of PCNA by p21 interferes with the movement of DNA polymerase-δ along the DNA strand (Flores-Rosas et al., 1994; Waga et al., 1994). Interestingly, p21 does not inhibit DNA synthesis that is necessary for DNA repair (Li et al., 1994). The PCNA-binding and cdk inhibitor domains of the p21 protein are distinct (Chen et al., 1995; Luo et al., 1995; Warbrick et al., 1995). Thus mammalian cells appear to have evolved a mechanism to coordinate DNA repair with cell cycle arrest in response to DNA damage (see also Chap. 4, Sec. 4.4.7). This allows time to repair damaged DNA before the error becomes fixed in the genome during subsequent replicative cycles. That p21, while important, is not the only effector of cell cycle arrest in response to DNA damage is demonstrated by the G1 arrest of gamma-irradiated cells from knockout mice that lack p21 (Brugarolas et al., 1995; Deng et al., 1995). Failure to dephosphorylate the inhibitory phosphorylation sites of cdk4, and an increase in the association of p27 with target cdks have been observed during UV-irradiation-induced G1 arrest of different cell types (Poon et al., 1995; Terada et al., 1995).

7.2.4 The Cell Cycle and Cancer

Increasing evidence suggests that the cyclins, cdks, and cdk inhibitors are either themselves targets for genetic change in cancer or are disrupted secondarily by other oncogenic events (see Hunter and Pines, 1994, and Sherr, 1996, for review). The development and progression of cancer involve processes that abort differentiation, prevent cellular senescence—thereby allowing cellular immortalization, and abrogate sensitivity to growth-inhibitory cytokines. Loss of sensitivity to growth-inhibitory signals can result from changes in the positive regulators, the cyclins, or from functional loss of the cdk inhibitors. In addition, one of the hallmarks of malignant cells is genetic instability: malignant cells have developed the ability to bypass the restriction on entrance to S phase normally imposed by damaged DNA and thereby accumulate genetic changes that promote the selective outgrowth of cells with a proliferative advantage.

Overexpression of cyclins is seen in many tumors (see Hunter and Pines, 1994; Bates and Peters, 1995, and references therein). In human breast carcinomas and cell lines, aberrant cyclin E and A expression has been reported and high cyclin E levels may predict a poor prognosis. Amplification of the *cyclin E* gene has also been observed in colon carcinoma cells. Genetic changes in *cyclin D* genes—including rearrangement, translocation, and amplification—are common in human cancers. The importance of D-type cyclins in steroid-induced mammary epithelial cell growth was demonstrated by the finding that cyclin D1 knockout mice fail to undergo pregnancy-induced mammary gland proliferation (Sicinski et al., 1995). Moreover, in transgenic mice, overexpression of cyclin D1, under the control of the mouse mammary tumor virus long terminal repeat, results in mammary hyperplasia and adenocarcinomas (Wang et al., 1994). Overexpression of cyclin D1 with or without gross genetic change has been demonstrated in up to 45 percent of breast cancers. In addition, the cdc25 phosphatases, which activate cdks by dephosphorylating inhibitory sites, are also overexpressed in some human tumors (Galaktionov et al., 1995).

Genes of the *INK4* family, such as *p16*, are commonly mutated in human tumor cell lines and in some primary tumors (Hunter and Pines, 1994; Sherr and Roberts, 1995). Germline mutations in the *p16* gene confer susceptibility to melanoma and mutant *p16* alleles encode defective inhibitor proteins (Koh et al., 1995; Liu et al., 1995; Lukas et al., 1995; Ranade et al., 1995). Mutations in the *p15* and *p18* genes have been found in human tumor-derived cell lines, raising the possibility that all *INK4* family members may be regarded as tumor suppressor genes (see Chap. 5, Sec. 5.5). Findings in p16 knockout mice support a tumor suppressor role for this INK4 protein (Serrano et al., 1996). The p16 knockout mice are prone to tumor development, and cell lines derived from such mice undergo spontaneous immortalization with high frequency.

Disruption of the pathways regulating pRb activity and phosphorylation is a common theme in human neoplasia (see Chap. 4, Sec. 4.5.2, and Bates and Peters, 1995, for review). Overexpression of cyclin D or of its partner cdk4, or inactivation of p15 or p16, or of pRb itself, through mutation or other genetic events, have at least one common outcome: loss of the restraining effect of functional pRb on the transition from G1 to S phase.

Mutation of the genes encoding the KIP family members p21 and p27 are infrequent in human tumors, but there is increasing evidence that the function of these inhibitors is altered at the level of gene expression or protein stability. One consequence of *p53* mutation is the disruption of the p53/p21 response that coordinates DNA repair with cell cycle arrest, leading to the accumulation of genetically altered cells. Also, there is evidence that in some advanced malignancies, such as melanomas, downregulation of p21 protein expression occurs even when the *p53* gene is wild-type (Maelandsmo et al., 1996). Reduction in p27 protein has been observed in primary human breast and colon carcinomas, and its loss appears to correlate with increased tumor grade and poor patient prognosis (Catzavelos et al., 1997; Loda et al., 1997; Porter et al., 1997). Thus, in a number of human malignancies, the function of the cdk inhibitor may be abrogated in the absence of gene mutation. The *KIP2* locus encoding p57 lies on chromosome 11p15, a site that is rearranged or deleted in many human cancers. The possibility that *p57* may be the tumor suppressor gene at this locus is under investigation.

7.3 APOPTOSIS AND CELLULAR SENESCENCE

Development and differentiation during embryogenesis and tissue homeostasis in the mature organism require a balance of responses to proliferative stimuli and to growth-inhibitory signals. One of the physiologic processes that helps to maintain homeostasis is programmed cell death, or *apoptosis*. In addition, one of the limits to tissue growth is the proliferative arrest resulting from aging of a cell population or organism known as *cellular senescence*. These processes are reviewed below with emphasis on their relevance to cancer.

7.3.1 Apoptosis

There are two major mechanisms of cell death: necrosis and apoptosis. Necrosis is a passive response to injury in which cells swell and lyse; the release of cellular contents into the intercellular space elicits an inflammatory response. In contrast, apoptosis involves the activation of a genetic program during which cells lose viability before they lose membrane integrity, and no inflammatory response is produced.

Apoptosis is the process by which multicellular organisms eliminate cells produced in excess during embryonic and adult development or cells that are functionally abnormal, maldeveloped, or harmful. Examples include the elimination of more than 50 percent of developing neurons, regression of interdigital webs in humans, and fusion of the palate.

During turnover of normal adult tissue, apoptosis is involved in shedding of cells from the skin and intestine, regression of mammary tissue postlactation, and loss of ovarian follicles. Apoptosis is involved in immune development to eliminate self-reactive lymphocytes. During many types of viral infections, the infected cell activates its own suicide program to shut down cellular metabolism, thereby preventing the formation of new virus particles. In cells that have sustained injury, with disruption of physiologic processes or DNA damage, activation of apoptosis minimizes the risk of perpetuating or expanding aberrant, mutated, or transformed cells.

Apoptotic cells have a characteristic ultrastructural appearance (Fig. 7.5A). There is nuclear fragmentation and chromosomal condensation, followed by shrinkage of the cell and loss of contact with neighboring cells. Subsequently there is ruffling and blebbing of the cell membrane, followed by cellular fragmentation with the formation of apoptotic bodies (containing parts of the chromatin enclosed in cellular membranes), which are then phagocytosed by neighboring cells. At a molecular level, there is movement of calcium from endoplas-

mic reticulum to the cytoplasm and activation of one or more endonucleases, which cleave DNA at specific sites between nucleosomes, leading to fragments whose molecular sizes are multiples of about 180 base pairs. When the DNA of such cells is subjected to gel electrophoresis, this may lead to a characteristic ladder-like appearance (Fig. 7.5B). Apoptotic cells may be recognized by their morphologic appearance or by the appearance of these characteristic DNA ladders.

The above techniques are specific but not very sensitive: more commonly used assays are based on recognition of DNA cleavage or degradation by flow cytometry (Darzynkiewicz et al., 1994). Since apoptosis leads to activation of endonucleases and breaks in DNA, a population of cells in which a proportion are undergoing apoptosis will have a DNA histogram in which apoptotic cells have a peak with a DNA content less than that of G1 cells (due to loss of DNA during fixation and staining). More sensitive methods, such as in situ nick translation or the TUNEL assay (terminal deoxynucleotidyl transferase–mediated d-UTP transferase nick-end labeling) involve labeling of the cut ends of DNA with a

A Normal cell   Apoptotic cell   Fragmentation

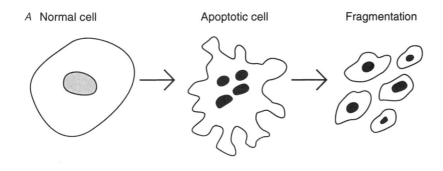

B DNA ladder

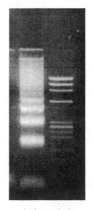

(1)   (2)

Fig. 7.5. *A.* Schematic diagram to illustrate the morphologic appearance of an apoptotic cell. Note condensation of chromatin to form apoptotic bodies and blebbing of the cell membrane. Fragmentation of the cell into membrane-bound fragments occurs subsequently. *B.* DNA ladder in apoptotic cells (lane 1). One of the final steps in the degradation phase of apoptosis involves endonuclease activation. DNA is cleaved at discrete ~180 base-pair intervals, and this gives rise to a DNA "ladder" when the DNA is subjected to gel electrophoresis. Molecular weight markers are shown in lane 2.

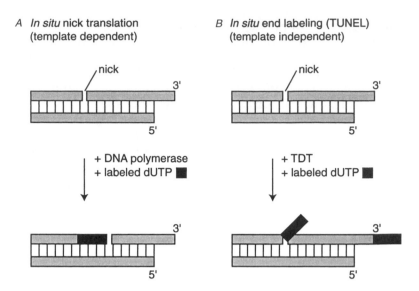

A *In situ* nick translation
   (template dependent)

B *In situ* end labeling (TUNEL)
   (template independent)

Fig. 7.6. Principles of (A) in situ nick translation and (B) the TUNEL assay for quantitating apoptotic cells. The nucleotide dUTP, labeled with fluorescein, biotin, or other marker that can be detected by using flow cytometry, is added to the breaks in DNA strands found in apoptotic cells. In (A), synthesis takes place using the opposite strand as a template; in (B), dUTP is added by the enzyme terminal deoxynucleotide transferase (TDT). (TUNEL = TDT-mediated dUTP nick-end labeling.)

fluorescent marker (e.g., biotin-conjugated dUTP; Fig. 7.6). These quantitative and sensitive methods are preferred to the assessment of apoptosis by morphologic criteria or by DNA ladders (Fig. 7.5) but will show variation with time after an apoptotic stimulus, as cells pass through the various stages of apoptotic death (Potten, 1996).

Apoptosis is brought about by mechanisms that are highly conserved from nematodes to humans (see Steller 1995, and Vaux and Stasser, 1996, for reviews). The machinery for cell death is present in all cells and can be activated without the need for de novo synthesis. Different stimuli, some of which are tissue-specific, may activate many different signaling pathways, which converge on a common effector mechanism. It is helpful to distinguish three phases of apoptosis: the *induction* or triggering phase; followed by the *effector phase*, during which the cell becomes irreversibly committed to death; and finally the *degradation phase* (Fig. 7.7; Bright and Khar, 1994; Kroemer et al., 1995; Vaux and Strasser, 1996).

7.3.2 Induction of Apoptosis

Cells in many tissues require hormones or growth factors to maintain survival and/or proliferation. Lack of these survival signals leads to apoptosis of many cell types. During development, this prevents the inappropriate migration and proliferation of progenitor cells in the wrong environment; for example, developing neurons require neurotropic factors. In some cell types, direct death signals can be transmitted through the interaction of cytokines with cell surface receptors (Cleveland and Ihle,

1995; Nagata and Golstein, 1995). An important example of this is the interaction of cytokines with cell-surface receptors, which leads to apoptosis of T-cell subsets, thereby modulating immune responses. When the Fas receptor on a T lymphocyte interacts with its ligand, the activated receptor then binds to signaling proteins via highly conserved sites of protein/protein interaction called *death domains,* which initiate intracellular signals leading to apoptosis.

Apoptosis is also activated when a cell receives confusing growth-regulatory signals in which both "stop" and "go" signals are triggered simultaneously. For example, the activation of the proto-oncogene *c-myc*, which usually provides a proliferative signal, may lead to apoptosis in the absence of an appropriate growth factor. Another paradoxical signal for apoptosis is the overexpression of G1 cyclins or dysregulation of other cell cycle components. The study of apoptosis is confusing because genes involved in normal proliferation can become triggers of apoptosis if activated inappropriately.

A major trigger of apoptosis is cellular injury (Kroemer et al., 1995). Anticancer drugs as well as ionizing and UV radiation cause a variety of types of damage to cells, including various types of lesions in DNA. Following such injury, many cells have been observed to undergo apoptosis; this process requires the involvement of p53 (Canman and Kastan, 1995). The observation of apoptosis after various types of anticancer treatment has stimulated much research into methods of enhancing the apoptotic process selectively in order to increase the responsiveness of tumor cells to treatment (see also Chap. 17, Sec. 17.2.8). The potential success of this re-

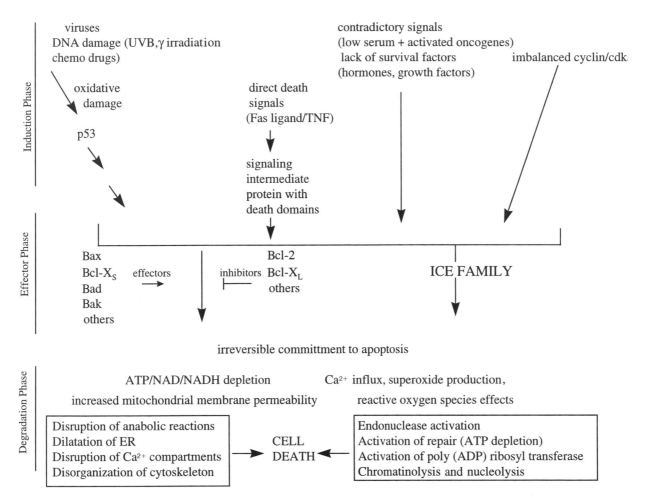

Fig. 7.7. The process of apoptosis. Multiple stimuli can initiate induction of apoptosis. This is followed by an effector phase, which involves positive effectors, the ICE-family proteases. The balance of apoptotic inhibitors and effectors regulate apoptosis in certain cell types and following certain stimuli. The final or degradation phase ensues with irreversible commitment to cell death.

search depends on the subtle but important distinction between (1) apoptosis as a mechanism for eliminating cells that have already sustained lethal and irreversible damage (modification of apoptosis may then influence the timing of cell lysis, but not the overall number of cells that are killed) and (2) apoptosis as a mechanism that is activated by potentially reversible injury and which could then influence the number of the cells that will proceed to cell death and lysis (Smets, 1994). Thus, stimulation of apoptosis might influence decisions between cell death and survival *if* the pathway can be stimulated by levels of cellular damage that are potentially reversible. Unfortunately the majority of studies have only observed or quantitated apoptosis after treatment with anticancer agents and do not give information that allows assessment of whether the apop-

totic process is a cause or effect of lethal injury. A few studies have suggested the importance of apoptosis as a mechanism leading to lethal damage by demonstrating change in cellular sensitivity to damaging agents after transfection of genes such as *bax* or *bcl-2* (see Sec. 7.3.3) that up- or downregulate apoptotic pathways, respectively (e.g., Hu et al., 1995; Zanke et al., 1996), but others have found no influence on cell survival as assessed by a colony-forming assay (Yin and Schimke, 1995).

7.3.3 Regulation of Apoptosis

Studies of development in the nematode *Caenorhabtidis elegans* have led to the discovery of genes whose function is critical for programmed cell death during development (Ellis et al., 1991; Hengartner and

Horvitz, 1994). Two genes, *ced-3* and *ced-4,* have been found to encode essential effectors of apoptosis. While the function of *ced-4* remains unknown, *ced-3* encodes a cysteine protease, indicating that apoptosis is dependent on proteolytic cleavage of one or more essential substrates. Another gene, *ced-9,* encodes a product that inhibits apoptosis. Inactivating mutations of *ced-9* result in death of the organism, suggesting that apoptosis is an active process that must be controlled and inhibited for cell survival.

Mammalian cells contain several *ced-3* homologues that appear to be effectors of apoptosis (Vaux and Strasser, 1996; White, 1996). These include interleukin 1β converting enzyme (ICE), which plays a role in immune cell apoptosis; CPP35 or prICE, which cleaves and inactivates poly(ADP-ribose) polymerase, a DNA repair enzyme; and a variety of other proteins. These cysteine proteases (known as *ICE proteases* or *caspases*) are all activated by cleavage of precursor molecules and by the formation of heterotetramers—i.e., the joining of four subunits of different family members. This capacity for heterogeneity may allow activity against a variety of substrates and increase the complexity of apoptotic signaling pathways. Programmed cell death can be inhibited by protease inhibitors. Although the ICE proteases are ubiquitously expressed, their enforced overexpression following transfection triggers apoptosis, suggesting that a threshold level of expression may be required for induction of apoptosis. Activation of ICE proteases is not needed for all forms of apoptosis. For example, developmental cell death and radiation-induced death of lymphocytes do not involve these proteases.

The first of the negative regulators of apoptosis to be identified in mammalian cells was the *bcl-2* gene (reviewed in Korsmeyer, 1995; Vaux and Strasser, 1996; and White, 1996), which is translocated and overexpressed in human B-cell follicular lymphomas. The *bcl-2* gene shares sequence homology with *C. elegans ced-9,* and it can compensate for *ced-9* mutation in *C. elegans.* Several *bcl-2* homologues have been cloned. *Mcl-2* acts like *bcl-2* and protects against apoptosis. Another gene, *bcl-x,* encodes two proteins: Bcl-x$_L$ (L = long) inhibits apoptosis, while Bcl-x$_S$ (S = short), the shorter protein product, stimulates apoptosis. Four other homologues Bax, Bak, Nbk1/Bik1, and Bad, all antagonize Bcl-2 and promote apoptosis. These proteins interact via highly conserved domains, forming homo- or heterodimers. The ratio of activator/inhibitor determines whether induction or inhibition of apoptosis occurs; thus a predominance of Bax/Bax dimers induces apoptosis, while Bcl-2/Bax dimers do not. However, overexpression of *bcl-2* does not inhibit apoptosis in all cell types, nor does it inhibit all different triggers in any one cell type.

During apoptosis, there is a rapid and sustained increase in intracellular calcium, an increase in mitochondrial membrane permeability with consequent loss of membrane potential, breakdown of energy metabolism, uncoupling of the respiratory chain, release of mitochondrial calcium, increased production of superoxide anions, and depletion of glutathione (Kroemer et al., 1995). Bcl-2 is bound to mitochondrial membranes, as are its antagonists, Bax and Bcl-x$_S$; in at least some cell types, this binding is essential for function of Bcl-2. Bcl-2 has pleiotropic effects that include inhibition of calcium efflux from the endoplasmic reticulum, blocking of the transport of p53 from nucleus to cytoplasm, and enhancement of the mitochondrial membrane potential and synthesis of ATP.

Not only is there a multiplicity of different stimuli that trigger apoptosis, but lineage-specific signaling pathways exist and multiple ICE-family effectors and Bcl-2-like inhibitors confer diversity and lineage specificity to effector mechanisms. Nonetheless, all apoptotic triggers converge on a final pathway (the degradation phase), when cells reach the point of irreversible commitment to death. Activation of the ICE proteases, calcium influx, and loss of mitochondrial membrane potential result in depletion of ATP and NAD/NADH, changes in intracellular signaling, oxidative damage to cellular membranes, disruption of intracellular compartments, dilatation of the endoplasmic reticulum, cross-linking of cytoplasmic proteins, and cell shrinkage. Within the nucleus there is activation of endonucleases, especially the Ca^{2+}/Mg^{2+}-dependent endonuclease, which cleaves DNA at nucleosomal cross-linker regions. Activation of DNA repair enzymes further depletes energy stores of NAD and ATP. Calmodulin may play a role in this process, as its antagonists inhibit DNA fragmentation. Finally, cells undergo fragmentation, with the formation of apoptotic bodies and engulfment by neighboring cells (Fig. 7.5).

7.3.4 Apoptosis and Cancer

Defects in genes that control apoptosis and the rescue of cells normally destined for destruction can promote cancer development or result in autoimmune disease. In contrast, excessive activation of apoptosis is involved in the pathogenesis of neurodegenerative diseases, myocardial infarction, and

AIDS. Many cancer cells have reduced ability to undergo apoptosis in response to both physiologic stimuli and to DNA damage. Loss of the ability to respond to DNA damage with either cell cycle arrest and repair or activation of apoptosis results in one of the hallmarks of the malignant cell: genetic instability. In addition, cancer cells tolerate marked dysregulation of cell cycle proteins, such as the overexpression of cyclins, without undergoing apoptosis, as would their nontransformed counterparts. Increased production of Bcl-2 protein is observed in many human tumors and correlates with a poor prognosis in carcinomas of the colon and prostate and in neuroblastoma. Overexpression of Bcl-2 or Bcl-x$_L$ proteins may also confer resistance to chemotherapeutic drugs. Because induction of apoptosis by DNA damage requires wild-type p53, the mutational inactivation of p53, which occurs very commonly in human cancer, abrogates at least one cellular pathway for elimination of genetically aberrant cells.

An increased understanding of the molecular controls regulating apoptosis might ultimately generate novel and more effective treatments for cancer. Nonspecific activators of apoptosis would be of limited benefit because of their potential to induce cell loss in many tissues. Manipulation of tumor cells with decreased ability to undergo apoptosis might lead to partial restoration of growth control and/or increased sensitivity to therapeutic agents.

7.3.5 Cellular Senescence

Normal cells grown in tissue culture will divide a finite number of times, even if passaged serially to prevent depletion of nutrients or crowding. They eventually reach a point where they remain viable but cease proliferation (Hayflick, 1965). They can remain in a nonproliferative state for a prolonged period. This is referred to as *proliferative senescence* and is thought to correlate with cellular aging in vivo. In contrast, many cell lines derived from advanced cancers can proliferate indefinitely in tissue culture. The loss of cellular senescence after malignant transformation of cells in tissue culture is thought to reflect the same process that occurs during cancer development and progression.

Telomeres, composed of protein and simple DNA sequences, cap the ends of chromosomes and protect them from recombination and degradation. The enzyme *telomerase* is required to replicate the telomeric DNA prior to cell division. In embryonic cells, germ cells, and certain mature cells such as lymphocytes, which maintain replicative capacity throughout adult life, the telomerase gene is active. However, in most somatic cells in vivo, telomerase is turned off. Telomeric DNA is lost every time somatic cells divide, presumably because of the inability of DNA polymerase to fully replicate the ends of a linear DNA template and because the telomerase enzyme, which elongates telomeric DNA, is inactive in most somatic cells. The shortening of telomeres as cells age is thought to act as a mitotic clock, regulating the number of divisions a cell may undergo and triggering cellular senescence. As a cell population ages, telomeres shorten to the point that they can no longer stabilize chromosome ends, leading to the formation of unstable dicentric chromosomes. It is postulated that cells recognize shortened telomeres as "damaged" DNA, with a resultant increase in the cell cycle inhibitor p21 (reviewed in Bacchetti and Counter, 1995). Indeed, p21 was cloned as a gene upregulated in senescent cells (Noda et al., 1994).

In many immortal and malignant cell lines, telomerase is active and lengthening of telomeres is observed. The molecular mechanisms that cause the loss of the senescence checkpoint and induction of telomerase in cancers are largely unknown. However, telomerase might be an appropriate target for anticancer therapy, since inhibition of this enzyme might restore senescence to cancer cells, eventually resulting in inhibition of tumor growth (see Chap. 15, Sec. 15.5.3)

7.4 ASSESSMENT OF CELL KINETICS

7.4.1 Tritiated Thymidine and Autoradiography

Cell proliferation in vitro and in vivo has been studied extensively by using autoradiography to detect uptake of radioactive thymidine into cellular DNA. Autoradiographs are prepared by coating thin sections of tissue or cell monolayers on a glass microscope slide with a photographic emulsion and exposing them in light-tight boxes (usually for 1 to 4 weeks) followed by development and fixation. The cell nuclei that have incorporated the isotope during thymidine exposure can then be identified. The proportion of labeled cells at a short interval after administration of tritiated thymidine (the *labeling index*) is a measure of the proportion of cells that were in S phase. All of the basic concepts of cell kinetics have been derived from experiments using tritiated thymidine and autoradiography. This technique has the advantage of allowing studies of morphologically distinct cell populations in situ (Steel,

1977), but it is rather laborious and has been largely replaced by flow cytometry (see Sec. 7.4.2).

Thymidine labeling has been used to estimate the cell-cycle time T_c and the duration of individual phases of the cell cycle. In the *percent-labeled-mitoses* (PLM) method, serial biopsies (or serial specimens from identical animals) are taken at intervals after a single injection of ³H-thymidine, and the proportion of mitotic cells that are labeled is estimated from autoradiographs prepared from these biopsies (see Steel, 1977, for details). While this method is technically difficult, PLM is one of the few methods that has allowed estimation of the duration of different cell cycle phases in human tumors and normal tissues (see Sec. 7.6)

In many normal tissues of the adult, only a small proportion of the cells is actively proliferating. Of the remaining cells, many are either differentiated or quiescent. Examples of the latter include stem cells in the bone marrow (Sec. 7.5.1), cells in skin that participate in wound healing after damage, and hepatocytes that proliferate after partial hepatectomy. These noncycling cells that retain their capacity for proliferation are referred to as a G0 population (Fig. 7.1). Most tumors also contain nonproliferating cells, and the term *growth fraction* was defined by Mendelsohn (1960) as the proportion of cells in the tumor population that is proliferating. Growth fraction can be determined by thymidine labeling and autoradiography (Steel, 1977), but alternative (and now preferred) methods for estimation of the growth fraction are based on distinguishing proliferating and nonproliferating cells by the presence or absence of specific enzymes or antigens. These proliferation-dependent markers may be detected by flow cytometry, as described in Sec. 7.4.3. Although approximate, the estimate of growth fraction is useful, since most anticancer drugs are more toxic to proliferating cells (see Chap. 15, Sec. 15.2.4) and growth fraction therefore indicates the proportion of tumor cells that might be sensitive to cycle-dependent chemotherapy.

Some quiescent tumor cells may be able to return to a proliferative state if their local environment changes, as might occur after tumor treatment, and such nonproliferating cells may be a cause of tumor resistance to cycle-dependent chemotherapy. The molecular stimuli that lead to initiation of DNA synthesis and passage through the cell cycle are described in Sec. 7.2.

The frequent occurrence of extensive necrosis and of apoptotic cells in tumors and the ability of tumor cells to metastasize from a primary tumor suggest that there may be considerable cell death or loss from tumors. The rate of cell loss from tumors can be estimated by comparing the rate of cell production (from assessment of the labeling index or fraction of S phase cells by flow cytometry) with the rate of tumor growth. The overall rate of cell production may be characterized by the potential doubling time of the tumor (T_{pot}), which is the expected doubling time of the tumor in the absence of cell loss. The value of T_{pot} is usually much shorter than the measured volume doubling time because of extensive cell loss in human tumors (Steel, 1977).

Normal tissues, such as bone marrow or intestine, contain a limited population of stem cells and other precursor cells, which are defined by their potential for regenerating all or part of the population. There is indirect evidence that many tumors also contain a relatively small population of stem cells (Sec. 7.6.2.). The existence of stem cells is documented through clonogenic assays that allow them to express their proliferative potential by forming colonies of progeny in an appropriate environment. Information analogous to the labeling index may be obtained for stem cells by comparing colony formation by untreated cells and by cells treated with high-specific-activity ³H-thymidine (the *"thymidine suicide method;"* Becker et al., 1965). Those cells that are synthesizing DNA at the time of thymidine administration will be killed by radiation damage from the high dose of tritium, leading to a reduction in the number of colonies: thus proliferative rate of the stem cells is related to the reduction in number of colonies that are formed. Drugs specific for the S phase of the cell cycle, such as hydroxyurea or methotrexate (see Chap. 15, Sec. 15.2.4), may be used instead of ³H-thymidine. This method fails to quantitate stem cells that do not generate colonies under the experimental conditions of the clonogenic assay, but it remains one of the few means of estimating proliferation within stem cell populations.

7.4.2 Principles of Flow Cytometry

The study of cell kinetics has been facilitated by the use of flow cytometry to determine cellular DNA content, which has the advantage over autoradiography of speed and automation. A schematic illustration of a flow cytometer is shown in Fig. 7.8. A single-cell suspension is prepared and cells are stained with a fluorescent dye whose binding (to DNA) is proportional to DNA content. Cells are then directed in single file through a laser beam to excite

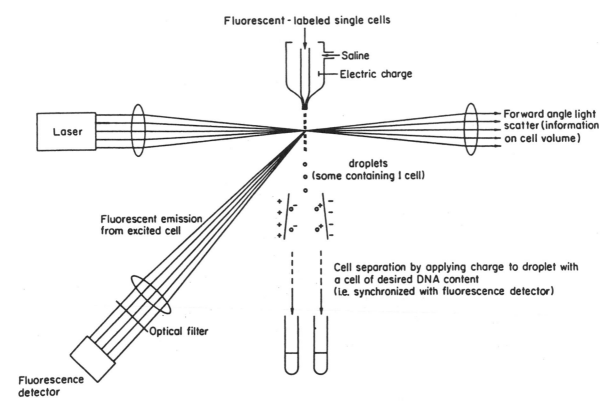

Fig. 7.8. The principle of flow cytometry and cell sorting. Single cells stained with a fluorescent dye whose uptake is proportional to DNA content are directed through a laser beam. Fluorescence measurements give a distribution of DNA content, and forward angle light scatter gives information about cell volume. Charge may be applied to droplets containing cells of different DNA content, so that they may be deflected in an electrostatic field and sorted.

the DNA-specific dye, and the fluorescence emission is collected and displayed as a fluorescence distribution. The technique allows enumeration of cells containing different quantities of fluorescent dye, and thus different amounts of DNA. More sophisticated instruments are capable of sorting cells with different fluorescence intensities for further biochemical and/or morphologic studies (Fig. 7.8).

Several fluorescent dyes have been used to stain DNA, including ethidium bromide, propidium iodide, acridine orange, mithramycin, and Hoechst 33342. Acridine orange can be used to separate and sort cells on the basis of both DNA content (green fluorescence, from staining double-stranded DNA) and RNA content (red fluorescence, from staining single-stranded RNA). Acridine orange has also been used to discriminate between G1 cells (which have abundant RNA) and nonproliferating subpopulations (which have low RNA content). Most dyes require fixation of the cells to allow access of dye to the DNA, although selected DNA specific dyes (e.g.,

Hoechst 33342) can enter viable cells; the Hoechst stain is a prototype for vital dyes that are minimally toxic to the cells. Use of vital DNA stains allows isolation of different cell populations according to DNA content by fluorescence-activated cell sorting. Numerous other reagents are available, including fluorescence-labeled antibodies against cellular antigens, which allow separation of cells according to expression of specific proteins. Often, fluorescent reagents are applied concurrently or sequentially to allow for analysis or separation of cells on the basis of two or more criteria (such as the expression of a specific protein and DNA content). Information about cell size may be obtained from analysis of scattered light. Multiparameter analyses are particularly useful in the study of heterogeneous tissue samples.

The application of flow cytometry to studies of cell cycle distribution requires analysis of a fluorescent DNA distribution (Fig. 7.9) to provide estimates of the proportion of cells with 2N DNA content (i.e., G1 and most nonproliferating cells), 4N

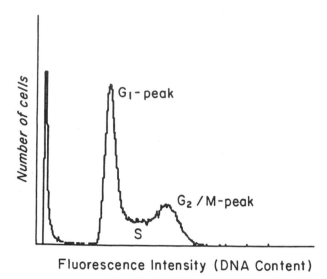

Fig. 7.9. DNA distribution for a human bladder cancer cell line produced by flow cytometry. Cells were stained with acridine orange. The peak at the origin represents cellular debris.

DNA content (G2 and mitotic cells) and intermediate DNA content (S phase cells). DNA distributions are analyzed by computer, using a number of mathematical models that allow estimation of the proportion of cells in each phase of the cycle. In tumors, the presence of aneuploidy (i.e., a G1-phase DNA content different from that of normal cells) and of variable DNA content among G1 cells complicates analysis of DNA distributions and the estimation of cell-cycle parameters. The proportion of S phase cells obtained from a DNA distribution is analogous to the thymidine labeling index and gives a broad indication of the proliferative rate.

Flow cytometry can be applied to the study of fixed tissue that is stored in paraffin blocks. A technique for dissolving the paraffin, followed by dispersion and staining of the cells, was developed by Hedley and his colleagues (reviewed in Hedley, 1989). This technique provides a useful retrospective analysis of the relationship of kinetic parameters of human tumors to subsequent outcome of treatment of the patients (see Sec. 7.6.4).

7.4.3. Analysis of Cell Kinetics by Flow Cytometry

Flow cytometry can be used to estimate cell-cycle phase distribution, growth fraction, and kinetic properties of cell populations. Minimally toxic nonradioactive precursors, such as 5-bromodeoxyuridine (BrdUrd), are incorporated into the newly synthesized DNA and can be recognized by flow cytometry using commercially available monoclonal antibodies. Application of a DNA stain such as propidium iodide allows one to distinguish cells with an intermediate DNA content (>2N and <4N) that are or are not actively synthesizing DNA at the time of exposure. The method may be used to study the proliferative rate of an unperturbed cell population or to identify a population of cells that has been arrested during the S phase following a genotoxic insult.

Administration of BrdUrd to an unperturbed cell population leads to the labeling of a cohort of cells that is originally in S phase and then moves through the cell cycle. Application of a DNA stain (e.g., propidium iodide) at intervals after administration of BrdUrd, with two-parameter flow cytometry to recognize both propidium iodide and BrdUrd in DNA using a fluorescence-labeled antibody, thus allows this cohort of cells to be followed as it passes around the cell cycle. This method is analogous to the older PLM technique using ^{3}H-thymidine and autoradiography. It is possible to obtain estimates of potential doubling time (T_{pot}) and the duration of S phase (T_s) from a single biopsy of a human tumor after intravenous injection of BrdUrd (Fig. 7.10; Wilson et al., 1988; Begg et al., 1990). Interest in this method has been stimulated by recognition of the importance of cell proliferation between treatments as a potential cause of failure of radiotherapy to eradicate tumors, and similar effects may limit cell killing with chemotherapy. Clinical trials are being performed to determine whether rapidly proliferating tumors (as defined by a short T_{pot} using the above method) are better treated by giving radiation treatments in a shorter overall treatment time (see Chap. 14, Sec. 14.4.1).

Several methods allow proliferating and nonproliferating cells to be distinguished by flow cytometry. Nonproliferating cells usually synthesize less RNA than proliferating cells in G1 phase, and staining with acridine orange gives equal green (i.e., DNA) fluorescence but greater red (i.e., RNA) fluorescence for cells in G1 phase as compared with quiescent cells. A variety of cellular antigens [e.g., Ki-67; proliferating cell nuclear antigen (PCNA)] appear to be expressed uniquely in cycling cells and can be recognized by fluorescence-labeled antibodies. The Ki-67 antigen (Gerdes et al., 1984) has been used most often as a marker for proliferating cells. Expression of proliferation-associated antigens by human cancer cells may provide useful information about prognosis. The development of monoclonal antibodies that recognize specific cyclins expressed at different times during the mitotic cycle (see Sec.

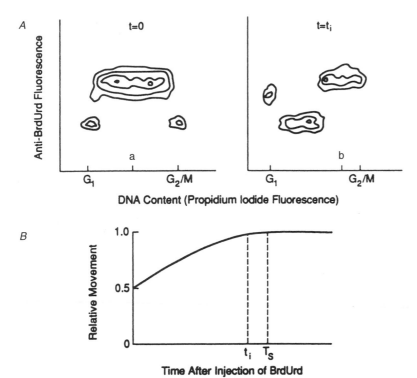

Fig. 7.10. Use of BrdUrd and flow cytometry to estimate the duration of DNA synthesis, T_s. *A.* Distribution of cells with or without incorporated BrdUrd (recognized by a fluorescent monoclonal antibody) versus DNA content immediately after injection of BrdUrd, and at time t_i later. BrdUrd-labeled cells are initially in S phase and then move through G2 and M phase to appear in G1 after cell division. *B.* To estimate T_s, the relative movement (RM) of the cohort of cells labeled with BrdUrd is plotted against time. RM is defined as the mean difference in DNA content of BrdUrd-containing cells (ignoring those that have already divided) and G1 cells (i.e., b–a on the horizontal axes of panel *A*), divided by the mean difference in DNA content of G2/M-phase and G1-phase cells (Begg et al., 1985). RM increases almost linearly with time from a value of about 0.5 at $t = 0$ to a value = 1.0 at time T_s, so that T_s can be calculated by extrapolation from the RM (from DNA content) of the BrdUrd-containing cells at time t_i.

7.2.2) may allow further analysis of cell kinetic parameters by flow cytometry and of their value as markers of prognosis.

Analysis of DNA distributions does not provide information about the proliferative status of *clonogenic cells*, such as stem cells, in normal tissues or tumors. However, cells can be sorted on the basis of their DNA content after staining with nontoxic fluorescent drugs, thus allowing subsequent study of their clonogenic capacity and other properties. This method can be used after treatment with radiation or anticancer drugs to provide information about the cell cycle distribution of clonogenic cells that survive such treatment. Unfortunately, currently available vital stains such as Hoechst 33342 are sometimes cytotoxic; these toxic effects depend on the cell population and may be complicated by interactions of the dye with radiation or anticancer drugs.

An alternative method for studying the cell kinetics of clonogenic cells involves the combined use of flow cytometry and *centrifugal elutriation*. Centrifugal elutriation separates cells on the basis of size and density in a continuous-flow centrifuge, and since cells increase in volume as they pass through the cell cycle, it can lead to separation of viable cells in different phases. Replicate samples of these separated cells can then be studied for colony formation and for DNA distribution using flow cytometry. This method has been used to study the cycle-dependent effects of drugs and radiation on clonogenic cells in experimental tumors (e.g., Grdina et al., 1980; Keng et al., 1990).

7.4.4 Other Applications of Flow Cytometry

Flow cytometry is playing an increasing role in the diagnosis and histologic classification of tumors. About 70 percent of human tumors contain cells with abnormal DNA content. The detection of a small number of malignant cells in an effusion or biopsy that contains mainly nonmalignant (inflammatory) cells is often difficult with conventional histology and light microscopy. If the tissue is dispersed and stained with a DNA stain, subsequent flow cytometry can detect a small population of malignant aneuploid cells. Technical refinements may lead to use of this technique as an alternative to conventional cytology for detection of cervical, bladder, and other types of cancer.

The ploidy status of a tumor is often described by the DNA index, which is the ratio of the DNA content of tumor cells in G1 phase to that in normal diploid cells. Tumors may be aneuploid with a DNA index greater than one and may contain subpopulations with differing DNA content. Diploid tumors tend to have a better prognosis than aneuploid tumors (see Sec. 7.6.4).

Flow cytometry is being used to sort individual chromosomes from cells based on fluorescent probes that recognize specific sequences of human chromosomes (Monard and Young, 1995). This flow cytometric modification of fluorescence in situ hybridization (FISH; see Chap. 3, Sec. 3.4.4) is a powerful technique that allows the rapid classification of chromosomes in aneuploid tumors and can recognize translocations of chromosomes and their associated genes.

The increasing availability of monoclonal antibodies that can be fluorescence-labeled makes flow cytometry a powerful tool for defining the distribution of antigenic properties among the cells of a population. The method is already in wide use to define subtypes of human leukemia and lymphoma, using fluorescence-labeled monoclonal antibodies directed against surface antigens. The method is useful as a guide to treatment, since different subtypes of leukemia and lymphoma are responsive to different types of treatment.

Flow cytometry may aid in the diagnosis of B-cell lymphomas, which are sometimes difficult to distinguish from benign lymphoid reactions by light microscopy. An important difference is that most lymphomas are clonal (i.e., derived from a single cell, see Sec. 7.6.2) and therefore express only one type of immunoglobulin. In particular, B cells express either κ or λ light chains on their cell surface, but not both. When nonclonal populations of lymphocytes are stained with fluorescent antibodies that recognize only κ or only λ light chains, the fluorescence distributions are similar. If, however, a malignant clone is present that expresses only κ chains, the fluorescence distributions of the lymphoid population stained with anti-κ antibody will be different from that stained with anti-λ antibody. This method has been shown to be sufficiently sensitive to detect 5 to 10 percent of malignant monoclonal B cells among an otherwise polyclonal population (Ault, 1979).

Flow cytometry is being used to define a number of phenotypic properties that may be important for the prognosis or treatment of different types of cancer. Examples include receptors for growth factors and protein products of oncogenes. The method can be applied to detect markers of drug resistance, such as P-glycoprotein (see Chap. 17, Sec. 17.2.4), or to assess the uptake of fluorescent drugs (e.g., doxorubicin) into cells. Because flow cytometry samples a large number of individual cells, it has the advantage of providing a distribution of phenotypic properties in the cell population and can identify variant subpopulations. This is particularly impor-

tant in studies of therapeutic resistance, since a small resistant subpopulation may regenerate the tumor following treatment.

7.5 CELL PROLIFERATION IN NORMAL TISSUES

Thymidine labeling or flow cytometry may be used to compare the overall rate of cell proliferation in a variety of normal tissues (Table 7.2). Although this classification is based on estimates of the labeling index in mice, more limited data in humans indicate that the relative rates of proliferation in different tissues are similar to those in the mouse, although absolute rates of cellular proliferation tend to be slower in humans.

The classification of Table 7.2 is of interest because the side effects of chemotherapy that are common to many drugs (e.g., myelosuppression, mucositis, hair loss, and sterility) are observed in rapidly proliferating tissues, reflecting the greater activity of most anticancer drugs against proliferating cells (see Chap. 15, Sec. 15.2.4). Acute effects of radiation injury are also observed in these tissues. Detailed discussion of the cell kinetics of normal tissue is beyond the scope of this book, but hemopoietic cells in the bone marrow and epithelial cells in the intestine are described as examples of renewal tissues in which the pattern of cell proliferation is an important determinant of anticancer therapy.

7.5.1 Hemopoietic Cells and Growth Factors

Studies of morphologically recognizable cells in bone marrow and blood have established an orderly progression of differentiation from myeloblasts to polymorphonuclear granulocytes, from pronormoblasts to red blood cells, and from megakaryocytes to platelets (Fig. 7.11). Characterization of

Table 7.2. Proliferative Rates of Selected Normal Tissues in Adults

Rapid	Slow	None
Bone marrow	Lung	Muscle
GI mucosa	Liver	Bone
Ovary	Kidney	Cartilage
Testis	Endocrine glands	Nerve
Hair follicles	Vascular endothelium	

Note: Acute side effects of chemotherapy occur commonly in rapidly proliferating tissue.

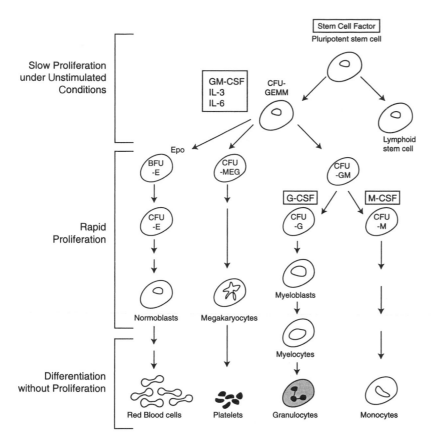

Fig. 7.11. Schematic diagram of the differentiation of hemopoietic precursor cells in the bone marrow, leading to the production of red blood cells, platelets, granulocytes, and monocytes. Various cells are stimulated to proliferate and/or differentiate by the growth factors IL-3, GM-CSF, G-CSF, M-CSF, erythropoietin (EPO), stem cell factor, and others (see Table 7.3); only their main target cells are indicated here. Under normal conditions, the early precursor cells proliferate slowly, intermediate precursors proliferate rapidly (in the megakaryocytic series there is nuclear replication without cell division) to expand the population, and later precursors of the functional cells differentiate without further cell division.

the earlier bone-marrow precursor cells shown in Fig. 7.11 has evolved from experiments in which it was found that conditioned medium (i.e., medium exposed to other cell populations) could stimulate proliferation and/or differentiation of cells in bone marrow, leading to production of more mature cells of a certain type (e.g., erythrocytes or granulocytes). Subsequently, the stimulant molecules were purified and their genes were cloned and sequenced (Table 7.3; Moore 1995).

The presence of a hemopoietic stem cell was inferred by the presence of common clonal markers in cells of both the granulocytic and lymphoid series (see also Sec. 7.6.2). Stem cells may be recognized by the expression on their cell surface of the CD34 antigen and the tyrosine kinase receptors known as c-kit and Flk-2/Flk-3; unlike other CD34-positive early precursor cells that are committed in their pathway of differentiation, stem cells do not express other antigens that are related to differentiation (Messner, 1995). These surface properties may be used to enrich stem cells and other early precursors from samples of bone marrow or peripheral blood by fluorescence-activated cell sorting. The pluripo-

tential stem cell may undergo self-renewal or may produce progeny that are either early precursor cells for lymphocytes or cells referred to as CFU-GEMM, which under appropriate conditions in culture will form colonies (CFU = colony-forming unit) containing cells of the granulocyte (G), erythroid (E), megakaryocyte (M), and monocyte (M) series. Further proliferation and differentiation produces precursor cells whose progency are bone-marrow cells of a given lineage (Fig. 7.11).

Growth factors that act on hemopoietic cells include a growing number of polypeptides referred to as *interleukins*, some of which are important in various types of immunological response (see Chap. 11, Sec. 11.3.5). Several of these growth factors act in concert to stimulate stem cells to proliferate, including stem-cell factor (also known as Kit-ligand), IL-1, IL-3, and IL-6 (Moore, 1995; Table 7.3). Considerable clinical experience has been obtained with the recombinant growth factors, granulocyte-macrophage colony-stimulating factor (GM-CSF), and granulocyte colony-stimulating factor (G-CSF). Both of these growth factors have been shown to decrease the duration and extent of myelosuppression after chemotherapy, and

Table 7.3. Selected Hemopoietic Growth Factors and the Target-Cell Population That Is Stimulated[a]

Growth Factor	Target-Cell Population
Stem-cell factor (Kit ligand)	Bone marrow stem cells
Interleukin 1 (IL-1)	Stimulates stromal cells to produce other factors (IL-6, GM-CSF, G-CSF)
Interleukin 3 (IL-3) Interleukin 6 (IL-6) Granulocyte macrophage colony-stimulating factor (GM-CSF)	Early multipotential cells (CFU-GEMM and others; see Fig. 7.11)
Granulocyte colony-stimulating factor (G-CSF)	Early cells in granulocytic series (CFU-G)
Erythropoietin (Epo)	Early red cell precursors (BFU-E, CFU-E)

[a]The interaction of growth factors to stimulate different types of cells is complex, and several growth factors have auxiliary effects to stimulate other types of precursor cells.

G-CSF is used widely to lower the incidence of infection and hospitalization (Chap. 15, Sec. 15.4.1). The growth factors GM-CSF, G-CSF, and erythropoietin may also influence stem cell proliferation, but they exert greater activity to stimulate committed precursor cells, as indicated in Table 7.3.

The hormone erythropoietin, which is produced by the kidney, is a relatively specific stimulant of red blood cell precursors. Aberrant production of erythropoietin by rare types of kidney cancer can cause polycythemia (excess red blood cells), while decreased production in renal disease may explain the anemia that usually accompanies kidney failure. Administration of recombinant erythropoietin is proving useful in the treatment of certain types of anemia, including those associated with malignancy.

Within cell lineages, thymidine-labeling studies have demonstrated a high rate of cell proliferation of the recognizable immature cells, with estimates of the labeling index (LI) for human myeloblasts ranging from about 30 to 75 percent. Estimates of cell-cycle time obtained by using the percent-labeled-mitoses technique have confirmed that recognizable precursors of granulocytes and red cells are among the most rapidly proliferating cells in the human body, with a mean duration of S phase (T_s) and mean cell cycle time (T_c) of about 12 and 24 h, respectively (Stryckmans et al., 1966; Todo, 1968). The more mature cells in each series undergo differentiation without proliferation (Fig. 7.11). The thymidine suicide method (Sec. 7.4.1) has been used to study the cell kinetics of early bone-marrow precursors. Stem cells and other early precursor cells proliferate quite slowly under resting conditions (Messner, 1995), and their more rapidly proliferating progeny provide replacement for the normal loss of mature cells, as shown in Fig. 7.11. However, stem cells may proliferate rapidly to restore the bone-marrow population following depletion of more mature forms (e.g., by cancer chemotherapy) or after bone-marrow ablation and transplantation.

The pattern of proliferation and differentiation in the bone marrow provides an explanation for the decrease in mature granulocytes at 10 to 14 days after cycle-active chemotherapy and their recovery by 21 to 28 days. The rapidly proliferating intermediate precursor cells (Fig. 7.11) are most likely to be killed by chemotherapy. Effects on cells in the peripheral blood are not seen immediately because the later-maturing cells are nonproliferating and tend to be spared by chemotherapy. Recovery occurs when earlier precursors are stimulated to proliferate (see also Chap. 15, Sec. 15.4.1). The proliferative stimulus to early precursor cells that follows loss of the mature functional cells is mediated in part by the growth factors described above.

7.5.2 Intestine

The functional part of the small intestine consists of numerous villi that project into the lumen and provide a large absorptive surface (Fig. 7.12). The villi are lined by a single layer of differentiated epithelial cells that do not proliferate. Apoptotic cell death accounts for the high rate of loss of these cells. These cells are replaced by upward migration of cells lining crypts, which lie between and at the base of the villi, where there is a rapid rate of cell proliferation. Cell division also takes place in crypts in the large intestine, but here the surface is flatter and without villi. Cell proliferation is not uniform over the zone of proliferation but occurs more slowly at the bases of the crypts (Fig. 7.12). Slowly proliferating cells in this region appear to be analogous to bone-marrow stem cells in that they act as precursors for the entire crypt and surrounding villi.

In a few studies (e.g., Lipkin et al., 1963) serial biopsies of human intestine have been taken through a colonoscope or peroral tube after injection of tritiated thymidine. These studies have shown values for the labeling index of crypts in the large intestine in the range of 12 to 18 percent and have allowed the derivation of percent-labeled-mitoses curves that suggest a short cell cycle time of 1 to 2 days. Thus, there is also a high rate of cell proliferation in the human intestine. Some cycle-de-

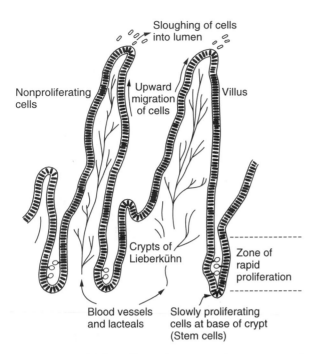

Fig. 7.12. Model for cell proliferation and migration in the small intestine. Slowly proliferating cells in the bases of the crypts probably act as stem cells for the entire cell population. Other cells in the lower two-thirds of the crypts proliferate rapidly, with nuclei of mitotic cells visible in the lumens of the crypts. Cells migrate up the villi to replace those sloughed into the lumen.

pendent drugs (e.g., cytosine arabinoside) may cause severe mucosal irritation of the intestine and diarrhea, although toxicity to this organ is less often dose-limiting than that to the bone marrow.

The in vivo signals that regulate cell renewal in the intestine are not known. However, studies of a rat jejunal crypt-cell line have shown that it is growth inhibited by TGF-β1 and that it produces this growth factor and expresses receptors for it (Barnard et al., 1989). In the rat intestine, TGF-β1 is maximally expressed by the terminally differentiated cells at the tip of the villus and acts to arrest crypt cells in the G1 phase through the activation of cdk inhibitors (Sec. 7.2.3); damage to the villi would remove this inhibitory stimulus, thus allowing increased proliferation of cells at the base of the crypt and recovery of the crypt-villus unit.

7.6 TUMOR GROWTH AND CELL KINETICS

7.6.1. Growth of Tumors

Tumor growth can be determined by measuring tumor volume as a function of time. Most commonly, this is done by making caliper measurements of at

least two orthogonal diameters and by assuming that the tumor is ellipsoid in shape. Exponential growth of tumors will occur if the rates of cell production and of cell loss or death are proportional to the number of cells present in the population. Exponential growth implies that the time taken for a tumor to double its volume is constant and often leads to the false impression that the rate of tumor growth is accelerating with time (Fig. 7.13). Increase in the diameter of a human tumor from 0.5 to 1.0 cm may escape detection, whereas increase in the diameter of a tumor from 5 to 10 cm is more dramatic and is likely to cause new clinical symptoms.

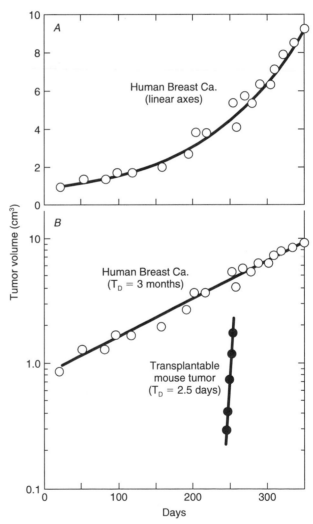

Fig 7.13. Growth curves for a lung metastasis from a human breast cancer. *A.* Plotted on linear axes. *B.* Same data plotted using a logarithmic scale for tumor volume. (Data of RP Hill and RS Bush, unpublished. Included with permission.) A growth curve for a rapidly growing transplantable tumor in the mouse is included in (*B*) for comparison. T_D = volume doubling time.

Both require three volume doublings; during exponential growth they will occur over the same period of time.

Estimates of the growth rates of untreated human tumors have been limited by the following constraints: (1) Only tumors that are unresponsive to therapy can ethically be followed without treatment, and limited data are available from older studies. (2) Accurate measurements can be made only on tumors from selected sites. The majority of studies have examined lung metastases using serial x-rays, although newer radiologic techniques have expanded the range of sites in which tumor volume can be estimated accurately. There have been few measurements of the growth of primary tumors. (3) The limited observation period between the time of tumor detection and either death of the host or the initiation of some form of therapy represents only a small fraction of the history of the tumor's growth (Figs. 7.14 and 7.15).

Despite these limitations, there are many published estimates of the growth rate of human tumors. Steel (1977) reviewed published measurements of the rate of growth of 780 human tumors, and estimates of volume doubling time for several types of tumor are summarized in Table 7.4. A few general conclusions may be stated:

1. There is wide variation in growth rate, even among tumors of the same histologic type and site of origin.
2. Representative mean doubling times for lung metastases of common tumors in humans are in the range of 2 to 3 months.

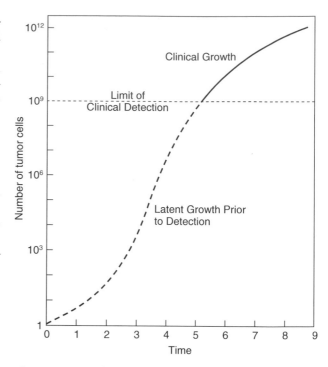

Fig. 7.15. Hypothetical growth curve for a human tumor, showing the long latent period prior to detection. Tumors may show an early lag phase and progressive slowing of growth at large size.

3. There is a tendency for childhood tumors and adult tumors that are known to be responsive to chemotherapy (e.g., lymphoma, cancer of the testis) to grow more rapidly than unresponsive tumors (e.g., cancer of the colon).
4. Metastases tend to grow more rapidly than the primary tumor in the same patient.

Superficial tumors may be detected clinically when they contain about 1 billion (10^9) cells; tumors of internal organs are likely to escape detection until they are considerably larger (Fig. 7.14). There is indirect evidence that many tumors arise from a single cell (see Sec. 7.6.2.), and a superficial tumor of 1 g (containing about 10^9 cells) will have undergone about 30 doublings in volume prior to clinical detection. (Note that, because of cell loss, this will involve more than 30 consecutive divisions of the initial cell.) After 10 further doublings in volume, the tumor would weigh about 1 kg (10^{12} cells), a size that may be lethal to the host. Thus, the range of size over which the growth of a tumor may be studied represents a rather short and late part of its total growth history (Figs. 7.14 and 7.15). There is evidence (e.g., for breast cancer) that the probability of metastatic spread increases with the size of the

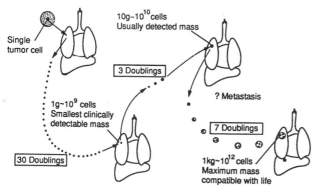

Fig. 7.14. A human solid tumor must undergo about 30 to 33 doublings in volume from a single cell before it achieves a detectable size at a weight of 1 to 10 g. Metastases may have been established prior to detection of the primary tumor. Only a few further doublings of volume lead to a tumor whose size is incompatible with life. (Adapted from Tannock, 1983.)

Table 7.4. Volume Doubling Time (T_D) for Representative Human Tumors

Tumor Type	Number of Tumors	Volume Doubling Time[a], weeks
Primary lung cancer		
Adenocarcinoma	64	21
Squamous cell carcinoma	85	12
Anaplastic carcinoma	55	11
Breast cancer		
Primary	17	14
Lung metastases	44	11
Soft tissues metastases	66	3
Colon/rectum		
Primary	19	90
Lung metastases	56	14
Lymphoma		
Lymph node lesions	27	4
Lung metastases of		
Carcinoma of testis	80	4
Childhood tumors	47	4
Adult sarcomas	58	7

[a]Geometric mean values.

Source: Adapted from Steel, 1977.

primary tumor, but the long preclinical history of the tumor may allow cells to metastasize prior to detection, so that "early" clinical detection may be expected to reduce but not to prevent the subsequent appearance of metastases.

The growth rate of a tumor in its preclinical phase can only be estimated indirectly. In patients, one may study the time to appearance of recurrent tumors after treatment that is curative in only some of the patients, so that growth in others may be assumed to derive from a small number of residual cells (Shackney et al., 1981). These studies support the concept that growth is more rapid in the preclinical phase of a disease such as breast cancer, but there is little evidence for deceleration of growth during the clinical phase of rapidly progressive malignancies such as Wilms' tumor or Burkitt's lymphoma.

Deceleration of growth of large tumors is probably due to increasing cell death and decreasing cell proliferation as tumor nutrition deteriorates (see Sec. 7.6.3). Also, tumors often contain a high proportion of nonmalignant cells such as macrophages, lymphocytes, and fibroblasts, and the proliferation and migration of these cells will influence changes in tumor volume. Tumor growth may also be slow at very early stages of development (Fig. 7.15). Tumor

cells may have to overcome immunologic and other host defense mechanisms, and they cannot expand to a large size until they have induced proliferation of blood vessels to support them (see Chap. 9, Sec. 9.3.1).

7.6.2 Stem Cells and Clonality

Renewal tissues such as bone marrow and intestinal mucosa represent a hierarchy of cells produced by cell division and differentiation from a small number of stem cells (Sec. 7.5). Most tumors arise in renewal tissues, and there is substantial evidence that many tumors contain a limited population of stem cells with the capacity to regenerate the tumor after treatment. Other cells in the tumor population may have lost the capacity for cell proliferation (e.g., through differentiation) or have only limited potential for cell proliferation (analogous to morphologically recognizable precursor cells in bone marrow, such as myelocytes) (Fig. 7.16; Mackillop et al., 1983). The following evidence supports the validity of a stem-cell model for human tumors:

1. There is evidence (described below) that cells within many different types of tumor are derived clonally from a single cell.
2. Tissue-specific differentiation occurs in tumors, and an inverse relationship has been observed

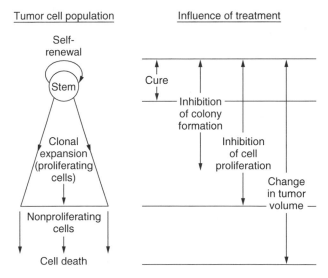

Fig. 7.16. The stem-cell model has important implications for cancer treatment. Curative treatment requires eradication of stem cells, whereas changes in cell proliferation or in tumor volume depend respectively on many or all of the cells in the tumor. Assessment of the effects of treatment against stem cells requires the use of a colony-forming assay. (Adapted from Mackillop et al, 1983.)

between indices of cell proliferation and differentiation. There is evidence that differentiated cells (which cannot generate a tumor on transplantation) are derived from undifferentiated cells that can generate tumors when transplanted into new hosts (Pierce and Speers, 1988). This relationship is similar to that observed in normal renewing tissues.

3. Cells from human tumors may generate colonies in a semisolid medium such as dilute agar provided that an adequate nutrient environment (including essential growth factors) is provided (Hamburger and Salmon, 1977, Courtenay et al., 1978). The proportion of cells that generate colonies is low (typically <1 percent) suggesting a low proportion of tumor stem cells (Davidson et al., 1992). This low colony-forming efficiency might be due, however, to the imperfect microenvironment provided by the tissue culture medium.

4. Experience with radiation therapy suggests that in many human tumors only a small proportion of the cells has the ability to repopulate the tumor. Successful achievement of local control in several types of human tumor with moderate doses of radiation therapy would be expected only if a small fraction of the tumor cells were stem cells that must be killed by the radiation (Moore et al., 1983).

Evidence for the monoclonal origin of human tumors is provided by the observation that a unique identifying feature (a clonal marker) may be found in all of the constituent cells. Clonal markers include chromosomal rearrangements such as the Philadelphia chromosome in chronic myelogenous leukemia (see Chap. 4, Sec. 4.3.2), uniquely rearranged immunoglobulins or T-cell receptors expressed by B-cell lymphomas or multiple myelomas and T-cell lymphomas respectively (see Chap. 11, Sec. 11.2.6), and an enlarging array of molecular markers whose detection has been facilitated by the availability of gene sequencing.

Evidence for the monoclonal origin of several types of malignancy has accrued from analysis of X-linked genes or gene products in cells from tumors in women who are heterozygous at these genetic loci. One of the X chromosomes becomes inactivated at random in all cells of females during early life. The normal tissues of heterozygous females are therefore mosaics that contain approximately equal number of cells in which one or the other (but not both) of the two alleles of a gene on the X chromo-

somes are expressed. However, if the tumors in such individuals arise from a single antecedent cell, all the tumor cells will express only one allele of the gene, which can be studied by molecular probes or by analysis of the gene product. This method has been used extensively by Fialkow and colleagues (e.g., Fialkow, 1974), who studied isoenzymes of glucose-6-phosphate dehydrogenase in malignant cells of heterozygous black females (Fig. 7.17). Several other polymorphic genes on the X chromosome have now been studied in tumors and normal tissues by analysis of restriction fragment length polymorphisms (RFLPs; Chap. 3, Sec. 3.3.5). These techniques have been used to demonstrate clonality in

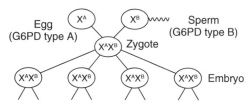

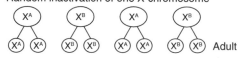

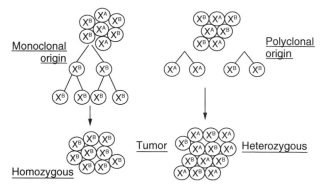

Fig. 7.17. The use of X-linked markers to study clonality in tumors. *A.* Females have random inactivation of an X-chromosome during development, and the cells then breed true. Subjects who are heterozygous for an X-linked enzyme (e.g., G6PD) have normal tissues that are heterozygous for production of the isoenzymes. *B.* A tumor originating in a single cell will produce only one isoenzyme, whereas a tumor of multicellular origin will produce both types. Molecular probes for other X-linked genes have allowed expansion for this method to a wide variety of tumors.

at least 95 percent of the wide range of tumors that have been examined (Fialkow, 1974; Vogelstein et al., 1987). Fearon et al. (1987) demonstrated clonal origin of 30 colonic adenomas (non-malignant or premalignant tumors) and 20 colonic carcinomas using analysis of X-linked genes; they also found a second clonal marker, loss of chromosome 17p sequences (Chap. 4, Sec. 4.5.4) in most of the carcinomas but not in the adenomas. This type of analysis has suggested that sequential selection of clonal populations occurs during progression from benign to premalignant to malignant tumors. The continued accrual of genetic changes in subpopulations probably leads to the phenotypic heterogeneity observed among the cells of most tumors (see Chap. 10, Sec. 10.1).

Although one explanation for the above results is that tumors originate in a single cell, the results prove only that the tumor cells present at the time of observation had a common antecedent cell; this could also occur in tumors that arose from multiple transformed cells if one of their progeny developed a sufficient growth advantage such that its descendants became dominant in the tumor.

The stem cell model has major implications for the treatment of human tumors. When the aim of treatment is cure or long-term control, then therapy must be directed toward eradication of stem cells, since only these cells maintain the potential to regenerate the tumor population (Fig. 7.16; Mackillop et al., 1983). If stem cells represent a small subpopulation of the total cells in some tumors, as suggested by the results of treatment with radiotherapy, then short-term changes in tumor volume may not reflect the effects of treatment on stem cells. Rather, stem cell effects must be evaluated by placing the cells in an environment where they may express their potential to generate a large number of progeny— that is, a colony-forming assay.

Although stem cells in tumors have by definition a high (infinite?) capacity for cell proliferation and are responsible for tumor regeneration after treatment, they are not necessarily proliferating rapidly in the untreated tumor (compare, for example, slowly proliferating bone marrow stem cells described in Sec. 7.5.1). The proliferative status of clonogenic tumor cells is important in determining their response to chemotherapy (see Chap. 15, Sec. 15.2.3). Assessment of this status by the thymidine suicide method (Sec. 7.4.1) has suggested a variable but often high rate of proliferation among the clonogenic cells of the few tumors that have been studied (Minden et al., 1978; Shimizu et al., 1982).

7.6.3 Cell Proliferation in Tumors

Typical values for thymidine labeling index or percent S phase cells are in the range of 3 to 15 percent for many types of human solid tumors. The rate of cell proliferation is usually less than that of some cells in normal renewing tissues such as the intestine or bone marrow. Higher rates of cell proliferation are evident in faster-growing malignancies, including some lymphomas.

Values of the labeling index (LI) for human leukemia are lower than those of the granulocyte and erythroid precursors in normal bone marrow. Thus, even in acute leukemia, accumulation of cells is not due to an increased rate of cell proliferation. Instead, there is defective maturation and the population of leukemic cells increases because the rate of cell proliferation (although slower than that of normal myeloblasts) exceeds the rate of cell death or removal from the population. That leukemia is caused primarily by a defect in cell differentiation and/or in pathways leading to cell death is further emphasized by the finding that the rate of proliferation of myeloblasts in the rapidly progressive acute myeloblastic leukemias (AMLs) is often slower than in chronic myelogenous leukemia (CML), where differentiation to more mature and partly functional cells occurs. In the aggressive preterminal phase of blast crisis in CML, differentiation is curtailed but proliferation of myeloblasts does not increase.

Information about the duration of the cell cycle and of its constituent phases in human tumors is available from a few early studies in which ^{3}H-thymidine was injected into patients and where serial biopsies allowed the generation of a percent-labeled-mitoses (PLM) curve. A larger number of estimates of the duration of S phase, T_s, and of the potential doubling time T_{pot}, have been derived more recently by taking a single biopsy after injection of BrdUrd (see Fig. 7.10). Representative data from these studies are shown in Table 7.5. Mean values for T_s tend to be in the range of 12 to 24 h. Typical values of mean cell-cycle time are in the range of 2 to 3 days, but this estimate is subject to uncertainty because the distribution of cell-cycle times is broad, and both the PLM and BrdUrd techniques tend to give information about the faster proliferating cells in the population.

The potential doubling times of human tumors may be estimated directly by using BrdUrd and flow cytometry (Sec. 7.4.3) or from measured values of T_s and LI. The potential doubling time T_{pot} reflects the proliferative capacity of cells in the absence of cell loss and may indicate the potential for proliferative recovery during prolonged treatment such as with radiotherapy. Values listed in Table 7.5 indicate considerable variability, but estimates of T_{pot} are much longer than estimates of mean cycle time T_c. This implies that many human tumors have a low growth fraction. If some of the slowly proliferating or non-proliferating cells in human tumors retain the properties of a tumor stem cell (i.e., they can repopulate the tumor if stimulated to divide), the low growth fraction may be a factor that contributes to the relative resistance of many slow-growing human tumors to cycle-active chemotherapy.

Estimates of mean values of T_{pot} in Table 7.5 are in the range of 4.5 to 20 days. In contrast, estimates of volume doubling time for common human tumors tend to be about 2 to 3 months (Table 7.4). It follows that the rate of cell loss in many human tumors is in the range of 75 to 90 percent of the rate of cell production.

Studies of human and animal tumors have demonstrated considerable heterogeneity in labeling and mitotic indices within different parts of the same tumor or its metastases. One of the factors that contributes to heterogeneity of cell proliferation is a variable degree of differentiation that may occur within the tumor: in general, there is an inverse relationship between differentiation and proliferative rates. A second factor is the generation of variant clonal subpopulations (see Sec. 7.6.2) with different proliferative capacities. A third and perhaps dominant factor is cell nutrition.

Necrosis occurs commonly in solid tumors, and both in human and experimental tumors an orderly relationship can sometimes be observed with the edge of a necrotic region being parallel to a tumor blood vessel and separated from it by a distance that in humans is commonly about 150 to 200 µm (Fig. 7.18; Thomlinson and Gray, 1955). In some tumors, this relationship may lead to the formation of either cylindrical cords of viable tissue with a central blood vessel and surrounding necrosis or to tumor nodules with a surrounding vascular network and central necrosis. These structures suggest that necrosis may occur when the concentration of essential nutrients that diffuse from tumor blood vessels has fallen to a critically low value, and/or when toxic breakdown products of cells have reached a critically high level. Static blood flow in tumor capillaries may also lead to necrotic regions of tumors. Apoptosis may be triggered by ischemia, although apoptotic cells are often distributed widely among the viable tumor cell population.

Table 7.5. Estimates of Mean Duration of S Phase (T_s), Cell-Cycle Time (T_c), and Potential Doubling Time (T_{pot}) for Selected Human Tumors[a]

| Tumor Type | Number of Estimates | Mean Values of | | | Range | Method |
		T_s, hour	T_c, days	T_{pot}, days		
Breast	6	21	2.5	20		PLM
Lung	6	20	4.5	—		PLM
	3	24	—	6	3–11	BrdUrd
Head/neck	4	20	2.5			
	47	11	—	4.5	2–15	IdUrd
Stomach	21	14	—	8		BrdUrd
Colon/rectum	10	17	3.0	5		PLM
	4	24	—	6.5	5–10	BrdUrd
Brain	15	15	—	12	6–27	BrdUrd
Melanoma	6	21	2.5	—		PLM
	2	9	—	5	3.5–7	BrdUrd
Lymphoma	7	12	2.0	—		PLM
Acute leukemia	17	22	2.5	9	6–18	PLM
	44	13	—	9	3–7	BrdUrd

[a]T_{pot} was calculated from T_s and concurrent LI using BrdUrd, IdUrd, or ^{3}H-thymidine incorporation.

Sources: Data obtained using the PLM method were reviewed in Steel (1977) and Tannock (1978). Data obtained by the BrdUrd/IdUrd method are from Wilson et al. (1988), Riccardi et al. (1989), and Begg et al. (1990).

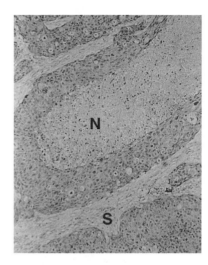

Fig. 7.18. Histologic section of a human lung cancer showing tumor cords between fibrous stroma (S) containing blood vessels and regions of necrosis (N). (Figure prepared by Dr RH Thomlinson, formerly of Mount Vernon Hospital, Northwood, England. Used with permission.)

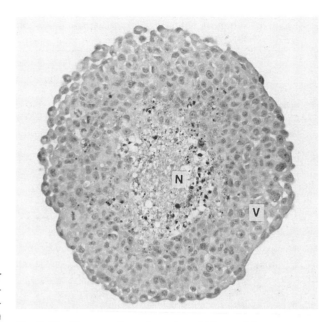

Fig. 7.19. Cross section of a spheroid formed from a tumor cell line derived from human bladder cancer, showing the viable rim (V) and central necrosis (N). (Courtesy of Dr. RM Sutherland.)

The presence of tumor cords or nodules has allowed study of cell proliferation in relation to the blood supply. Not surprisingly, well-nourished cells close to blood vessels have a more rapid rate of cell proliferation than poorly nourished cells close to a region of necrosis (e.g., Tannock, 1970). A similar gradient of cell proliferation is seen when tumor cells are grown as spheroids, which are multicellular aggregates grown in semisolid medium in vitro that resemble tumor nodules (Fig 7.19). Spheroids have a decreasing gradient of nutrient metabolites from their surface (Sutherland, 1988). The presence of slowly proliferating cells at a distance from functional blood vessels has implications for tumor therapy: such cells may be resistant to radiation because of hypoxia (see Chap. 13, Sec. 13.5.2) and to anticancer drugs because of their low proliferative rate (see Chap. 15, Sec. 15.2.4) and limited drug access. Exposure to hypoxia (or other nutrient deprivation) may also promote rapid progression of the tumor cells to a more malignant phenotype (see Chap. 13, Sec. 13.5.2).

Cell proliferation and cell death in tumors depend on tumor vasculature. Thus the rate of tumor growth is likely to depend on the rate of expansion of functional tumor blood vessels by angiogenesis. In experimental animals, the proliferation rate of capillary endothelial cells appears to be slower than that of surrounding tumor cells (Denekamp and Hobson, 1982), which may lead to decreasing tumor vasculature and slowing of growth in larger tumors.

The process of angiogenesis is discussed in Chap. 9, Sec. 9.3.

7.6.4 Cell Proliferation, Prognosis, and Therapy

The rate of cell proliferation in a human tumor is likely to influence both the natural history of the disease and its response to therapy. The technique of recovering cells from paraffin-embedded tissue stored in pathology departments, followed by analysis of DNA content using flow cytometry, has been used in a large number of studies to investigate the influence on prognosis of both the S phase fraction and the G1 phase DNA content (ploidy) of tumor cells (Hedley, 1989). A recent consensus conference about these techniques has emphasized the importance of quality control for flow cytometric methods (Hedley et al., 1993). However, for several types of tumor, both DNA index (i.e., the DNA content of G1 tumor cells relative to that of normal cells) and S phase fraction are prognostic, and these measures may give prognostic information that is additional to the traditional prognostic factors of tumor stage and grade (Table 7.6). In general, aneuploid tumors have a poorer prognosis than diploid tumors, and tumors with a more rapid rate of cell proliferation as reflected by a high S phase fraction or ^{3}H-labeling index have a poorer prognosis than tumors with a slower rate of cell proliferation,

Table 7.6. Prognostic Significance of Cellular DNA Content and S Phase Fraction Determined by Flow Cytometry for Selected Tumours

Tumor Type	Properties of	
	Aneuploid Tumors	Tumors with High S Phase Fraction
Bladder cancer	Correlates with higher grade (and poorer outcome) for superficial tumors	Equivocal studies
	Less useful for muscle-invasive tumors	
Breast cancer	Equivocal studies	Increased risk of recurrence and death for node-negative and node-positive patients (independent risk factor)
Colorectal cancer	Weak prognostic factor for poor survival	Prognostic factor for poor survival
	(Problem of quality control in studies)	
Prostate cancer	Prognostic factor for poor survival	Conflicting data
	(Independent risk factor in some studies)	
Non-Hodgkin's lymphoma	No proven utility	Strong prognostic factor for poor survival
Multiple myeloma	Prognostic factor for poor survival	No data
Acute leukemia	Conflicting data	Not prognostic

Source: Adapted from Hedley et al., 1993.

(e.g., Silvestrini et al., 1990). Estimation of the proportion of tumor cells that express proliferation-dependent antigens such as Ki-67 or PCNA has also demonstrated a relationship between more rapid cell proliferation and poorer prognosis in some but not all tumors that have been studied (Lipponen and Eskelinen, 1992; De Riese et al., 1993). Finally, increased expression of cyclins by human tumors or decreased expression of cyclin-dependent kinase inhibitors has been associated with poor prognosis (Esposito et al., 1997; Furihata et al., 1997; see also Sec. 7.2.4).

The relationship between proliferative parameters and response to treatment with chemotherapy is complex and may confound the relationship between proliferative rate and prognosis for tumors that are responsive to chemotherapy. There may be a higher chance of response to chemotherapy in malignancies with a rapid rate of cell proliferation, although intrinsic drug sensitivity of the cells is likely to be the major determinant of response. In contrast, malignancies with a rapid rate of cell pro-

liferation will grow more rapidly both in the absence of effective treatment and in recovery after partially effective therapy. A further confounding factor arises because most methods of assessing cell kinetics do not give information about proliferative rates of the stem cells in tumors, which are the important targets for curative therapy.

Many investigators have proposed that measurement of cell kinetic parameters following initial treatment of tumors might be used as a guide to optimization of subsequent scheduling of phase-specific anticancer drugs. Unfortunately, such studies are limited because they do not usually distinguish between the important surviving tumor stem cells and the (greater number of) cells that were sterilized by initial treatment and may remain intact for some time prior to their lysis. Heterogeneity in the cell-cycle phase distribution of both tumors and normal tissues is also likely to limit the potential of this approach, since any synchrony caused by initial treatment will be lost quite rapidly.

Estimates of proliferative rate in tumors prior to initiation of radiation therapy might find application in the optimization of schedules of fractionation. Radiation treatment is usually given over 5 to 7 weeks to improve tolerance of normal tissue, but proliferation of surviving tumor cells between radiation fractions decreases the probability of tumor control. Clinical trials are being conducted to determine whether accelerated fractionation (i.e., completion of radiotherapy within a shorter overall time period) will be more effective in eradicating rapidly proliferating tumors (Chap. 14, Sec. 14.4.1). Again, however, it is the proliferation of tumor stem cells that survive initial radiation treatments that is important, and this may not be reflected by the overall rate of proliferation prior to treatment.

7.7 SUMMARY

Cellular proliferation is regulated by extracellular signals such as the availability of nutrients and growth factors and signals mediated by cell-cell contact. Molecular events in G1 phase may trigger the synthesis of DNA and the orderly process of chromosome condensation and mitosis. Transitions from one cell cycle phase to another are governed by a series of cyclin-dependent kinases that bind to positive effectors, the cyclins, whose levels fluctuate during the cell cycle. These cyclin/cdk complexes can phosphorylate proteins such as pRb, which results in movement of the cells from G1 to S phase. There are two families of cdk inhibitors (KIP and INK4), which can cause cell cycle arrest by deactivating the cyclin/cdk complexes and may be triggered by a variety of molecular signals. Growth of tissues of multicellular organisms is also regulated by signals that stimulate cellular differentiation or cell death by apoptosis. Several of the molecular mechanisms that regulate the balance between cell proliferation and cell death may be disturbed in tumors.

Programmed cell death or apoptosis is a normal process for the elimination of unwanted cells in the maintenance of tissue homeostasis. Apoptosis may be stimulated by multiple signals including DNA damage (including that caused by therapeutic agents), lack of required growth stimulatory molecules, and imbalance of cell cycle regulatory molecules. Apoptosis is regulated by stimulatory (e.g., Bax, ICE) and inhibitory (e.g., Bcl-2) families of molecules; some cancer cells may have decreased ability to undergo apoptosis. Most normal cells can undergo only a finite number of cell division cycles before senescence; this process is due in part to lack

of the enzyme telomerase, which reproduces the DNA sequences at the ends of chromosomes (telomeres). The activation of telomerase in tumor cells may play an important role in their escape from senescence.

The mechanisms that inhibit cell cycle progression in response to (1) extrinsic DNA damage (such as that due to gamma or UV irradiation), (2) intrinsic "DNA damage" of telomere shortening, and (3) the action of growth-inhibitory cytokines, such as TGF-β, all act through common cdk inhibitors such as p21 and p27. Loss of cell cycle arrest, which normally allows time for repair after DNA damage, may contribute to genetic instability and the accumulation of genetic changes during the evolution of malignant cells. Events leading to loss of the ability to arrest the cell cycle in response to extrinsic DNA damage may result also in the progressive loss of responsiveness to growth-inhibitory cytokines that is commonly seen during malignant progression.

Information about the rate of cell proliferation in tissues has been derived from studies using thymidine autoradiography and flow cytometry. The proliferative rate of cells in different normal tissues varies widely and influences cellular sensitivity to anticancer drugs. Drug-sensitive tissues such as the bone marrow and intestine contain small numbers of slowly proliferating stem cells that can regenerate the tissue after damage. The processes of cell proliferation and differentiation are controlled by various growth factors; in the adult organism, cell production is balanced by cell death through apoptosis.

Human tumors have a wide range of growth rates, with typical volume doubling times of 2 to 3 months for common epithelial tumors. There is a long period of growth prior to clinical detection, which can explain metastatic spread prior to diagnosis. There is evidence that most tumors are clonal—i.e., derived from a single cell—although subsequent genetic changes lead to heterogeneity. Malignant tumors may also contain a subpopulation of stem cells that have the capacity for unlimited proliferation and are the important targets of cancer therapy. Analysis of cell proliferation within human tumors indicates the presence of some cells that are cycling quite rapidly (typical cell cycle time of 3 days), a low growth fraction, and a high rate of cell loss. A model of unrestrained proliferation is inappropriate for human tumors; rather, they may be compared with normal renewing epithelia but where a defect in homeostasis has led to an imbalance in the rates of cell production and cell loss. Proliferation of tumor cells may be limited by diffusion of nutrient

metabolites from tumor blood vessels and by proliferation of endothelial cells lining tumor blood vessels. A high rate of proliferation in tumors and the
presence of aneuploidy often indicates a poor prognosis.

REFERENCES

Adams PD, Kaelin WG: Transcriptional control by E2F. *Semin Cancer Biology* 1995; 6:99–108.

Ault KA: Detection of small numbers of monoclonal B lymphocytes in the blood of patients with lymphoma. *N Engl J Med* 1979; 300:1401–1405.

Bacchetti S, Counter CM: Telomeres and telomerase in human cancer (review). *Int J Oncol* 1995; 7:423–432.

Barnard JA, Beauchamp RD, Coffey RJ, et al: Regulation of intestinal epithelial cell growth by transforming growth factor type β. *Proc Natl Acad Sci USA* 1989; 1578–1582.

Bates S, Peters G: Cyclin D1 as a cellular proto-oncogene. *Semin Cancer Biol* 1995; 6:73–82.

Becker AJ, McCulloch EA, Siminovitch L, et al: The effect of differing demands for blood cell production on DNA synthesis by hemopoietic colony-forming cells of mice. *Blood* 1965; 26:296-308.

Begg AC, McNally NJ, Schrieve DC, Karcher M: A method to measure the duration of DNA synthesis and the potential doubling time from a single sample. *Cytometry* 1985; 6:620–626.

Begg AC, Hofland I, Moonen L, et al: The predictive value of cell kinetic measurements in a European trial of accelerated fractionation in advanced head and neck tumours: An interim report. *Int J Radiat Oncol Biol Phys* 1990; 19:1449–1453.

Bright J, Khar A: Apoptosis: programmed cell death in health and disease. *Biosci Rep* 1994; 14:67–81.

Brugarolas JC Gordon, J.I., Beach D, et al: Radiation-induced cell cycle arrest compromised by p21 deficiency. *Nature* 1995; 377:552–557.

Canman CE, Kastan M: Induction of apoptosis by tumor suppressor genes and oncogenes. *Cancer Biol* 1995; 6:17–25.

Catzavelos C, Bhattacharya N, Ung YC, et al: Decreased levels of the cell cycle inhibitor p27^{Kip1} protein: Prognostic implications in primary breast cancer. *Nature Med* 1997; 3:227–230.

Chen J, Jackson PK, Kirschner MW, et al: Separate domains of p21 involved in the inhibition of Cdk kinase and PCNA. *Nature* 1995; 374:386–388.

Cleveland JL, Ihle JN: Contenders in FasL/TNF death signalling. *Cell* 1995; 81:479–482.

Courtenay VD, Selby PJ, Smith IE, et al: Growth of human tumour cell colonies from biopsies using two soft-agar techniques. *Br J Cancer* 1978; 38:77–81.

Darzynkiewicz Z, Li X, Gong J: Assays of cell viability: Discrimination of cells dying by apoptosis. *Methods Cell Biol* 1994; 41:15–38.

Davidson SE, West CM, Hunter RD. Lack of association

between in vitro clonogenic growth of human cervical carcinoma and tumour stage, differentiation, patient age, host cell infiltration or patient survival. *Int J Cancer* 1992; 50:10–14.

Denekamp J, Hobson B: Endothelial-cell proliferation in experimental tumours. *Br J Cancer* 1982; 46:711–720.

Deng C, Zhang P, Harper JW, et al: Mice lacking p21CIP1/WAF1 undergo normal development, but are defective in G1 checkpoint control. *Cell* 1995; 82:675–684.

De Riese WT, Crabtree WN, Allhoff EP, et al: Prognostic significance of Ki-67 immunostaining in nonmetastatic renal cell carcinoma. *J Clin Oncol* 1993; 11:1804–1808.

Ellis RE, Yuan R, Horvitz RH: Mechanisms and functions of cell death. *Annu Rev Cell Biol* 1991; 7:663–698.

Esposito V, Baldi A, DeLuca A, et al: Prognostic role of the cyclin-dependent kinase inhibitor p27 in non-small cell lung cancer. *Cancer Res* 1997; 57:3381–3385.

Fearon ER, Hamilton SR, Vogelstein B: Clonal analysis of human colorectal tumors. *Science* 1987; 238:193–197.

Fero ML, Rivkin M, Tasch M, et al: A syndrome of multiorgan hyperplasia with features of gigantism, tumorigenesis and female sterility in p27^{KIP1}-deficient mice. *Cell* 1996; 85; 733–744.

Fialkow PJ: The origin and development of human tumors studied with cell markers. *N Engl J Med* 1974; 291:26–35.

Florenes VA, Bhattacharya N, Bani MR, et al: TGF-β mediated G1 arrest in a human melanoma cell line lacking p15^{INK4B}: evidence for cooperation between p21^{Cip1} and p27^{Kip1}. *Oncogene* 1996; 13:2447–2457.

Flores-Rosas H, Kelman Z, Dean FB, et al: Cdk-interacting protein 1 directly binds with proliferating cell nuclear antigen and inhibits DNA replication catalyzed by the DNA polymerase-δ holoenzyme. *Proc Natl Acad Sci USA* 1994; 91:8655–8659.

Furihata M, Ohtsuki Y, Sonobe H, et al: Cyclin A overexpression in carcinoma of the renal pelvis and ureter including dysplasia: Immunohistochemical findings in relation to prognosis. *Clin Cancer Res* 1997; 3: 1399–1404.

Fynan TM, Reiss M: Resistance to inhibition of cell growth by transforming growth factor-beta and its role in oncogenesis. *Crit Rev Oncogen* 1993; 4:493–540.

Galaktionov K, Lee A, Eckstein J, et al: Cdc25 phosphatases as potential human oncogenes. *Science* 1995; 269:1575–1577.

Gerdes J, Lemke H, Barsch H, et al: Cell cycle analysis of a cell proliferation-associated human nuclear antigen defined by monoclonal antibody Ki-67. *J Immunol* 1984; 133:1710–1715.

Grdina DJ, Sigdestad CP, Peters LJ: Cytotoxic effect in vivo of selected chemotherapeutic agents on synchronized murine fibrosarcoma cells. *Br J Cancer* 1980; 42: 677–683.

Hall M, Bates S, Peters G: Evidence for different modes of action of cyclin-dependent kinase inhibitors: p15 and p16 bind to kinases, p21 and p27 bind to cyclins. *Oncogene* 1995; 11:1581–1588.

Hamburger AW, Salmon SE: Primary bioassay of human tumor stem cells. *Science* 1977; 197:461–463.

Hannon GJ, Beach D: p15^{INK4B} is a potential effector of TGF-β-induced cell cycle arrest. *Nature* 1994; 371:257–261.

Hara E, Smith R, Parry D, et al: Regulation of p16^{CDKN2} expression and its implications for cell immortalization and senescence. *Mol Cell Biol* 1996; 16:859–867.

Hartwell L: Defects in a cell cycle checkpoint may be responsible for the genomic instability of cancer cells. *Cell* 1992; 71:543–546.

Hayflick L: The limited in vitro lifetime of diploid cell strains. *Exp Cell Res* 1965; 37:614–636.

Hedley DW: Flow cytometry using paraffin-embedded tissue: Five years on. *Cytometry* 1989; 10:229–241.

Hedley DW, Shankey VT, Wheeless LL. DNA cytometry consensus conference. *Cytometry* 1993; 14:471–500.

Hengartner MO, Horvitz RH: The ins and outs of programmed cell death during C. elegans development. *Philos Trans R Soc Lond Ser B* 1994; 345:243–246.

Hengst L, Reed S: Translational control of p27^{Kip1} accumulation during the cell cycle. *Science* 1996; 271:1861–1864.

Howard A, Pelc SR: Nuclear incorporation of p32 as demonstrated by autoradiographics. *Exp Cell Res* 1951; 2:178–187.

Hu Z-B, Minden MD, McCulloch EA: Direct evidence for the participation of bcl-2 in the regulation by retinoic acid of the Ara-C sensitivity of leukemic stem cells. *Leukemia* 1995; 9:1667–1673.

Hunter T, Pines P: Cyclins and cancer II: Cyclin D and cdk inhibitors come of age. *Cell* 1994; 79:573–582.

Jiang H, Lin J, Su Z, et al: Induction of differentiation in human promyelocytic HL-60 leukemia cell activates p21, WAF1/CIP1, expression in the absence of p53. *Oncogene* 1994; 9:3397–3406.

Keng PC, Allalunis-Turner J, Siemann DW: Evaluation of cell subpopulations isolated from human tumor xenografts by centrifugal elutriation. *Int J Radiat Oncol Biol Phys* 1990, 18:1061–1067.

King RW, DesRaies RJ, Peters J-M, Kirschner MW: How proteolysis drives the cell cycle. *Science* 1996; 274:1652–1659.

Kiyokawa H, Kineman RD, Manova-Todorova KO, et al: Enhanced growth of mice lacking the cyclin-dependent kinase inhibitor function of p27^{KIP1}. *Cell* 1996; 85:721–732.

Koff A, Ohtsuki M, Polyak K, et al: Negative regulation of G1 in mammalian cells: Inhibition of cyclin E-dependent kinase by TGF-β. *Science* 1993; 260:536–539.

Koh J, Enders G, Dynlacht BD, et al: Tumour-derived p16 alleles encoding proteins defective in cell cycle inhibition. *Nature* 1995; 375:506–510.

Korsmeyer SJ: Regulators of cell death. *Trends Genet* 1995; 11:101–105.

Kouzarides T: Transcriptional control by the retinoblastoma protein. *Semin Cancer Biol* 1995; 6:91–98.

Kroemer G, Petit P, Zamzami N, et al: The biochemistry of programmed cell death. *FASEB J* 1995; 9:1277–1287.

LaBaer J, Garrett M, Stevenson L, et al: New functional activities for the p21 family of CDK inhibitors. *Genes Dev* 1997; 11:847–862.

Li R, Waga S, Hannon G, et al: Differential effects by the p21 CDK inhibitor on PCNA-dependent DNA replication and repair. *Nature* 1994; 371:534–537.

Lipkin M, Bell B, Sherlock P: Cell proliferation kinetics in the gastrointestinal tract of man. I. Cell renewal in colon and rectum. *J Clin Invest* 1963; 42:767–776.

Lipponen PK, Eskelinen MJ: Cell proliferation of transitional cell bladder tumours determined by PCNA/cyclin immunostaining and its prognostic value. *Br J Cancer* 1992; 66:171–176.

Liu L, Lassam N, Slingerland J, et al: Germline p16^{INK4A} mutation and protein dysfunction in a family with inherited melanoma. *Oncogene* 1995; 11:405–412.

Loda M, Cukor B, Tam SW, et al: Increased proteasome-dependent degradation of the cyclin-dependent kinase inhibitor p27 in aggressive colorectal carcinomas. *Nature Med* 1997; 3:231–234.

Lukas J, Parry D, Aagaard L, et al: Retinoblastoma-protein-dependent cell-cycle inhibition by the tumor suppressor p16. *Nature* 1995; 375:503–506.

Luo Y, Hurwitz J, Massague J: Cell-cycle inhibition by independent CDK and PCNA binding domains in p21^{Cip1}. *Nature* 1995; 375:159–161.

MacKillop WJ, Ciampi A, Till JE, Buick RN: A stem cell model of human tumor growth: Implications for tumor cell clonogenic assays. *J Natl Cancer Inst* 1983; 70:9–16.

Maelandsmo GM, Holm R, Fodstad O, et al: Cyclin kinase inhibitor p21$^{WAF1/CIP1}$ in malignant melanoma: Reduced expression in metastatic lesions. *Am J Pathol* 1996; 149:1813–1822.

Massague J: The transforming growth factor-β family. *Annu Rev Cell Biol* 1990; 6:597–641.

Matsuoka S, Edwards MC, Bai C, et al: p57^{KIP2}, a structurally distinct member of the p21^{CIP1} Cdk inhibitor family, is a candidate tumor suppressor gene. *Genes Dev* 1995; 9:650–662.

Mendelsohn ML: The growth fraction: A new concept applied to tumors. *Science* 1960; 132:1496.

Messner HA: Assessment and characterization of hemopoietic stem cells. *Stem Cells* 1995; 13(suppl 3):13–18.

Minden MD, Till JE, McCulloch EA: Proliferative state of blast cell progenitors in acute myeloblastic leukemia (AML). *Blood* 1978; 52:592–600.

Monard SP, Young BD: Chromosome analysis by flow cytometry. In: Verma RS, Babu A eds. *Chromosomes, Principles and Techniques*, 2d ed. New York: McGraw-Hill; 1995.

Moore JV, Hendry JH, Hunter RD: Dose-incidence curves for tumour control and normal tissue injury, in relation to the response of clonogenic cells. *Radiother Oncol* 1983; 1:143–147.

Moore MAS: Hematopoietic reconstruction: New approaches. *Clin Cancer Res* 1995; 1:3–9.

Morgan DO: Principles of Cdk regulation. *Nature* 1995; 374:131–134.

Moses HL: TGF-β regulation of epithelial cell proliferation. *Mol Reprod Dev* 1992; 32:179–184.

Nagata S, Golstein P: The Fas death factor. *Science* 1995; 267:1449–1456.

Nakayama K, Ishida N, Shirane M, et al: Mice lacking p27^{KIP1} display increased body size, multiple organ hyperplasia, retinal dysplasia, and pituitary tumors. *Cell* 1996; 85:707–720.

Noda A, Ning Y, Venable SF, et al: Cloning of senescent cell-derived inhibitors of DNA synthesis using an expression screen. *Exp Cell Res* 1994; 211:90–98.

Pardee AB: G$_1$ events and regulation of cell proliferation. *Science* 1989; 246:603–608.

Parker SB, Eichele G, Zhang P, et al: p53-independent expression of p21^{CIP1} in muscle and other terminally differentiating cells. *Science* 1995; 267:1024–1028.

Parry D, Bates S, Mann DJ, Peters G: Lack of cyclin D-Cdk complexes in Rb-negative cells correlates with high levels of p16$^{INK4/MTS1}$ tumour suppressor gene product. *EMBO J* 1995; 14: 503–511.

Petrocelli T, Poon R, Drucker D, et al: UVB irradiation induces p21$^{Cip1/WAF1}$ and mediates G1 and S phase checkpoints. *Oncogene* 1996; 12:1387–1396.

Pierce GB, Speers WC: Tumors as caricatures of the process of tissue renewal: Prospects for therapy by directing differentiation. *Cancer Res* 1988; 48:1996–2004.

Polyak K, Kato JY, Solomon MJ, et al: p27^{Kip1}, a cyclin-Cdk inhibitor, links transforming growth factor-β and contact inhibition to cell cycle arrest. *Genes Dev* 1994; 8:9–22.

Poon R, Toyoshima H, Hunter T: Redistribution of the CDK inhibitor p27 between different cyclin-CDK complexes in the mouse fibroblast cell cycle and in cells arrested with lovastatin or ultraviolet light. *Mol Biol Cell* 1995; 6:1197–1213.

Porter PL, Malone KE, Heagerty PJ, et al: Expression of cell-cycle regulators p27^{KIP1} and cyclin E, alone and in combination, correlate with survival in young breast cancer patients. *Nature Med* 1997; 3:222–225.

Potten CS: What is an apoptotic index measuring? A commentary. *Br J Cancer* 1996; 74:1743–1748.

Ranade K, Hussussian CJ, Sikorski RS, et al: Mutations associated with familial melanoma impair p16^{INK4} function. *Nature Genet* 1995; 10:114–116.

Reed SI, Bailly E, Dulic V, et al: G1 control in mammalian cells. *J Cell Sci* 1994; suppl 18:69–73.

Reynisdottir I, Polyak K, Iavarone A, et al: Kip/Cip and Ink4 Cdk inhibitors cooperate to induce cell cycle arrest in response to TGF-β. *Genes Dev* 1995; 9: 1831–1845.

Riccardi A, Danova M, Dionigi P, et al: Cell kinetics in leukemia and solid tumours studied with *in vivo* bromodeoxyuridine and flow cytometry. *Br J Cancer* 1989; 59:898–903.

Sandhu C, Bhattacharya N, Daksis J: Transforming growth factor beta stabilizes p15^{INK4B} protein, increases p15^{INK4B}-cdk4 complexes, and inhibits cyclin D1-cdk4 association in human mammary epithelial cells. *Mol Cell Biol* 1997; 17:2458–2467.

Serrano M, Hannon GJ, Beach D: A new regulatory motif in cell cycle control causing specific inhibition of cyclin D/Cdk4. *Nature* 1993; 366:704–707.

Serrano M, Lee H-W, Chin L, et al: Role of the INK4a locus in tumor suppression and cell mortality. *Cell* 1996; 85:27–37.

Shackney SE, McCormack GW, Cuchural GJJ: Growth rate patterns of solid tumours and their relation to responsiveness to therapy: An analytical review. *Ann Intern Med* 1981; 89:107–121.

Sherr CJ: G1 phase progression: Cycling on cue. *Cell* 1994; 79:551–555.

Sherr CJ: Cancer cell cycles. *Science* 1996; 274:1672–1677.

Sherr CJ, Roberts JM: Inhibitors of mammalian G$_1$ cyclin-dependent kinases. *Genes Dev* 1995; 9:1149–1163.

Shimizu T, Motoji T, Oshimi K, et al: Proliferative state and radiosensitivity of human myeloma stem cells. *Br J Cancer* 1982; 45:679–683.

Sicinski P, Donaher JL, Parker SB, et al: Cyclin D1 provides a link between development and oncogenesis in the retina and breast. *Cell* 1995; 82:621–630.

Silvestrini R, Daidone MG, Valagussa P, et al: ^{3}H-thymidine-labeling index as a prognostic indicator in breast cancer. *J Clin Oncol* 1990; 8:1321–1326.

Skapek SX, Rhee J, Spicer DB, et al: Inhibition of myogenic differentiation in proliferating myoblasts by cyclin D1-dependent kinase. *Science* 1995; 267: 1022–1024.

Slingerland JM, Hengst L, Pan C-H, et al: A novel inhibitor of cyclin/Cdk activity detected in TGF-β arrested epithelial cells. *Mol Cell Biol* 1994; 14:3683–3694.

Smets LA: Programmed cell death (apoptosis) and response to anti-cancer drugs. *Anticancer Drugs* 1994; 5:3–9.

Solomon MJ: Activation of the various cyclin/cdc 2 protein kinases. *Curr Opin Cell Biol* 1993; 5:180–186.

Steel GG: *Growth Kinetics of Tumours: Cell Population Kinetics in Relation to the Growth and Treatment of Cancer.* Oxford, England: Clarendon Press; 1977.

Steinman RA, Hoffman B, Iro A, et al: Induction of p21(WAF1/CIP1) during differentiation. *Oncogene* 1994; 9:3389–3396.

Steller H: Mechanisms and genes of cellular suicide. *Science* 1995; 267:1445–1449.

Stryckmans P, Cronkite EP, Fache J, et al: Deoxyribonucleic acid synthesis time of erythropoietic and granulopoietic cells in human beings. *Nature* 1966; 211: 711–720.

Sutherland RM: Cell and environment interactions in tumour microregions: The multicell spheroid model. *Science* 1988; 240:177–184.

Tannock IF: Population kinetics of carcinoma cells, capillary endothelial cells, and fibroblasts in a transplanted mouse mammary tumor. *Cancer Res* 1970; 30:2470–2476.

Tannock IF: Cell kinetics and chemotherapy: A critical review. *Cancer Treat Rep* 1978; 62:1117–1133.

Tannock IF: Biology of tumor growth. *Hosp Pract* 1983; 18:81–93.

Terada Y, Tatsuka M, Jinno S, et al: Requirement for tyrosine phosphorylation of Cdk4 in G1 arrest induced by ultraviolet irradiation. *Nature* 1995; 376:358–362.

Thomlinson RH, Gray LH: The histological structure of

some human lung cancers and the possible implications for radiotherapy. *Br J Cancer* 1955; 9:539–549.

Thompson FH, Emerson J, Olson S et al: Cytogenetics of 158 patients with regional or disseminated melanoma: subset analysis of near diploid and simple karyotypes. *Cancer Genet Cytogenet* 1995; 83:93–104.

Todo A: Proliferation and differentiation of hematopoietic cells in hematologic disorders: In vivo radio-autographic study of leukemia including erythroleukemia. *Acta Haemat Jpn* 1968; 31:947–966.

Vaux DL, Strasser A: The molecular biology of apoptosis. *Proc Natl Acad Sci USA* 1996; 93:2239–2244.

Vogelstein B, Fearon ER, Hamilton SR, et al: Clonal analysis using recombinant DNA probes from the X-chromosome. *Cancer Res* 1987; 46:4806–4813.

Waga S, Hannon GJ, Beach D, et al: The p21 inhibitor of cyclin-dependent kinases controls DNA replication by interaction with PCNA. *Nature* 1994; 369: 574–578.

Wang QM, Jones JB, Studzinski GP: Cyclin-dependent kinase inhibitor p27 as a mediator of the G1-S phase block induced by 1,25-dihydroxyvitamin D_3 in HL-60 cells. *Cancer Res* 1996; 56:264–267.

Wang TC, Cardiff RD, Zukerberg L, et al: Mammary hyperplasia and carcinoma in MMTV-cyclin D1 transgenic mice. *Nature* 1994; 369:669–671.

Warbrick E, Lane DP, Glover DM, Cox LS: A small peptide inhibitor of DNA replication defines the site of interaction between the cyclin-dependent kinase inhibitor p21WAF1 and proliferating cell nuclear antigen. *Curr Biol* 1995; 5:275–282.

White E: Life, death, and the pursuit of apoptosis. *Genes Dev* 1996; 10:1–15.

Wilson GD, McNally NJ, Dische S, et al: Measurement of cell kinetics in human tumours in vivo using bromo-deoxyuridine incorporation and flow cytometry. *Br J Cancer* 1988; 58:423–431.

Xiong Y, Zhang H, Beach D: Subunit rearrangement of the cyclin-dependent kinases is associated with cellular transformation. *Genes Dev* 1993; 7:1572–1583.

Yin DX, Schimke RT: BCL-2 expression delays drug-induced apoptosis but does not increase clonogenic survival after drug treatment in HeLa cells. *Cancer Res* 1995; 55:4922–4928.

Zanke BW, Baidreau K, Rubie E, et al: The stress-activated protein kinase (SAPK/JNK) pathway mediates cell death following cis-platinum or heat induced injury. *Curr Biol* 1996; 6:606–613.

8

Chemical and Radiation Carcinogenesis

Allan B. Okey, Patricia A. Harper, Denis M. Grant, and Richard P. Hill

8.1 INTRODUCTION

8.2 BIOLOGICAL PROCESSES IN CHEMICAL CARCINOGENESIS
8.2.1 Multistep Carcinogenesis
8.2.2 Metabolism of Carcinogens
8.2.3 Genetic Polymorphisms of Carcinogen-Metabolizing Enzymes
8.2.4 DNA Adducts and DNA Repair
8.2.5 Targets of Chemical Carcinogens

8.3 IDENTIFICATION OF CARCINOGENS AND ASSESSMENT OF RISK
8.3.1 In Vitro Assays for Carcinogens
8.3.2 Bioassays in Animals
8.3.3 Challenges in Identifying Human Carcinogens
8.3.4 Molecular Epidemiology
8.3.5 Assessment and Management of Risk

8.4 CHEMOPREVENTION OF CANCER
8.4.1 Agents That Alter Bioactivation of Carcinogens
8.4.2 Blocking Agents
8.4.3 Suppressive Agents and Hormone Manipulations
8.4.4 Human Chemoprevention Trials

8.5 RADIATION CARCINOGENESIS
8.5.1 Cell Transformation by Radiation
8.5.2 Mechanisms of Radiation Transformation
8.5.3 Carcinogenesis by Ionizing Radiation in Animals
8.5.4 Human Data on Carcinogenesis by Ionizing Radiation
8.5.5 Ultraviolet Carcinogenesis

8.6 SUMMARY

REFERENCES

8.1 INTRODUCTION

Human cancer is the consequence of interactions among many factors, including exposure to xenobiotic ("foreign") chemicals and radiation. This chapter discusses mechanisms by which chemicals and radiation may act as carcinogens and how knowledge of these mechanisms might be exploited to improve human health through prevention or intervention.

The hypothesis that chemicals can cause cancer is at least as old as Percival Pott's observation in 1775 that scrotal cancer was linked to soot exposure in English chimney sweeps. In the late nineteenth century the German physician Rehn noted that cancer of the urinary bladder was frequent in workers exposed to aromatic amines in the dye industry.

In 1918, Yamagiwa and Ichikawa produced tumors by repeated painting of coal tar on the skin of rabbits. This breakthrough provided the foundation for the isolation, identification, synthesis, and biological testing of a host of chemical carcinogens. Most chemicals that were identified as carcinogens in early research are products or by-products of industrial-technological processes (Fig. 8.1). For example, benzo[*a*]pyrene (BP) and related polycyclic aromatic hydrocarbons (PAHs) arise from partial combustion of petroleum or tobacco; benzidine and other aromatic amines were present in the workplace, as was vinyl chloride. Many other chemical carcinogens occur as "natural" products in foodstuffs or in the environment. Notable examples include aflatoxin B1, a potent liver carcinogen formed by molds that contaminate improperly stored grains, and 2-amino-3-methylimidazo[4,5-*f*]quinoline (IQ), a heterocyclic amine derived

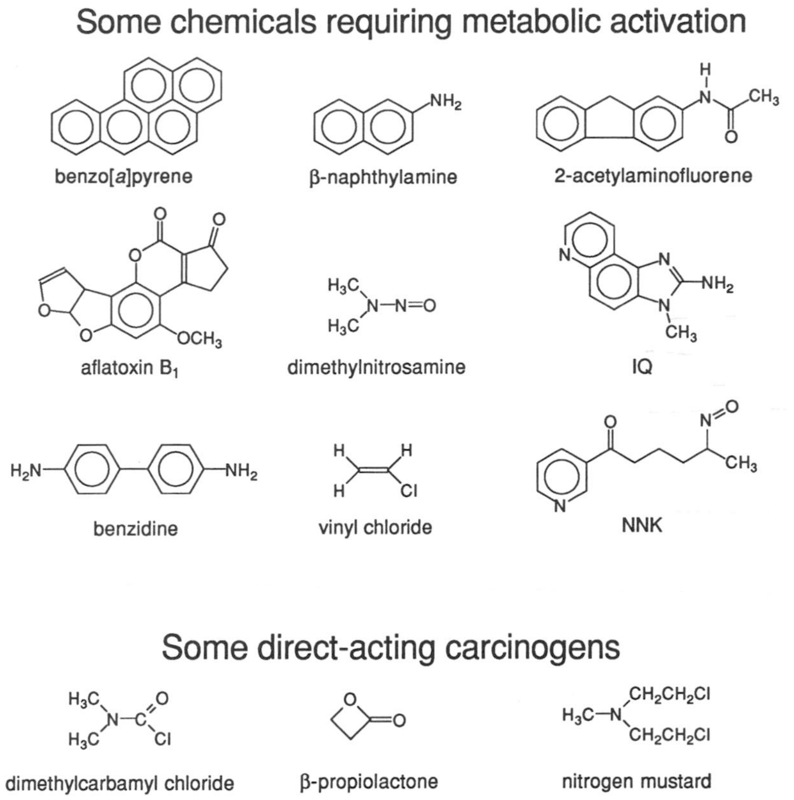

Some chemicals requiring metabolic activation

benzo[a]pyrene

β-naphthylamine

2-acetylaminofluorene

aflatoxin B$_1$

dimethylnitrosamine

IQ

benzidine

vinyl chloride

NNK

Figure 8.1. Structures of some established chemical carcinogens that require metabolic activation (*top*) or act directly (*bottom*). IQ = 2-amino-3-methylimidazo[4,5-*f*]quinoline; NNK = 4-(methylnitrosamino)-1-(3-pyridyl)-1-butanone.

Some direct-acting carcinogens

dimethylcarbamyl chloride

β-propiolactone

nitrogen mustard

from amino acids during high-temperature cooking. Thus, chemical carcinogens originate from both industrial and natural processes.

Both ultraviolet (UV) and ionizing radiation are environmental carcinogens. Skin cancer is prevalent in people with high levels of sun exposure. Recognition of the role of UV radiation in the induction of this disease and the degradation of the ozone layer, which absorbs UV in sunlight, has led to promotion of reduced levels of sun exposure (tanning) and more extensive use of sunscreen preparations. Studies of populations exposed to ionizing radiation (e.g., medical x-rays, atomic weapons, radon in houses) have shown an increased risk of cancer. These effects are dependent on radiation dose, and risk factors for cancer induction have been determined. On the basis of these risk factors, acceptable levels of environmental radiation exposure have been set for people working with radiation.

8.2 BIOLOGICAL PROCESSES IN CHEMICAL CARCINOGENESIS

8.2.1 Multistep Carcinogenesis

Experiments performed in the 1940s and 1950s led to a multistep model that divided the neoplastic process into three stages: (1) initiation, (2) promo-

tion, and (3) progression (Foulds, 1954). Initiation is the process whereby the chemical or its reactive metabolite causes a permanent change in the DNA of a target cell. Promotion is an experimentally defined process thought to involve epigenetic events that selectively influence the proliferation of the initiated cell. The third stage, progression, describes the stepwise development of a cancer cell as it acquires additional heritable changes leading to malignancy and metastatic potential. Chemical compounds can initiate, promote, and cause progression in the generation of a cancer.

Initiation An initiated cell is one in which a chemical carcinogen has interacted with DNA to produce a mutation, often a single base alteration, in the genome. At least three cellular functions are important in initiation, namely carcinogen metabolism, DNA repair, and cell proliferation. Metabolism may activate or inactivate the chemical carcinogen, DNA repair may either correct or introduce an altered base into the genome, and cell proliferation is necessary to produce heritable changes in the genome. Initiation is irreversible, but not all initiated cells will go on to establish a tumor, since many will die through the normal process of programmed cell death, or apoptosis. An initiated cell is not a tumor cell, since it has not acquired any autonomy of growth. The DNA alteration may remain undetected throughout the life of the organism unless further events stimulate the development of a clinically detectable neoplasm.

Tumor Promotion Chemical carcinogens usually interact with DNA in target tissues to produce covalent adducts that modify gene expression or the function of a gene product. One group of chemicals, known as *tumor promoters*, contributes to carcinogenesis by nongenotoxic mechanisms. Tumor promoters usually influence the proliferation of initiated cells, resulting in a focal proliferation of the preneoplastic cells and the formation of benign focal lesions such as papillomas, nodules, or polyps. Many of these lesions will regress, but a few cells may acquire additional mutations and progress to a malignant neoplasm. Active promotion is not always necessary, however, and cancer can result solely from the accumulation of genetic damage. The effects of a tumor promoter on multistage carcinogenesis are well illustrated by studies in mouse skin (Fig. 8.2). A single low dose of an initiating agent such as benzo[*a*]pyrene, applied directly to the skin, usually does not give rise to a tumor or other visible abnormality. When low doses of benzo[*a*]pyrene are fol-

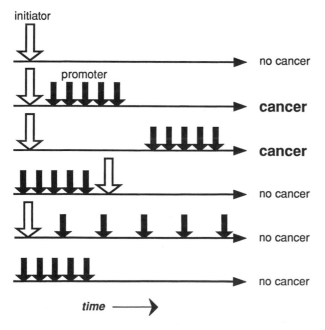

Figure 8.2. Outcome of various sequences of experimental exposure to initiating agents and promoting agents in mouse skin.

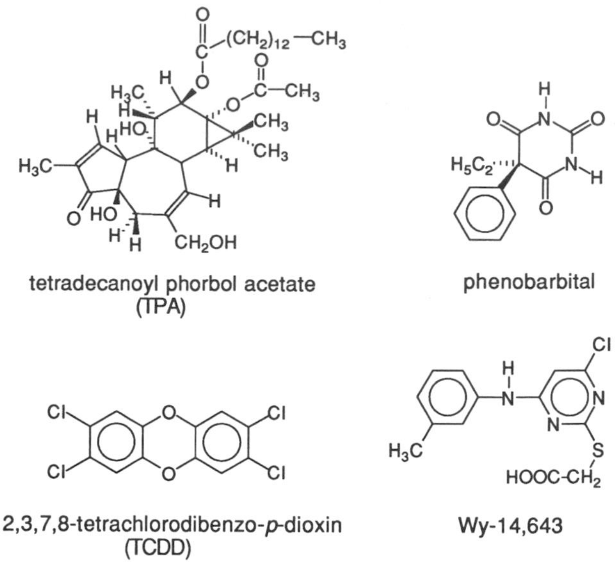

Figure 8.3. Chemical structures of some known promoting agents.

lowed by repeated doses of a promoting agent (e.g., croton oil), a large number of papillomas form and ultimately carcinomas develop. No tumors develop if only the promoting agent is applied or if the promoting agent is applied before the initiator. Tumors are induced, however, if the application of the promoting agent is delayed for several months after the initiator, but only when the intensity of the promoter exceeds a certain threshold.

Examples of tumor-promoting agents are shown in Fig. 8.3. The diterpene phorbol ester tetradecanoyl phorbol acetate (TPA), the active component in croton oil, is a potent tumor promoter in the mouse skin carcinogenesis model. Phenobarbital, certain chlorinated hydrocarbons such as 2,3,7,8-tetrachlorodibenzo-*p*-dioxin, and the peroxisome proliferator Wy-14,643 are effective promoters of liver carcinogenesis. Unlike initiators, most promoters do not form electrophilic species. They do not bind covalently to DNA and usually do not cause mutations or show genotoxicity in a variety of short-term tests, including the Ames test (see Sec. 8.3.1). Promotion is considered to be reversible up to a certain stage if the promoting agent is withdrawn. There is no single unifying mechanism to explain the activities of the various tumor-promoting agents, but in general, they appear to cause a transient increase in cell division and to decrease apoptosis, thus offering a selective growth advantage to initiated cells.

Tumor Progression During progression, tumors acquire the ability to grow, invade local tissue, and establish distant metastases. A major hallmark of progression is karyotypic instability. Chromosomes in tumors are often broken, and segments are translocated to other chromosomes, are present in multiple copies, or are partially or totally deleted. In parallel with these structural changes there are mutations in cellular oncogenes and/or tumor suppressor genes. These mutations probably reflect an ongoing selection for cells suited to neoplastic growth and may, in turn, enhance karyotypic instability. The acquisition of these mutations could result from an alteration in the function of oncogenes/tumor suppressor genes or from further exposure to a chemical carcinogen. Thus many chemicals that cause initiation will also cause progression. Some chemicals may affect only the transition of a cell from promotion to progression, but the experimental demonstration of such progressor agents is difficult; putative progressor agents (with no initiator activity) include benzene, benzoyl peroxide, and 2,5,2',5'-tetrachlorobiphenyl.

The classic model of initiation, promotion, and progression represents a convenient conceptual framework for the understanding of carcinogenesis. However, analysis of tumor development at the molecular level indicates that multiple changes in the genome are necessary for tumorigenesis. For example, studies on colorectal malignancies (Fearon and Vogelstein, 1992) have shown that alterations in at least four genes on different chromosomes must occur (see Chap. 4, Fig. 4.16). The number of genes that must be altered to produce a metastatic tumor is not known and may vary for both tissue and tumor type. Moreover, it is unknown whether mutations must be acquired in a particular temporal sequence or whether tumorigenesis proceeds simply with the accumulation of genetic defects (see also Chap. 4, Secs. 4.2 and 4.5).

8.2.2 Metabolism of Carcinogens

Genotoxic carcinogens have a wide diversity of chemical structures (Fig. 8.1), but all of them share one common feature: chemical reactivity. They are electrophilic (i.e., they attract electrons) either directly or via enzymatic conversion (Fig. 8.4) into metabolites that are positively charged, electron-deficient chemical species. Reactive electrophiles interact readily with negatively charged, electron-rich groups on biological molecules such as proteins and nucleic acids, forming covalent adducts. Covalent adducts with bases in DNA, if not enzymatically repaired prior to the next cycle of DNA replication, may lead to errors in DNA replication and hence to the fixation of nucleotide substitutions or frameshift mutations. If such mutations occur within the coding regions of genes involved in cell growth or differentiation, then dysfunction of the gene products may contribute to development of a malignant phenotype.

The majority of genotoxic carcinogens require enzymatic bioactivation (Miller and Miller, 1981). The catalysts for these reactions are the products of several multigene families of biotransforming or "drug-metabolizing" enzymes that convert lipophilic compounds into water-soluble metabolites that can be more efficiently excreted in urine or bile. The physiologic role of these catalysts is to defend organisms against chemical insults from the environment, and they have evolved both multiplicity and catalytic promiscuity to ensure that chemicals with widely divergent structures will undergo biotransformation. Biotransformation usually leads to inactivation of potentially harmful environmental chemicals; however, carcinogens possess structures that lead to their inadvertent biotransformation to electrophiles, with the potential to react with DNA. Because biotransformation can result in the production of a large number of metabolites from a single

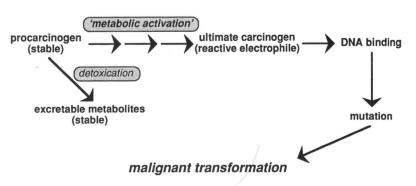

Figure 8.4. A general scheme illustrating the competition between pathways of procarcinogen detoxication and metabolic activation to reactive, DNA-binding electrophiles.

chemical via multiple competing pathways, the ultimate effect of carcinogen exposure in a particular individual is likely to depend on competing activation and detoxication pathways, which may be influenced by both genetic and environmental factors.

Drug-metabolizing enzymes belong to either the phase I or phase II category. Phase I enzymes (such as mono-oxygenases, oxidases, reductases, dehydrogenases, and esterases) introduce or unmask functional groups on the parent substrate. One of the most important of the phase I enzyme systems is the cytochrome P450 mono-oxygenase superfamily, consisting of several membrane-bound hemoproteins that catalyze the oxidation of carbon, nitrogen, and sulfur atoms in chemical molecules to produce hydroxylated metabolites. Oxidation by P450 enzymes has the potential to produce either inherently unstable electrophiles, such as epoxides, or stable hydroxylated compounds that may serve as substrates for further conjugation by transferase enzymes. Loss of chemical leaving groups can then lead to electrophile generation. Table 8.1 lists some human isoforms of cytochrome P450 implicated in pathways of carcinogen activation. Formation or unmasking of hydroxyl groups on chemicals may also be mediated by peroxidases, flavin-dependent mono-oxygenases, aldehyde and amine oxidases, and various esterases.

Many of the phase II biotransforming enzymes play dual roles in that they can both detoxify and activate procarcinogens. These enzymes, which include the UDP-glucuronosyltransferases, sulfotransferases, methyltransferases, glutathione-S-transferases, and acetyltransferases, can catalyze the addition ("conjugation") of bulky, often water-soluble substituents onto oxidase-generated hydroxyl groups on chemical molecules. In general, reactions catalyzed by conjugating enzymes are detoxifying, since their products can be excreted. However, the transferases may also contribute to bioactivation because the products formed are unstable and can break down spontaneously into DNA-reactive electrophiles.

With a few exceptions (such as acylating agents and unsaturated aldehydes), both directly acting carcinogens and those requiring prior metabolic activation interact ultimately with DNA by three general types of reaction chemistry (Dipple, 1995). These reactions involve transfer of (1) an alkyl group, (2) an arylamine group, or (3) an aralkyl group, as shown in Fig. 8.5. For chemicals that require metabolic activation to be carcinogenic, different types of biotransformations lead to reactive metabolites of the above classes (Fig. 8.5). For example, oxidation on carbon atoms (usually catalyzed by isoforms of cytochrome P450) can produce alkylating or aralkylating agents, while oxidation or reduction on nitrogen atoms produces arylaminating agents. Conjugation of C-hydroxyl or N-hydroxyl or direct carbon conjugation produces suitable leaving groups to result in chemical species that aralkylate, arylaminate, and alkylate, respectively. These chemical processes are described below.

Alkylation: Dialkylnitrosamines and Aflatoxin B1
Alkylating agents are those that lead to addition of an alkyl group (e.g., R-CH_2^+) to electron-rich sites in DNA; they are produced by hydroxylation of an aliphatic (nonaromatic) carbon atom in a chemical molecule. This process is most commonly mediated by isoforms of cytochrome P450 in a reaction that involves loss of a hydrogen ion (Guengerich, 1992). For N-nitroso compounds, which may be found in certain foods, beverages, cosmetics, and rubber products as well as being formed endogenously by nitrosation of amines and amides, cytochrome P450–mediated hydroxylation of the carbon adjacent to the nitroso group leads to spontaneous loss of the hydroxyalkyl group as an aldehyde. Tautomerization of the resultant primary nitrosamine to a diazonium hydroxide and spontaneous decomposition produces a carbonium ion, which is the ultimate alkylating agent. This process is illustrated in Fig. 8.6 for the CYP2E1-mediated bioactivation of dimethylnitrosamine. Larger N-nitroso compounds such as the tobacco smoke–derived NNK (Fig. 8.1) are activated primarily by other P450 isoforms such as CYP1A2. Aflatoxin B1 (AFB1) is also bioactivated by cytochrome P450 isoforms to an alkylating agent, by hydroxylation at an unsaturated C-C bond to yield a reactive epoxide metabolite (Fig. 8.7). Two

Table 8.1. Major Cytochrome P450 Enzymes Involved in Carcinogen Activation or Detoxification and Key Carcinogens That They Metabolize

---

CYP1A1: benzo[a]pyrene; 6-nitrochrysene

CYP1A2: 2-acetylaminofluorene; NNK; aflatoxin B1; β-naphthylamine; 4-aminobiphenyl protein pyrolysis products [IQ; MeIQ; GluP-1; etc.]

CYP1B1: 7,12-dimethylbenz[a]anthracene

CYP2E1: benzene; chloroform; vinyl chloride; dimethylnitrosamine

CYP3A4: aflatoxin B1; 6-aminochrysene; 1-nitropyrene

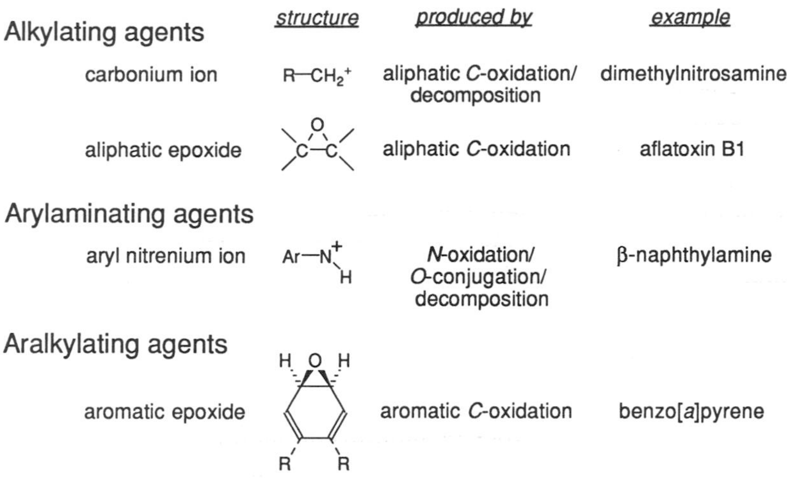

Alkylating agents

	structure	*produced by*	*example*
carbonium ion	R—CH₂⁺	aliphatic *C*-oxidation/ decomposition	dimethylnitrosamine
aliphatic epoxide	(epoxide structure)	aliphatic *C*-oxidation	aflatoxin B1

Arylaminating agents

aryl nitrenium ion	Ar—N⁺H	*N*-oxidation/ *O*-conjugation/ decomposition	β-naphthylamine

Aralkylating agents

aromatic epoxide	(aromatic epoxide structure)	aromatic *C*-oxidation	benzo[*a*]pyrene

Figure 8.5. Classes and structures of DNA-binding reactive electrophiles and the enzyme reactions that can produce them.

different isoforms of cytochrome P450, CYP1A2 and CYP3A4, are capable of catalyzing this reaction in humans, and there is disagreement concerning which form is more relevant for the human carcinogenicity of AFB1.

Arylamination: Aromatic Amines and Amides Aromatic amines and amides—as well as aminoazo dyes, nitroaromatics, and heterocyclic amine food-pyrolysis products—interact with DNA subsequent to formation of highly electrophilic aryl nitrenium ions (Ar-NH⁺). The latter are generated by cleavage of the bond between the nitrogen atom of an aryl-amino group and an oxygen atom generated initially by cytochrome P450–mediated *N*-hydroxylation and then modified to a good leaving group by

conjugation with either acetate, sulfate, or glucuronic acid, as shown for the aromatic amine ß-naphthylamine in Fig. 8.8. Competing metabolic pathways may be important in determining which DNA-reactive metabolites are formed in sufficient quantities to produce genotoxicity (Fig. 8.8). Oxidation by prostaglandin-H-synthase; conjugation by UDP-glucuronosyltransferases, sulfotransferases, and acetyltransferases; and deconjugation by glucuronidases, sulfatases, and deacetylases are all reactions that may compete or cooperate to produce ei-

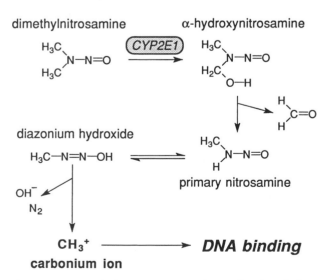

Figure 8.6. Metabolic activation pathway for dimethylnitrosamine.

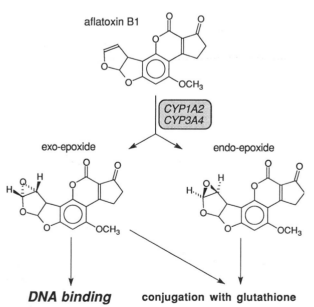

Figure 8.7. Metabolic activation pathway for aflatoxin B1.

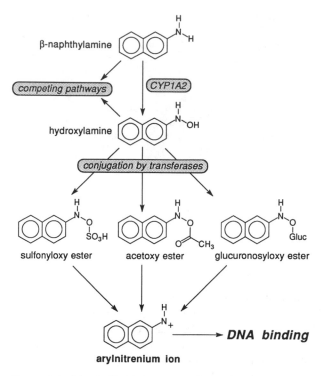

Figure 8.8. Metabolic activation pathway for the aromatic amine β-naphthylamine.

ther stable excretable metabolites or compounds that progress toward the ultimate DNA-binding species.

Aralkylation: Polycyclic Aromatic Hydrocarbons
Polycyclic aromatic hydrocarbons (PAHs) and related compounds are capable of transferring an aralkyl (aromatic alkyl) group to DNA. In the case of PAHs such as benzo[*a*]pyrene (Fig. 8.9), this is accomplished by generation of an electrophilic diol-epoxide metabolite. As with aromatic amines and amides, bioactivation of PAHs involves multiple enzymatic steps. Benzo[*a*]pyrene, for example, is converted by the P450 enzyme CYP1A1 to a 7,8-epoxide, which is hydrolyzed by epoxide hydrolase to the 7,8-dihydrodiol. This metabolite is then further oxidized by CYP1A1 to the 7,8-diol-9,10-epoxide, which is resistant to further metabolism by epoxide hydrolase and is sufficiently electrophilic to attack bases of DNA. Although important exceptions exist, it is common for the bioactivation of procarcinogens into their ultimate carcinogenic metabolites to require more than one enzyme-catalyzed step.

Figure 8.9. Metabolic activation pathway for the polycyclic aromatic hydrocarbon benzo[a]pyrene.

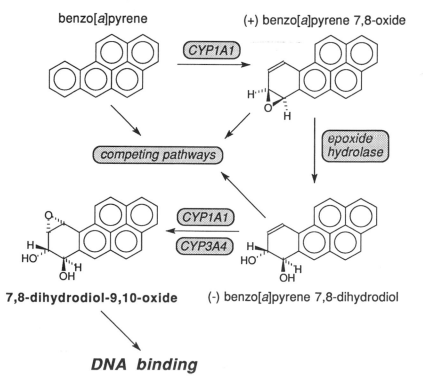

8.2.3 Genetic Polymorphisms of Carcinogen-Metabolizing Enzymes

There is interindividual variation, much of it genetically based, in several of the enzyme systems that activate and detoxify procarcinogens (Nebert et al., 1996). Epidemiologic studies have provided evidence that genetic defects of drug-metabolizing enzymes may be associated (albeit usually weakly) with altered susceptibility to chemically induced cancers. For example, there is an association between the "slow acetylator" phenotype, produced by allelic variants at the arylamine N-acetyltransferase 2 (NAT2) gene locus, and the incidence of bladder carcinoma. Allelic variation at the NAT1 gene locus (regulated independently from NAT2) may also play a role in predisposition to bladder cancer, and the NAT2 rapid acetylator phenotype may be associated with an increased risk for colorectal cancer. The NAT1 and NAT2 enzymes are involved in activation and detoxification of aromatic and heterocyclic amine procarcinogens.

Several studies have indicated that the "extensive metabolizer" phenotype for the polymorphic cytochrome P450 isoform CYP2D6 may be a risk factor for smoking-induced lung cancer. However, there are no known cigarette-derived carcinogens that are efficiently metabolized by CYP2D6 in vivo, although the human CYP2D6 enzyme can metabolize the N-nitroso compound NNK (Fig. 8.1) with low efficiency in vitro. Similarly, CYP2C19, the polymorphic S-mephenytoin hydroxylase, is defective in 3 to 5 percent of Caucasians and up to 20 percent of Asians, but no known carcinogens have yet been shown to be either activated or detoxified by it. The cytochrome P450 isoform CYP2E1 is known to metabolize several low-molecular-weight procarcinogens such as benzene, nitrosamines, and carbon tetrachloride, but it is unclear whether any of the known sequence polymorphisms within the CYP2E1 gene alter the activity of this enzyme sufficiently to affect risk for cancers caused by exposure to such agents. Finally, although CYP1A2 is required for the first step in the bioactivation of aromatic amines, it has not yet been demonstrated that differences in enzyme activity due to genetic defects within the CYP1A2 gene are able to alter cancer risk.

Although many epidemiologic studies of polymorphism of drug metabolism and cancer risk indicate only small increases in relative risk, this might be expected from the multifactorial nature of the disease. The effects of a carcinogen are influenced by multiple metabolic pathways as well as by DNA repair and cell cycle control, so that variation in a single bio-transformation pathway can be expected to produce only weak associations with cancer incidence. Combining multiple risk factors could provide stronger relative risks. For example, individuals with a combination of a null variant of the glutathione S-transferase-mu gene and an allelic variant of the cytochrome P450 CYP1A1 gene have been shown to have a 9-fold increase in relative risk for lung cancer, which jumps to a 41-fold elevation when stratified by smoking history (Nakachi et al., 1993).

8.2.4 DNA Adducts and DNA Repair

As indicated in Fig. 8.10, the three types of DNA-reactive chemical agents discussed above tend to produce distinctive adduct patterns, which are the result of differing reaction chemistries with particular atoms on the individual DNA bases (Pegg, 1984; Dipple, 1995). Highly ionic alkylating agents tend to bind to the exocyclic oxygen atoms on DNA bases, while less ionic species bind to ring nitrogen atoms such as N7 of deoxyguanosine. Arylaminating agents produce predominantly C8 deoxyguanosine adducts, although these may be formed by rearrangement subsequent to initial attack at the more nucleophilic N7 atom. Thus initial reactivity with N7 of deoxyguanosine may be a common feature of both alkylating and arylaminating agents.

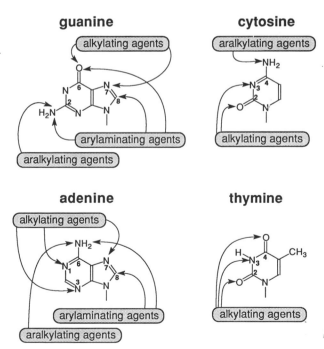

Figure 8.10. Sites of substitution on the four DNA bases by the three main chemical classes of genotoxic carcinogens. (Adapted from Dipple, 1995.)

Polycyclic aralkylating agents appear to produce different adducts by binding to the exocyclic nitrogen atoms of adenine and guanine bases.

The generation of adducts to bases in DNA affects the fidelity of DNA replication and can result in base substitutions. Several mechanisms have evolved that repair DNA and restore the original nucleotide sequence (Fig. 8.11). These include (1) direct repair of the DNA adduct, (2) excision and replacement of the modified base, (3) excision and replacement of a nucleotide sequence containing the modified base, and (4) repair of mismatched bases arising from mispairing during the replication of chemically modified DNA. These mechanisms are discussed in detail in Chap. 4, Sec. 4 (see also Friedberg et al., 1995; Sancar, 1995), but aspects of DNA repair that are relevant to chemical carcinogenesis are summarized below.

In direct repair, the bond between the adduct and nucleotide is broken, there is direct removal of small alkyl substituents, and the normal DNA configuration is re-created. Synthetic (exogenous) methylating agents such as N-methyl-N'-nitro-N-nitrosoguanidine (MNNG), N-methyl-N-nitrosourea (MNU), and dimethylnitrosamine, or natural (endogenous) agents such as S-adenosylmethionine can alkylate DNA at several sites to produce O-alkylated and N-alkylated products. The most important lesion biologically is probably the O^6 methylated derivative of guanine, O^6-meG (Fig. 8.10), which can pair with thymine and result in a mutagenic transi-

tion of G:C to A:T when DNA is replicated. Such damage can be repaired by the enzyme O^6-methyl-guanine-DNA methyltransferase (MGMT), which selectively removes methyl groups from the O^6 position of guanine as well as adducts such as O^6-ethylG, O^6-butylG, and O^4-methylthymine (see Chap. 4, Sec. 4.4.3). In several types of cancer, oncogene activation results from a transition of G:C to A:T, consistent with failure to repair the alkylation of guanine. Targeted overexpression of MGMT in the thymus protected transgenic mice against the development of thymic lymphomas induced by exposure to MNU (Dumenco et al, 1993). Targeted expression of human MGMT in bone marrow also protected mice against the myelosuppressive effects of the chemotherapeutic agent chloroethylnitrosourea (Maze et al., 1996).

Nonbulky base adducts that do not distort the DNA helix are substrates for base excision repair (see Chap. 4, Sec. 4.4.5). These adducts include 3-methyladenine, 7-methyladenine, O^2-hydroxymethylcytosine, or 8-hydroxyguanine residues produced by methylating agents such as MNU. Recently, repair by base excision has been shown for other chemically induced lesions, such as the ethonopurine derivative formed by vinyl chloride (Seeberg et al., 1995).

Bulky DNA adducts such as acetylaminofluorene-guanine or benzo[a]pyrene-guanine, or thymine-psoralen and guanine-cisplatin, may inhibit DNA replication and/or result in DNA polymerase preferentially filling the noninstructive site with adenine. If this occurs opposite a guanine adduct, thymine will pair with the adenine during the next round of DNA replication, resulting in a G-to-T transversion. Such bulky adducts are removed by nucleotide excision repair (see Chap. 4, Sec. 4.4.5). Nucleotide excision repair has a very broad substrate range, making it able to recognize and remove a large number of lesions (Sancar, 1994), including apurinic/apyrimidinic sites, N^6-methyladenine, and O^6-methylguanine (Huang et al., 1994). It may also serve as a backup repair mechanism for alkylation damage.

Chemically damaged bases such as O^6-meG do not necessarily block DNA replication but may result in an O^6-meG-T mismatch, thereby activating DNA mismatch repair (see Chap. 4, Sec. 4.4.4). Mismatch repair removes the incorrect base specifically from the newly synthesized daughter strand of DNA. Since O^6-meG is in the parental strand during replication, DNA mismatch repair is inefficient in repairing this adduct; it removes the thymine from the

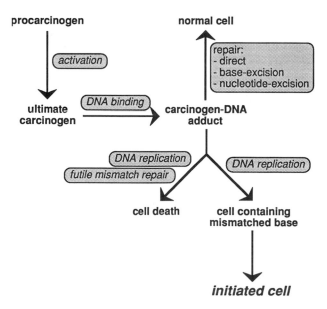

Figure 8.11. Possible outcomes following adduct formation.

daughter strand, but leaves O^6-meG in the parental strand. Subsequent repair synthesis reintroduces the mismatched thymine and causes futile cycling of removal/replacement of thymine, leading to eventual cell death. Transgenic mice deficient in the mismatch repair gene Msh-2 are tolerant to the toxic effects of simple methylating agents such as MNNG (deWind et al., 1995), possibly as the result of the pairing of O^6-meG with T in the first round of replication. A deficiency in mismatch repair may therefore allow survival of genetically damaged cells and predispose to cancer.

8.2.5 Targets of Chemical Carcinogens

The relevant targets for mutagenesis by carcinogens include proto-oncogenes and tumor suppressor genes. When proto-oncogenes are activated by a mutational event, signals for cell growth are increased, but for tumor suppressor genes, which regulate cell growth negatively, relevant mutations result in a loss of function (see Chap. 5). Usually at least two independent mutational events are required for deregulation of cell growth and subsequent malignant transformation. Commonly found mutations in chemically induced tumors in rodents are those that activate the *ras* family of oncogenes. For example, rat mammary tumors induced by a single dose of methyl nitrosourea (MNU) contain H-*ras* genes that have been activated by a single point mutation (G-to-A transition) at codon 12 of the gene (Zhang et al., 1991). In papillomas and carcinomas induced in mouse skin by 7,12-dimethyl-benz[*a*]anthracene, there is an activating mutation in codon 61 (A-to-T transversion) of the H-*ras* gene (Quintanilla et al., 1986).

Mutations in the tumor suppressor gene p53 are present in more than 50 percent of human tumors. The sites of mutation are not random but occur at discrete "hot spots" (see Chap. 5, Sec. 5.5.2). Mutational hot spots probably occur for two different reasons: (1) because of the high efficiency of adduct formation and the low efficiency of DNA repair at that site and (2) because specific regions of the gene are critical for its function. Different hot spots can be found in different cells or tissue types. For example, in liver cancers from southern China or southern Africa, where there are high incidences of both hepatitis B virus and exposure to aflatoxin B1, p53 mutations occur most frequently at codon 249. The reactive diol-epoxide metabolite of benzo[*a*]pyrene, when added to human cells in culture, preferentially forms adducts with guanine in

codons 157, 248, and 273 of the p53 gene, in the same positions where mutational hot spots are found in human lung cancer. This correspondence between the adduct hot spots and the clinically observed mutational hot spots strengthens the etiologic link between smoking and lung cancer (Denissenko et al., 1996). The clonal expansion of a cell that ultimately forms a tumor suggests that cells expressing a mutant p53 have a growth advantage. Thus sites where mutations occur frequently in tumors may be presumed to identify regions of the molecule important in p53 function (Greenblatt et al., 1994).

Not all carcinogens are genotoxic. When administered chronically, a number of chemicals induce tumor formation but demonstrate no evidence of interaction with DNA. Some compounds that have nongenotoxic carcinogenic activity might act as promoters for spontaneously initiated cells, but not all nongenotoxic carcinogens can be demonstrated to have promoting activity. These carcinogens probably act through a variety of mechanisms, which include (1) dysregulation of cell growth, either directly or through sustained tissue damage and subsequent cell proliferation; (2) increased oxygen stress, resulting in generation of reactive oxygen species leading to DNA damage; and (3) disruption of receptor-mediated cell-signaling processes.

8.3 IDENTIFICATION OF CARCINOGENS AND ASSESSMENT OF RISK

Establishing that a given chemical is a human carcinogen is a difficult and protracted process. Humans are exposed to a multitude of drugs and environmental agents, and there is a long latent period between exposure and tumor appearance. The most productive approach has involved astute clinical observation combined with carefully designed epidemiologic and laboratory studies (Table 8.2).

8.3.1 In Vitro Assays for Carcinogens

Rodent bioassays (see Sec. 8.3.2) are expensive, time-consuming, and impractical as an initial screen of the thousands of chemicals that need to be assessed for carcinogenic potential. Early studies were thus based on the development of assays for cell transformation. These assays were developed initially for fibroblasts, which are relatively easy to grow in culture, but they have also been applied to epithelial cell cultures. Most studies of cell transformation in vitro have used cell lines that will grow indefinitely in culture if subcultured

Table 8.2. Assays for Carcinogens

Long-term assays
   Clinical observation and epidemiology
   Bioassays in laboratory animals, principally rodents

Short-term assays
   Detection of DNA damage:
      Covalent adducts of the test compound with DNA
      after metabolic activation DNA strand breakage
   Detection of chromosomal damage:
      Chromosomal abnormalities by cytogenetics
      Sister chromatid exchange
      Micronucleus frequency
      Sperm abnormalities
   Detection of mutational events:
      Bacterial mutagenesis (Ames *Salmonella* assay, etc.)
      Sex-linked mutations and reciprocal translocations in
        Drosophila
   Unscheduled DNA synthesis in cells in culture
   Neoplastic transformation of mammalian cells in culture

under appropriate conditions; i.e. they are immortalized and do not senesce like cells from primary explants (see Chap. 7, Sec. 7.3.5). However, they do not form tumors when reinjected into syngeneic or immune-compromised mice. Such cell lines, when grown in tissue culture, exhibit contact inhibition of growth; i.e., they stop dividing when they come into close proximity with one another but remain viable. Occasionally in rodent cells (but rarely in human cells) a spontaneous change occurs that causes the cells to lose contact inhibition, so that they continue to proliferate by

spreading over adjacent cells and piling up. Such transformed cells form colonies or foci that can be distinguished and counted when stained. When cells from such foci are isolated, cloned, expanded, and reinjected back into syngeneic or immune-compromised mice, they often form tumors. Some of the properties of transformed fibroblasts are compared with those of immortalized (normal) fibroblasts in Table 8.3.

Transformed foci can be induced by treatment of the cells with many carcinogenic chemicals (as well as by radiation), or by oncogenic viruses and transfection of oncogenes (see Sec. 8.5.1 and Chap. 5, Sec. 5.4.1); thus focus-forming assays are quite suitable for screening putative carcinogens. Cell-transformation assays are time-consuming, however, and thus many shorter-term tests have been developed that are based on the premise that carcinogens are mutagenic. A wide variety of organisms has been used in these tests, including bacteria, fungi, mammalian cells, and insects (Ames et al., 1990; Shelby et al., 1990; Zeiger et al., 1990). End points include DNA damage, mutation, and chromosomal aberration (Table 8.2).

Perhaps the most widely used short-term assay is the Ames assay (Fig. 8.12). In devising this test, Ames selected mutant *Salmonella typhimurium* strains that are unable to synthesize the essential amino acid histidine and are therefore unable to grow if it is absent from the culture medium. Exposure of these bacteria to chemical mutagens can result in reversion of the mutation back to histidine independence in a

Table 8.3. A Comparison of the Properties of Normal and Transformed Fibroblasts

Normal Fibroblasts	Transformed Fibroblasts
Will not form tumors in mice	Form tumors when implanted into syngeneic or immune-deprived mice
Grow attached to plastic or glass (anchorage-dependent)	Grow in suspension or in semisolid media such as agar
Growth is inhibited by contact with other cells (contact inhibition)	Loss of contact inhibition allows piling up into colonies or foci
Require serum containing hormones and growth factors	Reduced dependence on growth factors or serum
Remain viable if growth is arrested by lack of serum	Cells die if inhibited from growing
Contain well-organized actin filaments	Show disorganization of actin filaments
Do not cause fibrinolysis	May cause fibrinolysis through secretion of plasminogen activator

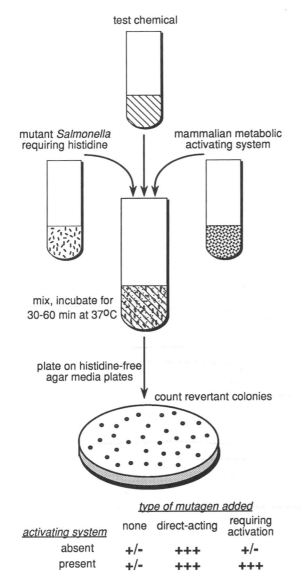

test chemical

mutant *Salmonella*
requiring histidine

mammalian metabolic
activating system

mix, incubate for
30-60 min at 37°C

plate on histidine-free
agar media plates

count revertant colonies

	type of mutagen added		
activating system	none	direct-acting	requiring activation
absent	+/-	+++	+/-
present	+/-	+++	+++

Figure 8.12. Detection of mutagenic chemicals in *Salmonella typhimurium* (Ames test). (Adapted from Pitot and Dragan, 1996.)

small number of cells; consequently they regain the ability to grow in histidine-deficient medium. The number of "revertant" colonies that grow on agar plates after chemical exposure is thus a measure of the mutagenic potency of the test compound in producing the reversion to histidine independence. Since many chemicals must be bioactivated in order to be mutagenic or carcinogenic, the assay is usually conducted in the presence of mammalian liver enzymes to bioactivate the procarcinogen.

Recently, transgenic animals (see Chap. 3, Sec.

3.3.12) carrying readily retrievable mutational targets have been developed for in vivo mutational testing. After exposure of the animal to the potential chemical mutagen, it is possible to retrieve the mutational target (usually either the LacI or the LacZ gene) and determine mutational frequencies as well as the nature of the mutation(s). These animals provide valuable information regarding tissue and organ specificity. Unlike the Ames assay, this approach is expensive and is used as a secondary assay after a chemical has been established as a mutagen through a primary screen in microorganisms.

Most of the chemical agents known to be important carcinogens in humans are mutagenic in assays of bacterial mutagenesis and cause cytogenetic changes in rodent bone marrow (Table 8.4). Many mutagens are also carcinogenic; however, most of the chemicals that are mutagenic in short-term assays have not been shown to be carcinogenic in humans. Assessment of the carcinogenic potential of nongenotoxic chemicals is particularly difficult, since there is no apparent common mechanism on which to base large-scale routine screening assays for chemicals that are not mutagenic.

8.3.2 Bioassays in Animals

While data from human epidemiologic studies (see Chap. 2) are required to establish human carcinogenicity, bioassays in rodents serve as a useful surrogate for attempting to detect potential human carcinogens. Testing for carcinogenicity of chemicals in rodents is often criticized because these tests frequently employ doses far in excess of the probable human exposure. At high doses (usually the "maximum tolerated dose," or MTD), cytotoxic effects of the test chemical can confound the outcome by causing necrosis and regenerative proliferation in some tissues, especially liver. However, most chemicals that induce tumors at high dose will also induce some tumors at lower doses in studies using larger numbers of animals.

High doses are used in animal tests for the practical reasons of improving the signal-to-noise ratio (i.e., induced-tumor incidence to spontaneous-tumor incidence) and reducing the number of animals required. Most animal models can detect tumor incidences of about 5 percent, but not as low as 1 percent. In a human population an increase in total tumor incidence of even 1 percent would be unacceptable. Carcinogenic activity in a rodent assay

Table 8.4. Mutagenicity in Bacteria and Rodent Bone Marrow
of Selected Known Human Carcinogens

	Salmonella Mutagenicity	Rodent Bone Marrow Cytogenetic Effects
Organic compounds		
Aflatoxins	+	+
Azathioprine	+	+
4-aminobiphenyl	+	+
2-naphthylamine	+	+
Phenacetin	+	+
Benzene	−	+
Benzidine	+	+
Chlorambucil	+	+
Cyclophosphamide	+	+
Melphalan	+	+
Methyl-CCNU	+	+
Mustard gas	+	+
Vinyl chloride	+	+
Complex mixtures		
Tobacco smoke	+	ND
Smokeless tobacco	+	+
Betel quid and tobacco	+	+
Coal tars and coal-tar pitches	+	+
Soots	+	ND
Metals and fibers		
Arsenic compounds	−	+
Chromium compounds	+	+
Asbestos	−	ND

ND = no data

Source: Adapted from Barrett 1993.

does not prove that a particular chemical will be a carcinogen in humans, but it does identify the chemical as a potential human carcinogen.

In laboratory animals it has been demonstrated empirically that the incidence of cancer caused by several chemical agents increases with dose (Fig. 8.13). Figure 8.13 also shows that carcinogenic potency can differ between two closely related compounds. In this example, benzo[*a*]pyrene is about tenfold less potent than 3-methylcholanthrene. Some generalizations concerning the quantitative relationship between exposure and responses to carcinogens are as follows:

1. A single exposure to certain chemical carcinogens is sufficient to induce tumors in a high proportion of the animals. A dramatic example is the induction of mammary carcinoma in female rats. As rats approach sexual maturity, any one of several polycyclic aromatic hydrocarbons (e.g., benzo[*a*]pyrene, benz[*a*]anthracene, 7,12-dimethylbenz[*a*]anthracene; ibenz[*a,h*]anthracene, 3-methylcholanthrene) is capable of producing mammary carcinomas in over 90

percent of exposed animals after a single oral dose.

2. Tumor production is often enhanced if chemical exposure is repeated. Repeated exposures also

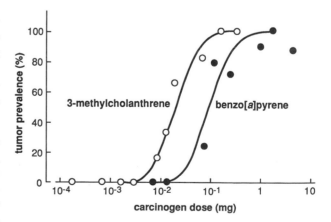

Figure 8.13. Dose-response curves for 3-methylcholanthrene (3-MC) and benzo[a]pyrene (BP) in male C3H mice. The carcinogens were injected subcutaneously and sarcomas arising at the site of a single injection were counted. (Adapted from Bryan and Shimkin, 1943.)

may shorten the latency period—i.e., the time between the first application of the agent and the eventual appearance of a tumor. This has been shown for induction of liver tumors in rodents treated with nitrosamines. Mechanistically, repeated exposure may enhance the probability that the required sequence of mutations will accumulate during the multistage process of carcinogenesis.

3. Tumor susceptibility varies widely among different animal species exposed to the same dose of the same chemical carcinogen. For example, rats are much more susceptible to liver tumors from feeding of aflatoxins than are mice. These variations in susceptibility may be due to differences in the activity of enzyme pathways that activate or detoxify chemical carcinogens. Genetically based diversity in metabolism and response to carcinogens can even exist across different strains within the same laboratory species and among different individuals in the human population.

4. Dose-response curves may not be identical in different tissues that are susceptible to a given carcinogen, even within the same animal. Figure 8.14 presents data from a large-scale dose-response study (about 24,000 mice) of the carcinogen 2-acetylaminofluorene (2-AAF). The prevalence of liver tumors in these animals begins to rise at doses considerably below the dose where a significant increase in bladder cancer is observed. However, the curve for induction of bladder cancer is much steeper than the response in liver, such that at higher doses of 2-AAF, bladder

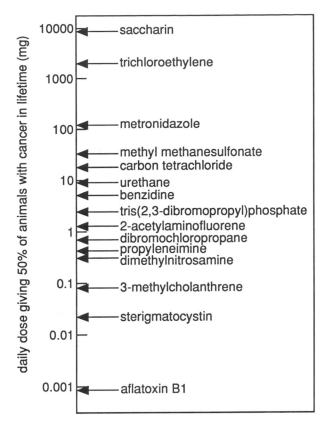

Figure 8.15. The range of carcinogenic potencies for various chemicals. The values shown on the y axis indicate the amount of daily intake that is required to produce cancer in 50 percent of test animals over a lifetime of exposure. Note that the scale is logarithmic. (Adapted from data compiled by Ames, as cited in Maugh, 1978.)

tumors occur in nearly twice as many animals as do liver tumors. Hence the definition of which tissue is at "greatest risk" depends upon which region of the dose-response curve is being examined (i.e., on the level of exposure). The difference in response between bladder and liver has been attributed not to pharmacokinetic differences in carcinogen distribution or adduct formation but to increased cell proliferation in bladder (but not liver) at the higher doses of 2-AAF (Cohen and Ellwein, 1991).

5. There is an extraordinarily broad range of potencies among different chemical carcinogens. As shown in Fig. 8.15, less than 1 μg/day of aflatoxin B1 is sufficient to produce tumors in 50 percent of rats after a lifetime of exposure, whereas compounds such as trichloroethylene or saccharin require more than 1 g/day to produce the same incidence of tumors. It may be more productive to view carcinogenicity as a spectrum

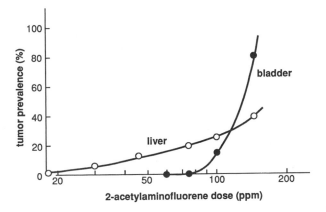

Figure 8.14. Dose-response curves for induction of liver and bladder tumors in female mice treated with 2-acetylaminofluorene; the tumor assessment was after treatment for 18 to 33 months. (Replotted from data in Cohen and Ellwein, 1991.)

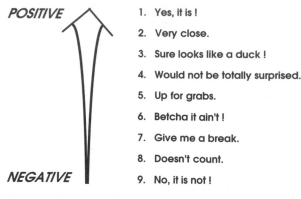

POSITIVE

1. Yes, it is !
2. Very close.
3. Sure looks like a duck !
4. Would not be totally surprised.
5. Up for grabs.
6. Betcha it ain't !
7. Give me a break.
8. Doesn't count.

NEGATIVE

9. No, it is not !

Figure 8.16. A classification scheme for carcinogens acknowledging the difficulty of distinguishing between "carcinogens" and "noncarcinogens." (Adapted from a report of the Toxicology Forum, Washington, D.C., 1991.)

relating to potency rather than an absolute property. Scientists in the Toxicology Forum have presented a classification scheme (Fig. 8.16) that acknowledges (in a lighthearted but not frivolous manner) that there is a spectrum of carcinogenicity for chemicals rather than only two categories of "yes, it is" versus "no, it is not."

8.3.3 Challenges in Identifying Human Carcinogens

Even after a particular chemical has been shown to be mutagenic by in vitro tests or to be carcinogenic in laboratory animals, the following problems make it difficult to determine whether or not that chemical causes cancer in humans:

1. The time interval between exposure to a potential carcinogen and the clinical detection of a tumor may be 10 to 20 years in humans. This lengthy "latent period" makes it difficult to link the disease to exposure to a particular agent.
2. It is often difficult to quantify the level of exposure, especially when it may have occurred decades before the disease. Most chemical residues and biomarkers of exposure have limited persistence (weeks to months) after exposure ends.
3. Humans are exposed to a multitude of chemicals and other potentially carcinogenic agents (viruses, ionizing radiation, etc.). These complex exposure patterns can confound attempts to attribute the disease to a particular agent.
4. People may differ widely from one another in their susceptibility to specific chemical carcino-

gens as a result of genetic variation at several loci, including those encoding genes involved in pathways of metabolic activation and detoxification of carcinogens (Sec. 8.2.3).
5. The statistical power for detecting carcinogens in epidemiologic studies is low unless the population studied is very large or unless there is a dramatic increase in tumor incidence at a particular anatomic site (see Chap. 2, Sec. 2.2.3).

Reduction of risk first requires that the factors contributing to risk be identified. These factors may be external forces, or they may be part of the makeup of the target organism. A systematic, stepwise approach is employed by regulatory agencies such as the Environmental Protection Agency (EPA) in the United States, which, in order to determine risk, integrates the multiple factors that interact in human carcinogenesis (Fig. 8.17).

Risk assessment is an attempt to quantify the probability of adverse effects, including cancer, from chemical exposure. The identification of suspect carcinogens and the extent of human exposure to them is a necessary prelude to the more quantitative assessment of risk. The assessor also needs some measurement of the relationship between the level of exposure and the biological response. To predict and prevent human harm, the dose-response assessment may rely heavily upon data from laboratory animals, despite the numerous caveats that apply in any attempt to extrapolate animal carcinogenesis data to humans.

8.3.4 Molecular Epidemiology

In estimating the dose-response component in risk assessment, an alternative to relying on cancer incidence in animals is to use surrogate biochemical end points rather than cancer outcomes per se. The molecular epidemiologic approach combines traditional cancer epidemiology with mechanistic information gained from studies in laboratory animals and from in vitro molecular models. For example, the carcinogen dose received by individuals might be quantified through measurement of biomarkers of exposure or responses such as adduct formation or mutational frequency in accessible cells and tissues. Figure 8.18 illustrates that the level of benzo[a]pyrene adducts in DNA in lung tissue of smokers is highly correlated with the activity of cytochrome P4501A1 (CYP1A1) in the same tissue. In other studies CYP1A1 induction has been correlated with the extent of smoke exposure. An increase in lung CYP1A1 activity signifies exposure to polycyclic

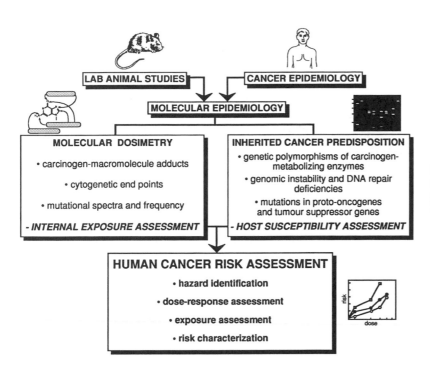

Figure 8.17. Strategy for using multiple approaches to assess chemical carcinogens for their risk of causing human cancer. (Adapted from Harris, 1991, 1993.)

aromatic hydrocarbons and may also portend an increase in adduct formation and risk of lung cancer (see also Sec. 8.2.3). Although this type of study is informative, the requirement for lung biopsy makes it suited primarily to studies in subjects with pre-existing disease.

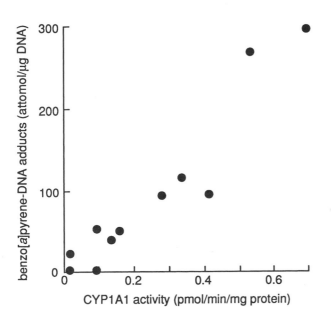

Figure 8.18. Correlation between cytochrome P4501A1 activity and formation of benzo[a]pyrene diol-epoxide adducts to DNA in lung samples from human lung cancer patients. (Adapted from Alexandrov et al., 1992.)

Biomarkers of exposure and response can sometimes be determined by minimally invasive tests in currently healthy subjects. For example, a hemoglobin-bound adduct of 4-aminobiphenyl is markedly elevated in smokers compared with nonsmokers, and this relatively simple measurement using peripheral blood may provide an integrated measure of smoke exposure over the previous period of about 4 months (Harris, 1991). A drawback of such studies is the required assumption that markers of exposure over a relatively recent time interval bear some relationship to initiating exposures which may have occurred decades earlier. This is problematic, for example, in attempting to correlate biomarkers of carcinogen exposure to cancer incidence in former smokers.

A major goal of molecular epidemiology is to identify individuals with elevated cancer risk due to heritable predisposing factors such as polymorphisms in carcinogen-metabolizing enzymes, genomic instability, or germline mutations in tumor suppressor genes (see Sec. 8.2.3; Chap. 4, Sec. 4.5.2 and 4.5.3; and Chap. 5, Sec. 5.5). To this end, molecular epidemiology asks three questions: (1) What is the inherent susceptibility of this individual? (2) What was the effective internal exposure of this individual to the carcinogen in question? and (3) What was the health outcome given the individual's genetic background and internal exposure? An attempt is then made to quantify risk.

8.3.5 Assessment and Management of Risk

Risk management applies the risk assessment, along with identification of sources of carcinogens, to the creation of regulations designed to eliminate or reduce sources and exposure. This process is an amalgam of science, societal values, economics, and political realities. The example of cigarette smoke illustrates that it can be difficult to achieve reduction in risk even when the risk factors and mechanisms are well known.

Permissible exposure ("negligible risk") has been set by some regulatory agencies as the level that would result in less than one additional case of cancer for every million people exposed. The determination of this "safe" exposure level is very difficult. Experiments in various laboratory animals have demonstrated that tumor incidence rises as exposure to chemical carcinogens is increased (Figs. 8.13 and 8.14). Humans also show increases in cancer risk with increased exposure to carcinogens. For example, data in Fig. 8.19 demonstrate that the relative risk of lung cancer in the United Kingdom, the United States, and Japan rises as the number of cigarettes smoked per day increases. Cigarette smoking

involves repeated delivery of a high dose of multiple chemical carcinogens directly to a susceptible tissue. In addition to this type of high-exposure situation, chronic involuntary human exposure to low levels of potential chemical carcinogens from proximity to smokers, occupation, or environment is of major concern. This may involve intake of only trace amounts per day of the suspected carcinogen from food, air, or water. A key practical challenge regarding carcinogen dose-response curves and human health is how to interpret the tumorigenic response at very low exposure levels. In practice, the risk from low-level exposure must be estimated by extrapolation downward from higher dose ranges where measurable responses (in animals or by molecular assays) can be observed in populations of achievable size.

Very often there is uncertainty about the shapes of the response curves at low doses due to the poor signal-to-noise ratio in the region where infrequent tumor responses are being superimposed upon a background of "spontaneous" tumors. When plotted against the logarithm of the dose, the standard pharmacologic response curve to xenobiotic chemicals is sigmoidal. Sigmoidal curves (Fig. 8.13) with shallow initial slopes at the lowest doses imply that there may be a "threshold" below which the increase in risk is insignificant. Several mathematical models attempt to define the tumor response at low exposure levels (Pitot and Dragan, 1996). The conservative position adopted by many regulatory agencies is that the carcinogenic dose-response curve is linear back to zero; i.e., there is some finite cancer risk even at the lowest doses, implying that even a single molecule of a carcinogen could cause cancer (albeit with very low probability).

New approaches to setting "safe" levels of exposure or for determining whether or not "thresholds" exist take into account the mechanisms by which the carcinogen acts as well as the protective mechanisms that animals have evolved to deal with foreign chemicals. It has been proposed that for genotoxic carcinogens (where the initiating event of somatic mutation is irreversible), the presumption should be made that there is no distinct threshold. In contrast, nongenotoxic carcinogens may in certain cases act via receptor-mediated mechanisms and thereby induce responses that, in principle, are reversible upon withdrawal of the agent. Thus, for nongenotoxic agents, there might exist a practical threshold below which there is no discernible harm (Cohen and Ellwein, 1991). For both genotoxic and nongenotoxic carcinogens it is plausible that host defense mechanisms will be more effective at lower

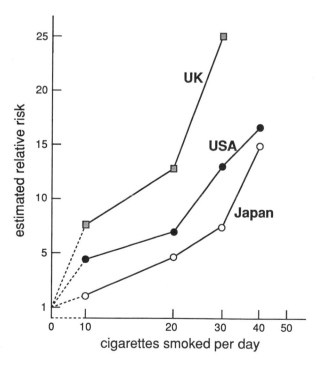

Figure 8.19. Dose-response relationship between the amount smoked and the risk of lung cancer in men from cohort studies from the United Kingdom, the United States, and Japan. (Replotted from data in Wynder and Hoffmann, 1994.)

exposure levels so that the probability of tumor formation is less than that predicted from linear extrapolation from higher doses. The debate about thresholds, no-effect levels, and the degree of cancer risk from low-level exposure applies to radiation and other carcinogens (Sec. 8.5; Goldman, 1996). At present, "quantitative risk assessment is . . . more mathematical extrapolation and scientific intuition than a rigorous science" (Harris, 1991).

8.4 CHEMOPREVENTION OF CANCER

Several clinical trials have been conducted or are in progress which attempt to reduce the risk of human cancer through administration of chemopreventive agents. These trials are based on experience with animal models, where sometimes dramatic reductions in cancer risk have been achieved through use of chemical preventive agents. Chemopreventive agents have been classified according to their primary site of action in the pathogenesis of cancer (Wattenberg, 1993) as follows: (1) agents that prevent carcinogen bioactivation, (2) agents that prevent potential carcinogens from reaching or reacting with target sites ("blocking agents"), and (3) agents that suppress neoplastic development after exposure ("suppressive agents").

8.4.1 Agents That Alter Bioactivation of Carcinogens

As described in Sec. 8.2.2, many procarcinogens are activated to their ultimate carcinogenic forms by various species of cytochrome P450. Chemicals that can inhibit P450 enzymes might, therefore, be effective anticarcinogens, and inhibition of P450 enzymes can reduce chemically induced cancers in laboratory animals (reviewed in Yang et al., 1994). For example, diallyl sulfide, a compound from garlic, can selectively inhibit the P450 microsomal enzymes CYP2B1 and CYP2E1, thereby interfering with both the bioactivation of NNK and the subsequent development of lung cancer in rodents. Phenethyl isothiocyanate, a component of some vegetables, also protects against NNK-induced lung tumors. Isothiocyanates may have a dual mechanism to suppress tumor formation: they can inhibit phase I "activating enzymes" (P450s) while simultaneously inducing some phase II conjugating enzymes (see below).

Indiscriminate inhibition of the full spectrum of P450 enzymes would not be useful as a chemopreventive strategy, since P450s are the major pathways by which humans and other animals eliminate a wide range of potentially harmful xenobiotic chemicals. Rather, it would be necessary (and challenging) to identify very selective inhibitors that could prevent bioactivation of specific chemical agents under defined high-risk circumstances.

Inhibitors of P450 enzymes can protect against chemically induced cancers, but so can some P450 inducers. This apparent paradox is due to competing roles of P450 enzymes in bioactivating procarcinogens into reactive metabolites that bind to DNA and their effect to enhance overall clearance of procarcinogens and carcinogens from the body. For example, P450 induction in liver can protect animals exposed to procarcinogens by the oral route because the high P450 activity in liver accomplishes "first-pass clearance" of the carcinogen (see Chap. 16, Sec. 16.2.1), so that exposure of susceptible peripheral tissues is reduced (Okey, 1992). Induction of a specific enzyme, P4501A2, is currently undergoing clinical trials to increase the clearance of the natural steroid estradiol-17β, with the goal of reducing breast cancer risk (see Sec. 8.4.3).

8.4.2 Blocking Agents

Natural products of plant origin such as vitamin E (α-tocopherol) and vitamin C (ascorbic acid) have antioxidant properties and can inhibit chemical mutagenesis in cell culture and some chemically induced cancers in laboratory animals (reviewed in Wattenberg, 1985; Bertram et al., 1987). It also has been shown that synthetic phenolic antioxidants such as the food preservatives butylated hydroxytoluene (BHT) and butylated hydroxyanisole (BHA) can be highly effective anticarcinogens in laboratory animals (O'Brien, 1994). Antioxidants act as scavengers of reactive metabolites and reduce the probability that the metabolites will bind to DNA and initiate tumors. In addition to nonenzymatic scavengers, there are several enzyme systems that carry out conjugation of reactive metabolites, thereby inactivating them and facilitating their excretion. Enzymes with this function include glutathione S-transferases that conjugate reactive metabolites with the abundant intracellular tripeptide glutathione (see also Chap. 17, Sec. 17.2.6), and UDP-glucuronosyltransferases, which conjugate reactive metabolites with glucuronic acid. Genetic deficiencies in UDP-glucuronosyltransferases in rats lead to an increased sensitivity to genetic damage from the tobacco carcinogens NNK and benzo[a]pyrene (Kim and Wells, 1996). Some of these transferases can be induced by products of plant origin such as sulforaphane from broccoli (Zhang et al., 1994), by environmental chemicals such as polycyclic aromatic hydrocarbons and dioxins, and by antioxidants such as BHA (O'Brien, 1994).

Induction of conjugating enzymes can be highly protective of animals against major chemical carcinogens. However, as described in Sec. 8.2.2, the conjugating enzymes occasionally function as bioactivating systems that convert unreactive precursors into toxic or carcinogenic products, as in the bioactivation of methylene chloride by glutathione S-transferases and of hydroxylated metabolites of aromatic amines by several enzyme systems. Thus, whether enzyme induction (or enzyme inhibition) is beneficial or detrimental depends upon which chemical agent is the main threat. Unfortunately, manipulations that protect from one class of carcinogens might increase the risk from some other chemical class. Generally, however, a high level of phase II enzymes protects from chemical carcinogenesis in laboratory animals and perhaps in people.

8.4.3 Suppressive Agents and Hormone Manipulations

Agents that suppress tumor development after exposure to carcinogens include nonsteroidal anti-inflammatory agents such as indomethacin as well as retinoids and other agents that influence cell differentiation and proliferation. Since hormonal regulation of growth and differentiation might play an important role in breast and prostate cancer, various natural steroid hormones or synthetic steroid antagonists have been tested as chemopreventive agents in animal models. For example, dehydroepiandrosterone (DHEA), a weak androgen that may be converted to estrogens (see Chap. 12, Sec. 12.2.1), has been highly effective in inhibiting spontaneous and chemically induced tumor formation at several sites in rodent models (Shibata et al., 1995).

An agent that has shown promise in preventing hormone-dependent tumors is indole-3-carbinole (I3C), which is found in broccoli, brussels sprouts, and other cruciferous vegetables. In animal studies, I3C protects from chemically induced mammary cancers and spontaneous endometrial carcinomas. I3C induces cytochrome P4501A2, a form that hydroxylates estradiol-17β and leads to lower circulating estrogen levels in both rodents and humans; it may thereby reduce the risk of estrogen-dependent tumors (Michnovicz and Bradlow, 1991). The protective effect of I3C may be due more to the removal of hormonal support later in the process of tumor progression than to a reduction in adduct formation in the earliest phases of carcinogenesis. I3C is now entering clinical trials in women who are judged to be at high risk for breast cancer.

Another chemopreventive strategy that is being investigated in a large clinical trial uses the estrogen antagonist tamoxifen. Tamoxifen is widely employed in the therapy of hormone-dependent breast cancers, and its proposed use as a prophylactic agent is based on observation of a reduced incidence of tumors in the opposite breast of treated patients (see Chap. 12, Sec. 12.4.1). Tamoxifen is relatively free of adverse effects, but recent studies have indicated that it may be bioactivated to genotoxic products. Tamoxifen can cause hepatic carcinomas in rats (Jordan, 1995) and increase the incidence of endometrial cancer in women; these findings have generated concern about the possible increased risk of inducing new cancers if large populations of healthy women were to be given tamoxifen as a chemopreventive agent.

8.4.4 Human Chemoprevention Trials

The success of cancer chemoprevention in laboratory animals has led to several clinical studies aimed at reducing human cancer by administration of various chemical agents (Greenwald, 1996). The candidate recipients of chemopreventive agents fall into two principal categories: (1) the general population and (2) individuals who may be at high risk due to genetic predisposition or heightened levels of exposure. For the general population, the preferred chemopreventive agents will be from "anticancer" diets rich in fruits and vegetables. Specific compounds that are active chemopreventive agents in animal studies have been isolated and identified from various plant sources, and these might be developed as pharmaceuticals for use in high-risk populations.

N-acetylcysteine (NAC), an antioxidant, free-radical scavenger, and precursor of reduced glutathione, is a successful blocking agent of carcinogenesis in animal models and is also used clinically as an antidote to acute drug toxicity such as hepatic damage from overdoses of acetaminophen. A relatively safe agent, NAC is being tested as an anticarcinogen in several human chemoprevention trials (De Flora et al., 1995). Beta-carotene and synthetic retinoids seemed, from animal studies, to have great promise as chemopreventive agents against human cancer. However, the results from human trials with beta-carotene have been disappointing and have led to an apparent increase in lung cancer in two trials (Omenn et al., 1996). Oltipraz, a synthetic dithiolthione related to compounds in cruciferous vegetables, was developed originally as an antischistosomiasis drug and was later shown to be a successful anticarcinogen against aflatoxins in animal studies. It appears to exert its effects by inhibiting P450 enzymes and by stimulating conjugating enzymes such as glutathione S-transferases and glucuronosyl transferases. Oltipraz is being tested in China to determine if it will reduce the incidence of hepatocellular carcinoma related to aflatoxin exposure.

In order to monitor the success of chemoprevention trials in humans, it is important to assess short-term intermediate markers rather than relying solely upon very long term cancer outcomes in treated groups versus control populations (Castonguay, 1992). Intermediate assays include the quantitation of chromosomal breakage via the "micronucleus assay" in exfoliated epithelial cells from the oral cavity or urogenital tract (Rosin, 1993) and quantitation of DNA adducts of aflatoxin or other carcinogens in nucleic acids excreted in urine (Groopman et al., 1996).

Any chemical used prophylactically in an attempt to prevent cancer will require continuous administration and may induce toxicity or the risk of other cancers, as cited above in the example of tamoxifen. Chemopreventive agents must pose very low risks to health.

8.5 RADIATION CARCINOGENESIS

8.5.1 Cell Transformation by Radiation

The development of experimental models to examine and predict the carcinogenic effects of exposures to ionizing radiation has been based on concepts similar to those described above for the study of chemical carcinogens, particularly the multistep carcinogenesis model. Cell transformation assays (see Sec. 8.3.1) provide the opportunity to examine mechanisms of radiation carcinogenesis in a well-controlled system, and a range of different cells has been studied. A general procedure for studying cell transformation by radiation in vitro is illustrated for murine 10T1/2 cells (fibroblasts) in Fig. 8.20. Cells are plated at low cell density to measure radiation cell killing (Chap. 13, Sec. 13.3.4) and at higher density, so that approximately 300 to 400 cells per dish will survive the treatment. These latter cells are then left to grow to confluence, which requires 11 to 13 divisions. At this time no foci are seen; but if the dishes are maintained with appropriate media changes for 4 to 6 weeks after confluence, discrete foci of transformed cells can be counted after appropriate staining of the dishes. These foci are identified by their dense multilayer structure, their basophilic staining, and the random orientation of the

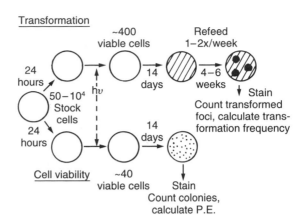

Figure 8.20. A general procedure for studying cell transformation in vitro. (Key: hυ = treatment with radiation.)

spindle-shaped cells. Similar results have been obtained with fresh explants of fibroblasts from hamster embryos, so it is not necessary for rodent cells to be immortalized before they become susceptible to radiation-induced transformation (Borek et al., 1978).

Transformed foci arise at a frequency that is dependent on radiation dose, and the frequency of transformation can be increased by known tumor promoters such as croton oil or phorbol esters (see Sec. 8.2.1). Many experiments have shown that cell proliferation is important for expression of the transformed phenotype, and it has been observed that, for a given radiation dose, the yield of foci per dish is approximately the same over orders of magnitude in the number of cells plated (Little, 1994). This finding has been interpreted to indicate that at least two steps are involved in radiation transformation: (1) An initial radiation-induced event that occurs in a large fraction of the cells, and (2) a second rare event that occurs in only a few of the descendants of the irradiated cells. Studies have shown that this second event has the characteristics of a mutation in that it occurs at a constant frequency per cell per generation during the growth of the cells to confluence (Little, 1994). Similar findings have been reported for radiation transformation of rat mammary cells growing in vivo (Kamiya et al., 1995).

In vitro focus assays are much more difficult to establish for human cells than for rodent cells, although transformation of primary human cells by radiation has been reported (e.g., Wazer et al., 1994). The reason appears to be that human cells are highly resistant to immortalization (Namba et al., 1996). Once immortalization is induced, transformation may occur fairly readily, although the frequencies of both spontaneous and radiation-induced transformation may be lower by one or two orders of magnitude as compared with rodent cells (Redpath et al., 1987; Band, 1995; Reinhold et al., 1996).

Using the assay illustrated in Fig. 8.20, the spontaneous transformation frequencies in rodent 10T1/2 cells are 10^{-4} to 10^{-5} per viable cell or lower. When such cells are irradiated with x- or γ-radiation and plated and their survival and transformation frequencies are measured, results as illustrated in Fig. 8.21 are obtained. The number of transformants per irradiated cell increases with dose over the range where little cell killing occurs (i.e., the shoulder of the survival curve; see Chap. 13, Sec. 13.4.1). At higher doses, as cell killing increases, the observed number of transformed foci decreases. Thus there is an optimum dose for maximal transformation (as has been seen for tumor induction in animal and humans; see Sec. 8.5.3). Plotting transformants per surviving cell, as in Fig. 8.21, indicates that the number of transformants increases for doses up to about 4 Gy and then plateaus, remaining constant up to about 12 Gy. When high linear energy transfer (LET) radiation is used (i.e., neutrons, α-particles), the cells are more efficiently killed (see Chap. 13, Sec. 13.5.1), and they are more efficiently transformed than by low-LET radiation (i.e., x- or γ-rays); thus the relative biological effectiveness (RBE) of high-LET radiation for transformation is also greater than unity (Miller et al., 1995). Also, as for cell survival, the RBE for cell transformation by high-LET radiation increases at low doses.

When low-LET radiation is given as a series of fractions, cell survival is higher as compared with equivalent single doses because of the repair of sublethal damage (see Chap. 13, Sec. 13.5.4). For cell transformation the results are more complex, since at doses less than about 1 Gy per fraction, fractionation of the dose may increase the number of transformants per irradiated cell, while at doses above 1 Gy per fraction, it reduces transformation relative to the same single dose of radiation (Hall and Miller, 1981). Fractionation or protraction of high-LET radiation does not decrease its ability to transform cells. In fact, some data indicate that fractionation of neutron exposures enhances their transforming ability compared with acute single exposures to the same dose. Both of these enhancement effects appear to require the cells to be proliferating during or between the exposures, and it has been hypothe-

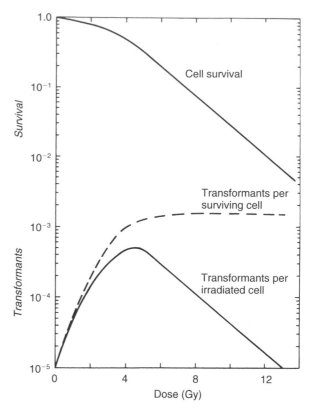

Figure 8.21. Typical results for cell survival, transformants per irradiated cell, and transformants per surviving cell for 10T1/2 cells exposed to low-LET ionizing radiation. When corrected for cell killing, the transformation frequency increases from a spontaneous level of 10^{-5} to a plateau value at 4 to 5 Gy of greater than 10^{-3}. (Adapted from Little, 1977.)

sized that they occur because there is a short time window in the cell cycle when the cells are very sensitive to transformation by radiation (Brenner et al., 1993; Elkind, 1996).

Ultraviolet (UV) radiation also causes transformation of cells, although the maximal levels of transformation appear to be lower by a factor of approximately 3 (Little, 1977). The efficiency of transformation as a function of wavelength (action spectrum) for mammalian cells is similar to that for formation of pyrimidine dimers (i.e., lesions in DNA where thymine or cytosine bases become crosslinked) (Rauth, 1986). This result strongly implicates initial damage to DNA as being a major factor in UV-induced mammalian cell transformation.

8.5.2 Mechanisms of Radiation Transformation

The relative sensitivity of cells to killing, transformation, or mutation can be compared following irradiation. The ratio of the frequency of a cell-killing event to a cell-transformation event to a (point) mutation event in a specific gene is approximately 1 to 10^{-2} to 10^{-4} for x- or γ-rays. Because the frequency of the transformation event is about 100 times higher than that for a point mutation in a specific gene, it has been argued that the target for transformation is larger than a single gene and smaller than a chromosome, perhaps involving more than one gene on one or more chromosomes (Goodhead, 1984). This is consistent with the observation that the majority of genetic damage to DNA caused by radiation is due to deletions, inversions, or chromosomal translocations rather than point mutations. Gene amplification is also induced by irradiation.

Contrary to the concept for carcinogenic chemicals that they cause a low-probability initiation event that results in DNA damage which is fixed in the genome by DNA replication (see Sec. 8.2), data for radiation transformation point toward a high-frequency initial step followed by a rare second step (see Sec. 8.5.1). Because of its high frequency, it has been suggested that the initial step in radiation transformation may involve a number of different genes or may be epigenetic in nature. The most important effect of radiation appears to be the induction of genetic instability (Murnane, 1996; Morgan et al., 1996), which then allows for a higher probability of "rare" mutations; these represent the second step(s) that, in turn, lead to malignant transformation. This concept is consistent with the observation that radiation tends to increase the incidence of the types of tumors arising naturally in the population—that for humans the increased incidence is seen primarily at ages when spontaneously arising tumors of the same type would occur and that radiation-induced tumors are not distinguishable from their naturally arising counterparts.

The mechanism(s) by which genetic instability is induced by radiation and maintained in the population are uncertain but probably include (1) mutations in genes involved in control of DNA synthesis or DNA repair, such as the mismatch repair system; (2) the induction of chromosome instability; and (3) persisting aberrant production of oxygen radicals, which can damage DNA (Morgan et al., 1996; Hampson, 1997; Suzuki, 1997). Irradiated cells demonstrate a higher incidence of mutations and chromosome instability for many generations after irradiation both in vitro and in vivo (Wright, 1997; Caron et al., 1997). Such instability appears to have a genetic component, since there are differences in the susceptibility of bone marrow cells to the induction of chromosome instability among different strains of mice and among different people. Similarly it has been observed that differences in the susceptibility of different strains of mice to radiation-induced mammary cancer are a direct result of differences in the sensitivity of the mammary epithelial cells to transformation (Ullrich et al., 1996).

One suggestion for how chromosome instability might perpetuate itself is a bridge-breakage-refusion cycle, which repeats at every cell division (Kaplan et al., 1997). This arises because radiation can break chromosomes and, during their repair, some can rejoin such that they contain two centromeres (dicentrics). When a cell divides, a dicentric chromosome has a 50 percent probability of being pulled to opposite poles of the metaphase plate and forming a chromosome bridge during anaphase, which eventually breaks and has to be rejoined (re-fused), with the possibility of recreating the dicentric. Even if the dicentric chromosomes are separated normally at metaphase (both centromeres on the same chromosome are pulled to the same pole), the same event will arise at the next mitosis. There is evidence that such a mechanism may be involved in radiation-induced gene amplification (Ma et al., 1993). Since the probability of observing dicentrics in cells is dose-dependent, this mechanism is consistent with evidence that initiation in radiation transformation is not an all-or-nothing event but rather that the degree of initiation is dose-dependent (Kennedy, 1997).

The ultimate mechanism by which radiation induces malignant transformation is likely the activation of (proto)oncogenes or inactivation of tumor suppressor genes. Since DNA lesions associated with ionizing radiation are primarily deletion, translocation, or inversion of DNA sequences, the inactivation of a tumor suppressor gene or inactivation of regulatory sequences would be a likely effect of the initial radiation event (Cox, 1994). However, chromosome breakage followed by faulty repair and translocation or amplification of DNA segments are also possible mechanisms by which activation of proto-oncogenes can occur (Chap. 5, Sec. 5.4). Some of the specific changes in oncogenes and tumor suppressor genes that have been observed in radiation-induced tumors are described in the next section.

8.5.3 Carcinogenesis by Ionizing Radiation in Animals

Single doses of low-LET radiation in the range of 0.25 to 8 Gy given to the whole body can increase the frequency of malignant and benign tumors in irradiated animals (Fry and Storer, 1987). A variety of animals have been studied, including dogs, monkeys, and rats, but the most intensive studies have been done with mice. In an experiment in which 12,000 female mice were irradiated with doses of 0.1 to 4 Gy of γ-rays and then followed for their lifetimes, autopsies and histologic examinations indicated relative tissue sensitivities for tumor induction as shown in Table 8.5 (Storer, 1982). The order of sensitivities of these tissues is not the same for all animals or even all strains of mice. Because tissues are not equally sensitive to radiation, it has been argued that the initial damage, which is uniformly produced at the tissue level, must be subject to a number of host factors that contribute to the overall process of cancer induction. These include levels of repair enzymes, rate of cell proliferation, endocrine function, and immune competence. An example illustrating the potential complexity of such host factors is the induction of thymic lymphoma in C57Bl mice by small whole-body doses of radiation (1.75 Gy) given weekly for 4 weeks. In this system, there is evidence for the activation of a unique leukemia virus, Rad LV, which interacts with target cells in the thymic environment (Weissman, 1985). Induction of tumor viruses, however, does not appear to be a general mechanism of radiation carcinogenesis.

Specific genetic changes have been observed in radiation-induced tumors. A particular oncogene (K-*ras*) was found to be activated through a single base change in mouse lymphomas induced by γ-radiation (Guerrero et al., 1984). Animal studies have also implicated mutations in the *ret* gene in thyroid cancer; this has also been observed in humans (Takahashi, 1995). The induction of acute myeloid leukemia in mice has been shown to involve specific

abnormalities in chromosome 2 (Rithidech et al., 1995; Bouffler et al., 1996). For solid tumors, there have been a number of studies of the role of *p53* mutations; both positive and negative results have been obtained (Selvanayagam et al., 1995; Jin et al., 1996). However, both *p53* knockout mice and mice carrying a mutant *p53* transgene are highly susceptible to radiation-induced tumors, which strongly suggests a role for *p53* in radiation carcinogenesis (Lee et al., 1994).

Many human leukemias and lymphomas appear to involve translocations or amplifications that can activate oncogenes, whereas many human solid tumors demonstrate *p53* (tumor suppressor) gene mutations. It is not known whether such mutations are an early primary event in radiation carcinogenesis or arise as a result of initial induction of genetic instability. The induction of leukemias and lymphomas in the Japanese A-bomb survivors occurred soon after exposure, and this may suggest a more direct action of radiation-induced DNA lesions for these cancers. In contrast, the induction of solid tumors occurred at much later times, more similar to the spontaneous occurrence of these tumors, and may involve a more complex sequence of genetic changes (Cox, 1994).

The dose dependence for tumor induction differs for different tissues, but for single acute doses of low-LET radiation given to the whole body, the relationship between tumor induction and dose appears to be sigmoid (Fig. 8.22, curve A). At low doses there is little induction, but as the dose increases, there is a steep increase in the number of tumors, followed by saturation or even a decrease at high doses. Factors that influence this dose-response curve are as follows:

1. Many strains of mice have a spontaneous level of occurrence of the specific tumor under study (in this hypothetical example, 10 percent) even in the absence of radiation. Spontaneous tumors may complicate the assessment of tumor induction at low doses, since radiation-induced tumors cannot be distinguished from them.
2. The induction curve for a specific tumor might have a low threshold dose, so that the rate of tumor production could appear to be linear with dose.
3. As the dose of radiation increases, cell killing will increase, leading to a maximal rate of tumor induction and a decrease in incidence at higher doses.
4. There is a latent period between radiation treatment and tumor detection. Thus an increase in

Table 8.5. Relative Tissue Sensitivities of RFM Female Mice to the Induction of Cancer by Radiation[a]

High Sensitivity	Moderate Sensitivity	Low Sensitivity
Thymus	Pituitary	Bone
Ovary	Uterus	Skin
	Breast	Stomach
	Myelopoietic tissue (myeloid leukemia)	Liver
		GI tract
	Lung	
	Haderian gland	

[a]Twelve thousand mice were irradiated at 10 weeks of age and followed for their lifetimes. High, moderate, or low sensitivity was defined as significant induction of tumors over controls at 0.25, 0.5–1.5, or greater than 1.5 Gy, respectively.

Source: Adapted from Storer, 1982.

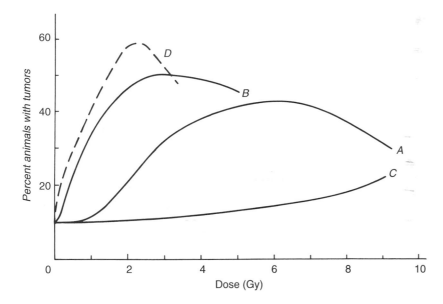

Figure 8.22. Schematic diagram of induction of a specific tumor type in mice exposed to various doses of ionizing radiation given to the whole body based on a review of a number of different in vivo results. *Curve A:* Tumors induced by single acute doses of low-LET radiation. *Curve B:* Tumors induced by single acute doses of high-LET radiation. *Curve C:* Tumors induced by fractionated doses (e.g., 1 Gy/day) of low-LET radiation. *Curve D:* Tumors induced by fractionated doses (e.g., 0.5 Gy/day) of high-LET radiation.

the frequency of tumors at a certain time after irradiation may represent an effect on the absolute level of tumor incidence, an earlier occurrence of tumors, or both.

Tumor induction for a single dose of high-LET radiation (such as neutrons or alpha particles) given to the whole body is, in general, more efficient than for low-LET radiation (x- or γ-rays). This is illustrated for neutron irradiation in Fig. 8.22, curve *B*, which indicates a small low-dose "threshold" portion, so tumor induction appears to be almost linear with dose. The curve continues to a maximum, which illustrates that a higher proportion of tumors occurs at a lower dose than for low-LET radiation and then decreases. In Fig. 8.22, 3.3 Gy of low-LET radiation produces 35 percent tumor induction, while a single dose of 1.1 Gy of neutrons produces the same effect. Therefore the RBE of neutrons relative to the low-LET radiation would be approximately 3.0. The RBE for neutrons (or other high- LET radiations), although greater than 1, is dependent on dose and increases as dose decreases. This effect is accounted for in risk assessment by multiplying dose received from high-LET sources by a "quality factor" (usually assumed to be 10) to convert it to an "equivalent" dose of low-LET radiation.

Other than exposures due to accidents and nuclear explosions, most radiation exposures of concern to humans involve fractionated or low dose-rate irradiation. Most studies of fractionated low-LET radiation have shown a reduction of tumor incidence for a given total dose, as illustrated by

Fig. 8.22, curve *C*, presumably because fractionation allows for extensive repair of damage and results in reduced carcinogenic effect. Continuous irradiation at a low dose rate gives a curve similar to curve *C*. In contrast, fractionating high-LET radiation or exposure at low dose rates has little effect on tumor induction, producing the same results as for single acute doses (Fig. 8.22, curve *B*), or it is more efficient in causing tumor induction (Fig. 8.22, curve *D*). Lack of repair of damage after high-LET radiation means that fractionation or prolonging the time for radiation delivery is of little or no benefit in reducing the probability of tumor induction.

8.5.4 Human Data on Carcinogenesis by Ionizing Radiation

For human populations, information on the carcinogenic risks of radiation exposure has been derived from many sources, including occupational exposures (e.g., radiologists and uranium miners), therapeutic exposures (e.g., unavoidable treatment of normal tissues in cancer therapy or treatment of ankylosing spondylitis), and accidental exposures. However, the majority of the information is from the studies of the A-bomb survivors in Hiroshima and Nagasaki, who were exposed in Japan in 1945, and from studies of exposures during medical x-ray examinations, particularly of pregnant women, which resulted in fetal exposure to irradiation. These groups of people were exposed to acute doses of irradiation; thus extrapolation of the risks to low levels of continuous exposure has relied on more limited information from occupational exposures and on experimental studies and modeling. The exposure of large numbers of people to radioactive fallout from the accident at the nuclear power plant in Chernobyl in 1986 may provide further information about the risks associated with this type of exposure. Initial studies have indicated high levels of thyroid tumors in exposed children (Rytomaa, 1996; Robbins, 1997). Experience with the A-bomb survivors indicates that it will be many years before the full extent of these risks will be known.

Radiation risk is defined as the increase in the number of cancer deaths over that expected for an unirradiated population. Excess absolute risk is expressed as the increased number of cancers per person exposed per sievert [1 sievert (Sv) is equivalent to 1 Gy of x- or γ-radiation]. Excess relative risk is the increase in cancers above that expected in an unirradiated population expressed as a fraction of the level in the unirradiated population.

Information about the A-bomb survivors is based on a leukemia registry established soon after the bombing and on a life-span study of more than 120,000 individuals living in the two cities that was initiated in 1950. Of these individuals, approximately 93,000 were A-bomb survivors and 27,000 were not in the cities at the time of the bombing. Detailed dosimetry (DS86) for about 87,000 of these individuals has been performed. The first evidence of a carcinogenic effect was an increase in the incidence of leukemias, due to the short latent period of this malignancy. The risk rose rapidly in the first 5 to 10 years after exposure and then declined, so that after 25 years there is little excess risk (Preston et al., 1994). Subsequently, the risk of solid cancers in many organs has also been found to be significantly increased. The excess relative risk for all solid cancers has been constant from 15 to 40 years after exposure for people over age 20 at the time of exposure. For those exposed at younger ages, the excess relative risk is greater than for the older ages, but it has declined over time (Thompson et al., 1994).

The results of an analysis of the incidence of hematologic malignancies (leukemia, lymphoma, and multiple myeloma) over the period 1950–1987 have been reported recently (Preston et al., 1994). The authors estimated an excess relative risk at 1 Sv for all leukemias of 3.9. The details for different leukemias, lymphoma, and multiple myeloma are shown for comparison to the risk of solid tumors in Fig. 8.23. One concern with this analysis is that it does not include (leukemia) cases that arose in the first 5 years after exposure because of the inade-

quacy of information for these early years. The authors have estimated that if these cases had been included, the average leukemia risk estimate would likely increase by 10 to 15 percent (to an excess relative risk at 1 Sv of 4.3–4.5).

The incidence of solid tumors in a cohort of about 80,000 people in the A-bomb life-span study has also been reported recently (Thompson et al., 1994). In this group, 8613 solid cancers were diagnosed between 1958 and 1987, of which 4327 were in the exposed group (dose, >10 mSv) and 4286 in the nonexposed group (dose, <10 mSv). The estimated excess relative risk for all solid cancers at 1 Sv is 0.63. The excess absolute risk is estimated to be about 30 per 10^4 person-year Svs. The excess relative risk for tumors of individual organs, estimated for a dose of 1 Sv, is shown in Fig. 8.23. Females demonstrate a higher excess relative risk than males for lung cancer and cancers of the urinary system. The risk for breast cancer is higher than that calculated for western populations, which is likely due to the low incidence of breast cancer in Japan (Doll, 1995).

There was no recorded effect of irradiation in utero in studies of A-bomb survivors, but studies of children irradiated in utero with medical x-rays from about 1940 to 1975 have consistently demonstrated an increased risk of cancer induction, with an overall excess relative risk of about 1.5 for leukemias and solid tumors (Doll and Wakeford, 1997). The relative risk is related to the number of x-ray exposures (films taken) and hence to dose received by these children and has declined with year of birth as the dose per film declined. For the period from about 1960 onward, most of the doses would have been equal to or less than 10 mGy and the relative risk is about 1.3. This leads to an estimate of excess risk of cancer of about 6 percent per Gy, with 40 percent of this risk (2.5 percent per Gy) being due to leukemia (Doll and Wakeford, 1997).

Little reliable information is currently available about the increased risk factor for high-LET radiation or about dose-rate effects for low-LET radiation for humans, but information on dose rate may develop from studies of the victims of the Chernobyl accident. There is also little reliable information about internally ingested isotopes. An important source of such exposure is radioactive radon gas in houses (radon is a decay product of radium). Studies of miners have shown that exposure to radon causes an increased risk of lung cancer (Darby et al., 1995; Lubin et al., 1995) that is roughly proportional to dose, but the analysis is confounded by a number of factors, particularly smoking. Lubin et al.

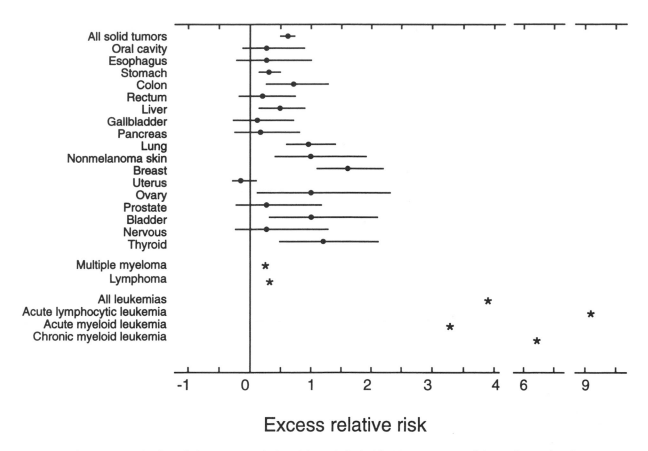

Figure 8.23. A plot of the excess relative risk at 1 Sv (with 95 percent confidence intervals where given) for induction of cancers in the A-bomb survivors. The data (*solid circles with error bars*) for solid tumors are from Thompson et al. (1994). The data for leukemias, lymphoma, and myeloma (stars) are estimated, based on fitting a linear-quadratic model to the data, and are from Preston et al. (1994).

(1995) have provided a formula for extrapolating these data to the general public and have estimated that the proportion of lung cancer deaths attributable to radon exposure in U.S. homes is 10 percent for men and 12 percent for women. It is less for smokers and greater for nonsmokers.

Extrapolation from the available data to estimate carcinogenic risk of low doses of radiation presents similar problems to those described in Sec. 8.3.5 for exposure to chemicals, as illustrated schematically in Fig. 8.24. The increase in tumor incidence is plotted as a function of an acute single dose of radiation (Storer, 1982; Kohn and Fry, 1984), and the problem is how to make an extrapolation. Three possibilities are a linear fit to the data (curve *A*), a linear quadratic curve (curve *B*), or a threshold linear curve (curve *C*). The linear curve *A* assumes that any dose of radiation has the potential to induce cancer and that risk of cancer induction is directly proportional to dose. This extrapolation implies that the increase in tumor number is the same for 100,000 persons each receiving a dose of 0.01 Gy of radiation as it is for 10,000 people receiving 0.1 Gy each. The recent analysis of tumor incidence in the A-bomb survivors suggests that a linear extrapolation is a valid assumption for all tumors except leukemia, for which a linear quadratic fit (curve *B*) was significantly better (Preston et al., 1994; Thompson et al., 1994). Curves *B* and *C* of Fig. 8.24 are more consistent with data from animals, but the shape of the low-dose portion of the curve varies from one experimental system to another.

Estimates based on linear extrapolation (Fig. 8.24, curve *A*) of the atomic bomb data, and on other more limited data from pooled results of various partial body exposures, give a population weighted average lifetime excess risk of cancer (except leukemia) from an acute dose of whole body irradiation of 1.6 to 2.4 percent per person per 0.2 Sv, depending on whether the excess risk for exposure

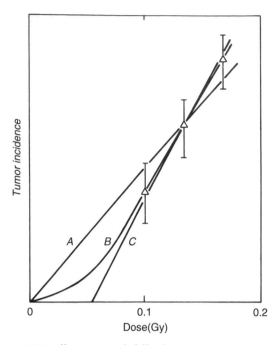

Figure 8.24. Illustration of difficulties in extrapolation of limited data at high doses in humans to a low-dose region where no data exist. Hypothetical data for tumor incidence versus dose are shown by the triangles with error bars. *Curve A*: Best fit linear curve. *Curve B*: A linear-quadratic fit to the data. *Curve C*: A threshold-linear fit to the data.

at young ages remains constant through life or declines with age (Doll, 1995). For lung cancer risk, it has been estimated that smoking one to nine cigarettes per day is equivalent to receiving a dose of 3.4 Sv or to living for 30 years in a home with a very high radon concentration (Boice and Lubin, 1996). These levels can be compared to average natural background levels of 2 to 3 mSv per year for radiation exposure.

8.5.5 Ultraviolet Carcinogenesis

There is a correlation between latitude (average sun exposure) and the incidence of malignant tumors of the skin, with the tumors tending to occur on sun-exposed areas, such as the face. Genetic background is also a determining factor, especially low skin pigmentation (among persons of Celtic, Scottish, or Welsh background, for example), since this contributes to an increase in the effective dose delivered to the cells at risk in the basal layer of the epidermis. Chronic exposure to sunlight is required for carcinogenesis, suggesting the need for multiple interactions of UV radiation with the target cells.

Because of the limited penetration of UV light through tissue, studies of the carcinogenic effect of UV radiation in animals have been limited to induction of tumors in skin (De Gruijl and Forbes, 1995). Studies of UV carcinogenesis have focused on exposures classed as UV-C, UV-B, and UV-A, corresponding to wavelengths of 200 to 290 nm, 290 to 320 nm, and greater than 320 nm, respectively. Because of filtering of UV light by the ozone layer, wavelengths shorter than 290 nm (UV-C) are believed to play little role in the exposure of the human population to solar radiation. The most effective range of wavelengths for skin carcinogenesis is UV-B, and its effect may become enhanced as the ozone layer is depleted.

Early studies of the UV induction of skin tumors were carried out on the ears of albino rats and mice. The induced tumors were a mixture of fibrosarcomas and squamous cell carcinomas. More recent experiments using hairless mice and lower doses produced mainly squamous cell carcinomas. If low daily doses of UV are given to mice over weeks to months, then, as the daily dose and dose rate increase, the latency time for initial tumor appearance decreases and the rate of tumor induction increases. A given total dose of UV radiation appears to be more effective as a carcinogen when administered at a lower exposure rate or as a fractionated course, in contrast to results with low-LET ionizing radiation. The relationship between tumor induction and wavelength in hairless mice has been found to peak at about 290 nm, similar to that observed for cell transformation in vitro and for the induction of skin erythema (sunburn) in humans. The relationship for induction of tumors (squamous and basal cell carcinomas) in humans is predicted to be similar (De Gruijl and Forbes, 1995). Melanoma in humans is also strongly associated with intermittent sun exposure (and with a history of sunburn) (see Chap. 2, Sec. 2.5.3), but there is no good animal model for studying the characteristics of the induction of this disease (Elwood, 1996).

Ultraviolet radiation is a complete carcinogen in that it can induce tumors by itself, as does ionizing radiation, but tumor incidence can be enhanced by promotors. In experiments in which multiple UV doses were given to induce known numbers of pyrimidine dimers (i.e., cross-linked thymine or cytosine bases in DNA) in the target basal layer of the skin, a clear relationship was obtained between the number of dimers induced and the subsequent incidence of tumors (Fry and Ley, 1983). In these experiments there was an appreciable dose range where no tumors were induced, followed by a significant increase with UV dose to the basal layer. Treatment of UV-irradiated animals with the tumor promoter 12-O-tetradecanoyl-phorbol-13-acetate (TPA) converted this curvilinear response to a linear no-threshold-type response. A high frequency of UV-induced tumors in mice demonstrate point mutations in the *p53* gene, and these mutations are primarily C-to-T transitions (Kress et al., 1992; Kanjilal et al., 1993). More than 50 percent of skin cancers in humans (both squamous and basal cell carcinomas) also have characteristic *p53* mutations (Brash et al., 1991; Ziegler et al., 1993). Many of these mutations are CC-to-TT transitions, which are characteristic of misrepair or lack of repair of pyrimidine dimers (Daya-Grosjean et al., 1995). In contrast, mutations of the *ras* gene are a rare event in UV-induced tumors (Khan et al., 1996).

Tumors induced by UV radiation in mice tend to be strongly immunogenic. Repeated UV irradiation of mice induces not only sarcomas but also an immunologic change that inhibits the ability of an irradiated mouse to reject transplanted syngeneic tumors induced by UV radiation (Kripke, 1990). Ultraviolet radiation has a profound effect on cutaneous immunity, inducing a reduction in the number of Langerhans cells, which play a role as cutaneous antigen-presenting cells; it also results in increased levels of suppressor T lymphocytes, which act against a common UVB-induced antigen (see Chap. 11, Sec. 11.3.3). Suppression of the induction of an immune response to UV-induced tumors can be transferred from one animal to another by these suppressor T cells. Thus the dose-response relationship for UV induction of tumors may be complex because these relationships for cancer induction and immune suppression may not be the same and the appearance of tumors will be mediated by both effects. Similar transient immune effects have been observed in humans following UV exposure (Streilein et al., 1996), and data have indicated that Australians (who have a high average sun exposure) undergoing immunosuppressive therapy for renal transplants have a higher frequency of squamous cell tumors of the skin than those in the general population (Hardie et al., 1980). Immunosuppression may allow previously initiated cells to express their malignant phenotype, as in animals.

in the capacity to repair DNA alters cancer risk, as does variation in enzymes that activate or detoxify carcinogens. Methods to identify carcinogens rely on the premise that most carcinogens are genotoxic. Based on knowledge of the mechanisms by which carcinogens act, it may be possible to manipulate biochemical or cellular defense mechanisms to reduce cancer risk, and a number of clinical trials are in progress. However, at present the most effective method to reduce the human cancer burden is through reduction of exposure—especially to such high-risk agents as tobacco smoke.

Ionizing and UV radiation can both give rise to tumors, but quite different initial DNA lesions probably initiate the process of carcinogenesis for these two types of radiation. For ionizing radiation, the critical damage probably leads to instability of the DNA, and this, in turn, leads to an increased probability of errors in DNA replication occurring in subsequent cell cycles. Alterations in DNA can then lead to expression or activation of oncogenes or inactivation of tumor suppressor genes. Ionizing radiation induces tumors in different tissues with different efficiencies, implying the existence of a variety of host factors. Carcinogenesis induced by UV requires multiple doses of UV radiation. Tumor induction increases with total dose and has a wavelength dependence similar to that for sunburn and induction of pyrimidine dimers in DNA. Many skin tumors contain mutations in the *p53* gene that are compatible with misrepair or lack of repair of pyrimidine dimers. Besides its effect in initiating carcinogenesis, UV can also reduce host immunity to UV-induced tumors. This effect of UV on antitumor immunity does not appear to have a parallel in carcinogenesis by ionizing radiation.

The risk of cancer in humans exposed to moderate doses of ionizing radiation (up to 4 Gy) has been estimated from studies of the Japanese A-bomb survivors. Most tissues are affected, but the relative risk varies. Estimates of risk for low doses of radiation and for low exposures to chemical carcinogens spread over long periods of time are made by extrapolation of data relating to risk after larger (usually acute) doses. There is considerable uncertainty about these extrapolated estimates of risk.

8.6 SUMMARY

Most chemical carcinogens form adducts with bases in DNA either directly or, more often, after metabolic activation. Cancers arise from multiple sequential unrepaired lesions at specific sites in oncogenes or tumor suppressor genes. Genetic variation

REFERENCES

Alexandrov K, Rojas M, Castegnaro M, et al: An improved fluorometric assay for dosimetry of benzo[*a*]pyrene diol epoxide-DNA adducts in smoker's lungs: Comparisons with total bulky adducts and aryl hydrocarbon hydroxylase activity. *Cancer Res* 1992; 52:6248–6253.

Ames BN, Profet M, Gold L: Dietary pesticides (99.9% all natural). *Proc Natl Acad Sci USA* 1990; 87:7777–7781.

Band V: Preneoplastic transformation of human mammary epithelial cells. *Semin Cancer Biol* 1995; 6:185–192.

Bertram JS, Kolonel LN, Meyskens FL Jr: Rationale and strategies for chemoprevention of cancer in humans. *Cancer Res* 1987; 47:3012–3031.

Boice JD, Lubin JH: Lung cancer risks: Comparing radiation with tobacco. *Radiat Res* 1996; 146:356–357.

Borek C, Hall EJ, Rossi HH: Malignant transformation in cultured hamster embryo cells produced by x-rays, 460-kev monoenergetic neutrons and heavy ions. *Cancer Res* 1978; 38:2997–3005.

Bouffler SD, Breckon G, Cox R: Chromosomal mechanisms in murine radiation acute myeloid leukemogenesis. *Carcinogenesis* 1996; 17:655–659.

Brash DE, Rudolph JA, Simon JA, et al: A role for sunlight in skin cancer: UV-induced p53 mutations in squamous cell carcinoma. *Proc Natl Acad Sci USA* 1991; 88:10124–10128.

Brenner DJ, Hall EJ, Randers-Pehrson G, Miller RC: Mechanistic considerations on the dose-rate/LET dependence of oncogenic transformation by ionizing radiation. *Radiat Res* 1993; 133:365–369.

Bryan WR, Shimkin MB: Quantitative analysis of dose-response data obtained with three carcinogenic hydrocarbons in strain C3H male mice. *J Natl Cancer Inst* 1943; 3:503–531.

Caron RM, Nagasawa H, Yu Y, et al: Evidence for a role for genomic instability in radiation-induced mutagenesis. *Radiat Oncol Invest* 1997; 5:119–123.

Castonguay A: Methods and strategies in lung cancer control. *Cancer Res* 1992; 52:2641s–2651s.

Cohen SM, Ellwein LB: Genetic errors, cell proliferation, and carcinogenesis. *Cancer Res* 1991; 51:6493–6505.

Cox R. Molecular mechanisms of radiation oncogenesis. *Int J Radiat Biol* 1994; 65:57–64.

Darby SC, Whitley E, Howe GR, et al: Radon and cancers other than lung cancer in underground miners: A collaborative analysis of 11 studies. *J Natl Cancer Inst* 1995; 87:378–383.

Daya-Grosjean L, Dumaz N, Sarasin A: The specificity of p53 mutation spectra in sunlight induced human cancers. *J Photochem Photobiol B-Biol* 1995; 28:115–124.

De Flora S, Cesarone CF, Balansky RM, et al: Chemopreventive properties and mechanisms of *N*-acetylcysteine: The experimental background. *J Cell Biochem Suppl* 1995; 22:33–41.

De Gruijl FR, Forbes PD: UV-induced skin cancer in a hairless mouse model. *Bioessays* 1995; 17:651–660.

Denissenko MF, Pao A, Tang M-S, Pfeifer GP: Preferential formation of benzo[*a*]pyrene adducts at lung cancer mutational hotspots in p53. *Science* 1996; 274:430–432.

deWind N, Dekker M, Berns A, et al: Inactivation of the mouse Msh2 gene results in mismatch repair deficiency, methylation tolerance, hyperrecombination, and predisposition to cancer. *Cell* 1995; 82:321–330.

Dipple A: DNA adducts of chemical carcinogens. *Carcinogenesis* 1995; 16:437–441.

Doll R: Hazards of ionizing radiation: 100 years of observations on man. *Br J Cancer* 1995; 72:1339–1349.

Doll R, Wakeford R. Risk of childhood cancer from fetal irradiation. *Br J Radiol* 1997; 70:130–139.

Dumenco L, Allay E, Norton K, Gerson S: The prevention of thymic lymphomas in transgenic mice by human O6-alkylguanine-DNA transferase. *Science* 1993; 259:219–222.

Elkind MM: Enhanced risks of cancer from protracted exposures to X- or gamma rays: A radiobiological model of radiation induced breast cancer. *Br J Cancer* 1996; 73:133–138.

Elwood JM: Melanoma and sun exposure. *Semin Oncol* 1996; 23:650–666.

Fearon ER, Vogelstein B: A genetic model for colorectal tumorigenesis. *Cell* 1992; 61:759–761.

Foulds L: The experimental study of tumor progression: A review. *Cancer Res* 1954; 14:327–339.

Friedberg EC, Walker GC, Siede W: *DNA Repair and Mutagenesis*. Washington, DC: ASM Press; 1995.

Fry RJM, Ley RD: Ultraviolet radiation carcinogenesis. In: Slaga TJ, ed. *Mechanisms of Tumor Promotion*. Boca Raton, FL: CRC Press; 1983:vol II:73–96.

Fry RJM, Storer JB: External radiation carcinogenesis. *Adv Radiat Biol* 1987; 13:31–90.

Goldman M: Cancer risk of low level exposure. *Science* 1996; 271:1821–1822.

Goodhead DT: Deductions from cellular studies of inactivation, mutagenesis and transformation. In: Boice JD, Fraumeni JF, eds. *Radiation Carcinogenesis: Epidemiology and Biological Significance*. New York: Raven Press; 1984:369–385.

Greenblatt MS, Bennett WP, Hollstein M, Harris CC: Mutations in the p53 tumor suppressor gene: Clues to cancer etiology and molecular pathogenesis. *Cancer Res* 1994; 54:4855–4878.

Greenwald P: Chemoprevention of cancer. *Sci Am* 1996; 275:96–99.

Groopman JD, Wang J-S, Scholl P: Molecular biomarkers for aflatoxins: From adducts to gene mutations to human liver cancer. *Can J Physiol Pharmacol* 1996; 74:203–209.

Guengerich FP: Metabolic activation of carcinogens. *Pharmacol Ther* 1992; 54:17–61.

Guerrero I, Villasante A, Corces V, Pellicer A: Activation of a c-K-ras oncogene by somatic mutation in mouse lymphoma induced by gamma radiation. *Science* 1984; 225:1159–1169.

Hall EJ, Miller RC. The how and why of in vitro oncogenic transformation. *Radiat Res* 1981; 87:208–233.

Hampson R: Selection for genomic instability by DNA damage in human cells: Unstable microsatellites and their consequences for tumorigenesis. *Radiat Oncol Invest* 1997; 5:111–114.

Hardie IR, Strong RW, Hartley LCJ, et al: Skin cancer in Caucasian renal allograft recipients living in a sub-tropical climate. *Surgery* 1980; 87:177–180.

Harris CC: Chemical and physical carcinogenesis: Advances and perspectives for the 1990s. *Cancer Res* 1991; 51:5023s–5044s.

Harris CC: p53 at the cross roads of molecular carcinogenesis and risk assessment. *Science* 1993; 262:1980–1981.

Huang J-C, Hsu DS, Kazantsev A, Sancar A: Substrate spectrum of human excinuclease: Repair of abasic sites, methylated bases, mismatches, and bulky adducts. *Proc Natl Acad Sci USA* 1994; 91:12213–12217.

Jin Y, Burns J, Garte SJ, Hosselet S: Infrequent alterations of the p53 gene in rat skin cancers induced by ionizing radiation. *Carcinogenesis* 1996; 17:873–876.

Jordan VC: Tamoxifen for breast cancer prevention. *Proc Soc Exp Biol Med* 1995; 208:144–149.

Kamiya K, Yasukawa-Barnes J, Mitchen JM, et al: Evidence that carcinogenesis involves imbalance between epigenetic high frequency initiation and suppression of promotion. *Proc Natl Acad Sci USA* 1995; 92:1332–1336.

Kanjilal S, Pierceall WE, Cummings KK, et al: High frequency of p53 mutations in UV-induced murine skin tumors: Evidence for strand bias and tumor heterogeneity. *Cancer Res* 1993; 53:2961–2964.

Kaplan MI, Limoli CL, Morgan WF: Perpetuating radiation-induced chromosome instability. *Radiat Oncol Invest* 1997; 5:124–128.

Kennedy AR: Evidence suggesting that the dose-response relationship for radiation-induced transformation in vitro is due to the degree of initiation in individual cells. *Radiat Oncol Invest* 1997; 5:144–149.

Khan SG, Mohan RR, Katiyar SK, et al: Mutations in ras oncogenes: Rare events in ultraviolet B radiation–induced mouse skin carcinogenesis. *Mol Carcinog* 1996; 15:96–103.

Kim PM, Wells PG: Genoprotection by UDP-glucuronosyltransferases in peroxidase dependent, reactive oxygen species-mediated micronucleus initiation by the carcinogens 4-(methylnitrosoamino)-1-(3-pyridyl)-1-butanone and benzo[a]pyrene. *Cancer Res* 1996; 56:1526–1532.

Kohn HI, Fry RJM: Radiation carcinogenesis. *N Engl J Med* 1984; 310:504–511.

Kress S, Sutter C, Strickland PT, et al: Carcinogen specific mutational pattern in the p53 gene in ultraviolet-B radiation induced squamous cell carcinomas of mouse skin. *Cancer Res* 1992; 52:6400–6403.

Kripke ML: Effects of UV radiation on tumor immunity. *J Natl Cancer Inst* 1990; 82:1392–1396.

Lee JM, Abrahamson JL, Kandel R, et al: Susceptibility to radiation carcinogenesis and accumulation of chromosomal breakage in p53 deficient mice. *Oncogene* 1994; 9:3731–3736.

Little JB: Radiation carcinogenesis in vitro: Implications for mechanisms. In: Hiatt HH, Watson JD, Winston JA, eds. *Origins of Human Cancer: Book B. Mechanisms of Carcinogenesis.* Cold Spring Harbor, NY: Cold Spring Harbor Laboratory; 1977:923–939.

Little JB: Changing views of cellular radiosensitivity. *Radiat Res* 1994; 140:299–311.

Lubin JH, Boice JD, Edling C, et al: Lung-cancer in radon-exposed miners and estimates of risk from indoor exposure. *J Natl Cancer Inst* 1995; 87:817–827.

Ma C, Martin S, Trask B, Hamlin JL: Sister-chromatid fusion initiates amplification of the dihydrofolate reductase gene in Chinese hamster cells. *Genes Dev* 1993; 7:605–620.

Maugh TH II: Chemical carcinogens: How dangerous are low doses? *Science* 1978; 202:37–41.

Maze R, Carney JP, Kelley MR, et al: Increasing DNA repair methyltransferase levels via bone marrow stem cell transduction rescues mice from the toxic effects of 1,3-bis(2-chloroethyl)-1-nitrosourea, a chemotherapeutic alkylating agent. *Proc Natl Acad Sci USA* 1996; 93:206–210.

Michnovicz JJ, Bradlow HL: Altered estrogen metabolism and excretion in humans following consumption of indole-3-carbinole. *Nutr and Cancer* 1991; 16:59–66.

Miller EC, Miller JA: Searches for ultimate chemical carcinogens and their reactions with cellular macromolecules. *Cancer* 1981; 47:2327–2345.

Miller RC, Marino SA, Brenner DJ, et al: The biological effectiveness of radon-progeny alpha particles: II. Oncogenic transformation as a function of linear energy transfer. *Radiat Res* 1995; 142:54–60.

Morgan WF, Day JP, Kaplan MI, et al. Genomic instability induced by ionizing radiation. *Radiat Res* 1996; 146:247–258.

Murnane JP: Role of induced genetic instability in the mutagenic effects of chemicals and radiation. *Mutat Res* 1996; 367:11–23.

Nakachi K, Imai K, Hayashi S, Kawajiri K: Polymorphisms of the CYP1A1 and glutathione S-transferase genes associated with susceptibility to lung cancer in relation to cigarette dose in a Japanese population. *Cancer Res* 1993; 53:2994–2999.

Namba M, Mihara K, Fushimi K: Immortalization of human cells and its mechanisms. *Crit Rev Oncogen* 1996; 7:19–31.

Nebert DW, McKinnon RA, Puga A: Human drug-metabolizing enzyme polymorphisms: Effects on risk of toxicity and cancer. *DNA Cell Biol* 1996; 15:273–280.

O'Brien PJ: Antioxidants and cancer. *Adv Exp Med Biol* 1994; 366:215–239.

Okey AB: Enzyme induction in the cytochrome P450 system. In: Kalow W, ed. *Pharmacogenetics of Drug Metabolism.* New York: Pergamon Press; 1992:549–608.

Omenn GS, Goodman GE, Thornquist MD, et al: Risk factors for lung cancer and for intervention effects in CARET, the beta-carotene and retinol efficacy trial. *J Natl Cancer Inst* 1996; 88:1550–1559.

Pegg AE: Methylation of the O^6 position of guanine in DNA is the most likely initiating event in carcinogenesis by methylating agents. *Cancer Invest* 1984; 2:223–231.

Pitot HC III, Dragan YP: Chemical carcinogenesis. In: Klessen CD, ed. *Casarett & Doull's Toxicology; The Basic Science of Poison,* 5th ed. New York: McGraw-Hill; 1996:201–267.

Preston DL, Kusumi S, Tomonaga S, et al: Cancer incidence in atomic bomb survivors. Part III: Leukemia, lymphoma and multiple myeloma, 1950–1987. *Radiat Res* 1994; 137(Suppl):S68–S97.

Quintanilla M, Brown K, Ramsden M, Balmain A: Carcinogen specific mutation and amplification of Ha-ras during mouse skin carcinogenesis. *Nature* 1986; 322: 78–80.

Rauth AM: The induction and repair of ultraviolet light damage in mammalian cells. In: Burns FJ, Upton AC, Silini G, eds: *Radiation Carcinogenesis and DNA Alterations.* New York: Plenum Press; 1986:212–226.

Redpath JL, Sun C, Colman M, Stanbridge EJ: Neoplastic transformation of human hybrid cells by gamma radiation: A quantitative assay. *Radiat Res* 1987; 110:468-472.

Reinhold DS, Walicka M, Elkassaby M, et al: Malignant transformation of human fibroblasts by ionizing radiation. *Int J Radiat Biol* 1996; 69:707–715.

Rithidech K, Bond VP, Cronkite EP, et al: Hypermutability of mouse chromosome 2 during development of x-ray–induced murine myeloid leukemia. *Proc Natl Acad Sci USA* 1995; 92:1152–1156.

Robbins J: Lessons from Chernobyl: The event, the aftermath fallout: Radioactive, political, social. *Thyroid* 1997; 7:189–192.

Rosin MP: Genetic alterations in carcinogenesis and chemoprevention. *Environ Health Perspect* 1993; 101: 253–256.

Rytomaa T: Ten years after Chernobyl. *Ann Med* 1996; 28: 83–87.

Sancar A: Mechanisms of DNA excision repair. *Science* 1994; 266:1954–1956.

Sancar A: DNA repair in humans. *Annu Rev Genet* 1995; 29:69–105.

Seeberg E, Eide L, Bjoras M: The base excision repair pathway. *Trends Biochemical Sci* 1995; 20:391–397.

Selvanayagam CS, Davis CM, Cornforth MN, Ullrich RL: Latent expression of p53 mutations and radiation-induced mammary cancer. *Cancer Res* 1995; 55: 3310–3317.

Shelby MD, Zeigler E: Detection of human carcinogens by *Salmonella* and rodent bone marrow cytogenetics tests. *Mutat Res* 1990; 234:257–261.

Shibata M-A, Hasegawa R, Imaida K, et al: Chemoprevention by epiandrosterone and indomethecin in a rat multiorgan carcinogenesis model. *Cancer Res* 1995; 55:4870–4874.

Storer JB: Radiation carcinogenesis. In: Becker FF ed. *Cancer: A Comprehensive Treatise,* 2d ed. New York: Plenum Press; 1982; 1:629–659.

Streilein JW, Taylor JR, Vincek V, et al: Relationship between ultraviolet radiation-induced immunosuppression and carcinogenesis. *J Invest Dermatol* 1994; 103 (suppl 5):107S–111S.

Suzuki K: Multistep nature of x-ray-induced neoplastic transformation in mammalian cells: Genetic alterations and instability. *J Radiat Res* 1997; 38:55–63.

Takahashi M: Oncogenic activation of the ret protooncogene in thyroid cancer. *Crit Rev Oncogenesis* 1995; 6: 35–46.

Thompson DE, Mabuchi K, Ron E, et al: Cancer incidence in atomic bomb survivors: Part II. Solid tumors, 1958–1987. *Radiat Res* 1994; 137 (suppl):S17–S67.

Ullrich RL, Bowles ND, Satterfield LC, Davis CM: Strain-dependent susceptibility to radiation-induced mammary cancer is a result of a difference in epithelial cell sensitivity to transformation. *Radiat Res* 1996; 146:353–355.

Wattenberg LW: Chemoprevention of cancer. *Cancer Res* 1985; 45:1–8.

Wattenberg LW: Prevention-therapy-basic science and the resolution of the cancer problem. *Cancer Res* 1993; 54:5284–5295.

Wazer DE, Chu Q, Liu XL, et al: Loss of p53 protein during radiation transformation of primary human epithelial cells. *Mol Cell Biol* 1994; 14:2468–2478.

Weissman IL: Thymic lymphocyte differentiation and thymic leukemogenesis. *Int J Radiat Oncol Biol Phys* 1985; 11:57–64.

Wright EG: Radiation-induced genomic instability in haemopoetic cells: Implications for radiation pathology. *Radiat Oncol Invest* 1997; 5:115–118.

Wynder EL, Hoffmann D: Smoking and lung cancer: Scientific challenges and opportunities. *Cancer Res* 1994; 54:5284–5295.

Yang CS, Smith TJ, Hong J-Y: Cytochrome P-450 enzymes as targets for chemoprevention against carcinogenesis and toxicity: Opportunities and limitations. *Cancer Res* 1994; 54:1982s–1986s.

Zeiger E, Haseman JK, Shelby MD, et al: Evaluation of four in vitro genetic toxicity tests for predicting rodent carcinogenicity: Conformation of earlier results with 41 additional chemicals. *Environ Mol Mutagen* 1990; 16(suppl. 18):1–14.

Ziegler A, Leffell DJ, Kunala S, et al: Mutation hotspots due to sunlight in the p53 gene of nonmelanoma skin cancers. *Proc Natl Acad Sci USA* 1993; 90:4216–4220.

Zhang R, Haag JD, Gould MN: Quantitating the frequency of initiation and cH-ras mutation in in situ N-methyl-N-nitrosourea-exposed rat mammary gland. *Cell Growth and Differ* 1991; 2:1–6.

Zhang Y, Kensler TW, Cho C-G, et al: Anticarcinogenic activities of sulforaphane and structurally related synthetic norbornyl isothiocyanates. *Proc Natl Acad Sci USA* 1994; 91:3147–3150.

9

The Extracellular Environment and Cancer

Shoukat Dedhar, Gregory E. Hannigan, Janusz Rak, and Robert S. Kerbel

9.1 INTRODUCTION
    9.1.1 The Extracellular Matrix and Its Interactions with Cells

9.2 CELL ADHESION MOLECULES
    9.2.1 Integrins
    9.2.2 Signal Transduction by Integrins
    9.2.3 Integrins in Tumor Progression and Metastasis
    9.2.4 Cadherins
    9.2.5 Adhesion Molecules of the Immunoglobulin Superfamily
    9.2.6 Carcinoembryonic Antigen
    9.2.7 CD44 Hyaluronate-Binding Proteins

9.3 TUMOR ANGIOGENESIS
    9.3.1 Dependence of Tumors on Blood Supply
    9.3.2 Angiogenic Growth Factors and Growth-Factor Receptors
    9.3.3 Inhibitors of Tumor Angiogenesis
    9.3.4 Tumor Angiogenesis as a Prognostic Indicator

9.4. SUMMARY

REFERENCES

9.1 INTRODUCTION

In the earlier chapters of this book, emphasis was placed on various ways that the normal function of individual cells is dysregulated during the carcinogenic process. In the current chapter, the interaction of cells both with other cells and with the extracellular environment is discussed in the context of malignant transformation and tumor progression. The chapter includes detailed discussion of the role of cell adhesion molecules in mediating cellular migration and growth and of the process of tumor-induced angiogenesis, which is essential for the progressive growth of a tumor. Possibilities for a therapeutic strategy based on inhibiting angiogenesis are also addressed.

9.1.1 The Extracellular Matrix and Its Interactions with Cells

During embryonic development, cells often move from one location to another in the embryo, which requires dissociation from their neighbors and reassociation with new neighbors. Such movements also take place during normal physiologic processes such as lymphocyte trafficking, wound healing, and homeostasis and are altered in pathologies such as inflammation, thrombosis, and tumor cell invasion and metastasis. The molecular bases for these biologic phenomena depend on the expression and function of a variety of cell adhesion molecules that mediate the interaction of cells with components of the extracellular matrix (ECM) and with other cell-surface receptors.

Most mammalian cells are in contact with an ECM whose composition and structure vary during development and differ for different cell types and their locations. For example, each cell in an epithelial cell layer has a specialized lateral, apical, and basal border, and the interactions of these cells with the basement membrane is instrumental for the formation and maintenance of the epithelial cell sheet and its polarized differentiated state. The basement membrane is a highly structured, specialized form of ECM and is composed of laminin, type IV collagen, entactin/nidogen, and heparan sulfate proteoglycan. In addition, smaller amounts of fibronectin, vitronectin, and chondroitin sulfate proteoglycans are also found in some basement membranes. There are at least seven forms of laminin, which vary in the composition of their subunits and are found in tissue-specific basement membranes (Burgeson et al., 1994). In contrast to epithelial cells, mesenchymal cells are not attached to each other or to a basement membrane but are surrounded by an ECM of quite different composition. Typical components are the interstitial collagens, types I to III, elastin, proteoglycans, fibronectin, and vitronectin. In more specialized tissue-specific ECMs, there are other components such as tenascin, thrombospondin, and osteopontin.

A large number of structural and functional domains have been identified in ECM proteins. These include the arginine-glycine-aspartic acid (RGD; single-letter amino acid code R = arginine, G = glycine, D = aspartic acid) cell attachment and integrin recognition motif (Fig. 9.1). Functionally active RGD motifs have been found in fibronectin, vitronectin, tenascin, osteopontin, thrombospondin, fibrinogen, and von Willebrand factor (Hynes, 1992). Fibronectin also contains a distinct attachment site for cells (mostly leukocytes) expressing the integrin $\alpha_4\beta_1$ (see Sec. 9.2). This site, present in the IIICS module and called CS-1, is present in a region of fibronectin distinct from the RGD motif (Fig. 9.1). Laminin also contains at least

two distinct non-RGD cell attachment sites, which are localized in distal regions of the molecule and exhibit cellular specificity and interaction with different receptors (Timpl, 1989). In addition to cell-attachment domains, ECM proteins have domains that recognize other components of the ECM, including collagen, heparin, and elastin. Through these interaction domains, proteins of the ECM can form a highly organized three-dimensional matrix in which the proteins can associate with each other and with cells.

Interaction between cells and the ECM is essential for cell survival and cell growth (Fig. 9.2), and the ECM can regulate the differentiation of a variety of cell types (Hay, 1984). These cellular cues are provided by the ECM through direct interactions of the components of the ECM with specific cell-surface receptors, and they require signal-transduction events. Depriving cells of such interactions results in the induction of apoptosis in epithelial and endothelial cells (e.g., Boudreau et al., 1995), or in cell-cycle arrest in fibroblasts (Fang et al., 1996). A common property of malignant cells is that they can continue to survive and proliferate in the absence of interactions with the ECM. Thus, such cells may be independent of the constraints of the ECM on cell survival (Fig. 9.2).

Components of the ECM can interact specifically with growth factors, especially basic fibroblast growth factor (bFGF) and transforming growth factor β (TGF-β) (see Chap. 6, Sec. 6.2). Basic FGF binds to heparin and to heparan sulfate proteoglycans (HSPG) via the glycoaminoglycan moi-

FIBRONECTIN

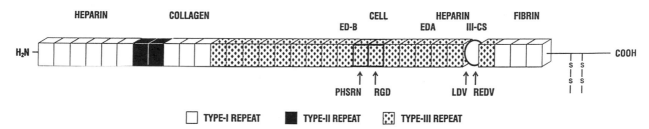

TYPE-I REPEAT   TYPE-II REPEAT   TYPE-III REPEAT

Figure 9.1. Model of the structure of fibronectin. Fibronectin is composed of three types of repeating modules, designated type I, type II, and type III. The ED-A, ED-B, and IIICS modules can be present or absent in some forms of fibronectin as a result of alternative splicing. Fibronectin is a homodimer with the two chains linked by an interchain disulfide bond at the carboxy terminus. Fibronectin can bind to various proteins as well as to cells and these domains are indicated at the top. The cell binding domain consists of the RGD (arginine-glycine-aspartic acid) cell-recognition sequence, which mediates cell adhesion to fibronectin in synergy with an adjacent sequence PHSRN (proline-histidine-serine-arginine-asparagine). Another cell-binding site present in the IIICS domain functions independently of the central cell binding region found in the type III repeat. This site contains two cell-recognition sequences, LDV (leucine-aspartic acid-valine) and REDV (arginine-glutamic acid-aspartic acid-valine).

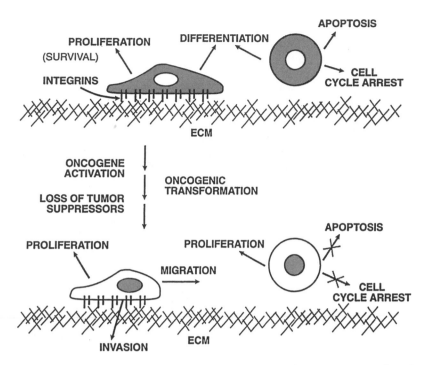

Figure 9.2. The interaction of cells with the ECM results in integrin-mediated signal transduction and promotion of cell survival (*shown at top left*). In the absence of such signals (*shown at top right*), fibroblasts undergo cell-cycle arrest in late G1 phase and endothelial and epithelial cells undergo apoptosis. Oncogenic transformation (*lower part of figure*) results in the integrin-mediated promotion of cell migration and basement membrane invasion as well as anchorage-independent cell growth.

ety of HSPG, and the growth factor can be released by heparitinase or by plasmin. Release of bFGF by plasmin may be important, since plasminogen activator is often produced by cancer cells. TGF-β binds to proteoglycans such as betaglycan and decorin, but the interactions occur via the protein cores of these proteoglycans. Fibronectin can also bind TGF-β, although the binding site has not yet been identified.

During tumor invasion and metastasis (Fig. 9.3; see also Chap. 10, Sec. 10.4), intimate interactions occur between tumor cells and components of the ECM. The interaction of cell-surface receptors on the tumor cells with ECM proteins induces the expression and secretion of proteases (metalloproteinases), which then degrade the ECM components, allowing for the invasion of the tumor cells through the matrix (basement membrane). Degraded components of the ECM (e.g., fibronectin fragments) can then trigger further induction of protease genes, resulting in a positive feedback loop

that further facilitates invasion and proliferation (Werb et al., 1989). The release of growth factors upon degradation of the ECM probably also facilitates tumor cell growth.

9.2 CELL ADHESION MOLECULES

Most mammalian cells express on their surface a diverse and versatile array of cell adhesion molecules (CAMs). The CAMs mediate the attachment of cells to the ECM and/or mediate interactions with the same (homotypic) or different (heterotypic) types of cells. Most of the CAMs are transmembrane proteins with extracellular and intracellular domains, but some are anchored in the plasma membrane by an L-terminal glycophosphatidyl-inositol moiety. Several families of CAMs have been identified and their primary structures have been elucidated. The generic structures of the CAMs which have been implicated in oncogenesis are shown in Fig. 9.4, and these are discussed in the following sections.

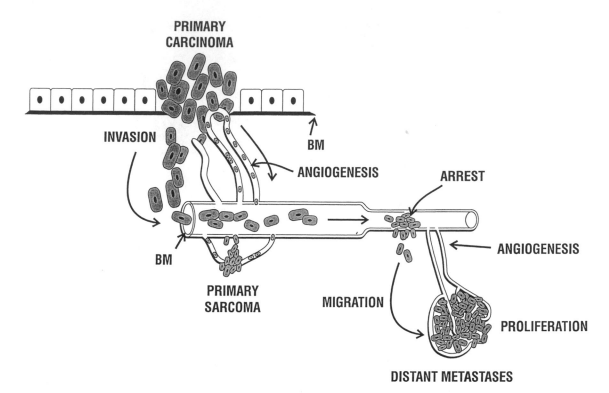

Figure 9.3. A model of the major steps of metastasis. Anchorage-independent growth of epithelial cells results in the formation of a primary carcinoma. The tumor induces the growth of blood vessels into the tumor by angiogenesis. Some cells separate from the primary tumor, invade through the basement membrane, enter the vasculature, and eventually arrest in capillaries, where they extravasate out of the blood vessels into the underlying connective tissue at the metastatic site; there, further cell growth and angiogenesis results in the formation of metastatic tumor growth. Angiogenesis may not be as critical for the invasion and metastasis of sarcomas, as these tumors arise in the stroma in close vicinity to blood vessels. The activity of a variety of adhesion molecules has been implicated in most of the steps in this metastatic cascade.

9.2.1 Integrins

Integrins are expressed in all cell types and are involved in the regulation of cellular functions during embryonic development, wound healing, inflammation, hemostasis, bone resorption, apoptosis, cell proliferation, tumor cell growth, and metastasis. They make up a family of widely expressed transmembrane receptors for proteins of the ECM, such as fibronectin, laminin, vitronectin, and collagens as well as for other plasma membrane proteins.

Integrins are obligate heterodimers, comprising noncovalently associated α and β subunits, each of which spans the plasma membrane and typically possesses a short (30 to 50 amino acids) cytoplasmic domain (Fig. 9.4). Receptor diversity and versatility in ligand binding is determined by the extracellular domains, through the specific pairing of 9 β and 16 α subunits, to form a family of at least 24 recognized heterodimers (Fig. 9.5). Further diversity is achieved by expression of alternatively spliced variants of the subunits. The extracellular domains of both α and β subunits contain a metal (M^{2+}) ion-dependent adhesion site (MIDAS), which is a sequence of approximately 200 amino acid residues required for binding to the integrin ligand.

The cytoplasmic domains of both α and β integrin subunits have been shown to be evolutionarily conserved (α subunits >85 percent amino acid identity, β subunits > 75 percent amino acid identity) among vertebrate species and in *Drosophila* (Hemler, 1991), implying conservation of function. In β subunits, an

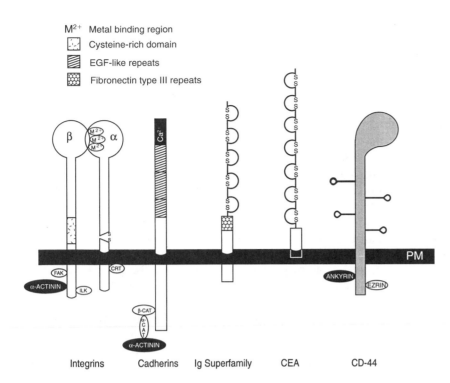

Figure 9.4. Major families of cell adhesion molecules (CAMs). The following structural motifs are depicted: fibronectin type III repeats; cystein-rich domain; EGF-like repeats. Ω = immunoglobulin loops; ◦— = glycosaminoglycan chains. CAT = catenin; FAK = focal adhesion kinase; ILK = integrin linked kinase; CRT = calreticulin; PM = plasma membrane.

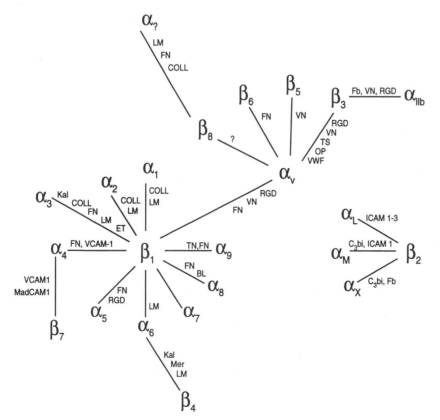

Figure 9.5. The integrin receptor family. A schematic representation of various $\alpha\beta$ integrin heterodimers and the ligands they interact with: COLL = collagen; FN = fibronectin; LM = laminin; ET = entactin; Kal = kalikrein; Mer = merosin; BL = basal lamina; VCAM = vascular cell adhesion molecule; ICAM = intercellular adhesion molecule; Fb = fibrinogen; VN = vitronectin; TS = thrombospondin; OP = osteopontin; VWF = von Willebrand factor; RGD = arginine-glycine-aspartic cid; MadCAM = mucosal address in cell adhesion molecule; TN = tenascin; C_3bi = breakdown product of the third component of complement.

NPXY motif (N = asparagine, P = proline, Y = tyrosine, X = any residue) and surrounding residues regulate β_1 and β_3 affinity for ligands, and a highly conserved α-subunit motif, KXGFFKR (K = lysine, G = glycine, F = phenylalanine, R = arginine) acts to regulate integrin function. An intracellular Ca^{2+} binding protein, calreticulin, interacts with this highly conserved membrane-proximal KXGFFKR sequence. This interaction is dynamic and has been shown to be important in the maintenance of the ligand-binding competency of the integrin (Coppolino et al., 1995).

The cytoplasmic domain of the β_1 subunit is thought to interact directly with components of the actin cytoskeleton, such as α actinin and talin, localizing via these interactions to focal adhesion plaques (FAPs) (Hannigan and Dedhar, 1996), which form cytoplasmically at points of contact between integrins and the ECM. These focal adhesion plaques represent the submembranous termini of actin stress fibers, indicating that integrins provide a structural bridge, linking the ECM and the actin cytoskeleton. Integrins are also found at other contact points between cells and the extracellular matrix, where they might act to mediate cell migration (Huttenlocher et al., 1995).

In addition to structural proteins, focal adhesion plaques contain a number of protein tyrosine kinases (such as the focal adhesion kinase p125[FAK], src, and csk) and ser/thr kinases (such as protein kinase Cα). One of these, p125[FAK], has been reported to bind in vitro to peptides representing the cytoplasmic domain of β_1 integrin (Schaller and Parsons, 1994), although physiologic confirmation of this interaction is lacking. Studies with chimeric integrin subunits (i.e., integrins engineered to contain different cytoplasmic domains) have shown that the β_1 cytoplasmic domain is required for integrin-induced phosphorylation of p125[FAK] (Clark and Brugge, 1995) and that the β_1 cytoplasmic domain is both necessary and sufficient for binding to cytoskeletal proteins to form focal adhesion plaques. Phosphorylation of the β_1 cytoplasmic domain on either the single serine residue or tyrosine residues renders the integrin inactive and unable to bind to focal adhesion plaques (Hynes, 1992). Phosphorylation-dephosphorylation of the β_1 subunit therefore plays an important role in the regulation of integrin function. The presence of regulatory protein kinases in focal adhesion plaques indicates that these structures probably also function as integrin signal-transduction complexes (reviewed in Clark and Brugge, 1995).

9.2.2 Signal Transduction by Integrins

Adherent cells require signals initiated by soluble mitogens and by adhesion for appropriate regulation of cell growth. These requirements have been particularly well characterized in fibroblasts, which will not proliferate in suspension (Otsuka and Moskowitz, 1975; Benecke et al., 1978). In addition to providing a physical link between ECM and the cytoskeleton, binding of integrins to their ligands elicits a variety of intracellular signaling events that are implicated in the regulation of cell shape and motility as well as cellular growth, survival, and differentiation. These include stimulation of protein kinase C activity, modulation of Na^+/H^+ antiporter activity, which influences cellular pH, and elevation of intracellular free Ca^{2+} (Hynes, 1992; Clark and Brugge, 1995).

Integrin-initiated signals stimulate the phosphorylation of tyrosine of a number of cellular proteins (Fig. 9.6) and can result in the induction of transcription factors such as c-fos and c-jun and in the transcription of genes such as metalloproteinases (Werb et al., 1989). Tyrosine kinase activity is required for at least some of these responses, since inhibition of tyrosine phosphorylation blocks adhesion-induced gene expression (Lin et al., 1994) and localization of integrins to focal contact points (Parsons et al., 1994). Adhesion-dependent signals are required for the appropriate transit of fibroblasts through the G1/S boundary (Fang et al., 1996) acting in concert with the soluble mitogenic signals required for entry of quiescent cells into G1 (see Chap. 7, Sec. 7.2.1). Cells may also require signals from the ECM to exit G1, as well as for S phase transit. These results suggest multiple, cell type–specific differences in the adhesive inputs to cell-cycle regulation. In adherent cells, the acquisition of anchorage-independent growth is a hallmark of neoplastic transformation (Shin et al., 1975) and implies dysregulation in growth signals emanating from the site or sites of cell-ECM interaction (Fig. 9.2).

Recent work, using a variety of cell-culture systems, has suggested that β_1 integrin–induced tyrosine kinase activity can activate the mitogenic Ras mitogen–activated protein kinase (MAPK) cascade (Fig. 9.6.; see also Chap. 6, Sec. 6.3), thus indicating overlap between integrin- and growth factor–mediated signaling pathways (Clark and Brugge, 1995). Integrin signaling may hinge on the activity of the tyrosine kinase p125[FAK], which is itself tyrosine phosphorylated upon binding to β_1 and β_3 integrins. Adhesion of cells to the ECM stimulates the tyrosine

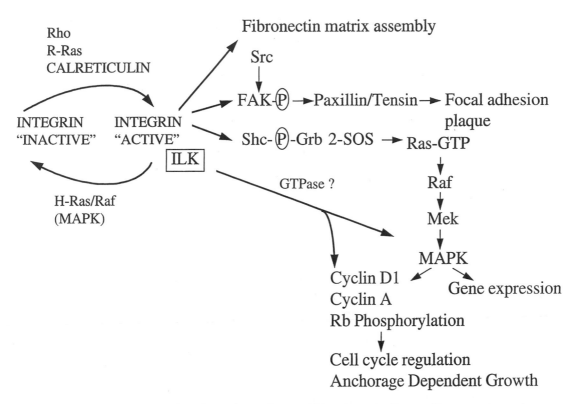

Figure 9.6. Integrin-mediated signal transduction. This schematic diagram illustrates the molecular basis of various responses to integrin activation and ligand binding. The major points illustrated are (1) all integrin receptors can exist in two states—"inactive" (i.e., unable to bind ligands), or "active" (i.e., capable of ligand binding). The interconversion of these two forms can be regulated by intracellular components and events. Some of these are shown here. The GTPases Rho and H-Ras can "activate" integrins, as can the calcium-binding protein calreticulin, which can bind directly to cytoplasmic domains of the α subunit of integrins. Activated H-Ras, or molecules stimulated by it such as Raf and mitogen-activated protein kinase (MAPK), can inactivate integrins. (2) Some "activated" integrins can participate in the assembly of a pericellular fibronectin matrix, resulting in constitutive occupation of integrin receptors by fibronectin. (3) Ligand-occupied integrins can stimulate several intracellular events, one of which is tyrosine phosphorylation of key signal-transducting proteins. The tyrosine phosphorylation of the focal adhesion kinase (FAK) regulates the formation of focal adhesion plaques, whereas the tyrosine phosphorylation of Shc activates the Ras-MAPK pathway (see also Chap. 6; Sec. 6.3.3). The newly-discovered integrin linked kinase (ILK), which binds directly to the β1 cytoplasmic domain of integrins, regulates the transit of cells from G1 into S phase by regulating the expression of cyclins D and A as well as retinoblastoma protein (Rb). Integrins can thus coordinate the regulation of extracellular matrix assembly, cytoskeletal organization, anchorage (adhesion)–dependent cell growth, and cellular responses to growth and inhibitory factors.

phosphorylation of paxillin and tensin, which are components of focal adhesion plaques (FAP); thus the focal adhesion kinase, FAK, and other FAP tyrosine kinases appear to regulate cytoskeletal reorganization in response to integrin engagement (Fig. 9.6).

Recently, a novel integrin-linked serine/threonine protein kinase, p59^{ILK}, which has a direct association with the cytoplasmic domain of β$_1$ integrin, has been identified (Hannigan et al., 1996). Overexpression of p59^{ILK} in epithelial cells induces anchorage-independent growth and malignant transformation, suggesting that the supranormal level of ILK activity is supplying growth signals normally provided by adhesion. The fact that p59^{ILK} complexes with β_1 and possibly β_3 integrin in vivo suggests that it functions as an integrin-specific signal transducer (Fig. 9.6).

The small GTP-binding protein Rho (see Chap. 6, Sec. 6.4.1) regulates ECM-dependent, as well as serum-dependent, cytoskeletal organization. The inactivation of Rho by ADP ribosylation inhibits activity of the focal adhesion kinase FAK, suggesting that Rho is also important in regulating activation of FAK by external stimuli. Perturbations in activation of Rho could be involved in malignant transformation due to the uncoupling of the integrin-Rho pathway. Indeed the constitutive inactivation of Rho results in altered cell adhesion to ECM and loss of actin polymerization in rat fibroblasts (McGlade et al., 1993); such cells have the morphologic phenotype of transformed cells. Further details of integrin "activation" and components involved in integrin-mediated signaling are shown in Fig. 9.6.

9.2.3 Integrins in Tumor Progression and Metastasis

The expression of integrin receptors is altered in malignant cells as compared with their normal counterparts, but the loss or gain of expression of a particular integrin has not been linked directly to malignant transformation. Rather, the changes in integrin expression seem to be tumor- as well as integrin-specific. In general, carcinomas (e.g., those of the breast, prostate, and colon) seem to lose expression of the integrins $\alpha_3\beta_1$, $\alpha_2\beta_1$, and $\alpha_5\beta_1$ while the expression of $\alpha_6\beta_1$ is maintained. It has been suggested that the integrin $\alpha_6\beta_1$ is involved in tumor invasion (Dedhar, 1995).

Functional studies involving gene transfer, anti-integrin antibodies, and adhesion-inhibiting peptides have demonstrated the potential for integrins to mediate tumor formation and metastasis. The expression of $\alpha_5\beta_1$ integrin in Chinese hamster ovary cells stimulated secretion of fibronectin and deposition of matrix in culture and suppressed tumor formation in nude mice. Transfection of an α_5 cDNA into α_5-deficient HT29 colon carcinoma cells rendered the cells dependent on fibronectin for growth, leading to the suggestion that an unoccupied $\alpha_5\beta_1$ receptor sends a growth-inhibitory signal to the cell, whereas an occupied $\alpha_5\beta_1$ receptor stimulates cell growth. Chemical transformation of human osteosarcoma cells (HOS) to a highly tumorigenic phenotype was associated with specific

increases in the expression of functional laminin ($\alpha_6\beta_1$), and collagen ($\alpha_2\beta_1$) receptors. A rhabdomyosarcoma cell line, transfected with a cDNA for the α_2 subunit, exhibited increased adhesion to collagen and laminin substrates in vitro and a marked increase in the number of lung metastases after intravenous or subcutaneous injection into nude mice. These results suggest that altered expression of, and perhaps signaling by, integrin α subunits may be important factors in the progression of some tumors (Dedhar, 1995).

The B16 murine melanoma model has been used to examine the potential role of integrins in tumor metastasis. A synthetic peptide containing the Arg-Gly-Asp (RGD) cell-binding peptide of fibronectin efficiently inhibits cell adhesion to fibronectin. Coinjection of this peptide with highly metastatic B16F10 cells into the tail veins of syngeneic mice inhibited experimental lung metastasis (see Chap. 10, Sec. 10.3.1) and resulted in prolonged survival of the injected mice, but it did not influence the ability of locally injected cells to form tumors. These experiments indicate the involvement of an integrin in mediating late stages of metastasis, most likely at the level of the interaction of tumor cells with pulmonary tissue (Akiyama et al., 1995). In another study, a cDNA for the α_4 integrin subunit was transfected into highly invasive, α_4-deficient B16a melanoma cells (Quian et al., 1994). Expression of $\alpha_4\beta_1$ integrin on the B16a cell surface resulted in a significant reduction in invasiveness into an extracellular matrix gel (Matrigel), and the suppression of pulmonary metastases in C57BL/6 mice. Specific suppression of spontaneous (from subcutaneous tumors), but not experimental metastases (from intravenous injection, see Chap. 10, Sec. 10.3.1) was seen with B16a-α_4 transfectants, and it was shown that α_4-expressing B16F10 cells do not form spontaneous metastases. These results suggest a minimum complexity for the involvement of integrin-ECM interactions in tumor progression, wherein one integrin (or lack of it, e.g., $\alpha_4\beta_1$) influences early invasive behavior, with a distinct RGD-sensitive integrin mediating subsequent tissue arrest and colonization.

As depicted in Fig. 9.3, a critical step in the metastatic spread of tumor cells is the active penetration of basement membrane and subsequent crossing of multiple tissue boundaries. Transformed cells are often defective in secreting fibronectin and laying down an organized matrix, and the increased production of metalloproteinases that degrade the basement membrane provides an invasive advantage to the tumor cells (reviewed in Stetler-Stevenson et al.,

1993). In human melanoma cells, occupation by ligand and antibody stimulation of the $\alpha_v\beta_3$ (vitronectin), but not $\alpha_5\beta_1$ (fibronectin) receptor have been shown to increase tumor cell invasiveness in vitro. These treatments did not alter adhesion of the melanoma cells to vitronectin or matrix, suggesting that, in these cells, reciprocal interaction of the matrix and tumor cell might be linked via $\alpha_v\beta_3$ integrin–mediated signal transduction. The $\alpha_v\beta_3$ integrin may also regulate tumor cell growth, since it was reported that melanoma cells selected for decreased $\alpha_v\beta_3$ expression had decreased ability to form tumors as compared with parental cells and that tumorigenicity was restored by transfer of an α_v cDNA into the β_3-expressing cells. Collectively, these data indicate that $\alpha_v\beta_3$ integrins may play a particularly important role in the development of metastatic melanoma (Nip and Brodt, 1995).

Angiogenesis, the growth of new blood vessels from preexisting capillaries, is required for the growth of primary or metastatic tumors beyond a few millimeters in diameter (see Sec. 9.3). Integrins have been shown to be positive mediators of angiogenesis. For example, migration of cultured endothelial cells on vitronectin and collagen was found to be mediated by $\alpha_v\beta_3$ and $\alpha_2\beta_1$ integrins, respectively. The expression of $\alpha_v\beta_3$ is increased in newly formed blood vessels, both in human wound granulation tissue and in chick chorioallantoic membranes treated with basic fibroblast growth factor, a positive angiogenic factor. The addition of tumor fragments to chorioallantoic membranes also induced angiogenesis, which, along with tumor proliferation, was selectively inhibited by either an anti-$\alpha_v\beta_3$ monoclonal antibody or specific peptide inhibitors of $\alpha_v\beta_3$ (Brooks et al., 1994a and b).

9.2.4 Cadherins

Cadherins are intercellular adhesion receptors. Adherent junctions and desmosomes are the two major forms of intercellular junction, required for maintenance of tissue architecture and for the differentiation of epithelial tissue. Distinct members of the cadherin family of cell adhesion receptors are principal constituents of each type of junction, mediating Ca^{2+}-dependent adhesion between similar cells. Many carcinomas display reduced intercellular adhesion and lose the characteristics of differentiated epithelium, suggesting a critical role for cadherins in the malignant progression of carcinoma. There are approximately 20 recognized cadherins and protocadherins, which are structurally related, integral

membrane proteins (see Fig. 9.4). E-cadherin, the major epithelial cadherin, contains four conserved extracellular domains, a fifth extracellular domain possessing conserved cysteine residues, a transmembrane domain, and a cytoplasmic domain (Takeichi, 1993). The most N-terminal of the extracellular cadherin conserved domains contains a histidine-alanine-valine amino acid triplet, which comprises the cell adhesion recognition sequence required for homophilic association (i.e., that between like cells). Calcium binding sites lie between adjacent extracellular domains 1 to 4. The cytoplasmic domain associates with cellular proteins, catenins, that act to link cadherins to the actin cytoskeleton as well as to signal-transduction components.

There is evidence that cadherins are involved in the suppression of tumor invasion and metastasis. This evidence derives from analyses of cadherin expression in tumors of variable differentiation status, gene transfer experiments, mutational analysis of cadherins in tumors, and the identification of a cadherin-associated protein (APC) as the product of a tumor suppressor gene (see below; see also Chap. 4, Sec. 4.5.4, and Chap. 5, Sec. 5.5.3). The role of the epithelial E-cadherin (also known as uvomorulin, L-CAM, or cell-CAM 120/80) has been particularly well studied with respect to the influences of intercellular adhesion on tumor development. In various carcinomas, expression of E-cadherin is low or absent in poorly differentiated, invasive tumors and tumor-derived cell lines. Also, epithelial cells become invasive (as demonstrated in invasion assays using collagen gels and embryonic heart tissue) when intercellular adhesion is disrupted by anti–E-cadherin antibodies. Furthermore, reversion of an invasive phenotype was achieved by transfection of E-cadherin cDNA into a human breast carcinoma line and into highly invasive *ras*-transformed cell lines derived from canine kidney and murine mammary tumors. In human basal cell carcinomas, which generally express normal E-cadherin levels and have low metastatic potential, reduced E-cadherin expression was found to be restricted to a subset of invasive tumors. Reduced or absent E-cadherin expression in poorly differentiated, invasive, or high-grade tumors has been reported for squamous cell carcinoma of the head and neck, basal cell carcinoma, female genital tract tumors, and carcinomas of the stomach, bladder, breast (particularly lobular type), colon, and lung (reviewed in Birchmeier and Behrens, 1994).

Genetic support for the concept that E-cadherin may be regarded as a tumor suppressor gene comes from studies documenting deletion of chromosome 16q22, encompassing the E-cadherin locus, in prostate, ovarian, breast, and hepatocellular carcinomas (reviewed in Hannigan and Dedhar, 1996). Also, mutations resulting in loss of extracellular domain residues in E-cadherin were found in 50 percent of diffuse-type gastric carcinomas. Somatic mutations, with and without loss of heterozygosity for the E-cadherin gene have also been described in a small fraction of endometrial and ovarian carcinomas.

Three endogenous proteins, of apparent molecular weights of 102, 88, and 80 kDa, have been demonstrated to interact directly or indirectly with cytoplasmic domains of cadherin. The 102-, 88-, and 80-kDa proteins are named catenins α, β, and γ, respectively. Molecular studies show that homophilic cell binding by E-cadherin requires association with β-catenin, mediated by a 72 amino acid region in the cadherin cytoplasmic domain. Interaction with α-catenin seems to be critical for the linkage of cadherin and β-catenin to actin filaments (Fig. 9.4), since the mutational loss of α-catenin, rather than downregulation of E-cadherin expression, was found to be correlated with reduced cell adhesion in a human lung carcinoma line. Moreover, transfection of a cDNA for α-catenin into nonadhesive carcinoma cells induced tight cell-cell adhesion and reversion to an epithelial morphology.

A surprising connection between cadherins, catenins, and tumor progression was made with the observation that the APC (adenoma polyposis coli) tumor suppressor protein (see Chap. 4, Sec. 4.5.4) and β-catenin form physiologic complexes. APC, β-catenin, and γ-catenin all possess domains comprising up to 13 repeats of a 42 amino acid motif. E-cadherin and APC compete in vivo for overlapping binding sites within the internal repeat domain of β-catenin, and each of these complexes associates with α-catenin through the N-terminal domain of β-catenin, while γ-catenin (plakoglobin) can substitute for β-catenin in either of the cadherin or APC complexes.

The existence of mutually exclusive cadherin-catenin and APC-catenin complexes suggests that APC does not function directly in cadherin-mediated adhesion. Mutations in APC, which are associated with the formation of adenomas, cluster within the β-catenin binding region, yielding truncated APC peptides that are unable to bind to β-catenin. Thus, the chronology and the molecular data suggest that APC mutations are not directly linked with the alterations in cadherin expression or function that are associated with invasive carcinomas. Expression of a dominant-negative N-cadherin mutant protein, lacking the extracellular domain, which leads to reduced E-cadherin expression in the intestinal crypts of transgenic mice, leads to the development of multiple intestinal adenomas. Intriguingly, these lesions are similar to those resulting from a germline mutation of the murine APC homologue; the Min mouse model of multiple intestinal neoplasia (Su et al., 1992). These results suggest that a dynamic equilibrium between complexed and free cytoplasmic β-catenin may play a role in regulatory interactions involving APC signaling and cadherin function.

9.2.5 Adhesion Molecules of the Immunoglobulin Superfamily

Members of the immunoglobulin superfamily (IgG superfamily) are also involved in cell-cell adhesion. However, these interactions are independent of divalent cations such as Ca^{2+}, in direct contrast to the adhesion mediated by cadherins. The first of the cell adhesion molecules to be described was the neural cell adhesion molecule (N-CAM), but it is clear that there is a large family of similar molecules. The non-lymphocyte members of this family typically express a number of immunoglobulin-related domains proximal to repeats of fibronectin type III domains (Fig. 9.4). This latter domain was first described in fibronectin, but it also occurs in cytokine receptors and in several ECM proteins. Well-characterized members of the IgG superfamily of CAMs include N-CAM, contactin, myelin-associated glycoprotein (MAG), DCC (deleted in colorectal carcinoma), intercellular adhesion molecules (I-CAMs), and vascular cell adhesion molecule (V-CAM). Some of these adhesion receptors mediate interactions between similar cells, in particular those expressed in the nervous system—e.g., N-CAM (Hynes and Lander, 1992)—although N-CAM can also bind to heparan sulfate proteoglycans in the extracellular matrix. Others, expressed on activated endothelial cells (I-CAM-1, I-CAM-2, and V-CAM) or on lymphocytes (I-CAMs), mediate heterophilic interactions (i.e., those between different types of cell) and bind to integrin receptors on adjacent cells.

Some members of the IgG superfamily of cell-cell adhesion receptors have been implicated in oncogenesis, most notably DCC, a candidate tumor suppressor gene located at 18q21.1 (Chap. 4, Sec. 4.5.4). The *DCC* gene encodes a protein of 1447 amino acids that shares overall structural similarity with N-CAM, thus identifying DCC as a member of the immunoglobulin (Ig) superfamily of cell adhesion molecules. The presence of Ig-like domains and fibronectin type III repeats in the extracellular domain suggests strongly that DCC is a receptor, mediating specific intercellular or cell-matrix interactions. Allelic loss of *DCC* in a variety of carcinomas is consistent with DCC affecting late events in tumor formation and indicates that its tumor suppressor role is not restricted to colonic epithelium.

Recently, direct evidence for the role of *DCC* as a tumor suppressor gene has been obtained from transfection studies in human epithelial cells. Transformation of human papillomavirus-immortalized keratinocytes by nitrosomethylurea (NMU) results in allelic loss of *DCC,* with concomitant loss of DCC expression and the acquisition of a malignant phenotype (Klingelhutz et al., 1993). Transfection of a full-length cDNA for DCC into these NMU-transformed cells resulted in high levels of expression of the DCC protein and suppression of the malignant phenotype. Importantly, DCC expression was not detectable in tumors that grew from revertant cells. Expression of variant forms of DCC on the cell surface from truncated cDNAs, which encode proteins lacking most of the cytoplasmic domain, did not suppress the tumorigenic phenotype, suggesting that the cytoplasmic domain of DCC mediates intracellular protein interactions important in epithelial cell differentiation and suppression of malignant transformation.

9.2.6 Carcinoembryonic Antigen

Carcinoembryonic antigen (CEA) (Fig. 9.4) is a cell-surface glycoprotein member of the Ig superfamily, which can function in epithelial cells to mediate Ca^{2+}-independent, homotypic cell adhesion (Benchimol et al., 1989). The extracellular N-terminal domain of CEA contains an IgV-like domain of 107 amino acid residues that is required for binding to CEA molecules on other cells. Extensive mapping and inhibition studies with monoclonal antibodies against various parts of the CEA molecule have suggested that homophilic adhesion results from two bonds formed between anti-parallel CEA molecules. None of the CEA family members contain cytoplasmic or transmembrane domains but are anchored in the external plasma membrane by a C-terminal, glycophosphatidyl-inositol moiety. CEA is overproduced in most colon carcinomas (Shuster et al., 1980), as well as other carcinomas, and 10- to 100-fold elevated serum levels of CEA indicate a poor prognosis in patients with adenocarcinomas of colon, breast, and lung. There are conflicting reports as to whether these increases in serum CEA represent increased release to the vasculature or cellular overproduction.

In vitro, CEA mediates homophilic binding of human colon adenocarcinoma cells, with kinetics of cell aggregation correlating directly with levels of CEA production by the cells. Antibodies to the N-terminal domain block the adhesion of colon carcinoma cells and normal colonic cells to immobilized CEA. Freshly isolated intestinal crypt cells express CEA on their surface, and treatment of these cells with a phosphoinositide-specific phospholipase C markedly reduces surface CEA expression and eliminates cellular adhesion to CEA. These studies indicate that CEA can mediate adhesion in intestinal epithelium, and the high levels of basolateral CEA expression seen in fetal colonic epithelium are consistent with a developmental role for CEA in intercellular adhesion. The expression of CEA in colon carcinomas may thus reflect a fetal pattern of expression that is disruptive of tissue architecture and differentiation. Quantitative in situ hybridization analyses (see Chap. 3, Sec. 3.4.6) using probes to the mRNA for CEA and immunoelectron microscopic localization of CEA protein have shown that CEA mRNA and protein levels are increased at the invading front of tumors, suggesting that free CEA may act as an antiadhesive factor to facilitate cell migration and perhaps help protect tumors from host defenses.

Although the mechanism(s) by which CEA contributes to progression of tumors is obscure, overexpression of CEA contrasts with the mutational inactivation, or functional downregulation, of other CAM-mediated intercellular adhesion systems that may occur in tumors. Thus, progression to advanced carcinoma may require a nonrandom, temporally regulated series of events involving downregulation of the expression and function of one subset of CAMs and upregulation or increased expression levels of others.

9.2.7 CD44 Hyaluronate-Binding Proteins

CD44 is a cell-surface glycoprotein (see Fig. 9.4), identified as the major receptor mediating cellular interactions with hyaluronate, a glycosaminoglycan component of the extracellular matrix (Arrufo et al., 1990). CD44 is widely expressed and exists in multiple forms with variable glycosylation. The N-terminal extracellular region mediates binding to hyaluronate through a disulfide bond–stabilized loop structure. All CD44 isoforms contain a cytoplasmic domain, which may link CD44 to actin filaments through interactions with ankyrin, ezrin, and moesin. The extracellular domain is encoded in part by a group of 10 exons (v1 through v10), which are variably expressed in all but "standard" CD44s and define the different CD44 isoforms. Alternative splicing of the mRNA to produce these variable isoforms (CD44v) is regulated in a tissue-specific manner or by antigen activation in lymphocytes. The tissue-restricted expression of CD44v isoforms presumably accounts for the involvement of CD44 in a wide variety of functions, including mediation of lymphocyte adhesion to endothelial cells of venules, cell migration, cytokine release, T cell activation and adhesion, and metastasis.

The metastasis-promoting ability of one CD44v isoform is of particular interest, as it may reflect the aberrant expression and regulation of a physiologic CD44v function. Transfection of the cDNA for this particular CD44v, which codes for a 162 amino acid insertion in the extracellular domain, resulted in the acquisition of a metastatic phenotype by rat pancreatic carcinoma cells (Gunthert et al., 1991). Subsequent studies have confirmed the metastasis-associated expression of specific CD44v in human carcinoma cell lines as well as a positive correlation between levels of CD44v expression and the metastatic potential of human melanoma cells. Western blot analyses of primary colon carcinomas and carcinoma cell lines demonstrated very low expression of another isoform known as CD44H, which contrasts with high expression levels in normal colonic mucosa. Transfection of a cDNA for CD44H into the colon carcinoma cells restored CD44H expression and inhibited the tumor-forming potential of these cells. Thus, it may be that both loss of CD44H expression and concomitant gain of CD44v expression are required in the development of metastatic colorectal carcinoma.

9.3 TUMOR ANGIOGENESIS

9.3.1 Dependence of Tumors on Blood Supply

The formation of new blood vessel capillaries from existing blood vessels is a normal and physiologic process similar to many of the steps of tumor-cell invasion. This process is known as angiogenesis: it involves activation of endothelial cells of a mature vessel, localized degradation of the surrounding basement membrane, the movement of adjacent vascular endothelial cells through such a breach, and their subsequent migration into the surrounding connective tissue stroma, where they proliferate and eventually form tubular structures. These can join with other similar structures to form a network of new blood vessels.

Angiogenesis is a normal part of early embryonic development, of formation of the corpus luteum in the ovary, and of healing of wounds. It is also a necessary component of the progressive growth of solid tumors (Folkman, 1976), since cells in solid tumors must receive the necessary oxygen and nutrients to survive and grow. Solid tumors up to about 1 to 2 mm in diameter can obtain required nutrients by passive diffusion from blood vessels in surrounding tissue. Growth beyond this "occult" size requires sustained angiogenesis (Folkman, 1976).

Although the growth of solid tumors is dependent on angiogenesis for the generation of a vascular network, tumor blood vessels show many differences as compared with those of most normal tissues. Tumor vessels are often dilated or leaky, and nonfunctional. Moreover, blood flow is often erratic, with stasis or even reversal of blood flow within individual vessels (Less et al., 1991; Helmlinger et al., 1997). As a result there is frequently imperfect delivery of nutrient metabolites such as oxygen to tumor cells and impaired clearance of the products of metabolism. Cells distant from functional blood vessels tend to become hypoxic, and their microenvironment is often acidic due to impaired clearance of lactic acid and carbonic acid (due to production of CO_2 by metabolism; Tannock and Rotin, 1989; Newell et al., 1993). The rate of cell proliferation decreases with increasing distance from functional blood vessels, presumably because of a lack of metabolic energy to support passage through the cell cycle (Tannock, 1970; see also Chap. 7, Sec. 7.6.3). Impaired clearance of fluid from tumors (due to a lack of lymphatic vessels) leads also to increased interstitial pressure within the extracellular matrix (Jain, 1994).

Each of the above factors may have important consequences for cancer treatment. Hypoxic cells are known to be resistant to radiation (see Chap. 13, Sec. 13.5.2). Cells within solid tumors may also be protected from the effects of chemotherapy because of poor delivery of drugs via the imperfect vascular supply. Also, there has been shown to be poor penetration of several drugs through tumor tissue, both because of the large intercapillary distance and as a result of the raised interstitial pressure in tumors (Jain, 1994; see also Chap. 15, Sec. 15.3.4).

9.3.2 Angiogenic Growth Factors and Growth-Factor Receptors

Folkman (1971) proposed that tumor cells could produce a *tumor angiogenesis factor* (TAF) that diffuses into the microenvironment and initiates the process of tumor angiogenesis. Once new blood vessels penetrate a microscopic primary tumor or distant metastasis, the lesions acquire the potential to grow into larger and potentially life-threatening macroscopic tumors. He reasoned that the phenomenon of tumor dormancy, whereby small tumors remain roughly the same size for prolonged periods, could be explained by their failure to produce sufficient quantities of TAF to induce tumor angiogenesis (Folkman, 1971).

Direct evidence for the existence of angiogenic growth factors secreted by tumor cells was inferred from experiments in which small, multicellular tumor fragments were implanted on the cornea of the rabbit eye and observed to induce the formation of new blood vessels (Fig. 9.7; Folkman, 1976). Only when the tumor pieces were penetrated by the new vessels did they expand and show rapid and highly significant increases in volume. The first angiogenic growth factor that was purified and characterized was basic fibroblast growth factor (bFGF; Folkman and Klagsbrun, 1987). Since then several other growth factors have been isolated or identified that have the ability to induce or facilitate tumor angiogenesis, as summarized in Table 9.1.

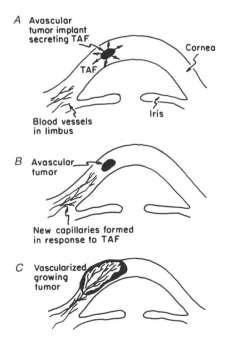

Figure. 9.7. Experiment to demonstrate that tumor tissue may stimulate the growth of blood vessels through secretion of tumor angiogenesis factor (TAF). A piece of tumor implanted into the avascular cornea of a rabbit eye grows to a maximum size of 1 to 2mm until blood vessels are stimulated to invade into it from the surrounding limbus. (Adapted from Folkman, 1976.)

There are some features of bFGF that have cast doubt on its ability to function as a primary and *direct-acting* angiogenic growth factor in vivo (Risau, 1996). For example, bFGF receptors are readily detectable on endothelial cells grown in tissue culture; however, their presence on endothelial cells in vivo has been difficult to demonstrate (Risau, 1996). Thus the demonstrated role of bFGF as an enhancer of angiogenesis might be mediated via a cytokine network—i.e., through its ability to induce the action of another growth factor. Such a molecule is vascular endothelial growth factor (VEGF), also known as vascular permeability factor (VPF).

VEGF/VPF was detected initially as a factor secreted by tumor cells into tissue culture medium or ascites fluid in vivo, which caused normal blood vessels to become hyperpermeable (Senger et al., 1983). The factor was identified as a heparin-binding protein of molecular weight 34 to 42 kDa, and was termed VPF. It was later demonstrated that VPF also stimulated endothelial cell division (Connolly et al., 1989). Independently, several groups isolated a secreted protein that had selective mitogenic activity for cultured endothelial cells, which they called VEGF (Ferrara and Henzel, 1989; Gospodarowicz et al., 1989). On the basis of amino acid and cDNA sequence analysis, it is now known that VEGF and VPF are the same protein (Thomas, 1996), and VEGF is now the more common term used to describe this growth factor.

VEGF is a homodimeric heparin-binding glycoprotein that exists in at least four isoforms because of alternative splicing of the primary mRNA transcript. The isoforms are designated $VEGF_{121}$, $VEGF_{165}$, $VEGF_{189}$, and $VEGF_{206}$, according to the number of amino acids the protein contains (Ferrara, 1995; Thomas, 1996). One of the features that sets VEGF apart from other putative angiogenesis growth factors, such as bFGF, is its selectivity as a mitogen for endothelial cells. This is due in part to the presence of two high-affinity cell-surface receptors, called Flk-1 (in mice) or KDR (in humans), and Flt-1, on "activated" endothelial cells. These receptors are also referred to as *VEGFR2* and *VEGFR1*, respectively. Both are tyrosine kinases (see Chap. 6, Sec. 6.3.1), having seven extracellular immunoglobulin-like globular domains and an intracellular kinase domain (Ferrara, 1995; Terman and Dougher-Vermazen, 1996).

VEGF receptors are not detectable in endothelial cells of resting, mature blood vessels or in most other cell types in the body, and it is thought that high levels of expression on endothelial cells may be

Table 9.1. Angiogenic Growth Factors

Factor	Properties	Receptor
Vascular endothelial growth factor/vascular permeability factor (VEGF/VPF)	Endothelial mitogen, survival factor, and permeability inducer produced by many types of tumor cells	Flk-1/KDR Flt-1 (both present on activated endothelium)
Placental growth factor (PlGF)	Weak endothelial mitogen	Flt-1
Basic fibroblast growth factor (bFGF/FGF-2)	Endothelial mitogen, angiogenesis inducer, and survival factor; inducer of Flk-1 expression	FGFR1-4
Acidic fibroblast growth factor (aFGF/FGF-1)	Endothelial mitogen and angiogenesis inducer	FGFR1-4
Fibroblast growth factor 3 (FGF-3/Int-2)	Endothelial mitogen and angiogenesis inducer	FGFR1-4
Fibroblast growth factor 4 (FGF-4/Hst/K-FGF)	Endothelial mitogen and angiogenesis inducer	FGFR1-4
Transforming growth factor α (TGF-α)	Endothelial mitogen and angiogenesis inducer; inducer of VEGF expression	EGFR
Epidermal growth factor (EGF)	Weak endothelial mitogen; inducer of VEGF expression	EGFR
Hepatocyte growth factor/scatter factor (HGF/SF)	Endothelial mitogen and angiogenesis inducer	c-MET
Transforming growth factor β (TGF-β)	In vivo acting angiogenesis inducer or endothelial growth inhibitor; inducer of VEGF expression	TGF-βR I, II, III
Tumor necrosis factor α (TNF-α)	In vivo acting angiogenesis inducer. Endothelial mitogen (low concentrations) or inhibitor (high concentrations); inducer of VEGF expression	TNFR-55 (TNFR-75?)
Platelet-derived growth factor (PDGF)	Mitogen and motility factor for endothelial cells and fibroblasts; in vivo angiogenesis inducer	PDGFR
Granulocyte colony-stimulating factor (G-CSF)	In vivo acting angiogenesis-inducing factor with some mitogenic activity for endothelial cells	G-CSFR
Pleiotrophin	Angiogenesis inducing pleiotrophic growth factor	proteoglycan
Thymidine phosphorylase (tP)/platelet-derived endothelial cell growth factor (PD-ECGF)	In vivo acting angiogenesis factor	The mode of action remains unclear
Angiogenin	In vivo acting angiogenesis inducer with RNase activity	170-kDa angiogenin receptor
Proliferin	35-kDa angiogenesis-inducing protein in mouse	unknown

induced by the presence of VEGF. That the presence of these receptors and their interactions with VEGF are necessary for angiogenesis is indicated by the observation that VEGF "knockout" mice (see Chap. 3, Sec. 3.3.12) do not survive as embryos but die as a result of severe developmental vascular abnormalities (Carmeliet et al., 1996; Ferrara et al., 1996). Indeed, even the absence of only one of the two VEGF alleles can cause a severe defect in embryonic angiogenesis (Carmaliet et al., 1996; Ferrara et al., 1996). This could be due in part to the function of VEGF as a differentiation and a survival factor to prevent apoptosis of endothelial cells in newly

formed capillaries (Alon et al., 1995) as well as its function as a mitogenic growth factor.

A seminal role for VEGF in tumor angiogenesis is suggested by the following evidence (Klagsbrun and Soker, 1993):

1. VEGF is present in almost every type of human solid tumor. It is found in especially high concentrations around tumor blood vessels (primarily because it binds to VEGF receptors expressed by endothelial cells or to heparin sulfate proteoglycans in subendothelial basement membranes) and in (presumed) hypoxic areas of the tumor

parenchyma that are distal from blood vessels (Senger et al., 1994; Shweiki et al., 1992). Hypoxia is a potent inducer of VEGF, primarily by a process involving increased stability of mRNA (Stein et al., 1995): this may represent an adaptive, compensatory response by cells and tissues to obtain more oxygen.

2. VEGF receptors are detected in blood vessels within or near tumors.

3. Various VEGF antagonists such as monoclonal neutralizing antibodies can suppress the growth of VEGF-expressing solid tumors in mice (Ferrara, 1995) but lack any such effect on tumor cells grown in cell culture where angiogenesis is not required. A similar suppressive effect on transplanted tumor growth can be achieved by blocking the signaling function of VEGF receptors in endothelial cells (Millauer et al., 1994).

4. VEGF, unlike other known angiogenic growth factors, is capable of inducing extracellular matrix in tumors (Senger et al., 1994). It does so by causing extravascular leakage of plasma proteins such as fibrinogen, which can then be converted into a cross-linked fibrin gel in the tumor. This vascular permeability–dependent provisional matrix may be critical for a sustained angiogenic response (Senger et al., 1994).

In addition to hypoxia, a number of cytokines can upregulate VEGF production, including known angiogenic growth factors such as bFGF. Indeed, bFGF can act synergistically with VEGF to induce or upregulate endothelial cell proliferation in vitro and angiogenesis in vivo (Pepper et al., 1992; Asahara et al., 1995). Thus the ability of bFGF to function as a stimulator of angiogenesis may depend on its ability to induce and/or interact with a direct-acting angiogenic molecule such as VEGF. The same may be true for a number of other cytokines that induce or upregulate tumor angiogenesis, such as transforming growth factor α (TGF-α), acidic FGF, and TGF-β. If so, this would make VEGF (or VEGF receptors) an attractive therapeutic target for cancer treatment despite the redundancy of growth factors that may influence tumor angiogenesis (Bicknell and Harris, 1996).

Recent results suggest that oncogenes such as mutant *ras* can induce or enhance the expression of VEGF in tumor-cell populations (Grugel et al., 1995; Rak et al., 1995b). Thus, one of the ways in which oncogenes or overexpressed proto-oncogenes, which utilize Ras signaling pathways (see Chap. 6, Sec. 6.3.4), may contribute to the formation of solid tumors is by helping to stimulate angiogenesis. This

also has some therapeutic implications, since agents that inhibit the function of proteins encoded by mutant oncogenes (e.g., Ras farnesyltransferase inhibitors; see Chap. 15, Sec. 15.5.3) or certain proto-oncogenes (e.g., neutralizing antibodies to the EGF receptor or the neu/erbB-2 receptor tyrosine kinase) might inhibit tumor growth in vivo not only by a direct antiproliferative effect but also by suppressing tumor angiogenesis (Rak et al., 1995a; Viloria-Petit et al., 1997).

The gene knockout technology has revealed what appear to be several new key molecular mediators of angiogenesis—the "angiopoietins" and angiopoietin receptors, called Tie-1 and Tie-2/Tek. Like Flk-1/KDR and Flt-1, Tie-1 and Tie-2/Tek are receptor tyrosine kinases selective for endothelial cells. They are upregulated in newly formed blood vessels. As summarized in Table 9.2, targeted disruption of genes encoding VEGF, VEGF receptors, angiopoietin, or angiopoietin receptors all lead to embryonic lethality (Risau, 1994; Davis et al., 1996; Hanahan and Folkman, 1996; Hanahan, 1997). The most severe phenotype is associated with knockout of VEGF receptors as well as VEGF itself, reinforcing the notion that endothelial cell differentiation, survival, and proliferation mediated through this receptor system are essential for embryonal and most likely adult angiogenesis (including that induced at the tumor site; Hanahan, 1997; Risau, 1997). As in the case of VEGF receptors, disruption of the genes encoding Tie-1 and Tie-2/Tek in mouse embryos results in profound defects in blood vessel formation and functional integrity. Similar phenotypes are also observed in the absence of angiopoietin-1, the ligand for the Tie-2/Tek receptor, or upon overexpression of a transgene encoding its natural antagonist, angiopoietin-2. Apparently angiopoietin-1 is involved in blood vessel maturation and maintenance, whereas angiopoietin-2 reverses this process and thereby may facilitate the proangiogenic effect of VEGF (Davis et al., 1996; Folkman and D'Amore, 1996; Hanahan, 1997). Recently evidence has been obtained to show that tumor angiogenesis can be inhibited by blocking the function of the Tie-2/Tek receptor on endothelial cells, with a soluble form of the receptor (Lin et al., 1997).

9.3.3 Inhibitors of Tumor Angiogenesis

Attempts to uncover suppressors of angiogenesis began with a search for endogenous angiogenesis inhibitors, which led to the extraction of a substance from cartilage (an avascular tissue), this substance was molecularly characterized many years later

Table 9.2. Key Molecular Regulators of Blood Vessel Formation as Defined by Gene Knockout Studies

Molecule	Function	Gene Knockout Phenotype	Relevance to Tumor angiogenesis
VEGF/VPF	Polypeptide growth factor that mediates survival and differentiation of endothelial cells	Embryonic lethal (both homo- and heterozygotes) Impaired endothelial cell differentiation and angiogenesis	Elevated levels expressed in tumor parenchyma
Flt-1 (VEGFR-1)	VEGF receptor tyrosine kinase	Embryonic lethal Disorganized assembly of endothelial cells	Expression induced in tumor blood vessels. Flt-1 antagonists inhibit tumor angiogenesis
Flk-1/KDR (VEGFR-2)	VEGF receptor tyrosine kinase	Embryonic lethal Lack of endothelial cell differentiation and angiogenesis	Expression induced in tumor blood vessels. Flk-1 antagonists inhibit tumor angiogenesis
Angiopoietin-1	Polypeptide factor that maintains capillary integrity	Embryonic lethal Defective complexity of the vasculature, poor interaction between endothelial cells and vessel wall	Unknown
Angiopoietin-2	Physiologic antagonist of angiopoietin-1	Unknown	Unknown
Tek/Tie-2	Angiopoietin-1/2 receptor tyrosine kinase	Embryonic lethal Defective blood vessel complexity and structure	Expression induced in tumor blood vessels. Tie-2 antagonists inhibit tumor angiogenesis
Tie-1	Receptor tyrosine kinase (ligand unknown)	Embryonic lethal Impaired integrity of capillaries, edema, hemorrhage	Expression elevated in tumor blood vessels
TGF-β1	Polypeptide growth factor	Defect in angiogenesis in 50% of homozygotes	Expressed in tumors
PDGFR-β	Receptor tyrosine kinase	Perinatal hemorrhage, lack of pericytes (similar phenotype in the case of PDGF-B ligand)	Expressed in tumors
Tissue factor	Polypeptide active in the coagulation cascade	Embryonic lethal Vascular abnormalities, deficient recruitment of pericytes and smooth muscle cells	Expressed in tumors
RasGAP	Signaling cofactor of Ras (activating GTPase activity)	Embryonic lethal Abnormal vessel branching, edema	May regulate responses of endothelial cells to tumor angiogenic factors

(Moses and Langer, 1991). Called CDI for cartilage-derived inhibitor, it is a member of the family of tissue inhibitors of metalloproteinases (TIMPs). The ability of CDI to inhibit angiogenesis is thought to be related primarily to its suppression of various proteases involved in endothelial cell migration dur-ing the formation of vessel "sprouts" (Moses and Langer, 1991).

It was discovered subsequently that a combination of certain batches of commercial heparin and corti-sone acetate could block bFGF-dependent angio-genesis in both in vitro and in vivo assays (Folkman et al., 1983). This led to research on "angiostatic" steroids and heparin fragments or their analogues, which together could strongly inhibit angiogenesis (Moses and Langer, 1991; Auerbach and Auerbach, 1994). More recently, other exogenous agents that inhibit angiogenesis have been discovered, some of which are listed in Table 9.3. This list includes agents that are not directly toxic to cells, but angiogenesis may also be inhibited by conventional chemotherapeutic drugs such as paclitaxel and vinblastine (Baguley et al., 1991; Dordunoo et al., 1995; Kerbel and Hawley, 1995; Pluda, 1997).

The antiangiogenic mode of action of most of the exogenous or endogenous antiangiogenic agents is unknown. One possible exception to this are blocking antibodies (or peptide antagonists) to defined molecular targets expressed by "activated" endothelial cells in newly formed vessels such as the cell-surface $\alpha_v\beta_3$ integrin—i.e, the "vitronectin" receptor. As discussed above (Sec. 9.2.3) anti-$\alpha_v\beta_3$ blocking antibodies or peptide antagonists can cause regression of newly formed blood vessels by induction of endothelial cell apoptosis (Brooks et al., 1994b; Brooks, 1996). Detailed reviews of the role of adhesion molecules in regulating angiogenesis have been published (Bischoff, 1995; Brooks, 1996). The inhibitory effects of $\alpha_v\beta_3$ antagonists on endothelial cell growth and survival is most likely due to a form of apoptosis known as *anoikis* (Meredith and Schwartz, 1997). This refers to disruption of the ability of normal cells (in this case endothelial cells) to interact with surrounding basement membrane/extracellular matrix structures. Such adhesion receptor (e.g., integrin-mediated) interactions appear to be vital for endothelial cell differentiation and remodeling of new blood vessels, and hence their survival. These interactions illustrate the critical importance of endothelial cell adhesion receptors for a fundamental property of solid tumors—namely, induction of angiogenesis.

Current research is again focused on endogenous inhibitors (see Table 9.3), many of which are proteolytically cleaved fragments of various proteins, including platelet factor 4, plasminogen, fibronectin, prolactin, thrombospondin, and epidermal growth factor (Gupta et al., 1995; Chen et al., 1995). Interest in these inhibitors has been stimulated by the discovery of *angiostatin*, a 38-kDa fragment of plasminogen (O'Reilly et al., 1994). Various proteolytic enzymes, produced either by tumor cells or host cells, are presumed to generate angiostatin from plasminogen (Dong et al., 1997). Since many of these endogenous inhibitors appear to be proteolytically cleaved fragments of larger proteins, it is possible that certain proteases may function to inhibit the growth of solid tumors even though some of these same proteases might also have the potential to enhance tumor cell invasion through degradation of components of the extracellular matrix.

There is evidence that some endogenous inhibitors of angiogenesis are regulated by the presence of wild-type tumor suppressor genes (see Chap. 5, Sec. 5.5). For example, *p53* regulates expression of thrombospondin and of a *glioma-derived angiogenesis inhibitory factor* (GD-AIF) (Dameron et al., 1994; Van Meir et al., 1994). Hence, inactivation of the *p53* gene may result in a loss of inhibition of angiogenesis, so that a combination of inactivation of *p53* with induction of angiogenic stimulators, such as the induction of VEGF by an activated mutant *ras* oncogene, as discussed earlier, could induce and "drive" angiogenesis in parallel with malignant transformation. The induction (and maintenance) of tumor angiogenesis appears to be the outcome of a change in the relative balance of stimulators and inhibitors of angiogenesis (as illustrated in Fig. 9.8), and both oncogenes and tumor suppressor genes can have regulatory effects on the expression of these angiogenic regulators (Bouck, 1990; Rak et al., 1995a; Bouck et al., 1996; Hanahan and Folkman, 1996; Volpert et al., 1997).

Antiangiogenesis is a therapeutic approach that might circumvent the problem of acquired anticancer drug resistance (Chap. 17, Sec. 17.2.1) in cancer treatment that occurs as a result of the genetic instability of tumor cells—hence their ability to give rise to mutant subpopulations (Kerbel, 1991, 1997). If (normal) endothelial cells in newly formed tumor-associated blood vessels are targeted for therapy, the relative genetic stability of their genome should prevent or delay the development of drug resistance. Indeed, recent studies have shown that repeated cycles of therapy in tumor-bearing mice with a direct acting inhibitor of angiogenesis called *endostatin* do not lead to acquired resistance, whereas resistance rapidly developed to the conventional antitumor agent cyclophosphamide (Boehm et al., 1997). Another significant potential advantage of an anti-endothelial/angiogenic strategy in treating solid tumors is that it could bypass the physiologic barriers to achieving effective drug penetration from blood vessels through tissue in solid tumors, which occurs partly as a result of their high interstitial pressures (Jain, 1994; see also Chap. 15, Sec. 15.3.4).

The clinical use of inhibitors of tumor angiogenesis is at an early stage and is likely to require chronic administration to obtain a significant antitumor effect (Pluda, 1997). This type of therapy is an exam-

Table 9.3. Inhibitors of Angiogenesis

Inhibitor	Characteristics and Mode of Action
Endogenous Inhibitors of Angiogenesis	
Angiostatin	Systemically acting angiogenesis inhibitor. Plasminogen fragment generated by proteolytic action of elastase. Inhibits endothelial cell proliferation by unknown mechanism.
Endostatin	Systemically acting angiogenesis inhibitor. Proteolytic fragment of collagen XVIII, a component of perivascular extracellular matrix. Inhibits endothelial cell proliferation and angiogenesis by unknown mechanism.
Platelet factor 4 (PF4)	Inhibits angiogenesis by interference with bFGF receptor. An active fragment can be generated by N-terminal cleavage. In clinical trials as an antiangiogenic agent.
Prolactin (16-kDa fragment)	Inhibits angiogenesis, by bFGF and VEGF induced proliferation of endothelial cell (S-phase arrest).
EGF fragment	Inhibits EGF and laminin–dependent endothelial cell motility and angiogenesis.
Thrombospondin-1 (TSP-1)	TSP-1 (fragment) binds to CD36 on endothelial cells and inhibits angiogenesis by a mechanism possibly involving proliferation, migration, and cell survival.
Interferon α (IFN-α)	Inhibits angiogenesis by antimitotic and antimigratory effect on endothelial cells and in part by blockade of bFGF production by parenchymal cells. In clinical trials as an antiangiogenic agent.
Interferon β (IFN-β)	Inhibits endothelial cell migration and proliferation.
Interferon γ (IFN-γ)	Inhibits endothelial cell proliferation and migration.
Interleukin 12 (IL-12)	Inhibits angiogenesis by stimulation of IFN-γ and interferon-inducible-protein-10 (IP-10) production. In clinical trials as an antiangiogenic agent
Tissue inhibitors of metalloproteinases (TIMP1-3, CDI)	Block dissolution of the extracellular matrix and endothelial cell invasion by inhibiting metalloproteinases.
Proliferin-related protein (PRP)	Inhibits directed migration of mouse endothelial cells.
2-Methoxy estradiol	Inhibits endothelial proliferation and angiogenesis by unknown mechanism.
Exogenous Inhibitors of Angiogenesis	
TNP-470 (AGM1470)	Synthetic analog of fumagillin; fungal inhibitor of endothelial cell proliferation and angiogenesis. In clinical trials as an antiangiogenic agent.
Pentosan polysulfate	Inhibits paracrine action of heparin-binding angiogenic growth factors (bFGF, VEGF). In clinical trials as an antiangiogenic agent.
Tecogalan	Sulfated bacterial polysaccharide peptidoglycan complex that is inhibitory for endothelial cell proliferation, particularly in combination with tamoxifen.
Batimastat (BB-94)	Synthetic inhibitor of metalloproteinases. Inhibits endothelial cell invasion. In clinical trials.
Marimastat (BB2516)	Synthetic, oral inhibitor of metalloproteinases. Inhibits endothelial cell invasion. In clinical trials.
Suramin	Interferes with multiple endothelial functions and bFGFR activity.
CM101	Streptococcal polysaccharide; binds specifically to activated endothelial cells and induces vascular inflammation.
Vitaxin	Humanized anti αvβ3 antibody. Prevents ligation of αvβ3 integrin causing endothelial apoptosis.
Vitamin D3 analogues	Inhibit angiogenesis by unknown mechanism.
Thalidomide	Originally used as a sedative and to treat leprosy. Teratogenic, antiangiogenic (epoxide metabolite). In clinical trials as an antiangiogenic agent.
Minocycline	A tetracycline with antiangiogenic activity.

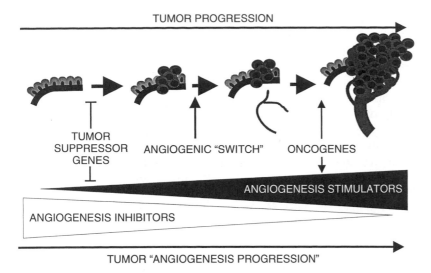

TUMOR PROGRESSION

TUMOR
SUPPRESSOR
GENES

ANGIOGENIC "SWITCH"

ONCOGENES

ANGIOGENESIS STIMULATORS

ANGIOGENESIS INHIBITORS

TUMOR "ANGIOGENESIS PROGRESSION"

Figure 9.8. Shift in the balance between angiogenesis inhibitors and stimulators during tumor progression. Accumulation of genetic defects during the course of cancer progression likely affects the production of angiogenesis regulators by cells of the tumor parenchyma. As a result of such quantitative and qualitative changes, the balance between angiogenesis inhibitors and stimulators changes gradually in favor of the latter. Angiogenesis is initiated after a threshold of proangiogenic activity is reached. With further genetic alterations in tumor cells, the angiogenic phenotype may become increasingly severe.

ple of an anticancer strategy aimed at *controlling* the disease rather than eradicating it. Despite chronic treatments, toxic side effects in treated animals have not usually been a serious problem, but adverse effects on fertility and healing of wounds might be expected. Ideally there should be a very high degree of specificity for tumor-associated blood vessels. While there is increased expression of various markers on activated endothelial cells in tumors such as the $\alpha_v\beta_3$ integrin and the Flk-1/KDR receptor tyrosine kinases for VEGF, it is uncertain whether they convey a sufficient degree of tumor specificity, although experiments in mice are encouraging (Boehm et al., 1997).

9.3.4 Tumor Angiogenesis as a Prognostic Indicator

A clinical application of research in tumor angiogenesis could be its use as an independent prognostic indicator (Weidner et al., 1991). Many blood vessels in tumors are too small to be detected in normal histologic sections stained with hematoxylin and eosin. However, if such sections are immunohistochemically stained with antibodies that detect antigenic determinants expressed exclusively or preferentially by vascular endothelial cells, the blood vessels can be seen and counted. It has been shown that primary tumors such as breast, prostate, and lung carcinoma contain localized zones of high vascular density, so-called vascular hot spots. When the number of vessels is counted in such hot spots, a strong correlation is frequently noted between high vessel density and poor prognosis as measured by recurrence-free survival or overall survival (Weidner et

al., 1991). Such correlations imply a relationship between angiogenesis and metastasis. A correlation has also been reported for VEGF expression and vascular density in breast cancer (Toi et al., 1995). These observations highlight another important feature of solid tumors: namely, that vascular endothelial cells can represent up to 10 percent or more of the cell mass in a solid tumor and can themselves be a rich source of cytokines and other growth or survival factors. Such endothelial cell–derived factors would have an excellent opportunity to influence the growth of adjacent tumor cell populations (Rak et al., 1994, 1996), in addition to having fundamental effects on the supply of essential nutrients and removal of toxic products of tumor metabolism.

9.4 SUMMARY

This chapter illustrates some of the molecular and cellular means by which tumor cells can interact with their immediate extracellular environment. These interactions depend heavily on the contribution of a wide range of adhesion receptors, such as integrins and constituents of the extracellular matrix, and can have a profound effect on the behavior of tumors. Studies with integrins, in particular, have demonstrated the role of cell adhesion molecules in signal transduction and in the control of cell growth and differentiation. The dependence that tumors have on their extracellular environment is perhaps best illustrated by the impact of angiogenesis on the processes of tumor development, tumor dormancy, termination of the dormant state, and the formation of distant metastases. Other aspects of the extracellular environment that can have a major impact on tumor growth and response to therapy include the formation of a tissue stroma in solid tumors, leukocyte endothelial interactions, and the impact that tissues in different organ sites can have on the metastatic process. The reductionist approach to studying cancer in simple cell-culture systems has tended to downplay or ignore the impact that the dynamic interaction of the tumor cell with its extracellular environment can have on the fundamental biology of cancer. Recent progress made in the fields of cell adhesion (including integrins) and extracellular matrix and in tumor angiogenesis highlights an increasing appreciation of the role of the extracellular environment in cancer.

REFERENCES

Akiyama SK, Olden K, Yamada KM. Fibronectin and integrins in invasion and metastasis. *Cancer Metastasis Rev* 1995; 14:173–189.

Alon T, Hemo I, Itin A, et al: Vascular endothelial growth factor acts as a survival factor for newly formed retinal vessels and has implications for retinopathy of prematurity. *Nature Med* 1995; 1:1024–1028.

Arrufo A, Stamenkovic I, Melnick M, et al: CD44 is the principal cell surface receptor for hyaluronate. *Cell* 1990; 61:1303–1313.

Asahara T, Bauters C, Zheng LP, et al: Synergistic effect of vascular endothelial growth factor and basic fibroblast growth factor on angiogenesis in vivo. *Circulation* 1995; 92:365–371.

Auerbach W, Auerbach R: Angiogenesis inhibition: A review. *Pharm Ther* 1994; 63:265–311.

Baguley BC, Holdaway KM, Thomsen LI, et al: Inhibition of growth of colon 38 adenocarcinoma by vinblastine and colchicine: Evidence for a vascular mechanism. *Eur J Cancer* 1991; 51:482–487.

Benchimol S, Fuks A, Jothy S, et al: Carcinoembryonic antigen, a human tumor marker, functions as an intercellular adhesion molecule. *Cell* 1989; 57:327–334.

Benecke BJ, Ben-Ze'ev A, Penman S: The control of mRNA production, translation and turnover in suspended and reattached anchorage-dependent fibroblasts. *Cell* 1978; 14:931–939.

Bicknell R, Harris AL: Mechanisms and therapeutic implications of angiogenesis. *Curr Opin Oncol* 1996; 8:60–65.

Birchmeier W, Behrens J: Cadherin expression in carcinomas: Role in the formation of cell junctions and the prevention of invasiveness. *Biochim Biophys Acta* 1994; 1198:11–26.

Bischoff J: Approaches to studying cell adhesion molecules in angiogenesis. *Trends Cell Biol* 1995; 5:69–74.

Boehm T, Folkman J, Browder T, O'Reilly, MS: Antiangiogenic therapy of experimental cancer does not induce acquired drug resistance. *Nature* 1997; 390:404–407.

Bouck N: Tumor angiogenesis: The role of oncogenes and tumor suppressor genes. *Cancer Cells* 1990; 2: 179–185.

Bouck N, Stellmach V, Hsu SC: How tumors become angiogenic. *Adv Cancer Res* 1996; 69:135–174.

Boudreau N, Sympson CJ, Werb Z, Bissell MJ: Suppression of ICE and apoptosis in mammary epithelial cells by extracellular matrix. *Science* 1995; 267:891–893.

Brooks PC: Cell adhesion molecules in angiogenesis. *Cancer Metastasis Rev* 1996; 15:187–194.

Brooks PC, Clark RAF, Cheresh DA: Requirement of vascular integrin $\alpha_v\beta_3$ for angiogenesis. *Science* 1994a; 264:569–571.

Brooks PC, Montgomery AMP, Rosenfeld M, et al: Integrin $\alpha_v\beta_3$ antagonists promote tumor regression by inducing apoptosis of angiogenic blood vessels. *Cell* 1994b; 79:1157–1164.

Burgeson RE, Chiquet R, Deutzmann P, et al: A new nomenclature for the laminins. *Matrix Biol* 1994; 14:209–211.

Carmeliet P, Ferreira V, Breier G, et al: Abnormal blood vessel development and lethality in embryos lacking a single VEGF allele. *Nature* 1996; 380:435–439.

Chen C, Parangi S, Tolentino MJ, et al: A strategy to discover circulating angiogenesis inhibitors generated by human tumors. *Cancer Res* 1995; 55:4230–4233.

Clark EA, Brugge JS: Integrins and signal transduction pathways: The road taken. *Science* 1995; 268:233–239.

Connolly DT, Heuvelman DM, Nelson R, et al: Tumor vascular permeability factor stimulates endothelial cell growth and angiogenesis. *J Clin Invest* 1989; 84: 1470–1478.

Coppolino M, Leung-Hagesteijn C, Dedhar S, et al: Inducible interaction of integrin $\alpha_2\beta_1$ with calreticulin: Dependence on the activation-state of the integrin. *J Biol Chem* 1995; 270:23132–23138.

Dameron KM, Volpert OV, Tainsky MA, et al: Control of angiogenesis in fibroblasts by p53 regulation of thrombospondin-1. *Science* 1994; 265:1582–1584.

Davis S, Aldrich TH, Jones PF, et al: Isolation of angiopoietin-1, a ligand for the TIE2 receptor, by secretion-trap expression cloning. *Cell* 1996; 87:1161–1169.

Dedhar S: Integrin-mediated signal transduction in oncogenesis: An overview. *Cancer Metastasis Rev* 1995; 14: 165–172.

Dong Z, Kumar R, Yang X, et al: Macrophage-derived metalloelastase is responsible for the generation of angiostatin in Lewis lung carcinoma. *Cell* 1997; 88:801–810.

Dordunoo SK, Jackson JK, Arsenault LA, et al: Taxol encapsulation in poly (E-caprolactone) microspheres. *Cancer Chemother Pharmacol* 1995; 36:279–282.

Fang F, Orend G, Watanabe N, et al: Dependence of cyclin E-CDK2 kinase activity on cell anchorage. *Science* 1996; 271:499–502.

Ferrara N: The role of vascular endothelial growth factor in pathological angiogenesis. *Breast Cancer Res Treat* 1995; 36:127–137.

Ferrara N, Henzel WJ: Pituitary follicular cells secrete a novel heparin-binding growth factor specific for vascular endothelial cells. *Biochem Biophys Res Commun* 1989; 161:851–858.

Ferrara N, Carver-Moore K, Chen H, et al: Heterozygous embryonic lethality induced by targeted inactivation of the VEGF gene. *Nature* 1996; 380:439–442.

Folkman J: Tumor angiogenesis: Therapeutic implications. *N Engl J Med* 1971; 285:1182–1186.

Folkman J: The vascularization of tumors. *Sci Am* 1976; 234:58–73.

Folkman J: Clinical applications of research on angiogenesis. *N Engl J Med* 1995; 333:1757–1763.

Folkman J: Tumor angiogenesis: A possible control point in tumor growth. Ann Intern Med 1995; 82:96–100.

Folkman J, D'Amore PA: Blood vessel formation: What is its molecular basis? (comment). *Cell* 1996; 87:1153–1155.

Folkman J, Klagsbrun M: Angiogenic factors. *Science* 1987; 235:442–447.

Folkman J, Langer R, Linhardt RJ, et al: Angiogenesis inhibition and tumor regression caused by heparin or a heparin fragment in the presence of cortisone. *Science* 1983; 221:719–725.

Gospodarowicz D, Abraham JA, Schilling J: Isolation and characterization of a vascular endothelial cell mitogen produced by pituitary-derived folliculo stellate cells. *Proc Natl Acad Sci USA* 1989; 86:7311–7315.

Grugel S, Finkenzeller G, Weindel K, et al: Both v-Ha-ras and v-raf stimulate expression of the vascular endothelial growth factor in NIH 3T3 cells. *J Biol Chem* 1995; 270:25915–25919.

Gunthert U, Hofmann M, Rudy W, et al: A new variant of glycoprotein CD44 confers metastatic potential to rat carcinoma cells. *Cell* 1991; 65:13–24.

Gupta SK, Hassel T, Singh JP: A potent inhibitor of endothelial cell proliferation is generated by proteolytic cleavage of the chemokine platelet factor 4. *Proc Natl Acad Sci USA* 1995; 92:7799–7803.

Hanahan D : Signaling vascular morphogenesis and maintenance. *Science* 1997; 277:48–50.

Hanahan D, Folkman J: Patterns and emerging mechanisms of the angiogenic switch during tumorigenesis. *Cell* 1996; 86:353–364.

Hannigan GE, Dedhar S: Adhesion molecules in tumor growth and metastasis. In: Paul LC, ed. *Targeting Cell Adhesion Molecules for a Therapeutic Application.* New York: Marcel Decker; 1996.

Hannigan GE, Leung-Hagesteijn C, Fitz-Gibbon L, et al: Regulation of cell adhesion and anchorage-dependent growth by a new β1-integrin-linked protein kinase. *Nature* 1996; 379:91–96.

Hay EC: Cell matrix interaction in the embryo: Cell shape, cell surface, cell skeleton and their role in differentiation. In: Trelstadt RL, *The Role of the Extracellular Matrix in Development.* New York: Liss; 1984:1–31.

Helmlinger G, Yuan F, Dellian M, Jain RK: Interstitial pH and pO_2 gradients in solid tumors in vivo: High resolution measurements reveal a lack of correlation. *Nature Med* 1997; 3:177–182.

Hemler, M: Structures and functions of VLA proteins and related integrins. In: Mecham RP, McDonald JA, eds.

Receptors for Extracellular Matrix. New York: Academic Press; 1991: 255–299.

Huttenlocher A, Sandborg R, Horwitz A: Adhesion in cell migration. *Curr Opin Cell Biol* 1995; 7:697–706.

Hynes RO: Integrins: Versatility, modulation, and signaling in cell adhesion. *Cell* 1992; 69:11–25.

Hynes RO, Lander AD: Contact and adhesive specificities in the associations, migrations, and targeting of cells and axons. *Cell* 1992; 68:303–322.

Jain RK : Barriers to drug delivery in solid tumors. *Sci Am* 1994; 271:58–65.

Kerbel RS: Inhibition of tumor angiogenesis as a strategy to circumvent acquired resistance to anti-cancer therapeutic agents. *Bio Essays* 1991; 13:31–36.

Kerbel RS: A cancer therapy resistant to resistance. *Nature* 1997; 390:335–336.

Kerbel RS, Hawley RG: Interleukin 12: Newest member of the antiangiogenesis club. *J Natl Cancer Inst* 1995; 87:557–559.

Klagsbrun M, Soker S: VEGF/VPF: The angiogenesis factor found? *Curr Biol* 1993; 3:699–702.

Klingelhutz AJ, Smith PP, Garrett LR, McDougall JK: Alteration of the DCC tumor-suppressor gene in tumorigenic HPV-18 immortalized human keratinocytes transformed by nitrosomethylurea. *Oncogene* 1993; 8: 95–99.

Less JR, Skalak TC, Seick EM, Jain RK: Microvascular architecture in a mammary carcinoma: Branching patterns and vessel dimensions. *Cancer Res* 1991; 51: 265–273.

Lin P, Polverini P. Dewhirst M, Shan S, Rao PS, Peters K: Inhibition of tumor angiogenesis using a soluble receptor establishes a role for Tie2 in pathologic vascular growth. J Clin Invest 1997; 100:2072–2078

Lin TH, Yurochko A, Kornberg L, et al: The role of protein tyrosine phosphorylation in integrin mediated gene induction in monocytes. *J Cell Biol* 1994; 126: 1585–1593.

McGlade J, Brunkhorst B, Anderson D, et al: The amino terminal region of GAP regulates cytoskeletal structure and cell adhesion. *EMBO J* 1993; 12:3073–3081.

Meredith JEJ, Schwartz MA: Integrins, adhesion and apoptosis. *Trends Cell Biol* 1997; 7:146–151.

Millauer B, Shawver LK, Plate KH, et al: Glioblastoma growth inhibited *in vivo* by a dominant-negative Flk-1 mutant. *Nature* 1994; 367:576–579.

Moses MA, Langer R: Review: Inhibitors of angiogenesis. *Biotechnology* 1991; 9:630–634.

Newell K, Franchi A, Pouyssegur J, Tannock I: Studies with glycolysis-deficient cells suggest that production of lactic acid is not the only cause of tumor acidity. *Proc Natl Acad Sci USA* 1993; 90:1127–1131.

Nip J, Brodt P: The role of the integrin vitronectin receptor, αbβ3 in melanoma metastasis. *Cancer Metastasis Rev* 1995; 14:241–252.

O'Reilly MS, Holmgren L, Shing Y, et al: Angiostatin: A novel angiogenesis inhibitor that mediates the suppression of metastases by a Lewis lung carcinoma. *Cell* 1994; 79:315–328.

Otsuka H, Moskowitz MJ: Arrest of 3T3 cells in G1 phase by suspension culture. *J Cell Physiol* 1975; 87:213–220.

Parsons JT, Schaller MD, Hildebrand J, et al: Focal adhesion kinase: Structure and signalling. *J Cell Sci* 1994; 18:109–113.

Pepper MS, Ferrara N, Orci L, et al: Potent synergism between vascular endothelial growth factor and basic fibroblast growth factor in the induction of angiogenesis in vitro. *Biochem Biophys Res Commun* 1992; 189:824–831.

Pluda JM: Tumor-associated angiogenesis: Mechanisms, clinical implications, and therapeutic strategies. *Semin Oncol* 1997; 24:203–218.

Quian F, Vaux DL, Weissman I: Expression of the integrin α4β1 on melanoma cells can inhibit the invasive stage of metastasis formation. *Cell* 1994; 77:335–347.

Rak J, Filmus J, Kerbel RS: Reciprocal paracrine interactions between tumor cells and endothelial cells: The "angiogenesis progression" hypothesis. *Eur J Cancer* 1996; 32A:2438–2450.

Rak J, Filmus J, Finkenzeller G, et al: Oncogenes as inducers of tumor angiogenesis. *Cancer Metastasis Rev* 1995a; 14:263–277.

Rak J, Mitsuhashi Y, Bayko L, et al: Mutant *ras* oncogenes upregulate VEGF/VPF expression: Implications for induction and inhibition of tumor angiogenesis. *Cancer Res* 1995b; 55:4575–4580.

Rak J, St. Croix B, Kerbel RS: Consequences of angiogenesis for tumor progression, metastasis and cancer therapy. *Anticancer Drugs* 1995c; 6:3–18.

Rak JW, Hegmann EJ, Lu C, et al: Progressive loss of sensitivity to endothelium-derived growth inhibitors expressed by human melanoma cells during disease progression. *J Cell Physiol* 1994; 159:245–255.

Risau W: Angiogenesis and endothelial cell function. *Arzneimittelforschung* 1994; 44:416–417.

Risau W: What, if anything, is an angiogenic factor? *Cancer Metastasis Rev* 1996; 15:149–151.

Risau W: Mechanisms of angiogenesis. *Nature* 1997; 386:671–674.

Schaller MD, Parsons JT: Focal adhesion kinase and associated proteins. *Curr Opin Cell Biol* 1994; 6:705–710.

Senger DR, Brown LF, Claffey KP, et al: Vascular permeability factor, tumor angiogenesis and stroma generation. *Invasion Metastasis* 1994; 95:385–391.

Senger DR, Galli S, Dvorak AM, et al: Tumor cells secrete a vascular permeability factor that promotes accumulation of ascites fluid. *Science* 1983; 219:983–985.

Shin S-I, Freedman VH, Risser R, et al: Tumorigenicity of virus-transformed cells in nude mice is correlated specifically with anchorage-independent growth in vitro. *Proc Natl Acad Sci USA* 1975; 72:4435.

Shuster J, Thompson DMP, Fuks A, et al: Immunologic approaches to the diagnosis of disease. *Prog Exp Tumor Res* 1980; 25:89–139.

Shweiki D, Itin A, Soffer D, et al: Vascular endothelial growth factor induced by hypoxia may mediate hypoxia-initated angiogenesis. *Nature* 1992; 359:843–845.

Stein I, Neeman M, Shweiki D, et al: Stabilization of vascular endothelial growth factor mRNA by hypoxia and hypoglycemia and coregulation with other ischemia-induced genes. *Mol Cell Biol* 1995; 15:5363–5368.

Stetler-Stevenson WG, Aznavoorian S, Liotta LA: Tumor cell interactions with the extracellular matrix during invasion and metastasis. *Annu Rev Cell Biol* 1993; 9:541–573.

Su LK, Kinzler KW, Vogelstein B, et al: Multiple intestinal neoplasia caused by a mutation in the murine homolog of the APC gene. *Science* 1992; 256:668–670.

Takeichi M: Cadherins in cancer: Implications for invasion and metastasis. *Curr Opin Cell Biol* 1993; 5:806–811.

Tannock IF: Population kinetics of carcinoma cells, capillary endothelial cells, and fibroblasts in a transplanted mouse mammary tumor. *Cancer Res* 1970; 30:2470–2476.

Tannock IF, Rotin D: Acid pH in tumors and its potential for therapeutic exploitation. *Cancer Res* 1989; 49:4373–4384.

Terman BI, Dougher-Vermazen M: Biological properties of VEGF/VPF receptors. *Cancer Metastasis Rev* 1996; 15:159–163.

Thomas KA: Vascular endothelial growth factor, a potent and selective angiogenic agent. *J Biol Chem* 1996; 271:603–606.

Timpl R: Structure and biological activity of basement membrane proteins. *Eur J Biochem* 1989; 180:487–502.

Toi M, Inada K, Suzuki H, et al: Tumor angiogenesis in breast cancer: Its importance as a prognostic indicator and the association with vascular endothelial growth factor expression. *Breast Cancer Res Treat* 1995; 36:193–204.

Van Meir EG, Polverini PJ, Chazin VR, et al: Release of an inhibitor of angiogenesis upon induction of wild type *p53* expression in glioblastoma cells. *Nature Genet* 1994; 8:171–182.

Viloria Petit AM, Rak J, Hung MC, Rockwell P, Goldstein N, Kerbel, RS: Neutralizing antibodies against epidermal growth factor and ErbB-*2/neu* receptor tyrosine kinases down-regulate vascular endothelial growth factor production by tumor cells *in vitro* and *in vivo*: Angiogenic implications for signal transduction therapy of solid tumors. *Am J Path* 1997; 151:1523–1530.

Volpert OV, Dameron KM, Bouck N: Sequential development of an angiogenic phenotype by human fibroblasts progressing to tumorigenicity. *Oncogene* 1997; 14:1495–1502.

Weidner N, Semple JP, Welch WR, et al: Tumor angiogenesis and metastasis—Correlation in invasive breast carcinoma. *N Engl J Med* 1991; 324:1–8.

Werb Z, Tremble PM, Behrendtsen O, et al: Signal transduction through the fibronectin receptor induces collagenase and stromelysin gene expression. *J Cell Biol* 1989; 109:877–889.

10

Tumor Progression and Metastasis

Ann F. Chambers and Richard P. Hill

10.1 TUMOR PROGRESSION AND HETEROGENEITY
    10.1.1 Clinical Tumor Progression
    10.1.2 Clonal Evolution
    10.1.3 Molecular Genetics of Tumor Progression
    10.1.4 Tumor Heterogeneity

10.2 METASTASIS
    10.2.1 The Spread of Cancer
    10.2.2 Metastases of Human Tumors
    10.2.3 Metastatic Inefficiency

10.3 EXPERIMENTAL APPROACHES IN THE STUDY
OF METASTASIS
    10.3.1 In vivo Assays for Metastatic Ability
    10.3.2 Intravital Videomicroscopy in the Study of Metastasis
    10.3.3 In vitro Assays for Properties Associated
        with Metastatic Ability
    10.3.4 Selection of Cell Populations with Specific
        Metastatic Properties
    10.3.5 Organ Specificity
    10.3.6 Clonal Populations and Heterogeneity

10.4 STEPS IN THE METASTATIC PROCESS
    10.4.1 Detachment from the Primary Tumor
    10.4.2 Host Defense Mechanisms
    10.4.3 Arrest and Extravasation
    10.4.4 Establishment of a New Growth

10.5 MOLECULAR MECHANISMS OF METASTASIS
    10.5.1 Cell Adhesion Molecules
    10.5.2 Proteolytic Enzymes
    10.5.3 Oncogenes and Metastasis
    10.5.4 Metastasis-Associated Genes

10.6 STRATEGIES FOR ANTIMETASTATIC THERAPY

10.7 SUMMARY

REFERENCES

10.1 TUMOR PROGRESSION AND HETEROGENEITY

10.1.1 Clinical Tumor Progression

Cancer is not a static disease. Many tumors show a tendency toward increasing malignancy with time. In some tumors (e.g., melanoma, colon cancer, cervical cancer) there appears to be an orderly progression from benign tissue to noninvasive, premalignant lesions (e.g., carcinoma in situ of the cervix) to frank malignancy. In other cases, this is less clear; it is possible that the tumor has passed through less malignant stages before detection, but, alternatively, highly malignant tumors may arise de novo, without passing through less malignant stages. The pathologic and clinical criteria for degree of progression are in part specific to a given type of tumor. In general, however, tumors that are confined to a local site and have well-differentiated cells are at the benign end of the spectrum, progressing to locally invasive tumors. Tumors with poorly differentiated cells that have spread beyond the local site and have seeded metastases represent the malignant end of the spectrum. Increasing numbers and kinds of chromosomal abnormalities, often specific for the tumor type, accompany tumor progression (see Chap. 4, Sec. 4.3).

10.1.2 Clonal Evolution

Forty years ago Foulds defined tumor progression as "the acquisition of permanent, irreversible qualitative changes in one or more characteristics of a neoplasm" that lead to the tumor becoming more au-

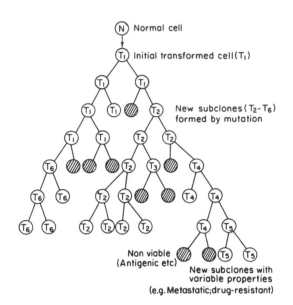

Figure 10.1. Schematic illustration showing the clonal evolution of tumors. New subclones arise by mutation. Many of these may become extinct (indicated by shading), but others may have a growth advantage and become dominant. All of the subclones (indicated by T_2 to T_6) may share common clonal markers, but many of them have new properties leading to heterogeneity.

tonomous and malignant (for reviews see Heppner and Miller, 1998; Klein, 1998). In 1986, Nowell proposed that such changes arise because cancer cells tend to be genetically unstable and described a conceptual model to explain the process of tumor progression (Fig. 10.1). The key features of this model are the generation of variant (mutant) cells within a tumor and the selection and outgrowth of the more autonomous cells to become dominant subclones in the population, leading to progression of the tumor to increasing malignancy. More recent studies have demonstrated that the growth and development of the various subclones of cells within a tumor are subject to constraints associated with interactions among the cells and with the extracellular environment (reviewed by Heppner and Miller, 1998). Thus the normal homeostatic mechanisms that control cell proliferation in the body are not completely lost in a tumor but rather the cells in the various subclones may become increasingly less responsive to them. These findings are consistent with the original concepts of Foulds that there are many different paths to malignancy. Although there is evidence that cells within most tumors are derived from a single cell (Chap. 7, Sec. 7.6.2), mutation, selection, and clonal expansion result in heterogeneity for many properties. Changes in the properties of clonally derived cells due to differentiation and to the

influence of the variable microenvironment in tumors contribute further to heterogeneity. Tumors are thus evolving cell populations with properties that continue to change as they grow.

10.1.3 Molecular Genetics of Tumor Progression

Genetic instability of tumor cells may arise as a result of genetic and/or epigenetic changes. Epigenetic changes such as methylation of cytosine bases in DNA can modify the expression of genes and are an important mechanism for "silencing" genes during normal differentiation (see Chap. 4, Sec. 4.2.1). There is substantial evidence that tumor cells have aberrant methylation patterns which modify gene expression. For example, hypermethylation in the promoter region can serve to inactivate certain tumor suppressor genes (for review see Baylin et al., 1998).

Genetic changes may occur by various mechanisms, including point mutation, deletion, gene amplification and translocation. A cell is continually exposed to both external (see Chap. 8) and internal stresses, such as reactive oxygen species, that may cause DNA damage, and there are inherent errors made by DNA polymerases whenever DNA is being replicated. Normally such damage is either repaired by the various DNA repair mechanisms in the cell (see Chap. 4, Sec. 4.4) or damaged cells are induced to undergo apoptosis (Chap. 7, Sec. 7.3). However, these mechanisms are not 100 percent efficient, leading to a natural frequency of mutation in cells (Simpson, 1997).

Many cancer cells appear to have an increased frequency of mutation (a "mutator phenotype"—see Loeb, 1998) due both to deficiencies in their ability to repair lesions in DNA and/or decreased activation of apoptosis, so that mutated cells may survive and proliferate. Deficiencies of mismatch repair have been demonstrated in tumor cells from patients with non-polyposis colon cancer (see Chap. 4, Sec. 4.4.4). Inactivation of this repair system is characterized by microsatellite instability (i.e., changes in the short repetitive sequences that are distributed throughout the genome of all cells). This deficiency in mismatch repair [also referred to as the *replication error repair* (*RER*) negative phenotype] can result in up to a 1000-fold increase in the mutation frequency. Thus failures in DNA repair, either due to random chance or due to mutations in the repair genes themselves, are likely to allow mutation or alteration in the expression of the many oncogenes and tumor suppressor genes that have been associated with different human cancers (see Chaps. 4–6).

The finding that the p53 protein is mutated or inactivated in a high percentage of human cancers is consistent with its role in controlling the response of cells to DNA damage (see Chap. 5, Sec. 5.5.2; Chap. 13, Sec. 13.3.2). Normal p53 participates in cellular signaling that leads to cessation of proliferation of cells that have sustained damage to their DNA, or to cell death by apoptosis (Chap. 7, Sec. 7.3). In human cancers, mutations have been observed primarily (80–90 percent) in the DNA binding region of the p53 protein (exons 5–8); such binding is required for its function as a transcription factor. Up to seven mutation hot spots have been identified (Greenblatt et al., 1994). These hot spots are detected in cancers because of the importance of these regions to the function of the protein, but these regions may also be more difficult to repair or they may be particularly vulnerable to a specific carcinogenic insult, as in skin cancers induced by UV radiation (see Chap. 8, Secs. 8.2.5 and 8.5.5). There is recent evidence that the hypoxic microenvironment which occurs in many solid tumors can stimulate mutation of genes (see Chap. 13, Sec. 13.5.2), and it may also allow the selective survival of cells with p53 mutations, thus contributing to progressive changes in the malignant phenotype (Graeber et al., 1996).

That multiple changes must occur in cells during tumor development and progression is well illustrated by the model established by Vogelstein and colleagues to describe the changes that occur in the progression of colon cancer (see Chap. 4, Sec. 4.5.4; Kinzler and Vogelstein, 1996). This model forms a paradigm which is being applied to other cancers, such as breast, and head and neck tumors (Califano et al., 1996; Shackney and Sharkey, 1997). An extensive review of cytogenetic changes in human solid tumors has suggested that epithelial and neurogenic tumors tend to display deletions of genetic material, suggesting inactivation of tumor suppressor genes, whilst sarcomas and hemopoietic tumors tend to exhibit rearrangements (translocations), consistent with inappropriate or aberrant expression of growth-promoting genes or genes associated with apoptosis (Rodriguez et al., 1994). A molecular description of tumor progression thus envisages that each type of cancer will progress in stages and that the genetic changes (e.g., mutations in specific oncogenes, loss of specific tumor suppressor genes) accompanying this progression will have features that are unique to each type of cancer.

10.1.4 Tumor Heterogeneity

As predicted by the Nowell model, cells within animal and human tumors demonstrate considerable heterogeneity in their properties. This heterogeneity extends to almost any property that can be assessed and includes morphology, karyotype, surface markers, biochemical products, cell proliferation ability, metastatic ability, and sensitivity to therapeutic agents. The model thus also offers an explanation for the development in tumors of drug resistance following chemotherapy (or other therapy), owing to the selection of those cells present in the tumor that are resistant to the treatment (see Chap. 17, Sec. 17.2). Because metastases may arise from a small subset of cells within a primary tumor, histologic or biochemical characterization of the tumor does not always give a reliable picture of the properties (and propensity to metastasize) of all the cells within the tumor. This property of tumors has made it difficult to determine the cellular and molecular properties necessary for metastatic spread, since the bulk of the tumor population may not reflect the properties of the individual cells responsible for the metastases.

10.2 METASTASIS

The generation of the cells within a cancer, which have the ability to disseminate and form new foci of growth at noncontiguous sites (i.e., to form metastases), represents its most malignant characteristic and can be thought of as the final stage of tumor progression. Tumors that have metastasized are generally more difficult to treat successfully than those that have not spread, making it important to clarify how cancer cells metastasize and to determine the underlying genetic changes that make this behavior possible.

10.2.1 The Spread of Cancer

Cancer cells can spread along tissue planes and into various tissue spaces and cavities, but the two major routes of metastatic spread are via lymphatic vessels or blood vessels. Indeed, for the purpose of clinical staging, metastases are subdivided into two groups: those in regional lymph nodes, which are usually regarded as having disseminated via the lymphatic circulation, and those that arise at more distant sites and organs, which have usually spread via the blood vascular system (Fig. 10.2). These two routes were once thought to be independent, but these two circulation systems are widely interconnected and cannot be regarded as independent routes of spread.

Different types of tumors have different patterns of spread. Tumors of the head and neck, for example, usually spread initially to regional lymph nodes and, only when more advanced, to distant sites; thus

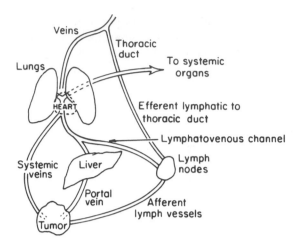

Figure 10.2. The major routes by which cancer cells can spread from a primary tumor are through the lymphatic or blood vessels. These two systems are interconnected, as illustrated. The vascular drainage for tumors of the GI tract is usually via the portal circulation, whereas for tumors at other sites in the body drainage is via the systemic veins. (Adapted from Sugarbaker, 1981.)

localized therapy that includes treatment of regional neck nodes can be curative. In contrast, tumors of the breast can spread early to distant sites. Involvement of axillary lymph nodes at the time of primary treatment for breast cancer is correlated with the presence of distant metastases, but about 25 percent of patients with no evidence of lymph node disease at the time of primary treatment are later found to have widespread metastases. Thus, the lack of lymph-node metastases does not rule out the possibility that the cancer has disseminated via the blood vascular system. Factors that predict metastatic spread in breast cancer include poor dif-

ferentiation and presence of tumor cells in the blood vessels (or lymphatics) in the primary tumor. It is possible to detect very small numbers of tumor cells (1 in 10^5–10^6) in lymph nodes or blood using PCR (see Chap. 3, Sec. 3.3.7) to amplify tumor-cell specific DNA markers. Histologic detection of a high density of new blood vessels (angiogenesis) in breast and other tumors has been associated with poor prognosis and increased likelihood that the patient will subsequently develop metastases (Weidner et al., 1992). These vessels provide nutrients for further growth of the tumor and also access to the circulation, facilitating metastasis (see also Chap. 9, Sec. 9.3). Recent studies have also suggested that the tumor microenvironment, in particular hypoxia (see Chap. 13, Sec. 13.5.2), may select for more aggressive tumor-cell phenotypes, which are more likely to metastasize (Hockel et al., 1996; Graeber et al., 1996).

10.2.2 Metastases of Human Tumors

Clinical observations (Sugarbaker, 1981; Plesnicar, 1989) have indicated that metastases from certain types of tumors tend to occur in specific target organs (see Table 10.1). While lungs, liver, lymph nodes, bone, and brain are the most common sites of spread, observation of the spread of cancer to specific sites led Paget (1889) to propose the "soil and seed" hypothesis, in which he postulated that differential tumor-cell/host-organ interactions can occur, that are more or less favorable for metastatic development. The alternate, although not mutually exclusive, hypothesis is that "organ preference" can be explained largely on the basis of hemodynamic considerations: i.e., the number of metastases that develop in an organ is related to the number of tu-

Table 10.1. Clinical Metastasis to Specific Target Organs

Primary Tumor	Common Distant Secondary Sites
Clear-cell carcinoma of the kidney	Lung, bone, adrenal
Gastrointestinal carcinomas	Liver
Prostatic carcinoma	Bone
Small-cell carcinoma of the lung	Brain, liver, bone marrow
Melanoma in the skin	Liver, brain, bowel
Melanoma in the eye	Liver
Neuroblastoma	Liver, adrenal
Carcinoma of breast	Bone, brain, adrenal, lung, liver
Follicular carcinoma of thyroid	Bone, lung

mor cells delivered to that organ by the blood and the number that are arrested in the capillaries (Fig. 10.3). In fact, both theories are correct, in that circulating cancer cells need first to arrest in the small vessels of an organ (often the first capillary bed that they encounter) but will grow only if the organ provides a suitable growth environment for the particular tumor cells.

Sugarbaker (1981) reviewed data on the dissemination of human cancers, obtained either from autopsies or from studies of the initial development of metastatic lesions in treated patients. Data from autopsies demonstrated the concept of organ specificity (Table 10.1), but the site of initial metastasis tended to be the organ containing the first capillary bed encountered (first-pass organ) by the cells after their release from the tumor (Fig. 10.3). For tumors whose blood supply drains into the systemic veins, this would be the lung, while for tumors whose venous drainage is into the portal system (gastrointestinal cancers), it would be the liver. These findings suggest that there are sites of initial metastatic development from which further metastases are spread to other (tumor-specific) organs. The development of metastases as sequential tertiary or quaternary growths is illustrated by the metastatic patterns observed at autopsy in patients with colorectal cancer (liver only, liver plus lung, or liver and lung

plus other organs; Weiss, 1990). Alternatively, the observations may reflect the trapping of most tumor cells in the first-pass organ, so that relatively few viable cells reach the arterial circulation, in which they can be distributed to all parts of the body. Thus, even if the probability that a tumor cell will survive and initiate a metastasis in the first-pass organ is very much lower than that for another (tumor-specific) organ, the large number of cells trapped could result in an overall higher chance of metastasis formation in the first-pass organ. Molecular mechanisms responsible for organ-specific growth are discussed in Secs. 10.4 and 10.5.

10.2.3 Metastatic Inefficiency

The establishment of metastases by tumor cells appears to be a very inefficient process. Blood samples taken from cancer patients during or just after surgery often contain large numbers of tumor cells, yet the patients do not always develop metastatic disease. Glaves et al. (1988) took samples of blood from the renal vein in 10 patients just prior to surgery for renal cell carcinoma and estimated that tumor cells were being released at rates of 10^7 to 10^9 cells per day. Two of the patients had no evidence of metastatic disease 30 and 55 months after the surgery. Similarly, patients with peritoneovenous shunts for malignant ascites have shown no evidence that release of large numbers of tumor cells into the blood increases the number of metastases observed (Tarin et al., 1984). Studies in animals have shown that many viable tumor cells are released into the circulation but that few circulating cells are able to form metastases. By collecting blood samples from the sole efferent vessel of a carcinoma growing in the rat ovary, a tumor that forms very few metastases, Butler and Gullino (1975) estimated that about 1 million tumor cells were released every 24 h. Similar results have been obtained from the shedding of cells into lymphatic vessels (Carr and Carr, 1980). Glaves (1983), who sampled blood from the right ventricles of mice, estimated that between 10^7 and 10^8 viable cells are shed into the blood during the growth of transplantable B16 melanomas and Lewis lung tumors (approximately 20 days), but these cells gave rise to less than 100 lung metastases per mouse. Furthermore, in the large number of experiments in which tumor cells have been introduced directly into the circulation of mice or rats, it is rare that more than 1 percent of such cells form tumor nodules. More commonly, the efficiency is two or more orders of magnitude lower.

The inefficiency of the metastatic process leads naturally to the question of whether metastasis is a

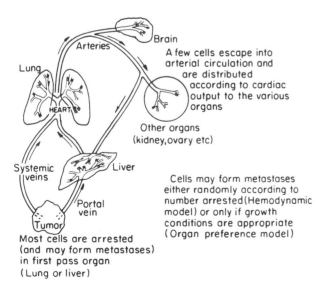

Figure 10.3. The vascular spread of tumor cells results in most of the cells being delivered initially to the lung or (for gastrointestinal tumors) the liver, where they are likely to be arrested in the capillary bed. If the cells traverse the capillary bed of the first-pass organ, they can be distributed to the other organs where they may be similarly trapped.

random or a specific process. A small subpopulation of the cells in a tumor might express properties that give the cells a higher probability of being able to form metastases, or all tumor cells might have an equal probability of forming metastases but only a few manage to survive through the various stages of the process (Fig. 10.4; see also Chap. 9, Fig. 9.3). There is substantial evidence that specific cellular properties are associated with the formation of metastases, including the observation of organ preference and the isolation of specific gene products associated with metastasis (see Secs. 10.3.5 and 10.5.4). In contrast, support for the random nature of the metastatic process derives from extensive studies which have failed to demonstrate that cells obtained from metastases are consistently more metastatic than cells from the parent tumor. Such a result would be expected if cells from metastases

were expressing a stable phenotype that predisposed them to form metastases (see Weiss, 1990, for review). It is sometimes possible to select cell populations with increased metastatic ability in mice by serial passaging of tumor cells from metastasis to metastasis, but these populations rarely achieve a metastatic efficiency greater than 1 to 2 percent. The probable explanation for these observations is that metastatic phenotypes can be unstable and that both random and specific elements are involved in the metastatic process.

10.3 EXPERIMENTAL APPROACHES IN THE STUDY OF METASTASIS

10.3.1 In vivo Assays for Metastatic Ability

Studies of metastatic potential have usually been performed in rodents because of the availability of a wide range of tumor systems that are syngeneic to inbred strains of animals. In addition, rodents (and especially laboratory mice) provide the opportunity for testing of human tumor cells in immune-deficient hosts [e.g., athymic *nude* mice; SCID (severe combined immune deficient) mice]. Chick embryos have also been used to test tumorigenic and metastatic properties because of the natural immune deficiency of the developing embryo.

Two types of assays are commonly used (Fig. 10.5), both in rodents and chick embryos. Spontaneous metastasis assays model the full metastatic process by the implantation of tumor cells to allow formation of an artificial primary tumor from which cells can spread to form metastatic tumors in target organs such as lung or liver. In such an assay, it is possible to remove the local tumor surgically or to ablate it with radiation, allowing sufficient time for cells seeded from a local tumor to form macroscopically detectable metastases. While this procedure allows more time for metastases to grow, it may also lead to acceleration of the growth of the metastases if they have been retarded by inhibitory substances (e.g., angiogenesis inhibitors) produced by the primary tumor (see Chap. 9, Sec. 9.3.3).

Recent studies have demonstrated that the local site of growth of an implanted tumor may influence its capacity to seed spontaneous metastases (Fidler, 1990; Radinsky, 1995). Tumors that are transplanted (and grow) in orthotopic sites (tissue of the same pathologic type as the tumor) are more likely to seed metastases than tumors grown in ectopic sites. This applies particularly to human tumor xenografts in nude mice, for which subcutaneous implantation and growth rarely gives rise to metastases. The

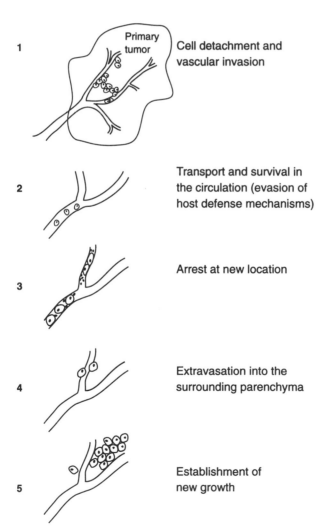

1   Primary tumor   Cell detachment and vascular invasion

2   Transport and survival in the circulation (evasion of host defense mechanisms)

3   Arrest at new location

4   Extravasation into the surrounding parenchyma

5   Establishment of new growth

Figure 10.4. Schematic illustration of the various stages of the metastatic process.

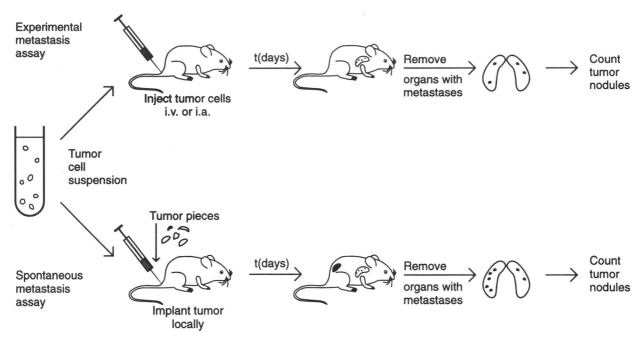

Figure 10.5. Schematic representation of experimental and spontaneous metastasis assays in mice.

mechanisms underlying these effects are unknown but may relate to the ability of the tumor cells to respond to organ-specific factors. The expression of genes that influence malignancy can be dramatically different for tumor cells transplanted into ectopic versus orthotopic sites, and expression of these genes can contribute to the metastatic behavior displayed by the tumor (Radinsky, 1995). For example, the dense fibrous capsule that often forms around subcutaneously transplanted tumors may also restrict release of cells from the tumor.

It is also possible to use a spontaneous metastasis assay to examine the ability of cells to form lymphatic metastases by implanting the cells into the hind footpad of the animal. Such primary tumors will often spread to the popliteal lymph node, which can easily be examined for tumor growth.

In the experimental metastasis (or colonization) assay (see Fig 10.5), tumor cells are injected directly into the arterial or venous blood circulation and allowed to disseminate and arrest at various sites. The choice of injection route will determine the organ in which the cells are most likely to be arrested. For example, injection into the tail vein of a mouse will target the cells to the lung microcirculation, while injection into the spleen or a mesenteric vein will target cell arrest to the liver. These organs will often be the main sites of tumor nodule formation but are not necessarily the only sites at which metastases may form. This assay allows direct quantitation of

the number of tumor nodules formed in relation to the number of cells injected (seeded) into the first-pass organ.

There are inherent difficulties in the above assays. In particular, they do not examine individual metastatic properties of the cells; rather, they examine the end result of a combination of properties. An experimental metastasis assay tests the ability of cells to survive in the circulation, arrest in a target organ, avoid host defenses, invade a new organ, and establish a new tumor growth. The spontaneous metastasis assay tests all these properties plus the ability to initiate tumor growth at the local site and to invade and disseminate into blood vessels. Although many properties are required for metastasis formation, one specific property may represent a "rate-limiting step," which controls the frequency of metastasis formation. It is possible that this rate-limiting property may vary for different tumors. Because the assays measure only the end point of whether metastatic tumors are present or not at the end of the assay, they cannot determine what the rate-limiting step is for a given experiment. The metastasis assays described above allow the determination of the effect on metastatic capacity of various genetic and molecular manipulations and permit an association between cellular properties, specific molecules or therapeutic strategies, and metastatic ability. These traditional assays can be likened to a "black box" where the input (numbers, types of injected cells, experimental manipulations) and output (numbers of metastatic tumors) are known. Conclusions about steps in the metastatic process have often been derived from logical inference rather than observation. This concern has recently been addressed using the technique of intravital videomicroscopy, in which individual steps in the process are observed as they occur. In addition, various in vitro assays have been used to clarify the nature of the molecular processes that occur in the various steps of metastatic tumor formation.

10.3.2 Intravital Videomicroscopy in the Study of Metastasis

Intravital videomicroscopy (IVVM) is a technique (see Fig. 10.6) that permits dynamic study of events in the metastatic process (Chambers et al., 1995). In this procedure, an anesthetized mouse is placed on the stage of an inverted microscope, with an organ for study (e.g., liver, muscle) surgically exposed so that the organ is viewed from below. Alternatively, chicken embryo chorioallantoic membrane can be viewed with this procedure. Lighting is provided by oblique fiberoptic illumination, which provides sufficient contrast to permit clear views of the microcirculation of the organ. Steps in the metastatic process are observed and quantified following injection of cancer cells (fluorescently labeled to permit unambiguous identification). Rather than simply providing confirmatory visual evidence for many of the previous inferences about the metastatic process, results from IVVM have sometimes produced unexpected results that are changing concepts about how metastasis occurs (see Sec. 10.4.3). In particular, the findings from IVVM suggest that extravasation may be a relatively easy step, with ability to grow in the new organ environment following extravasation providing the primary rate-limiting restrictions to the formation of metastases.

10.3.3 In vitro Assays for Properties Associated with Metastatic Ability

In vitro assays to model the steps that occur in metastasis include assays to measure the ability of cells to adhere to, migrate on, or invade into basement membrane. Such assays have the advantages of permitting study of these processes in isolation; they also permit identification of molecules associated with the ability to carry out these processes (for reviews, see Liotta et al., 1991; Chambers and Tuck, 1993; Jiang et al., 1994). The basic concepts of tumor cell attachment to and invasion through endothelial cell monolayers and their basement membrane–like matrix are illustrated in Fig. 10.7 and discussed in Sec. 10.4.3. The invasive ability of tumor cells can be measured by assays that assess the ability of the cells to pass through barriers of basement membrane proteins (e.g., Matrigel or pieces of human amnion membrane). These assays measure cellular ability to adhere to, degrade, and mi-

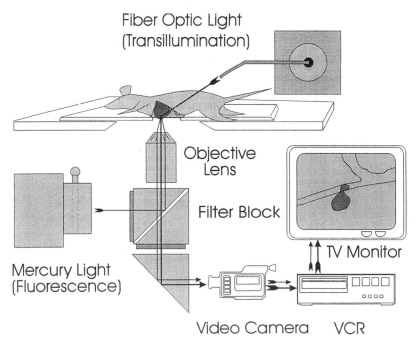

Figure 10.6. Schematic diagram of the IVVM procedure for studying steps of metastasis in vivo. Fluorescently labeled tumor cells are injected into the circulation of an experimental animal (chick embryo, mouse). At various times after injection, organs are exposed and placed intact on the coverslip over the objective lens of an inverted microscope. Lighting is provided by oblique transillumination using a fiberoptic source and/or episcopic fluorescent illumination. Images are viewed using a videocamera and monitor, and are recorded for subsequent analysis. The technique can be used for observing chick chorioallantoic membrane, mouse liver (*insert*), or other organs. (Modified from Chambers et al., 1995.)

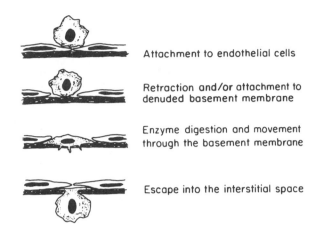

Attachment to endothelial cells

Retraction and/or attachment to
denuded basement membrane

Enzyme digestion and movement
through the basement membrane

Escape into the interstitial space

Figure 10.7. Schematic representation of the processes involved in extravasation of a tumor cell through the wall of a capillary. (Adapted from Nicolson, 1982.)

grate through the protein matrix. These abilities can be further differentiated by in vitro assays that measure adhesion to specific extracellular matrix proteins, activity of proteases, and motility either alone or toward chemotactic substances.

10.3.4 Selection of Cell Populations with Specific Metastatic Properties

Cells with increased or decreased probability of generating metastases may be selected from experimental tumors, as would be predicted by Nowell's hypothesis. The now classical example is the selection of the B16F10 cell population from B16 mouse melanoma cells by Fidler (1973). The procedure (Fig. 10.8) involved serial passage of the cells through animals, with selection at each stage for cells that had formed lung metastases. The cells from the lung metastases were grown in culture to expand their number before being reinjected into animals. After 10 such passages, a population of cells was obtained (termed B16F10 cells) that was about 10 times as efficient at forming experimental lung metastases after intravenous injection as the starting B16F1 cell population. Interestingly these cells were not more capable of forming metastasis in a spontaneous metastasis assay, suggesting that the selection process might have selected against invasive properties necessary for initial escape from the primary tumor. Other investigators have also been successful, using similar approaches, in selecting cell populations from a number of experimental tumors that have enhanced metastatic (colonizing) ability in a variety of organs including lung, liver, ovary, and brain. However, such selection procedures do not always yield cells with increased metastatic ability (Ling et al., 1985; Stackpole et al., 1991), leading to

the suggestion that some properties that contribute to metastatic ability may not be stably maintained within the tumor cell population during the selection procedures and that they may function transiently to promote metastasis.

A range of in vitro attributes that may be related to various stages of the metastatic process have also been used to select for cells that, when tested in vivo, were found to have altered metastatic ability. These procedures have included detachment from monolayers, resistance to lysis by lymphocytes, resistance to lectin-mediated toxicity, attachment to collagen, and the ability to invade various tissues maintained in organ culture. In one such experiment (Hart, 1979), B16 melanoma cells were placed inside an excised mouse bladder suspended in semi-solid agar with tissue-culture medium. Cells that were capable of migrating through the bladder wall and growing in the agar were selected, and the process was repeated sequentially six times (see Fig. 10.8). The cell line obtained (called B16BL6) is highly invasive and more efficient at forming spontaneous metastases than unselected B16 cells, but it is not more efficient in a colonization assay.

10.3.5 Organ Specificity

The concept of organ specificity of metastatic development, derived from autopsy studies (see Sec.

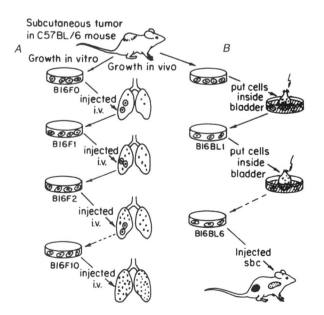

Figure 10.8. Procedures used for selecting highly metastatic cell populations from B16 melanoma cells. The B16F10 cells were selected by passaging the cells 10 times through the lungs of mice, while the B16BL6 cells were selected by requiring them to invade 6 times through the walls of mouse bladders.

10.2.2), is supported by investigations using animal tumor models. Cell populations that form a large number of metastatic deposits in one organ (e.g., the lung following intravenous injection of the cells) are not necessarily capable of doing so in another (e.g., the liver following intraportal injection). It has been possible to obtain populations of cells that have enhanced ability to form metastases in specific organs by serially selecting cells from metastases in these organs. Furthermore, it has been shown that cells forming metastases preferentially in the lung will "home" to a lung lobe even when it is transplanted ectopically into a subcutaneous site; such cells do not form metastases in other organs that are transplanted ectopically (Hart and Fidler, 1981). Organ specificity may reflect selection of cells for differential ability to respond to and grow in the microenvironment of a particular organ (Nicolson, 1988, Nicolson and Menter, 1995).

10.3.6 Clonal Populations and Heterogeneity

Fidler and Kripke (1977) cloned B16 melanoma cells by plating them in vitro at limiting dilution so that any growth could be expected to originate from a single cell. A number of clones were isolated and expanded in culture and the cells were tested for their ability to form experimental metastases (see Fig. 10.9). Variability in metastatic ability for cells from a single clone was found to be much less than that observed when cells from different clones were compared. These results indicated wide heterogeneity in metastatic ability between the different clones, and limited experiments in which subclones were isolated and tested suggested that the individual clones "bred true" in terms of metastatic ability.

These findings, which demonstrate wide variation between clonal populations, have been interpreted to indicate that the parental tumor population is heterogeneous and that the cloning procedure reveals this heterogeneity. Subsequent studies of the metastatic properties of clonally derived populations have often shown them to be relatively unstable. Experiments reported by Hill et al. (1986) suggest that much of the heterogeneity observed between clones is the result of stochastic generation of metastatic variant cells during clonal growth. These authors found that cells capable of forming experimental metastases were generated spontaneously during the growth of the cloned populations, so that clones grown to larger sizes contained proportionally more cells capable of forming experimental metastases (Fig. 10.10). To explain these results, they postulated a "dynamic heterogeneity" model in which cells can acquire metastatic properties because of heritable phenotypic changes, but that these changes are unstable (i.e., such properties are acquired and lost over the course of 10 to 30 cell divisions). Thus, a growing clonal population initially accumulates metastatic variant cells but increasingly tends to establish a dynamic equilibrium between a small subpopulation of highly metastatic (variant) cells and a majority of essentially non-metastatic cells (see Ling et al., 1985, for review).

The "dynamic heterogeneity" model is similar in concept to the "transient metastatic compartment" model (Weiss, 1990), which proposes that, while all viable tumor cells have metastatic potential, some may have a capacity that is temporarily enhanced by differing metabolic or cell-cycle states, by random epigenetic events, or by other physiologic variations

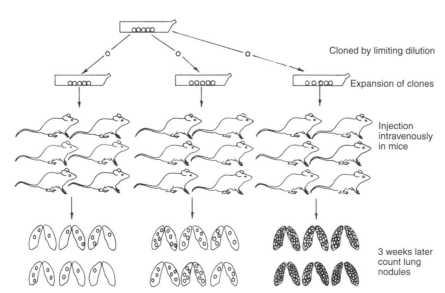

Cloned by limiting dilution

Expansion of clones

Injection intravenously in mice

3 weeks later count lung nodules

Figure 10.9. Clonal heterogeneity is demonstrated by establishing a series of clones from a tumor-cell population and, after expansion, testing them for metastatic ability. Although there is some variability in the number of nodules observed in different animals injected with cells from the same clone, there is much greater variability between the clones.

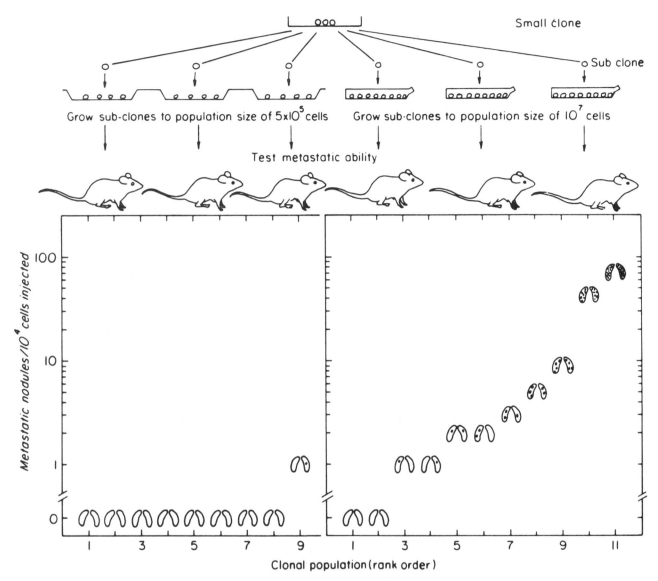

Figure 10.10. The generation of metastatic variant cells in clones of B16F1 melanoma cells. A small clone was subcloned and the subclones were grown to carefully controlled population sizes before the cells were tested for metastatic ability using an experimental metastasis assay. Although the same number of cells was injected into each animal, many more metastases were observed in the mice injected with cells from the larger clones. (Adapted from Hill et al., 1984.)

associated with growth of a tumor. These two models emphasize the idea that specific phenotypes need not be expressed stably to enhance metastasis formation.

10.4 STEPS IN THE METASTATIC PROCESS

10.4.1 Detachment from the Primary Tumor

The sequential steps in metastasis formation are illustrated in Fig. 10.4. These steps have been inferred from the in vivo and in vitro assays described above (Sec. 10.3). Metastatic cells must detach from

the primary tumor mass, and the site of initial detachment will likely influence whether the initial route of spread is via the lymphatic or venous system. Detachment or shedding of cells into blood vessels may occur as a result of prior invasion of the tumor mass into vessels or because the abnormal vasculature of some tumors may permit passage of cells into the circulation. Most in vitro studies of this process have examined penetration through membranes from the endothelial cell side (i.e., extravasation rather than intravasation; see Fig. 10.7), but it is generally assumed that similar mechanisms are involved. Detachment of cancer cells from the primary tumor mass may involve decreased expression of adhesion molecules (e.g. cadherins) involved in the "homotypic" adhesion of cells to one another (see Chap. 9, Sec. 9.2).

10.4.2 Host Defense Mechanisms

Immunologic mechanisms (see Chap. 11, Secs. 11.3 and 11.4) are involved in defense against development of metastases from experimental tumors and possibly also from human tumors. Tumors induced in animals by chemical carcinogens or viruses or resulting from exposure to ultraviolet (UV) light can be highly immunogenic and, although they grow locally, they rarely metastasize. It has been shown that cytotoxicity mediated by T lymphocytes inhibits metastases by such tumor cells, both by establishing an inverse correlation between the degree of immunogenicity and metastatic ability and by demonstrating that immunosuppressive procedures can increase the metastatic ability of the tumor cells. These observations explain why many experimental tumors are poorly metastatic, but their relevance to human tumors or spontaneous tumors in animals is unclear, since few such tumors elicit this type of strong immune rejection response. There is evidence that some human tumors may elicit weaker immunologic responses mediated by various cytokines and by nonspecific effector cells such as natural killer (NK) cells. These processes might inhibit metastasis formation. Using transplanted rodent tumor cells, Hanna (1984) has shown that there is an inverse correlation between the activity of NK cells in the host animal and the metastatic ability of injected tumor cells. Studies by Greenberg et al, (1987) demonstrated that NK cells acted in the first few days after intravenous injection of H-*ras*-transformed fibroblasts into mice to regulate seeding and early growth of metastases. Experiments with human tumor cells growing in immune-deprived mice have also indicated that NK cells can play a role in the reduction of metastases, and studies in patients have also been supportive of such an effect (Brittenden et al., 1996).

10.4.3 Arrest and Extravasation

Early hypotheses about rate-limiting steps in metastasis suggested that the majority of cancer cells in the circulation would be killed by hemodynamic forces and that only a small proportion of the remaining cells would extravasate successfully. Ex-

travasation was considered to be a major rate-limiting step in the metastatic process. Experimental studies in which radiolabeled tumor cells were injected into the systemic or portal veins indicated that the majority of cells are arrested initially in the lung or liver capillaries, respectively. This finding has been confirmed by studies using intravital videomicroscopy (IVVM; see Sec. 10.3.2). Cells from most solid tumors are large relative to capillaries and thus tend to lodge in the first capillary bed encountered. This physical arrest is accompanied by deformation of the tumor cell in proportion to the blood pressure in the particular organ (little deformation of cells in low-pressure organs such as liver and larger deformation in high-pressure organs such as muscle; see Fig. 10.11).

Experiments with radiolabeled cells have suggested that most cells are lost from this initial site of arrest over the first few hours due to rapid cell death, based on the observation of the rapid loss of radioactivity from the site of arrest. This conclusion has not been supported by IVVM, at least for metastasis to mouse liver and chick embryo chorioallantoic membrane. In these organs the vast majority of injected cells remain intact and succeed in extravasating over the first 24 h or so after injection (Chambers et al., 1995). The reason for these apparently contradictory results is currently unknown.

Studies in which different numbers of tumor cells have been injected intravenously into mice have indicated that the efficiency of metastasis formation per cell injected increases when very large numbers ($\sim 10^6$) of cells are injected (Hill et al., 1986). Similarly, injection of small clumps of tumor cells results in increased efficiency of metastasis formation, in support of the hypothesis that physical trapping in small blood vessels is the major mechanism leading to arrest of cells (Thompson, 1974).

The arrest of tumor cells in the small blood vessels of organs has sometimes been associated with thrombus formation involving the interaction of the cells with platelets and leukocytes, although the IVVM studies indicate that this is not a requirement for metastasis. The importance of thrombus formation in the development of metastasis is controversial. Administration of anticoagulants can reduce the number of metastases after intravenous injection (experimental metastases) but has little effect on formation of spontaneous metastases (Hilgard, 1984; see also Sec. 10.6). It is possible that adhesive interactions between tumor cells and endothelial cells lining the capillaries, which may occur after the arrest of the cells, initiate a signal-transduction pathway (see Chap. 9, Sec. 9.2) that promotes

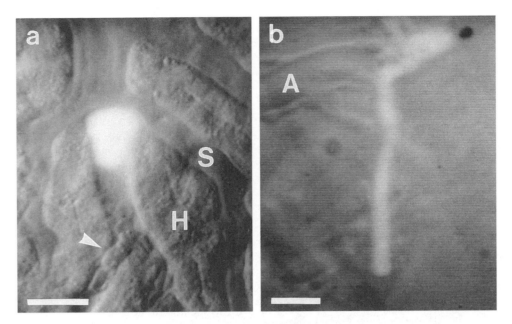

Figure 10.11. Initial arrest of fluorescently labeled cancer cells in mouse liver (a) and cremaster muscle (b). In liver, cells are arrested by size restriction on entering liver sinusoids (S) from the terminal portal venule and are only slightly deformed by the portal pressure: H = hepatocyte. In muscle (b), cells are also arrested by size restriction in vessels but are deformed considerably by the higher blood pressure in this organ. A = arteriole. Bar = 20 μm. (Modified from Morris et al., 1993.) (Photograph courtesy of EE Schmidt.)

metastasis, presumably by inducing expression of genes important to the next steps of the metastatic process.

Following arrest of cells in the microcirculation, they may extravasate (escape from the circulation into host tissue). This procedure has been described in vitro (Nicolson, 1982) and is illustrated in Fig. 10.7. The tumor cell extends pseudopodia into the endothelial cell junctions or induces endothelial cell retraction, allowing access to the basement membrane. These projections, referred to as *invadopodia*, may contain concentrations of proteases and adhesive molecules that facilitate extravasation and migration. Alternatively, the cells may attach directly to regions of denuded basement membrane. The subendothelial basement membrane is usually a better adhesive substrate for tumor cells than the endothelial cell surface, so that trauma and inflammation, which may lead to denudation of the basement membrane, can facilitate tumor cell attachment. Adhesion to basement membrane involves binding to membrane components such as laminin, fibronectin, vitronectin, type IV collagen, and proteoglycans (Liotta, 1986; Nicolson, 1988). This binding appears to be mediated by cell-surface receptors, many of which are part of the integrin family (Chap. 9, Sec. 9.2). The next step is digestion of the basement membrane by various proteolytic enzymes produced by the tumor cells (and perhaps by normal cells in the vicinity). Many different proteolytic enzyme activities have been found to be released by tumor cells growing in vitro (see Sec. 10.5.2), although the exact role of these enzymes in vivo remains uncertain.

In vivo studies of extravasation using IVVM have been reported by Chambers et al., 1995. Examples of extravasated cells are shown in Fig. 10.12. While the details of the process of extravasation remain poorly understood, the majority of arrested cells seem to be able to extravasate, even cells with reduced proteolytic capability (Koop et al., 1994) or nonmalignant fibroblasts (Koop et al., 1996), suggesting that this process is not a major barrier to the metastatic process. Following extravasation, a fraction of the cells have been reported to preferentially migrate and adhere to the outer surface of arterioles, where they begin to proliferate (Koop et al., 1996).

10.4.4 Establishment of a New Growth

The regulation of growth of tumor cells after extravasation is complex and, as noted above, appears to make a major contribution to metastatic inefficiency

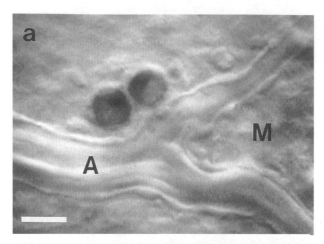

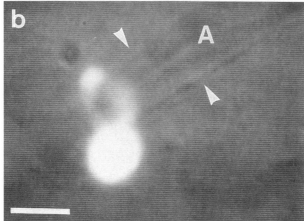

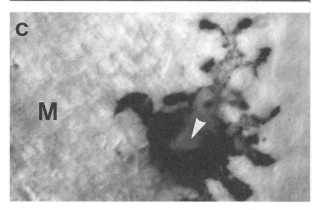

Figure 10.12. Extravasated cells in chick embryo chorioallantoic membrane, viewed by IVVM. Melanotic cells 24 h after intravenous injection (a) which extravasated and then divided, remaining near arteriole A. Fluorescently labeled, extravasated fibroblast, 3.5 h after injection (b), shown with projections extending around outer surface of arteriole. Three-day-old melanotic micrometastasis (c), which formed around an arteriole (*arrowhead*). Bars = 20 μm. (Photographs courtesy of S Koop and EE Schmidt.)

and organ-specific growth. The appropriateness of the growth conditions in a *specific* organ for a *particular* tumor cell is an important aspect of Paget's "soil

and seed" hypothesis to explain organ specificity of metastases (Paget, 1889). Most experimental studies have concentrated on cellular properties (the seed) and only recently have specific organ properties (the soil) received attention. Cells are known to require specific growth factors for proliferation (see Chap. 6, Secs. 6.2 and 6.3), although as discussed in Chap. 9 (Sec. 9.1.1), cellular interactions with the extracellular matrix (ECM) are also important. A number of soluble organ-derived factors have been identified that show some specificity for stimulation of the proliferation, in vitro, of tumor cells that preferentially metastasize to that particular organ (Nicolson, 1988). For example, melanoma cells that metastasize to brain may respond to neurotrophins produced by normal brain cells (Nicolson and Menter, 1995). There are also factors known to inhibit cell proliferation (e.g., TGF-β), and these may also play a role in organ-specific metastasis.

Tumor cells are less dependent on exogenous growth factors than normal cells, and there is evidence that the more autonomous the cells, the more capable they are of forming tumors in animals (e.g., nude mice) and of metastasizing. For many tumor cells, lack of dependence on an exogenously produced growth factor is a result of autocrine production of such factors and/or modification of response to such factors (see Chap. 6, Secs. 6.2 and 6.3). For example, during progression of melanoma, a switch from a requirement for exogenously supplied growth factors to independence from this requirement has been reported (Lu and Kerbel, 1994). Similarly, there is evidence that as tumor cells progress to greater malignancy, they may switch from being growth inhibited by TGF-β to being growth-stimulated by TGF-β (Wright et al., 1993; Lu and Kerbel 1994)

An important aspect of the growth of a metastasis is the ability of the tumor cells to induce angiogenesis (growth of new blood vessels). Several growth factors, particularly basic fibroblast growth factor (bFGF) and vascular endothelial growth factor (VEGF), are angiogenic and stimulate endothelial cell growth and morphologic differentiation (see Chap. 9, Sec. 9.3.2). Without such angiogenesis, a tumor would be unable to grow larger than a few millimeters in diameter because of limited diffusion of essential nutrients to the tumor cells. Recently it has been reported that there are factors that can suppress the formation of metastases by preventing their angiogenesis (Chap. 9, Sec. 9.3.3). These inhibitory factors may be generated by the primary tumor.

10.5 MOLECULAR MECHANISMS OF METASTASIS

The evidence that metastatic properties of cells are heritable, at least in the short term, suggests that genetic changes may be involved. The question of whether metastatic phenotypes are dominant or recessive has been studied using cell hybrids with a variety of different fusion partners (Chap. 3, Sec. 3.4.2). Results of these studies (as discussed in Ling et al., 1985) have suggested that nonmetastatic cells can acquire metastatic properties by fusing with normal cells, possibly as a result of modified immunogenicity, but this is not a universal finding. Results involving fusions of tumor cells with different metastatic properties have also been equivocal. As discussed in previous sections, several classes of molecules have been associated with various steps of the metastatic process. Two broad classes of "effector" molecules have been repeatedly implicated in contributing to metastatic ability: adhesion molecules and proteolytic enzymes. An understanding of the contributions of specific members of these classes of molecules to steps in metastasis will be important in understanding the molecular nature of the metastatic process as well as for providing reasonable targets for the development of antimetastatic therapy. A second level of understanding is also important; that of clarifying the molecular regulation of these and other "effector" molecules, such as those involved in stimulation or inhibition of the growth of metastatic cells. Oncogenes, tumor suppressor genes, and a range of other genes have been implicated at this level as genes whose products are ultimately involved in the regulation of gene expression. Many of these changes have been identified by comparisons of metastatic versus nonmetastatic cells (see Secs. 10.5.3 and 10.5.4).

10.5.1 Cell Adhesion Molecules

Tumor cells interact with each other as well as with host cells and with molecules of the extracellular matrix during tumor growth and metastasis (see Chap. 9, Secs. 9.1 and 9.2). These interactions depend upon several classes of molecules expressed on the cell surface, including integrins and cadherins, and the ligands that bind to these molecules. While these molecules were originally named *adhesion molecules*, it is now clear that they have multiple functions including the initiation of signal transduction (see Chap. 9, Sec. 9.2.2). The formation and breaking of adhesive bonds between tumor cells and their environment during steps in metastasis may, therefore, provide information to the cell about its environment and lead to changes in the expression of specific genes that determine cell proliferation, invasion, or other processes.

10.5.2 Proteolytic Enzymes

A series of tissue barriers—e.g., basement membrane, interstitial connective tissue—are traversed by tumor cells during the steps of the metastatic process. Members of all five classes of naturally occurring proteinases [serine-, cysteine-, aspartyl-, threonine-, and matrix metallo-proteinases (MMPs)] have been associated with increased aggressiveness of tumor cells and have been implicated functionally in steps in metastasis (for reviews, see Stetler-Stevenson et al., 1993; Mignatti and Rifkin, 1993; Sloane et al., 1994; Chambers and Matrisian, 1997). Plasminogen activator [urokinase type (uPA)], which acts on plasminogen in the blood to release plasmin, was one of the first proteinases associated with malignant cells. This enzyme and the various MMPs (which include type IV collagenases and stromelysin) and the lysosomal cysteine proteinases cathepsins B and L (for reviews, see Liotta et al., 1991; Jiang et al., 1994; Sloane et al., 1994; MacDougall and Matrisian, 1995) are usually secreted in a latent form. They are activated by the action of other proteases or possibly by environmental conditions such as acidity. Recent evidence implicates plasminogen activator and plasmin as major players in the activation of MMPs (see Mazzieri et al., 1997). Concerted action by these and perhaps other enzymes is required to degrade the basement membrane and extracellular matrix and allow escape of the tumor cell into the interstitial space. Inhibitors of these enzymes have been identified and can be produced by malignant and normal cells; examples are plasminogen activator inhibitor (PAI), TIMP-1 and TIMP-2 (tissue inhibitors of MMPs) (Stetler-Stevenson, 1990; DeClerck and Imren, 1994), and stefin A, which inhibits the action of cysteine proteinases (Sloane et al., 1990).

Under normal physiologic conditions, proteolysis is under strict control with the activated proteinases and their inhibitors in balance; but when malignant cells invade tissues, this balance is disturbed, allowing uncontrolled invasion. The important role of inhibitors is illustrated by the work of Khokha et al. (1989), who demonstrated that downregulation of TIMP-1 activity in murine fibroblasts, using transfected antisense RNA (see Chap. 3, Sec. 3.3.11), resulted in increased invasive capacity and ability to form tumors that metastasized in nude mice. Similarly, increased levels of TIMP-1 or TIMP-2 can reduce the invasive and metastatic abilities of malignant cells (see DeClerck and Imren, 1994, for review). Recent studies with IVVM have shown that cells genetically altered to overexpress TIMP-1 have reduced metastatic ability but have unimpaired ability to extravasate in vivo (Koop et al., 1994), suggesting that TIMP/MMP balance may also play an important role in the postextravasation growth of metastases, perhaps through the release of growth factors bound to the ECM.

10.5.3 Oncogenes and Metastasis

Some nonmetastatic tumor cell lines and some immortalized (nontumorigenic) fibroblast cell lines can be converted into metastatic tumor cell lines by transfection with activated oncogenes (see Chambers and Tuck, 1993, for review). Most of the studies have involved the H-*ras* oncogene transfected into cells such as NIH/3T3 or C$_3$H10T1/2 cells, both immortalized fibroblast lines. It has been demonstrated that the level of expression of the p21^{ras} protein is correlated with metastatic ability, both by testing clonal isolates with different p21 expression and by transfecting the *Ras* gene attached to an inducible promoter. The *Ras* gene was also implicated when transfection of DNA from human tumors into NIH/3T3 cells was found capable of inducing tumorigenicity and metastatic ability (Chap. 5, Sec. 5.4.1). Other oncogenes that can induce a metastatic phenotype in immortalized fibroblasts include v-*src* and v-*mos,* while mutant forms of *myc* and *p53* can cause cells that are already tumorigenic to become metastatic.

Transfection of the H-*ras* oncogene can cause pleiotropic changes in cells, many of which could be involved in the metastatic process (see Table 10.2); particularly important may be those associated with increased protease secretion. It has been demonstrated that transfection of the *E1A* oncogene from adenovirus 2 into H-*ras*-transformed NIH/3T3 cells can reduce the metastatic ability of such cells and that their secretion of collagenase type IV activity is also reduced. This effect may be consistent with the trans-activating activity (ability to influence the expression of other genes) of *E1A*. It was also found that the cells had increased levels of *nm23* mRNA, a metastasis-associated gene (see Sec. 10.5.4). A study by Su et al. (1993) also reported that transfection with the *Ras* oncogene caused metastatic behavior and reduced expression of nm23 in rat embryo fibroblasts. When these cells were subsequently trans-

Table 10.2. Examples of *Ras*-induced Cellular Properties Possibly Related to Metastasis

- Increased type IV collagenase activity
- Increased plasminogen activator activity
- Increased cathepsin-L activity
- Increased secretion of osteopontin
- Altered membrane glycoproteins
- Altered cytoskeleton
- Decreased sensitivity to NK-cell cytolysis

fected with the *k-rev* tumor suppressor gene, there was reduced metastatic potential and an increase in the expression of nm23. There were also changes in other metastasis-related genes, including MMPs, TIMPs, osteopontin, and transin. Recent work has also demonstrated that H-*ras* can upregulate the expression of vascular endothelial growth factor (VEGF) in malignant cells, thus potentially facilitating angiogenesis (see Chap. 9, Sec. 9.3.2).

Many protein products of oncogenes serve as broad-function signal-transducing molecules, including those that act as nuclear transcription factors (see Chaps. 5 and 6). In a recent study, Guo et al. (1995) reported that metastatic cells produced increased levels of a nuclear protein that bound to a Ras-responsive promoter element. Such regulatory proteins may contribute to the regulation of the complex phenotypic behavior that results in metastatic ability.

10.5.4 Metastasis-Associated Genes

A number of different groups have attempted to identify genes controlling metastatic behavior using techniques of subtractive hybridization of cDNA libraries (see Chap. 3, Sec. 3.3.9) obtained from pairs of metastatic and nonmetastatic cell lines. A small number of genes, some known and some novel, have been isolated (see Table 10.3). The first five genes in the table are poorly (or not) expressed in the metastatic pair of the cell lines from which they were isolated, while the others have increased expression. Many of the genes appear to be associated with the growth characteristics of the cells and possibly promote the growth of individual or small groups of cells during the early stages of metastatic growth. Others appear to be associated with the earlier stages of the metastatic process in terms of cell adhesiveness and invasive capacity.

One of the most studied metastasis-associated genes is *nm23,* a gene isolated by Steeg et al. (1988). There are two similar genes in rodent (*nm23-1* and

Table 10.3. Metastasis-Associated Genes Identified by Screening c-DNA Libraries from Metastatic and Nonmetastatic Cells

Gene Identified	Protein Function/Homology
Decreased Expression in Metastatic Cells	
nm23	NDP kinase, Transcription factor (?) Signal transduction
wdm-1	?
wdm-2	NAD(P)H menadione reductase
KAI-1	CD-82, membrane glycoprotein
KiSS-1	Signal transduction (SH3 binding domain)
Increased Expression in Metastatic Cells	
pLm59	Acidic ribosomal protein
pGm21	Elongation factor-1
Stromelysin (transin)	Metalloproteinase
mts-1	Calcium-binding protein
st-3 (stromelysin-3)	Metalloproteinase
pMeta-1	Cell adhesion molecule
Tiam-1	GDP/ GTP exchange protein signal transduction
Osteopontin	Cell adhesion molecule

nm23-2) and human (*nm23-H1* and *nm23-H2*) cells, which encode proteins of about 17-kDa and are about 90 percent identical. The gene was isolated from rodent tumor cells and low expression of the gene product, particularly nm23-1, was initially associated with increased metastatic potential, suggesting that the *nm23* gene may be a metastasis suppressor gene. Transfection of the gene, under the control of various promoters, resulted in the loss of metastatic ability (both experimental and spontaneous) in cell lines with high levels of gene expression (Leone et al., 1991). There is evidence that expression, of *nm23-H1* may be associated with metastatic potential of a variety of human tumors, particularly breast cancers (Hennessy et al., 1991), but both up- and downregulation of the gene have been observed in different tumor types (see Table 10.4). The *nm23* gene has been found to have homology with the *awd* (abnormal wing disks) gene in Drosophila and appears to be involved in cellular development and differentiation in both flies and rodents. Both the human and rodent protein products have nucleoside diphosphate (NDP) kinase activity, but the level of activity does not obviously correlate with the effect on metastasis. The gene product has some features similar to a transcription factor and may play a role in c-*myc* expression, although this remains to be clearly established. It has also been demonstrated that the gene product may play a role in the response of cells to TGF-β, in that cells with low levels of nm23 can be stimulated to grow by TGF-β while cells with high levels of nm23 are insensitive to such stimulation (see MacDonald et al., 1995, for review). This observation is consistent with the results discussed earlier, indicating that as tumor cells progress to greater malignancy, they may switch from being growth-inhibited by TGF-β to being growth-stimulated.

Another gene identified by subtractive hybridization is the stromelysin-3 (*st-3*) gene (Basset et al., 1990). This gene was found to be overexpressed in a cDNA library obtained from an invasive human breast cancer relative to that from a benign fibroadenoma. The gene is a member of the MMP

Table 10.4. nm23 Expression and Malignancy in Human Tumors

Tumor Type	Number of Studies	Trend
Breast Cancer	11	
Melanoma	2	Decreased expression in more
Hepatocellular Cancer	3	malignant (metastatic) cancers
Gastric Cancer	3	
Ovarian Cancer	2	
Pancreatic Cancer	1	Increased expression in more
Neuroblastoma	2	malignant cancers
Colorectal Cancer	4	
Lung Cancer	2	No correlation of expression
Thyroid Cancer	5	with malignancy
Prostate Cancer	5	

Source: Modified from De La Rosa et al., 1995.

family. The gene was found to be expressed only in the stromal cells surrounding the tumor cells, not in the tumor cells themselves and not in stromal cells at a distance from the invasive carcinoma cells. These observations suggest that the tumor cells produce a diffusible substance that induces expression of the *st-3* gene in the stromal cells, thereby enhancing the invasion of the tumor cells.

10.6 STRATEGIES FOR ANTIMETASTATIC THERAPY

The term *antimetastatic drug* is reserved ideally for a compound that may inhibit the process of tumor dissemination through mechanisms other than direct toxicity to tumor cells. The process of metastasis involves several steps (Fig. 10.4) that include vascular invasion from the primary tumor, circulation through the blood, arrest in a new capillary bed, invasion through the blood vessel wall, and growth in the new site, which depends on angiogenesis (see Chap. 9, Sec. 9.3). Several types of drug may influence this process and have led to reduction in metastases in experimental animals (Goldfarb and Brunson, 1992; Dickson et al., 1996).

Metastasis depends on the arrest of circulating tumor cells, and many anticoagulant and antiplatelet drugs have been assessed for their ability to inhibit metastases. The coumarin family of drugs (e.g., warfarin), which cause anticoagulation by inhibiting synthesis of clotting factors, appears to have moderate but consistent effects in reducing metastases in animal systems, including those from established tumors. Reduction of pulmonary metastasis can be prevented by giving factor VII, which may, therefore, be important in preventing arrest of circulating tumor cells (Francis et al., 1992). Warfarin has been reported to inhibit metastases in patients, but a large trial of its use in patients with lung, colon, head and neck, and prostate cancer led to little or no improvement in survival (Zacharski et al., 1984). Aspirin and dipyridamole, which have long been known to inhibit platelet aggregation, have only minor effects on formation of metastases. Recently, more potent inhibitors of platelet aggregation have been tested, including calcium-channel blockers, antiplatelet antibodies, the prostaglandin PG-I$_2$ (also known as prostacyclin), nafazatrom, forskolin, and the protease inhibitor leupeptide, which inhibits thrombus formation. Each of these agents can induce a large decrease in lung metastases after intravenous injection of tumor cells or a decrease in metastases from transplanted tumors, although this is not observed

for all tumors. One of the more promising agents is the prostacyclin analogue cicaprost, which has a longer half-life than prostacyclin. This agent inhibits tumor cell-induced platelet aggregation, tumor-cell adhesion to endothelial cells and to the subendothelial matrix, and endothelial cell retraction; it has pronounced antimetastatic action for a series of spontaneously metastasizing rodent tumors (Schneider et al., 1994, 1996).

Invasion of tumor cells, both from the primary tumor into the circulation and from the circulation into a secondary site, provides an alternative target for antimetastatic therapy. Invasion requires breakdown of the matrix that surrounds tumor cells or normal cells in the secondary site. Many tumors produce MMPs and genes that encode tissue inhibitors of MMPs (TIMPs) have been proposed as tumor (or metastasis) suppressor genes. For this reason a number of synthetic inhibitors of MMPs are being evaluated for antitumor and antimetastatic properties (e.g., Wang et al., 1994; DeClerck and Imren, 1994). These agents may also exert effects on tumor growth and metastasis through inhibition of angiogenesis (see Chap. 9, Sec. 9.3.3). Proteolysis by tumor cells is mediated by urokinase-type plasminogen activator present on their membrane, and inhibitors of this enzyme have been shown to have a profound effect to reduce metastasis in an experimental system (Crowley et al, 1993; Fazioli and Blasi, 1994). Agents that inhibit breakdown of tissue matrix are undergoing clinical evaluation.

A major limitation to the clinical use of therapy to prevent metastasis formation is the presence of microscopic metastases prior to detection and treatment of the primary tumor. Prevention of secondary metastases (i.e., metastases from metastases) might be useful in palliation, but the potential for increased cure through the use of antimetastatic agents is limited to patients in whom metastases are seeded after diagnosis and prior to eradication of the primary tumor. Tumor cells are known to enter the circulation at the time of surgery, and the prostacyclin analogue cicaprost was able to decrease metastatic spread when given around the time of excision of mammary tumors in rodents (Schneider et al., 1996). However, seeding at the time of surgery is probably the sole source of metastases for only a small proportion of patients.

Recently an approach to "control" rather than "cure" metastases has been proposed (see Schipper et al., 1993a, b; Kohn and Liotta, 1995). It is known that malignant cells often have dysregulated signal transduction pathways whose normal function is to transmit information to the cell about its environment and to elicit an appropriate, controlled, and transient response (see Chap. 6, Sec. 6.7). One approach to control metastatic growth is to attempt to regain control of this information transfer by, for example, interfering with an altered signal transduction pathway (Levitzki, 1994). This might be achieved by blocking *Ras* oncogene-mediated signals (Gibbs et al., 1994) or by calcium-mediated signaling (Kohn and Liotta, 1995). By regulating the "regulatory pathway," induction of the various "effector genes," such as proteases and adhesion molecules, would be prevented. A second approach is to prevent growth of metastases by blocking angiogenesis, since by preventing the expansion of micrometastases beyond a small size, their clinical effects might be held in check (for detailed discussion see Chap. 9, Sec. 9.3.3).

10.7 SUMMARY

Metastasis is the major cause of death due to cancer, and it occurs primarily by dissemination of tumor cells through the lymphatic and blood vessels. In humans there is evidence for organ-site specificity in the development of metastases from particular types of primary tumors, and cells that have specific organ-site preferences for metastatic development have been selected from tumors in animals. Isolation of cloned cell populations from rodent tumors has demonstrated wide heterogeneity in metastatic potential between clonal populations. The metastatic phenotype of such clonal populations, however, has usually been found to be unstable.

Several major steps are involved in the process of metastasis, including the ability to invade into and out of blood vessels, to survive in the circulation, and to arrest and grow at a new site. Extensive studies have identified a range of properties (particularly those relating to cell adhesion and secretion of proteolytic enzymes) that may be involved in the process of metastasis, but identification of specific biochemical properties that characterize all metastatic cells has proved elusive. On the contrary, many different cellular biochemical changes seem capable of producing phenotypes that increase the ability of tumor cells to form metastases. Despite the evidence for specificity in metastatic development, metastasis is an inefficient process and may depend to some extent on random survival factors associated with traversing the various stages of the metastatic process. The development of metastatic potential may be viewed as one of the late stages of the process of tumor progression. While the details of the genetic changes that contribute to

metastatic ability remain incompletely understood, a number of possible therapeutic targets have been identified that may in future provide the possibility of regulating the formation of metastases and their consequences for the patient.

REFERENCES

Basset P, Bellocq JP, Wolf C, et al: A novel metalloproteinase gene specifically expressed in stromal cells of breast carcinomas. *Nature* 1990; 348:699–704.

Baylin SB, Herman JG, Graff JR et al: Alterations in DNA methylation: A fundamental aspect of neoplasia. *Adv Cancer Res* 1998; 72:141–196.

Brittenden J, Heys SD, Ross J, Eremin O: Natural killer cells and cancer. *Cancer* 1996; 77:1226–1243.

Butler TP, Gullino PM: Quantitation of cell shedding into efferent blood of mammary adenocarcinoma. *Cancer Res* 1975; 35:512–516.

Califano J, van der Riet P, Westra W: Genetic progression model for head and neck cancer: Implications for field cancerization. *Cancer Res* 1996; 56: 2488–2492.

Carr I, Carr J: Experimental lymphatic invasion and metastases. In: Weiss L, Gilbert HA, eds. *Lymphatic System Metastases*. Boston: Hall; 1980:41–75.

Chambers AF, Matrisian LM: Changing views of the role of matrix metalloproteinases in metastasis. *J Natl Cancer Inst* 1997; 89:1260–1270.

Chambers AF, Tuck AB: *Ras*-responsive genes and tumor metastasis. *Criti Rev Oncog* 1993; 4:95–114.

Chambers AF, MacDonald IC, Schmidt EE, et al: Steps in tumor metastasis: New concepts from intravital videomicroscopy. *Cancer Metastasis Rev* 1995; 14:279–301.

Crowley CW, Cohen RL, Lucas BK, et al: Prevention of metastasis by inhibition of the urokinase receptor. *Proc Natl Acad Sci USA* 1993; 90:5021–5025.

DeClerck YA, Imren S: Protease inhibitors: Role and potential therapeutic use in human cancer. *Eur J Cancer* 1994; 30A:2170–2180.

De la Rosa A, Williams RL, Steeg PS: Nm23/nucleoside diphosphate kinase: Toward a structural and biochemical understanding of its biological functions. *Bioessays* 1995; 17(1):53–62.

Dickson RB, Johnson MD, Maemura M, Low J: Anti-invasion drugs. *Breast Cancer Res Treat* 1996; 38:121–132.

Fazioli F, Blasi F: Urokinase-type plasminogen activator and its receptor: New targets for anti-metastatic therapy? *Trends Pharmacol Sci* 1994; 15:25–29.

Fidler IJ: Selection of successive tumour lines for metastasis. *Nature New Biol* 1973; 242:148–149.

Fidler IJ: Critical factors in the biology of human cancer metastasis. *Cancer Res* 1990; 50:6130–6138.

Fidler IJ, Kripke ML: Metastasis results from preexisting variant cells within a malignant tumor. *Science* 1977; 198:893–895.

Francis JL, Carty N, Amirkhosravi M, et al: The effect of

warfarin and factor VII on tissue procoagulant activity and pulmonary seeding. *Br J Cancer* 1992; 65:329–334.

Gibbs JB, Oliff A, Kohl NE: Farnesyltransferase inhibitors: Ras research yields a potential cancer therapeutic. *Cell* 1994; 77:175–178.

Glaves D: Correlation between circulating cancer cells and incidence of metastases. *Br J Cancer* 1983; 48:665–673.

Glaves D, Huben RP, Weiss L: Haematogenous dissemination of cells from human renal adenocarcinomas. *Br J Cancer* 1988; 57:32–35.

Goldfarb RH, Brunson KW: Therapeutic agents for treatment of established metastases and inhibitors of metastatic spread: Preclinical and clinical progress. *Curr Opin Oncol* 1992; 4:1130–1141.

Graeber TG, Osmanian C, Jacks T, et al. Hypoxia-mediated selection of cells with diminished apoptotic potential in solid tumours. *Nature* 1996; 379:88–91.

Greenberg AH, Egan SE, Jarolin L, et al: Natural killer cell regulation of implantation and early lung growth of H-*ras*-transformed 10T1/2 fibroblasts in mice. *Cancer Res* 1987; 47:4801–4805.

Greenblatt MS, Bennett WP, Hollstein M, Harris CC: Mutations in the *p53* tumor suppressor gene: Clues to cancer etiology and molecular pathogenesis. *Cancer Res* 1994; 54:4855–4878.

Guo X, Zhang YP, Mitchell DA, et al: Identification of a ras-activated enhancer in the mouse osteopontin promoter and its interaction with a putative ETS-related transcription factor whose activity correlates with the metastatic potential of the cell. *Mol Cell Biol* 1995; 15:476–487.

Hanna, N: Role of natural killer cells in host defense against cancer metastasis. In: Nicolson GL, Milas L, eds. *Cancer Invasion and Metastasis: Biologic and Therapeutic Aspects.* New York: Raven Press; 1984:309–319.

Hart IR: The selection and characterization of an invasive variant of the B16 melanoma. *Am J Pathol* 1979; 97:587–600.

Hart IR, Fidler IJ: Role of organ selectivity in the determination of metastatic patterns of B16 melanoma. *Cancer Res* 1981; 41:1281–1287.

Hennessy C, Henry JA, May FEB, et al: Expression of the anti-metastatic gene *nm23* in human breast cancer: An association with good prognosis. *J Natl Canc Inst* 1991; 83:281–285.

Heppner GH, Miller FR: The cellular basis of tumor progression. *Int Rev Cytology* 1998; 177:1–56.

Hilgard P: Anticoagulants and tumor growth: Pharmacological considerations. In: Nicolson GL, Milas L, eds. *Cancer Invasion and Metastasis: Biologic and Therapeutic Aspects.* New York: Raven Press; 1984:353–360.

Hill RP, Chambers AF, Ling V, Harris IF: Dynamic heterogeneity: Rapid generation of metastatic variants in mouse B16 melanoma cells. *Science* 1984; 224:998–1001.

Hill RP, Young SD, Cillo C, Ling V: Metastatic cell phenotypes: Quantitative studies using the experimental metastasis assay. *Cancer Rev* 1986; 5:118–151.

Hockel M, Schlenger K, Aral B, et al: Association between tumor hypoxia and malignant progression in advanced cancer of the uterine cervix. *Cancer Res* 1996; 56:4509–4515.

Jiang WG, Puntis MCA, Hallett MB: Molecular and cellular basis of cancer invasion and metastasis: Implications for treatment. *Br J Surg* 1994; 81:1576–1590.

Khokha R, Waterhouse P, Yagel S, et al: Anti-sense RNA-induced reduction in murine TIMP levels confers oncogenicity in Swiss 3T3 cells. *Science* 1989; 243:947–950.

Kinzler KW, Vogelstein B: Lessons from hereditary colorectal cancer. *Cell* 1996; 87:159–170.

Klein G: Foulds' dangerous idea revisited: The multistep development of tumors 40 years later. *Adv Cancer Res* 1998; 72:1–23.

Kohn EC, Liotta LA: Molecular insights into cancer invasion: Strategies for prevention and intervention. *Cancer Res* 1995; 55:1856–1862.

Koop S, Khokha R, Schmidt EE, et al: Over-expression of metalloproteinase inhibitor in B16F10 cells does not affect extravasation but reduces tumor growth. *Cancer Res* 1994; 54:4791–4797.

Koop S, Schmidt EE, MacDonald IC, et al. Independence of metastatic ability and extravasation: Metastatic *ras*-transformed and control fibroblasts extravasate equally well. *Proc Natl Acad Sci USA* 1996; 93:11080–11084.

Leone A, Flatow U, King CR, et al: Reduced tumor incidence, metastatic ability and cytokine responsiveness of nm-23-transfected melanoma cells. *Cell* 1991; 65:25–35.

Levitzki A: Signal-transduction therapy: A novel approach to disease management. *Eur J Biochem* 1994: 226:1–13.

Ling V, Chambers AF, Harris JF, Hill RP: Quantitative genetic analysis of tumor progression. *Cancer Metastasis Rev* 1985; 4:173–192.

Liotta LA: Tumor invasion and metastases—Role of the extracellular matrix. *Cancer Res* 1986; 46:1–7.

Liotta LA, Steeg PS, Stetler-Stevenson WG: Cancer metastasis and angiogenesis: An imbalance of positive and negative regulation. *Cell* 1991; 64:327–336.

Loeb LA: Cancer cells exhibit a mutator phenotype. *Adv Cancer Res* 1998; 72:25–56.

Lu C, Kerbel RS: Cytokines, growth factors and the loss of negative growth controls in the progression of human cutaneous malignant melanoma. *Curr Opin Oncol* 1994: 6:212–220.

MacDonald NJ, de la Rosa A, Steeg PS: The potential roles of nm23 in cancer metastasis and cellular differentiation. *Eur J Cancer* 1995; 31A:1096–1100.

MacDougall JR, Matrisian LM: Contributions of tumor and stromal matrix metalloproteinases to tumor progression, invasion and metastasis. *Cancer Metastasis Rev* 1995; 14:351–362.

Mazzieri R, Masiero L, Zanetta L, et al. Control of type IV collagenase activity by components of the urokinase-plasmin system: A regulatory mechanism with cell-bound reactants. *EMBO J* 1997; 16:2319–2332.

Mignatti P, Rifkin DB: Biology and biochemistry of proteinases in tumor invasion. *Physiol Rev* 1993; 73:161–195.

Morris VL, MacDonald IC, Koop S, et al. Early interactions of cancer cells with the microvasculature in mouse liver and muscle during hematogenous metastasis: Videomicroscopic analysis. *Clin Exp Metastasis* 1993; 11:377–390.

Nicolson GL: Cancer metastasis: Organ colonization and the cell-surface properties of malignant cells. *Biochim Biophys Acta* 1982; 695:113–176.

Nicolson GL: Organ specificity of tumor metastasis: Role of preferential adhesion, invasion and growth of malignant cells at specific secondary sites. *Cancer Metastasis Rev* 1988; 7:143–188.

Nicolson GL, Menter DG: Trophic factors and central nervous system metastasis. *Cancer Metastasis Rev* 1995; 14:303–321.

Nowell P: Mechanisms of tumor progression. *Cancer Res* 1986; 46:2203–2207.

Paget S: The distribution of secondary growths in cancer of the breast. *Lancet* 1889; 1:571–573.

Plesnicar S: Mechanisms of development of metastases. *Crit Rev Oncog* 1989; 1:175–194.

Radinsky R: Modulation of tumor cell gene expression and phenotype by the organ-specific metastatic environment. *Cancer Metastasis Rev* 1995; 14:323–338.

Rodriguez E, Sreenantaiah C, Chaganti RSK: Genetic changes in epithelial solid neoplasia. *Cancer Res* 1994; 54:3398–3406.

Schipper H, Goh CR, Wang TL: Rethinking cancer: Should we control rather than kill? Part 1. *Can J Oncol* 1993a; 3:207–216.

Schipper H, Goh CR, Wang TL: Rethinking cancer: Should we control rather than kill? Part 2. *Can J Oncol* 1993b; 3:220–224.

Schneider MR Schirner M, Lichtner RB, Graf H: Antimetastatic action of the prostacyclin analogue cicaprost in experimental mammary tumors. *Breast Cancer Res Treat* 1996; 38:133–141.

Schneider MR, Tang DG, Schirner M, Horn KV: Prostacyclin and its analogues: Antimetastatic effects and mechanisms of action. *Cancer Metastasis Rev* 1994; 13:349–364.

Shackney SE, Sharkey TV: Common patterns of genetic evolution in human solid tumors. *Cytometry* 1997; 29:1–27.

Simpson AJ: The natural somatic mutation frequency and human carcinogenesis. *Adv Cancer Res* 1997; 71:209–240.

Sloane BF, Moin K, Lah TT: Regulation of lysosomal endopeptidases in malignant neoplasia. In: TG Pretlow, TP Pretlow, eds. *Biochemical and Molecular Aspects of Selected Cancers.* New York: Academic Press; 1994:411–466.

Sloane BF, Moin K, Krepela E, Rozhin J: Cathepsin B and its endogenous inhibitors: The role in tumor malignancy. *Cancer Metastasis Rev* 1990; 9:333–352.

Stackpole CW, Alterman AL, Valle EF: B16 melanoma variants selected by one or more cycles of spontaneous metastasis to the same organ fail to exhibit organ specificity. *Clin Exp Metastasis* 1991; 9:319–332.

Steeg PS, Bevilacqua G, Kopper L, et al: Evidence for a novel gene associated with low tumor metastatic potential. *J Natl Cancer Inst* 1988; 80:200–204.

Stetler-Stevenson WG: Type IV collagenases in tumor invasion and metastasis. *Cancer Metastasis Rev* 1990; 9:289–303.

Stetler-Stevenson WG, Liotta LA, Kleiner DR Jr: Extracellular matrix 6: Role of matrix metalloproteinases in tumor invasion and metastasis. *FASEB J* 1993; 7:1434–1441.

Su ZZ, Austin VN, Zimmer SG, Fisher PB: Defining the critical gene expression changes associated with expression and suppression of the tumorigenic and metastatic phenotype in Ha-ras-transformed cloned rat embryo fibroblast cells. *Oncogene* 1993; 8:1211–1219.

Sugarbaker EV: Patterns of metastasis in human malignancies. *Cancer Biol Rev* 1981; 2:235–278.

Tarin D, Price JE, Kettlewell MG, et al: Clinicopathological observations on metastasis in man studied in patients treated with peritoneovenous shunts. *Br Med J Clin Res Ed* 1984; 288:749–751.

Thompson SC: The colony-forming efficiency of single cells and cell aggregates from a spontaneous mouse mammary tumour using the lung colony assay. *Br J Cancer* 1974; 30:332–336.

Wang X, Fu X, Brown PD et al: Matrix metalloproteinase inhibitor BB-94 (Batimastat) inhibits human colon tumor growth and spread in a patient-like orthotopic model in nude mice. *Cancer Res* 1994; 54:4726–4728.

Weidner N, Folkman J, Pozza F, et al: Tumor angiogenesis: A new significant and independent prognostic indicator in early-stage breast cancer. *J Natl Cancer Inst* 1992; 84:1875–1887.

Weiss L: Metastatic inefficiency. *Adv Cancer Res* 1990; 54:159–211.

Wright JA, Turley EA, Greenberg AH: Transforming growth factor beta and fibroblast growth factor as promoters of tumor progression to malignancy. *Crit Rev Oncogen* 1993; 4:473–492.

Zacharski LR, Henderson WG, Rickles FR, et al: Effect of warfarin anticoagulation on survival in carcinoma of the lung, colon, head and neck, and prostate: Final Report of VA Cooperative Study #75. *Cancer* 1984; 53:2046–2052.

11

Immunology Related to Cancer

David Spaner, Laszlo Radvanyi, and Richard G. Miller

11.1 INTRODUCTION

11.2 BIOLOGY OF THE IMMUNE RESPONSE
    11.2.1 Innate Immunity
    11.2.2 Acquired Immunity
    11.2.3 Specificity and Clonal Selection
    11.2.4 Time Course of an Immune Response
    11.2.5 Self-Nonself Discrimination and Immunoregulation
    11.2.6 Antibodies, Immunoglobulin Receptors, and B-Cell Activation

11.3 CELL-MEDIATED IMMUNITY
    11.3.1 Transplantation Immunity
    11.3.2 The Major Histocompatibility Complex

11.3.3 T Lymphocytes
11.3.4 The T-Cell Receptor
11.3.5 Activation of T Lymphocytes: Inter- and Intracellular Signaling
11.3.6 Geography of T-Cell Activation
11.3.7 Natural Killer Cells

11.4 TUMOR IMMUNITY
    11.4.1 Tumor Antigens
    11.4.2 Immune Surveillance
    11.4.3 Failure of the Immune Response

11.5 SUMMARY

REFERENCES

11.1 INTRODUCTION

The immune system is composed of cells and secreted molecules that respond in a coordinated fashion to foreign substances in the body. Most of us have suffered from one or more of the common childhood diseases caused by viruses, such as measles, mumps, or chickenpox. Our immune systems recognized these viruses as foreign and provided a response that eradicated the foreign pathogen. The response against one disease is specific and, in order to eliminate another disease, a separate immune response must be generated. Usually, a person gets a disease such as mumps only once, despite being exposed to it from his or her own children, implying that during the first exposure to the disease, the individual develops an ability to eradicate a second infection before any clinical symptoms become manifest. Thus, the immune response has both specificity and memory.

The ability to manipulate the immune response under controlled conditions is one of the major goals of immunology as a scientific discipline. One of the best examples of this is vaccination. Here, protection against an infectious disease is conferred artificially by injection of a small dose of a nonviable or nonpathogenic form of the infectious agent. Vaccination has been successful in eradicating smallpox and in limiting the effects of many other infectious diseases. Immunization represents perhaps the single most effective intervention of medical science to date.

If a foreign agent can be recognized by the immune system, it is said to be *antigenic,* and if the immune system can also mount an immune response against it, the agent is said to be *immunogenic.* Not all antigens are immunogenic. Under some circumstances an antigenic material can induce a state in which the immune response against the antigen is suppressed. This state is called *tolerance* and is important in preventing the immune system from reacting against the body's own cells and tissues. Suppression of the immune response against self-antigens (called *self-tolerance*) is a continual process throughout life, and a breakdown in these control measures leads to autoimmune diseases. Mechanisms that induce tolerance in the immune system can prevent an immune response against an antigen or suppress an ongoing immune response. Thus, along with specificity and memory, another feature of the immune system is self-tolerance.

Many investigators have proposed that tumor cells carry antigens that can be recognized as being foreign to the body and that one of the major functions of the immune system is to eliminate such cells before they can form large tumors. This process, known as *immune surveillance*, has been ineffective in a patient with progressive cancer. As described in this chapter, the protective measures that suppress self-reactivity in the immune system (i.e., that induce self-tolerance) may represent a major barrier in the immune system's ability to eradicate tumor cells.

In the following sections, the components of the immune system and its biological properties are described. This knowledge is then applied to a description of how the immune system responds against cancer and why it fails to eradicate many tumors.

11.2 BIOLOGY OF THE IMMUNE RESPONSE

11.2.1 Innate Immunity

The first line of defense against invading pathogens consists of a group of cells and factors making up the natural or innate immune system. Innate immunity is nonspecific and present at all times in normal individuals. Vertebrate animals have also evolved a more specific type of immunity called the *acquired* or *adaptive* immune system; acquired immunity requires stimulation to function and is specific. Both systems cooperate through cellular interactions and soluble mediators called *cytokines*.

The components of the innate immune system include the polymorphonuclear white blood cells or granulocytes, natural killer or large granular lymphocytes (see Sec. 11.3.7), and macrophages. Physical barriers (e.g., the skin and intestinal mucosa) inhibit entry of foreign substances into the blood and are also part of the innate immune system. Granulocytes are of three main types: neutrophils, eosinophils, and basophils. These cells are stimulated by cytokines to act as phagocytes that engulf foreign material or release toxic oxygen radicals that penetrate and kill target cells through oxidative damage. Cells of the innate immune system are the first to be attracted from the bloodstream to sites of infection by substances called *chemokines*, which are

released from damaged cells and tissues. There, macrophages and natural killer cells secrete cytokines, which not only stimulate the action of granulocytes but also attract other cells, including lymphocytes, to the area. These cytokines include members of the interferon (IFN) family, tumor necrosis factor (TNF) family, and interleukins such as IL-12. The innate immune system acts as a first line of defense while an acquired immune response is mounted (Fearon and Locksley, 1996).

Vaccination protocols often require that the injected immunogen be mixed with an "adjuvant" such as alum. The role of the adjuvant appears to be to activate the innate system to provide cytokines that aid in the activation of the acquired immune system. Injection of Bacille Calmette-Guérin (BCG) into melanoma nodules in the skin will often stimulate immunologic rejection of the tumor at that site but rarely of nodules at other sites (Rosenberg and Rapp, 1976). Here, BCG appears to be acting as an adjuvant.

11.2.2 Acquired Immunity

The acquired immune system operates through a system of antigen-specific receptors that control the specificity and memory of the immune system; it is largely responsible for the recognition and eradication of foreign antigens. It has several components, including T and B lymphocytes and a specialized group of cells called *antigen-presenting cells* (APCs). Although all cells in the body have the capacity to present antigens on their surfaces, only certain hemopoietic cells are "professional" APCs capable of fully activating lymphocytes and inducing an immune response. These cells include dendritic cells, Langerhans cells in the skin, macrophages, and activated B lymphocytes.

The ability to mount an antigen-specific secondary immune response immediately after exposure to an antigen can be transferred from a previously immunized animal to a naive or unimmunized animal. This procedure has been used to define two major types of acquired immunity; *humoral immunity*, in which serum alone can transfer the response, and *cell-mediated immunity*, in which lymphocytes must be transferred. The humoral response is mediated by soluble molecules called *antibodies* that are secreted by plasma cells, produced by the proliferation and differentiation of B lymphocytes following cooperation with one type of T lymphocytes (known as helper T cells or T_h cells). In cell-mediated immunity, the effectors include cytotoxic T lymphocytes (CTLs), which kill infected cells by recognizing a foreign antigen on their surface.

11.2.3 Specificity and Clonal Selection

Specificity in the immune response is manifest by antigen receptors on lymphocytes that bind to small parts of proteins or polysaccharides called *epitopes*. Each receptor recognizes a unique epitope. Recognition that lymphocytes possess receptors for specific antigens led to the development of the *clonal selection hypothesis* (Fig. 11.1), which provided a testable model of how a specific immune response might be generated. The clonal selection hypothesis argues that every T and B cell carries preformed antigen receptors of a single specificity and that recognition of a particular foreign antigen triggers the outgrowth of specific cells (Burnet, 1959; Talmage, 1986). Some of these clonal cells differentiate into effector cells and memory cells. The result is that each individual contains many different lymphocyte clones, each of which has arisen from a single precursor cell that recognizes a distinct epitope. If there is no T or B cell with a receptor capable of binding a particular foreign epitope, there will be no immune response against that epitope. Many experiments have confirmed the validity of the clonal selection hypothesis.

The immune system is required to generate a large number of different receptors able to recognize diverse epitopes. In a normal adult, the immune "repertoire" is composed of at least 10^7 different receptor specificities at any one time. The diversity of this repertoire is achieved through a ge-netic mechanism involving gene rearrangement, which takes place during development and is described in Secs. 11.2.6 and 11.3.4.

11.2.4 Time Course of an Immune Response

The time course of a normal immune response is illustrated in Fig. 11.2. There is first a lag phase during which the antigen load increases to a certain threshold level (e.g., a virus replicates in the body), yet no measurable response is detected. This is followed by an activation phase during which antigen-presenting cells (APCs) present various antigenic epitopes to lymphocytes. The epitopes are not necessarily immunogenic and the response may be shut down, leading to tolerance (see Sec. 11.2.5); this can occur in the response against tumor cells. Lymphocyte activation is then followed by a measurable response involving the proliferation of antigen-specific clones of lymphoid cells, which rise to some peak level and then fall to a level approaching baseline (Fig. 11.2). The decline in an immune response usually occurs after the antigen has been cleared and the source of stimulation eliminated. However, the process can also be controlled by a feedback mechanism involving regulatory lymphocytes whose function is to secrete cytokines such as IL-10 and transforming growth factor β (TGF-β), which dampen the immune response. These cells, usually specialized T cells, are called *suppressor* (T_s) cells (Bloom et al., 1992).

In a normal immune response, lymphocytes become activated for a brief period of time, undergo clonal expansion, perform their effector function, and return to a quiescent state. Many lymphocytes also die during an immune response through a highly regulated process called *apoptosis* or *programmed cell death* (see Chap. 7, Sec. 7.3) and are eliminated from the body. Some T lymphocytes develop into long-lived *memory cells*, which allow rapid activation of the immune response after re-exposure to the same antigen.

The initial activation step requires that the lymphocyte receive two signals (Fig. 11.3). Signal 1 is occupation of the antigen-specific receptor by the epitope to which it binds, which for B cells may be part of an intact protein but for T cells is made up of peptide fragments presented in association with molecules of the major histocompatibility complex on an APC (see Sec. 11.3.2). Signal 2 is binding of a "costimulatory" receptor to its ligand on the APC. This receptor is not clonally distributed, as is the antigen specific receptor. It is typically CD28 on T cells and CD40 on B cells (June et al., 1994; Noelle,

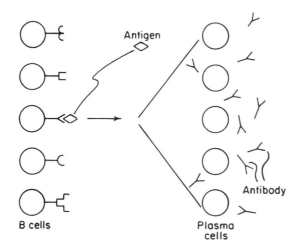

Figure 11.1. Clonal selection. Each T and B lymphocyte carries an antigen receptor of single specificity. Recognition of a particular foreign antigen triggers proliferation and maturation of lymphocytes, which carry receptors that recognize the antigen leading to antigen-specific cytotoxic T cells, or (as illustrated in the figure) to plasma cells that secrete specific antibodies.

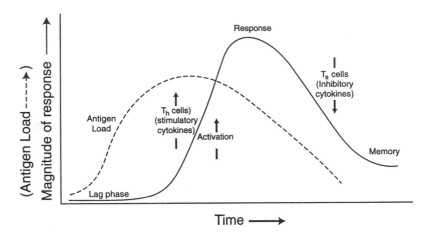

Figure 11.2. Time course of an immune response. After exposure to a foreign antigen, there is a lag phase during which antigen load increases to a threshold level. During the activation phase, antigen presented on antigen-presenting cells (APCs) leads to activation and maturation of specific lymphocytes, stimulated by secretion of cytokines by T-helper (T_h) cells. A subsequent decline in the immune response occurs after clearance of antigen and is mediated by inhibitory cytokines secreted by T-suppressor (T_s) cells and/or the programmed cell death of effector lymphocytes. Specific memory cells remain, which allow more rapid response upon re-exposure to the same antigen.

1996). Its ligand (B7 for T cells) is found only on APCs and distinguishes them from other cells that can present signal 1. In the absence of signal 2, the lymphocyte does not undergo activation. In fact, signals to the T-cell receptor (signal 1) in the absence of adequate costimulation (signal 2) have been found to induce an antigen-specific lymphocyte to enter an unresponsive state (called *anergy*) or even to die by apoptosis (Schwartz, 1996). Given both signal 1 and signal 2, the lymphocyte undergoes *blast transformation* (designated L* in Fig. 11.3), during which the genes required for proliferation become activated. At the same time, the lymphocyte expresses growth factor receptors (GFRs); if the corresponding growth factors (GFs) are present, they will enable the lymphocyte to enter cell cycle and proliferate. Proliferation is required to expand antigen-specific populations of effector cells, memory cells, and immunoregulatory cells. Proliferation continues until differentiation factors (DFs) are encountered, which cause it to stop and immunologic effector function to be expressed (Fig. 11.3). In the absence of GFs, there is no growth and the lymphocyte may die. Growth factors are provided by T_h cells, one example being IL-2. Differentiation factors are also typically provided by T_h cells, one example being interferon γ (IFN-γ). There are large numbers of GFs and DFs that interact in a compli-

cated way, which is only partially understood. By producing these factors, T_h cells act as the major regulators of the magnitude of an immune response (see also Sec. 11.3.5).

The mechanisms that lead to differentiation of T lymphocytes into memory cells (T_m cells) and how they survive and circulate in the body for long periods of time are not known with certainty. T_m cells have less stringent requirements for activation than naive T cells; they respond to a wider variety of cells presenting a given antigen and can be stimulated by lower levels of a stimulating antigen.

11.2.5 Self-Nonself Discrimination and Immunoregulation

One of the most critical functions of the immune system is to distinguish foreign antigens from self antigens and to prevent self antigens from being immunogenic (*self tolerance*). For example, humans have B cells that can recognize both bovine and chicken albumin; antibodies can be produced which distinguish between them. These two albumins are not very different from each other or from human albumin. It seems likely that the process that produces B cells capable of recognizing and distinguishing between bovine and chicken albumin will also produce B cells capable of recognizing human

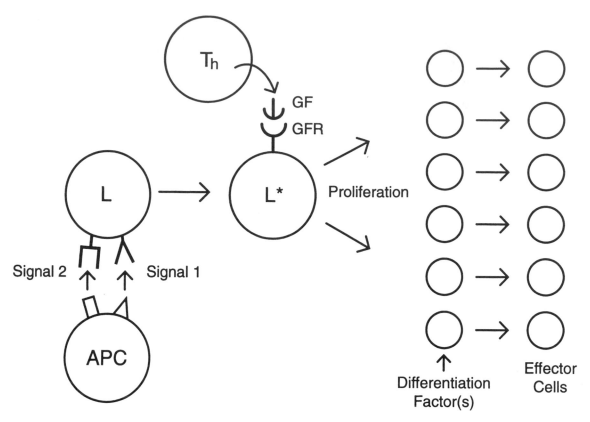

Figure 11.3. Schematic diagram of lymphocyte (L) activation. Initial activation requires two signals: signal 1 is occupation of the antigen-specific receptor, and signal 2 is binding of a costimulatory molecule. For T cells, both are presented on an antigen-presenting cell (APC), as shown, but for B cells, signal 1 may come from an antigenic site of an intact protein. The activated lymphocyte (L*) expresses growth factor receptors (GFRs) and undergoes a proliferative response under the influence of growth factors (GFs) produced by T-helper (T$_h$) cells. Differentiation factors (DFs) induce maturation into lymphoid effector cells (i.e., cytotoxic T lymphocytes or antibody-producing plasma cells).

albumin. These cells, if present, are normally not activated by human albumin in the circulation. One is said to be "tolerant" of self.

Self tolerance is not an innate feature of lymphocytes. Instead, it is learned during the development of immature lymphocytes into mature lymphocytes. Immature T and B cells go through a critical period immediately after expressing antigen-specific receptors on their surfaces, when strong engagement of the receptor causes their apoptotic death. This takes place in the bone marrow (B cells) or thymus (T cells), in which normally only self epitopes will be found. Thus self-reactive cells are eliminated. Surviving lymphocytes mature and are exported to the periphery (von Boehmer, 1988). The signal required for survival is also delivered through the antigen re-

ceptor. For T cells, this process of *positive selection* ensures they can only respond to peptides presented by the MHC molecules present during their development. The result is that the peripheral T-cell receptor repertoire is *MHC restricted.*

The above mechanism for inducing tolerance (known as *central tolerance*) does not eradicate all self-reactive lymphocytes. The bone marrow and thymic environments can induce tolerance only to self antigens that are expressed in these organs (Bonomo and Matzinger, 1993). Many mature T cells carry antigen receptors capable of responding to self antigens found elsewhere in the body. For example, a sample of peripheral blood from any individual will contain T lymphocytes reactive against myelin basic protein (MBP), a major component of the myelin sheath surrounding neurons of the central nervous system. Addition of MBP to a culture of peripheral blood mononuclear cells in vitro will generate a measurable immune response (Wucherpfennig and Strominger, 1995). The polyclonal T-cell response to a foreign agent with multiple epitopes may result in the expansion of clones with receptors that are cross-reactive against self-antigens (Oldstone, 1987). Alternatively, some resting self-reactive T cells may become activated because of the rich supply of cytokines available during an immune response; these bystander responses can also be a source of self-reactivity (Tough et al., 1996).

A number of mechanisms have evolved to prevent potentially self-reactive peripheral T cells from mounting a functional immune response against self antigens. Some of these mechanisms of *peripheral tolerance* are thought to include the following (Schwartz, 1993):

1. Lack of production of T or B cells capable of recognizing the antigen (or "holes in the receptor repertoire")
2. Presence of the antigen in immunologically privileged sites to which circulating lymphocytes do not usually traffic
3. Induction of unresponsiveness or *anergy*, a process in which a self-reactive cell is silenced by an internal biochemical mechanism (see Sec. 11.3.5)
4. Programmed cell death of self-reactive lymphocytes
5. Active suppression of an anti-self response by suppressor lymphocytes that secrete regulatory cytokines
6. Expression of the self antigen in very small amounts, below the threshold required for lymphocyte activation

Failure of the immune system's ability to engage mechanisms of peripheral tolerance results in autoimmune disease. Autoimmune diseases may be organ-specific, such as juvenile-onset diabetes, in which insulin-secreting beta islet cells of the pancreas are destroyed, and multiple sclerosis, in which the myelin sheath insulating the nerves is destroyed. They also include some systemic diseases such as rheumatoid arthritis and systemic lupus erythematosus, which are characterized by high levels of antibody against DNA and common intracellular proteins.

Some of the mechanisms of peripheral tolerance listed above play a role in downregulating a normal immune response after a foreign antigen has been cleared from the system. They can also cause the immune response to be shut down prematurely instead of being activated fully. Nonself components, which should be recognized as foreign by the immune system and destroyed, are then treated as self and are not attacked because of the engagement of a tolerance mechanism that halts lymphocyte activation. Infection with HIV leading to AIDS or with hepatitis B virus leading to chronic liver disease (and sometimes to liver cancer) are examples of diseases where the immune system becomes activated against the foreign agent but then shuts down prematurely owing to the induction of peripheral tolerance mechanisms. If developing tumors have antigens that can be recognized as nonself, it is conceivable that the same factors leading to peripheral tolerance in the immune system also cause failure to mount an effective immune response against cancer (see also Sec. 11.4.3).

11.2.6 Antibodies, Immunoglobulin Receptors, and B-Cell Activation

The basic structure of an antibody molecule is shown in Fig. 11.4. It is composed of four polypeptide chains: two identical large chains referred to as *heavy (H) chains* and two identical small chains re-

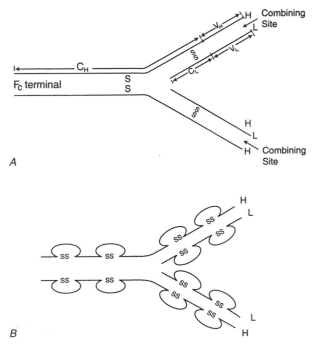

Figure 11.4. *A.* Structure of an antibody molecule (IgG). *B.* Structure of an antibody molecule indicating the presence of domains.

ferred to as *light* (*L*) *chains*. They are joined together by disulfide bonds, as indicated in Fig. 11.4. The antibody molecule has two identical sites capable of recognizing and binding to the antigen that the molecule can recognize. Analysis of the amino acid sequence of many different antibody molecules has shown that each chain consists of a *constant* or *C* region showing relatively little variation and a *variable* or *V* region showing substantial variation. Further analysis has shown that the antigen-combining (binding) site is made up of elements from V regions of both the H and L chains (V_H and V_L). Thus, the V regions of the molecule determine its specificity (Fig. 11.4), while the C region determines its biological function. There are a limited number of different C (F_c) regions that determine the class of antibody. These classes differ in the location in the body in which they are produced and/or in their ability to mediate various biological functions (Table 11.1).

Antibody molecules function in three different ways to elicit the lysis of foreign cells, such as bacteria and fungi, or to facilitate their uptake into host effector cells (Fig. 11.5). First, antibodies can bind to target cells, leaving a coat of antibody molecules over the cell surface—a process called *opsonization*. Phagocytic cells express receptors to the constant F_c portion of the antibody molecules and may engulf the target cell. Second, classes of antibody molecules such as IgM and a subclass of IgG called IgG2b

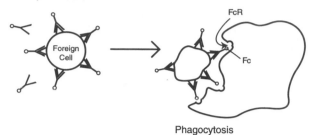

A Opsonization

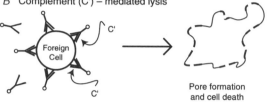

Phagocytosis

B Complement (C') – mediated lysis

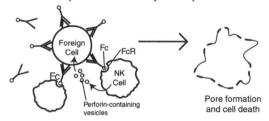

Pore formation
and cell death

C Antibody-directed cellular cytotoxicity

Pore formation
and cell death

Figure 11.5. Processes by which antibodies may lead to lysis of foreign cells. *A.* Opsonization. Specific antibodies coat the foreign cell; antibody F_c portions may then bind to F_c receptors (F_cRs) on phagocytes, and the foreign cell is phagocytosed. *B.* Activation of complement which includes enzymes that cause pore formation in the target cells. *C.* Certain cells, including natural killer (NK) cells, express F_c receptors, which bind to the F_c portion of antibodies, followed by secretion of perforin and granzymes from lytic granules, which cause pore formation in the foreign cell.

Table 11.1. Class of Antibody

Class	Mean Adult Serum Level, mg/mL	Physiologic Function
IgM	1.0	First antibody produced in primary response Fixes complement Good opsonin[a] and agglutinin
IgG	12.0	Produced after IgM in primary response Fixes complement Good opsonin[a] Can cross placenta
IgA	1.8	Localized protection in secretions
IgD	0.03	Function unknown Little secreted Mostly cell-bound
IgE	0.0003	Stimulates mast cells Mediates allergic reactions

[a]Opsonins coat bacteria to facilitate their phagocytosis.

interact via their C regions with the complement system after binding to antigen on the cell surface. The complement system includes a group of enzymes that form pores in a target cell, causing it to lose its membrane integrity and die. Third, certain cells (including natural killer or NK cells) have F_c receptors (FcRs); recognition by the antibody-F_cR complex triggers the secretion of the contents (perforin and granzymes) of cytoplasmic granules that lyse the target cell. This type of killing is termed *antibody-directed cellular cytotoxicity*. These processes can also lead to lysis of tumor cells following recognition of a tumor antigen by an antibody, although cell-mediated immune responses are more important in antitumor immunity (see Secs. 11.3 and 11.4).

There is considerable homology in the amino acid sequences of V_L, C_L, and V_H components of antibody molecules, suggesting that they all evolved from duplicated copies of a single primitive gene. Analysis of C_H suggests that it consists of three such duplicated genes: each encodes a single polypeptide "domain" having a characteristic loop structure formed by disulfide bonds (Fig. 11.4) and referred to as the *immunoglobulin domain*. This domain is also present in other proteins expressed on the surface of lymphocytes and various hemopoietic cells. Examples include the T-cell receptor (see Sec. 11.3.4), the CD4, CD8, CD28, and CD45 antigens, and the cellular adhesion molecule (CAM) group of proteins (see Chap. 9, Sec. 9.2.5). Collectively, these proteins are called the *immunoglobulin superfamily*.

Antibodies with a single specificity are secreted by plasma cells. Much of our knowledge of the structure of antibody molecules has been derived from studies of the protein (myeloma protein) secreted by plasma-cell tumors (called *myelomas*). Plasma cells are mature end-stage cells that have a relatively short life span. Antigenic stimulation of B cells results in a complex series of interactions leading to their activation, proliferation, and differentiation into plasma cells. Each B cell is programmed in its DNA to make an antibody molecule of a single specificity.

The surface antigen receptor on B cells is a transmembrane protein that carries the same immunoglobulin domains and V_L and V_H domains as the antibody that the cell secretes. This B-cell receptor (BCR), called *surface immunoglobulin* (sIg), is associated with a number of additional protein complexes in the plasma membrane that transduce the antigenic signal (see Chap. 6, Sec. 6.6).

Immature B cells carry multiple copies of various antibody gene segments arranged in a "germline configuration." Diversity is produced through a process of gene rearrangement that takes place as the cells develop into mature lymphocytes. One member of each gene family encoding a given segment of the antibody molecule is selected, forming a single gene coding for a complete receptor chain (Tonegawa, 1983; Fig. 11.6). The same process of gene rearrangement occurs during T-lymphocyte development in the thymus gland (see Sec. 11.3.4). Receptor gene rearrangement appears to be largely a random and undirected process, yet it is remarkably successful in producing T and B cells capable of recognizing a vast array of foreign antigens. Variation in the V region is largely restricted to a few small regions. Determination of the three-dimensional structure of an antibody molecule complexed to an antigen has revealed that the highly variable portions of V regions are precisely the parts of the molecule in direct contact with antigen (Amit et al., 1986).

An important additional source of antibody diversity comes from an incompletely understood muta-

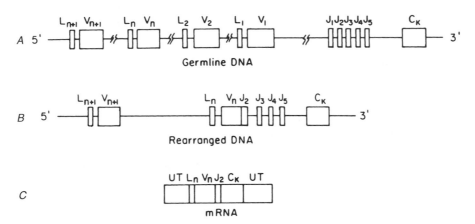

Figure 11.6. Illustration of gene rearrangement to provide antibody molecules of single specificity. *A.* The germline state of DNA; there are a series of V genes each with its own leader (L), a series of J genes, and a single C_K gene. *B.* DNA in a B lymphocyte: gene V_n has been translocated immediately adjacent to J_2. *C.* The whole sequence L_n to C_K plus some untranslated tails (UT) have been transcribed into mRNA. All introns, as well as J_3 to J_5 have been spliced out. The leader sequence is translated but later cleaved off. The illustration applies to the antibody light chain gene, but a similar process of rearrangement occurs in genes encoding the antibody heavy chain and components of the T-cell receptor.

tional mechanism that arises once a B cell has been activated. During proliferation in specialized areas of lymph nodes called *germinal centers,* an extremely high rate of mutation occurs in the rearranged V genes of the activated B-cell clone in precisely those regions already known to be most variable. This process, known as *somatic hypermutation,* results in the production of some receptors with increased affinity for the antigen. B cells in the germinal centers compete for survival signals from persistent antigen on follicular dendritic cells, which are required to prevent apoptosis. Cells with increased affinity have a competitive advantage and are selected to become memory or plasma cells (Nossal, 1992). Somatic hypermutation of the B-cell receptor can cause an increase of 1000-fold or more in the affinity of the antibodies produced.

During an immune response, a broad spectrum of antibody molecules will be produced that differ in both the amino acid sequence of their V region and in the affinity with which they recognize the antigen. Each of the unique amino acid sequences is referred to as an *idiotype.* Sometimes an idiotype can be recognized as an antigen by the immune system, which will make an antibody against it (i.e., an anti-idiotypic antibody). Similarly, the V regions of the T- cell receptor can be presented as antigens by T cells and can also generate anti-idiotypic antibodies. Anti-idiotypic antibodies may be important in immunoregulation, although this remains controversial. Lymphomas frequently arise from clonal populations of activated lymphocytes carrying specific idiotypes, and antibodies against these idiotypes can be used for therapeutic benefit (see Chap. 18, Sec. 18.4.1).

11.3 CELL-MEDIATED IMMUNITY

11.3.1 Transplantation Immunity

Understanding of cell-mediated immunity, involving antigen-specific T cells rather than antibody molecules, has developed from studies of the rejection of transplanted tissue. If a normal tissue (e.g., skin) is transplanted from one unrelated human to another, it is almost always rapidly rejected by an immunologic process. This occurs because the donor and host carry different alleles of genes coding for normal components of the cell surface which are recognized by the immune system; these are called *histocompatibility (H) antigens.* There are a very large number of H antigens; some can lead to a very strong immune rejection response. Tumor cells transferred from one individual to another will be rejected because they express the normal H antigens of the donor. However, the tumor cells may also have some unique cell-surface components that may be immunogeneic (see Sec. 11.4).

Histocompatibility antigens were discovered in experiments in which skin or tumors were transplanted from one mouse to another. Such transplants between outbred mice were almost always unsuccessful. However, if breeding techniques were used to produce mice that were genetically identical, the transplant would "take," and a transplanted tumor would grow to kill the new host. The standard protocol for creating a new inbred mouse strain is to select a brother and sister from a litter, mate them, select a brother and a sister from the ensuing litter, mate them, and so forth. After about twenty generations of inbreeding in this manner, the probability of a genetic locus remaining heterozygous is less than 1 percent (Klein, 1986). Transplants of tissue can be made between mice of the same inbred strain, since they share the same transplantation antigens; this is referred to as *syngeneic* transplantation. Transplants of tissue between mice of different inbred strains (known as *allogeneic* transplants) almost invariably fail unless special measures are taken to prevent immunologic rejection. Transplants from one parent to an F_1 hybrid between two strains usually succeed because the F_1 carries all the H antigens of both parents. These last three statements embody the "laws" of transplantation.

The identification of transplantation antigens was facilitated by the breeding of congenic mice that were genetically similar at all but one genetic locus, which conveyed resistance to transplantation (Klein, 1986). Over fifty histocompatibility (transplantation antigen) genes that confer transplant rejection have been discovered by the breeding of congenic strains. One locus (called H-2 and now known to be a genetic complex) was found to be very much stronger than all the others and is now called the *major histocompatibility complex* (MHC). All other loci are referred to as *minor H* loci. Identifying the components of and understanding the function of the MHC has been central to our current understanding of T cells and cell-mediated immunity.

The MHC antigens in humans have been identified. It was found that the sera of patients who had previously rejected a kidney transplant contained antibodies that reacted against the leukocytes from the blood of the kidney donor. Similarly, sera of multiparous women contain antibodies against leukocytes of the father. Thus, as with mice, humans have alloantigens that cause the production of allospecific antibodies to transplanted donor cells and a cellular immune response that leads to rejection of donated tissues. Using alloantisera collected from immunized volunteers, multiparous women, and transfusion and transplant recipients, at least six genetic loci encoding MHC antigens have been identified in humans. The human MHC products are also termed *human leukocyte antigens* (HLA) because of their initial identification on leukocytes using allospecific antibodies. Molecular genetic techniques of gene cloning and sequencing have identified many different HLA isotypes belonging to each of the six loci (Trowsdale et al., 1991).

Differences in MHC antigens are potent barriers to transplantation. In an outbred population such as humans, syngeneic transplants can be performed only between identical twins. Advances in HLA typing methods have allowed the identification of individuals that are matched in the most highly expressed HLA loci. The success of organ and bone marrow transplants is increased by HLA matching between donor and host. Bone marrow transplantation has had a major impact on the treatment of leukemia.

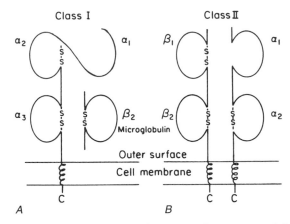

Figure 11.7. Structure of the major histocompatability complex. *A.* Class I molecules are found on the surface of most cells. They are composed of two noncovalently linked chains, α and β. The α chain, also known as the heavy or H chain, is composed of three domains and a C-terminal transmembrane portion. The β chain has a single domain and is referred to as β2 microglobulin. *B.* Class II molecules are found only on specialized cells of the immune system. They are composed of two noncovalently associated chains, α and β, each with two domains and a C-terminal transmembrane portion.

11.3.2 The Major Histocompatibility Complex

The genes encoding products of the major histocompatibility complex (MHC) can be grouped into three different classes. Class I MHC products are glycoproteins expressed on the surface of most cells, whereas class II MHC products are glycoproteins expressed constitutively only on antigen-presenting cells (APCs). Class III MHC products form part of the complement system and include some cytokines such as tumor necrosis factor-α (TNF-α).

In the mouse, there are three different genes coding for three class I products called K, D, and L (or H-2K, H-2D, and H-2L). Class II products are coded for in a subregion of the MHC locus designated as the I region. Two class II isotypes (I-A and I-E) are expressed on the surface of some immunocompetent cells of mice. In humans, there are three different class I loci, HLA-A, HLA-B, and HLA-C, and three different class II products, referred to as HLA-DP, HLA-DQ, and HLA-DR. Proteins encoded by the class I and II genes in mice and humans are similar in structure. Both are transmembrane heterodimers. The class I protein (Fig. 11.7A) consists of a transmembrane heavy (H) chain of approximately 45,000 molecular weight containing three extracellular domains. It associates noncovalently

with a β_2-microglobulin light chain of 12,000 molecular weight. For class II, two transmembrane chains called α (32,000 molecular weight) and β (28,000 molecular weight) are found in association (Fig. 11.7B); each consists of two domains. Both class I and class II proteins are members of the immunoglobulin superfamily; all membrane-proximal domains are homologous to the basic immunoglobulin domain (see Fig. 11.4).

In addition to having two or more loci of the class I and II genes, the MHC has an added degree of complexity called *allelic polymorphism*. Two or more different forms of a gene at a given genetic locus are called *alleles*. Polymorphic alleles can either be homozygous, when the same allele is expressed on both chromosomes (one from either parent), or heterozygous, when the two alleles are different. In outbred populations, such as wild mice or humans, the MHC loci are usually heterozygous with multiple alleles.

Most of the polymorphism in these MHC molecules occurs in the outermost extracellular domains, [i.e., the α_1 and α_2 domains of class I and the α_1 and β_1 domains of class II (Fig. 11.7)], which form the floor and flanking regions of a binding cleft involved in binding and presenting antigenic peptides to T lymphocytes (Bjorkman et al., 1987; Brown et al.,

1993). There are two α-helices in the peptide-binding groove of class II MHC molecules, which form a pocket open-ended on both ends, whereas the peptide-binding pocket in class I is closed on both ends. The result is that class II molecules bind significantly longer peptide fragments (15 to 18 amino acids in length) than class I molecules (8 to 11 amino acids). Note that particular alleles of a given class I or II locus will bind different peptides because of differences in structure of the binding cleft. Thus, different peptides binding to different MHC subtypes will yield different three-dimensional structures for recognition by the T-cell receptor on T lymphocytes. Moreover, a given peptide antigen may be efficiently bound and presented by one MHC subtype for T-cell binding but not another subtype. A result of this polymorphism is that immune responses to a given antigen vary between different individuals (humans) or inbred strains (mice): some strains produce antibodies to the antigen, while others given the same antigen do not (Benaceraff and McDevitt, 1972). Cellular immune responses controlled by CTLs recognizing class I antigens are also found to have strain-to-strain variation.

These differences in MHC-peptide interactions and T-cell responses caused by MHC polymorphism can convey benefit to the immune system. During an immune response to an infectious agent, certain "dominant" peptide epitopes are generated and presented to the immune system by APCs (Vanderlugt and Miller, 1996). The polymorphic nature of class I and II MHC molecules ensures that within a population containing many allelic forms of MHC, at least some of these peptides are immunogenic and capable of stimulating humoral and cell-mediated immunity. Subtypes of HLA may have been selected in different areas of the world in accordance with how efficiently they presented dominant epitopes from various endemic pathogens in order to confer protective immunity.

Peptides become associated with class I and II MHC via different pathways (Germain, 1994). Class I MHC proteins present peptides from intracellular proteins that have been produced by a cytoplasmic protease complex called the *proteosome* (Koopman et al, 1997). Class I H chain is produced from mRNA on the rough endoplasmic reticulum and extruded into the lumen of the endoplasmic reticulum. Here, the newly formed class I molecules are loaded with peptide fragments from intracellular proteins that have also been transported into the lumen of the endoplasmic reticulum by a specific group of transport proteins called TAPs (ATP-dependent trans-

porters associated with antigen processing) (Elliott, 1997; Fig. 11.8A). Peptides loaded onto class I molecules must be very short, in the range of 8 to 11 amino acids in length, and must also have particular amino acids in particular positions in order to bind with high affinity. Both peptides from proteins degraded during normal metabolic functioning and peptides generated from infectious agents can be presented. The peptide-loaded class I H chains become associated with β_2 microglobulin and are further glycosylated in the Golgi apparatus. They are then inserted into the plasma membrane (Fig. 11.8A). Some class I protein is not loaded with peptide in the endoplasmic reticulum (called *empties*). However, these empties are usually unstable at the cell surface and their function is unclear. The antigen processing and presentation pathway is quite rapid and efficient in most cells; inflammatory cytokines such as interferon γ (IFN-γ) increase the activity of this process.

Since class I MHC molecules are constitutively expressed on most somatic cells, presentation of intracellular peptides on class I MHC molecules can be considered a way for cells to reveal their intracellular contents to the immune system. The presence of foreign antigens would result in a peptide-MHC complex that could be recognized by a T cell and initiate an immune response.

Although class II MHC molecules are usually found only on specialized cells of the immune system such as APCs and epithelial cells of the thymus gland, some tissues can express class II molecules after exposure to inflammatory cytokines such as IFN-γ and TNF-α (Bottazzo et al., 1983). Vascular endothelium, intestinal epithelium, melanocytes, and astrocytes and Schwann cells of the central nervous system are examples. The function of class II MHC molecules is to present extracellular antigens to T cells. Class II MHC molecules are also synthesized in the endoplasmic reticulum. They are prevented from binding to peptides because they associate with a molecule called the *I* (*invariant*) *chain* which blocks access to the binding cleft (Germain, 1994). Extracellular proteins are taken up via fluid-phase endocytosis into vesicles, which fuse with and eventually bind to secretory vesicles that contain the class II MHC–I chain complexes. In the acidic milieu of the fused vesicles, the I chain dissociates and proteases cleave the proteins into peptides. If they have particular amino acids in the right position, the peptides are loaded into the free binding cleft of the class II MHC molecules and shuttled to the cell surface (Fig. 11.8B).

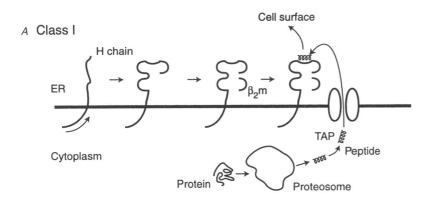

A Class I

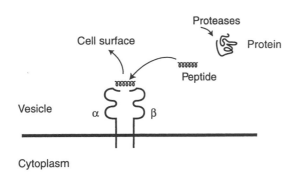

B Class II

Figure 11.8. Schematic of presentation of peptides on antigen-presenting cells in association with MHC molecules. *A.* Intracellular peptides are transported into the endoplasmic reticulum (ER) and interact with H chains of class I MHC molecules. Peptides of 8 to 11 amino acids are produced by the proteosome and are transported into the ER by transport proteins (TAPs). They may fit in the closed polymorphic peptide-binding groove formed by α-helices and are then presented on the cell surface. *B.* Extracellular proteins are ingested in vesicles and broken down into peptides. The vesicles fuse with transport vesicles from the endoplasmic reticulum, where peptides of 15 to 18 amino acids may fit in the open polymorphic peptide-binding pocket formed by α-helices of the α and β chains of class II MHC molecules. They are then presented on the cell surface.

The variation in peptide binding by different MHC molecules is likely to impose important limitations to the potential use of CTLs in immunotherapy of cancer. Cytotoxic T lymphocytes reactive against tumor antigens will recognize them in association with specific class I MHC products; the response is said to be *MHC-restricted*. Given that the MHC is extremely polymorphic, it is unlikely that CTLs from one individual would kill tumor cells from a second, even if the two tumors had the same tissue of origin and shared common tumor-specific antigens.

11.3.3 T Lymphocytes

Mature, postthymic T lymphocytes serve various functions in the adaptive immune system. In cell-mediated immunity, CTLs kill target cells infected with intracellular pathogens whose antigens are presented as foreign peptides by class I MHC proteins. Cytotoxic T lymphocytes may also kill tumor cells that present nonself antigens through a variety of mechanisms that are described in Sec. 11.4.2.

Most CTLs are distinguished by expressing the CD8 coreceptor on their surfaces. The second major class of T cells, the T-helper (T_h) cells, express a surface coreceptor called CD4, which binds to class II MHC. CD4 strengthens the interaction between the T-cell receptor and the antigenic complex on the APC. The main function of T_h cells is the secretion of cytokines required for the proliferation and differentiation of antigen-activated CD4$^+$ and CD8$^+$ T cells, and B cells. A variety of cytokines are secreted by activated CD4$^+$ and some CD8$^+$ T cells. Proteins expressed on the surface of T_h cells also serve as ligands for important signaling complexes on B cells such as CD40; CD40 signaling is required for cell survival in germinal centers of the spleen and lymph nodes, where B-cell proliferation and hypermutation take place. Mutations impairing the function of CD40 are responsible for X-linked hyperimmunoglobulin M (IgM) syndrome in humans, which is characterized by a loss of IgG production and humoral immunity (Noelle, 1996).

A further level of complexity in T-lymphocyte biology is based on the fact that T_h cells are divided into (at least) three categories—T_h1, T_h2, and T_h0—on the basis of the cytokines they secrete (Mosmann and Coffman, 1989). T_h1 cells secrete IL-2, IL-3, IFN-γ, TNF-α, TNF-β, and granulocyle macrophage colony-stimulating factor (GM-CSF). These cytokines facilitate cell-mediated or CTL-based immunity and the production of immunoglobulin G isoforms that can interact with the complement system to lyse target antigen-bearing cells (see Table 11.1). T_h2 cells secrete IL-3, IL-4, IL-5, IL-10, IL-13, TNF-α, and GM-CSF. These T_h2 cytokines are not involved in cell-mediated immunity, but rather generate immunoglobulin secretion. T_h1 cells and CTLs require IL-2 for proliferation, while T_h2 cells utilize IL-4. The third category of CD4$^+$ T cells, T_h0, secrete mixtures of both T_h1 and T_h2 lymphokines.

Once an immune response is biased to make T_h1 cells, production of T_h2 cells is actively suppressed by the T_h1 cytokines and vice versa. Thus primary immune responses in vivo can be dominated by a T_h1 or a T_h2 cytokine profile that can profoundly affect the immune response. For example, responses to some parasitic infections (e.g., *Leishmania major*) are skewed toward a T_h2 phenotype (antibody response) in some mouse strains while being predominately of a T_h1-type (CTL response) in other strains. Mice that mount a T_h1 response rapidly reject the *Leishmania* and survive; those that mount a T_h2 response succumb to the disease (Bretscher et al., 1992). In humans, a number of autoimmune diseases such as systemic lupus erythematosus (SLE) and allergic reactions are associated with a predominance of T_h2-secreted cytokines. It is possible that this skewing toward T_h1 or T_h2 responses against certain antigens has evolved as a protective mechanism. Antibody-mediated (T_h2) responses are inherently weaker and usually less immediately deleterious for the host than T_h1-mediated responses, since they cannot generate CTLs or the secretion of complement-fixing antibodies. However, T_h2 responses may be deleterious in the long term, as indicated by the morbidity and mortality associated with SLE and some chronic viral infections. For example, recent evidence suggests that chronic infection with HIV leading to acquired immunodeficiency syndrome (AIDS) results from a dominant T_h2 response which prevents the host from mounting a protective CTL response against the virus (Clerici and Shearer, 1994). Whether an individual mounts a predominantly T_h1 or T_h2 response against a given antigen depends on the antigen, the antigen dose, and (unknown) genetically determined elements in the individual. Professional APCs at different sites may direct T-helper cells to either T_h1 or T_h2 responses. For example, APCs in the spleen promote T_h1 responses, whereas those in the mesenteric nodes promote T_h2 responses (Everson et al., 1996).

A final category of T cells, less well defined, includes immunoregulatory cells (also called *suppressor* or T_s cells), which secrete cytokines such as IL-10, IL-4, and TGF-β, which inhibit the generation of CTLs. Cells from both the CD4$^+$ and CD8$^+$ subsets can have suppressor-like properties. T_s cells can inhibit cell-mediated immune responses and prevent reactivity against self antigens. However, they may also be harmful if they shut down cell-mediated immune responses against foreign antigens. Activated T cells, can also induce tolerance by acting as "deletional APC" or "veto cells" that present antigen to other activated T cells (Miller, 1986). Here, CTL precursors are inactivated, perhaps through a death process, after contact with a veto cell.

11.3.4 The T-Cell Receptor

The T-cell receptor (TCR) consists of two disulfide-linked transmembrane protein subunits belonging to the immunoglobulin superfamily of proteins (Hedrick et al., 1984; Yanagi et al., 1984; Fig. 11.9A). The TCR is expressed in two forms: $\alpha\beta$ and $\gamma\delta$. The $\alpha\beta$ TCR is expressed on 90 to 95 percent of the T cells (called $\alpha\beta$ T cells) found in the blood, thymus, lymph nodes, and spleen. The other type of T cells (called $\gamma\delta$ T cells) are rare in the circulation and in lymphoid organs but are present in very large numbers in the epidermis and intestinal epithelium, such that the total number of $\gamma\delta$ T cells greatly exceeds the total number of $\alpha\beta$ T cells (Raulet, 1989). Their function remains speculative. The following sections focus on $\alpha\beta$ T cells.

The α and β subunits of the TCR are characterized by having one or two major looplike structures in the extracellular amino-terminal half of the protein formed by disulfide bridges. The α and β subunits are also held together near the outer surface of the plasma membrane by an intersubunit disulfide bridge, which adds stability to the complex. Like antibody molecules (Sec. 11.2.6), $\alpha\beta$ TCR molecules have enormous diversity and recognize a very large number of antigens presented by MHC molecules on APCs. The loop closest to the amino-terminus (N) in the extracellular region of each TCR subunit contains the variable (V) regions that bind antigen. The second, inner looplike structure in both α and β subunits consists of the TCR constant (C) regions. The V and C regions are connected by a joining region, or J segment in the case of the α

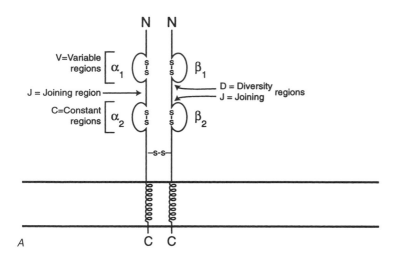

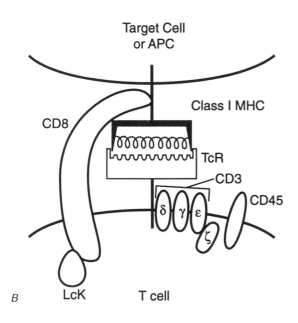

Figure 11.9. Structure of the T-cell receptor. *A.* The αβ form of the T-cell receptor (TCR) is composed of two chains, α and β, each of about 45 kDa molecular weight and held together by a disulfide bond. Each chain contains two domains and a C-terminal transmembrane portion. The N-terminal α_1 and β_1 domains contain antigen recognition sequences and are highly variable. The α_2, β_2, and transmembrane portions are nearly invariant (C region). The domains are linked by joining (J) regions and in the β chain by an additional diversity (D) region. *B.* Engagement of the TCR initiates signaling. The TCR has a short cytoplasmic tail, and other proteins—including the CD3 complex, ζ, CD4 or CD8, Lck, and CD45—are involved in signal transduction.

subunit, while in the β subunit both a J segment and a diversity or D region are present (Fig. 11.9*A*). The gene encoding the TCR is rearranged during T-cell maturation in the thymus: V regions in the germline configuration recombine with J and D regions to code for a mature αβ TCR capable of recognizing antigen in the context of MHC protein. This process of gene rearrangement [called *V(D)J recombination*] is analogous to that which leads to diversity in the generation of immunoglobulin molecules (see Fig. 11.6). A major difference is that T-cell receptors do not undergo somatic mutation during an immune response.

The cytoplasmic tails of both α and β subunits of the TCR consist of only short stretches of 3 to 4 amino acids, so that the TCR cannot participate directly in intracellular signaling. In mature peripheral T cells the TCR complex is always associated with two sets of transmembrane signaling proteins—the CD3 complex and the ζ family, each of which has more extensive (30 to 40 amino acids) intracytoplasmic domains (Fig. 11.9*B*; Janeway, 1992). The CD3 complex consists of three different proteins, ε, γ, and δ, each having N-terminal extracellular domains whose ligands (if any) are unknown. The ε subunit is the main intracellular signaling molecule, and associates with either the γ or δ subunits via disulfide bonds at the cell surface. The ζ family is almost entirely intracellular and consists of three proteins. All three can form homodimers as well as heterodimers via disulfide bridges outside the main CD3 complex. Antibodies to either CD3ε or the ζ chain can activate T cells without engagement of the TCR and generate a similar signaling cascade to that following antigen binding, suggesting that the CD3 and ζ protein complexes are the major signaling moieties in the TCR complex (Irving and Weiss, 1991).

In addition to the CD3 complex, the TCR is associated with one of the two coreceptor proteins that functionally distinguish the two major T-cell subsets, CD4 or CD8. The CD4 and CD8 complexes bind to the α_2 domain of class II MHC molecules and the α_3 domain of class I MHC molecules, respectively. Following antigen binding, they are drawn into the TCR-CD3 complex and increase the avidity of binding of the TCR to the peptide-MHC complex. They then also participate in intracellular signaling by associating with a tyrosine kinase called p56 Lck that phosphorylates a number of substrates during T-cell activation (Fig. 11.9B; Janeway, 1992; see also Chap. 6, Sec. 6.6, and Fig. 6.11).

One other important signaling protein involved in T-cell activation is CD45, a transmembrane protein having intrinsic tyrosine phosphatase activity in its intracytoplasmic region (Fig. 11.9B; Justement, 1997). CD45 is also a member of the immunoglobulin superfamily of receptors (Chap. 6, Sec. 6.6.1). A potential ligand for CD45 has not been identified. Two main isoforms of CD45 are expressed on the surface of human T lymphocytes and correlate with the developmental and activation state of the T cell. The main human isoform, CD45RA, is expressed mainly on naive, previously unactivated T cells and is downregulated following T-cell activation and proliferation. In contrast, a lower-molecular-weight isoform in humans, CD45RO, is found only on the surface of activated T cells and is especially prominent on both resting and proliferating memory cells. CD45 plays a crucial role during T-cell activation by dephosphorylating a negative regulatory tyrosine residue in the carboxyl-terminal end of members of the Src family of kinases such as p56 Lck, which are required for TCR signaling (see following section and Chap. 6, Sec. 6.6.1).

11.3.5 Activation of T Lymphocytes: Inter- and Intracellular Signaling

The central feature of a primary immune response is the induction and modulation of lymphocyte proliferation following antigen-receptor engagement. Multiple signals are required for the efficient activation of CTLs following antigen presentation by APCs; these are indicated schematically in Fig. 11.10. The interaction of APCs with CD4$^+$ T-helper (T$_h$) cells induces the secretion of IL-2 and IFN-γ. T$_h$ cells and activated macrophages also secrete TNF-α. Specific CTL precursors become activated through TCR recognition of antigen on class I MHC molecules in association with costimulation; IL-2 is then necessary for the expansion of antigen-specific clones. Following expansion of the CD8$^+$ clone, IFN-γ and TNF-α are required for the differentiation of mature CTLs capable of lysing cells carrying the target antigen (Fig. 11.10). The nature and timing of the cytokine signals are critical to this process: lack of IL-2 usually aborts development of CTLs; in the absence of IFN-γ, there is significant proliferation but no functional CTLs are produced. However, release of IFN-γ at too early a stage induces terminal differentiation before the CTL clone has undergone expansion.

Once activated, both CTLs and T$_h$ cells can be maintained as cell lines in tissue culture by restimulating them regularly with a fresh source of APCs carrying the appropriate antigen and (for CTLs) by providing a source of IL-2. Large quantities of recombinant cytokines such as IL-2 are now available, and the culture of CTLs that may react with antigens expressed on human tumors is being investigated as an approach to immunotherapy (see Chap. 18, Sec. 18.3).

The activation of T lymphocytes by APCs requires the interaction of two major signaling pathways (see Figs. 11.3 and 11.10). These are (1) primary signals generated through the TCR complex and its associated coreceptors (CD4 and CD8 complexes), as described in Sec. 11.3.4, and (2) secondary or "costimulatory" signals generated through the CD28 complex on the surface of T lymphocytes. CD28 signaling is necessary to turn on the full extent of lymphokine secretion (e.g., IL-2, IFN-γ) by CD4$^+$ T$_h$ cells in order to trigger lymphocyte proliferation and differentiation.

Signal 1 (transmembrane signaling through the TCR-CD3 complex) leads to (Berridge, 1997): (1) activation of tyrosine kinases associated with the TCR-CD3 complex and its coreceptors, causing tyrosine phosphorylation of intracellular substrates; (2) activation of phospholipase C-γ (PLC-γ), which leads to the production of the second messengers inositol triphosphate and diacylglycerol, which in turn, raise intracellular calcium and stimulate protein kinase C; and (3) activation of the p21 ras sig-

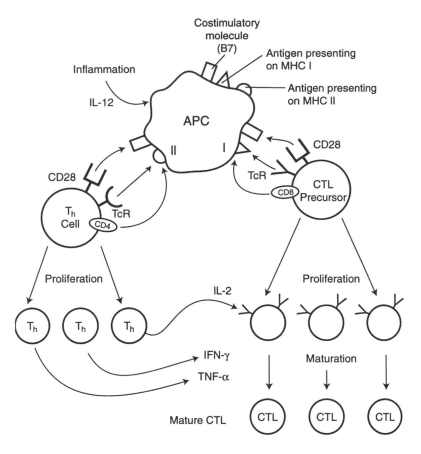

Figure 11.10. Activation of cytotoxic T lymphocytes (CTLs). Presentation of antigens on MHC molecules of antigen-presenting cells (APCs) is stimulated by cytokines such as IL-12. Dual signals with the T-cell receptor (TCR) and the CD28 receptor for costimulatory molecules cause antigen-specific activation of both T-helper (T_h) cells expressing CD4 and CTL precursors expressing CD8. Proliferation of CTLs requires IL-2 produced by T_h cells, and their maturation requires other cytokines including IFN-γ and TNF-α. A complex series of other signaling complexes on T cells lead to secretion of other stimulatory or inhibitory cytokines which regulate the immune response.

naling pathway leading to the activation of the *mitogen-associated protein kinase* (MAPK) cascade, which consists of a series of serine/threonine phosphorylation events (see Chap. 6; Fig. 6.4). Signals generated through the TCR-CD3 complex activate a number of nuclear transcription factors responsible for secretion of cytokines (e.g., IL-2) and expression of growth factor receptors (e.g., IL-2R) required for T-cell proliferation.

Signal 2 (CD28 costimulation) also involves a series of tyrosine phosphorylation events in the cell, which turn on a transcription factor called CD28RC (Rudd, 1996). CD28RC cooperates with a number of other transcription factors generated via TCR signaling and strongly augments the production of IL-2 and other cytokines, such as IFN-γ and TNF-α.

The CD28 complex is expressed as a homodimer (44,000 molecular weight) with a cytoplasmic domain capable of interacting with a number of signaling proteins including tyrosine kinases. In mice, it is expressed on all $CD4^+$ and $CD8^+$ T cells, while in humans it is found on all $CD4^+$ T cells and approximately half of all $CD8^+$ T cells (June et al., 1994). CD28 signaling is induced by the interaction of the CD28 complex with a member of the B7 family of

proteins expressed on professional APCs. The expression of these proteins is tightly regulated and can be turned off by cytokines such as IL-10 (Pretolani and Goldman, 1997). The need for two signals, together with the limited expression of the B7 counterreceptor for CD28, places a severe restriction on when and where a productive immune response against a given antigen can be generated. It also places a severe restriction on the generation of antitumor immune responses, since most tumor cells and other nonprofessional APCs do not express the B7 family of proteins.

A number of other cell-surface complexes on T lymphocytes—such as Thy 1.2, CD2, CD5, and CD7—have also been found to mediate activation signals that can trigger cytokine secretion and T-cell proliferation. These complexes require the presence of a functional CD3 complex in order to initiate signaling, and signals induced by ligand binding of CD2 or Thy 1.2 are similar to those induced by engagement of the TCR. These alternative activation pathways may serve to augment T-cell activation through the TCR or may induce activation of T cells in an antigen-independent manner (Bierer and Burakoff, 1989). This may be important in responses against tumor cells, some of which express the ligand for CD2 called *leukocyte functional antigen-3* (LFA-3; Wingren et al., 1995).

The development of "gene targeted mutagenesis," by which the expression of specific genes can be "knocked out" in mice (see Chap. 3, Sec. 3.3.12), has further delineated the importance of the various molecules and signaling pathways involved in T-cell activation. This technology has made possible the production of mice lacking the expression of a variety of T-cell and signaling proteins, including CD4, CD8, CD28, IL-2, IL-4, IL-10, TAP-1, $\beta2$ microglobulin, Lck, and class II MHC molecules (Mittrucker et al., 1995). Work with knockout mice has not only confirmed the importance of the various signaling pathways described above but also uncovered new pathways involved in control of the cellular immune response.

11.3.6 Geography of T-Cell Activation

Naive T cells circulate in the blood and lymphatics and can be activated only when they encounter antigen on antigen presenting cells (APCs) in the secondary lymphoid organs such as the spleen and lymph nodes. After activation, T cells proliferate and differentiate into effector and memory T cells. These cells leave the secondary lymphoid organs and traffic back to the site where an effector response takes place. Not only do lymph nodes serve as repositories for lymphocytes and APCs, but they also facilitate interactions between these cell types. Antigens are picked up by APCs, especially dendritic cells, at sites of inflammation; this process induces the migration of the cells to local lymph nodes where they attach to a protein matrix. T cells entering the lymph nodes are able to survey the APCs attached to the matrix and become activated when a specific T-cell receptor binds to a target antigen. Thus the lymphoid organs are sites where foreign antigens are presented to T cells within a structural framework that ensures maximal contact with APCs and allows for high local concentrations of cytokines that are required for T-cell proliferation and differation. The amount of stimulating antigen required for an optimal response is also controlled in the secondary lymphoid organs. In the presence of too much antigen, which may occur at the effector site, T cells may die (Zinkernagel et al., 1997).

Activation of lymphocytes in specific lymphoid organs helps to imprint the location of the effector site. T cells activated in draining lymph nodes of the skin tend to home back to the skin, where the path-

ogenic insult was located, whereas T cells activated in mesenteric lymph nodes home back to the intestine. One mechanism for this specific homing is thought to involve the upregulation of a class of molecules called *selectins*, which recognize molecules called *addressins* (Salmi and Jalkanen, 1997). For example, the cutaneous leukocyte antigens (CLA) are upregulated on T cells activated in lymph nodes draining the skin, and direct effector T cells to inflammatory sites by binding to E-selectin on cutaneous endothelial cells. Naive T cells home to peripheral lymph nodes by their expression of L-selectin, which binds mainly to the addressin Gly-CAM-1 on the high endothelial venules of the lymph nodes (Salmi and Jalkanen, 1997).

The above discussion applies to the overwhelming majority of circulating T cells expressing the $\alpha\beta$ form of the T-cell receptor (see Sec. 11.3.4). T cells expressing the $\gamma\delta$ form of the receptor are almost all fixed in epithelial tissue. It has been hypothesized that they respond to epithelial stress by the secretion of cytokines that mobilize APCs and initiate a response by circulating T cells expressing the $\alpha\beta$ receptor (Boismenu et al., 1996).

Activation of tumor-specific T cells is also most likely to take place in draining lymph nodes (Kundig et al., 1995). Leukemias and other hematologic malignancies may localize in multiple lymph nodes. For solid tumors, either living or dead cells may enter the nodes through lymphatics, where tumor antigens are taken up by APCs and presented to T cells (see Chap. 18; Fig. 18.1). Alternatively, tumor antigens may be shed at the primary site and picked up by local macrophages or dendritic cells that carry them to the draining lymph nodes, where they can activate a response. Failure of these processes to occur—for example, in slowly growing nonnecrotic tumors—may prevent the immune system from recognizing the presence of the tumor—even if it expresses nonself antigens, until it has achieved a large size.

11.3.7 Natural Killer Cells

Natural killer (NK) cells stand on the border between the innate and acquired immune systems. They exhibit spontaneous cytotoxic activity against many virus-infected and tumor cells. They release factors that aid the activation of the acquired immune system and also stimulate their own activation and proliferation. How NK cells recognize their targets is only now becoming clear (Kumar et al., 1997). It appears that they can adhere to most myelolymphoid cells (and perhaps other cells) via an activation receptor [ligand(s) unknown] and cause lysis unless an inhibitory receptor on the NK cell is engaged by a ligand on the potential target cell. This ligand is associated with class I MHC molecules, and the population of NK cells from an individual has multiple different inhibitory receptors recognizing different class I MHC molecules. A particular NK cell will have at least one (and perhaps several) receptors recognizing one (or more) self class I MHC alleles. Thus lysis of target cells by NK cells is prevented by recognition of a self marker, class I MHC. A peculiar consequence of this mechanism for regulating NK lysis is that NK cells from the progeny of inbred parental mouse strains A and B will kill targets from either parent. Targets of parent A are killed because they lack MHC class I antigens of parent B, which are necessary to inhibit NK cells that carry the "B strain" inhibitory receptor, and vice versa. Thus NK cells can lead to graft rejection when allogeneic bone marrow is transplanted, not because the bone marrow carries foreign antigens (whose presence might trigger rejection by T cells) but because the bone marrow lacks self MHC markers of the host (Ljunggren and Karre, 1990).

Many tumors, particularly myelolymphoid tumors, are good NK targets. Cells in at least some of these tumors have low or absent expression of one or more class I MHC molecules. Other tumors that are good NK targets have apparently normal expression of class I MHC molecules; it is not known why they are targets.

If one takes human peripheral blood lymphocytes and incubates them in vitro with very high levels of IL-2, some proliferate and differentiate into aggressive killer cells with NK-like activity. These are referred to as LAK (lymphokine-activated killer) cells and develop from both NK cells and T cells. When LAK cells are generated from a cancer patient and reinfused into the patient, there is sometimes evidence of tumor regression. However, there are also very toxic side effects that have limited the widespread application of the procedure (Rosenberg, 1988).

11.4 TUMOR IMMUNITY

In order for the immune system to respond to a tumor, it must recognize tumor antigens that are viewed as nonself—i.e., that differ from antigens expressed by normal tissues in the same individual. The evidence for such antigens and the effects of immune responses induced by them are summarized in the present section. Approaches to immunotherapy, and other biological mechanisms that

might lead to tumor destruction are described in Chap. 18.

11.4.1 Tumor Antigens

Tumor antigens may be either intracellular components that are broken down into peptides 8 to 11 amino acids in length and presented in the peptide-binding cleft of MHC class I molecules or slightly larger extracellular components that are shed from tumor cells and presented on MHC class II molecules (Sec. 11.3.2). It is expected that tolerance will have developed to all such peptides from normal cells. However, the expanding knowledge of molecular properties of tumors indicates that various proteins may be mutated or otherwise modified during tumor development. Some of the possible categories of tumor antigens include the following (see also Chap. 18, Sec. 18.1):

1. *Point mutations in oncogenes or tumor suppressor genes (see Chap. 5, Secs. 5.4 and 5.5).* Some transforming events are caused by point mutations. Peptides derived from the region of the protein that includes the resulting amino acid change would be novel compared with peptides derived from the normal protein. If these altered peptides can bind to class I MHC molecules, they may be recognized by T cells. For example, point mutations in the p53 gene can lead to activation of some T cells (Theobald et al., 1995).

2. *Chromosomal rearrangements.* The breakpoint region of the rearranged gene will encode a novel peptide structure that has not been encountered previously by the immune system. If a peptide that includes the breakpoint can bind to a class I molecule, it may also trigger a T-cell response. Peptides from the *bcr-abl* transcript that is characteristic of chronic myelogenous leukemia (see Chap. 4, Sec. 4.3.2, and Chap. 5, Sec. 5.4.4) have been able to stimulate T-cell responses (Bocchia et al., 1996).

3. *Adult expression of developmental genes.* Some genes are expressed only during embryonic development and not in adult life. Consequently, either the immune system never encountered peptides derived from these gene products or the original state of tolerance may wane with time. During oncogenesis, some of these fetal antigens may be re-expressed and become tumor antigens. Some human tumor antigens fall into this category. The MAGE-1 gene is present but not expressed in normal cells, but is expressed in some melanoma cells. It was found to be a tumor anti-

gen by studying T-cell clones reactive against melanoma cells. The cDNA from a melanoma expression library was transfected into APCs that did not otherwise stimulate the T cells. The melanoma antigens were then determined from those genes that caused proliferation. A peptide encoded by the third exon of the MAGE-1 gene bound to the HLA-A1 protein and stimulated the T-cell clones (Van der Bruggen et al., 1991).

4. *Overexpression of adult genes.* Some proteins are normally expressed at levels too low for peptides derived from them to activate T cells. Upregulation of protein levels during malignant transformation may increase the number of presenting MHC molecules on the cell surface to a level sufficient for T-cell activation. This number has been shown to be of the order of 100 (Christinck et al., 1991). An example of a protein that may be a tumor antigen by this mechanism is the HER-2/neu gene in breast cancer (see Chap. 5, Sec. 5.4.3).

5. *Changes in carbohydrate structures.* Some tumors express altered carbohydrate structures (Ragupathi, 1996). These changes are potentially recognizable by some T cells, especially those expressing the γδ form of the T-cell receptor (Sieling et al., 1996). They may also be recognized by immunoglobulins.

A list of some human tumor antigens that have been associated with an antitumor immune response is provided in Chap. 18, Table 18.1.

11.4.2 Immune Surveillance

If tumors express tumor-specific antigens that can be presented to T cells, then many potential cancers might be eradicated prior to their clinical detection. This theory of immune surveillance has long been the topic of heated discussion. Proponents argue that mutations leading to malignant transformation are common, and that without immune surveillance, cancer would be a much more common disease. Opponents point out that although the incidence of cancer is increased in immune-suppressed individuals such as recipients of organ transplants, this increase is largely limited to lymphoid tumors, which might arise as a result of mutagenic effects of the immunosuppressive therapy itself.

Although the extent of immune surveillance remains unknown, it is clear that some tumors are immunogenic in the original host in the sense that they present antigenic determinants that can be recognized by receptors on T and/or B cells. Many solid tumors contain infiltrating lymphocytes. Cytotoxic T lymphocytes that have been activated in draining lymph nodes to recognize tumor antigen(s) may traffic back to the growing tumor. This localization may depend on recognition of tumor antigens (probably an inefficient process) or upregulation of adhesion molecules and vascular addressins on endothelial cells at the tumor site (see Sec. 11.3.6). Within the tumor, activated CTLs may kill tumor cells by several mechanisms (Fig. 11.11):

1. *Granule exocytosis.* Granules in CTLs and NK cells contain a number of proteins, including perforin and proteases of the granzyme family. When T cells or NK cells bind their targets, the contents of these granules are released into the region of cell contact. Perforin polymerizes in the membrane of the target tumor cells, forming pores. It is thought that during the repair of these pores, the granzymes are internalized by pinocytosis. They subsequently cleave cytoplasmic molecules that control apoptosis, causing a proteolytic cascade resulting in cell death (Kagi et al., 1996).

2. *Fas-Fas ligand interactions.* Activated T cells express the Fas ligand. Target tumor cells that express the Fas antigen (a protein that can signal cells to undergo cell death) are induced to undergo apoptosis upon binding to the Fas ligand (Nagata, 1997).

3. *Tumor necrosis factor.* Tumor necrosis factor (TNF) is a member of the same gene superfamily as Fas, and TNF secreted by T cells can cause the death of cells expressing TNF receptors (Korner and Sedgwick, 1996).

4. *Recruitment of T-helper cells.* Activated T_h cells that are recruited to the tumor site secrete a number of inflammatory cytokines. For example, IL-2 increases the number of CTLs and also activates NK cells. IL-4 and IL-5 can activate mast cells and eosinophils. GM-CSF can activate macrophages and granulocytes which can, in turn, help to clear tumor cells. TNF-α secreted by T_h cells may be directly toxic to tumor cells, as described above (Geppert and Lipsky, 1989).

11.4.3 Failure of the Immune Response

The clinical presence of a growing tumor implies that the tumor has evaded the immune response. Mechanisms by which a tumor surveillance system might fail include the following:

1. *Hiding from the immune response.* Even if the tumor is antigenic and T cells reactive to the tumor antigen are present, unless both are simultaneously

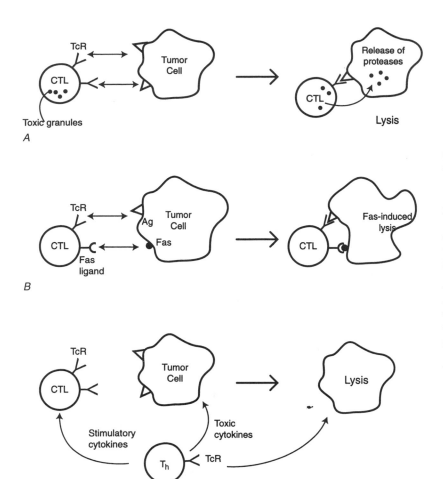

Figure 11.11. Mechanisms by which cytotoxic T lymphocytes (CTLs) might kill tumor cells. *A.* CTLs that recognize tumor cells may secrete cytotoxic granules whose contents penetrate into them. *B.* CTLs express the Fas ligand, which can convey signals to undergo apoptosis to tumor cells expressing the Fas antigen. Tumor necrosis factor (TNF) is a member of the same gene family as Fas and may cause death of tumor cells in a similar way. *C.* Activation of T-helper (T_h cells) will lead to secretion of cytokines that stimulate CTLs, and also cytokines (e.g., TNF-α) that may be directly toxic to tumor cells.

localized to secondary lymphoid organs, a functional immune response will not take place. As described in Sec. 11.3.6, this mechanism may be relevant for solid tumors that grow because the immune system is ignorant of their presence (Zinkernagel et al., 1997). In addition, the poor vasculature of many solid tumors prevents the efficient migration of APCs and lymphocytes into the tumor.

2. *Downregulation of class I MHC expression.* Many examples of tumors with decreased expression of class I MHC molecules have been described. The mechanisms include downregulation or complete loss of class I MHC expression. Obviously such tumors are unlikely to be recognized by CD8[+] T cells, although they should then become targets for NK cells (Möller and Hammerling, 1992).

3. *Elaboration of immune-suppressive factors by tumor cells.* Some tumors secrete immunosuppressive factors that can downregulate a local immune response. For example, some gliomas secrete TGF-β, which decreases T-cell proliferation and cyto-

toxicity (Siepl et al., 1988). Local downregulation of the immune response may explain animal experiments in which challenges with low numbers of tumor cells are rejected by animals with a preexisting tumor burden of the same cells, suggesting that the main tumor is growing in the face of adequate effector cells (North, 1984). Some tumors may also secrete a factor that leads to changes in the CD3 component of the T-cell receptor complex (see Sec. 11.3.4), causing impaired signal transduction (Ochoa and Longo, 1995). Soluble antigens released by tumors may also bind to the T-cell receptor and block its interaction with antigen that is presented on APCs. Recently, some tumors have been shown to express Fas ligand, described above as a molecule used by CTLs to kill targets. The tumor can then turn the tables and kill Fas-expressing CTLs (Strand et al., 1996).

4. *Biasing towards an inappropriate response.* Since perforin-dependent cytotoxic T cells that arise from a T_h1 response are likely the major effectors of an

antitumor response, a T_h2 response may be ineffective. A humoral response may even produce antibodies that can bind antigenic sites on the tumor and block access to effector cells. The local cytokine milieu at the time of the initial response to the tumor determines whether a T_h1 or T_h2 response will develop (Sec. 11.3.3). If, for whatever reason, there is a significant presence of IL-4 or IL-10, a largely ineffective T_h2 response will develop, whereas the presence of IL-12 biases toward an effective T_h1 response.

5. *Induction of anergy in tumor reactive T cells.* Most tumor cells are poor APCs because they lack costimulatory molecules on their surfaces. Although, as described above, it is unlikely that naive tumor-reactive T cells will encounter tumor cells outside the costimulatory-rich environment of the secondary lymphoid organs, recognition of tumor antigens without costimulation may cause T-cell anergy or even programmed cell death of T cells and prevent the induction of an immune response. This mechanism may have some relevance for hemopoietic malignancies (Cardoso et al., 1996).

6. *High-dose suppression of an immune response.* If the tumor can attain a sufficient mass, it may be able to downregulate the subsequent immune response. This may occur because the response of a T-cell clone to increasing concentrations of antigen follows a bell-shaped curve. At low doses of antigen, responses are low because of inadequate stimulation through the T-cell receptor. At medium doses, responses are optimal. At high antigenic doses, proliferative responses are decreased because of the process of activation-induced cell death (Russell, 1995). Teleologically, the property of T cells to shut down their responses in the presence of large amounts of antigen may be an attempt to avoid the deleterious effects of prolonged release of large amounts of toxic cytokines. The immune response can also become exhausted (Moskophidis et al., 1993). Normally the immune response favors the induction of effector cells at the site of inflammation and memory cells in secondary lymphoid organs. Effector cells are often terminally differentiated cells that die in situ. If the antigen load is initially very high, all the activated T cells may differentiate into effectors that die after an initial attempt to clear the tumor, and no antigen-specific memory cells remain. Without memory cells, newly developing T cells from the thymus will recognize tumor antigens as self and become tolerant to them.

The relative importance of the above mechanisms in leading to tumor growth in the face of a potential immune rejection response remains unknown. However, the extensive advances in understanding the molecular basis for the immune response, summarized in the present chapter, are leading to multifaceted attempts to use immunologic manipulation in tumor therapy. These approaches are described in Chap. 18.

11.5 SUMMARY

There has been a rapid increase in knowledge about the genetic and molecular basis by which the immune system can mount a rejection response against antigens recognized as different from those in normal tissues (i.e., nonself). Both B and T lymphocytes express receptors on their surfaces that are encoded from rearranged genes; these can allow recognition of a large number (more than 10^7) of antigenic structures. B cells recognize conformational epitopes on intact proteins. T cells recognize antigens degraded into peptides that can complex with MHC molecules on a cell surface. Antigen-specific recognition, together with signals from costimulatory molecules, causes an intracellular signaling cascade that influences transcription factors in the cell nucleus. These transcription factors cause the expression of various genes, including those that produce cytokines, and result in differentiation and proliferation of lymphoid cells to produce effectors of the immune response—i.e., plasma cells that produce antibodies and cytotoxic T lymphocytes. Additional mechanisms lead to tolerance to self antigens and control the strength and type of immune response against given antigens.

Malignant transformation is accompanied by mutation of oncogenes or tumor suppressor genes and/or by other changes in expressed proteins in malignant cells. These changes can lead to production of tumor antigens that are presented on MHC molecules and recognized by the immune system as nonself. Some tumors may be eradicated by the immune system before they become evident clinically in a process known as *immune surveillance.* Tumors that grow use a number of mechanisms to evade or inhibit the immune response, but they may still be amenable to therapy based on immunologic manipulation.

REFERENCES

Amit AG, Mariuzza RA, Phillips SE, et al: Three-dimensional structure of an antigen-antibody complex at 2.9 Å resolution. *Science* 1986; 233:747–753.

Benaceraff B, McDevitt HO: Histocompatibility linked immune response genes. *Science* 1972; 175:273–279.

Berridge MJ: Lymphocyte activation in health and disease. *Crit Rev Immunol* 1997; 17:155–178.

Bierer BE, Burakoff SJ: T-lymphocyte activation: The biology and function of CD2 and CD4. *Immunol Rev* 1989; 111:267–294.

Bjorkman PJ, Saper MA, Samraoui B, et al: Structure of the human class I histocompatibility antigen. *Nature* 1987; 329:506–512.

Bloom BR, Modlin RL, Salgame P: Stigma variations: Observations on suppressor T cells and leprosy. *Annu Rev Immunol* 1992; 10:453–488.

Bocchia M, Korontsvit T, Xu Q, et al: Specific human cellular immunity to bcr-abl oncogene-derived peptides. *Blood* 1996; 87:3587–3592.

Boismenu R, Feng L, Xia YY, et al: Chemokine expression by intraepithelial gamma delta T cells: Implications for the recruitment of inflammatory cells to damaged epithelia. *J Immunol* 1996; 157:985–992.

Bonomo A, Matzinger P: Thymus epithelium induces tissue-specific tolerance. *J Exp Med* 1993; 177:1153–1164.

Bottazzo GF, Pujol-Borrell R, Hanafusa T, et al: Role of aberrant HLA-DR expression and antigen presentation in induction of endocrine autoimmunity. *Lancet* 1983; 2:1115–1119.

Bretscher PA, Wei G, Menon JN, Bielefeldt-Ohmann H: Establishment of stable, cell-mediated immunity that makes "susceptible" mice resistant to *Leishmania* major. *Science* 1992; 257:539–542.

Brown JH, Jardetzky TS, Gorga JC, et al: Three-dimensional structure of the human class II histocompatibility antigen HLA-DR1. *Nature* 1993; 364:33–339.

Burnet FM: *The Clonal Selection Theory of Acquired Immunity.* Cambridge, England: Cambridge University Press; 1959.

Cardoso AA, Schultze JL, Boussiotis VA, et al: Pre-B acute lymphoblastic leukemia cells may induce T-cell anergy to alloantigen. *Blood* 1996; 88:41–48.

Christinck ER, Luscher MA, Barber BH, Williams DB: Peptide binding to class I MHC on living cells and quantitation of complexes required for CTL lysis. *Nature* 1991; 352:67–70.

Clerici M, Shearer GM: The Th1-Th2 hypothesis of HIV infection: New insights. *Immunol Today* 1994; 15:575–581.

Disis ML, Cheever MA: HER-2/neu protein: A target for antigen-specific immunotherapy of human cancer. *Adv Cancer Res* 1997; 71:343–371.

Elliott T: Transporter associated with antigen processing. *Adv Immunol* 1997; 65:47–109.

Everson MP, McDuffie DS, Lemak DG, et al: Dendritic cells from different tissues induce production of different T cell cytokine profiles. *J Leuk Biol* 1996; 59: 494–498.

Fearon DT, Locksley RM: The instructive role of innate immunity in the acquired immune response. *Science* 1996; 272:50–53.

Geppert TD, Lipsky PE: Antigen presentation at the inflammatory site. *Crit Rev Immunol* 1989; 9:313–362.

Germain RN: MHC-dependent antigen processing and peptide presentation: Providing ligands for T lymphocyte activation. *Cell* 1994; 76:287–299.

Grosser N, Thompson DM: Tube leukocyte adherence inhibition assay for the detection of anti-tumour immunity. *Int J Cancer* 1976; 18:58–66.

Hedrick SM, Cohen DI, Nielsen EA, Davis MM: Isolation of cDNA clones encoding T cell–specific membrane-associated proteins. *Nature* 1984; 308:149–153.

Irving BA, Weiss A: The cytoplasmic domain of the T cell receptor zeta chain is sufficient to couple to receptor-associated signal transduction pathways. *Adv Immunol* 1997; 66:1–65.

Janeway CA Jr: The T cell receptor as a multicomponent signalling machine: CD4/CD8 coreceptors and CD45 in T cell activation. *Annu Rev Immunol* 1992; 10: 645–674.

June CH, Bluestone JA, Nadler LM, Thompson CB: The B7 and CD28 receptor families. *Immunol Today* 1994; 15:321–331.

Justement LB: The role of CD45 in signal transduction. *Adv Immunol* 1997; 66:1–65.

Kagi D, Ledermann B, Burki K, et al: Molecular mechanisms of lymphocyte-mediated cytotoxicity and their role in immunological protection and pathogenesis in vivo. *Annu Rev Immunol* 1996; 14:207–232.

Klein J: *Natural History of the Major Histocompatibility Complex.* New York: Wiley; 1986.

Koopmann JO, Hämmerling GJ, Momburg F: Generation, intracellular transport and loading of peptides associated with MHC class I molecules. *Curr Opin Immunol* 1997; 9:80–88.

Korner H, Sedgwick JD: Tumor necrosis factor and lymphotoxin: Molecular aspects and role in tissue-specific autoimmunity. *Immunol Cell Biol* 1996; 74:465–472.

Kumar V, George T, Yu YYL, et al: Role of murine NK cells and their receptors in hybrid resistance. *Curr Opin Immunol* 1997; 9:52–56.

Kundig TM, Bachmann MF, DiPaolo C, et al: Fibroblasts as efficient antigen-presenting cells in lymphoid organs. *Science* 1995; 268:1343–1347.

Ljunggren H-G, Karre K: In search of the "missing self": MHC molecules and NK cell recognition. *Immunol Today* 1990; 11:237–244.

Miller RG: The veto phenomenon and T-cell regulation. *Immunol Today* 1986; 7:112–114.

Mittrucker HW, Pfeffer K, Schmits R, Mak TW: T-lymphocyte development and function in gene-targeted mutant mice. *Immunol Rev* 1995; 148:115–150.

Möller P, Hämmerling G: The role of surface HLA-A,B,C molecules in tumour immunity. *Cancer Surv* 1992; 13:101–128.

Moskophidis D, Lechner F, Pircher H, Zinkernagel RM: Virus persistence in acutely infected immunocompetent mice by exhaustion of antiviral cytotoxic effector T-cells. *Nature* 1993; 362:758–761.

Mosmann TR, Coffman RL: TH1 and TH2 cells: different patterns of lymphokine secretion lead to different functional properties. *Annu Rev Immunol* 1989; 7:145–173.

Nagata S: Apoptosis by death factor. *Cell* 1997; 88:355–365.

Noelle RJ: CD40 and its ligand in host defence. *Immunity* 1996; 4:415–419.

North RJ: The murine antitumor immune response and its therapeutic manipulation. *Adv Immunol* 1984; 35:89–155.

Nossal GJ: The molecular and cellular basis of affinity maturation in the antibody response. *Cell* 1992; 68:1–2.

Ochoa AC, Longo DL: Alteration of signal transduction in T cells from cancer patients. *Imp Adv Oncol* 1995; pp 43–54.

Oldstone MB: Molecular mimicry and autoimmune disease. *Cell* 1987; 50:819–820.

Pretolani M, Goldman M: IL-10: A potential therapy for allergic inflammation? *Immunol Today* 1997; 18:277–280.

Ragupathi G: Carbohydrate antigens as targets for active specific immunotherapy. *Cancer Immunol Immunother* 1996; 43:152–157.

Raulet DH: The structure, function and molecular genetics of the gamma/delta T cell receptor. *Annu Rev Immunol* 1989; 7:175–207.

Rosenberg SA: The development of new immunotherapies for the treatment of cancer using Interleukin-2. A review. *Ann Surg* 1988; 208:121–135.

Rosenberg SA, Rapp HJ: Intralesional immunotherapy of melanoma with BCG. *Med Clin North Am* 1976; 60: 419–430.

Rudd CE: Upstream-downstream: CD28 cosignaling pathways and T cell function. *Immunity* 1996; 4:527–534.

Russell JH: Activation-induced death of mature T cells in the regulation of immune responses. *Curr Opin Immunol* 1995; 7:382–388.

Salmi M, Jalkanen S: How do lymphocytes know where to go: Current concepts and enigmas of lymphocyte homing. *Adv Immunol* 1997; 64:139–218.

Schwartz RH: Models of T cell anergy: Is there a common molecular mechanism? *J Exp Med* 1996; 184:1–8.

Schwartz RH: Immunological tolerance. In Paul WE ed. *Fundamental Immunology*, 3d ed. New York: Raven Press; 1993: 677–732.

Sieling PA, Catterjee D, Porcelli SA, et al: CD1-restricted T cell recognition of microbial lipoglycan antigens. *Science* 1995; 269:227–230.

Siepl C, Bodmer S, Frei K, et al: The glioblastoma-derived T cell suppressor factor/transforming growth factor beta 2 inhibits T cell growth without affecting the interaction of interleukin 2 with its receptor. *Eur J Immunol* 1988, 18:593–600.

Strand S, Hofmann WJ, Hug H, et al: Lymphocyte apoptosis induced by CD95 (APO-1/Fas) ligand-expressing tumor cells—A mechanism of immune evasion? *Nature Med* 1996; 2:1361–1366.

Talmage DW: The acceptance and rejection of immunological concepts. *Annu Rev Immunol* 1986; 4:1–11.

Theobald M, Biggs J, Dittmer D et al: Targeting p53 as a general tumor antigen. *Proc Natl Acad Sci USA* 1995; 92:11993–11997.

Tonegawa S: Somatic generation of antibody diversity. *Nature* 1983; 302:575–581.

Tough DF, Borrow P, Sprent J: Induction of bystander T cell proliferation by viruses and type I interferon in vivo. *Science* 1996; 272:1947–1950.

Trowsdale J, Ragoussis J, Campbell RD: Map of the human MHC. *Immunol Today* 1991; 12:443–446.

Van der Bruggen P, Traversari C, Chomez P, et al: A gene encoding an antigen recognized by cytolytic T lymphocytes on a human melanoma. *Science* 1991; 254: 1643–1647.

Vanderlugt CJ, Miller SD: Epitope spreading. *Curr Opin Immunol* 1996; 8:831–836.

von Boehmer H: The developmental biology of T lymphocytes. *Annu Rev Immunol* 1988; 6:309–326.

Wingren AG, Parra E, Varga M, et al: T cell activation pathways: B7, LFA-3, and ICAM-1 shape unique T-cell profiles. *Crit Rev Immunol* 1995; 15:235-253.

Wucherpfennig KW, Strominger JL: Molecular mimicry in T cell–mediated autoimmunity: Viral peptides activate human T cell clones specific for myelin basic protein. *Cell* 1995; 80:695–705.

Yanagi Y, Yoshikai Y, Leggett K, et al: A human T cell—specific cDNA clone encodes a protein having extensive homology to immunoglobulin chains. *Nature* 1984; 308:145–149.

Zinkernagel RM, Ehl S, Aichele P, et al: Antigen localisation regulates immune responses in a dose- and time-dependent fashion: A geographical view of immune reactivity. *Immunol Rev* 1997, 156:199–209.

12

Hormones and Cancer

Paul E. Goss and Lesley M. Tye

12.1 INTRODUCTION
    12.1.1 Types of Hormones
    12.1.2 Inter- and Intracellular Signaling

12.2 STEROID HORMONES
    12.2.1 Structure and Classification of Steroid Hormones
    12.2.2 Transport of Steroid Hormones
    12.2.3 Steroid Hormone Receptors
    12.2.4 Quantitation of Steroid Receptors
    12.2.5 Interaction of Steroid Hormones and Growth Factors

12.3 CARCINOGENESIS AND HORMONES
    12.3.1 Risk Factors for Breast Cancer

12.3.2 Experimental Models for Breast Cancer
12.3.3 Risk Factors for Prostate Cancer
12.3.4 Experimental Models for Prostate Cancer
12.3.5 Hormonal Interactions with Oncogenes

12.4 PHARMACOLOGIC APPLICATIONS OF HORMONES IN CANCER
    12.4.1 Treatment of Breast Cancer
    12.4.2 Resistance to Endocrine Therapy
    12.4.3 Treatment of Prostate Cancer
    12.4.4 Prostate Cancer and Androgen Resistance

12.5 SUMMARY

REFERENCES

12.1 INTRODUCTION

12.1.1 Types of Hormones

In multicellular organisms, no single cell lives in an isolated environment. The major components that integrate body functions include the following: (1) *The nervous system,* which includes both electrical and chemical signals to communicate between the brain and peripheral organs or between organs in reflex circuits. (2) *The immune system,* which uses cytokines and antibodies for cell-to-cell communication to protect the organism against both external (invasive pathogens) and internal (malignant and stress) threat. (3) *The endocrine system,* which incorporates hundreds of different hormones to achieve its integrating functions. Organs and cells in these systems all express and secrete molecules to coordinate cell-to-cell signaling. Although each of these systems has distinct features, the development and survival of the multicellular organism depends upon their functioning in a coordinated and cooperative manner.

The endocrine system was thought originally to consist only of discrete endocrine glands. This con-

cept is now referred to as the *classical endocrine system.* Hormonal substances were found later to be expressed in organs other than these discrete endocrine glands; thus the term *diffuse endocrine system* was coined. For example, the steroid hormone estrogen is produced in the ovary, but it has also been shown to be produced in other tissues such as the placenta and in adipocytes (Simpson et al., 1994).

Hormones modulate the expression of growth factors, oncogenes, tumor suppressor factors, cytokines, and other components involved in signal transduction, cell-cycle checkpoints, and cell death (apoptosis) (White 1996); thus they are actively involved in the processes of cell proliferation and differentiation. Abnormal expression of hormones may lead either directly or indirectly to tumor initiation and progression.

Hormones can be categorized structurally into two broad groups: nonsteroid and steroid. Nonsteroid hormones include peptides or amino acid derivatives and range from complex polypeptides such as luteinizing hormone to small peptides (e.g., angiotensin) and derivatives of single amino acids such as catecholamines. Nonsteroid hormones are unable to penetrate the cell membrane directly. Instead, they act through receptors and signal transduction across the plasma membrane. Thus, the binding of, for example, peptide hormones to their receptors generates or increases the level of activator substances (e.g., cAMP, diacylglycerol, or calcium-calmodulin), which are referred to as *second messengers*. These molecules, in turn, activate a protein kinase, which initiates a signal transduction pathway leading eventually to modification of the DNA binding protein(s) in the nucleus and regulation of transcription of mRNA from the target gene(s) (Meyer and Habener, 1993; Chap. 6, Sec. 6.3). In contrast to this mechanism of peptide hormone action, steroid hormones (because they are more lipophilic) generally enter cells by simple diffusion. They bind to specific receptors, which are then activated; and the steroid receptor complex translocates into the nucleus, where it binds to DNA and in doing so regulates transcription of mRNA.

12.1.2 Inter- and Intracellular Signaling

The term *endocrine signaling* relates to hormone production by a discrete endocrine gland and the transport of this hormone via the circulation to distantly located, phenotypically different cells, which are acted upon by the hormone. *Exocrine signaling* involves some type of "external" secretion such as sweat, milk, or bile, which are produced by a gland and excreted via a duct in response to a hormonal stimulus. *Paracrine signaling* occurs when a substance released by one cell influences phenotypically different neighboring cells. This type of signaling is generally important in homeostasis—for example, in the stimulation of tissue proliferation in response to injury and stress. Abnormal expression of paracrine molecules (i.e., cytokines or growth factors) is associated with the initiation and progression of tumors (see also Chap. 6, Sec. 6.7.1). A variation on paracrine signaling involves *juxtacrine factors*, which are growth regulatory molecules that are exposed on a cell surface and modulate adjacent cells through contact. If a cell responds to a molecule that is produced either by that cell or by the same cell type, this is described as *autocrine signaling*. Many growth factors act in this fashion. For example, cultured cells often synthesize and release growth factors that stimulate their own proliferation. *Intracrine signaling* occurs when molecules produced by a cell act directly on that cell without cellular release. These various mechanisms are indicated conceptually in Fig. 12.1.

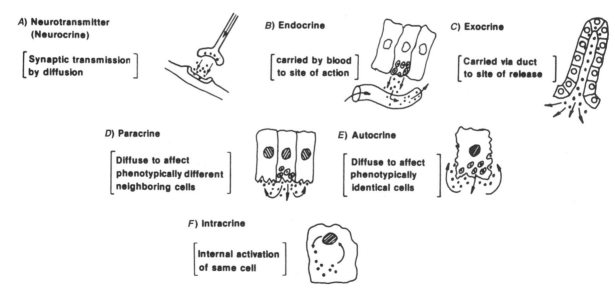

Figure 12.1. Different types of humoral signals. *A.* Neurotransmission, in which signals are transmitted by a diffusible substance at synapses between nerves or between nerve and muscle. *B.* Endocrine, in which hormones are carried by blood to their site of action. *C.* Exocrine, in which substances are released into a duct. *D.* Paracrine, in which mediators diffuse to influence neighboring cells that are phenotypically different. A variation on paracrine signaling involves juxtacrine factors, which are growth-regulatory molecules that are exposed on a cell surface and modulate adjacent cells through contact. *E.* Autocrine, in which growth factors act on the cells that produce them, as well as on neighboring cells. *F.* Intracrine, in which growth factors act on the producing cell without release from the cell.

All of the above types of cellular signaling work in concert to control the development of an organ. For example, the normal growth and differentiation of the mammary gland is influenced by endocrine hormones, paracrine factors contributed by breast stromal cells, and autocrine molecules generated by breast epithelial cells (Dickson and Lippman, 1995).

The same molecule can act in more than one type of cell-to-cell signaling. For example, catecholamine hormones, such as dopamine, norepinephrine, and epinephrine, may function both as neurotransmitters, acting in a paracrine manner on adjacent cells, and as systemic endocrine hormones, acting on distantly located cells or tissue. Another example is epidermal growth factor (EGF), which can be considered a peptide hormone. Membrane-bound EGF can bind to and signal an adjacent cell by direct contact. However, it may also be cleaved by a protease and act as an endocrine signal on distantly located cells.

In addition to the heterogeneity of function at a cellular level, a single hormone may have functions in multiple organs and the function of a single organ may require many hormones. An example of the former is testosterone, which is involved in the induction of male differentiation of the Wolffian ducts, growth of the male urogenital tract, induction of spermatogenesis, growth of beard and body hair, and multiple other functions. An example of the latter is the control of lactation, which involves at least seven hormones: prolactin, placental lactogen, glucocorticoids, thyroxine, estrogen, progesterone, and oxytocin. These diverse functions are due to the fact that different cells are programmed to respond differently to hormones at different stages of development.

A review of nonsteroid hormones is beyond the scope of this chapter. However, tumors of the breast and prostate are highly dependent on steroid hormones, and these two endocrine tumors are used here to exemplify the role of steroid hormones in cell growth and differentiation, in carcinogenesis, and in the treatment and prevention of cancer. Cellular mechanisms of hormonal resistance will also be discussed.

12.2 STEROID HORMONES

12.2.1 Structure and Classification of Steroid Hormones

Steroid hormones are synthesized from cholesterol within the smooth endoplasmic reticulum of specialized cells in the adrenal cortex, testis, ovary, and placenta; they are released as they are synthesized. All naturally occurring steroid hormones share a common chemical structure called the *steroid nucleus*. Additional chemical groups bound to the steroid nucleus confer the functional specificity of glucocorticoids, mineralocorticoids, progestins, estrogens, and androgens (Fig. 12.2). Each of the functional groups of steroid hormones is described briefly below, but emphasis is placed on estrogens and androgens, the principal hormones involved in the development and treatment of breast and prostate cancers.

Glucocorticoids have multiple physiologic functions. Cortisol is the major glucocorticoid and is synthesized in the adrenal cortex under the modulation of the hypothalamic/pituitary/adrenal axis. Briefly, environmental stress signals the limbic area of the central nervous system, which, in turn, signals the hypothalamus to release corticotropin releasing factor (CRF). This then stimulates the anterior pituitary gland to release adrenocorticotropic hormone (ACTH), which circulates to the adrenal cortex and enhances the synthesis and release of cortisol by the zona fasciculata (middle layer). Cortisol has a direct negative feedback effect on the hypothalamus (CRF formation) and anterior pituitary (ACTH formation; Fig. 12.3).

Several synthetic glucocorticoids (e.g., hydrocortisone, prednisone, and dexamethasone, in increasing order of potency) are used in the management of patients with cancer. These agents may have direct antitumoral effects (i.e., antilymphocytic effects) in lymphocytic leukemias, myelomas, and lymphomas. They may reduce the number of T cells (perhaps by inhibiting the transcription of the gene for interleukin 2, a potent T-cell growth factor) and inhibit B-cell activation and proliferation. Glucocorticoid-mediated immunosuppression may involve nuclear factor kappa B (NF-κB), a regulator of the immune system and inflammation genes. Dexamethasone has been shown to induce the transcription of IκBα—the cytoplasmic inhibitor of NF-κB—and thus the translocation of NF-κB to the nucleus. This decrease in nuclear NF-κB would decrease cytokine secretion and thus block the activation of the immune system (Scheinman et al., 1995). The anti-inflammatory effects of glucocorticoids may contribute to control of pain and reduction of edema in the CNS if brain metastases are present. They are used also to prevent nausea and vomiting associated with chemotherapy by acting directly on the vomiting center in the central nervous system.

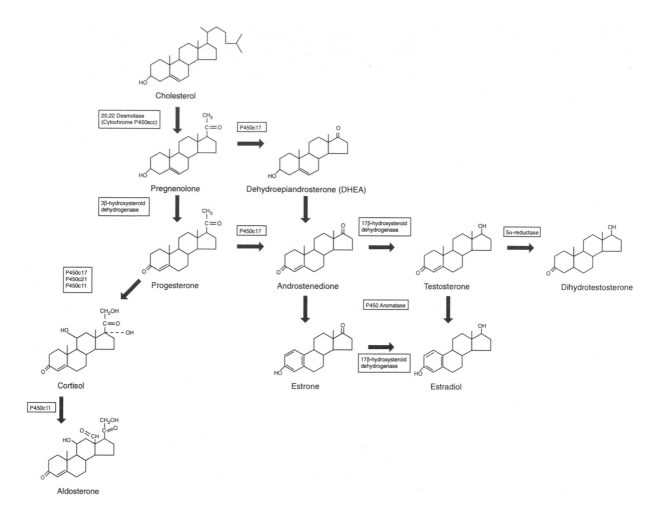

Figure 12.2. The steroid biosynthesis pathway for some of the major steroids such as gluco-corticoids (cortisol), mineralocorticoids (aldosterone), progestins (progesterone), estrogens (es-trone, estradiol), and androgens (androstenedione, testosterone, dehydroepiandrosterone). The enzymes that catalyze the reactions are shown in rectangular boxes. P450c17 catalyzes three reactions: 11β-hydroxylase, 18-hydroxylase, and 18-methyloxidase.

Mineralocorticoids are essential for the maintenance of electrolyte balance and extracellular fluid volume. Aldosterone, the major mineralocorticoid, is produced in the adrenal cortex and acts mainly on the distal tubules of the kidney to promote the reabsorption of sodium. Metastases from solid tumors (e.g., breast, lung cancers) may destroy the adrenal cortex, resulting occasionally in hypoaldosteronism. Treatment is then required with a synthetic mineralocorticoid such as 9α-fluorocortisol (fludrocortisone).

Progestins are involved in the preparation of the uterus for pregnancy and the breast for lactation; they are also important hormones in the normal development of the breast. The major progestin is progesterone, which is produced predominantly in the ovary, under hypothalamus/pituitary control, and plays a major role in the menstrual cycle. Progesterone also induces cell differentiation in tissues such as the uterus and tends to arrest the proliferative effects of estrogenic stimulation. This is modulated through the regulation of growth-factor and cell-cycle genes, as described in Sec. 12.2.5. In the breast, progesterone causes the alveolar cells to proliferate and enlarge. Because progestins play a major role in the normal development of the breast and the cyclic preparation of the breast for pregnancy and lactation, they are important in the control of cell growth and differentiation. Progestins and antiprogestins have been used in the treatment

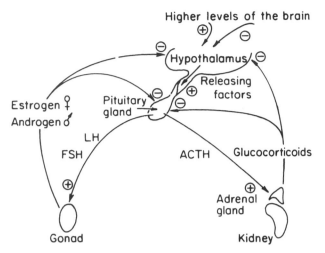

Figure 12.3. Schematic illustration of the complex feedback loops that act to control production of glucocorticoids and sex hormones by the adrenal gland and gonads.

of cancer, especially uterine and breast cancer (see Sec. 12.4.1).

Estrogens are responsible for the development of most of the secondary female sexual characteristics. The principal estrogen, 17β-estradiol, is produced predominantly in the parafollicular cells of the ovary in premenopausal women. Its production is under hypothalamus/pituitary control through the coordinated stimulation of luteinizing hormone (LH) and follicle-stimulating hormone (FSH) and negative feedback inhibition by estrogens (Fig. 12.3).

Luteinizing hormone induces the synthesis of a constant supply of androstenedione (estrogen precursor) by the stromal cells of the ovary, while FSH stimulates the conversion of these precursors into estrogen by the parafollicular cells. This reaction involves aromatization, as estrogens have an aromatic ring structure (i.e., a 6-carbon ring with 3 double bonds, Fig. 12.2), and the enzyme catalyzing this reaction is therefore referred to as *aromatase* (estrogen synthetase).

After menopause, ovarian estrogen production ceases, and subsequently estrogen is derived primarily from the aromatization in peripheral tissues of adrenal androgens to estrone, with some estrone being subsequently converted to 17β-estradiol, a more potent estrogen. Thus, in postmenopausal females, plasma levels of estrone are higher than those of 17β-estradiol. In addition, obese postmenopausal females tend to have even higher serum levels of estrone, which is probably explained by the fact that adipocytes are a major site of aromatization (Cauley

et al., 1989; Zhao et al., 1995). Obesity (associated with higher levels of estrogen) appears to increase the risk of breast cancer in postmenopausal women (see Sec. 12.3.1).

Estrogens develop and maintain the breast and uterus by promoting specific cellular proliferation and growth. Estrogens can induce the expression of the progesterone receptor (PR). Together, both hormones appear to regulate other genes such as growth factors and cell cycle–associated genes to promote cell proliferation. They are also thought to play important roles in the induction and maintenance of mammary gland tumors (Dickson and Lippman, 1995). Epidemiology, animal models, and therapeutic effects underscore the central importance of estrogens in breast cancer. These items are dealt with in later sections .

Androgens are responsible for most of the secondary male sexual characteristics. The major source of androgens is the testis, but a small contribution (10 to 15 percent of total circulating androgens) is made by the adrenal gland. The most important androgen, testosterone, is produced primarily by interstitial Leydig cells in the testis. This process is under pituitary/hypothalamic control, with luteinizing hormone (LH) stimulating the synthesis and release of testosterone (Fig. 12.3). Although the serum levels of LH may fluctuate, the production of testosterone is quite constant in the adult male.

In some of its target tissues, testosterone may be metabolized by the enzyme 5α-reductase to a more potent androgen, dihydrotestosterone (DHT), which is required for hormonal effects to occur in certain tissues. For example, DHT plays a role in the normal growth, development, and maintenance of the prostate gland (Klein, 1992) as well as in the development of secondary sexual characteristics. The major adrenal androgens are dehydroepiandrosterone (DHEA) and its sulfate (DHEA-S). A smaller amount of androstenedione is also produced. These adrenal androgens are weak androgens but can be converted to testosterone in extraglandular tissues. Adrenal androgen production contributes to adolescent growth and is important in maintaining normal anabolic function throughout life without giving rise to masculinization. Androgens stimulate growth of prostatic tumors, and their removal or inhibition plays an important role in the therapy of this malignancy (see Sec. 12.4.3).

12.2.2 Transport of Steroid Hormones

Steroid hormones are hydrophobic molecules that are released into the bloodstream immediately after synthesis. These molecules circulate either free or bound to transport proteins with half lives ranging from 30 to 90 min. The bound and unbound fractions are in a dynamic equilibrium determined by the amount of hormone, the amount of binding protein, and the binding affinity of the hormone for the protein. The half-life in plasma and the activity of a steroid hormone can be modulated by its interaction with its transport protein(s). For example, most circulating 17β-estradiol is bound to two plasma proteins: sex hormone binding globulin (SHBG)(37 percent) and albumin (63 percent), with only 1 to 2 percent being "free" (Dunn et al., 1981). It is the free fraction that is considered biologically active, although the uptake of bound hormone may play a role in some cell types.

Factors that influence SHBG levels will influence indirectly the amount of bound versus free 17β-estradiol and thus affect the biologic expression of this molecule. For example, estrogens stimulate SHBG production, whereas obesity, androgens, and progestins are known to suppress it (Anderson, 1974). Pharmacologic agents such as the antiestrogen tamoxifen and dietary substances such as flaxseed have been shown to increase SHBG (Thompson, 1995). The resulting alteration in the bound to unbound 17β-estradiol fraction likely has biological implications for the use of these agents in the treatment and/or prevention of breast cancer (see Sec. 12.4.1) Drugs that compete with a hormone for binding with the transport molecule may also increase hormone activity by increasing the amount of active unbound hormone.

12.2.3 Steroid Hormone Receptors

Steroid hormones enter most cells by diffusion, although active uptake may occur in some cells. In target cells, the hormone binds to its receptor, which is a large protein molecule located in both the cytoplasmic and nuclear fractions of the cell. Steroid hormone receptors belong to a superfamily of nuclear receptor proteins. To date more than 150 members of the family have been identified, and these span a diversity of animal species from worms to insects to humans (Mangelsdorf et al., 1995). Figure 12.4 shows the general structure of the receptor, while Fig. 12.5 shows a schematic comparison of a number of important family members. These share a common structure and conserved functional domains. The most important and conserved domain is domain C, also called the DNA- binding domain. This domain targets the receptor to the target genes via binding to the hormone response element (HRE), which is a short regulatory nucleotide sequence located at the 5' end of various responsive genes. The DNA-binding domain is 66 to 68 amino acids in length and includes nine cysteine residues. Eight of these cysteine residues are incorporated into two "zinc fingers," in which a zinc ion is linked to two pairs of cysteines (Fig. 12.6). This zinc-finger motif also occurs in many other DNA- binding transcription factors (see Chap. 6, Sec. 6.3.6). This region also has weak constitutive dimerization activity.

The other domains of the steroid receptors are the variable *N*-terminal region (A/B; trans-activating domain), which is thought to optimize the tran-

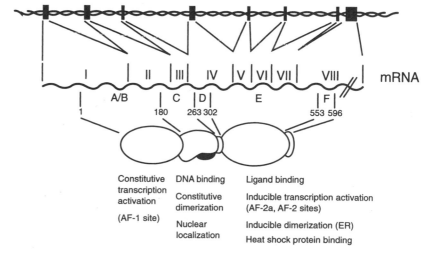

Figure 12.4. Schematic representation of the estrogen receptor, a protein belonging to the steroid nuclear receptor superfamily. The top portion of this diagram shows the genomic organization of the estrogen receptor. Exons are indicated by black boxes. The middle section of the figure shows the structure of the spliced mRNA with the amino acid numbers corresponding to the boundaries of the various functional domains of the protein, indicated at the base of the diagram. Various activities that have been described for each domain are noted. See Sec. 12.2.3 for further details. (Adapted from Wolf and Fuqua, 1995.)

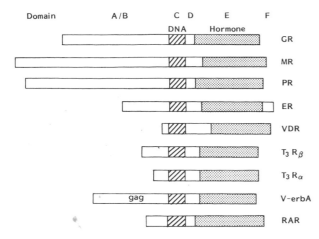

Figure 12.5. Comparison of members of the steroid receptor "superfamily." Each receptor can be divided into four to five regions. The relative lengths of the regions are shown by the size of the boxes. Region A/B is hypervariable with little homology of amino acid sequences between members. This region is thought to optimize the transcriptional activation capability of the receptor and contains AF-1, a constitutively active transcription activation region. Region C, the DNA-binding region, has extensive homology and includes two zinc-finger motifs. It is postulated that the variability of the amino acid sequences in this region determines the specificity of the interaction between the receptor and hormone response element. This region also has weak constitutive dimerization activity. Region D, the variable hinge region, contains the sequences necessary for nuclear localization, which must be present for the receptor to remain within the nucleus in the absence of ligand. Region E is the ligand-binding region and has significant homology among receptors with similar ligands. In addition to the ligand binding, this region is also the site for the binding of heat-shock protein and has AF-2a and AF-2 ligand-inducible transcription activation regions. F = variable C terminal region; GR = glucocorticoid receptor; MR = mineralocorticoid receptor; PR = progesterone receptor; ER = estrogen receptor; VDR = vitamin D receptor; T₃Rβ and T₃Rα = thyroid hormone receptors; T_3R_β and T_3R_α = thyroid hormone receptors; V-erbA = product of the viral oncogene; RAR = retinoic acid receptor. (Adapted from Evans, 1988.)

scriptional activation capability of the receptor (AF-1 is a constitutively active transcription activation region in this domain); a variable hinge region (D; contains sequences necessary for nuclear localization, which must be present for the receptor to remain within the nucleus in the absence of ligand); a conserved ligand-binding domain (E; AF-2a and AF-2 are ligand-inducible transcription activation regions in this domain; it also includes the ligand-dependent dimerization region and the site for binding to heat-shock protein); and a variable C-ter-

minal region (F), to which no specific function has been assigned (Fig. 12.4).

In the inactive state, the steroid hormone receptor is believed to be complexed with a 90-kDa heat-shock protein that masks the DNA binding site and prevents interaction of the receptor with the hormone response element. In the presence of the hormone "ligand," the heat-shock protein is released and the receptor becomes activated. The binding of steroid to its receptor molecule results in structural change leading to dimerization, which converts the receptor from an inactive to an active conformation (Fig. 12.7). The "activated" or "transformed" receptor-steroid complex has a high binding affinity for the hormone response element, and the binding of the receptor-hormone complex to this element generally results in gene activation—i.e., the enhancement of the transcription of the gene by RNA polymerase to produce messenger RNA (mRNA) and ultimately protein. In some cases, receptor gene interaction causes gene activity to be decreased rather than increased.

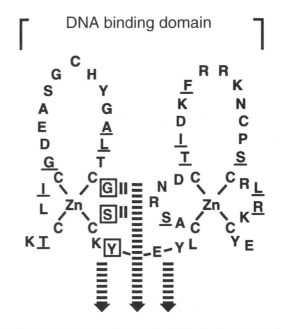

Figure 12.6. Zinc fingers in the DNA-binding domain of the androgen receptor—a hypothetical model. Each letter refers to an amino acid in the DNA-binding domain of the androgen receptor. Note that each zinc ion is linked to four cysteine residues. The zinc-finger motif also occurs in many other DNA-binding transcription factors. (Adapted from Liao, 1994.)

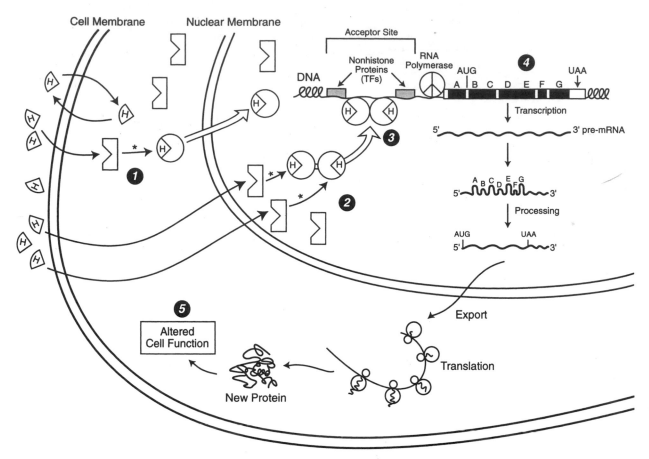

Figure 12.7. Molecular pathway of steroid hormone action. 1. Hormone (H) binds to receptor. Heat-shock protein is released, leading to structural change in receptor. 2. Dimerization occurs and receptor is activated. 3. Receptor-hormone complex has high affinity for the hormone response element of DNA and binds to this region. 4. Gene activation occurs. 5. Resulting gene product alters cell function, growth, and/or differentiation. (Adapted from Clarke et al., 1992.)

The intracellular concentration of steroid receptors is important in determining the responsiveness of the "target cell." For example, both the prostate and the uterus contain receptors for progesterone, estrogen, and androgen, but the *relative concentrations* are very different. Consequently, the uterus is primarily a target organ for estrogens and progestins, while the prostate is primarily influenced by androgens. Cellular receptor levels can be up- and downregulated by a reduction in the level of receptor mRNA by either reduced synthesis or increased degradation. For example, the enzyme protein kinase C (PKC) has been implicated in the downmodulation of estrogen receptor (ER) mRNA. Stimulation of ER-positive breast cancer cells with 12-O-tetradeconylphorbol-13-acetate, an activator of PKC, has been shown to cause destabilization of ER mRNA (Tzukerman et al., 1991).

Upregulation of steroid receptors may have clinical implications. For example, the upregulation of a steroid receptor followed by exposure of the cell to hormone occurs when T cells undergo *programmed cell death* (apoptosis) in response to glucocorticoids. Apoptosis can result from the rise or fall in the level of hormones; for example, the death of uterine endometrial cells at the beginning of menstruation is initiated by the fall in progesterone and 17β-estradiol levels. Steroids may regulate steroid receptors other than their own. For example, 17β-estradiol increases the level of progesterone receptors by increasing mRNA concentration and thus the rate of protein synthesis. However, progesterone may suppress the synthesis of the ER and may therefore modulate the synthesis of its own receptor through this mechanism (Clarke et al., 1992).

The specificity of the ligand-binding domain determines which hormone(s) bind(s) to a receptor (Fig. 12.5). Because there is a high degree of homology between the ligand-binding domains of some receptors, there is some degree of cross-reaction between these receptors and hormones of different classes. For example, progestins often have androgenic effects because they bind with fairly high affinity to the androgen receptor. Additionally, the specific amino acid sequences of the DNA binding domain, operating through the hormone response element, determine which target genes are activated. "Chimeric" receptors have been constructed—for example, a 17β-estradiol–binding domain linked to a glucocorticoid receptor DNA-binding domain. Activation of such receptors with 17β-estradiol results in transcription of glucocorticoid-inducible genes but not of estrogen-inducible genes (Green and Chambon, 1986). Because of the very high homology between the DNA-binding domains of receptors for progesterone and glucocorticoids, it is thought that these receptors may activate a common hormone response element.

Receptor mutations may result in altered hormonal activity, which, in turn, may result in altered end-organ function and/or be important in carcinogenesis and cancer treatment. For example, Taplin et al. (1995) showed that in 5 of 10 patients with metastatic androgen-independent prostate cancer, the androgen receptor genes had point mutations, all in the ligand-binding domain. Functional studies showed that two of these mutant androgen receptors could be activated by progesterone and estrogen.

12.2.4 Quantitation of Steroid Receptors

The determination of the estrogen receptor (ER) and progesterone receptor (PR) status in breast cancer is of clinical significance, since receptor status helps to predict the likelihood of response to endocrine therapy (Muss, 1992). For example, in patients who are both ER- and PR-positive, response rates to initial endocrine therapy of approximately 70 percent are observed, compared to response rates of ≤10 percent in patients who are ER- and PR-negative (Osborne, 1991). Also, postmenopausal patients with an ER-positive primary tumor will generally receive adjuvant tamoxifen (an antiestrogen), as in this setting tamoxifen has been shown to increase disease-free and overall survival (Fisher et al., 1989; see Sec. 12.4.1).

Until recently, the most widely used assay for steroid receptors was the dextran-coated charcoal method (Fig. 12.8), which involves the incubation of radiolabeled hormone with a cytosol preparation (supernatant from tumor tissue that has been homogenized and ultracentrifuged). Dextran-coated charcoal is added to adsorb unbound hormone, and the receptor-bound radiolabeled hormone remains in the supernatant and can be quantitated. A tumor is considered generally to be ER- and/or PR-positive if the receptor content is greater than 10 fmol of receptor per milligram of cytosol protein, although the threshold values for positivity have ranged from 3 to 20 fmol/mg protein in different laboratories. This variability has led to variations in tumor receptor classification (i.e., one laboratory considering the tumor receptor-negative and the other receptor-positive) and may explain why some "receptor-negative" tumors respond to hormonal therapy. The method requires relatively large amounts of fresh or fresh-frozen tissue and cannot identify the cellular origin of the receptors. Furthermore, a small quantity of ER-positive tumor cells in a tissue specimen may lead to a false-negative result owing to dilution by the relatively large volume of nontumor tissue present.

Monoclonal antibodies to a number of receptors have been developed and immunocytochemical assays are now used in routine quantitation of steroid receptors (Fig. 12.8). These antibodies are available in commercial kits, and this method has several advantages over the radioligand binding method. It can be used on smaller tissue specimens, is faster, and does not require the use of radiolabeled compounds. Also, false-negative results do not occur as a result of the receptor being occupied by tamoxifen or estrogen. Depending on the epitope to which the antibody has been raised, immunocytochemical methods do not require a functional receptor, whereas the dextran-coated charcoal method does. One method in which monoclonal antibodies are employed is the ER enzyme immunoassay, in which beads, coated with anti-ER are incubated with a cytosol preparation. Any ER present binds to the beads, and the supernatant is then removed. Anti-ER conjugated with molecules that acquire color upon exposure to a developing agent is then added, and this conjugate binds to any ER present. Unbound conjugate is removed and the beads are incubated with a developing agent. The intensity of the color is proportional to the concentration of ER in the sample and is measured spectrophotometrically and compared with a standard curve. Again, a value less than 10 fmol/mg protein is generally considered negative. Immunocytochemical assay results for ERs and PRs have been shown to correlate with the older

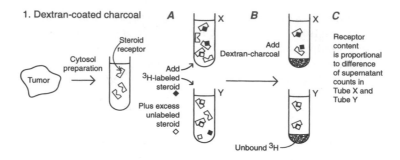

1. Dextran-coated charcoal

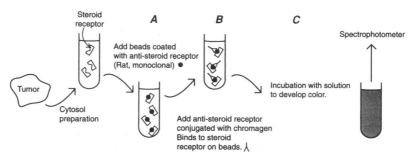

2. Immunocytochemical

3. Immunohistochemical: Avidin-biotin-peroxidase complex method

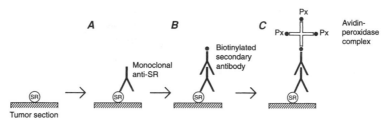

Figure 12.8. Methods for detection and quantification of steroid receptors in tumor tissue.

1. The dextran-coated charcoal method. *A.* Tumor tissue is homogenized and ultracentrifuged and the supernatant (cytosol) incubated with a known quantity of ^{3}H-labeled steroid with or without excess unlabeled steroid. *B.* Dextran-coated charcoal is added to adsorb unbound steroid. *C.* The receptor-bound ^{3}H steroid remains in the supernatant and can be quantitated by the difference in ^{3}H counts between the two tubes and expressed per milligram of cytosolic protein.

2. The immunocytochemical method. *A.* Tumor tissue is homogenized and ultracentrifuged and the supernatant (cytosol) incubated with beads coated with monoclonal antisteroid receptor (anti-SR). Standards are also run containing known amounts of SR. Steroid receptor present in the sample binds to the beads and the supernatant is removed. *B.* Anti-SR, which is conjugated to a chromogen, is added and binds to any SR present. *C.* Unbound conjugate is removed, the beads are incubated with a developing agent, and the intensity of color is read in an spectrophotometer. Color intensity is proportional to the concentration of SR in the sample.

3. The immunohistochemical avidin-biotin-peroxidase complex method. Thin sections of tumor are cut from formalin-fixed, paraffin-embedded biopsy specimens. *A.* Section is exposed to a monoclonal antibody specific for the steroid receptor (SR) being assessed and binds to it. *B.* Section is exposed to a second biotinylated antibody specific for the first antibody and binds to it. *C.* Avidin-peroxidase complex is added, followed by a chromogen, and color appears where the SR is located.

biochemical detection methods. Again, however, one disadvantage is that a tissue homogenate is required, so that morphologic correlation with the presence of carcinoma cells is not possible.

Immunohistochemical methods permit direct correlation of histology with receptor status (Fig. 12.8). There are commercially available antibodies that will bind to receptors in formalin-fixed, paraffin-embedded tissue sections. The most commonly used technique is the avidin-biotin-peroxidase method; however, there are other "sandwich" immunohistochemical techniques. These stain the nucleus predominately and permit testing of small paraffin-embedded tumors and cytologic samples. This technique has the advantage of determining whether the receptor measured is within tumor cells. It can also show receptor heterogeneity within samples (see Sec. 12.4.2). ER immunocytochemical assay (ER-ICA) results are generally reported simply as positive or negative, although semiquantitative methods have been used. Positive results are generally reported when more than 10 percent of nuclei stain positively; this has been found to correlate with the threshold of 10 fmol/mg protein used for the dextran-coated charcoal method of receptor analysis.

12.2.5 Interaction of Steroid Hormones and Growth Factors

There are three principal differentiated cell types of the mammary gland: stromal fibroblasts, myoepithelial cells, and epithelial cells. The majority of breast development, proliferation, and differentiation studies have focused on the epithelium because it is dynamic, undergoing repetitive periods of proliferation and apoptosis in premenopausal women. Both ERs and PRs are expressed in a proportion of epithelial cells of the terminal duct lobular unit of the breast (Ricketts et al., 1990; Battersby et al., 1992). It is hypothesized that estrogen and progesterone working concordantly regulate the growth of breast tissues, in part by regulating the stimulatory and inhibitory autocrine/intracrine/paracrine growth factor pathways (Murphy, 1994; Dickson and Lippman, 1995). Most of the data examining the function of growth factors have been generated from in vitro models using cultured immortalized human epithelial or cancer cells, and only recently have in vivo studies been undertaken in transgenic mouse models (see Chap. 3, Sec. 3.3.12). These studies have demonstrated the complexity of the underlying hormone/growth factor relationships associated with normal breast tissue and tumor initiation.

Breast tumors, in addition to displaying steroid receptors, frequently express epidermal growth factor (EGF) receptors. Epidermal growth factor, members of the transforming growth factor families (e.g. TGF-α), and amphiregulin (an EGF-related and heparin-binding growth factor) bind to the EGF receptor, which activates a specific tyrosine kinase. High levels of EGF receptor in breast tumors correlate with a poor prognosis and are often accompanied by low levels of (or absent) ER, suggesting a link between the EGF receptor and hormone independence. Interestingly, estrogen can modulate the ability of human mammary epithelial cells to respond to EGF. It has also been observed that ER-positive breast cancer cell lines express higher levels of amphiregulin than ER-negative cell lines and that estrogen treatment increases amphiregulin levels (Normanno et al., 1994). Receptors with extensive homology to the EGF receptor, referred to as *HER-2/neu* or *c-erbB-2*, have been identified in breast tumors and are found amplified or overexpressed in approximately 30 percent of breast cancers. In general, these tumors tend to be hormone-unresponsive (ER- and PR-negative), have higher proliferative and invasive rates, and have a poorer clinical prognosis (Fitzpatrick et al., 1984; Klijn et al., 1992).

Estrogen may stimulate tumor growth by the production of proteases, which activate precursors of other growth factors such as TGF-α. An estrogen-induced increase in TGF-α expression in vitro has been shown to be mediated through the ER, as it can be blocked by administration of the antiestrogen tamoxifen (Murphy and Dotzlaw, 1989). Elevated expression of TGF-α is associated with endocrine resistance, but the mechanism associated with this observation is as yet unknown (Nicholson et al., 1994). Overexpression in tumor biopsies of another transforming growth factor, TGF-β, has been shown to be associated with clinical progression of breast cancer (Gorsch et al., 1992). This appears paradoxical, since treatment of epithelial tissue (malignant or normal) in vitro with TGF-β is usually growth-inhibitory, but some malignant cells have been found to be stimulated by this growth factor.

The cellular enzyme protein kinase C (PKC) has been found to be overexpressed in ER-negative and drug-resistant breast cancers. Protein kinases are involved in the phosphorylation of cellular proteins, and phosphorylation of specific sites on the ER may lead to inactivation of ER function. Treatment of ER-positive breast cancer with a PKC activator has been shown to cause a downregulation of ER (Saceda et al., 1991; Tzukerman et al., 1991). Other studies suggest that phosphorylation of both the ER and PR at different sites may constitutively activate these receptors and that this phosphorylation can be induced by growth factors such as insulin-like growth factor I(IGF-I) (Aronica and Katzenellenbogen, 1993). An overview of the influence of estrogen and progesterone on release of growth factors and expression of their receptors in breast cancer cells or cell lines is given in Table 12.1. The control of mammary gland growth and differentiation is thus extremely complex, and a greater understanding of the interplay between hormones and growth factors and their relationship to the development of malignancy is needed.

12.3 CARCINOGENESIS AND HORMONES

Hormones are likely to influence carcinogenesis, since they are known to have profound effects on cellular differentiation. Abnormalities of hormonal pathways may also stimulate cellular proliferation and accelerate the occurrence of "somatic genetic errors"—i.e., by increasing mitotic activity, DNA replication, and cell division, which may occur before DNA repair is complete (see Chap. 4, Sec. 4.4). Thus although hormones themselves are not genotoxic, they may lead to an increased level of mutations. The influence of hormones on carcinogenesis has been extensively studied as related to breast and prostate cancers; these are discussed below in relation to data from epidemiologic studies and animal models.

12.3.1 Risk Factors for Breast Cancer

Risk factors for breast cancer are summarized in Table 12.2 and are outlined below (Bernstein and Ross, 1993: Hulka et al., 1994).

Table 12.1. Effects of Estrogen and Progestin on Expression of Growth Factors and Their Receptors in Breast Cancer Cells and Cell Lines

	Effects of Exposure to	
	Estrogen	Progestin
Growth Factor		
Epidermal growth factor (EGF)	—	↑[a]
Transforming growth factor α (TGF-α)	↑[b]	↑[a]
Transforming growth factor β (TGF-β)	↓[a, b]	↓[a]
Amphiregulin (member of EGF family, binds to EGF-R)	↑[b]	—
Insulin-like growth factor II (IGF-II)	↑[a] ↓[e] ↑[f]	—
Receptor Content		
EGF receptor (EGF-R)	↑[b, c, g]	↑[a, d]
IGF-I receptor	↑[c]	↓[a]
ER	↑[a] ↓[b, i]	↓[a, b]
PR	↑[b]	↓[h]

[a]T-47D cell line.

[b]MCF-7 cell line.

[c]Rat uterus.

[d]ZR75 cell line.

[e]T61 xenograft.

[f]MCF-7 xenograft.

[g]BT474 cell line.

[h]T-47Dco cell line (estrogen insensitive; PR rich).

[i]Effect is dependent upon prior growth history of cells (T-47D cells have low ER and high PR content, whereas MCF-7 cells have high ER and low PR content).

Table 12.2. Hormonally Related Epidemiologic Risk Factors for Breast Cancer

| Factor | Risk Group | | Relative Risk[a] |
	Low	High	
Sex	Male	Female	183
Oophorectomy	Age < 35	No	2.5
Age at menarche	≥ 14 years	≤ 11 years	1.5
Age at first birth	< 20 years	≥ 30 years	1.9
Parity	≥ 5	Nulliparity	1.4
Age at natural menopause	< 45 years	≥ 55 years	2.0
Obesity (BMI),[b]	< 22.9	> 30.7	1.6
Oral contraceptive use	Never	Ever	1.0
	Never	≥ 4 years use before first pregnancy	1.7
Estrogen replacement therapy	Never	Current	1.4
	Never	> 15 years	1.3
Dense mammogram[c]	None	≥ 75% density	5.3

[a]Using low-risk group as a reference.

[b]Body mass index (kg/m²).

[c]Boyd et al., 1995.

Source: Adapted from Hulka et al., 1994.

Age at Menarche Early menarche (≤ 11 years of age) and *late menopause* (age ≥ 55 years) are associated with a slight increase in breast cancer risk. Early menarche and late menopause increase the lifetime exposure of the breast to ovarian hormones, which may explain these findings. A cohort of Finnish girls followed through puberty and into adulthood found that early menarche (defined as before age 12) was associated with significantly higher estradiol levels in adolescence and with higher estradiol levels in the follicular (not luteal) phase in women aged 21 to 31 years (Vikho and Apter, 1984). The women with early menarche had 30 percent lower sex hormone binding globulin (SHBG) levels than those women with menarche starting after age 13 (Apter et al., 1989), but other reports have not found evidence of an effect of age at menarche on estrogen levels.

Parity The younger the age of a woman at the time of her first pregnancy, the lower the risk of breast cancer. Additionally, the completion of a full-term pregnancy also lowers the risk of breast cancer. The mechanism(s) underlying these observations are not fully understood. During early pregnancy, there is extensive proliferation of ductal, alveolar, and lob-

ular tissues plus stem-cell differentiation in the terminal ducts and lobules (Russo et al., 1982). Thus the induction of stem-cell differentiation might make the breast less susceptible to carcinogenesis, and pregnancy would confer a "protective" effect. There are data to suggest that parity may affect estrogen levels or estrogen bioavailability. Bernstein et al. (1985) compared plasma and urinary hormone levels of nuns with those of their parous (biological) sisters and found that the parous women had shorter menstrual cycles and that their serum estradiol levels on the 11th day of their menstrual cycle were 22 percent lower. Additional studies have shown that SHBG-binding capacity is 10 to 12 percent higher in parous versus nulliparous premenopausal women (Bernstein et al., 1985; Moore et al., 1987). No relation was seen between SHBG and number of births, and in postmenopausal women there was no effect of parity on SHBG levels (Moore et al., 1987).

Obesity Obesity in postmenopausal women may increase the risk of breast cancer, perhaps related to increased estrogen production via peripheral aromatization. Recently, Toniolo et al. (1995) showed increased serum levels of estrone and 17β-estradiol (both total and free) and a lower percent of 17β-estradiol bound to SHBG in postmenopausal women who subsequently developed breast cancer. As obesity is associated with decreased SHBG production, the increase in breast cancer risk in obese postmenopausal women might be related to the increased bioavailability of these hormones (Moore et al., 1987).

Age   The incidence of breast cancer increases with age, but the rate of increase is more rapid for women under age 50. This is likely associated with ovarian activity, which produces sex steroids to drive breast cell proliferation during the menstrual cycle. After menopause, the incidence of breast cancer increases, but at a slower rate. This increase may reflect genetic damage that occurred during the premenopausal period.

Race/Ethnicity   A number of studies have been performed to assess whether populations with a low rate of breast cancer (such as those in many parts of Asia) have lower levels of estrogens. Studies comparing estrogen levels of premenopausal western women with premenopausal Asian women living in Japan or China or those who were recent immigrants to Hawaii have in general found lower estrogen levels in Asian women. However, when people from countries with low breast cancer incidence move to western countries, they slowly assume a western rate of breast cancer, suggesting a dietary influence (see Chap. 2, Sec. 2.3.2). African American women have a higher incidence of breast cancer than Caucasian American women. It was reported recently that healthy African American women have more metabolites with estrogen agonist activity in their urine than do Caucasian American women (Taioli et al., 1996).

Dense Mammogram   A recent study by Boyd et al. (1995) demonstrated increased risk for breast cancer in women with dense mammograms. It has been established that estrogens influence breast density and that a reduction in estrogen decreases breast density (Spicer et al., 1994). Thus the interaction between mammographic density and estrogen stimulation is important in understanding the basis of this increased risk.

Dietary Components

Fat   Differences in breast carcinoma mortality rates in different countries and their correlation with dietary fat consumption have led to the hypothesis that a fat-rich diet may increase breast cancer risk. Currently a large clinical trial is ongoing in Canada to assess the effects of a low-fat diet on breast density in women at increased breast cancer risk by virtue of having dense mammograms.

Fiber   Case-control studies from various countries have shown breast cancer risk to be decreased by a high intake of dietary fiber, although two large prospective studies in the United States found no association. Various mechanisms for this have been postulated—most related to estrogen effects; for example, a high-fiber diet may reduce circulating estrogen levels by reducing the enterohepatic recirculation of estrogen (see Stoll, 1996, for review). It has been observed that mammalian lignans and isoflavinoid phytoestrogens, synthesized in the intestine from plant precursors, affect hormone metabolism and thus might have a protective role in breast cancer. Flaxseed is a plant species that is high in prelignan content. Mammalian lignans are produced from flaxseed precursors by the action of bacterial flora in the colon, the major lignans being enterolactone and enterodiol. These compounds are structurally similar to tamoxifen, diethylstilbestrol, and estradiol. These lignans have a wide range of biologic activities, which include stimulation of SHBG synthesis, growth-inhibitory and antiproliferative effects, ability to bind to estrogen receptor, aromatase inhibition, antiangiogenesis activity, and antioxidative effects (Thompson, 1995). Thus flaxseed and its lignans antagonize the effects of estrogen and therefore have a potential role in breast cancer prevention and treatment. Ingestion of 25 g/day of flaxseed is being studied in several settings to assess its potential as a breast cancer preventative.

Oral Contraceptives   Numerous case-control and several prospective studies have been performed to assess the relationship between exposure to oral contraceptives and risk of breast cancer. Evaluation of these data is complicated by issues such as differences in the hormonal composition of the oral contraceptives used and changing patterns of use. There is, however, no consistent evidence to suggest that the use of oral contraceptives has a major impact on the risk of breast cancer. Oral contraceptives function by inhibiting gonadotrophin secretion, which, in turn, reduces the synthesis of ovarian sex steroids; this potential benefit might be offset by the sex-steroid components of the oral contraceptive (Spicer et al., 1995).

Hormone Replacement Therapy Hormone replacement therapy (HRT) is given to postmenopausal women to decrease menopausal symptoms, as well as the risk of osteoporosis and cardiovascular disease. Epidemiologic studies of HRT appear to indicate that any increase in breast cancer risk is modest, with estimates of 1.3- to 2-fold (Hulka et al., 1994). These estimates of risk depend upon duration of use, age, and menopausal status. It has been shown that in women on 0.625 mg of conjugated estrogens, the SHBG-bound estrogen is approximately twice as high as that of a postmenopausal woman not on HRT (Pike et al., 1993). In women with a strong family history of breast cancer, the risk appears higher, with relative risks of four- to sixfold (see Isaacs and Swain, 1994, for review). There are insufficient data on risks from the combined effects of estrogen plus progestin replacement therapy, but given the proliferative effects of progesterone on breast tissue, the risk might be greater with the combination.

If the abnormalities in hormone pathways lead directly or indirectly to carcinogenic events, sex steroid antagonists could block the induced breast cell proliferation, thus reducing breast cancer incidence rates by inhibiting or deferring the development of cancer. For example, the antiestrogen tamoxifen (see Sec. 12.4.1) is effective not only in the treatment of metastatic breast cancer and in reducing recurrence in the adjuvant setting but also in decreasing the incidence of new cancers in the opposite breast. Large randomized, placebo-controlled trials are in progress to assess the effects of tamoxifen on the incidence of breast cancer in women who are at increased risk for contracting the disease.

The gene encoding human aromatase (*CYP19*) is expressed in ovary, placenta, and adipose tissue, and each tissue has a different type of promoter region (Simpson et al., 1994). Aromatase activity in adipose tissue in breast quadrants has been correlated with tumor site and mutations in the human *CYP19* gene (O'Neill et al., 1988; Shozu et al., 1991). Overexpression of *int-5/aromatase* in mammary glands of transgenic mice results in the induction of hyperplasia and nuclear abnormalities, which are indicative of preneoplastic changes (Tekmal et al., 1996). Thus the control of the aromatase gene in breast tissue may play an important role in breast carcinogenesis.

12.3.2 Experimental Models for Breast Cancer

Animal models of breast cancer have been widely used to study various aspects of breast cancer biology (Gould, 1995). These are diverse, including chemically and virally induced tumors, transgenic mouse models, and human tumor xenografts. Established breast cancer models have contributed to our understanding of the various factors—e.g., endocrinologic and immunologic—influencing both normal mammary gland development and breast carcinogenesis. These models permit investigation to further our understanding of the processes involved in breast cancer initiation, promotion, and progression.

Chemically Induced Mammary Tumorigenesis The two most widely used experimental systems for the study of rat mammary tumorigenesis are those in which tumors are induced in the Sprague-Dawley rat by administration of either 12-dimethylbenz(a)-anthracene (DMBA) or *N*-methyl-*N*-nitrosourea (NMU). Most tumors develop within 20 weeks of exposure. These models are useful for looking at early events in the process of chemical carcinogenesis and for studying malignant progression. The DMBA-induced tumors have a relatively low incidence of activated *ras* expression (25 percent), whereas 75 percent or more of NMU-induced tumors express mutant *ras* gene; ras proteins mediate cellular proliferation signals from stimulated growth factor receptors—e.g., the EGF receptor (see Chap. 6, Sec. 6.3.4; Zhang et al., 1990). Therefore, use of the NMU model might slant mechanistic studies towards *ras*-mediated events, and *ras* mutations occur in less than 10 percent of human breast tumors (Bos, 1989). Both the DMBA- and NMU-induced mammary tumor models have been used extensively in assessing antiestrogen efficacy in both the treatment and prevention of breast cancer. For example, in both models, tamoxifen and other antiestrogens administered after carcinogen exposure but before tumor appearance were shown to delay tumor appearance until the withdrawal of therapy (Lindsey et al., 1981). These models have also been used to assess the efficacy of new pharmaceutical agents such as aromatase inhibitors.

Virally Induced Rodent Models Mammary tumors may be induced by polyomavirus, adenovirus type 9, and the murine mammary tumor virus (MMTV), which is discussed in greater detail below. MMTV is a nonacute transforming RNA-containing virus that induces breast cancer in mice (Hynes et al., 1984; Morris et al., 1990). This agent is a biological carcinogen that induces somatic mutations by acting as an insertional mutagen, causing deregulation of expression of adjacent cellular genes (designated the *Int* loci) in mammary cells. To identify affected cellular genes, the viral genome has been used as a molecular tag, and using this approach six *Int* loci (*Int1/Wnt1*, *Int2/Fgf3*, *Wnt3*, *Hst/k-Fgf4*, *Wnt10b*, and *Fgf8*) have been identified in mammary tumors of MMTV-infected transgenic mice (see Callahan, 1996, for review). Examination of the human homologues of these genes as targets for somatic mutations during breast carcinogenesis is under way. It is probable that multiple factors are necessary for the development of breast cancers and multiple somatic mutations may be involved in this process. The MMTV–mouse model system provides an experimental approach to identify genes and signaling pathways that, when altered by mutations, contribute to the deregulation of normal mammary gland development and subsequent mammary tumorigenesis. The MMTV model has also been used to study possible mechanisms by which steroid hormones may influence gene expression in target cells.

The mouse models have some limitations relative to human breast cancer, as there are species differences; for example, the histopathology of mouse mammary tumors does not correspond to the most frequent forms of human breast tumors (invasive ductal carcinomas). It is also uncertain whether the genetics of mouse mammary tumorigenesis is directly relevant to human breast cancer since, for example, *Wnt1* and *Wnt3* do not appear to be rearranged or amplified in invasive ductal carcinomas of the human breast; while *Fgf3/FGf4* are frequently coamplified in invasive ductal carcinomas, whether they are expressed as a consequence is a controversial matter (Vande Vijver et al., 1989; Callahan et al., 1993; Roelink et al., 1993). Human homologues of the other *Int* genes have not as yet been tested for genetic alterations in breast cancer. Since the *Int6* type of viral insertion can be functionally similar to LOH (loss of heterozygosity; see Chap. 4, Sec. 4.5.3 and Chap. 5, Sec. 5.5.1), identification of genes affected by this mutation may direct us to genes which may be candidates for mutations in human breast cancer.

Human breast tissue xenografts are used widely to study breast cancer. This process involves grafting human breast cancer cell lines into immune-deficient animals, such as athymic nude mice or mice homozygous for the severe combined immune deficiency (SCID) mutation (see Chap. 15, Sec. 15.3.2). The three most widely used hormone-dependent human breast cancer xenografts are the MCF-7, ZR-75-1, and T-47D cell lines. All three were derived

from malignant effusions in postmenopausal women and require estrogenic supplementation for tumorigenesis in nude mice. The estrogen-induced growth is inhibited by antiestrogen administration. Several other breast cancer cell lines are used as xenografts to mimic the spectrum of human breast tumor characteristics, including hormone-independence; hormone unresponsiveness (the majority of these are ER-negative, e.g., MDA-MB-231); drug resistance (e.g., MCF-7^{ADR}, a cell line that overexpresses the pg170 product of the human *MDR1* gene, described in Chap. 17, Sec. 17.2.4; MCF-7^{ADR} cells are ER-negative and resistant to antiestrogens); and metastatic models [(e.g., two ER-negative cell lines, MDA-MB-231 and MDA-MB-435, produce locally invasive tumors with metastases reproducibly found in the lungs and other organs (see Clarke, 1996, for review)].

While xenograft models have some limitations, similarities between these models and clinical breast cancer are substantial, and the histology of these xenografts often reflects that of human adenocarcinomas. Since the cell lines are already transformed, xenograft models are of limited value for looking at early events in breast carcinogenesis.

Transgenic animal models (see Chap. 3, Sec. 3.3.12) have been used to study the impact of various genetic manipulations on breast cancer development. Experiments with transgenic animals often use promoters—such as the mouse mammary tumor virus long-terminal repeat (MMTV-LTR) promoter/enhancer, the whey acidic protein promoter (WAP), and the β-lactoglobulin promoter—to target oncogenes to the mammary gland. WAP and β-lactoglobulin promoter are from milk-specific genes and cause expression of transgenes in the later stages of pregnancy and during lactation. MMTV is active in the virgin mammary gland, has increased expression during pregnancy, and causes expression of transgenes in other tissues. Several studies have been performed using transgenic mice that overexpress *erbB-2* in the mouse mammary gland, which leads to the appearance of breast tumors in female mice (Guy et al., 1992). The corresponding *HER2/neu* gene has been found to be amplified and/or overexpressed in human breast cancers (see Sec. 12.3.5). Another example is transgenic mice with enhanced expression of cyclin D1, a cell-cycle regulatory gene (see Chap. 7, Sec. 7.2.2, and Sec. 12.3.5, below). These mice develop mammary gland hyperplasias at young age and adenocarcinomas after about 18 months (see Amundadottir et al., 1996, for review). Overexpression of cyclin D1 mRNA is seen in approximately 45 percent of human breast cancer samples (Buckley et al., 1993). Also, the expression of this gene is known to be induced by estrogen and progesterone, as demonstrated using the T-47D model (Musgrove et al., 1993). It is now believed that cyclin D1 is involved in the mediation of mitogenic response to growth factors and hormones. The current generation of bi- or tritransgenic animals may provide additional information on how the various genes may interact and may determine which pathways are important for tumorigenesis.

12.3.3 Risk Factors for Prostate Cancer

There is substantial evidence that androgens are involved in the etiology of prostate cancer (Key, 1995; Klein, 1995). For example, the factors outlined below influence the risk of disease (see also Table 12.3).

Castration Prostate cancer does not occur in persons whose testes were removed before puberty, which indicates that an intact hormonal environment is important for the development of prostate cancer (Huggins and Hodges, 1941). Supportive data come from the low incidence of prostate cancer in males with elevated estrogen levels—for example, cirrhotic patients (Robson, 1966). These patients have decreased hepatic estrogen metabolism and frequently have testicular atrophy and gynecomastia.

Sexual Behavior There is a slight increase in relative risk (~1.3) for early age at first intercourse, for multiple sexual partners (~1.2), and for history of sexually acquired infection (~1.9). These observations suggest a relationship between increased sexual activity, increased hormonal stimulation (androgen), and prostate cancer risk, although an infectious agent might also be implicated in this increased risk.

Vasectomy In a review by Key (1995), a summary relative risk of 1.54 (nine studies) was determined. The slight increase in risk associated with vasectomy remains controversial, as the results from studies vary. Several studies have reported changes in hormonal status following vasectomy, although others have not confirmed these findings.

Age The incidence of prostate cancer increases with age. Changes that occur with age include a decline in serum testosterone levels and an increase in the incidence of benign prostatic hyperplasia, but neither of these factors appear to be related to the development of prostate cancer.

Race/Ethnicity The incidence of prostate cancer varies among populations. African Americans have a higher age-specific incidence and prostate cancer death rate than Caucasian Americans. Epidemiologic studies demonstrate that black men generally present at a younger age with higher grade and stage

Table 12.3. Hormonally Related Epidemiologic Risk Factors for Prostate Cancer

Factor	Risk Group	Relative Risk
Obesity	More obese	1.25[a]
Dietary fat	Higher-fat diet	1.31[a]
Smoking	Yes	1.16[a]
Sexual behavior	Early age at first intercourse	1.31[a]
	Multiple sexual partners	1.24[a]
	History of sexually acquired infection	1.86[a]
Vasectomy	Yes	1.54[a]
Age	>55 years	—
Race (age-adjusted)	Black	1.8[b]
Family history	One first-degree relative	2.0[c]
	One first- and one second-degree relative	8.8[c]

[a]Summary of relative risks (data summarized from multiple studies); Key, 1995.

[b]Morton, 1994.

[c]Klein, 1995.

Source: Adapted from Morton, 1994; Key, 1995; and Klein, 1995.

disease and have markedly decreased survival as compared with white men (see Morton, 1994, for review). These observations support the argument that there may be a difference in the biology of prostate cancer in black men. Several studies have found that black men have higher testosterone levels than white men. The racial difference in serum testosterone levels appears age-related; it is higher in younger black men (versus white) and similar to that in white men by ages 40 to 50 years. Thus, at the time many prostate cancers appear, circulating androgen levels in black and white men are similar. This does not exclude the possibility that the early elevated exposure to androgens may be a factor in the observed elevated prostate cancer risk in black men.

Diet An association between a high-fat diet and the development of prostate cancer has been demonstrated in several studies. Observed international differences (for example, men in Japan and Taiwan have much lower rates of clinical prostate cancer than men in western countries) suggest that diet might influence the etiology of this disease (Berg, 1975; Graham et al., 1983). Reductions in total dietary fat have been shown to reduce circulating androgen levels (Hill et al., 1979).

Obesity Obesity appears to be associated with a slight increase in risk for prostate cancer (~1.3). This might be associated with the physiologic impact of obesity on sex steroid metabolism or with a particular pattern of diet.

Sex Hormone Levels There are conflicting data concerning sex hormone levels and prostate cancer. Studies assessing prediagnostic serum hormone levels found that lower levels of dihydrotestosterone and higher testosterone : dihydrotestosterone (DHT) ratio and androstenedione levels were related to an increased risk of prostate cancer (Nomura et al., 1988; Barrett-Connor et al., 1990; Hsing and Comstock, 1993). Since blood hormone levels do not correlate well with hormone levels in the prostate (Rose et al., 1984), testosterone : DHT ratios in plasma provide an indirect measure of the metabolic activity within the prostate; but other studies have not confirmed these serum hormone correlations. Differences in 5α-reductase activity (converts testosterone to DHT), as measured by the presence of androgen metabolites, have been observed, with young black and white men having significantly higher levels of androgen metabolites than young Japanese men (Ross et al., 1992).

Smoking Association of cigarette smoking with prostate cancer risk is controversial. A review of 20 studies (10 of which reported an increase in prostate cancer risk) found a summary relative risk of 1.16 (Key, 1995). Cigarette smoking has been shown to be associated with high circulating testosterone levels in middle-aged men (Dai et al., 1981).

12.3.4 Experimental Models for Prostate Cancer

Although prostate cancer is one of the leading causes of cancer-related mortality, the biology of this disease is poorly understood. There are few established animal cell lines or models for prostate cancer as opposed to breast cancer, where there are 100 to 150 different cell lines. Various technical reasons account for this: Prostate cancer rarely arises spontaneously in animals and is difficult to grow in culture or as xenografts. Some laboratory models of prostate cancer have been developed and include rodent models, human cell lines, xenografts, and transgenic mouse models.

Rodent Models The transplantable Dunning (R3327) rat tumor arose spontaneously in 1961 and is one of the oldest and best-studied animal models for prostate cancer. This tumor is very slow-growing and resembles a well-differentiated prostate adenocarcinoma. The R3327 tumor has given rise to a number of sublines with varying hormonal sensitivity, histopathology, and metastatic potential (Isaacs et al., 1986; Figure 12.9). The H subline (R3327H) is slow-growing, well-differentiated, androgen-sensitive, and contains 5α-reductase as well as androgen, estrogen, and progesterone receptors. This subline rarely metastasizes but randomly undergoes progression to androgen independence in that if rats are castrated or treated with hormonal agents (e.g., antiandrogens), the tumor regresses, but a proportion of the cells are androgen-insensitive; after initial growth inhibition, the tumor relapses from hormonal control and tumor growth resumes. This tumor is now referred to as the R3327H1 subline and has a similar pattern of growth and hormone responsiveness as the disease in humans. Following serial transplantation into castrated rats, the A subline was discovered. This line is a squamous cell cancer; it is androgen-independent, lacks androgen receptors and the 5α-reductase enzyme, and grows 10 times faster than the H subline. These models have been used to provide information on the mechanisms involved in the development of androgen independence. A variety of sublines have been developed, including G, AT-1, and AT-2 (all arising

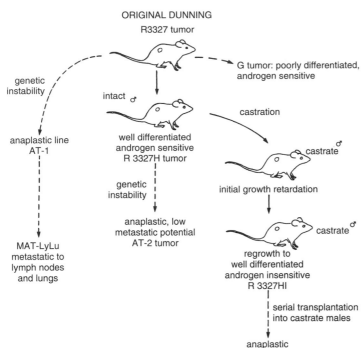

ORIGINAL DUNNING
R3327 tumor

G tumor: poorly differentiated, androgen sensitive

genetic instability

intact ♂

anaplastic line AT-1

well differentiated androgen sensitive R 3327H tumor

castration

castrate ♂

initial growth retardation

genetic instability

anaplastic, low metastatic potential AT-2 tumor

castrate ♂

MAT-LyLu metastatic to lymph nodes and lungs

regrowth to well differentiated androgen insensitive R 3327HI

serial transplantation into castrate males

anaplastic

Figure 12.9. The transplantable Dunning prostatic carcinoma model has been used widely as a model for the human disease. Transplantation of the original tumor into intact males leads to an androgen-sensitive tumor (R3327H) with a subpopulation of androgen-insensitive cells that can grow to form androgen-independent tumors in castrated animals (R3327H1). Other sublines have developed, including anaplastic (AT-1 and AT-2) and metastatic (e.g., MAT-LyLu) lines. (Adapted from Isaacs et al., 1986.)

spontaneously and with low metastatic potential); MAT-LyLu, MAT-Lu (both arising from the AT-1 subline); and AT-3 (arising spontaneously and with high metastatic potential, generally metastasizing to lung and/or lymph nodes). These models have provided some information on the mechanisms of metastases, although the most common metastatic site for prostate cancer in humans is bone (see Royai et al., 1996, for review).

Another animal model is provided by the Shionogi mouse mammary tumor, which arose spontaneously in 1961 and is responsive to androgens after passage in male mice. Tumor shrinkage occurs after androgen ablation in this model; it has therefore been used to study mechanisms of androgen action on tumors. Other animal models of prostate cancer include the Noble rat prostate adenocarcinoma, the Pollard, and the ACI models.

Human Cell Lines The most commonly studied cell lines are PC-3, DU-145, and LNCaP. All three originate from metastatic lesions. PC-3 and DU-145 are poorly differentiated; they lack androgen receptors and 5α-reductase and do not produce prostate-specific antigen (PSA; tumor marker). LNCaP is the most commonly used cell line; it expresses PSA and prostatic acid phosphatase and is androgen-sensitive, although it has a mutated androgen receptor. The LNCaP cell line can be grown as xenografts in nude mice.

Appropriate models for prostate cancer are needed to provide an understanding of the clinical events occurring in prostate cancer, such as transition from androgen dependence to androgen independence. Additionally, as the molecular biology of this disease is studied, animals models may provide more information about which genes are important and how various genes interact during tumorigenesis.

12.3.5 Hormonal Interactions with Oncogenes

The primary oncogenic events in breast cancer occur at a cellular level. The development of tumors may (1) be influenced indirectly by hormonal pathways as outlined above or (2) be due to genetic changes that result in the development of a "hormone-dependent" cancer. Examples that link these two concepts are outlined below.

HER-2/neu/c-erbB-2 Proto-oncogene Amplification/overexpression of these proto-oncogenes has been found in 10 to 30 percent of breast tumor specimens (Dickson, 1995). The *HER-2/neu* product is a membrane tyrosine kinase receptor homologous to the EGF receptor. *HER-2/neu* amplification is thought to be an early lesion and is associated with absence of ER and PR and a poor prognosis in invasive breast cancers (Tsuda et al., 1989). Olsson et al. (1991) have reported that use of oral contraceptives before age 20 or use late in reproductive life leads to an increased risk of breast cancers with *HER-2/neu* amplification (odds ratio, 5.3). Treurniet et al. (1992) reported that breast-feeding and late age of first pregnancy both increase the risk of *HER-2/neu*-positive tumors. These studies suggest a hormonal influence on expression of this oncogene.

Int-2 and PRAD-1 Oncogenes Amplification and/or overexpression of the *Int-2* gene appears to be associated with ER-positive tumors with an aggressive course and poor prognosis (Lidereau et al., 1988). Olsson et al. (1991) reported that *Int-2* amplification in breast tumors was associated with progestin use and abortion before first full-term pregnancy. The *Int-2* gene is a member of the Fibroblast Growth Factor (FGF) gene family and is amplified in 4 to 23 percent of human breast carcinomas (Barrett-Lee, 1991). Since the amplified *Int-2* gene is not commonly expressed in breast cancers, another linked gene (i.e., a gene located close to the *Int-2* gene on the same chromosome) may be of more importance, and this gene may be *PRAD-1*. The *PRAD-1* gene product is cyclin D1, which is involved in control of the cell cycle (see Chap. 7, Sec. 7.2.2). Cyclin-D1 appears to be estrogen-regulated, since estradiol can induce cyclin-D1 and antiestrogens have been shown to downregulate cyclin D1 expression in the MCF-7 cell line (Watts et al., 1994; see also Sec. 12.3.2). These data again indicate a possible hormonal influence on the expression of these genes.

12.4 PHARMACOLOGIC APPLICATIONS OF HORMONES IN CANCER

12.4.1 Treatment of Breast Cancer

The finding in 1896 that oophorectomy could result in regression of skin metastases in women with breast cancer initiated the concept of endocrine treatment for breast cancer (Beatson, 1896). A number of factors predict the likelihood of response to endocrine therapy, of which hormone receptor status is the most important (Table 12.4). Patients with ER-positive/PR-positive disease have response rates of approximately 70 percent, versus < 10 percent in ER-negative/PR-negative disease (Muss, 1992). Thus, from a treatment perspective, quantitation of receptor level is of importance. However, the correlation between receptor positivity and hormone response is not exact, and these discrepancies may be explained in part by receptor variants. A number of ER variants have been identified, as discussed below (see Sec. 12.4.2). Correla-

Table 12.4. Factors Associated with the Response of Breast Cancer to Endocrine Therapy

Variable	Response, %
Estrogen and progesterone receptor	
ER+/PR+	70
ER+/PR−	30
ER−/PR+	40
ER−/PR−	< 10
Site of metastases	
Soft tissue	30–60
Bone	20–50
Lung/pleura	20–40
Liver	5–30
Menopausal status	
Premenopausal	30
Postmenopausal > 5 years	30–35
Perimenopausal	20
Age (years)	
30–39	20
40–49	30
50–59	30
60–69	37
≥ 70	46
Disease-free interval	
< 5 years	30–42
> 5 years	56
Prior response to endocrine therapy	
Yes	35–60
No	17–30

Source: From Muss, 1992, with permission.

tions between receptor positivity and patient characteristics were analyzed by Clark et al. (1984), who assayed biopsy specimens from approximately 3000 patients with primary breast cancer. They determined that 64 percent of premenopausal and 79 percent of postmenopausal patients had ER-positive tumors. Additionally, 62 percent and 80 percent of patients aged < 50 or ≥ 50 years, respectively, had ER-positive tumors. Both age and menopausal status were found to be significant predictors for ER positivity. It was also determined that 58 percent of premenopausal and 53 percent of postmenopausal patients had PR-positive tumors. There appeared to be no relationship between PR status and age or menopausal status; however, the probability of PR positivity was inversely correlated with the size of the primary tumor.

Ablation of ovarian function reduces the amount of estrogen available to bind to its receptor. This results in a reduction in the transcription of the estrogen-induced genes and thus suppression of tumor growth. Ablation of ovarian function can be achieved by surgical castration (oophorectomy), radiation therapy, or biochemical castration via use of LHRH analogues (leuprolide, goserelin acetate, buserelin acetate). This therapy is used in premenopausal females likely to respond to endocrine therapy.

Antiestrogens bind competitively to the estrogen receptor, thus inhibiting estrogen-induced proliferation. Antiestrogens may be grouped into two classes based upon structure: nonsteroidal and steroidal. Tamoxifen is a nonsteroidal antiestrogen (Fig. 12.10). Although not all of its mechanisms of actions are elucidated, tamoxifen competes with circulating estrogen to bind to the estrogen receptor (ER). It binds to the ligand-binding domain, inducing receptor activation. Although the tamoxifen-ER

17-β-estradiol

tamoxifen

ICI 182780 (steroidal antiestrogen)

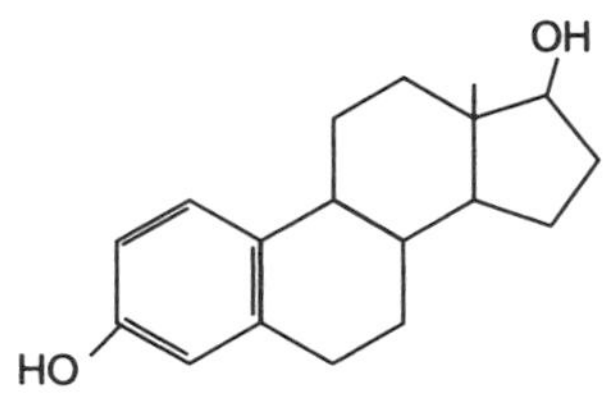

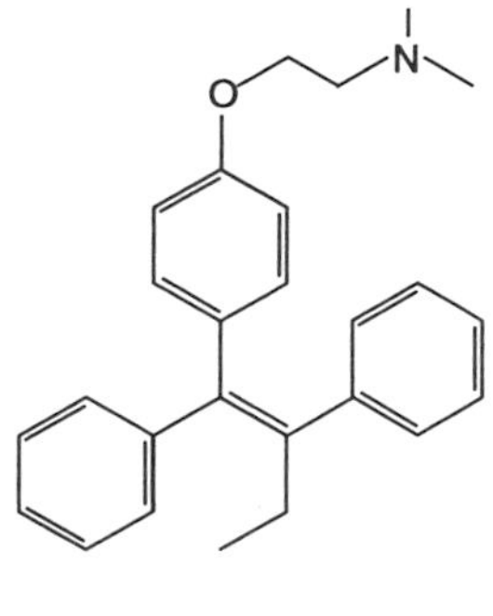

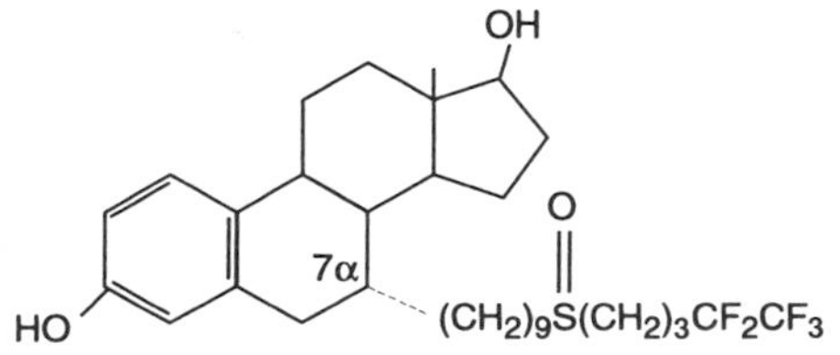

Figure 12.10. Structures of 17-β-estradiol, tamoxifen, and the steroidal antiestrogen ICI 182780.

complex binds to the estrogen response element (ERE) on target genes (see Sec. 12.2.3), it does not induce gene transcription and cell growth is inhibited (Fig. 12.11). The mechanism(s) by which the tamoxifen-ER-ERE complex is modulated may involve transcriptional factors or altered interaction with ER "accessory" proteins (Fuqua, 1994). Tamoxifen also has weak estrogen-agonist effects. In tissues such as uterus and bone, tamoxifen may have stronger agonist properties due to the presence of other proteins that augment transcriptional activation (Osborne et al., 1996). It is thought that binding of tamoxifen to the estrogen receptor augments transcription through the transcription-activating site AF-1, which is in the A/B domain of the ER (Fig. 12.4). AF-1 is constitutively active even in the absence of estrogen. Another transcription-activating site, AF-2, which is in the ligand-binding domain, is activated by estrogens and inhibited by binding of tamoxifen (Fig. 12.4). In hormone-responsive human breast cancer cells, tamoxifen was also found to decrease positive growth factor levels (e.g., TGF-α), and in human breast cancer in vivo following tamoxifen treatment, the expression of TGF-β$_1$, which is growth-inhibitory, was induced (Butta et al., 1992).

Given its low toxicity, tamoxifen is often given as first-line therapy to patients with hormone-responsive metastatic breast cancer (both pre- and postmenopausal patients). The rate of response achieved is comparable to that observed with other endocrine therapies (Haller et al., 1991). Tamoxifen use is associated with an increased risk (two- to threefold) of endometrial cancer (Fornander et al., 1989); in the laboratory it has been shown that tamoxifen can stimulate the growth of human endometrial carcinoma. This is likely related to its estrogen-agonist effects in this tissue. New nonsteroidal antiestrogens such as toremifine, droloxifene (3-hydroxy-tamoxifen), and trioxifene have estrogen agonist-versus-antagonist effects different from those of tamoxifen. Clinical trials are under way to assess whether these agents are superior to tamoxifen for efficacy and/or side effects.

Steroidal antiestrogens have been developed, such as 7α long-chain analogues of estradiol (Fig. 12.10), with the aim of decreasing estrogenic side effects, which are observed with nonsteroidal antiestrogens such as tamoxifen. These compounds bind to and block estrogen receptors, but they also inhibit receptor dimerization and DNA binding. In addition, they may promote estrogen receptor degradation; thus, by depleting estrogen receptors,

Figure 12.11. Diagram of estrogen/tamoxifen action in cells. Estrogen (E_2) or tamoxifen (TAM) binds to the hormone-binding domain of the estrogen receptor (ER), which dimerizes through protein : protein interactions. The ER dimer then binds to specific DNA sequences, termed *estrogen-response elements* of estrogen-responsive genes, thereby influencing gene expression. Depending on the ligand bound, either stimulation or inhibition of growth is seen. (From Fuqua, 1994, with permission.)

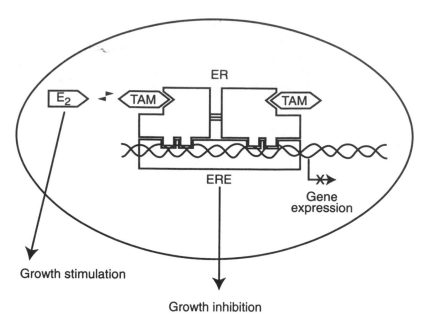

the steroidal antiestrogens may demonstrate a "pure" antiestrogen effect in their target tissues and inhibit tumor growth (Osborne et al., 1996).

Progestins/Antiprogestins   The mechanism of action of progestins is not well understood but may involve direct action on breast cancer cells and an indirect effect through the hypothalamus/pituitary/ovarian and pituitary/adrenal axes. At a molecular level, progestins bind to the progesterone receptor (PR) and the activated complex then binds the progesterone response element (PRE) on target genes, inducing gene transcription. It is known that estrogen can positively regulate PR expression (Clarke and Sutherland, 1990) and that presence of the PR improves the probability of tumor response to hormone therapy. The most common progestational agents used in breast cancer are megestrol acetate and medroxy-progesterone acetate. In randomized trials, these and other progestins appear to be equivalent in efficacy to tamoxifen and other endocrine agents, with reported response rates of 20 to 40 percent (Muss et al., 1985). Owing to side effects such as weight gain and fluid retention, megestrol acetate is generally used following tamoxifen as second- or third-line therapy for advanced disease. With the increasing use of tamoxifen in the adjuvant setting, this positioning may alter in the future.

The experimental antiprogestin RU486 (mifepristone) has been shown to bind to the PR and the resulting complex is activated and binds to the PRE

of the target genes. However, the conformation of the RU486-PR-PRE differs from that of the progestin complex and induction of gene transcription does not occur. In a phase II study of RU486 in 28 patients with untreated metastatic breast cancer, 3 partial responses were observed and toxic effects were generally mild to moderate (Perrault et al., 1996). The authors concluded that the data did not support the use of RU486 as a single agent in the management of breast cancer.

Murphy et al. (1994) demonstrated that growth of cultured T-47D human breast cancer cells could be inhibited by both progestins and antiprogestins. Their data suggest that these agents differentially regulate the expression of genes such as c-*myc*, c-*jun*, and c-*fos*, which are known to have important roles in growth and differentiation. Since the products of the *jun* and *fos* gene families can form homo- and/or heterodimers comprising AP-1 transcription factors (see Chap. 6, Sec. 6.3.6), progestins and antiprogestins may differentially regulate the expression of AP-1 transcription complexes. Additionally, progestins have been shown to transiently increase c-*myc* mRNA levels, c-*myc* being a proto-oncogene associated with growth modulation/differentiation. Antiprogestins have been shown to inhibit the progestin-induced effect on c-*myc* (Musgrove et al., 1991). These data indicate that progestins and antiprogestins, which are both growth-inhibitory in T-47D cells, differ in their mechanisms of action, although both work through binding to the PR.

Aromatase Inhibitors The mechanism of action of these agents is to reduce the synthesis of estrogens by inhibiting the aromatase enzyme complex; they are used in postmenopausal women, where estrogens are produced predominantly by the aromatization of adrenal androgens in the peripheral tissues (Goss and Gwyn, 1994). The most extensively studied aromatase inhibitor is aminoglutethimide, which gives response rates comparable to other endocrine therapies, albeit with greater toxicity. Aminoglutethimide also inhibits the conversion of cholesterol to pregnenolone by blocking the enzyme 20,22 desmolase (Fig. 12.2). Because this inhibition is early in the steroid biosynthesis pathway, hydrocortisone supplementation is necessary to avoid adrenal insufficiency. Since the side effects of aminoglutethimide are considerable, this agent is being replaced by more specific and potent inhibitors of aromatase, such as anastrozole, vorozole, letrozole, formestane (4-hydroxyandrost-4-ene-3,17-dione), and others. Another agent, liarozole, may be useful in breast cancer treatment. This agent, in addition to inhibiting aromatase, inhibits the synthesis of testosterone and the 4-hydroxylase enzyme responsible for the metabolism of retinoids. Toxicity is moderate and is "retinoid-like," involving predominately skin rashes. Aromatase inhibitors are not used in premenopausal women, as a functional hypothalamus/pituitary axis can lead to increases in gonadotrophins, subsequently increasing estrogen levels and overcoming aromatase inhibition. Elevated gonadotropin levels can, in turn, lead to ovarian enlargement and hyperstimulation.

12.4.2 Resistance to Endocrine Therapy

Resistance to endocrine therapy has been most studied for the antiestrogen tamoxifen. The primary mechanism responsible for tamoxifen resistance, either intrinsic or acquired, remains unknown, and it is probable that multiple mechanisms are involved in the emergence of tamoxifen resistance.

The presence of ERs and/or PRs in breast tumors is predictive of tumor sensitivity to endocrine therapy. However, this correlation is not exact, since a proportion of ER-positive tumors fail to respond initially to endocrine therapy. This is referred to as *intrinsic resistance*. Even tumors that respond initially to endocrine therapy will develop resistance over time, which may range from several weeks to several years (see Muss, 1992, for review). This is referred to as *acquired resistance*. In some instances resistance may occur due to loss of ER-positive cells; however, in most cases, expression of the ER is maintained (Encarnacion et al., 1993). It is proposed that breast tumors have subpopulations of cells—for example, those with normal or variant ERs. When treated with endocrine therapy such as tamoxifen, cells with normal ERs are growth-inhibited while those with ER variants may be unaffected. Thus, over time, the growth and emergence of subpopulations unresponsive to or stimulated by tamoxifen occurs. The hormone treatment itself provides the selective pressure that results eventually in the clinical observation of endocrine resistance (Horwitz, 1994).

Various ER variants have been found in breast cancer biopsies and breast cancer cell lines. For example, Fuqua et al. (1991) demonstrated the presence of an ER (ERδE5) that lacks a region in the ligand-binding domain (exon 5 deletion). This variant activated transcription in an estrogen-dependent gene construct in yeast cells in the *absence* of estrogen. Another variant, ERδE3, lacks exon 3, encoding the second zinc finger of the DNA-binding domain. This variant is nonfunctional, since this ER cannot bind to the estrogen response element (Fuqua et al., 1992). These mutants could lead to the clinical picture of an ER-positive breast cancer unresponsive to endocrine therapy. Progesterone receptor heterogeneity has also been detected, but its effect on responsiveness to hormone therapy is unknown. Roodi et al. (1995) investigated whether an ER-negative phenotype was the result of mutations in the coding region of the ER gene by examining the ER gene in various ER-positive and ER-negative breast tumors. They found few mutations, suggesting that the ER-negative phenotype is likely due to deficient ER expression at the transcriptional or posttranscriptional level.

A variety of mechanisms have been proposed for the development of acquired resistance to tamoxifen (Tonetti and Jordan, 1995; Wolf and Fuqua, 1995); these are discussed in relation to Fig. 12.12.

1. *Metabolism of tamoxifen* Tamoxifen is converted in the cell to two main metabolites, 4-hydroxytamoxifen (4HT; minor) and N-desmethyltamoxifen (NDT; major). 4HT is a potent antiestrogen that binds to the ER with high affinity; however, it is somewhat unstable and may isomerize to a less potent antiestrogen. The major metabolite, NDT, is a weak antiestrogen. Tamoxifen may also be metabolized to two estrogenic compounds, metabolite E and bisphenol. Alterations in tamoxifen metabolism in breast tumor cells could increase excretion or produce less active metabolites, thus reducing efficacy. The concept has

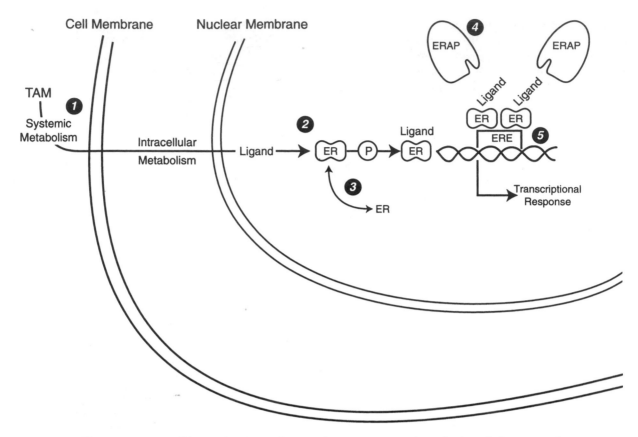

Figure 12.12. Possible mechanisms of tamoxifen resistance. Potential sites of alteration of the ER-mediated signal-transduction pathway resulting in tamoxifen (TAM) resistance. *1.* Metabolism of TAM to estrogenic compounds. *2.* Loss or mutation of the estrogen receptor (ER). *3.* Aberrant posttranslational modification of the ER. *4.* Alteration of other transcription factors or ER-associated proteins (ERAP). *5.* Alteration of the estrogen response element (ERE). P indicates phosphorylation. (From Tonetti and Jordan, 1995, with permission.)

been explored by quantitating the levels of tamoxifen and its metabolites in tamoxifen-stimulated and inhibited tumors. In this study, MCF-7 human breast cancer cells were implanted into athymic BALB/c mice, which were subsequently treated with tamoxifen as a model to study acquired resistance. It was reported that tamoxifen-stimulated tumors had significantly reduced levels of tamoxifen compared with tamoxifen-inhibited tumors. However, others were not able to reproduce this finding.

2. *Loss or mutation of the estrogen receptor* When tamoxifen binds to the ER, it forms a complex capable of interacting with the estrogen response element, but it does *not* activate the process of transcription. A mutation in the ER might confer tamoxifen resistance by allowing the tamoxifen-ER complex to activate the transcriptional

process. Catherino and Jordan (1995) transfected an ER mutated at codon 351 (obtained from a tamoxifen-stimulated human breast cancer cell line) into the ER-negative human breast cancer cell line MDA-MB-231 and were able to demonstrate that this mutant ER was activated by the binding of 4-hydroxytamoxifen (tamoxifen analogue) or estradiol. Although a variety of ER mutations have been identified, it does not appear that this is a major mechanism of tamoxifen resistance, as these mutations are present infrequently in human breast cancer. However, these data could suggest a possible mechanism for the observation of tumor regression that occurs infrequently after withdrawal of tamoxifen.

3. *Aberrant post-translational modification of the ER* Phosphorylation of specific serine residues within the N-terminal region of the A/B domain

of the ER may mediate hormone binding, DNA binding, and transcriptional activation. This phosphorylation is induced by estradiol and by 4-hydroxytamoxifen as well as by activators of protein kinases A and C. Resistance to tamoxifen might occur owing to a defect or alteration in the phosphorylation of the ER, and this could be related to a protein kinase abnormality. Activation of the protein kinase A pathway has been shown to increase the agonist activity of the tamoxifen-ER complex, and increased intracellular cAMP levels have been associated with increased transcription activity of an antiestrogen-ER complex. Increased cAMP levels may lead to tamoxifen-stimulated growth.

4. *Other transcription factors* Recent reports have identified several proteins that associate specifically with the ER-ligand-estrogen response element complex and influence transcriptional activation. There are three transcriptional activator sites: AF-1 (A/B domain, constitutive), AF-2a (recently discovered), and AF-2, which are in the ligand-binding domain and activated by the binding of hormone. A possible mechanism for tamoxifen resistance might involve alterations in specific receptor-associated proteins that may be required for effective transcriptional activation. Several ER-associated proteins that directly associate with the ER in the presence of estrogen but not in the presence of 4-hydroxytamoxifen have been isolated. Mutations within the ligand-binding domain have abolished the binding of these proteins. Thus a defect in any of these proteins might result in an alteration of the signal at the estrogen response element.

5. *Estrogen response element (ERE) modification* Modifications to the ERE (sequence variation, placement of multiple EREs; orientation) could influence the binding of the ligand-ER complex as well as the transcriptional response to the ligand. For example, the binding might be interpreted as agonistic rather than antagonistic.

12.4.3 Treatment of Prostate Cancer

Hormonal treatment of prostate cancer is based upon its marked sensitivity to androgen deprivation, as documented originally by Huggins and Hodges (1941), when they showed that surgical or medical (diethylstilbestrol) castration produced a dramatic reduction in cancer mass and clinical remissions. The aim of all current endocrine treatments for prostate cancer is to deprive the cancer of androgens (Fig. 12.13).

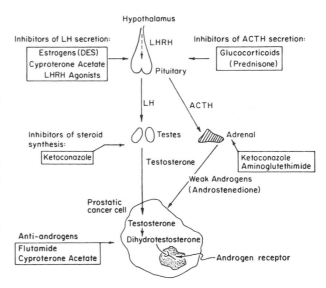

Figure 12.13. Sites of action for pharmacologic approaches to the treatment of prostate cancer. These approaches attempt to decrease androgen stimulation of prostatic cancer.

Androgen Ablation Ablative therapy reduces the amount of available androgen to bind to its receptor, resulting in a reduction in the transcription of the androgen-induced genes, which, in turn, suppresses tumor growth. About 70 to 80 percent of men with prostate cancer respond to initial treatment with androgen ablation, with a median duration of response of about 1 year. Ablation may be by surgical removal of the testes (orchiectomy) or by pharmacologic means using gonadotropin [luteinizing hormone releasing hormone (LHRH)] analogues. A bilateral orchiectomy reduces the circulating serum levels of testosterone by about 95 percent, to approximately 2 nmol/L within the first 24 h postsurgery. When administered initially, LHRH agonists (e.g., leuprolide, goserelin acetate, buserelin acetate) stimulate pituitary gonadotropin secretion for 4 to 5 days, after which gonadotropin secretion is suppressed. This causes testosterone levels to rise initially, then to decline, and low serum testosterone concentrations are observed within 2 to 3 weeks. Antiandrogens (see below) are often administered during the first few weeks of treatment to prevent flare of disease at this time. Continuous administration of these LHRH analogues inhibits LH and FSH release, leading to subsequent suppression of testosterone secretion, which is comparable to that obtained by surgical castration.

Estrogens act primarily by inhibiting the activity of the hypothalamic-pituitary axis through a negative feedback mechanism. This leads to a decline in the secretion of LH and, in turn, testicular testosterone synthesis and release, with testosterone reaching castrate levels within 10 to 14 days. In addition, estrogens may also have a direct effect on prostate tumors, since at high concentration they have been shown to inhibit DNA synthesis in prostate cancer cells (Altwein, 1983). Estrogens have comparable efficacy to orchiectomy or LHRH treatment, but because of unfavorable side effects (especially cardiovascular morbidity), they are no longer in common use. Diethylstilbestrol (DES) has been the most widely used synthetic estrogen in the treatment of prostate cancer.

Antiandrogens act by competing with androgens (testosterone; dihydrotestosterone) for binding to the androgen receptor, thus inhibiting androgen-induced effects. *Nonsteroidal* antiandrogens such as flutamide (Fig. 12.14), nilutamide, and bicalutamide are often described as "pure antiandrogens" since they have no endocrine side effects. When bound to the ligand-binding domain of the androgen receptor, receptor activation and subsequent DNA binding occurs but transcription is not induced. Since these agents bind to androgen receptors in the hypothalamus (as well as to target organs), they inhibit negative feedback of the hypothalamic-pituitary loop and there is a subsequent rise in LH secretion, resulting in an increased serum testosterone level. This may permit patients to remain sexually potent, but elevated testosterone levels may overcome the competitive blockade of the antiandrogen, with the resulting stimulation of tumor growth. Thus, the use of nonsteroidal antiandrogens as monotherapy is limited.

Steroidal antiandrogens such as cyproterone acetate (Figure 12.14) have a dual mechanism of action: They bind competitively to androgen receptors as noted above but also have progestational effects and inhibit LH release, thereby decreasing testicular secretion of testosterone.

Maximal androgen ablation remains a controversial issue in the hormonal therapy of prostate cancer. This concept espouses combined therapy (e.g., orchiectomy or LHRH analogue plus an antiandrogen) to reduce both testicular *and* adrenal androgens, since it is well established that prostate tissue can metabolize adrenal steroids (dehydroepiandrosterone, DHEA, DHEA-sulfate, and androstenedione) to dihydrotestosterone (Labrie et al., 1985). Some randomized trials have suggested that combined therapy may confer a survival benefit as compared to treatment with orchiectomy or LHRH agonist alone (e.g., Crawford et al., 1989), but a recent

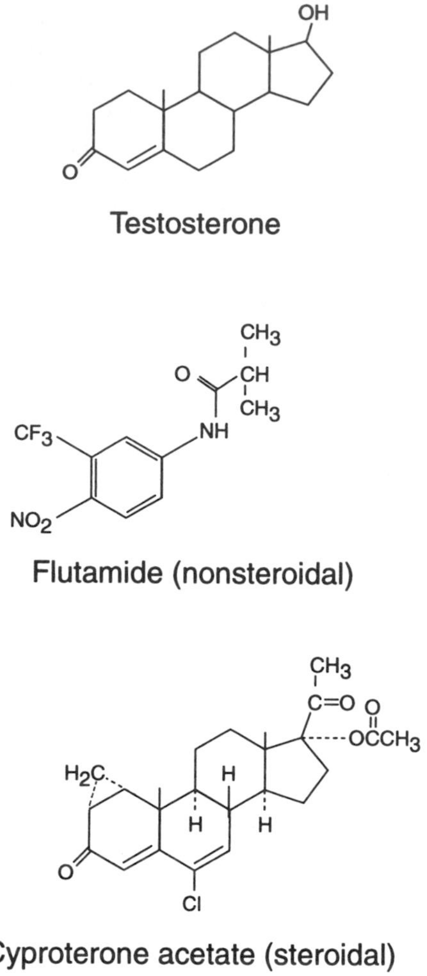

Figure 12.14. Structure of testosterone and nonsteroidal and steroidal antiandrogens.

patient-based meta-analysis of more than 22 randomized trials did not show a significant effect on overall survival (Prostate Cancer Trialists Collaborative Group, 1995). There has, however, been some criticism of the meta-analysis methodology, as the trials included in this analysis used different antiandrogen agents (nonsteroidal, steroidal) and dosage regimens (Labrie and Crawford, 1995; Waxman and Pandha, 1995).

Direct Inhibition of Androgen Synthesis Drugs that inhibit one or more essential enzyme(s) necessary for the synthesis of testosterone have been used in the treatment of advanced prostate cancer. They include ketoconazole and aminoglutethimide. Ketoconazole is a broad-spectrum oral antifungal agent; at higher doses, it interferes with the cytochrome P450 system involved in steroid biosynthesis, thereby inhibiting both testicular and adrenal androgen formation. It has led to some short-term responses after failure of other hormone-based therapies. Aminoglutethimide inhibits the conversion of cholesterol to pregnenolone (a steroid precursor) by blocking the 20-22-desmolase enzyme (Fig. 12.2), and it is also an aromatase inhibitor. This agent thereby inhibits the synthesis of glucocorticoids and mineralocorticoids as well as sex steroids. While aminoglutethimide may decrease the synthesis of androgens, its aromatase-inhibiting properties may have the unwanted side effects of increasing androgen activity by blocking conversion to estrogens. Glucocorticoid supplementation must be provided with aminoglutethimide, and these agents (prednisone, hydrocortisone) may lead to response in patients with prostate cancer due to feedback inhibition of ACTH with decreased stimulation of the adrenal cortex and decreased production of adrenal androgens.

5α-Reductase Inhibitors The enzyme 5α-reductase converts testosterone to the potent androgen dihydrotestosterone. Examples of 5α-reductase inhibitors include finasteride and episteride. These agents decrease prostatic volume and are useful in the management of benign prostatic hypertrophy (McConnell et al., 1993), but they appear to have only marginal efficacy against prostate cancer (Presti et al., 1992).

12.4.4 Prostate Cancer and Androgen Resistance

About 20 percent of prostate cancer patients are initially refractory to androgen-deprivation therapy and all tumors progress ultimately in spite of hormonal manipulation. Heterogeneity in human androgen receptor expression in prostate cancer is likely implicated in tumor progression. Prostate tumors may consist of clones of androgen-dependent and androgen-independent cells. Thus, hormonal treatment may lead to the selective outgrowth of androgen-resistant cells. This concept is supported by data from animal models (see Sec. 12.3.4).

Several mutant androgen receptors have been identified in prostate cancers. For example, Culig et al. (1993) demonstrated a change at position 715 (valine to methionine) in the ligand-binding domain and showed that this mutation enabled mutant androgen receptor to be activated by progesterone and the adrenal steroids dehydroepiandrosterone and androstenedione. Taplin et al. (1995) analyzed the androgen receptor genes for 10 patients with metastatic androgen-independent prostate cancer. All tumors expressed high levels of androgen-receptor gene transcripts, so that androgen independence was not related to loss of the androgen receptor. This supports work by Sadi et al. (1991) showing that loss of the androgen receptor occurs infrequently. Taplin et al. (1995) identified point mutations in 5 of the 10 tumors, and all mutations were in the ligand-binding domain. Functional studies were undertaken by transfection of two of the mutant androgen receptors [(Thr - Ser)^{877} and (His - Tyr)^{874}] into cell lines: These studies demonstrated that these two mutant receptors could be stimulated by the presence of estradiol and progesterone. The normal or "wild-type" androgen receptor is specific for androgens and only weakly stimulated by these hormones.

The above results suggest that mutant androgen-receptor genes that are functionally altered may be present in some patients with androgen-independent prostate cancer. However, other mechanisms are likely to be involved; for example, expression of the proto-oncogene *bcl-2* or of mutated *p53* has been shown to be associated with the emergence of androgen-independent prostate cancer (McDonnell et al., 1992; Bookstein et al., 1993).

The androgen-responsive human prostatic cell line LNCaP has been used as an in vitro model to examine the role of the androgen receptor (AR) in the control of cell proliferation in prostate cancer (see Sec. 12.3.4). LNCaP-S (androgen-stimulatory) cells were grown in an androgen-depleted medium. Over time (20 passages), the cells became more sensitive to lower concentrations of androgens, and the cells were referred to as LNCaP-I (intermediate); after an additional 20 passages, the cells were repressed by lower concentrations of androgens and termed LNCaP-R (androgen-repressed). The androgen receptor levels increased as the cells progressed from LNCaP-S to LNCaP-R (Kokontis et al., 1994). Under selective pressure (exposure to antiandrogen therapy), cells may thus adapt to lower androgen concentrations by increasing the transcription activity or steroid affinity of the androgen receptor and thereby may overcome the therapy. It has been suggested that proliferating prostate cancer cells that are hypersensitive to a low concentration of androgen may be repressed by moderate concentrations of androgen and that patients who have previously received hormonal therapy and have progressed might benefit from this approach. Clinical trials need to be performed to assess the viability of such a treatment approach.

The concept of *intermittent therapy* is based on the hypothesis that prostate tumor heterogeneity leads to the selective outgrowth of androgen-resistant cells in response to hormonal therapy. It is hypothesized that by giving intermittent hormonal treatment one would prevent or slow this selective pressure. There is evidence from animal models to suggest that intermittent therapy might delay progression to hormone resistance (Bruchovsky et al., 1990; Akakura et al., 1993). Clinical trials are in progress which compare intermittent with continuous androgen ablation therapy.

12.5 SUMMARY

Hormones are involved in cellular proliferation and differentiation. One hormone may have multiple functions, and multiple hormones may be required for one function. Nonsteroid hormones function through signal transduction (secondary messengers), whereas steroid hormones diffuse into cells and bind to specific receptors, which, when activated, bind to the hormone response element of specific genes and enhance their transcription. Steroid hormones are synthesized from cholesterol and have a common chemical structure—the steroid nucleus. The major classes of sex hormones are estrogens, progestins, and androgens. Steroid hormones circulate either free or bound to transport proteins, and their half-lives and activity may be modulated by interactions with their transport proteins. The free components are biologically active. Steroid receptors belong to a superfamily of nuclear receptor proteins having common structures and conserved functional domains, including (N terminal) A/B, transactivating; C, DNA-binding; D, hinge region; E, ligand-binding; and F, variable (C terminal). Receptor mutations may result in altered response to a hormonal signal.

Mammary gland proliferation and development is under a complex control process. It is hypothesized that estrogens have direct effects on mammary cells but also regulate their growth by regulating the stimulatory and inhibitory autocrine/paracrine growth-factor pathways. Endocrine therapy aims to deprive the hormone-sensitive tumor of stimulatory hormone(s) and thus cause tumor regression. This is done by (1) reducing the amount of hormone available to bind to its receptor or (2) inhibiting binding of the hormone to the receptor. In *breast cancer*, this may be achieved by ovarian ablation (surgical or biochemical, e.g., LHRH agonist); the use of antiestrogens (e.g., tamoxifen, which binds to the estrogen receptor, blocking estrogen action); progestational agents (direct or indirect pituitary/ovarian actions); or aromatase inhibitors (inhibiting the

synthesis of estrogens). In *prostate cancer*, this may be achieved by testicular ablation (surgical or biochemical, e.g., LHRH agonist); use of estrogens (DES; reduces LH release, and therefore testicular testosterone synthesis and release); or antiandrogens (blocking the binding of testosterone or dihydrotestosterone to the androgen receptor).

Endocrine resistance—either intrinsic or acquired—has been most studied for the antiestrogen tamoxifen. There are several hypotheses, which include alterations in antiestrogen metabolism, the estrogen receptor (loss or mutation or aberrant posttranslational modification), other transcription factors or estrogen receptor-associated proteins, or the estrogen response element. An understanding of the complexity of the mechanisms of hormonal resistance may lead to improvements in both prevention and treatment of breast and prostate cancer.

REFERENCES

Akakura K, Bruchovsky N, Goldenberg SL, et al: Effects of intermittent androgen suppression on androgen-dependent tumours. *Cancer* 1993; 71:2782–2790.

Altwein JE: Estrogens in the treatment of prostate cancer. In: Pavone-Macaluso M, Smith PH, eds. *Cancer of the Prostate and Kidney.* New York: Plenum Press; 1983:317.

Amundadottir LT, Merlino G, Dickson RB: Transgenic mouse models of breast cancer. *Breast Cancer Res Treat* 1996; 39:119–135.

Anderson DC: Sex-hormone-binding globulin. *Clin Endocrinol* 1974; 3:69–96.

Apter D, Reinila M, Vihko R: Some endocrine characteristics of early menarche, a risk factor for breast cancer, are preserved into adulthood. *Int J Cancer* 1989; 44:783–787.

Aronica SM, Katzenellenbogen BS: Stimulation of estrogen receptor–mediated transcription and alteration in the phosphorylation state of the rat uterine estrogen receptor by estrogen, cyclic adenosine monophosphate, and insulin-like growth factor-1. *Mol Endocrinol* 1993; 7:743–752.

Barrett-Connor E, Garland C, McPhillips JB, et al: A prospective, population-based study of androstenedione, estrogens and prostatic cancer. *Cancer Res* 1990; 50:169–173.

Barrett-Lee PJ: Growth factor expression in breast tissue. In: Stoll BA, ed. *Approaches to Breast Cancer Development.* The Netherlands: Kluwer; 1991:53–60.

Battersby S, Robertson BJ, Anderson TJ, et al: Influence of menstrual cycle, parity and oral contraceptive use on steroid hormone receptors in normal breast. *Br J Cancer* 1992; 65:601–607.

Beatson GT: On the treatment of inoperable cases of carcinoma of the mamma: Suggestions for a new method of treatment, with illustrative cases. *Lancet* 1896; 2:104–107.

Berg JW: Can nutrition explain the pattern of international epidemiology of hormone-dependent cancers? *Cancer Res* 1975; 35:3345–3350.

Bernstein L, Pike MC, Ross RK, et al: Estrogen and sex hormone-binding globulin levels in nulliparous and parous women. *J Natl Cancer Inst* 1985; 74:741–745.

Bernstein L, Ross RK: Endogenous hormones and breast cancer risk. *Epidemiologic Rev* 1993; 15:48–65.

Bookstein R, MacGrogan D, Hilsenbeck SG, et al: P53 is mutated in a subset of advanced-stage prostate cancers. *Cancer Res* 1993; 53:3369–3373.

Bos JL: *ras* oncogenes in human cancer: A review. *Cancer Res* 1989; 49:4682–4689.

Boyd NF, Byng JW, Jong RA, et al: Quantitative classification of mammographic densities and breast cancer risk: Results from the Canadian National Breast Screening Study. *J Natl Cancer Inst* 1995; 87:670–675.

Bruchovsky N, Rennie PS, Coldman AJ, et al: Effects of androgen withdrawal on the stem cell composition of the Shionogi carcinoma. *Cancer Res* 1990; 50:2275–2282.

Buckley MF, Sweeney KJE, Hamilton JA, et al: Expression and amplification of cyclin genes in human breast cancer. *Oncogene* 1993; 8:2127–2133.

Butta A, MacLennan K, Flanders KC, et al: Induction of transforming growth factor β_1 in human breast cancer in vivo following tamoxifen treatment. *Cancer Res* 1992; 52:4261–4264.

Callahan R: MMTV-induced mutations in mouse mammary tumors: Their potential relevance to human breast cancer. *Breast Cancer Res Treat* 1996; 39:33–44.

Callahan R, Cropp C, Merlo GR, et al: Genetic and molecular heterogeneity of breast cancer cells. *Clin Chim Acta* 1993; 217:63–73.

Catherino WH, Jordan VC: The biological action of cDNAs from mutated estrogen receptors transfected into breast cancer cells. *Cancer Lett* 1995; 90:35–42.

Cauley JA, Gutal JP, Kuller LH, et al: The epidemiology of serum sex hormones in postmenopausal women. *Am J Epidemiol* 1989; 129:1120–1131.

Clark GM, Osborne CK, McGuire WL: Correlations between estrogen receptor, progesterone receptor, and patient characteristics in human breast cancer. *J Clin Oncol* 1984; 2:1102–1109.

Clarke CL, Sutherland RL: Progestin regulation of cellular proliferation. *Endocr Rev* 1990; 11:266–301.

Clarke JH, Schrader WT, O'Malley BW: Mechanisms of action of steroid hormones. In: Wilson JD, Foster DW, eds. *Williams Textbook of Endocrinology*, 8th ed. Philadelphia: Saunders; 1992:35–90.

Clarke R: Human breast cancer cell line xenografts as models of breast cancer—The immunobiologies of recipient mice and the characteristics of several tumorigenic cell lines. *Breast Cancer Res Treat* 1996; 39:69–86.

Crawford ED, Eisenberger MA, McLeod DG, et al: A controlled trial of leuprolide with and without flutamide in prostatic carcinoma. *N Engl J Med* 1989; 321:419–424.

Culig Z, Hobisch A, Cronauer MV, et al: Mutant androgen receptor detected in an advanced-stage prostatic carcinoma is activated by adrenal androgens and progesterone. *Mol Endocrinol* 1993; 7:1541–1550.

Dai WS, Kuller LH, LaPorte RE, et al: The epidemiology of plasma testosterone levels in middle-aged men. *Am J Epidemiol* 1981; 114:804–816.

Dickson RB: The molecular basis of breast cancer. In Kurzrock R, Talpaz M, eds. *Molecular Biology in Cancer Medicine*. London, Martin Dunitz Ltd; 1995:241–272.

Dickson RB, Lippman ME: Growth factors in breast cancer. *Endocr Rev* 1995; 16:559–589.

Dunn JF, Nisula BC, Rodbard D: Transport of steroid hormones: Binding of 21 endogenous steroids to both testosterone-binding globulin and corticosteroid-binding globulin in human plasma. *J Clin Endocrinol Metab* 1981; 53:58–68.

Encarnacion CA, Ciocca DR, McGuire WL, et al: Measurement of steroid hormone receptors in breast cancer patients on tamoxifen. *Breast Cancer Res Treat* 1993; 26:237–246.

Evans RM: The steroid and thyroid hormone receptors superfamily. *Science* 1988; 240:889–895.

Fisher B, Costantino J, Redmond C, et al: A randomized clinical trial evaluating tamoxifen in the treatment of patients with node-negative breast cancer who have estrogen-receptor-positive tumors. *N Engl J Med* 1989; 320:479–484.

Fitzpatrick SL, Brightwell J, Wittliff J, et al: Epidermal growth factor binding by breast tumor biopsies and relationship to estrogen and progestin receptor levels. *Cancer Res* 1984; 44:3448–3453.

Fornander T, Rutqvist LE, Cedermark B, et al: Adjuvant tamoxifen in early breast cancers: Occurrence of new primary cancers. *Lancet* 1989; 1:117–120.

Fuqua SAW: Estrogen receptor mutagenesis and hormone resistance. *Cancer* 1994; 74:1026–1029.

Fuqua SAW, Fitzgerald SD, Chamness GC, et al: Variant human breast tumor estrogen receptor with constitutive transcriptional activity. *Cancer Res* 1991; 51:105–109.

Fuqua SAW, Fitzgerald SD, Allred DC, et al: Inhibition of estrogen receptor action by a naturally occurring variant in human breast tumors. *Cancer Res* 1992; 52:483–486.

Gorsch SM, Memoli VA, Stukel TA, et al: Immunohistochemical staining for transforming growth factor beta1 associates with disease progression in human breast cancer. *Cancer Res* 1992; 52:6949–6952.

Goss PE, Gwyn KMEH: Current perspectives on aromatase inhibitors in breast cancer. *J Clin Oncol* 1994; 12:2460–2470.

Gould MN: Rodent models for the study of etiology, prevention and treatment of breast cancer. *Semin Cancer Biol* 1995; 6:147–152.

Graham S, Haughey B, Marshall J, et al: Diet in the epidemiology of carcinoma of the prostate gland. *J Natl Cancer Inst* 1983; 70:687–692.

Green S, Chambon P: A superfamily of potentially oncogenic hormone receptors. *Nature* 1986; 324:615–617.

Guy CT, Webster MA, Schaller M, et al: Expression of the neu protooncogene in the mammary epithelium of transgenic mice induces metastatic disease. *Proc Natl Acad Sci USA* 1992; 89:10578–10582.

Haller DG, Fox KR, Schuchter LM: Metastatic breast cancer. In: Fowble B, Goodman RL, Glick JH, Rosato EF, eds. *Breast Cancer Treatment: A Comprehensive Guide to Treatment.* St. Louis: Mosby Year Book; 1991:403–455.

Hill P, Wynder EL, Garbaczewski L, et al: Diet and urinary steroids in black and white North American men and black South African men. *Cancer Res* 1979; 39: 5101–5105.

Horwitz KB: How do breast cancers become hormone resistant? *J Steroid Biochem Mol Biol* 1994; 49:295–302.

Hsing AW, Comstock GW: Serological precursors of cancer: Serum hormones and risk of subsequent prostate cancer. *Cancer Epidemiol Biomarkers Prev* 1993; 2:27–32.

Huggins C, Hodges CV: Studies of prostatic cancer. I. Effect of castration, estrogen and androgen injections on serum phosphatases in metastatic carcinoma of the prostate. *Cancer Res* 1941; 1:293–297.

Hulka BS, Edison LT, Lininger RA: Steroid hormones and risk of breast cancer. *Cancer* 1994; 74:1111–1124.

Hynes NE, Groner B, Michalides R: Mouse mammary tumor virus: Transcriptional control and involvement in tumorigenesis. *Adv Cancer Res* 1984; 41:155–184.

Isaacs CJD, Swain SM: Hormone replacement therapy in women with a history of breast carcinoma. *Hematol Oncol Clin North Am* 1994; 8:179–195.

Isaacs JT, Isaacs WB, Feita WF, et al: Establishment and characterization of seven Dunning rat prostatic cancer cell lines and their use in developing methods for predicting metastatic abilities of prostatic cancers. *Prostate* 1986; 9:261–281.

Key T: Risk factors for prostate cancer. In: *Preventing Prostate Cancer. Screening versus Chemoprevention.* Cold Spring Harbor, NY: Cold Spring Harbor Laboratory Press; 1995:63–77.

Klein EA: Prostate cancer: Current concepts in diagnosis and treatment. *Cleve Clin J Med* 1992; 59:383–389.

Klein EA: An update on prostate cancer. *Cleve Clin J Med* 1995; 62:325–338.

Klijn JG, Berns PM, Schmitz PI, et al: The clinical significance of epidermal growth factor receptor (EGF-R) in human breast cancer: A review on 5232 patients. *Endocr Rev* 1992; 13:3–17.

Kokontis J, Takakura K, Hay N, et al: Increased androgen receptor activity and altered c-myc expression in prostate cancer cells after long-term androgen deprivation. *Cancer Res* 1994; 54:1566–1573.

Labrie F, Crawford D: Anti-androgens in treatment of prostate cancer. *Lancet* 1995; 346:1030–1031.

Labrie F, Dupont A, Belanger A: Complete androgen blockade for the treatment of prostate cancer. In: De Vita VT, Hellman S, Rosenberg SA, eds. *Important Advances in Oncology.* Philadelphia: Lippincott; 1985: 193–217.

Liao S: Androgen action: Molecular mechanism and medical application. *J Formos Med Assoc* 1994; 93:741–751.

Lidereau R, Callahan R, Dickson C, et al: Amplification of the *int*-2 gene in primary human breast tumors. *Oncogene Res* 1988; 2:285–291.

Lindsey WF, Das Gupta TK, Beattie CW: Influence of the estrous cycle during carcinogen exposure on nitrosomethylurea-induced rat mammary carcinoma. *Cancer Res* 1981; 41:3857–3862.

Mangelsdorf DJ, Thummel C, Beato M, et al: The nuclear receptor superfamily: The second decade. *Cell* 1995; 83:835–839.

McConnell JD, Akakura K, Bartsch G, et al: Hormonal treatment of BPH. Proceedings of the Second International Consultation on Benign Prostatic Hyperplasia. Paris: SCI; 1993:418–436.

McDonnell TJ, Troncoso P, Brisbay SM, et al: Expression of the proto-oncogene bcl-2 in the prostate and its association with emergence of androgen-independent prostate cancer. *Cancer Res* 1992; 52:6940–6944.

Meyer TE, Habener JF: Cyclic adenosine 3',5'-monophosphate response element binding protein (CREB) and related transcription-activating deoxyribonucleic acid-binding proteins. *Endocr Rev* 1993; 14:269–290.

Moore JW, Key TJA, Bulbrook RD, et al: Sex hormone binding globulin and risk factors for breast cancer in a population of normal women who had never used exogenous sex hormones. *Br J Cancer* 1987; 56: 661–666.

Morris DW, Barry PA, Bradshaw HD Jr, et al: Insertion mutation of the *int*-1 and *int*-2 loci by mouse mammary tumour virus in premalignant and malignant neoplasms from the GR mouse strain. *J Virol* 1990; 64:1794–1802.

Morton RA Jr.: Racial differences in adenocarcinoma of the prostate in North American men. *Urology* 1994; 44:637–645.

Murphy LC: Antiestrogen action and growth factor regulation. *Breast Cancer Res Treat* 1994; 31:61–71.

Murphy LC, Dotzlaw H: Regulation of transforming growth factor α and transforming growth factor β messenger ribonucleic acid abundance in T-47D human breast cancer cells. *Mol Endocrinol* 1989; 3:611–617.

Murphy LC, Alkhalaf M, Dotzlaw H, et al: Regulation of gene expression in T-47D human breast cancer cells by progestins and antiprogestins. *Hum Reprod* 1994; 9(S1):174–180.

Musgrove EA, Hamilton JA, Lee CS, et al: Growth factor, steroid, and steroid antagonist regulation of cyclin gene expression associated with changes in T-47D human breast cancer cell cycle progression. *Mol Cell Biol* 1993; 13:3577–3587.

Musgrove EA, Lee CSL, Sutherland RL: Progestins both stimulate and inhibit breast cancer cell cycle progession while increasing expression of transforming growth factor α, epidermal growth factor receptor, c-fos and c-myc genes. *Mol Cell Biol* 1991; 11:5032–5043.

Muss HB: Endocrine therapy for advanced breast cancer: A review. *Breast Cancer Res Treat* 1992; 21:15–26.

Muss HB, Paschold EH, Black WR, et al: Megestrol acetate

versus tamoxifen in advanced breast cancer: A phase III trial of the Piedmont Oncology Association (POA). *Semin Oncol* 1985; 12:55–61.

Nicholson RI, McClelland RA, Gee JMW, et al: Transforming growth factor-α and endocrine sensitivity in breast cancer. *Cancer Res* 1994; 54:1684–1689.

Nomura A, Heilbrun LK, Stemmermann GN, et al: Prediagnostic serum hormones and the risk of prostate cancer. *Cancer Res* 1988; 48:3515–3517.

Normanno N, Ciardiello F, Brandt R, et al: Epidermal growth factor-related peptides in the pathogenesis of human breast cancer. *Breast Cancer Res Treat* 1994; 29:11–27.

Olsson H, Borg Å, Fernö M, et al: Her-2/*neu* and *INT-2* proto-oncogene amplification in malignant breast tumors in relation to reproductive factors and exposure to exogenous hormones. *J Natl Cancer Inst* 1991; 83:1483–1487.

O'Neill JS, Elton RA, Miller WR: Aromatase activity in adipose tissue from breast quadrants: A link with tumor site. *Br Med J Clin Res Ed* 1988; 296:741–743.

Osborne CK: Receptors. In: Harris JR, Hellman S, Henderson IC, Kinne DW, eds. *Breast Diseases*. Philadelphia: Lippincott; 1991:301–325.

Osborne CK, Elledge RM, Fuqua SAW: Estrogen receptors in breast cancer therapy. *Sci Am* 1996; 37:32–41.

Perrault D, Eisenhauer EA, Pritchard KI, et al: Phase II study of the progesterone antagonist mifepristone in patients with untreated metastatic breast carcinoma: A National Cancer Institute of Canada Clinical Trials Group study. *J Clin Oncol* 1996; 14:2709–2712.

Pike MC, Bestein L, Spicer DV: Exogenous hormones and breast cancer. In: Niederhuber JE, ed. *Current Therapy in Oncology*. St Louis: Mosby, 1993:292–303.

Presti JC Jr, Fair WR, Andriole GL, et al: Multicenter, randomized, double-blind, placebo controlled study to investigate the effect of finasteride (MK-906) on stage D prostate cancer. *J Urol* 1992; 148:1201–1204.

Prostate Cancer Trialists Collaborative Group. Maximum androgen blockade in advanced prostate cancer: An overview of 22 randomised trials with 3283 deaths in 5710 patients. *Lancet* 1995; 346:265–269.

Ricketts D, Turnbull L, Ryall G, et al: Estrogen and progesterone receptors in the normal female breast. *Cancer Res* 1991; 51:1817–1822.

Robson MC: Cirrhosis and prostatic neoplasms. *Geriatrics* 1966; 21:150–154.

Roelink H, Wang J, Black DM, et al: Molecular cloning and chromosomal localization to 17q21 of the human WNT3 gene. *Genomics* 1993; 17:790–792.

Roodi N, Bailey LR, Kao W-Y, et al: Estrogen receptor gene analysis in estrogen receptor–positive and receptor-negative primary breast cancer. *J Natl Cancer Inst* 1995; 87:446–451.

Rose DP, Laakso K, Sotarauta M, et al: Hormone levels in prostatic fluid from healthy Finns and prostate cancer patients. *Eur J Cancer Clin Oncol* 1984; 20:1317–1319.

Ross RK, Bernstein L, Lobo RA, et al: 5-alpha-reductase activity and risk of prostate cancer among Japanese and US white and black males. *Lancet* 1992; 339: 887–889.

Royai R, Lange PH, Vessella R: Preclinical models of prostate cancer. *Semin Oncol* 1996; 23(S14):35–40.

Russo J, Tay LK, Russo IH: Differentiation of the mammary gland and susceptibility to carcinogenesis. *Breast Cancer Res Treat* 1982; 2:5–73.

Saceda M, Knabbe C, Dickson RB, et al: Post transcriptional destabilization of estrogen receptor mRNA in MCF-7 cells by 12-O-tetradecanylphorbol-13-acetate. *J Biol Chem* 1991; 266:17809–17814.

Sadi MV, Walsh PC, Barrack ER: Immunohistochemical study of androgen receptors in metastatic prostate cancer: Comparison of receptor content and response to hormonal therapy. *Cancer* 1991; 67:3057–3064.

Scheinman RI, Cogswell PC, Lofquist AK, et al: Role of transcriptional activation of IKBα in mediation of immunosuppression by glucocorticoids. *Science* 1995; 270: 283–286.

Shozu M, Akasofu K, Harada T, et al: A new cause of female pseudohermaphroditism: Placental aromatase deficiency. *J Clin Endocrinol Metab* 1991; 72:560–566.

Simpson ER, Mahendroo MS, Means GD, et al: Aromatase cytochrome P450 the enzyme responsible for estrogen biosynthesis. *Endocr Rev* 1994; 15:342–355.

Spicer DV, Krecker EA, Pike MC. The endocrine prevention of breast cancer. *Cancer Invest* 1995; 13:495–504.

Spicer DV, Ursin G, Parisky YR, et al: Changes in mammographic densities induced by a hormonal contraceptive designed to reduce breast cancer. *J Natl Cancer Inst* 1994; 86:431–436.

Stoll BA: Diet and exercise regimens to improve breast carcinoma prognosis. *Cancer* 1996; 78:2465–2470.

Taioli E, Garte SJ, Trachman J, et al: Ethnic differences in estrogen metabolism in healthy women (correspondence). *J Natl Cancer Inst* 1996; 88:617.

Taplin M-E, Bubley GJ, Shuster TD, et al: Mutation of the androgen-receptor gene in metastatic androgen-independent prostate cancer. *N Engl J Med* 1995; 332: 1393–1398.

Tekmal RR, Ramachandra N, Gubba S, et al: Overexpression of *int-5/aromatase* in mammary glands of transgenic mice results in the induction of hyperplasia and nuclear abnormalities. *Cancer Res* 1996; 56:3180–3185.

Thompson LU. Flaxseed, lignans and cancer. In: Cunnane SC, Thompson LU, eds. *Flaxseed in Human Nutrition*. Champaign, IL: AOCS; 1995:219–235.

Tonetti DA, Jordan VC: Possible mechanisms in the emergence of tamoxifen-resistant breast cancer. *Anti-Cancer Drugs* 1995; 6:498–507.

Toniolo PG, Levita M, Zeleniuch-Jacquotte A, et al: A prospective study of endogenous estrogens and breast cancer in postmenopausal women. *J Natl Cancer Inst* 1995; 87:190–197.

Treurniet HF, Rookus MA, Peterse HL, et al: Differences in breast cancer risk factors to *neu*(c-erbB-2) protein overexpression of the breast tumor. *Cancer Res* 1992; 52:2344–2345.

Tsuda H, Hirohashi S, Shimosato Y, et al: Correlation between long-term survival in breast cancer patients and amplification of two putative oncogene-coamplification units: hst-1/*int*-2 and c-erbB-2/ear-1. *Cancer Res* 1989; 49:3104–3108.

Tzukerman M, Zhang XK, Pfahl M: Inhibition of estrogen receptor activity by the tumor promoter 12-O-tetradeconylphorbol-13-acetate: A molecular analysis. *Mol Endocrinol* 1991; 5:1983–1992.

Vande Vijver MJ, Petersen J, Mooi W, et al: Oncogene activations in human breast cancer. In: Furth M, Greaves M, eds. *Molecular Diagnostics of Human Cancer*. Cold Spring Harbor, NY: Cold Spring Harbor Laboratory Press; 1989:385–391.

Vihko R, Apter D: Endocrine characteristics of adolescent menstrual cycles: Impact of early menarche. *J Steroid Biochem* 1984; 20:231–236.

Watts CK, Sweeney KJ, Warlters A, et al: Antiestrogen regulation of cell cycle progression and cyclin D1 gene expression in MCF-7 human breast cancer cells. *Breast Cancer Res Treat* 1994; 31:95–105.

Waxman J, Pandha H: Anti-androgens in treatment of prostate cancer (letter). *Lancet* 1995; 346:1030.

White E: Life, death, and the pursuit of apoptosis. *Genes Dev* 1996; 10:1–15.

Wolf DM, Fuqua SAW: Mechanisms of actions of antiestrogens. *Cancer Treat Rev* 1995; 21:247–271.

Zhang R, Haag JD, Gould MN: Reduction in the frequency of activated ras oncogenes in rat mammary carcinomas with increasing *N*-methyl-*N*-nitrosourea doses or increasing prolactin levels. *Cancer Res* 1990; 50:4286–4290.

Zhao Y, Nichols JE, Bulun SE, et al: Aromatase P450 gene expression in human adipose tissue: Role of a Jak/STAT pathway in regulation of the adipose-specific promoter. *J Biol Chem* 1995; 270:16449–16457.

13

Molecular and Cellular Basis of Radiotherapy

Robert G. Bristow and Richard P. Hill

13.1 INTRODUCTION

13.2 INTERACTION OF RADIATION WITH MATTER
    13.2.1 Types of Radiation and Energy Deposition
    13.2.2 Linear Energy Transfer and Energy Absorption
    13.2.3 Sites of Radiation Damage within the Cell
    13.3.4 Ultraviolet Radiation

13.3 MOLECULAR AND CELLULAR RESPONSES
    TO IONIZING RADIATION
    13.3.1 Activation of Radiation-Response Genes
    13.3.2 Cell-Cycle Arrest
    13.3.3 Radiation-Induced Cell Death
    13.3.4 In vitro Assays for Proliferative Capacity
    13.3.5 In vivo Assays for Proliferative Capacity

13.4 MODELS OF RADIATION CELL SURVIVAL
    13.4.1 Radiation Survival Curves
    13.4.2 Target Theory

13.4.3 The Linear-Quadratic Model
13.4.4 Surviving Fraction following 2 Gy (SF2) and the
    Mean Inactivation Dose

13.5 FACTORS THAT INFLUENCE CELL SURVIVAL
    13.5.1 Radiation Quality and Relative
    Biological Effectiveness
    13.5.2 Oxygen Effect and Hypoxia in Tumors
    13.5.3 Cell-Cycle Position
    13.5.4 Molecular and Cellular Repair
    13.5.5 Adaptive Radiation Responses
    13.5.6 Oncogenes, Tumor Suppressor Genes,
    and Growth Factors

13.6 SUMMARY

REFERENCES

BIBLIOGRAPHY

13.1 INTRODUCTION

Since their discovery by Roentgen almost a century ago, x-rays have played a major role in modern medicine. The first recorded use of x-rays for the treatment of cancer occurred within about 1 year of their discovery. Subsequently there has been intensive study of x-rays and other ionizing radiations, and their clinical application to cancer treatment has become increasingly sophisticated. This chapter and Chap. 14 review the biological effects of ionizing radiation and the application of that knowledge to cancer treatment. The importance of ionizing radiation in the diagnosis and staging of cancer is not discussed because it is beyond the scope of this book.

The present chapter begins with a review of the physical properties of ionizing radiations and their interaction with targets within the cell membrane, cytoplasm, and nucleus. The effect of energy deposition in tissue is discussed next, with emphasis on the molecular pathways that are thought to control cellular proliferation following exposure to ionizing radiation. Finally, various genetic and epigenetic factors known to influence the effect of radiation on cells and therefore to alter the relative radiosensitivity of normal and tumor cells are described.

13.2 INTERACTION OF RADIATION WITH MATTER

13.2.1 Types of Radiation and Energy Deposition

X- and γ-rays constitute part of the continuous spectrum of electromagnetic (EM) radiation that includes radio waves, heat, and visible and ultraviolet (UV) light (see Fig. 13.1). All types of EM radiation can be considered as moving packets (quanta) of energy called *photons*. The amount of energy in each individual photon defines its position in the electromagnetic spectrum. For example, x- or γ-ray photons carry more energy than heat or light photons and are at the high-energy end of the EM spectrum. Individual photons of x-rays (but not UV light) are sufficiently energetic that their interaction with matter can result in the complete displacement of an electron from its orbit around the nucleus of an atom. Such an atom (or molecule) is left with a net positive charge and is thus an ion; hence the term *ionizing radiation*. Typical binding energies for electrons in biological material are in the neighborhood of 10 eV (electron volts). Thus photons with energies greater than 10 eV are considered to be ionizing radiation, while photons with energies of 2 to 10 eV are in the UV range and are nonionizing. An interaction that transfers energy but does not completely displace an electron produces an "excited" atom or molecule and is called an *excitation*.

When x-ray photons interact with tissue, they give up energy by one of three processes: the photoelectric effect, the Compton effect, or pair production (Johns and Cunningham, 1983). In the energy range most widely used in radiotherapy (100 keV to 20 MeV), the Compton effect is the most important mechanism leading to deposition of energy in biological materials. This energy-transfer process involves a billiard-ball type of collision between the photon and an outer orbital electron of an atom, with partial transfer of energy to the electron and scattering of the photon into a new direction. The electron (and the photon) can then undergo further interactions, causing more ionizations and excitations, until its energy is dissipated. All three of the interaction processes mentioned above result in the production of energetic electrons that, in turn, lose energy by exciting and ionizing target atoms and molecules and setting more electrons in motion.

An electron is a charged particle, and it is possible, with modern particle accelerators, to irradiate directly with electrons or with other charged particles such as those listed in Table 13.1. The deposition of energy in matter by moving charged particles is chiefly a result of electrical field interactions and depends both on the velocity and on the charge of the particle (see below). Detailed discussion of the mechanisms involved is given in Johns and Cunningham (1983). Neutrons have no charge and do not interact with atomic electrons to produce ionizations. They deposit energy by collision with nuclei, particularly hydrogen nuclei (protons), and thereby transfer their energy to create moving charged particles capable of both ionization and excitation.

Radiation dose is measured in terms of the amount of energy (joules) absorbed per unit mass (kg) and is quoted in grays (1 J/kg). It is not, however, the total amount of energy absorbed that is critical for the biologic effect of ionizing radiation. A whole-body dose of 8 grays (Gy) would result in the death (due to bone marrow failure) of many animals, including humans, yet the amount of energy deposited, if evenly distributed, would cause a temperature rise of only 1 to 3×10^{-3}°C. It is the size and localized nature of the individual energy-deposition events caused by ionizing radiations that is the reason for their efficacy in damaging biological systems.

13.2.2 Linear Energy Transfer and Energy Absorption

As a charged particle moves through matter, it transfers energy by a series of interactions that occur at random. Thus particles lose energy along their track

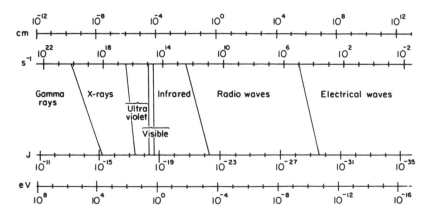

Figure 13.1. Electromagnetic spectrum showing the relationship of photon wavelength in centimeters (cm) to its frequency in inverse seconds (s^{-1}) and to its energy in joules (J) and electron volts (eV). The various bands in the spectrum are indicated. Slanted lines between bands indicate the degree of overlap in the definition of the various bands. (Adapted from Upton, 1982.)

Table 13.1. Linear Energy Transfer (LET) of Various Radiations

Radiation	LET, keV/μm
Photons	
^{60}Co (~1.2 MeV)	0.3
200-keV x-ray	2.5
Electrons	
1 MeV	0.2
100 keV	0.5
10 keV	2
1 keV	10
Charge particles	
Proton 2 MeV	17
Alpha 5 MeV	90
Carbon 100 MeV	160
Neutrons	
2.5 MeV	15–80
14.1 MeV	3–30

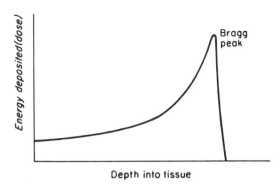

Figure 13.2. Schematic illustration of the energy deposition by a charged particle along its track in tissue. The particle has a high velocity at the left-hand side of the figure, but as it loses energy, it slows down until it comes to rest in the region of the Bragg peak.

as they traverse the target. The particle's energy loss $-dE$, along a portion of this track dx, is dependent on its velocity v, charge Z, and the electron density of the target ρ, as indicated by Eq. (13.1):

$$-\frac{dE}{dx} \alpha \frac{Z^2 \rho}{v^2} \qquad (13.1)$$

The efficiency with which different types of ionizing radiation cause biological damage varies, even though photons, charged particles, and neutrons ultimately all set electrons in motion. The important difference between different types of radiation is the average density of energy loss *along* the path of the particle. The average energy lost by a particle over a given track length is known as the *linear energy transfer* (LET). The units of LET are given in terms of energy lost per unit pathlength, e.g., keV/μm. Some representative values of LET for different particles are given in Table 13.1. From Eq. (13.1), it can be seen that as a particle slows down, it loses energy more and more rapidly and reaches a maximum rate of energy loss (the Bragg peak) just before it comes to rest (Fig. 13.2). The LET of a charged particle thus varies along the length of its track.

The concept of LET does not address the size of the individual energy-loss events that occur along the track of a particle. All radiations set electrons in motion, and the amount of energy lost per collision of a 20-keV electron with target molecules has a distribution as shown in Fig. 13.3. The discrete energy-

loss events are large relative to the energy required to break chemical bonds. Using the value 60 eV for the average energy-loss event (Fig. 13.3), the number of such events per unit path length can be calculated. The density of these discrete energy-loss events along the particle track increases with LET (Fig. 13.4).

The biological effect of a dose of radiation depends on its LET (see Sec. 13.5.1); it is therefore necessary to know the LET at each point in an irradiated volume to predict the biological response accurately. When EM radiation (e.g., 6-MV photons produced by a linear accelerator) is used to irradiate tissue, electrons are set in motion in the tissue, and because of their small mass (1/1860 of the mass of a proton), they are easily deflected and their track through the tissue is tortuous. Each electron

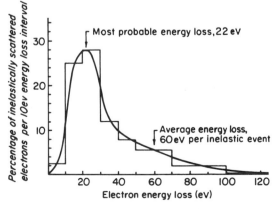

Figure 13.3. The distribution of "first-collision" energy loss for 20-keV electrons passing through a "biologically equivalent" solid. (Adapted from Rauth and Simpson, 1964.)

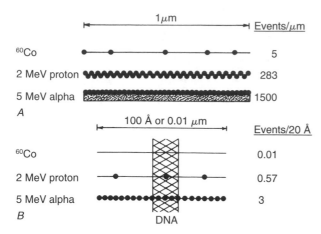

Figure 13.4. The frequency of primary energy-loss events along the tracks of various radiations of widely differing LETs. *A.* Schematic diagram of primary energy-loss events over a distance of 1 μm. *B.* The pattern of primary energy-loss over a distance of 0.01 μm or 100 Å. The cross-hatched region represents the dimensions of a DNA double helix.

track has a Bragg peak at its termination and a range of LET values along its track, but both the initiation and termination points of the electron tracks occur at random in the tissue, so that the LET spectrum is similar at all depths. A similar result occurs if the irradiation is with a primary electron beam. In contrast, if a beam of monoenergetic heavier-charged particles (e.g., protons, He or Ne nuclei) is used to irradiate the tissue, the tracks of the particles are much straighter because their much larger mass reduces the chance of significant deflection. The Bragg peak then occurs at a similar depth in the tissue for all particles. Thus, for each type of monoenergetic heavy-charged particle, there is a region in the tissue where a relatively large amount of energy is deposited. This feature of irradiation with heavy-charged particles makes them potentially attractive for some therapeutic applications (see Chap. 14, Sec. 14.4.4).

13.2.3 Sites of Radiation Damage within the Cell

The interactions leading to energy deposition in tissue occur very rapidly and generate chemically reactive free electrons and free radicals (molecules with unpaired electrons). Many different molecules in cells will be altered either as a result of *direct* energy absorption or as a result of energy transfer from one molecule to another, giving rise to *indirect* effects. Most of the energy deposited in cells is absorbed initially in water (because the cell is about 80 percent water), leading to the rapid production of reactive

radical intermediates (i.e., within 10^{-14} to 10^{-4} s), which, in turn, can interact with other molecules in the cell. The [OH·] radical, an oxidizing agent, is probably the most damaging. The cell contains naturally occurring thiol compounds such as glutathione, cysteine, and cysteamine, whose structures contain sulfhydryl (SH) groups that can react chemically with the free radicals to decrease their damaging effects.

The random nature of the energy-deposition events means that radiation-induced changes can occur in any molecule in a cell. Ward (1994) has described focal areas of DNA damage that arise because of the clustering of ionizations within a few nanometers of the DNA. These "multiply damaged sites" include combinations of single- or double-strand breaks in the sugar-phosphate backbone of the molecule, alteration or loss of DNA bases, and formation of cross-links between the DNA strands or between DNA and chromosomal proteins. It has been estimated that approximately 1×10^5 ionizations can occur within the cell per gray of absorbed radiation dose, leading to approximately 200 single-strand and 25 to 50 double-strand DNA breaks.

Ionizing radiation can also induce reactive oxygen species (e.g., peroxides), which can interact with proteins in the cell membrane, some of which may be involved in signal transduction. This can lead to apoptosis in certain cell types (e.g., endothelial cells) by activation in the membrane of a ceramide-sphingomyelin pathway (Fuks et al., 1995). Inhibition of specific biochemical processes in cells, such as DNA, RNA, or protein synthesis, respiration, or substrate metabolism, is also affected by irradiation but usually requires quite large doses of radiation of the order of 10 to 100 Gy.

Evidence to support the critical role of damage to DNA as the most crucial type of cellular damage in relation to cell killing is outlined in Table 13.2. A number of techniques—such as velocity sedimentation, filter elution, assays for chromosomal damage, and DNA electrophoresis—have been used to study specific DNA lesions caused by radiation (Whitaker et al., 1991; Fairbairn et al., 1995). Two techniques, fluorescence in situ hybridization (FISH; see Chap. 3, Sec. 3.4.4) and premature chromosome condensation (PCC), allow the quantification of single- or double-strand breaks (manifest as chromatid breaks or aberrant chromosomal forms) following doses of ionizing radiation as low as 1 Gy (Sasai et al., 1994). Other techniques, such as pulsed-field gel electrophoresis (PFGE), can facilitate the separation and quantitation of large DNA fragments secondary to single- or double-

Table 13.2. Evidence Supporting DNA as a Critical Target for Radiation-Induced Lethality

1. Microbeam irradiation demonstrates the cell nucleus to be much more sensitive than the cytoplasm.

2. Radioisotopes with short-range emissions (e.g., ^{3}H, ^{125}I) incorporated into the DNA cause cell killing at much lower absorbed doses than those incorporated into the cellular cytoplasm.

3. Incorporation of thymidine analogues (e.g., IUdR or BUdR) into DNA modifies cellular radiosensitivity.

4. The level of chromatid and chromosomal aberrations following ionizing radiation correlates well with cell lethality.

5. The number of unrepaired DNA double-strand breaks has been found to correlate with cell lethality following ionizing radiation in many cells.

6. For different types of radiation, cell lethality correlates best with the level of radiation-induced DNA double-strand breaks rather than with other types of damage.

7. The extreme radiosensitivity of some mutant cells is due to defects in DNA repair (see Chap. 4, Sec. 4.4).

strand DNA breaks following radiation damage (Table 13.3). The results from these assays suggest that cell survival following radiation is correlated with levels of either initial or residual DNA damage (Nunez et al., 1996; Schwartz et al., 1996a). Many lesions in DNA can be partially or completely repaired (Sec. 13.5.4 and Chap. 4, Sec. 4.4); thus the expression of DNA damage at the cellular level is complex. It is probable that unrepaired or incorrectly repaired double-strand breaks (dsb) are the critical lesions in DNA for cell lethality.

13.2.4 Ultraviolet Radiation

The measurement of UV dose is based on the exposure dose expressed as incident energy per unit area or J/m^2. In contrast to ionizing radiation, UV radiation (wavelength 200 to 400 nm) deposits energy in selected molecules that absorb energy in the range of 3 to 10 eV (Rauth, 1986). This is not enough energy to ionize these molecules, but it is enough to put them in a short-lived excited state and make them chemically reactive. In DNA in aqueous solution, absorption of photons with a wavelength in the range 200 to 300 nm results in the excitation of pyrimidine bases (thymine or cytosine) that can react with water to form pyrimidine hydrates or with a neighboring pyrimidine to give rise to pyrimidine dimers of the cyclobutane type

(thymine-thymine, cytosine-thymine, or cytosine-cytosine) as well as other linkages. Dimers formed in DNA are chemically stable, but the pyrimidine hydrates are unstable and can dehydrate, resulting in the restoration of the original pyrimidine or, in the case of cytosine, a deaminated derivative. Reaction of excited pyrimidines with other molecules such as amino acids can occur, and evidence for DNA-protein cross-links in cells exposed to UV irradiation has been obtained. Because of its chemical stability, the lesion that has been most extensively monitored in biological systems is the cyclobutane pyrimidine dimer. Pyrimidine dimers can be quantitated in mammalian cells by a variety of techniques, and at doses of biological interest, their production is linear with dose. At high doses, an equilibrium is established between dimer formation and reversal (see Chap. 4, Sec. 4.4.3) that is dependent on wavelength. Pyrimidine dimers appear to be formed at equal rates in all phases of the cell cycle. The initial lesions formed in biological material by ionizing and by UV radiation are quite different in their type and distribution throughout the cell. These differences are reflected in differences in the cellular and molecular behavior of cells exposed to these radiations.

When asynchronous populations of mammalian cells are exposed to UV irradiation and their colony-forming ability is determined (see Sec. 13.3.4), a survival curve that is qualitatively similar to curves for ionizing radiation is obtained (see Sec. 13.4.1). The relative effectiveness of different wavelengths of UV light to inactivate cell colony-forming ability has a close correspondence to the absorption spectrum of DNA. This spectrum is identical to the action spectrum for dimer formation. Lethal damage probably arises from an initial excitation of pyrimidine bases, with subsequent formation of dimers. However, the reaction of excited bases with other cellular components such as proteins might also explain the lethal effects of UV radiation. Surviving cells respond to a second dose of UV radiation as if they had not been exposed to the first dose if they are allowed to progress through their DNA synthesis phase between the doses of fractionated radiation (Rauth, 1986). Cells possess mechanisms for removing pyrimidine dimers (Chap. 4, Secs. 4.4.3 and 4.4.5), and presumably damage is repaired during the period of DNA synthesis. For many but not all cell lines, late S-phase cells are most resistant to UV radiation and there is increasing sensitivity through G2, M, and G1 to early S phase. This pattern differs from that seen with ionizing radiation (see Sec. 13.5.3).

Table 13.3. Assays for the Detection of DNA Damage Following Ionizing Radiation

Assay	Dose Range[a]	Technique	Limitations
1. Sucrose velocity sedimentation	ssb > 5 Gy dsb > 15 Gy	Larger DNA fragments sediment to a greater extent.	Insensitive to clinically relevant low radiation doses
2. Filter elution	ssb > 1 Gy (alkaline elution) dsb > 5 Gy (neutral elution)	Smaller DNA fragments elute more quickly through a filter of defined pore size.	Uncertain effects of DNA conformation, cell cycle, cell number, and lysis
3. Nucleoid sedimentation	ssb 1–20 Gy	Irradiated cells show altered DNA supercoiling within nucleus.	Uncertain which DNA lesion(s) are being detected.
4. Pulse-field gel electrophoresis (PFGE)	dsb > 2 Gy	Allows for resolution of DNA-dsb, which can be quantified by relative migration within the gel.	Uncertain effects of DNA conformation. High number of cells in S phase may bias results of assay.
5. Comet assay	ssb > 1 Gy (alkaline lysis) dsb > 2 Gy (neutral lysis)	Following lysis, individual nuclei are subjected to agarose gel electrophoresis. The DNA that moves out of the nucleus (head) to form the "tail" of the comet is quantitated to provide a measure of DNA damage.	Requires image analysis system to quantify DNA damage. Increased numbers of cells in S phase may bias assay.
6. Fluorescence in situ hybridization (FISH)	Doses > 1 Gy	Chromosome-specific probes, which can be detected with a fluorescent ligand, are used to identify radiation-induced translocations.	May be difficult to interpret in tumor cells that contain translocations prior to irradiation.
7. Premature chromosome condensation (PCC)	Doses > 1 Gy	An irradiated interphase cell is fused to a mitotic cell. The chromosomes in the interphase cell undergo premature condensation, allowing radiation-induced chromosome damage to be scored.	May be difficult to interpret in tumor cells that contain chromosome aberrations prior to irradiation.

[a]ssb = single-strand breaks; dsb = double-strand breaks.

Source: Adapted from Whitaker et al., 1991.

13.3 MOLECULAR AND CELLULAR RESPONSES TO IONIZING RADIATION

13.3.1 Activation of Radiation-Response Genes

Cellular damage to ionizing radiation can affect the expression of a number of genes involved in the response of cells to stress. Induction of the expression of early-response genes by ionizing radiation can be initiated by damage to the plasma membrane or to nuclear DNA. Many studies have reported that cellu-lar exposure to ionizing radiation is associated with the induction of transcription factors including the c-myc, p53, c-fos/c-jun, and nuclear factor-kappa B (NF-κB) proteins. These proteins bind to specific DNA sequences and can activate transcription of cy-tokine, growth factor, and cell cycle–related genes. Furthermore, irradiation can modify intracellular signaling through modification of the activity of ty-rosine kinases, MAP-kinases, SAP-kinases, and ras-associated proteins (see Chap. 6, Secs. 6.3 and 6.4;

Weichselbaum et al., 1994). Some early-response genes, such as the epidermal growth factor (*EGR-1*) gene, contain radiation-responsive regulatory domains in their promoter regions, which can facilitate their rapid induction by ionizing radiation (Hallahan et al., 1995).

Other genes induced by radiation include those encoding cell cycle–related proteins [e.g., growth arrest after DNA damage (GADD), p34^{cdc2}, cyclin B, p53], growth factors or cytokines [e.g., platelet-derived growth factor (PDGF), transforming growth factor α (TGF-α), basic fibroblast growth factor (bFGF), tumor necrosis factor (TNF)], and enzymes (e.g., plasminogen activator]. Liberation of inflammatory cytokines such as TNF and interleukin-1 (IL-1) by cells following radiation damage may lead to a continuing cascade of cytokine production, which may be responsible for the acute inflammation and late-onset fibrosis observed in some irradiated tissues (see Chap. 14, Sec. 14.2.2). There have also been recent reports of specific genes that are induced solely by ionizing radiation, although their function in relation to the radiation response of the cell is still largely unknown (Boothman, 1994). In summary, the cellular response to ionizing radiation is mediated not only by the direct damage to DNA but also by a complex interaction between a number of proteins located within the plasma membrane, cytoplasm, and nucleus of the cell.

13.3.2 Cell-Cycle Arrest

Mammalian cells respond to ionizing radiation by delaying their progression through the cell cycle. Such delays could allow for the repair of DNA damage in cells prior to undergoing either DNA replication or mitosis and could prevent the acquisition of genetic instability or mutant cellular phenotypes in future cell generations (Hartwell and Kastan, 1994). Early kinetic studies reported a rapid decrease in the mitotic index in an irradiated cell population, as both lethally damaged and surviving cells ceased to enter mitosis, while cells already in mitosis continued their cell-cycle progression. After a period of time, which depends on both the cell type and the radiation dose, surviving cells re-enter mitosis (Fig. 13.5); this time is known as the *mitotic delay*. Mitotic delay appears to be due largely to a block of cell-cycle progression in G2 phase, although cells in G1 and S phases are also delayed in their progres-

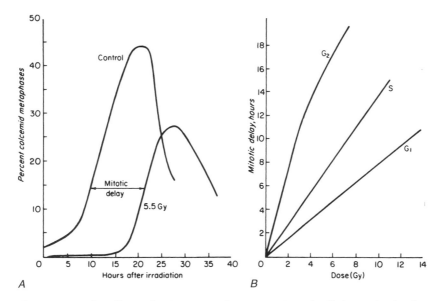

Figure 13.5. The effects of radiation on the progression of cells into mitosis after the treatment. *A.* At time zero, the cells are placed in medium containing colcemid, a drug that arrests cells in mitosis, and the percentage of cells that accumulate in mitosis is plotted as a function of time. The decline in the curves at late times is a result of cells escaping the drug-induced block or dying. The mitotic delay due to a radiation dose of 5.5 Gy displaces the curves for the radiation-treated cells to the right. *B.* Cells are irradiated when in different phases of the cell cycle and the mitotic delay observed is plotted as a function of radiation dose. (Adapted from Elkind and Whitmore, 1967.)

sion, albeit to a lesser extent. As a result of radiation-induced delays in the cell cycle, cell populations can be partially synchronized by irradiation. They may continue to experience delays in their progression through the next and subsequent cell cycles.

Control of the cell growth cycle has been discussed in Chap. 7, Sec. 7.2. The molecular basis for the G1 cell-cycle arrest following radiation damage appears to involve the p53 and retinoblastoma tumor suppressor (pRb) proteins. In normal cells, the pRb protein is found to be hypophosphorylated in the early part of the G1 phase but becomes hyperphosphorylated as the cells enter S phase. The hyperphosphorylation of the pRb protein is facilitated by cyclin-cdk complexes. Radiation-induced G1 arrest in normal cells appears to be dependent on increased expression of the normal p53 protein and is not usually observed in those cells that express a mutant p53 protein (Kastan et al., 1991). The p53-dependent G1 arrest response is reduced in cells derived from patients with the disorder ataxia telangiectasia (Canman et al., 1994). The gene that is mutated in ataxia telangiectasia (the *ATM* gene) has recently been cloned (Savitsky et al., 1995), and encodes a signal transduction protein that may be activated by DNA damage prior to the p53 protein response (see Chap. 4, Sec. 4.4.7; Morgan and Kastan, 1997).

Recent evidence suggests that the carboxy-terminal end of the p53 protein may recognize DNA damage in the form of single- or double-stranded DNA breaks (Jayaraman and Prives, 1995; Reed et al., 1995). The conformation of the p53 protein may thus be altered, facilitating its binding to specific DNA sequences and thereby activating a number of downstream genes including the *p21*$^{WAF1/CIP1}$ gene. The p21$^{WAF1/CIP1}$ protein acts as a potent inhibitor of the phosphorylation activity of the G1 cyclin-dependent kinases, so that the pRb protein remains hypophosphorylated and the cell arrests in the G1 phase (see Chap. 7, Sec. 7.2.3). In fibroblasts, irradiation may cause loss of reproductive potential by the induction of a permanent G1 phase arrest (reviewed by Little, 1994). However, the capacity for the p53 protein to mediate G1 arrest is reduced in human tumor cells, suggesting that other, as yet unidentified, G1-modulating factors may be important in the radiation-induced cell-cycle response of transformed cells (Li et al., 1995). In summary, it is now believed that the p53, p21$^{WAF1/CIP1}$, and pRB proteins interact in normal proliferating cells to cause arrest at the G1 checkpoint following ionizing radiation, as shown in Fig. 13.6 (Levine, 1997).

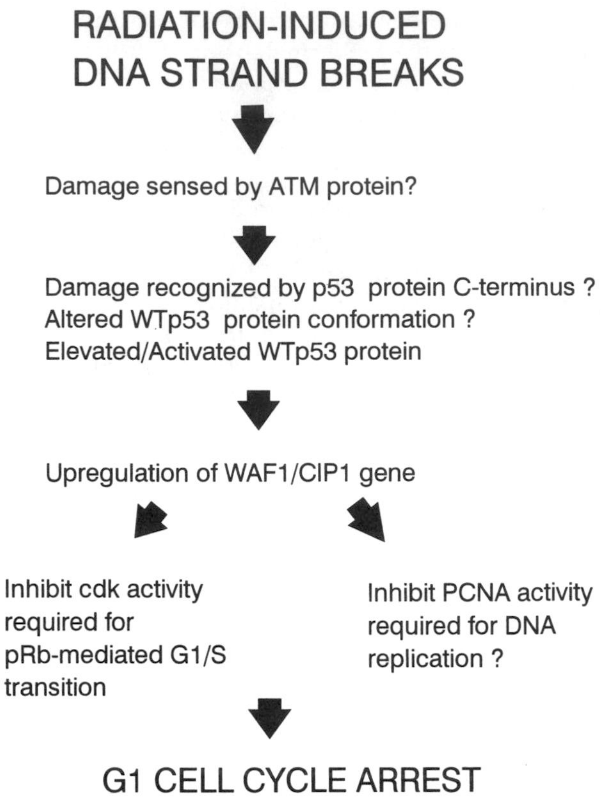

RADIATION-INDUCED DNA STRAND BREAKS

Damage sensed by ATM protein?

Damage recognized by p53 protein C-terminus ?
Altered WTp53 protein conformation ?
Elevated/Activated WTp53 protein

Upregulation of WAF1/CIP1 gene

Inhibit cdk activity required for pRb-mediated G1/S transition

Inhibit PCNA activity required for DNA replication ?

G1 CELL CYCLE ARREST

Figure 13.6. The wild-type p53–dependent DNA damage response pathway can be activated by DNA strand breaks leading to a G1 cell cycle arrest (or apoptosis) depending on cell type. The ATM ("mutated in ataxia telangiectasia") protein appears to act upstream of the p53 protein in mediating signals following radiation-induced DNA damage. Subsequent inhibition of cyclin-kinase activity by the p21$^{WAF1/CIP1}$ protein leads to hypophosphorylation of the pRb protein and G1 phase cell-cycle arrest. The exact role of the p53 protein as a modifier of the events required for DNA replication in cells remains to be defined but may involve activities associated with p21-mediated inhibition of PCNA (proliferating-cell nuclear antigen). WTp53-dependent apoptosis may occur through a separate pathway (not shown), involving the relative expression of bax and bcl-2 gene sequences (Chap. 7, Sec. 7.3). (Adapted from Bristow et al., 1996.)

The G2 phase of the cell cycle is under the control of the G2-associated cyclin-B and its catalytic partner, the p34^{cdc2} protein kinase (Chap. 7, Sec. 7.2.2). The duration of the G2 arrest following radiation damage is dose-dependent and can be decreased by pretreating cells with caffeine or with inhibitors of protein kinases prior to radiation (Bernhard et al., 1994b). Molecular alterations that have been associated with the onset and duration of the G2 delay following radiation treatment include (1) decreased expression or stability of the cyclin-B protein; (2) altered phosphorylation of the p34^{cdc2} protein; and (3) cytoplasmic sequestration of the cyclin-B protein, thereby preventing the formation of nuclear cyclin-B-p34^{cdc2} complexes (Maity et al., 1994; Metting and Little, 1995; Smeets et al., 1994). Several studies have also implicated the Ras and p53 proteins in the control of G2 arrest (Bernhard et al., 1994a; Levine, 1997). The cell-cycle arrest during S phase in irradiated cells is poorly understood, but probably involves inhibition of replicon initiation, which is required for DNA synthesis.

Several investigators have studied the relationship between cell-cycle arrest and loss of viability as assessed by a colony-forming assay (see Sec. 13.3.4). The length of the radiation-induced G2 delay has been reported to correlate with cell survival in rat and human cells that have been transfected with various oncogenes (Bernhard et al., 1994a; Su and Little, 1993). However, the length of G2 delay is quite similar among resistant and sensitive cells when they are irradiated with equitoxic doses of ionizing radiation (Nagasawa et al., 1994; Schwartz et al., 1996b). In contrast, the level of clonogenic radiation survival does not appear to be related to the duration of the radiation-induced G1 arrest phase in either human or rodent tumor cells that express a normal *p53* gene (Peacock et al., 1995; Li et al., 1995).

13.3.3 Radiation-Induced Cell Death

Inhibition of the continued reproductive ability of cells is an important consequence of the molecular and cellular responses to radiation, both because it occurs at relatively low doses (a few grays) and because it is the major aim of irradiation of malignant disease. A tumor is controlled if its stem cells (i.e., clonogenic cells) are prevented from continued proliferation. Most types of cells do not show morphological evidence of radiation damage until they attempt to divide. Following doses of less than about 10 Gy, lethally damaged cells may (1) undergo a permanent growth arrest such as that observed for fibroblasts, (2) undergo interphase death or lysis, or (3) undergo one or two abortive mitotic cycles and then finally undergo cell lysis. Cell lysis following irradiation can occur by apoptosis or necrosis. The biochemical and morphologic differences observed for cells undergoing these types of cell death have been reviewed in Chap. 7 (Sec. 7.3).

For the majority of normal and tumor cells, death secondary to mitosis-linked events accounts for most of the cell kill following irradiation. However, in some radiosensitive cells—notably lymphocytes, spermatocytes, thymocytes, and intestinal crypt cells—irradiation causes the cells to undergo an early (within a few hours) interphase death that can be associated with the biochemical and morphologic characteristics of apoptosis (i.e., cell membrane blebbing, the formation of nuclear apoptotic bodies, and specific DNA fragmentation patterns). Depending on the type of cell, the intracellular target(s) for the induction of the apoptotic response may be either the cell membrane or the DNA or both. The involvement of the cell membrane in triggering radiation-induced apoptosis is supported by the observation that ionizing radiation can initiate a sphingomyelin-dependent signaling pathway within the cell membrane of endothelial cells which, in turn, can induce apoptosis in the absence of DNA damage (Verheij et al., 1996). Furthermore, pre-incubation of cells with agents capable of altering either protein function or lipid peroxidation within the cell membrane can also modify the level of radiation-induced apoptosis (Fuks et al., 1995). The genetic events that control apoptosis have been described in Chap. 7 (Sec. 7.3); in hematopoietic and intestinal crypt cells, radiation can lead to upregulation of genes such as *bax*, which can facilitate apoptosis (Kitada et al., 1996), but the reasons why some cell types undergo extensive radiation-induced apoptosis within a few hours after irradiation while others do not remain to be elucidated.

Cells that do not undergo early apoptosis may do so at later times (> 12 h), but there is currently no clear understanding of whether the events leading to apoptotic death (early or late) are separate from events leading to loss of colony-forming ability (Hockenbery, 1995). Some studies have shown that the level of radiation-induced apoptosis does not correlate with eventual clonogenic cell survival as measured by colony-forming assays (Aldridge et al., 1995; Yin and Schimke, 1995). However, others suggest that for transformed rodent cells, radiation-induced apoptosis does predict for subsequent loss of colony-forming ability under the conditions of low-dose-rate irradiation or during a course of fractionated radiotherapy (Dewey et al., 1995). At present it is clear that the apoptotic pathway of cell death is an important mechanism by which cells can die following irradiation, but whether it has a cause and effect relationship to the loss of proliferative capacity is currently unknown.

13.3.4 In vitro Assays for Proliferative Capacity

A cell that retains unlimited proliferative capacity after radiation treatment is regarded as having *survived* the treatment, while one that has lost the ability to generate a "clone" or *colony* is regarded as having been killed, even though it may undergo a few divisions or remain intact in the cell population for a substantial period. This definition of cell death is independent of the proliferation rate of different cells either before or after irradiation. Furthermore, colony formation following irradiation is an important end point for radiobiologists and radiation oncologists, as it relates to a cell's ability to repopulate normal or tumor tissues following exposure to ionizing radiation. Assessing survival of cells after radiation thus depends on the demonstration that they retain the ability to produce a large number of progeny (i.e., to produce a colony). One of the commonest ways to assess cell survival is to use a clonogenic assay (Puck and Marcus, 1956; see Fig. 13.7*A*). In this assay, cells grown in culture are irradiated either before or after preparation of a suspension of single cells and plated at low density in tissue-culture dishes. Following irradiation, the cells are incubated for a number of days, and those that retain proliferative capacity divide and grow to form discrete colonies of cells. After incubation, the colonies are fixed and stained so that they can be counted easily.

Cells that do not retain proliferative capacity following irradiation (i.e., are killed) may divide a few times but form only very small "abortive" colonies. If a colony contains more than 50 cells (i.e., derived from a single cell by at least six division cycles), it is usually capable of continued growth and can be regarded as having arisen from a surviving cell. The plating efficiency (PE) of the cell population is calculated by dividing the number of colonies formed by the number of cells plated. Untreated cells rarely have a PE of 1 (more usually it is 0.5 to 0.8 for cells passaged for many generations). The ratio of the PE for the irradiated cells to the PE for control cells is calculated to give the fraction of cells surviving the treatment (*cell survival*). If a range of radiation doses is used, then these cell-survival values can be plotted to give a *survival curve*, such as the ones shown in Fig. 13.10. Cells taken directly from animal or human tumors can also be grown in culture, allowing the in vitro assay method to be extended to the study of the radiation sensitivity of tumor cells treated in vivo (see Fig. 13.7*B*). As the plating efficiency of untreated human tumor cells in culture is usually quite low (i.e., PE < 0.01), clonogenic assays for human tumor cells attempt to improve tumor cell clonogenicity by plating the cells into semisolid agarose or methylcellulose cultures supplemented with growth factors.

Nonclonogenic assays may also be used to determine the relative radiosensitivity of cells. These assays can be completed in a short period of time and used for those cells that do not produce well-defined colonies. Many of these assays are *growth assays,* which determine the number of viable cells at various times following irradiation in untreated and treated cell cultures. Cellular growth can be measured by a variety of methods including the *MTT assay,* in which cellular viability is measured by colorimetric assessment of the reduction of a tetrazolium compound. One growth assay that has been optimized for determining the radiosensitivity of human tumor cells is the cell adhesive matrix (CAM) assay, in which primary human tumor cells are plated di-

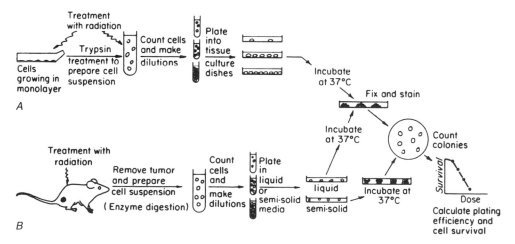

Figure 13.7. Schematic diagram of in vitro plating assays to assess cell survival. *A*. Assay for the radiation sensitivity of cells growing in culture. *B*. In vivo–in vitro assay for the sensitivity of tumor cells grown and irradiated in vivo.

rectly into culture dishes coated with a combination of cell-adhesive proteins (Baker et al., 1988). Although clonogenic survival remains the "gold standard" for determining the reproductive potential of cells following irradiation, data from growth assays can be informative provided that the acquisition and interpretation of the data are rigorous (Price and McMillan, 1994).

13.3.5 In vivo Assays for Proliferative Capacity

A number of assays are available for estimating the radiation survival of normal and tumor cells by transplantation of irradiated and control cells in vivo. For example, in the endpoint-dilution technique, cells from an irradiated tumor are diluted to different concentrations and implanted into new recipients (Fig. 13.8; Hewitt and Wilson, 1959). Clonogenic cells that survive radiation may proliferate to form solid tumors in vivo. The percent of tumors that develop can be plotted as a function of the cell number injected, and the number of cells required for 50 percent tumor takes (i.e., the TD_{50} value) is determined. The ratio of the TD_{50} value obtained for cells from untreated control tumors to that obtained for cells from radiation-treated tumors gives the cell survival. This technique has been adapted to the study of the radiosensitivity of the cells of a number of normal tissues (e.g., mammary gland, thyroid gland, liver) and for use in vitro (in multiwell plates) for cells that do not form colonies (Clifton, 1980; Jirtle et al., 1990).

Methods have been developed for assessing the ability of cells to form colonies in situ. The best-known of these is the spleen-colony method described in Chap. 15, Sec. 15.2.4, which has been used to assess both the radiation and drug sensitivity of bone marrow stem cells (e.g., McCulloch and Till, 1962). An analogous method, which has been used to examine radiation and drug sensitivities of the cells of solid tumors, is the lung-colony assay (Hill and Bush, 1969). Some ingenious colony-forming assays have been developed to study the radiation response of stem cells in situ in certain proliferative tissues, including skin, gastrointestinal tract, testis, cartilage, kidney, and certain tumors. An example is the technique used to study the sensitivity of individual crypt stem cells in the small intestine (Withers and Elkind, 1970; Fig. 13.9). Radiation doses sufficient to reduce the number of surviving crypt cells to a low level are given to groups of mice. The surviving cells grow rapidly to form regenerating crypts, which can be identified in histologic sections made about 3 to 4 days after radiation treatment. The fraction of crypts capable of regenerating can then be calculated and plotted as a function of radiation dose to give a survival curve for intestinal crypts. The number of cells in each crypt capable of regenerating the crypt (i.e., the crypt stem cells) is between 8 to 40 (Roberts et al., 1995). Consequently, crypt survival does not reflect individual cell survival unless radiation doses sufficient to reduce the probable number of stem-cell survivors to less than 1 per crypt are used. In this assay, the low-dose initial part of the

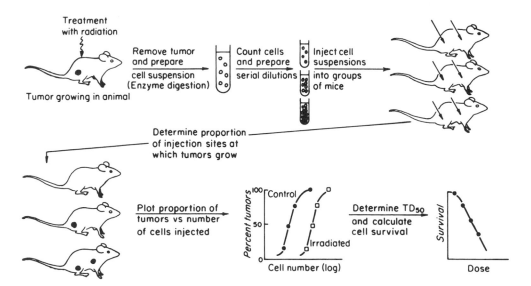

Figure 13.8. Schematic diagram of the application of the endpoint-dilution assay to determine the radiosensitivity of tumor cells treated in vivo.

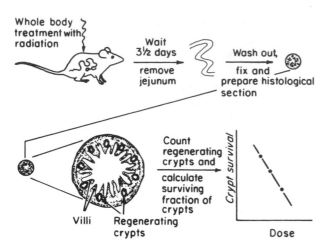

Figure 13.9. Schematic diagram describing the in situ assay used to determine the radiation sensitivity of individual crypt stem cells in the small intestine of a mouse.

cell-survival curve thus cannot be determined directly; only the final slope of the survival curve is obtained in this assay.

13.4 MODELS OF RADIATION CELL SURVIVAL

13.4.1 Radiation Survival Curves

The various techniques described above have been used to obtain survival curves for a wide range of malignant and normal cell populations. In general, for low-LET radiation (e.g., x- or γ-rays), these curves have the shape(s) illustrated in Fig. 13.10, in which cell survival is plotted on a log scale as a function of dose on a linear scale. At low doses, there is evidence of a shoulder region; but at higher doses, the curve either becomes steeper and straight so that survival decreases exponentially with dose (dotted line) or appears to be continually bending downward on a semilogarithmic plot (solid line). As illustrated, the accuracy of the data obtained is usually such that either shape could fit the data adequately over the first few decades of survival. Many different mathematical models have been used to produce equations that can fit survival-curve data within the limits of experimental error. Two of the more commonly used models are the *target-theory* and *linear-quadratic* models of cell survival.

13.4.2 Target Theory

The target-theory model of cell survival was based on the hypothesis that a number of critical targets had to be inactivated for cells to be killed. Cell killing by radiation is now recognized to be more

complex, but the equation and parameters derived from the model are still used to describe the shape of cell survival curves. The number of targets (dN) inactivated by a small dose of radiation (dD) should be proportional to the initial number of targets N and dD, so that

$$dN \propto N \cdot dD \quad \text{or} \quad dN = \frac{N \cdot dD}{D_0} \quad (13.2)$$

where $1/D_0$ is a constant of porportionality and the negative sign is introduced because the number of active targets N decreases with increasing dose. This equation can be integrated to give

$$N = N_0 \cdot e^{-\frac{D}{D_0}} \quad (13.3)$$

where N_0 is the number of active targets present at zero dose. If it is assumed that cells contain only a single target that must be inactivated for them to be killed, then the fractional survival (S) of a population of cells is represented by

$$S = \frac{N}{N_0} = e^{-\frac{D}{D_0}} \quad (13.4)$$

where N_0 and N are the initial and final number of cells surviving following a radiation dose D, respec-

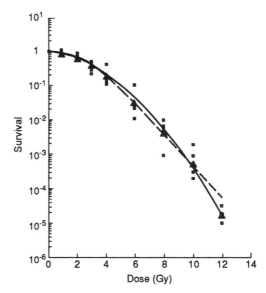

Figure 13.10. Survival data for a murine melanoma cell line treated with low-LET radiation. The survival is plotted on a logarithmic scale against dose plotted on a linear scale. The data from five independent survival experiments are shown as the small squares, with the geometric mean value at each dose shown as the large triangles. The survival curves shown are the result of fitting the data to target theory or linear quadratic models (Secs. 13.4.2 and 13.4.3). (Adapted from Bristow et al., 1990a.)

tively, and D_0 is a constant. This also represents the probability that any individual cell will survive the radiation dose D. Equation (13.4) gives a *single-hit, single-target* survival curve that is a straight line on a semilogarithmic plot originating at a surviving fraction of 1 at zero dose (Fig. 13.11, line a). Survival curves of this shape have been obtained for viruses and bacteria, for radiosensitive normal and malignant cells (i.e., cells in the bone marrow or lymphoma cells), and for many types of cells treated with high-LET radiation (see Sec. 13.5.1). The term D_0 represents the dose required to reduce the surviving fraction to 37 percent and is a measure of the slope of the line in Fig. 13.11. It can be shown mathematically that the radiation dose required to kill 90 percent of the initial number of cells, termed the D_{10} value, is equivalent to $2.3 \times D_0$ (where 2.3 is the natural logarithm of 10).

If, instead, it is assumed that a cell contains n identical targets, *each of which* must be inactivated (by a single hit) to cause cell death, then the *multitarget, single-hit* cell survival equation can be represented by

$$S = \frac{N}{N_0} = 1 - (1 - e^{-\frac{D}{D_0}})^n \quad (13.5)$$

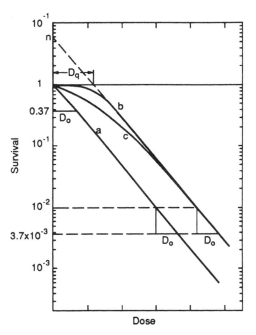

Figure 13.11. Survival curves defined by the single-hit and multitarget models of cell killing discussed in the text. Curve a. Single-hit (single-target) survival curve defined by Eq. (13.4). Curve b. Multitarget survival curve defined by Eq. (13.5). Curve c. Composite (two-component) survival curve resulting from both multitarget and single-hit components defined by Eq. (13.6). Also shown is how the parameters D_0, n, and D_q can be derived from the survival curves.

Again, this equation represents the probability that any individual cell will survive a dose D. A plot of this equation leads to a survival curve with a shoulder at low doses and a straight-line section on a semilogarithmic plot, as shown in Fig. 13.11, line b. The parameters D_0, n, and D_q can be determined for this curve as shown. At doses that are large compared to D_0 (i.e., $D \gg D_0$), Eq. (13.5) reduces to $S = n \exp(-D/D_0)$, which is similar to Eq. (13.4). The straight-line part of the survival curve thus extrapolates to a value n at zero dose and has a slope defined by D_0. As indicated previously, the D_0 value is the dose required to reduce cell survival from S to $0.37S$ in the *straight-line region* of the survival curve. The quasi-threshold dose D_q, is the dose at which the extrapolated straight-line section of the survival curve crosses the dose axis (survival = 1) and quantitatively describes the size of the shoulder. It can be calculated by $D_q = D_0 \times \ln n$. For this model, the size of the shoulder is regarded as giving an indication of the repair capacity of cells.

One limitation of Eq. (13.5) is that it predicts that a certain amount of damage must be accumulated in a cell before it is killed—i.e., that, at very low doses, the survival curve should be parallel to the dose axis or have an initial slope of zero. This is contrary to much experimental data, which indicate that, for cell populations irradiated with x- or γ-rays, the survival curve often has a finite initial slope (Fig. 13.11, curve c). This observation can be accommodated by modifying Eq. (13.5) to allow for an additional single-hit mechanism by which cells may be killed. Thus Eq. (13.5) would have an initial single-hit component added to give the following *two-component multitarget* model:

$$S = \frac{N}{N_0} = e^{-\frac{D}{D_S}} [1 - (1 - e^{-\frac{D}{D_0}})^n] \quad (13.6)$$

The extra parameter D_S defines the initial slope of the survival curve.* The single-hit component can be regarded as describing cell inactivation due to damage that is nonrepairable, while the rest of the equation describes cell inactivation due to accumulation of damage that is potentially repairable. This equation is the one that has been fitted to the data in Fig. 13.10 to give the dashed line.

The D_0 values for almost all mammalian cells are quite similar (about 1 to 2 Gy for irradiation with x- or γ-rays given under aerobic conditions), and there

---

*The final slope of the survival curve (D_0') is modified and is given by $D_0' = D_0 D_S / (D_0 + D_S)$.

are no consistent differences in D_0 value between malignant and normal cells. For low-LET radiations, the size of the shoulder varies considerably between different normal and tumor cell lines. For example, certain radiosensitive cell lines of bone marrow or fibroblast origin and derived from selected inherited radiosensitive syndromes (e.g., ataxia telangiectasia, Fanconi's anemia) have essentially no shoulder to their cell survival curves (i.e., $D_q = 0$). Larger shoulders ($D_q > 3$ Gy) have been observed for more radioresistant cells, including those transfected with combinations of oncogenes (see Sec. 13.5.6) and cell lines derived from human melanoma, renal cell carcinoma, and other tumors (see Chap. 14, Sec. 14.2.1).

13.4.3 The Linear-Quadratic Model

The linear-quadratic model of cell kill is based on the idea that multiple lesions, induced by radiation, interact in the cell to cause cell killing. The lesions that interact could be caused by a single ionizing track, giving a direct dependence of cell killing on dose, or by two or more separate tracks, giving a dependence of lethality on higher powers of dose. The assumption that two lesions must interact to cause cell killing gives an equation that can fit most experimental survival curves quite adequately, at least over the first few decades of survival, and is given by

$$S = N/N_0 = \exp(-\alpha D - \beta D^2) \qquad (13.7)$$

The parameters α and β are assumed to describe the probability of the interacting lesions being caused by energy-deposition events due to a single charged-particle track or by two independent tracks, respectively. The linear-quadratic equation defines a survival curve that is concave downward on a semilogarithmic plot and never becomes strictly exponential (see Figs. 13.10 and 13.12). However, the curvature is usually small at high doses. The α component can be regarded as describing cell inactivation by nonrepairable damage, while the β component describes cell inactivation by accumulation of repairable damage (see Fig. 13.12). The values for α and β vary considerably for different types of mammalian cells both in vitro and in vivo (see Chap. 14, Sec. 14.3.8). Typical values of α are in the range 1 to 10^{-1} Gy^{-1} and of β in the range 10^{-1} to 10^{-2} Gy^{-2}.

Alternative equations similar to the linear-quadratic equation can be derived by making various biological assumptions, e.g., concerning the capacity of cells to repair radiation damage and the effect of radiation treatment on that capacity (Foray et al.,

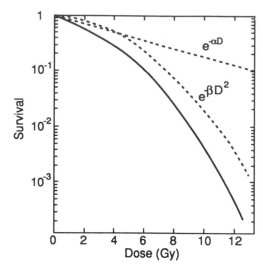

Figure 13.12. Survival curve (*solid line*) as defined by the linear-quadratic model of cell killing, Eq (13.7). The curves defined by the two components of the equation are shown separately as the dashed lines.

1996). It should be stressed that a good fit of a given equation to the survival data does not validate the underlying biological assumptions of the model.

13.4.4 Surviving Fraction Following 2 Gy (SF2) and the Mean Inactivation Dose

There is greater variation in the low-dose or shoulder region of the radiation survival curves obtained for mammalian cells as compared to the variation in the slopes of the high-dose region of the curve (e.g., Deacon et al., 1984; Fertil and Malaise, 1985). Measured or calculated radiobiologic parameters that describe the survival of cells following doses of 1 to 3 Gy reflect clinically relevant cell survival, given that the majority of clinical radiotherapy consists of daily fractions of 1 to 2.5 Gy. Two of these parameters are the surviving fraction of cells following a dose of 2 Gy (i.e., *the SF2 value*) and the value of α from a fit of radiation survival data to the linear-quadratic equation. In contrast to the SF2 or α parameters that describe radiation survival solely in the low-dose region of the curve, another parameter, the *mean inactivation dose* (MID), is defined as the integrated area under the entire radiation survival curve. The MID, therefore, describes cell survival in both the low- and high-dose regions of the curve (Malaise et al., 1987). Values for SF2 and MID among normal and malignant mammalian cells range between 0.1 to 0.8 and 1 to 4 Gy, respectively. The SF2 value is discussed in greater detail in Chap. 14 (Sec. 14.5.1) in relation to its potential use in predicting the clinical response of normal tissues and tumors to fractionated radiation treatments.

13.5 FACTORS THAT INFLUENCE CELL SURVIVAL

13.5.1 Radiation Quality and Relative Biological Effectiveness

The biological effect of radiation depends on its effective linear energy transfer (see Sec. 13.2.2). The difference in survival curves for x- or γ-rays (low-LET) and for fast-neutron (high-LET) irradiation is illustrated in Fig. 13.13. In general, both the slope and the shoulder of the survival curve are reduced for higher-LET radiation. The biological effectiveness of different types of radiation can be characterized by a parameter known as the *relative biological effectiveness* (RBE). The RBE is defined as the ratio of the dose of a standard type of radiation to that of the test radiation that gives the same biological effect. The standard type of radiation is usually taken as 200- or 250-kVp x-rays. Cobalt 60 γ-rays are also used as a standard for comparison studies, although their RBE relative to 250-kVp x-rays is about 0.9. Because the shoulder of the survival curve is reduced for high-LET radiation, the RBE varies with the dose or the survival level at which it is determined (see Fig. 13.13). Thus the RBE increases as the dose at which it is determined is reduced.

The relationship between the RBE and the LET for different types of radiation is complex (see Fig.

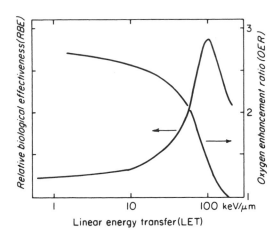

Figure 13.14. Illustration of the dependence of the RBE (*left-hand axis*) and the OER (*right-hand axis*) on the LET of the radiation. The actual value of the RBE depends on the level of biological damage being examined.

13.14; Barendsen, 1968). The RBE rises to a maximum at an LET of about 100 keV/μm before declining again. The rise in RBE indicates that increasing the density of energy-deposition events increases the efficacy with which a given amount of energy deposited causes biological damage, but there is an optimum (~ 100 keV/μm) beyond which the extra energy deposited is wasted on cells that have already been killed (i.e., there is an "overkill" phenomenon). The reduction in the shoulder of the survival curve for higher-LET radiation also depends on the LET. At very high LET values (≥ 100 keV/μm), the shoulder on the survival curve is completely eliminated, indicating that, as the LET increases, an increasing proportion of the observed cell killing is due to nonrepairable damage.

13.5.2 Oxygen Effect and Hypoxia in Tumors

The biological effects of radiation are influenced by oxygen. There is some uncertainty about the exact mechanism involved, but it is believed to be because O_2 can interact with the radicals formed by the radiation resulting in products that are more difficult for the cell to repair. Cells irradiated in the presence of air are about three times more sensitive than cells irradiated under conditions of severe hypoxia (see Fig. 13.15A). The sensitizing effect of different concentrations of oxygen is shown in Fig. 13.15B. At very low levels of oxygen, the cells are resistant, but as the level of oxygen increases, their sensitivity rises rapidly to almost maximal levels at oxygen concentrations above about 20 μmol/L (equivalent oxygen partial pressure ~14 mmHg).

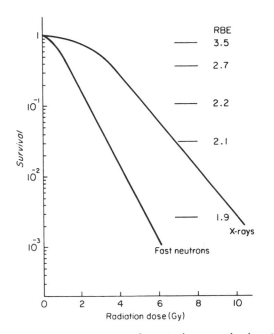

Figure 13.13. Comparison of survival curves for low-LET (x-ray) and high-LET (fast-neutron) irradiation. The RBE is calculated as indicated in the text and varies at different levels of survival.

The oxygen concentration at which the sensitizing effect is one-half of maximum (the K_m value) is about 5 μmol/L (3 to 4 mmHg). Most normal tissues have an average oxygen concentration equivalent to a partial pressure (P_{O_2}) of about 40 mmHg and are fully sensitive to radiation. Some tissues in the body may have lower P_{O_2} levels (e.g., liver, cartilage, brain), but many tumors contain a substantial proportion of cells that are hypoxic and hence are more resistant to radiation.

The degree of sensitization afforded by oxygen is characterized by the *oxygen enhancement ratio* (OER), which is defined (Fig. 13.15A) as the ratio of doses required to give the same biological effect in the absence or presence of oxygen. For radiation doses greater than about 3 Gy, the OER for a wide range of cell lines in vitro and for most tissues in vivo irradiated with x- or γ-rays (i.e., low-LET radiations), is in the range 2.5 to 3.3. For x- or γ-ray doses less than 3 Gy (i.e., in the shoulder region of the survival curve), the OER appears to be reduced in a dose-dependent manner. For example, for Chinese hamster ovary cells, the OER at a dose of 0.8 Gy was about 70 percent of its value at high doses (Palcic and Skarsgard, 1984). A reduction of the OER at low doses may be clinically important, since the individual treatments of a fractionated course of radiation are usually 2 Gy or less. The OER is also dependent on the LET, declining to a value of 1 for radiations with LET values greater than about 200 keV/μm (Fig. 13.14).

Experimental and clinical studies have provided both direct and indirect evidence for the presence of hypoxic cells in tumors. Early histomorphometric analyses in human and rodent tumors (Thomlinson and Gray, 1955; Moore et al., 1985) suggested that regions of viable cells exist in proximity to tumor blood vessels. In contrast, at increased distance from the blood vessels, regions of necrosis were observed (see Chap. 7, Fig. 7.18). The width of the viable regions of cells between the stroma and the necrotic areas (referred to as *tumor cords*) was found to be about 150 to 180 μm for human tumors or 80 to 100 μm for rodent tumors. These distances are equivalent to the calculated distance that oxygen would be expected to diffuse through the tumor. This implies that, at the edge of the necrotic regions, there could be viable cells at very low oxygen tensions. Among a variety of tumor types, the width of the viable regions of cells can vary quite widely, depending on the P_{O_2} in the vessel(s), the respiration rate of the viable cells, and other nutrient conditions in tumor microregions.

Further evidence for the presence of viable hypoxic cells in a tumor was provided by Powers and

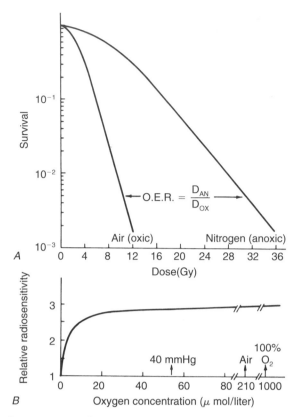

Figure 13.15. Effect of oxygen as a radiosensitizer. *A.* Survival curves obtained when cells are treated with low-LET radiation in the presence (air) or absence (nitrogen) of oxygen. The oxygen-enhancement ratio (OER) is calculated as indicated (D_{OX} = dose in air, D_{AN} = dose in nitrogen) and as described in the text. *B.* The relative radiosensitivity of cells is plotted as a function of oxygen concentration in the surrounding medium to illustrate the dependence of the sensitizing effect on oxygen concentration. (Adapted from Chapman et al., 1974.)

Tolmach (1964), who studied the radiation sensitivity of the cells of a solid lymphosarcoma growing subcutaneously in a mouse. The tumor was irradiated in situ and cell survival was assessed using an endpoint-dilution assay. The results are illustrated schematically in Fig. 13.16A. The survival curve was found to have two components; at low doses, the line is quite steep; but at high doses, it is much shallower. The difference in slope is a factor of approximately 3, suggesting that the two components may represent the survival of two subpopulations of cells—well oxygenated and hypoxic, respectively. This was confirmed by further studies, which demonstrated that cells which survived high doses of radiation were not intrinsically more resistant and that the relative position of the more resistant part of the survival curve (the tail) could be altered by modifying oxygen delivery to the tumor (Fig. 13.16B).

The proportion of hypoxic cells in tumors can be estimated (Fig. 13.16B) from the ratio (S_{air}/S_{anox}) of the cell survival obtained for tumors in air-breathing animals irradiated with a large dose to that obtained for tumors irradiated with the same dose under anoxic conditions (e.g., tumor blood supply clamped or animal killed prior to the irradiation). It is assumed that the tumors made deliberately anoxic contain 100 percent hypoxic cells and that the radiation survival curve for the naturally occurring hypoxic cells is the same as that for the cells made deliberately anoxic. The proportion of naturally occurring hypoxic cells in the lymphosarcoma studied by Powers and Tolmach was estimated to be about 1 percent using the above method. Most other tumors treated in air-breathing animals contain a larger proportion of hypoxic cells, in the range of 10 to 20 percent (Moulder and Rockwell, 1987; Rockwell and Moulder, 1990). These proportions represent the cells that are sufficiently hypoxic to be maximally resistant to irradiation (radiobio-

logically hypoxic); it is expected that there will also be a substantial proportion of cells in tumors that are at oxygen levels intermediate between radiobiologically hypoxic and well-oxygenated levels. A variety of techniques have provided evidence that hypoxic cells exist in human tumors and may affect the outcome of radiation therapy (see Table 13.4 and Chap. 14, Sec. 14.5.3).

Two mechanisms have been proposed to explain the existence of hypoxic cells in tumors (Fig. 13.17). The tumor "cord" model discussed earlier implies that hypoxic cells exist at the limits of the diffusion range of oxygen away from blood vessels. The hypoxic cells in such cords presumably remain hypoxic for a period of time, until division of cells closer to the blood vessels causes them to be pushed so far away from the vessel that they die and become necrotic (assumed to happen because of lack of oxygen and other nutrients). Such cells are often referred to as *chronically hypoxic cells,* although there is evidence that in rapidly growing tumors (doubling

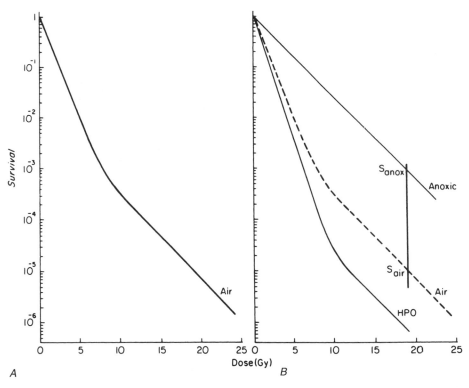

Figure 13.16. The influence of a subpopulation of hypoxic cells on the survival curve obtained for an irradiated tumor. *A.* Curve was obtained when the tumors were irradiated in situ in air-breathing animals and demonstrates two components with different slopes. *B.* Curves marked Anoxic and HPO were obtained when the animals were killed or given high-pressure oxygen to breathe prior to the irradiation, respectively. The broken line marked Air is from (*A*). The fraction of cells that were hypoxic in the tumor in air-breathing animals can be estimated as described in the text. (Modified from Powers and Tolmach, 1964.)

Table 13.4. Assays for Intratumoral Hypoxia

Technique	Principle	Advantages	Disadvantages
1. Histomorphometric assays	Measuring distances between blood vessels and zones of necrosis within histologic sections.	Simple. Can be combined with cryospectro-photometry to measure oxygen load of hemoglobin within frozen tissue sections	Indirect measure of tumor oxygenation. May not take into account changes in microregional blood flow.
2. Polarographic oxygen electrode assay	P_{O_2} electrode is advanced through tissue and electrode signals are processed by computer to produce P_{O_2} histograms.	Technically simple. Provides real-time and direct measurement of tissue P_{O_2}.	Invasive. Does not differentiate P_{O_2} values among necrotic and viable regions of tumors or between tumor and normal tissues.
3. DNA strand break assays	Use of alkaline comet assay to ascertain DNA strand breaks in irradiated tumor cells. Hypoxic cells exhibit less breaks than well-oxygenated cells.	Direct assay to measure DNA damage under hypoxic conditions.	Invasive. Subject to sampling errors and requires rapid (min) acquisition and processing of samples post-irradiation.
4. Hypoxic cell markers	The binding/uptake of radioactive or fluorescence-labeled hypoxic cell markers (nitroimidazoles) can be imaged by MRS, PET, SPECT, scintillation counting, ELISA, or microscopy, depending on the marker.	Hypoxic cells visualized at the cellular level or detection can be noninvasive with certain markers (i.e., [123]I 2-nitroimidazoles with SPECT scanning or [18]F 2-nitroimidazoles with PET scanning).	Requires injection or ingestion of hypoxic marker. Intensity of marker binding can be affected by inter-tumor metabolic factors.

Source: Data from Raleigh et al., 1996.

time of a few days), the length of time for which they survive under hypoxic conditions may be less than a day.

Another factor that can cause cells in tumors to become hypoxic is fluctuation in blood flow through tumor vessels. Regions of tumors supplied by one or more blood vessels may become hypoxic for short periods of time as a result of intermittent interruptions in blood flow, and cells may be hypoxic for only short periods of time (Fig. 13.17). Studies involving the intravenous injection of diffusable fluorescent dyes as markers of functional blood vessels and sophisticated measurements of microregional blood flow have given direct evidence for this effect in experimental tumors (Trotter et al., 1989; Chaplin and Hill, 1995). These two mechanisms for hypoxia may coexist in the same tumor (Chaplin et al., 1986).

Activation of cell signal-transduction pathways has been observed in cells exposed to hypoxia, particularly the activation of ras- and raf-associated pathways (Giaccia, 1996; Koong et al., 1994). Other proteins can also be activated in hypoxic cells, including proteins involved in transcriptional activation, cell-cycle control, angiogenesis, and the cellular processing of free radicals. For example, hypoxic cells may undergo a p53-independent, reversible G1/S cell-cycle arrest as a consequence of hypophosphorylation of the retinoblastoma protein (Graeber et al., 1994; Ludlow et al., 1993). Hypoxic conditions cause increased levels of the transcription factor HIF-1 (hypoxia-inducible factor), which increases the expression of a number of genes including vascular endothelial growth factor (VEGF), which is known to be an important mediator of tumor angiogenesis (Mazure et al., 1996).

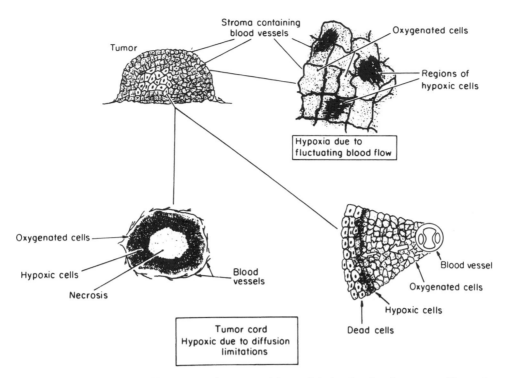

Figure 13.17. Schematic illustration of two possible models for the development of hypoxia in tumors. Hypoxia may arise as a result of diffusion limitations in the tumor cord model or as a result of fluctuating blood flow.

Studies utilizing oncogene-transfected rodent cells have suggested that mutant tumor cells which have acquired genetic resistance to hypoxia-mediated apoptosis may be preferentially selected during tumor progression (Graeber et al., 1996). Furthermore, genetic studies support the concept that the cells which are exposed to a hypoxic tumor environment are more likely to develop genomic instability and acquire mutant genotypes as compared with tumor cells growing in a non-hypoxic region of the tumor (Reynolds et al., 1996). These observations suggest that cells growing within hypoxic regions of tumors constitute an important target for cancer treatment, given their potential for both chemo- and radioresistance and their development of mutant phenotypes with increased angiogenic and metastatic potential (Young and Hill, 1990; Hockel et al., 1996).

13.5.3 Cell-Cycle Position

In a growing cell population, the cells will be distributed asynchronously throughout their growth cycle. Techniques have been devised that allow cell populations to be synchronized in one of the phases of the cell cycle; these include (1) the selective detach-

ment of mitotic cells from monolayers, (2) separation of cells on the basis of volume by centrifugal elutriation, (3) the introduction and subsequent removal of a metabolic block (e.g., nocodazole, aphidicolin, excess thymidine), (4) the use of agents (e.g., high-specific-activity H^3-thymidine or hydroxyurea) that kill cells exposed during the S phase of the cell cycle, and (5), direct sorting on the basis of DNA content using a vital DNA stain and fluorescence-activated cell sorting (see Chap. 7, Sec. 7.4).

Terasima and Tolmach (1961) used synchronized HeLa cells to show that cells in different phases of the cell cycle have different radiosensitivities. This is illustrated for Chinese hamster cells by the survival curves shown in Fig. 13.18A. If a single radiation dose is given to cells in different phases (i.e., a vertical cut is taken through the curves in Fig. 13.18A), then a pattern of cell survival as a function of cell-cycle position is obtained (Fig. 13.18B). Figure 13.18 shows that Chinese hamster cells in late S phase have the highest probability of survival after radiation (i.e., are the most resistant), and that cells in G2/M phases are the most sensitive. Although many cell lines appear to have a resistant period in S phase and a sensitive period in G2 phase following irradiation in vitro, other

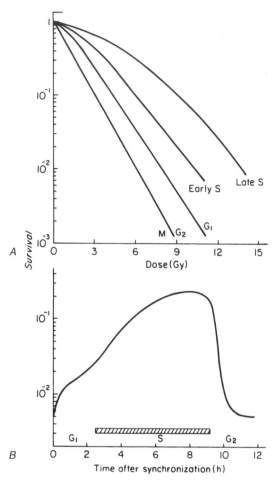

Figure 13.18. The effect of position in the cell growth cycle on cellular radiosensitivity. *A.* Survival curves for Chinese hamster cells irradiated in different phases of the cell cycle. *B.* Cells were selected in mitosis and irradiated with a fixed dose as a function of time of incubation after synchronization. The pattern of cell survival reflects the changing cellular sensitivity as the cells move through the cell cycle. (Adapted from Sinclair, 1968.)

cell lines have different patterns of sensitivity throughout the cell cycle. For example, some oncogene-transfected cells show increased resistance in the G2 phase, whereas other cells, including DNA repair-deficient cells, show similar sensitivity throughout all phases of the cell cycle (Cheong et al., 1993). Tumor cells growing and treated with radiation in vivo also demonstrate variations in radiosensitivity in different phases of the cell cycle (Grdina, 1980). The pattern of radiosensitivity throughout the cell cycle can be different for the same tumor cells growing in vivo or in vitro, indicating the influence of microenvironment on cell survival (Keng et al., 1984).

The varying radiosensitivity as a function of cell-cycle phase demonstrated in Fig. 13.18 means that

irradiating asynchronous populations will result in partial synchrony of the surviving cells, since those in the resistant phase(s) have a higher probability of survival than those in sensitive phases. The mitotic delay and the G2 block (see Sec. 13.3.2) will also tend to cause synchronization of the cell population. Thus, after irradiation, the surviving cells will progress into and/or be arrested in phases in which they would be more sensitive to a subsequent dose of radiation. Owing to the variable rate at which cells progress through the cycle, this synchrony will decay rapidly.

13.5.4 Molecular and Cellular Repair

The repair of cellular damage between radiation doses is the major mechanism underlying the clinical observation that a larger total dose can be tolerated when the radiation dose is fractionated. Elkind and Sutton (1960) showed that the shoulder of the survival curve for Chinese hamster cells reflects the accumulation of sublethal damage that can be repaired (Fig. 13.19). When the cells were incubated at 37°C for 2.5 h between the first and second radiation treatments, the original shoulder of the survival curve was partially regenerated, and it was completely regenerated when the cells were incubated for 23 h between the treatments—i.e., the horizontal displacement between the single-dose and split-dose curves was equivalent to the D_q value (Fig. 13.19*A*). When the interval between two fixed doses was varied (Fig. 13.19*B*), there was a rapid rise in survival as the interval was increased from zero (single dose) to about 2 h. This was followed by a decrease before the survival rose again to a maximum level after about 12 h. This pattern of recovery is due to two processes. *Repair of sublethal damage (SLDR)* accounts for the early rise in survival. Since cells that survive radiation tend to be synchronized in the more resistant phases of the cell cycle, their subsequent progression (inevitably into more sensitive phases) leads to a reduction in survival at 4 h. Continued repair and repopulation explain the increases in survival at later times. This pattern of SLDR has been demonstrated for a wide range of cell lines in vitro, using many of the assay procedures described in Sec. 13.3.4.

The repair capacity of the cells of many tissues in vivo has been demonstrated using either the cell-survival assays described in Sec. 13.3.5 or the functional assays described in Chap. 14 (Sec. 14.2.2). An increase in total dose is required to give the same level of biological damage when a single dose (D_1) is split into two doses (total dose D_2) with a time inter-

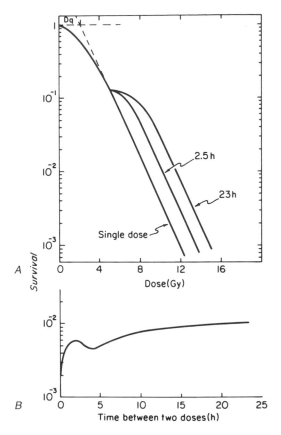

Figure 13.19. Illustration of the repair of sublethal damage that occurs between two radiation treatments. *A.* Survival curves for a single-dose treatment or for treatments involving a fixed first dose followed after 2.5 or 23 h of incubation (at 37°C) by a range of second doses. *B.* Pattern of survival observed when two fixed doses of irradiation are given with a varying time interval of incubation (at 37°C) between them. (Adapted from Elkind and Sutton, 1960.)

ponent repair model. In most tissues, repair is about 95 percent complete within 2 to 8 h (four half-times) of a radiation treatment. In human tissues, interpretable data are sparse, but it appears that repair half-times may be longer (1 to 3 h); thus it may require 4 to 12 h for most of the repair to occur (Thames et al., 1990). Many tissues irradiated in vivo demonstrate a larger amount of SLDR (as measured by values of D_2-D_1) than would be expected on the basis of D_q values observed for cell lines growing in culture; this may be due to the three-dimensional cell contact occurring in vivo, which may allow for increased repair (Olive and Durand, 1994).

Cell survival can also be increased by holding cells after irradiation under conditions of suboptimal growth (e.g., low temperature, nutrient deprivation, or density inhibition) as compared with cells maintained under optimal growth conditions. Radiation damage is thought to be repaired during the period that the cells are maintained under suboptimal growth conditions (Little, 1973; Malaise et al., 1989). Repair of this *potentially lethal damage* (PLDR) usually results in a change in the slope of the cell-survival curve and occurs over times similar to those required for SLDR. It is not known whether PLDR represents the expression of a different repair process from that which occurs in SLDR, but it has been suggested that PLDR may arise because of a competition for resources in the cell. If the cell is not called upon to progress through the cell cycle for a period of time after irradiation, it may be more able to mobilize resources for repair (of its DNA) that would otherwise be required for cell-cycle progression. This is consistent with the observation that some proteins are involved in both transcription and DNA repair (see Chap. 4, Sec. 4.4.7). PLDR can also occur in vivo. When some irradiated tumors or normal tissues are left in situ for a number of hours before excision and assay (by the in vivo-in vitro assay procedure described in Sec. 13.3.4), the survival level is often higher than after immediate excision and assay (Hahn et al., 1974; Mulcahy et al., 1980). This effect may be due to increased PLDR of normal cells or hypoxic or nutrient-deprived tumor cells in the G0 phase of the cell cycle during irradiation.

The underlying mechanism(s) responsible for the cellular repair processes described above are not well established but are presumed to relate to repair of DNA damage (see Chap. 4, Sec. 4.4). That DNA repair capacity can influence cellular radiosensitivity is indicated by the extreme radiosensitivity of cells from some patients with DNA repair deficiency syndromes such as ataxia telangiectasia and the re-

val between them (see Fig. 13.20). The difference in dose (D_2-D_1) is a measure of the repair by the cells in the tissue. The capacity of different cell populations to undergo SLDR is reflected by the width of the shoulder on their survival curve—i.e., the D_q or D_2-D_1 value. Thus survival curves for bone marrow cells have little to no shoulder ($D_q \sim 0$ Gy), and the cells demonstrate little or no repair, while other cells (e.g., jejunal crypt cells) demonstrate a large repair capacity (D_2-D_1 value of 4 to 5 Gy).

The process of sublethal damage repair (SLDR) is usually regarded as occurring as a single exponential function of time after irradiation, with a half-time for repair in the range 0.5 to 2.0 h for most cultured cells and rodent tissues, although there is evidence that repair kinetics in some tissues (e.g., spinal cord) may be better described by a two-com-

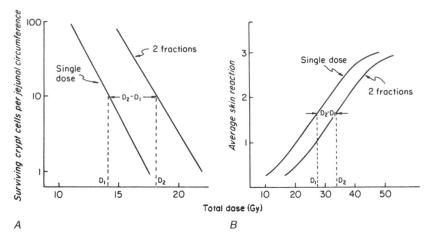

Figure 13.20. Repair of radiation damage in vivo. *A.* Survival curves for murine intestinal crypt cells γ-irradiated in situ with a single dose or with two equal fractions given 3 h apart. (Modified from Withers et al., 1974.) *B.* Average skin reaction following x-irradiation of mouse skin with a single dose or two fractions given 24 h apart. The technique used to determine these curves is described in Chap. 14, Sec. 14.2.2.

duced capacity for repair of DNA double-strand breaks among x-ray-sensitive mutant Chinese hamster ovary (CHO) cells and radiosensitive fibroblasts derived from severe combined immunodeficiency (SCID) mice (Jackson and Jeggo, 1995). The molecular components of DNA repair pathway(s) that may be responsible for mammalian normal and tumor cell radiosensitivity are under intensive study. Repair of DNA double-strand breaks appears to be an important component of postradiation DNA repair (see Chap. 4, Sec. 4.4.6). How well the extent, rate, or fidelity of the rejoining of DNA double-strand breaks correlates with clonogenic radiation cell survival varies as a function of the assay used for the analysis and the cell type under study (reviewed by Nunez et al., 1996).

13.5.5 Adaptive Radiation Responses

Following very low doses of radiation, mammalian cells may have an inducible radioprotective response that acts both in vitro and in vivo. This so-called *adaptive response* appears to be triggered by a threshold level of radiation damage (Marples and Joiner, 1993). For example, some mammalian cells appear to be hypersensitive to very low doses of ionizing radiation (0.01 to 0.3 Gy) as compared with higher radiation doses. Following doses of radiation greater than 1 Gy, this cell survival "hypersensitivity" is not observed, suggesting that a certain radiation dose threshold is required to activate mechanisms leading to maximal radiation cell survival for a given

cell line. Differences in the radiosensitivity of human tumor cells might be explained in part by the variation in the adaptive response observed for different human tumor cell lines (Lambin et al., 1996). The adaptive radiation response is also observed for irradiated normal skin and rodent kidney cells growing in vivo (Turesson and Joiner, 1996). For example, the use of multiple radiation fractions of less than 1 Gy can decrease the total dose required for the same biological effect in vivo by a factor of 2 to 4 (relative to that required with fractions of 2 Gy). The molecular mechanisms involved in the adaptive response are largely unknown but likely include the activation of some of the early-response genes discussed in Sec. 13.3.1.

13.5.6 Oncogenes, Tumor Suppressor Genes, and Growth Factors

Gene transfer studies have suggested that the aberrant expression of oncogenes or tumor suppressor genes may modify the intrinsic radiosensitivity of human or rodent cells. Increased radiation survival has been observed in selected cell lines following the transfection of a single oncogene, such as an activated *ras, src,* or *raf* oncogene (reviewed in Kasid et al., 1993). However, increased radioresistance is more commonly observed in cells transfected with an activated *ras* gene in combination with a nuclear co-operating oncogene, such as c-*myc* or mutant *p53* (McKenna et al., 1990; Bristow et al., 1994). Radioresistance may or may not occur among human tumor cell lines that acquire these genetic changes during the process of human tumor progression (reviewed in Bristow et al., 1996).

The loss of the G1 checkpoint in tumor cells might be expected to lead to a decreased period for DNA repair and hence result in increased cell killing following exposure to ionizing radiation. Most data, however, suggests that cells having altered p53 protein function (and an abrogated G1 checkpoint) acquire relative radioresistance in comparison with those cells having normal p53 protein function (reviewed in Bristow et al., 1996). The radioresistant phenotype has also been correlated with the level of expression of mutant p53 protein in transformed cells (Bristow et al., 1994). Acquired radioresistance may also result from the inactivation of normal p53 function by cellular proteins such as the HPV-E6 protein, which can bind to and degrade the normal p53 protein (Tsang et al., 1995). The underlying mechanisms might be related to the genetic instability observed among those cells lacking normal p53 function and the acquisition of genetic changes that lead to altered clonogenic survival, apoptosis, and/or DNA repair following radiation damage (Girinsky et al., 1995; Morgan and Murnane, 1995).

The radiosensitivity of cells may also be influenced by the addition of exogenous growth factors or hormones in receptor-positive cells before or after irradiation. For example, stem-cell factor (SCF), a growth factor that binds to the c-kit tyrosine kinase receptor, enhances the radiation survival of bone marrow progenitor cells and intestinal crypt cells when added to the culture system prior to irradiation (Leigh et al., 1995). SCF does not alter the radiosensitivity of human lymphoma and solid tumor cells growing as xenografts (Shui et al., 1995). However, modification of tumor-cell radiosensitivity has been reported for cells exposed to IL-1, insulin-like growth factor-1 (IGF-1), and epidermal growth factor (EGF), although the effect of each growth factor depends on cell type, growth conditions, and the relative expression of growth-factor receptors (Kwok and Sutherland, 1992; Laderoute et al., 1994; Jayanth et al., 1995). Furthermore, cells that usually undergo p53-dependent apoptosis can be diverted to undergo G1 cell-cycle arrest by the addition of cytokines, such as SCF, IL-3, or erythropoietin. This may allow DNA repair, so that these growth factors can act as cellular survival factors (Lin and Benchimol, 1995). These observations add support to the potential importance of signal transduction and its modification in determining the response of mammalian cells to ionizing radiation (Kasid et al., 1996; Pirollo et al., 1997).

13.6 SUMMARY

Ionizing radiation causes damage to cells and tissues by depositing energy as a series of discrete events. Different types of radiation have different abilities to cause biological damage because of the densities of the energy deposition events produced. The relative biological effectiveness (RBE) of densely ionizing (high-LET) radiation is greater than that of low-LET radiation. Radiation can cause damage to any molecule in a cell, but damage to DNA is most crucial in causing cell lethality expressed by loss of proliferative potential. Depending on cell type, cells may die by an interphase death (usually associated with an apoptotic morphology) or by mitosis-linked death, which can be associated with both apoptosis- and necrosis-linked pathways. The molecular events relating to G1- and G2-phase cell-cycle arrest following ionizing radiation appear to involve p53 and proteins associated with cell-cycle regulation. Several assay procedures have been developed for assessing the clonogenic capacity of both normal and malignant cells, and these have been used to obtain radiation survival curves for a wide range of different cell types. For x- and γ-rays, survival curves for most mammalian cells have a shoulder region at low doses, while at higher doses the survival decreases approximately exponentially with dose. No systematic differences are observed between normal and malignant cells. The slope of the high-dose region of the survival curve is quite similar for most mammalian cells, but there are differences in the clinically relevant, low-dose shoulder region.

Various factors can influence the response of cells to radiation treatment. These include LET, cell-cycle position, hypoxia, and the expression of certain oncogenes. Following treatment with low-LET radiation, cells can repair some of their damage over a period of a few hours; thus if the treatment is prolonged or fractionated, it is less effective than if given as a single acute dose. The accurate and timely rejoining of DNA double-strand breaks can be correlated to the relative radiation survival of both normal and tumor cells. Cells in S phase are often more resistant than cells in the G2/M phases, but there is variability between cell types. When cells are treated with low-LET radiation in the absence of oxygen, they require approximately three times as large a dose to produce a given level of cell killing as the dose required for cells irradiated in the presence of oxygen. Most experimental (and many human) tumors have been demonstrated to contain a substantial fraction of hypoxic cells that are resistant to radiation. There is an association between the aberrant expression of ras, raf and p53 proteins and cellular response to ionizing radiation. Accessibility to exogenous growth factors may also modify the intrinsic radiosensitivity of cells through alteration of intracellular signaling and cell-cycle arrest following DNA damage.

REFERENCES

Aldridge DR, Arends MJ, Radford IR: Increasing the susceptibility of the rat 208F fibroblast cell line to radiation-induced apoptosis does not alter its clonogenic survival dose-response. *Br J Cancer* 1995; 71:571–577.

Baker FL, Spitzer G, Ajani JA, Brock WA: Drug and radiosensitivity testing of primary human tumor cells using the adhesive-tumor-cell culture system (ATCCS). *Prog Clin Biol Res* 1988; 276:105–117.

Barendsen GW: Responses of cultured cells, tumours and normal tissues to radiations of different linear energy transfer. *Curr Top Radiat Res* 1968; 4:293–356.

Bernhard EJ, McKenna WG, Muschel RJ: Cyclin expression and G2 phase delay after irradiation. *Radiat Res* 1994a; 138:S64–67.

Bernhard EJ, Maity A, Muschel RJ, McKenna WG: Increased expression of cyclin B1 mRNA coincides with diminished G2-phase arrest in irradiated HeLa cells treated with staurosporine or caffeine. *Radiat Res* 1994b; 140:393–400.

Boothman DA, Majmider G, Johnson T: Immediate x-ray-inducible responses from mammalian cells. *Radiat Res* 1994; 138:S44–46.

Bristow RG, Hardy PA, Hill RP: Comparison between in vitro radiosensitivity and in vivo radioresponse of murine tumor cell lines: Part I. Parameters of in vitro radiosensitivity and endogenous cellular glutathione levels. *Int J Radiat Oncol Biol Phys* 1990a; 18:133–145.

Bristow RG, Hill RP: Comparison between in vitro radiosensitivity and in vivo radioresponse of murine tumor cell lines: Part II. In vivo radioresponse following fractionated treatment and in vitro/in vivo correlations. *Int J Radiat Oncol Biol Phys* 1990b; 18:331–345.

Bristow RG, Benchimol S, Hill RP: The p53 gene as a modifier of intrinsic radiosensitivity: Implications for radiotherapy. *Radiother Oncol* 1996; 40:197–223.

Bristow RG, Jang A, Peacock J, et al: Mutant p53 increases radioresistance in rat embryo fibroblasts simultaneously transfected with HPV16-E7 and/or activated H-ras. *Oncogene* 1994; 9:1527–1536.

Canman CE, Wolff AC, Chen CY, et al: The p53-dependent G_1 cell cycle checkpoint pathway and ataxia-telangiectasia. *Cancer Res* 1994; 54:5054–5068.

Chaplin DJ, Hill SA: Temporal heterogeneity in micro-regional erythrocyte flux in experimental solid tumours. *Br J Cancer* 1995; 71:1210–1213.

Chaplin DJ, Durand RE, Olive PL: Acute hypoxia in tumors: Implications for modifiers of radiation effects. *Int J Radiat Oncol Biol Phys* 1986; 12:1279–1282.

Chapman JD, Dugle DL, Reuvers AP, et al: Studies on the radiosensitizing effect of oxygen in Chinese hamster cells. *Int J Radiat Biol* 1974; 26:383–389.

Cheong N, Wang Y, Iliakis G: Radioresistance induced in rat embryo cells by transfection with the oncogenes H-ras plus v-myc is cell cycle dependent and maximal in S and G2. *Int J Radiat Biol* 1993; 63:623–629.

Clifton KH: Quantitative studies of the radiobiology of hormone-responsive normal cell populations. In: Meyn RE, Withers HR, eds. *Radiation Biology in Cancer Research.* New York: Raven Press; 1980:501–513.

Deacon J, Peckham M, Steel GG: The radioresponsiveness of human tumours and the initial slope of the cell survival curve. *Radiother Oncol* 1984; 2:317–323.

Dewey WC, Ling CC, Meyn R: Radiation-induced apoptosis: Relevance to radiotherapy. *Int J Radiat Oncol Biol Phys* 1995; 33:781–796.

Elkind MM, Sutton H: Radiation response of mammalian cells grown in culture: I. Repair of x-ray damage in surviving Chinese hamster cells. *Radiat Res* 1960; 13:556–593.

Elkind MM, Whitmore GF: *The Radiobiology of Cultured Mammalian Cells.* New York: Gordon and Breach; 1967:351–353.

Fairbairn DW, Olive PL, O'Neill KL: The comet assay: A comprehensive review. *Mutat Res* 1995; 339:37–59.

Fertil B, Malaise EP: Intrinsic radiosensitivity of human cell lines is correlated with radioresponsiveness of human tumors: Analysis of 101 published survival curves. *Int J Radiat Oncol Biol Phys* 1985; 11:1699–1707.

Foray N, Badie C, Alsbeih G, et al: A new model describing the curves for repair of both DNA double-strand breaks and chromosomal damage. *Radiat Res* 1996; 146:53–60.

Fuks Z, Haimovitz-Friedman A, Kolesnick, RN: The role of the sphingomyelin pathway and protein kinase C in radiation-induced cell kill. *Imp Adv Oncol* 1995; 19–31.

Giaccia AJ: Hypoxic stress proteins: survival of the fittest. *Semin Radiat Oncol* 1996; 6:46–58.

Girinsky T, Koumenis C, Graeber T, et al: Attenuated response of p53 and p21 in primary cultures of human prostatic epithelial cells exposed to DNA-damaging agents. *Cancer Res* 1995; 55:3726–3731.

Graeber T, Peterson J, Tsai W, et al: Hypoxia induces accumulation of p53 protein, but activation of a G1-phase checkpoint by low-oxygen conditions is independent of p53 status. *Mol Cell Biol* 1994; 14:6264–6277.

Graeber T, Osmanian C, Jacks T, et al: Hypoxia-mediated selection of cells with diminished apoptotic potential in solid tumours. *Nature* 1996; 379:88–91.

Grdina DJ: Variations in radiation response of tumor subpopulations. In: Meyn RE, Withers HR, eds. *Radiation Biology in Cancer Research.* New York: Raven Press; 1980:353–363.

Hahn GM, Rockwell S, Kallman RF, et al: Repair of potentially lethal damage in vivo in solid tumor cells after x-irradiation. *Cancer Res* 1974; 34:351–354.

Hallahan DE, Dunphy E, Virudachelam S, et al: C-jun and egr-1 participate in DNA synthesis and cell survival in response to ionizing radiation. *J Biol Chem* 1995; 270:30303–30309.

Hartwell LH, Kastan MB: Cell cycle control and cancer. *Science* 1994; 266:1821–1828.

Hewitt HB, Wilson CW: A survival curve for mammalian cells irradiated in vivo. *Nature* 1959; 183:1060–1061.

Hill RP, Bush RS: A lung colony assay to determine the radiosensitivity of cells of a solid tumor. *Int J Radiat Biol* 1969; 15:435–444.

Hockel M, Schlenger K, Aral B, et al: Association between tumor hypoxia and malignant progression in advanced cancer of the uterine cervix. *Cancer Res* 1996; 56:4509–4515.

Hockenbery D: Defining apoptosis. *Am J Pathol* 1995; 146:16–19.

Jackson SP, Jeggo PA: DNA double-strand break repair and V(D)J recombination: involvement of DNA-PK (review). *Trends Biochem Sci* 1995; 20:412–415.

Jayanth VR, Belfi CA, Swick AR, Varnes ME: Insulin and insulin-like growth factor (IGF-1) inhibit repair of potentially lethal radiation damage and chromosomal aberrations and alter DNA repair kinetics in plateau-phase A549 cells. *Radiat Res* 1995; 143:165–174.

Jayaraman L, Prives C: Activation of p53 sequence-specific DNA binding by short single strands of DNA requires the p53 C-terminus. *Cell* 1995; 81:1021–1029.

Jirtle RL, Anscher MS, Alati T: Radiation sensitivity of the liver. *Adv Radiat Biol* 1990; 14:269–311.

Johns HE, Cunningham JR: *The Physics of Radiology,* 4th ed. Springfield, IL: Charles C. Thomas; 1983:167–216.

Kasid U, Pirollo K, Dritschilo A, Chang E: Oncogenic basis of radiation resistance. *Adv Cancer Res* 1993; 61:195–233.

Kasid U, Suy S, Dent P, et al: Activation of Raf by ionizing radiation. *Nature* 1996; 382:813–816.

Kastan MB, Onyekwere D, Sidransky D, et al: Participation of p53 protein in the cellular response to DNA damage. *Cancer Res* 1991; 51:6304–6311.

Keng PC, Siemann DW, Wheeler KT: Comparison of tumour age response to radiation for cells derived from tissue culture or solid tumours. *Br J Cancer* 1984; 50:519–526.

Kitada S, Krajewski S, Miyashita T, et al: γ-radiation induces upregulation of Bax protein and apoptosis in radiosensitive cells in vivo. *Oncogene* 1996; 12:187–192.

Koong AC, Chen EY, Mivechi NF, et al: Hypoxic activation of nuclear factor-kappa B is mediated by a ras and raf signaling pathway and does not involve MAP kinase (ERK1 or ERK2). *Cancer Res* 1994; 54:5273–5279.

Kwok TT, Sutherland RM: Cell cycle dependence of epidermal growth factor induced radiosensitization. *Int J Radiat Oncol Biol Phys* 1992; 22:525–527.

Laderoute KR, Ausserer WA, Knapp AM, et al: Epidermal growth factor modifies cell cycle control in A431 human squamous carcinoma cells damaged by ionizing radiation. *Cancer Res* 1994; 54:1407–1411.

Lambin P, Malaise EP, Joiner MC: Might intrinsic radioresistance of human tumour cells be induced by radiation? *Int J Radiat Biol* 1996; 69:279–290.

Leigh BR, Khan W, Hancock SL, Knox SJ: Stem cell factor enhances the survival of murine intestinal stem cells after photon irradiation. *Radiat Res* 1995; 142:12–15.

Levine AJ: p53, the cellular gatekeeper for growth and division. *Cell* 1997; 88:323–331.

Li C-Y, Nagasawa H, Dahlberg WK, Little JB: Diminished capacity for p53 in mediating a radiation-induced G_1 arrest in established human tumor cell lines. *Oncogene* 1995; 11:1885–1892.

Lin Y, Benchimol S: Cytokines inhibit p53-mediated apoptosis but not p53-mediated G_1 arrest. *Mol Cell Biol* 1995; 15:6045–6054.

Little JB: Factors influencing the repair of potentially lethal radiation damage in growth-inhibited human cells. *Radiat Res* 1973; 56:320–333.

Little JB: Changing views of cellular radiosensitivity. (Failla Memorial Lecture) *Radiat Res* 1994; 140:299–311.

Lowe SW, Bodis S, McClatchey A, et al: P53 status and the efficacy of cancer therapy in vivo. *Science* 1994; 266:807–810.

Ludlow J, Howell R, Smith H: Hypoxic stress induces reversible hypophosphorylation of pRB and reduction in cyclin A abundance independent of cell cycle progression. *Oncogene* 1993; 8:331–339.

Maity A, McKenna WG, Muschel RJ: The molecular basis for cell cycle delays following ionizing radiation: A review. *Radiother Oncol* 1994; 31:1–13.

Malaise EP, Deschavanne PJ, Fertil B: The relationship between potentially lethal damage repair and intrinsic radiosensitivity of human cells. *Int J Radiat Biol* 1989; 56:597–604.

Malaise EP, Fertil B, Deschavanne PJ, et al: Initial slope of radiation survival curves is characteristic of the origin of primary and established cultures of human tumor cells and fibroblasts. *Radiat Res* 1987; 111:319–333.

Marples B, Joiner MC: The response of Chinese hamster V79 cells to low radiation doses: Evidence of enhanced sensitivity of the whole cell population. *Radiat Res* 1993; 133:41–51.

Mazure NM, Chen EY, Yeh P, et al: Oncogenic transformation and hypoxia synergistically act to modulate vascular endothelial growth factor expression. *Cancer Res* 1996; 56:3436–3440.

McCulloch EA, Till JE: The sensitivity of cells from normal mouse bone marrow to gamma radiation in vitro and in vivo. *Radiat Res* 1962; 16:822–832.

McKenna W, Weiss M, Endlich B, et al: Synergistic effect of the v-myc oncogene with H-ras on radioresistance. *Cancer Res* 1990; 50:97–102.

Metting NF, Little JB: Transient failure to dephosphorylate the cdc2-cyclin B1 complex accompanies radiation-induced G2-phase arrest in HeLa cells. *Radiat Res* 1995; 143:286–292.

Morgan SF, Kastan MB: p53 and ATM: Cell cycle, cell death and cancer. *Adv Cancer Res* 1997; 71:1–25.

Morgan WF, Murnane JP: A role for genomic instability in cellular radioresistance? *Cancer Metastasis Rev* 1995; 14: 49–58.

Moore JV, Hasleton PS, Buckley CH: Tumor cords in 52 bronchial and cervical squamous cell carcinomas: Inferences for their cellular kinetics and radiobiology. *Br J Cancer* 1985; 51:407–413.

Moulder JE, Rockwell S: Tumor hypoxia: Its impact on cancer therapy. *Cancer Metastasis Rev* 1987; 5:313–341.

Mulcahy RT, Gould MN, Clifton KH: The survival of thyroid cells: In vivo irradiation and in situ repair. *Radiat Res* 1980; 84:523–528.

Nagasawa H, Keng P, Harley R, et al: Relationship between γ-ray-induced G_2/M delay and cellular radiosensitivity. *Int J Radiat Biol* 1994; 66:373–379.

Nunez M, McMillan TJ, Valenzuela M, et al: Relationship between DNA damage, rejoining and cell killing by radiation in mammalian cells. *Radiother Oncol* 1996; 39:155–165.

Olive PL, Durand RE: Drug and radiation resistance in spheroids: Cell contact and kinetics. *Cancer Metastasis Rev* 1994; 13:121–138.

Palcic B, Skarsgard LD: Reduced oxygen enhancement ratio at low doses of ionizing radiation. *Radiat Res* 1984; 100:328–339.

Peacock JW, Chung S, Bristow RG, et al: The p53-mediated G_1 checkpoint is retained in tumorigenic rat embryo fibroblast clones transformed by the human papillomavirus type 16 E7 gene and EJ-*ras*. *Mol Cell Biol* 1995; 15:1446–1454.

Pirollo KF, Hao Z, Rait A, et al: Evidence supporting a signal transduction pathway leading to the radiation-resistant phenotype in human tumor cells. *Biochim Biophys Res Commun* 1997; 230:196–201.

Powers WE, Tolmach LJ: Demonstration of an anoxic component in a mouse tumor-cell population by in vivo assay of survival following irradiation. *Radiology* 1964; 83:328–336.

Price P, McMillan TJ: The use of non-clonogenic assays in measuring the responses of cells in vitro to ionising radiation. *Eur J Cancer* 1994; 30A:838–841.

Puck TT, Marcus PI: Actions of x-rays on mammalian cells. *J Exp Med* 1956; 103:653–666.

Raleigh JA, Dewhirst MW, Thrall DE: Measuring tumor hypoxia. *Semin Radiat Oncol* 1996; 6:37–45.

Rauth AM: The induction and repair of ultraviolet light damage in mammalian cells. In: Burns FJ, Upton AC, Silini G, eds. *Radiation Carcinogenesis and DNA Alterations.* New York: Plenum Press; 1986:212–226.

Rauth AM, Simpson JA: The energy loss of electrons in solids. *Radiat Res* 1964; 22:643–661.

Reed M, Woelker B, Wang P, et al: The C-terminal domain of p53 recognizes DNA damaged by ionizing radiation. *Proc Natl Acad Sci USA* 1995; 92:9455–9459.

Reynolds TY, Rockwell S, Glazer PM: Genetic instability induced by the microenvironment. *Cancer Res* 1996; 56: 5754–5757.

Roberts SA, Hendry JH, Potten CS: Deduction of the clonogen content of intestinal crypts: A direct comparison of two-dose and multiple-dose methodologies. *Radiat Res* 1995; 141:303–308.

Rockwell S, Moulder JE: Hypoxic fractions of human tumors xenografted into mice: A review. *Int J Radiat Oncol Biol Phys* 1990; 19:197–202.

Sasai K, Evans JW, Kovacs MS, Brown JM: Prediction of human cell radiosensitivity: Comparison of clonogenic assay with chromosome aberrations scored using premature chromosome condensation with fluorescence in situ hybridization. *Int J Radiat Oncol Biol Phys* 1994; 30:1127–1132.

Savitsky K, Bar-Shira A, Gilad S, et al: A single ataxia telangiectasia gene with a product similar to PI-3 kinase. *Science* 1995; 268:1749–1753.

Schwartz JL, Mustafi R, Beckett MA, Weichselbaum RR: DNA double-strand break rejoining rates, inherent radiosensitivity and human tumour response to radiotherapy. *Br J Cancer* 1996a; 74:37–42.

Schwartz JL, Cowan J, Grdina DJ, Weichselbaum RR: Attenuation of G2-phase cell cycle checkpoint control is associated with increased frequencies of unrejoined chromosome breaks in human tumor cells. *Radiat Res* 1996b; 146:139–143.

Shui C, Khan WB, Leigh BR, et al: Effects of stem cell factor on the growth and radiation survival of tumor cells. *Cancer Res* 1995; 55:3431–3437.

Sinclair WK: Cyclic X-ray responses in mammalian cells in vitro. *Radiat Res* 1968; 33:620–643.

Smeets MF, Mooren EHM, Begg AC: The effect of radiation on G_2 blocks, cyclin B expression and cdc2 expression in human squamous carcinoma cell lines with different radiosensitivities. *Radiother Oncol* 1994; 33:217–227.

Su LN, Little JB: Prolonged cell cycle delay in radioresistant human cell lines transfected with activated ras oncogene and/or simian virus 40 T-antigen. *Radiat Res* 1993; 133:73–79.

Terasima T, Tolmach LJ: Changes in the x-ray sensitivity of HeLa cells during the division cycle. *Nature* 1961; 190:1210–1211.

Thames HD, Bentzen SM, Turesson I, et al: Time-dose factors in radiotherapy: A review of the human data. *Radiother Oncol* 1990; 19:219–235.

Thomlinson RH, Gray LH: The histological structure of some human lung cancers and the possible implications for radiotherapy. *Br J Cancer* 1955; 9:539–549.

Trotter MJ, Chaplin DJ, Durand RE, Olive PL: The use of fluorescent probes to identify regions of transient perfusion in murine tumors. *Int J Radiat Oncol Biol Phys* 1989; 16:931–934.

Tsang NM, Nagasawa H, Li C, Little JB: Abrogation of p53 function by transfection of HPV16 E6 gene enhances the resistance of human diploid fibroblasts to ionizing radiation. *Oncogene* 1995; 10:2403–2408.

Turesson I, Joiner MC: Clinical evidence of hypersensitivity to low doses in radiotherapy. *Radiother Oncol* 1996; 40:1–3.

Upton AC: Physical carcinogenesis: radiation—history and sources. In: Becker FF, ed. *Cancer: A Comprehensive Treatise,* 2d ed. New York: Plenum Press; 1982:551–567.

Verheij M, Bose R, Lin XH, et al: Requirement for ceramide-initiated SAPK/JNK signalling in stress-induced apoptosis. *Nature* 1996; 380:75–79.

Ward JF: The complexity of DNA damage: Relevance to biological consequences. *Int J Radiat Biol* 1994; 66: 427–432.

Weichselbaum RR, Hallahan D, Fuks Z, Kufe D: Radiation induction of immediate early genes: Effectors of the radiation stress response. *Int J Radiat Oncol Biol Phys* 1994; 30:229–234.

Whitaker SJ, Powell SN, McMillan TJ: Molecular assays of radiation-induced DNA damage. *Eur J Cancer* 1991; 27:922–928.

Withers HR, Elkind MM: Microcolony survival assay for cells of mouse intestinal mucosa exposed to radiation. *Int J Radiat Biol* 1970; 17:261–267.

Withers HR, Mason K, Reid BO, et al: Response of mouse intestine to neutrons and gamma rays in relation to dose fractionation and division cycle. *Cancer* 1974; 34:39–47.

Young SD, Hill RP: Effects of reoxygenation on cells from hypoxic regions of solid tumors: Anticancer drug sensitivity and metastatic potential. *J Natl Cancer Inst* 1990; 82:371–380.

Yin DX, Schimke RT: *BCL*-2 expression delays drug-induced apoptosis but does not increase clonogenic survival after drug treatment in HeLa cells. *Cancer Res* 1995; 55:4922–4928.

BIBLIOGRAPHY

Elkind MM, Whitmore GF: *The Radiobiology of Cultured Mammalian Cells.* New York: Gordon and Breach; 1967.

Hall EJ: *Radiobiology for the Radiologist,* 4th ed. Philadelphia: Lippincott; 1995.

Johns HE, Cunningham JR: *The Physics of Radiology,* 4th ed. Springfield, IL: Charles C Thomas; 1983.

Potten CS, Hendry JH, eds: *Cell Clones: Manual of Mammalian Cell Techniques.* Edinburgh: Churchill-Livingstone; 1985.

Steel GG (ed): *Basic Clinical Radiobiology,* 2nd ed. London, England: Edward Arnold; 1997.

14

Experimental Radiotherapy

C. Shun Wong and Richard P. Hill

14.1 INTRODUCTION

14.2 DOSE RESPONSE AND THERAPEUTIC RATIO
    14.2.1 Tumor Control
    14.2.2 Normal Tissue Response
    14.2.3 Therapeutic Ratio

14.3 FRACTIONATION
    14.3.1 Repair
    14.3.2 Repopulation
    14.3.3 Redistribution
    14.3.4 Reoxygenation
    14.3.5 Low-Dose-Rate Irradiation
    14.3.6 Time and Dose Relationships
    14.3.7 Isoeffect Curves
    14.3.8 Models for Isoeffect

14.4 APPROACHES TO IMPROVING THE THERAPEUTIC RATIO
    14.4.1 Altered Fractionation Schedules
    14.4.2 Increase in Oxygen Delivery
    14.4.3 Sensitizers
    14.4.4 High-LET Radiation

14.5 PREDICTIVE ASSAYS
    14.5.1 Intrinsic Radiosensitivity of Tumor and Normal Cells
    14.5.2 Tumor-Cell Kinetics and Cell Death
    14.5.3 Hypoxia

14.6 SUMMARY

REFERENCES

BIBLIOGRAPHY

14.1 INTRODUCTION

In radiotherapy, the dose of radiation that can be delivered to a tumor is limited by the damage caused to surrounding normal tissues and the consequent risk of complications. Hence, therapeutic efficacy can be improved either by increasing the effective radiation dose delivered to the tumor relative to that given to surrounding normal tissues or by devising an approach that will increase the response of the tumor relative to that of the surrounding normal tissues. The former approach implies improvement in the physical aspects of radiation therapy. The introduction of high-energy x- and γ-ray treatment machines has been very effective in improving the results of treatment of patients with deep-seated tumors. Further improvements may be possible using more sophisticated treatment-planning methods to allow for conformal and stereotactic treatments that further limit the volume of normal tissues irradiated. The second approach involves exploiting biological factors that result in differences in the response of tumors and normal tissues to radiation therapy. The empiric development of multifractionated treatments, which involve giving fractions of about 1.8 to 2 Gy daily for 5 to 7 weeks, is an example of this approach. Exploration of possible ways to exploit the oxygen effect or to modify existing fractionation schedules may offer further improvements. Our current understanding of biological factors that may influence the outcome of radiation therapy is discussed in this chapter.

14.2 DOSE RESPONSE AND THERAPEUTIC RATIO

14.2.1 Tumor Control

The emphasis in the last chapter on the molecular and cellular effects of radiation treatment reflects the belief that, to a large extent, the response of tumors can be understood in terms of the response of the cells within those tumors. At the tissue level, tumor response to radiation treatment can be assessed by a number of techniques that do not measure tumor cell survival directly (Fig. 14.1). One such endpoint is growth delay, which is determined by measuring the size of untreated and irradiated tumors as a function of time to generate growth curves (Fig. 14.1A). The delay in growth is the difference in time for untreated and treated tumors to grow to a defined size. The time difference is a measure of tumor response and can be plotted as a function of radiation dose, as shown in Fig. 14.1B. The shape and position of this curve will be different for different treatments. The curve shown in Fig. 14.1B has a change in slope, which could be interpreted as indicative of the presence of a fraction of hypoxic cells in the tumor in analogy with the change in slope of the tumor-cell survival curve shown in Chap. 13 (Fig. 13.16A). At higher radiation doses, some tumors will be permanently controlled. If

groups of animals receive different radiation doses to their tumors, the percentage of controlled tumors can be plotted as a function of dose to give a dose-control curve, as shown in Fig. 14.1C.

Intrinsic to tumor growth is the concept that tumors contain a fraction of cells that have unlimited proliferative capacity (i.e., tumor stem cells; see Chap. 7, Sec. 7.6.2). To achieve tumor control, all the tumor stem cells must be killed. Thus, in the most fundamental terms, the dose of radiation required to control a tumor depends on only two parameters: (1) the radiation sensitivity of the stem cells and (2) their number. From a knowledge of the survival curve for the cells in a tumor, it is possible to predict the expected level of survival following a given single radiation dose. A simple calculation, using Eq. (13.5) in Chap. 13 and typical survival curve parameters for well-oxygenated cells ($D_0 = 1.3$ Gy, $D_q = 2.1$ Gy), indicates that a single radiation dose of 26 Gy might be expected to reduce the probability of survival of an individual cell to about 10^{-8}. For a tumor containing 10^8 stem cells, this dose would thus leave, on average, one surviving cell. Because of the random nature of radiation damage, there will be statistical fluctuation around this value. The statistical fluctuation expected from random cell killing by radiation follows a Poisson distribution; the probability (P_n) of a tumor having n surviving cells when the average number of cells surviving is a is given by

$$P_n = \frac{a^n e^{-a}}{n!} \qquad (14.1)$$

For tumor control, the important parameter is P_0, which is the probability that a tumor will contain no surviving stem cells (i.e., $n = 0$). From Eq. (14.1), we have

$$P_0 = e^{-a} \qquad (14.2)$$

so for $a = 1$, as in the example above, the probability of control would be $e^{-1} = 0.37$. Different radiation doses will, of course, result in different values of a. For example, for identical tumors each containing 10^8 cells, a dose that reduces the survival level to 10^{-9} will give $a = 0.1$ (i.e., 10 cells surviving in 100 tumors), with an expected probability of control of $e^{-0.1} = 0.90$. From such calculations, it is possible to construct a theoretical tumor control versus dose curve, which shows a sigmoid relationship (Fig. 14.2, solid lines).

The central solid curve in Fig. 14.2 represents a group of identical tumors each containing 10^8 tu-

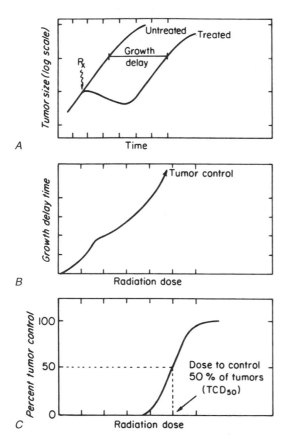

Figure 14.1. Illustration of two assays for tumor response. In A, growth curves for groups of treated and untreated tumors are shown and the measurement of growth delay indicated. B. Growth delay plotted as a function of radiation dose. At large doses some of the tumors may not regrow. The percentage of controlled tumors can be plotted as a function of dose, as in C.

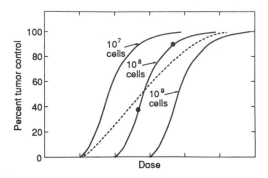

Figure 14.2. Percent tumor control plotted as a function of dose for single radiation treatments. Theoretical curves for groups of tumors containing different numbers of tumor stem cells are shown. The points on the curve labeled "10^8 cells" are derived as discussed in the text. The composite curve (*dashed*) was obtained assuming a group containing equal numbers of tumors with 10^7, 10^8, or 10^9 stem cells.

mor stem cells. For tumors containing 10^7 or 10^9 stem cells, the curves will be displaced (to smaller or larger doses, respectively) by a dose sufficient to reduce survival by a factor of 10. These dose-control curves illustrate that the dose of radiation required to control a tumor depends on the number of stem cells it contains (Hill and Milas, 1989). Thus a large tumor is likely to require a larger dose for control than a small tumor, assuming that in each there is the same proportion of stem cells.

In clinical practice, even tumors of the same size and histopathologic type are likely to vary in their proportion of stem cells. Thus a dose-control curve for a group of human tumors will be a composite of ones similar to those shown in Fig. 14.2: the slope of the composite dose-control curve will be less than

that for the individual groups of tumors (Fig. 14.2, dashed line). Fractionation of the radiation treatment and heterogeneity in the radiosensitivity of tumor stem cells (see below and Sec. 14.3) will also result in a decrease in the slope of the dose-control curve. Thus the slope of the dose-control curve derived from a clinical study is likely to be shallow because of tumor heterogeneity. It is therefore desirable to seek a way of assigning the tumors to more homogeneous groups, so that patients with differences in prognosis may be identified. This is a major motivation for attempts to develop predictive assays, as discussed in Sec. 14.5.

Studies of a wide range of cell lines derived from human tumors have shown intrinsic variations in radiation sensitivity (Deacon et al., 1984; Fertil and Malaise, 1985). Survival curves can vary considerably even for cells of similar histopathologic types (see Fig. 14.3), and it is the size of the shoulder of the curves that varies most widely. Even small differences in the shoulder region can be important, because they are likely to be magnified during the multiple fractionated daily doses of 1.8 to 2 Gy given in clinical radiotherapy (see Sec. 14.3.1). Figure 14.3 illustrates the variability in cell-survival curves for cell lines derived from different human melanomas (Fertil and Malaise, 1981). Survival following a dose of 2 Gy varies from about 0.2 to 0.9 (Fig. 14.3B). Consider a tumor for which survival following a dose of 2 Gy is 0.8. Assuming that each fraction of a multiple-dose treatment is equally effective and that there is no cell proliferation between dose fractions (an assumption that ignores some of the issues to be discussed in Sec. 14.3), the survival following 30 fractions of 2 Gy would be $0.8^{30} \approx 10^{-3}$. In contrast, for a tumor in which the

Figure 14.3. *A.* Survival curves for a number of different human melanoma cell lines. The lines were drawn to be continuously curving and conform to the linear-quadratic model (see Chap. 13, Sec. 13.4.3). *B.* The low-dose region of the curves is illustrated, demonstrating the range of survival values at 2 Gy. (Adapted from Fertil and Malaise, 1981.)

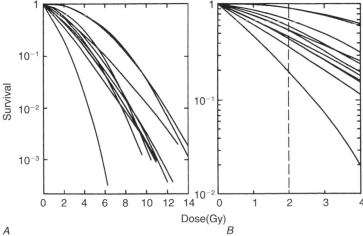

survival following 2 Gy is 0.6, survival after 30 fractions would be $0.6^{30} \approx 2 \times 10^{-7}$. Thus, small differences in survival at low doses can translate into very large differences during a course of fractionated treatment.

Estimates of the surviving fraction following a dose of 2 Gy for different human tumor cell lines growing in culture may be grouped according to histopathologic type and compared with the likelihood that such tumors will be controlled by radiation treatment (Table 14.1). There is a trend toward higher survival values for the cells from tumor groups expected to be less radiocurable, but there is a large range in each group. An analysis of the growth delay, induced by single radiation doses, in a range of different types of human tumors growing as xenografts in immune-deficient mice suggests a similar correlation (Rofstad, 1985). Results of studies correlating intrinsic tumor-cell radiosensitivity with clinical outcome are discussed further in Sec. 14.5.1.

The radiocurability of a tumor depends both on the radiosensitivity of the tumor stem cells (i.e., their underlying survival characteristics) and the number of such cells in the tumor. The terms *radiosensitive* and *radioresistant* have also been used to describe, respectively, tumors that regress rapidly or slowly after radiation treatment. This can be misleading, because the rate of regression may not correlate with the ability to cure a tumor with tolerable doses of radiation. A better term to describe a tumor that regresses rapidly after treatment is *radioresponsive*. The rate of response of a tumor depends on the proliferative rate of its cells, because most tumor cells express their radiation damage when they attempt mitosis (see Chap. 13, Sec. 13.3.3). Thus, a tumor that contains a large proportion of proliferating cells will tend to express radiation damage to its cells early and will regress rapidly. Although radioresponsive, the tumor may contain surviving stem cells that will be responsible for its recurrence.

14.2.2 Normal Tissue Response

As discussed in Chap. 13, Sec. 13.3.5, the sensitivity of the cells of a number of normal tissues can be determined directly using in situ assays. A comparison of survival curves obtained for the cells of a number of different normal tissues in mice and rats is shown in Fig. 14.4. Considerable variability in sensitivity is apparent and, again, most of the difference appears to be in the shoulder region of the survival curve.

Radiation treatment can cause loss of function in normal tissues. In renewal tissues, such as bone marrow or the gastrointestinal tract, loss of function may be correlated with loss of proliferative activity of stem cells. In other tissues, loss of function may occur through damage to more mature cells. The crudest functional assay is simply the determination of

Table 14.1. Values of the Surviving Fraction at 2 Gy for Human Tumor Cell Lines

Tumor Cell Type[a]	Number of Lines	Mean Survival at 2 Gy (range)
1. Lymphoma Neuroblastoma Myeloma Small-cell lung cancer Medulloblastoma	14	0.20(0.08–0.37)
2. Breast cancer Squamous cell cancer Pancreatic cancer Colorectal cancer Non-small-cell lung cancer	12	0.43(0.14–0.75)
3. Melanoma Osteosarcoma Glioblastoma Hypernephroma	25	0.52(0.20–0.86)

[a]Tumor types are grouped (1–3) approximately in decreasing order of their likelihood of local control by radiation treatment. (Modified from Deacon et al., 1984.)

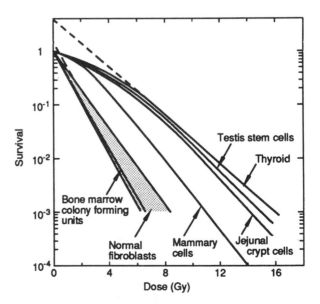

Figure 14.4. Survival curves for cells from some normal tissues. Most of the curves are for cells from rodent tissues, and the curves were produced using in vivo or in situ clonogenic assays, as described in Chap. 13. The range of values for normal human fibroblasts are for cultured cell lines. (Modified from Hall, 1988, and Fertil and Malaise, 1981.)

the dose of radiation given either to the whole body or to a specific organ that will cause lethality in 50 percent of the treated animals within a specified time (LD_{50}). The relationship between lethality and single radiation dose is usually sigmoidal in shape; some experimentally derived relationships for different normal tissues are shown in Fig. 14.5. Dose-response relationships for normal tissues are generally quite steep and well defined. There are, however, substantial differences in the doses required to achieve a given endpoint (e.g., LD_{50}) between different species of animals and even between different strains of the same species, largely because of differences in the ability of the animal to tolerate a given level of cell killing in the organ involved.

Some of the functional assays that have been used to assess the radiation response of normal tissues are listed in Table 14.2. Numerical scoring systems have been developed to assess damage in the skin and other tissues; these can be used to generate dose-response curves, as illustrated in Fig. 14.6. Another approach is to define a level of functional deficit and determine the percentage of irradiated animals that express at least this level of damage following different radiation doses. An example of such dose-response curves for radiation damage in the spinal cord, using forelimb paralysis as the endpoint is shown in Fig. 14.7. This approach results in sigmoidal curves similar to the percent lethality

Table 14.2. Functional Assays for Radiation Damage

Tissue	Assay Endpoint
Bone marrow	Depletion of different cell types
GI Tract	Weight loss, protein or electrolyte leakage
Lung	Breathing rate, CO uptake
Kidney	Urine output, EDTA clearance
Bladder	Urination frequency
Skin	Acute reactions, late deformities or skin contraction, hair loss, telangiectasia
CNS	Paralysis (spinal cord)

curves shown in Fig. 14.5. In these functional assays, the assumption is that the defined level of functional deficit corresponds to a decrease in the number of surviving target cells in the normal tissue to a specific level.

The effects of radiation treatment on normal tissues can be divided into early or acute responses, which occur within a few weeks of radiation treatment, and late responses, which may take many months to develop. Acute responses occur primarily in tissues with rapid cell renewal and where cell division is required to maintain the function of the organ. Since most cells express radiation damage during mitosis, there is early death and loss of cells killed by the radiation treatment. Following irradiation of skin, for example, the expression of radiation damage depends on the relative rates of cell loss and cell proliferation of the basal cells, and acute skin reactions occur more rapidly in murine (7 to 10 days) than in human skin (2 to 3 weeks). Following irradiation of the small bowel, if villus cells lost into the lumen are not replaced adequately by division of the surviving crypt cells (see Chap. 7, Sec. 7.5.2), acute injury occurs rapidly in both mice (4 to 7 days) and humans (8 to 10 days).

Late responses tend to occur in organs whose parenchymal cells divide infrequently (e.g., liver or kidney) or not at all (e.g., central nervous system or muscle) under normal conditions. Depletion of the parenchymal cell population due to entry of cells into mitosis, with the resulting expression of radiation damage and cell death, will thus be slow. Damage to the connective tissue and vasculature of the organ may also develop, leading to fibrosis and progressive impairment of its circulation. If the damage to the circulation is severe enough, secondary parenchymal cell death will occur due to nutrient deprivation. This loss of functional cells may induce other parenchymal cells to divide, causing further

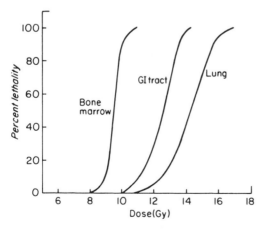

Figure 14.5. Three different curves indicating percent lethality plotted as a function of radiation dose for the same strain of mouse. The "bone marrow" and "GI tract" curves were obtained using whole-body irradiation and assessing lethality prior to day 30 or prior to day 7, respectively, since death due to damage to the GI tract occurs earlier than that due to bone marrow failure. The curve labeled "lung" was obtained by assessing lethality 180 days after local irradiation to the thorax.

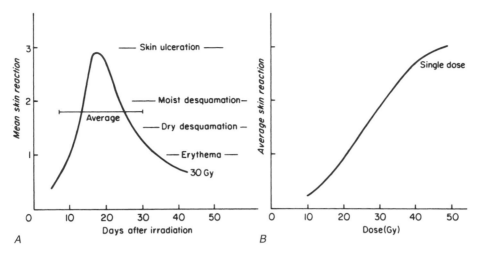

Figure 14.6. Assessment of the response of mouse skin to irradiation. *A.* The skin reaction (mean of a group of mice) assessed on an arbitrary scale, as indicated, is plotted as a function of time after a dose of radiation (30 Gy). *B.* The average reaction calculated over a certain time range (e.g., 7 to 30 days) is determined and plotted as a function of radiation dose.

cell death as they express their radiation damage. The end result may be functional failure of the organ involved. The relative importance of direct radiation damage to the parenchymal cells as compared with secondary damage due to connective tissue and vascular injury in causing specific late effects remains uncertain.

Division of the effects of radiation therapy into early and late responses has been based largely on functional and histopathologic endpoints, such that there is a latent period between radiation and the clinical or histopathologic expression of damage in late-responding normal tissues. At the biochemical and molecular level, there is increasing evidence to suggest that there is no latent period. In a number of late-responding normal tissues such as the brain (Hong et al., 1995) and lung (Fuks and Weichselbaum, 1992; Rubin et al., 1995), a cascade of cytokine expression has been observed within hours after irradiation, when there are no apparent functional or histopathologic changes. These cytokines have included transforming growth factor β, basic fibroblast growth factor, tumor necrosis factor, interleukin 1, and other growth factors associated with collagen deposition, fibrosis, inflammation, and aberrant vascular growth. These observations suggest a continuum of cytokines being upregulated postirradiation, which contributes to the histopathologic expression of late tissue injury (Hallahan, 1996).

Although mitosis-linked death has generally been regarded as the mode of radiation-induced cell

death in early-responding normal tissues, radiation-induced apoptosis has been detected in many cells and tissues, such as lymphoid, thymic, and hematopoietic cells; spermatogonia; and small bowel crypts (Wyllie et al., 1980; Potten, 1992). More recently, apoptosis has also been observed within hours after irradiation of a number of late responding normal tissues, such as the salivary glands (Stephens et al., 1991a), pulmonary endothelial cells (Fuks et al., 1994) and the central nervous sys-

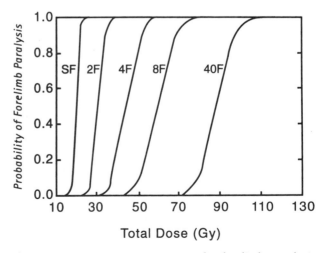

Figure 14.7. Dose response curves for forelimb paralysis following fractionated radiation treatments to the rat spinal cord. The fractions (F) were given once daily to allow for complete repair of radiation damage between fractions. SF = single fraction. (Redrawn from Wong et al., 1992.)

tem (Li et al., 1996; Shinohara et al., 1997). Apoptotic endpoints, however, have often not correlated with clonogenic survival or classical functional or histopathological end-points, and the relevance of apoptosis in radiation-induced early and late normal tissue damage remains to be established (Dewey et al., 1995; Meyn et al., 1996). However, these recent findings suggest opportunities to modulate the development of normal tissue injury following irradiation and hence to improve the therapeutic ratio in radiation therapy (Haimovitz-Friedman et al., 1996).

Although tissues may repair damage and regenerate after irradiation, previously irradiated tissues have a reduced tolerance for subsequent radiation treatments, indicating the presence of residual injury. The extent of residual injury appears to depend on the level of the initial damage (Wong and Hao, 1997) and is tissue-dependent, generally being greater for late- (Stewart et al., 1994) than for early-responding normal tissues (Terry et al., 1989).

14.2.3 Therapeutic Ratio

The choice of radiation dose to treat a given tumor is based on an assessment of the relative probabilities of tumor control and normal tissue complications. Whether a certain risk of developing complications is regarded as acceptable depends both on the tissue(s) and the severity of the damage involved, and it must be compared to the probability of benefit (eradicating the tumor) in order to determine the overall gain from the treatment. This gain can be estimated for an average group of patients,

but it may vary for individual patients depending on the particular characteristics of their tumors and the normal tissues at risk. The balance between the probabilities for tumor control and normal tissue complications gives a measure of the therapeutic ratio of a treatment.

Although the concept is expressed in mathematical terminology, the therapeutic ratio is ill defined in numerical terms. The concept is illustrated in Fig. 14.8, which shows theoretical dose-response curves for tumor control and normal tissue complications. Even tumors of identical size are likely to vary in the number of clonogenic stem cells (see Fig. 14.2) and heterogeneity of response to irradiation; thus the tumor-control curve tends to be shallower than that for normal tissue response. The therapeutic ratio is often defined as the percentage of tumor cures obtained at a given level of normal tissue complications (i.e., by taking a vertical cut through the two curves at a dose that is clinically acceptable). An approach more in keeping with the definition of other ratios, such as relative biological effectiveness (RBE) and oxygen enhancement ratio (OER), is to define the therapeutic ratio in terms of the ratio of radiation doses D_n/D_t required to produce a given percentage of complications and tumor control (usually 50 percent). It is then a measure of the horizontal displacement between the two curves. It remains imprecise, however, because it depends on the shape of the dose-response curves for tumor control and normal tissue complications.

The curves shown in Figure 14.8A depict a situation in which the therapeutic ratio is favorable, since the tumor-control curve is displaced to the left

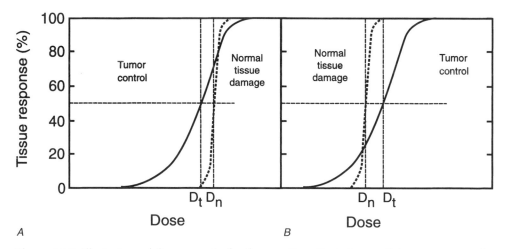

Figure 14.8. Illustration of the concept of a therapeutic ratio in terms of dose-response relationships for tumor control (*solid line*) and normal tissue damage (*thick dotted line*). See text for discussion of the two parts of the figure.

of that for normal tissue damage. The greater this displacement, the more radiocurable the tumor. Since the tumor-control curve is shallower than that for normal tissue damage, the therapeutic ratio tends to be favorable only for low and intermediate tumor-control levels. If the two curves are close together (see Fig. 14.8*B*) or the curve for tumor control is displaced to the right of that for complications, the therapeutic ratio is unfavorable, since a high level of complications must be accepted to achieve even a minimal level of tumor control.

14.3 FRACTIONATION

Clinical radiotherapy is usually given 5 days a week for 5 to 7 weeks as a series of daily fractions of about 2 Gy. The use of fractionated treatment arose from studies of French radiotherapists in the early part of the century. Seminal among the studies were those of Regaud (del Regato, 1976) who demonstrated that with fractionated treatment to a ram's testis, it was possible to achieve sterilization without significant damage to the scrotal skin; while with a single dose, it was difficult to obtain sterilization even after a dose sufficient to produce severe skin damage. Many empiric modifications of fractionation regimes evolved from these early studies, and there is now a consensus that the therapeutic ratio is improved by fractionation. Many of the underlying biological effects occurring during fractionated radiation treatment have been identified, and the improvement of the therapeutic ratio may be explained in terms of the biological response of tissue. The most important processes occurring during fractionated treatment are the "4 R's": repair, repopulation, redistribution, and reoxygenation. Each is described below.

14.3.1 Repair

The cellular and molecular mechanisms underlying the repair of radiation damage are discussed in Chap. 4, Sec. 4.4 and Chap. 13, Sec. 13.5.4. The shoulder on the survival curve after single radiation doses is indicative of the capacity of the cells to accumulate and repair radiation damage. If multiple doses are given with sufficient time between the fractions for repair to occur (2 to 24 h, depending on the cells or tissue involved; see Chap. 13, Sec. 13.5.4), survival curves for cells treated with fractionated irradiation will be similar to those illustrated in Fig. 14.9. The dashed lines in this figure represent the effective survival curves for different fractionated treatments. The effective slope depends on the size of the individual dose fractions,

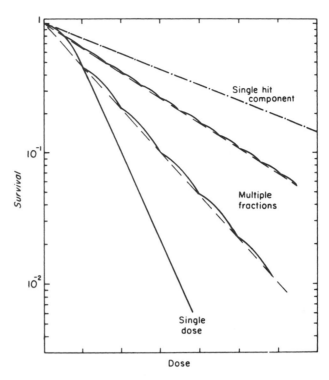

Figure 14.9. The influence of fractionating the radiation treatment on the shape of cell survival curves. When repair occurs between the fractions, the shoulder of the survival curve is repeated for every fraction. The curve labeled "single-hit component" is discussed in the text.

becoming shallower as the fraction size is reduced. This effect is also illustrated by the dose-response curves shown in Fig. 14.7 for forelimb paralysis of rats following irradiation with different numbers of fractions to the spinal cord, where the curves for higher numbers of fractions are displaced to higher total doses.

The single-dose survival curve for most cells has a finite initial slope apparently due to a (single-hit) nonrepairable damage component (Chap. 13, Sec. 13.4), so that there is a limit below which further reduction of the fraction size will no longer reduce the effective slope of the survival curve (see Fig. 14.9). At this limit, essentially all the repairable damage is being repaired between each fraction, so that the cell killing is due almost entirely to nonrepairable events. The fraction size at which this limit is reached is likely to be different for different cell populations.

When the size of the individual dose fractions is such that the survival is represented by the curvilinear shoulder region of the survival curve, as for most dose fractions used clinically, then repair will be maximal when equal-sized dose fractions are given. Thus, if a certain total dose is given with un-equal fraction sizes, it would be expected to produce more damage than the same total dose given in equal fraction sizes (see also Sec. 14.3.6).

14.3.2 Repopulation

In tumors and in normal tissues that contain proliferating cells, proliferation of surviving cells may occur during the course of fractionated treatment. Furthermore, as cellular damage and cell death occur during the course of the treatment, the tissue may respond with an increased rate of cell proliferation. The effect of this cell proliferation during treatment, known as *repopulation,* will be to increase the number of cells during the course of the treatment and reduce the overall response to irradiation. This effect is most important in early-responding normal tissues (e.g., skin, gastrointestinal tract) or in tumors whose stem cells are capable of rapid proliferation; it will be of little consequence in late-responding, slowly proliferating tissues (e.g., kidney), which do not suffer much early cell death and hence do not produce an early proliferative response to the radiation treatment. This effect of repopulation is illustrated in Fig. 14.10.

Repopulation is likely to be more important toward the end of a course of treatment, when sufficient damage has accumulated (and cell death occurred) to induce a regenerative response. The regenerative response in mouse skin during and following fractionated treatment with doses of 3 Gy is illustrated in Fig. 14.11. There is a period of about 10 days of treatment before significant repopulation occurs (2 to 4 weeks in humans), after which a rapid regenerative response is observed. Regenerative responses are probably important in reducing acute responses during split-course treatments.

Evidence that an "accelerated" repopulation effect can occur in human tumors during a course of fractionated therapy is shown in Fig. 14.12 (Withers et al., 1988). Here the total dose required to give 50 percent control of head and neck cancers for fractionation schedules of different overall duration is plotted as a function of the overall time of the treatment. The fractionation schedules have all been normalized to the same fraction size. For overall times less than about 3 to 4 weeks, there is little change in the dose required for 50 percent tumor control; at longer times, however, there is a substantial increase in the total dose required as the duration of treatment increases. This observation suggests that the initial part of the fractionated therapy has resulted in increased proliferation of the surviving tumor stem cells, which for head and neck tumors becomes apparent at 3 to 4 weeks after the start of the treatment. For individual tumors and other tumor types, it is likely that similar effects will occur at different times after the start of the treatment, depending on the cell kinetics of the tumor cells. Repopulation of tumor cells during a conventional course of radiotherapy is now believed to be an important factor influencing local tumor control in patients with head and neck or cervical cancer (Fowler and Lindstrom, 1992; Fyles et al., 1992). Repopulation is the biological rationale for accelerated fractionated radiation therapy (see Sec. 14.4.1). It may also be important in combined-modality treatment in which chemotherapy is given prior to irradiation, since tumor shrinkage, as a re-

Figure 14.10. Illustration of the effect of repopulation during fractionated treatment of skin or kidney. Treatment was a single dose or 16 equal fractions given in different overall times, as indicated. Acute skin response was assessed using a numerical scoring technique (as illustrated in Fig. 14.6) and kidney response was determined by reduction in EDTA clearance. For acute skin reactions, extending the time over which a course of 16 fractions is given results in an increase in the total dose required for a given level of effect. In contrast, for late response of kidney, there is no change in the isoeffective dose for 16 fractions regardless of whether the treatment is given over 20, 40 or 80 days. (Modified from Denekamp, 1986.)

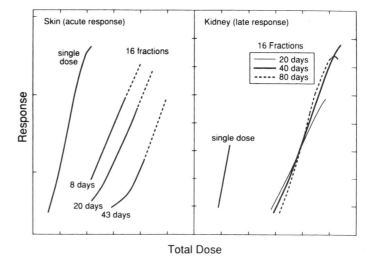

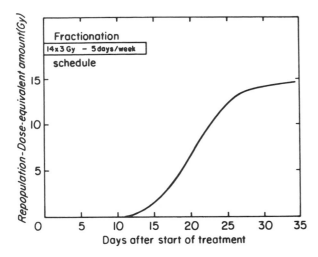

Figure 14.11. Illustration of the effect of the regenerative response in mouse skin that occurs during the course of a fractionated treatment. The repopulation that occurs is plotted in terms of the extra (single) radiation dose, required to be given at different times after the start of the 3-Gy/day schedule, in order to produce equivalent levels of acute skin reaction, assessed as described in Fig. 14.6. (Modified from Denekamp, 1973.)

sult of chemotherapy, might induce accelerated repopulation at an earlier stage of the radiation treatment (see Fig. 14.13).

14.3.3 Redistribution

Variation in the radiosensitivity of cells in different phases of the cell cycle results in the cells in the more resistant phases being more likely to survive a dose of radiation (see Chap. 13, Sec. 13.5.3). During a course of fractionated treatment, proliferating cells may move from one phase of the cell cycle to another between the radiation doses. Two effects can make the cell population more sensitive to a subsequent dose of radiation. First, some of the cells will be blocked in the G2 phase of the cycle (see Chap. 13, Sec. 13.3.2), which is usually a sensitive phase. Second, some of the surviving cells will redistribute into more sensitive parts of the cell cycle. Both effects will tend to make the whole population more sensitive to fractionated treatment as compared with a single dose. The effect of this process on cell sur-

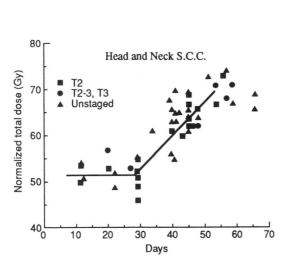

Figure 14.12. Estimated total doses of fractionated irradiation required to achieve 50 percent probability of tumor control for squamous cell carcinomas of the head and neck (various stages) plotted as a function of the overall treatment time. Each point is for a different group of patients and is obtained from published results. The actual doses used to treat the different groups of patients were normalized to a standard schedule of 2 Gy per fraction using the technique described in Sec. 14.3.8. (Modified from Withers et al., 1988.)

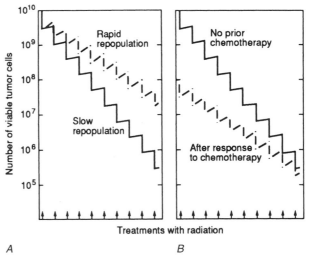

Figure 14.13. Schematic diagram illustrating the effect of repopulation in a tumor during a course of fractionated irradiation. Each radiation fraction is assumed to kill the same fraction of tumor cells. In *A*, the effect of different rates of repopulation is illustrated. In *B*, it is assumed that prior chemotherapy kills 99 percent of the cells but induces "accelerated" repopulation by the survivors. Response to radiation treatment alone (*solid line*) or radiation treatment following the chemotherapy (*dashed line*) is illustrated. The accelerated repopulation induced by the prior drug treatment rapidly negates the extra cell kill achieved by the drug treatment. (Redrawn from Tannock, 1989. With permission.)

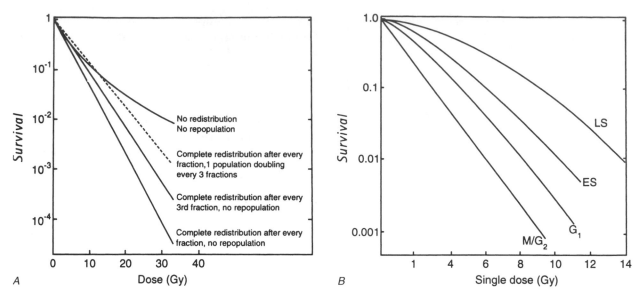

Figure 14.14. Theoretical survival curves calculated to illustrate the effect of redistribution on the level of cell killing following treatment with 2-Gy fractions. The curves in *A* were calculated using the data in *B* by assuming an asynchronous cell population containing 5 percent cells in M, 30 percent cells in G1, 25 percent cells in early S (ES), 25 percent cells in late S (LS), and 15 percent cells in G2. Redistribution and/or repopulation were assumed to occur as indicated on the individual lines. Two different rates of redistribution were assumed, giving the two lower curves. These curves can be compared to the upper curve, which was calculated assuming no redistribution. *B.* Survival curves for different phases of the cell cycle, reproduced from Fig. 13.18.

vival is shown in Fig. 14.14, where the effect has been calculated for a course of 2-Gy fractions given to Chinese hamster cells, using the survival curves for different phases of the cell cycle shown previously in Fig. 13.18. Since redistribution inevitably involves cell proliferation, the survival will also be influenced by repopulation, which reduces the effect of redistribution (Fig. 14.14). Both redistribution and repopulation are important only in proliferating cell populations. Also, not all cell lines show large differences in radiosensitivity between cells in different cell-cycle phases, and the effect of redistribution will be correspondingly less for these types of cells.

In many normal tissues (and probably in some tumors), stem cells can be in a resting phase (G0) but can be recruited into the cell cycle to repopulate the tissue (see Chap. 7, Secs. 7.5 and 7.6). There is some evidence that cells in cycle are slightly more sensitive to radiation than G0 cells, possibly because G0 cells may repair potentially lethal damage (Chap. 13, Sec. 13.5.4). Recruitment of resting cells into the proliferative cycle during the course of fractionated treatment, therefore, may tend to increase the sensitivity of the whole population. Neither recruitment nor redistribution would be expected to

have much influence on late responses, which occur predominantly as a result of injury to tissues in which the rate of proliferation is low.

14.3.4 Reoxygenation

The response of tumors to large single doses of radiation is dominated by the presence of hypoxic cells within them, even if only a very small fraction of the tumor stem cells are hypoxic (See Chap. 13, Sec. 13.5.2). Immediately after a dose of radiation, the proportion of the surviving cells that is hypoxic will be elevated. However, with time, some of the surviving hypoxic cells may gain access to oxygen and hence become *reoxygenated* and more sensitive to a subsequent radiation treatment. Reoxygenation can result in a substantial increase in the sensitivity of tumors during fractionated treatment. In Fig. 14.15 it is shown that the survival curve following fractionated irradiation for a tumor containing 10 percent hypoxic cells that do not reoxygenate would be dominated at higher doses by the radioresistant hypoxic cells. In contrast, the survival curve for a reoxygenating tumor-cell population lies close to the curve for a fully oxygenated population. This calculation considers only two popu-

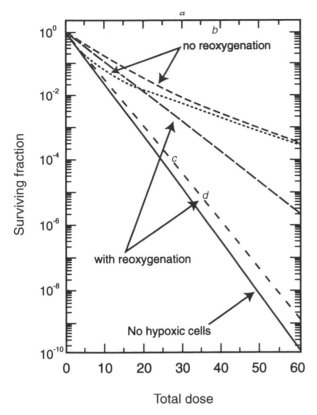

Figure 14.15. Theoretical survival curves calculated to illustrate the influence of reoxygenation on the level of cell killing in a tumor following treatment with 2-Gy fractions. It was assumed that the tumor initially had 10 percent hypoxic cells and either 90 percent well-oxygenated cells (lines *a* and *d*) or a proportion of well oxygenated cells and cells at intermediate oxygen concentrations calculated using a radial diffusion model (as described in Wouters and Brown, 1997) (lines *b* and *c*). It was assumed that reoxygenation was sufficient to maintain the same proportions among the surviving cells during the fractionated treatment. (Redrawn from Wouters and Brown, 1997.)

lations of cells, those that are fully oxygenated and those that are completely radiobiologically hypoxic. However, it is expected that there will also be many cells at intermediate oxygen levels in tumors, and a recent calculation by Wouters and Brown (1997) has emphasised their importance during reoxygenation. As seen in Fig. 14.15, it is the cells at intermediate oxygen concentrations that may come to dominate the survival curve when reoxygenation occurs during fractionated treatment.

Reoxygenation has been shown to occur in almost all rodent tumors that have been studied, but both the extent and timing of this reoxygenation are variable (see Fig. 14.16). Reoxygenation may result from increased or redistributed blood flow, reduced oxygen utilization by radiation-damaged cells, or

rapid removal of radiation-damaged cells so that the hypoxic cells become closer to functional blood vessels (Kallman, 1988). Large single doses of radiation were used to induce the reoxygenation in the animal tumors illustrated in Fig. 14.16; reoxygenation will probably be less extensive following smaller fractionated doses and the kinetics of the process may be different. Experimental studies with animal tumors using fraction sizes of 2 to 3 Gy are very limited but suggest that reoxygenation may not be sufficient to prevent the hypoxic cells from influencing the response of the tumor to the radiation treatment (Hill, 1986). Even though there is no direct evidence for reoxygenation of surviving hypoxic cells in human tumors, it is probably a major reason why fractionating treatment leads to an improvement in therapeutic ratio (as compared to single large doses) in clinical radiotherapy. Measurements of the oxygenation of tumors during fractionated radiotherapy have demonstrated improved oxygen status in some tumors, but at present these measurements do not distinguish between surviving cells and those already killed by the treatment (see Koh et al., 1995; Zywietz et al.,1995).

14.3.5 Low-Dose-Rate Irradiation

The effect of giving continuous low dose-rate irradiation is similar to that of reducing fraction size (see

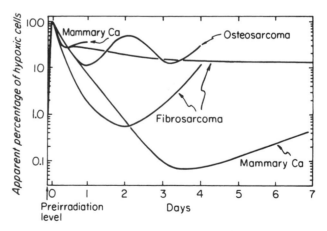

Figure 14.16. The apparent percentage of surviving cells, which were hypoxic in the tumor, is plotted as a function of time after a single radiation dose (10 to 15 Gy) given to a number of different rodent tumors. The initial (preirradiation) percentage of hypoxic cells was 1 to 15% for the different tumors, but immediately after the radiation dose, essentially all the surviving cells were hypoxic. As a function of time after the first radiation dose, second radiation doses were given to allow determination of the fraction of hypoxic cells among the survivors of the first dose. (Modified from Hill, 1986.)

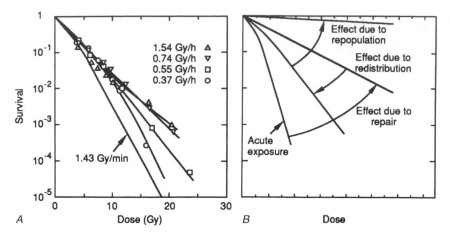

Figure 14.17. *A.* Survival curves for HeLa cells treated with γ-irradiation given at different continuous (low) dose rates. (Redrawn from Mitchell et al., 1979.) *B.* Schematic diagram to illustrate the influence, on the survival curve following continuous low dose-rate irradiation, of the processes of repair, redistribution and the G2 block, and repopulation. (Redrawn from Hall, 1988.)

Fig. 14.9). Dose rates above about 1 Gy/min can be regarded as acute (single-dose) treatment and result in survival curves similar to the curve for 1.43 Gy/min shown in Fig. 14.17A. At lower dose-rates, the processes of repair, repopulation, redistribution, and reoxygenation can occur during the course of the irradiation. Repair is the major factor and most of its effect occurs in the range of dose rates of 1.0 to 0.01 Gy/min. Below about 0.1 Gy/min, the effects of cell-cycle progression (redistribution and the G2 block) become apparent; below about 0.01 Gy/min, the effects of repopulation will start to become evident (Steel et al., 1986). These effects are illustrated schematically in Fig. 14.17B. There is a general trend to a shallower slope for the survival curve as the dose rate decreases, owing to repair and repopulation, but this trend is slowed or reversed by the effects of cell-cycle redistribution. The influence of dose rate on radiation response varies for different cell populations (or tissues) depending on the extent of the above processes for that cell line or tissue—e.g., bone marrow cells demonstrate a small sparing at a low dose rate because they have a low repair capacity. In tumors, reoxygenation during the course of the treatment will have an effect similar to that of redistribution—i.e., to oppose the trend to the shallower slope caused by repair and repopulation.

14.3.6 Time and Dose Relationships

Repair and repopulation can be expected to increase the total dose required to achieve a given level of biological damage (an isoeffect) in a course of fractionated radiation treatment. Redistribution and reoxygenation would be expected to reduce the total dose required for the isoeffect. Reoxygenation applies mostly to tumors (since they contain hypoxic cells), while repopulation and redistribution apply both to tumors and proliferating normal tissues. Repair is an important factor in the response of nearly all tissues. It is often difficult to dissect the influence of the individual factors. The relative importance of repair and repopulation was addressed in studies of the responses of pig skin to fractionated radiation (Fowler and Stern, 1963). Pig skin was chosen because it has a structure similar to that of human skin. The data, summarized in Table 14.3, show that the total radiation dose required to produce a given level of early skin reaction was substantially greater when the number of fractions was increased from 5 to 20 but delivered over a constant time of 28 days; in contrast, an increase in the duration of treatment from 4 to 28 days when the fraction number (5) remained constant required a smaller increase in total dose. These results suggest that repair of sublethal damage between fractions is more important than repopulation over the course of a 4-week treatment. If the fractionated treatment had been extended to longer times, the contribution of repopulation would have been greater for the early skin-reaction endpoint used in these studies. This effect also occurs in tumors, as illustrated in Fig. 14.12.

The finding that the biological effect of radiation depends on the fractionation schedule has impor-

Table 14.3. Single and Fractionated Doses Required for a Fixed Level of Acute Reaction in Pig Skin

Number of Fractions	Overall Time, days	Total Dose, Gy
1	<1	20
5	4	36
5	28	42
20	28	~60

Source: Adapted from Fowler and Stern (1963).

tant clinical implications for the planning of therapy. To obtain the maximum dose to a tumor while minimizing dose to surrounding normal tissue, the radiation oncologist will often use a number of overlapping radiation beams. The dose at any given location will be calculated by summing the doses given by the various individual beams, and the dose distribution will be represented by a series of isodose curves (like contours on a map) joining points that are expected to receive equal percentages of the dose at a particular point (usually within the tumor). These isodose lines must be viewed with caution, because the same total dose may not give the same biological effect if the doses delivered by the individual beams are of unequal size and they are not given in close temporal sequence. For example, it was noted in Sec. 14.3.1 that equal-sized dose fractions allow for maximum repair; thus, if different beams are delivered on different days, the surrounding normal tissues that receive unequal contributions from different beams would repair less of the radiation damage than the tumor where the contributions are equal. The biological effect would then be different at different points on the same isodose line. This is the radiobiological rationale of treating all fields daily where multiple fields are used to treat a tumor.

14.3.7 Isoeffect Curves

Different fractionation schedules that give the same level of biological effect can be presented in the form of an isoeffect curve, a concept introduced by Strandqvist (1944). The total dose used to treat tumors of the skin and lip was plotted against the overall treatment time, using logarithmic scales, and the fit to these data (Fig. 14.18A) represented the maximum total doses, given over different time periods, that could be tolerated by the skin. An isoeffect curve describing the response of pig skin to fractionated irradiation is shown in Fig. 14.18B

(Fowler, 1971). In this plot, the horizontal axis represents fraction number rather than time, since this is a more important variable over the time range involved (see Sec. 14.3.6). When the fraction number is increased, there is a concomitant decrease in the dose per fraction to maintain the isoeffect relationship. An isoeffect curve with total dose plotted as a function of dose per fraction is shown in Fig. 14.18C.

Experimental studies performed mainly in rodents have established isoeffect curves for different normal tissues using endpoints of either early or late radiation damage. Some of these isoeffect curves are shown in Fig. 14.19, with the broken lines representing early responses and the solid lines late responses. The isoeffect lines for late responses are steeper than those for early responses, i.e., a larger

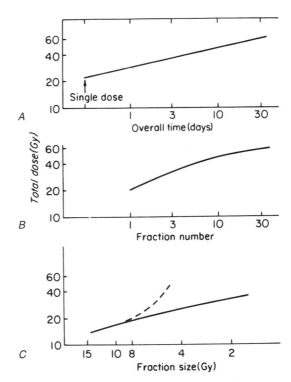

Figure 14.18. Isoeffect curves for fractionated treatments plotted in three different formats. *A.* Line plotted by Strandqvist (1944) to define normal tissue tolerance and control of carcinoma of the skin and lip using the axes of total dose and overall treatment time. *B.* Isoeffect curve for damage to pig skin plotted as total dose versus number of fractions. (Adapted from Fowler, 1971.) *C.* Isoeffect curves for the crypt cells of the mouse intestine plotted as total dose versus fraction size using an inverted scale. The solid line is for fractions given 3 h apart and the broken line for fractions given 24 h apart. (Adapted from Withers and Mason, 1974.)

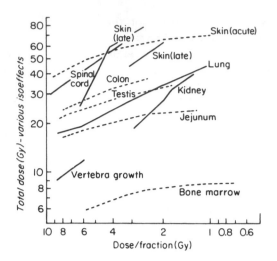

Figure 14.19. Isoeffect curves for a number of rodent tissues obtained using a variety of different cell survival or functional assays. The total dose required to obtain a fixed level of tissue damage is plotted as a function of the dose/fraction. The displacement of the curves on the vertical axis is a result of the fact that different isoeffective endpoints were used for the different tissues. (Modified from Thames et al., 1982.)

increase in total dose is required to give the same level of late toxicity as the dose per fraction is reduced and the number of fractions increased. This implies a greater capacity for the repair of damage in tissues where it is expressed late than for damage in tissues where it is expressed early after radiation treatment (Thames et al., 1982). The reasons for this difference remain unknown. The observation that late-responding normal tissues demonstrate greater effective repair capacity than early-responding normal tissues is a fundamental radiobiological principle underlying altered fractionation schedules using multiple daily fractions in clinical radiotherapy. This is discussed in more detail in Sec. 14.4.1.

14.3.8 Models for Isoeffect

A straight line on a log-log plot implies a power-law relationship; the isoeffect line drawn by Strandqvist (Fig. 14.18A) can be represented by the following relationship:

$$\text{Total dose} \propto (\text{time})^n \qquad (14.3)$$

where the exponent n is obtained from the slope of the line. Strandqvist's line gave $n \approx 0.3$, consistent with the "cube-root law" that was used by early radiotherapists as a guide to modifying fractionation schedules. Subsequently, Ellis (1969) developed the

concept of the nominal standard dose (NSD), in which he postulated that the total dose (D), tolerated by normal tissues, was related to the number of fractions (N) and overall treatment time (T) by the relationship:

$$D = (\text{NSD})\ N^{0.24} \cdot T^{0.11} \qquad (14.4)$$

This formula is similar to Eq. (14.3), but it emphasizes the importance of fraction number and is based on clinical data for cure of squamous cell carcinoma and for tolerance of skin. Modifications of the NSD equation have been proposed to describe the tolerance of different normal tissues and different organs (Kirk et al., 1971; Orton and Ellis, 1973; Ellis, 1985), but the original NSD equation and its related formulas are useful only in making minor changes to fractionation schedules without causing large changes in late normal-tissue damage.

The NSD equation and its modifications were applied quite widely in clinical radiotherapy until the introduction of the linear-quadratic (LQ) equation (Chap. 13, Sec. 13.4.3) to model isoeffect relationship in the early 1980s (Fowler, 1984, 1989). In using the LQ model, it is assumed that each fraction has an equal effect, thus for a fractionated regime (n fractions of size d):

$$\text{SF} = [e^{-(\alpha d + \beta d^2)}]^n \qquad (14.5)$$

or

$$-\ln \text{SF} = n\,(\alpha d + \beta d^2)$$

It is further assumed that if different fractionation regimes (e.g., n_1 fractions of size d_1 and n_2 fractions of size d_2) are isoeffective for a given tissue, they lead to the same surviving fraction (SF). Thus we have:

$$\text{Isoeffect } (E) = -\ln \text{SF} = n_1\,(\alpha d_1 + \beta d_1^2)$$
$$= n_2\,(\alpha d_2 + \beta d_2^2) \qquad (14.6)$$

Eq. (14.6) can then be simplified to give

$$\frac{n_1 d_1}{n_2 d_2} = \frac{\alpha/\beta + d_2}{\alpha/\beta + d_1} \qquad (14.7)$$

From this relationship, the constant α/β can be determined for the particular tissue involved and used in the equation to predict other isoeffective treatment schedules.

Data similar to those shown in Fig. 14.19 have been used to derive α/β values for different normal tissues in rodents. In general, it is found that late-responding tissues have α/β values in the range 2 to 4

Gy, while early-responding tissues have α/β values in the range 8 to 12 Gy. Data available for human tissues suggest values in the same ranges (Thames et al., 1990). Most experimental and human tumors appear to have α/β values similar to or greater than those for early-responding tissues. In fact, recent analysis of results for head and neck cancer suggests that α/β is large enough that, for a given total dose, there is little or no effect of using different fraction sizes in the range 1.5 to 3.5 Gy (Withers et al., 1995). Whether this result indicates low repair capacity in these tumors or whether it reflects the influence of reoxygenation or redistribution (which could give the same effect because both increase the sensitivity of tumors to fractionated irradiation) is unknown. One exception is melanoma, which may have an α/β value close to 1, implying high repair capacity (Thames et al., 1990).

There is no consideration of the effect of treatment time in the LQ model. In practice, this is a limitation that applies more to early normal tissue responses, which occur in proliferative tissues (and tumors), than to late normal tissue responses, which generally occur in tissues that have slowly proliferating parenchymal cell populations, and for which response to radiation is less influenced by the duration of fractionated treatment. In this model, it is also assumed that there is complete repair between the fractions, and predictions from the model may lead to serious overdosing when the interfraction interval is too short or where repair of sublethal damage is slow in the dose-limiting normal tissues (Ang et al., 1992; Kim et al., 1997; see Sec. 14.4.1). Modifications of the LQ model have been proposed to deal with the effects of overall treatment time (Newcombe et al., 1993) and of incomplete repair (Thames, 1989; Bentzen et al., 1996). The extrapolation of the LQ model to describe the effect of very small fraction sizes has also been problematic (Wong et al., 1992; Marples and Joiner, 1995). The LQ model suffers from similar problems to those that apply to empirical formulas such as NSD. Because appropriate clinical data are limited, it is difficult to verify the formulas over a wide range of treatment schedules; consequently extrapolations beyond the existing database must be undertaken with caution.

14.4 APPROACHES TO IMPROVING THE THERAPEUTIC RATIO

Most radiation treatments aimed at controlling a tumor are limited by the tolerance of the irradiated normal tissues. Improving the therapeutic ratio thus requires knowledge of the possible reasons for the failure of radiation treatment to control the tumor and/or of ways of increasing the tolerance of normal tissue. The preceding sections have discussed a number of radiobiological factors that could influence tumor control by, or normal tissue tolerance to, fractionated radiation treatment. Some of these factors are (1) the number of stem cells that a tumor contains, (2) the level of hypoxia in the tumor and the extent of reoxygenation, (3) the growth kinetics of the tumor and critical normal tissue cells, (4) the repair capacity of the cells, and (5) the intrinsic radiosensitivity of the cells. These factors are susceptible to manipulation to improve the therapeutic ratio.

14.4.1 Altered Fractionation Schedules

In Sec. 14.3.7, data were summarized that indicate a high capacity for repair of radiation damage in late-responding normal tissues (low α/β values) as compared with early-responding normal tissues and most tumors. This difference in repair capacity can be exploited to obtain a therapeutic gain by reducing the fraction size below that used conventionally (from about 2 Gy to 1 to 1.5 Gy) and increasing the number of fractions. The increase in dose that can be tolerated at the isoeffective level of late normal tissue damage should be greater than that required to maintain the same level of tumor control (i.e., the tumor would receive a larger biologically effective dose and hence the control rate should be higher). The larger number of fractions required must be given more than once per day if the treatment time is not to be prolonged. Such a treatment protocol is termed *hyperfractionation*. The time interval between the fractions must be sufficiently long to allow time for complete repair to occur. Repair kinetics have been estimated in a number of normal tissues, and half-times for repair ranged from 0.5 h in jejunum to 1 to 2 h in skin, lung, and kidney (see also Chap. 13, Sec. 13.5.4). Thus, repair can be considered to be complete in most normal tissues for an interfraction interval of 6 to 8 h. In the rodent spinal cord, it has been found that the effective repair half-time is greater than 2 h, so repair is not complete even with an interfraction interval of 8 h (Ang et al., 1992; Kim et al., 1997). Thus an increase in late morbidity would be expected when multiple fractions per day are given to fields that include the spinal cord, as was observed by Dische and Saunders (1989) in patients given three fractions per day. An increase in early normal tissue reactions would be expected with hyperfractionation versus conventional fractionation, since the larger α/β value for early-responding tissues implies a smaller change in the amount of repair as fraction size is reduced relative to that occurring in late-responding tissues. The increase in dose that can be tolerated can be calculated as discussed in Sec. 14.3.8, but the low reliability of current estimates of α/β for human tissues requires that such calculations be treated with caution.

The rationale for hyperfractionation does not consider reoxygenation. Since there is no change in overall treatment time, it is assumed that reoxygenation will not be much different than for a conventional fractionation scheme. Clinical trials of the strategy of using a larger total dose delivered by hyperfractionation have reported an increase in local control with no difference in late normal tissue damage (e.g., Horiot et al., 1992). These results support the hypothesis that an increase of total dose can be achieved by hyperfractionation without increasing the probability of late complications (see Peters et al., 1990, for further discussion).

Shortening of the overall treatment time might also improve the therapeutic ratio, since it will reduce the time for repopulation to occur in the tumor during treatment (Sec. 14.3.2). The tolerance of late-responding normal tissues should be little affected, since cell proliferation is slow within them. Reduced treatment time is achieved by giving more than one fraction per day with standard dose fractions of 1.8 to 2.5 Gy given 6 to 8 h apart to allow for repair; a strategy called *accelerated fractionation* (AF). Results of randomized trials with two such schedules compared against conventional fractionation (CF) for treatment of head and neck cancer have recently been reported. Both provided evidence supporting the importance of repopulation as a cause of treatment failure (Horiot et al., 1997; Dische et al., 1997). The combined hyperfractionated accelerated radiation therapy (CHART) study gave a reduced dose in the AF arm of the study but maintained the same tumor control level, with a slight reduction in late morbidity (Dische et al., 1997). The second study, which gave a similar total dose in both arms of the study, reported increased tumor control in the AF arm, but there was also increased late toxicity (Horiot et al., 1997). This latter effect may have been due to the short (4 h) interfraction interval in the AF arm, which was probably not sufficient to allow for complete repair between the fractions.

Accelerated fractionation is likely to be beneficial for rapidly repopulating tumors in sites where acutely responding tissues (which will also have less time for repopulation) would not become dose-limiting. Because of increased acute toxicity with accelerated fractionation schedules, it would be desirable to select patients most likely to benefit from it. An assay of tumor cell kinetics (Begg et al., 1990), which may have predictive value for the repopulation potential of tumors during therapy, is discussed in Sec. 14.5.2.

14.4.2 Increase in Oxygen Delivery

Hypoxic cells represent a radiation-resistant subpopulation in tumors that does not exist (or only to a very minor extent) in most normal tissues. Thus, the therapeutic ratio might be improved by reducing the influence of these cells on tumor response. Reoxygenation during fractionated radiotherapy reduces the influence of hypoxic cells, but reoxygenation is variable from tumor to tumor in animals. Recent work with oxygen electrodes has demonstrated that the oxygen status of human tumors can predict treatment outcome (see Sec. 14.5.3) and suggests that reoxygenation is inadequate for at least some tumors in humans.

A number of clinical studies have demonstrated the negative effect of anemia on prognosis (Bush, 1986); and in many centers, blood transfusions are used to maintain patients at normal hemoglobin levels during treatment. A small randomized study in patients with carcinoma of the cervix has shown a significant improvement of local control with blood transfusions (Bush, 1986). Experimental studies have suggested that low arterial oxygen tensions may also influence tumor response by affecting the level of hypoxia (Horsman et al., 1993). Carbon monoxide in cigarette smoke reduces the oxygen unloading capacity of the blood and may result in reduced tumor oxygenation (Siemann et al., 1978). Patients with head and neck cancer who continue to smoke during radiotherapy have been found to have decreased local control and survival after radiation treatment (Browman et al., 1993).

Oxygen delivery to tumor cells may be increased by giving animals or patients oxygen under hyperbaric conditions (200 to 300 kPa) (HPO) during radiation treatment. An increase in the dissolved oxygen concentration in blood plasma should result in greater diffusion of oxygen into the hypoxic regions. Studies with animal tumors have demonstrated that the use of HPO will indeed sensitize them to radiation, particularly when used with fractionated treatments (Suit et al., 1977). Clinical studies with HPO as an adjuvant to radiation therapy have demonstrated improvement in local tumor

Table 14.4. Summary of Clinical Trials Testing Sensitization of Hypoxic Cells

Sensitizing Agent	Number of Trials	Significant Benefit	Margin in Favor	No Benefit
Hyperbaric Oxygen	15	3	6	6
Misonidazole	39	4	4	31

Tumor Size	Number of Patients (Trials)	Percent Local Control		p Value
		Radiation Alone	Radiation plus Sensitizer	
Head and neck cancer	4064 (22)	40.6%	47.2%	0.00002
Cervical cancer	2292 (12)	59.6%	61.2%	0.014

[a]The upper part of the table gives results from individual trials while the lower part gives the results of a meta-analysis of all the suitable data (using HPO or hypoxic-cell radiosensitizers).

Sources: Top, adapted from Dische, 1989; bottom, data from Overgaard and Horsman, 1996. With permission.

control and survival for patients with cancers of the head and neck or cervix (see Table 14.4) but not for other sites (Henk et al., 1977; Watson et al., 1978).

Possible *biological* reasons why these trials failed to show a positive result include the following: (1) tumor control was not limited by hypoxic cells in many of the tumors, either because of effective reoxygenation or because some tumors contained few hypoxic cells, and (2) the extra oxygen was able to diffuse to only some hypoxic cells. The results of the positive trials indicate, however, the presence of hypoxic cells in some human tumors, and that reoxygenation is not sufficient in these tumors to prevent the hypoxic cells from influencing the probability of tumor control during fractionated radiation treatment. The introduction of a number of techniques, most notably the (Eppendorf) polarographic oxygen electrode, to measure the extent of hypoxia in tumors may allow better selection of patients likely to benefit from these therapeutic strategies (see Sec. 14.5.3).

Other possibilities for improving tumor oxygenation currently under investigation include artificial blood substitutes, such as perfluorocarbon emulsions or cross-linked hemoglobins, to increase the oxygen-carrying capacity of the blood and human erythropoietin to increase the hemoglobin concentration (Lavey and Dempsey, 1993). Nicotinamide has been shown to increase tumor perfusion and is being evaluated in combination with carbogen (95 percent O_2 and 5 percent CO_2) breathing to overcome tumor hypoxia (Chaplin et al., 1991; Zackrissen et al., 1994).

14.4.3 Sensitizers

An alternative approach to reduce the influence of tumor hypoxia involves the use of drugs that mimic the radiosensitizing properties of oxygen. These drugs, known as *hypoxic-cell radiosensitizers,* must diffuse to all parts of a tumor to be effective. Development of radiosensitizers was based on the idea that the radiosensitizing properties of oxygen are due to its electron affinity and that other compounds with this characteristic might act as sensitizers. A family of compounds, the nitromidazoles (Fig. 14.20), has been found to contain members that can sensitize hypoxic cells both in vitro and in animal tumors. The most extensively studied of these compounds is misonidazole (Overgaard, 1995), which can sensitize hypoxic cells in vitro in a dose-dependent fashion and does not sensitize oxygenated cells. The extent of the sensitization can be assessed in terms of a sensitizer enhancement ratio (SER), (Fig. 14.21), which is analogous to the OER discussed in Chap. 13, Sec. 13.5.2. Sensitizer enhancement ratios depend on the drug concentration in the tumor at the time of radiation. There is a good correspondence between the values obtained for tumors and the results from in vitro studies. If misonidazole is combined with fractionated radiation doses, the SER is reduced both because of reoxygenation occurring between the fractions (Hill, 1986) and because lower individual doses of the drug are tolerated when it is given as fractionated treatment.

A large number of sensitizers have been investigated, and nine have been evaluated in clinical tri-

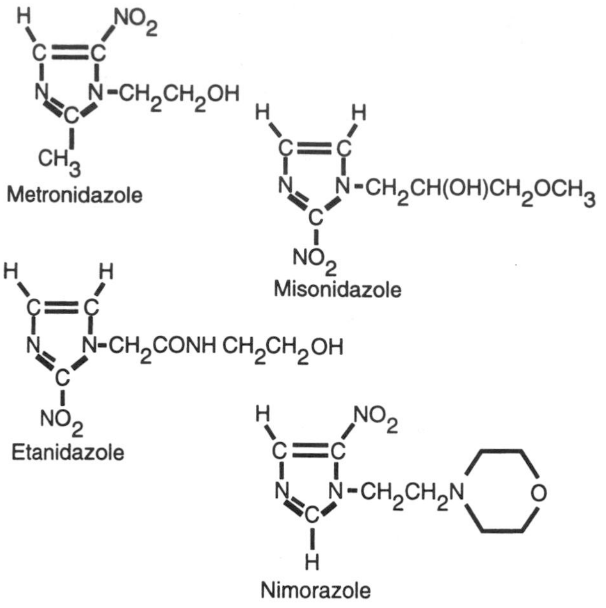

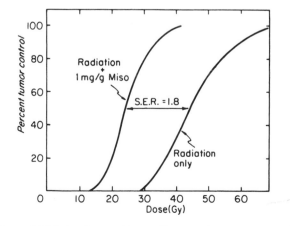

Figure 14.20. The structure of some hypoxic cell radiosensitizers that have been or are being studied in clinical trials.

als. Overall, results from the earlier trials using misonidazole have been disappointing (see Table 14.4). In addition, misonidazole was limited by a dose-dependent peripheral neuropathy (Overgaard and Horsman, 1996). More recent studies using drugs that are less toxic, such as etanidazole and nimorazole, revealed conflicting results. Whereas nimorazole has been associated with improved tumor control in head and neck cancer in the DAHANCA trial (Overgaard et al., 1998), benefit was not demonstrated in two multicenter trials for head and neck cancer using etanidazole (Chassagne et al., 1991; Lee et al., 1995). Although, most trials with nitroimidazoles have failed to demonstrate a benefit, a recent meta-analysis of results from over 7000 patients (see Table 14.4) included in 50 randomized trials indicated a small but significant improvement in local control (and survival), with most of the benefit attributed to an improved response in patients with head and neck cancer (Overgaard and Horsman, 1996). The apparent lack of clinical benefit in the individual trials may be due to the small numbers of patients included in most of these trials and not due to lack of the biological importance of tumor hypoxia. Predictive assays that determine oxygenation in individual tumors should allow a better selection of patients with hypoxic tumors who are more likely to benefit from hypoxic radiosensitizers (see Sec. 14.5.3).

Another approach to reducing the influence of hypoxia on the radiation response of tumors is to use bioreductive drugs that are toxic under hypoxic conditions. Complementary effects of radiation (against aerobic cells) and of drug (against hypoxic cells) might then increase the therapeutic ratio (Brown and Giaccia, 1994). Since normal tissues are generally well oxygenated and do not allow for activation of the bioreductive drug, it is expected that a therapeutic gain could be achieved. The principal bioreductive drugs of current clinical interest are mitomycin C and porfiromycin, which are quinones, and tirapazamine, an *N*-oxide (see Fig. 14.22). Mitomycin C has only modest selectivity toward hypoxic cells and requires extremely low oxygen levels for maximum cytotoxicity (Marshall and Rauth, 1988). Tirapazamine, however, is cytotoxic to hypoxic cells at much higher oxygen concentrations. It is metabolized to an oxidizing radical that produces DNA damage; in the presence of oxygen, it oxidizes back to the parent compound (Brown, 1993). Tirapazamine is currently being evaluated in clinical trials (Brown and Siim, 1996).

Anticancer drugs may also interact with radiation to cause increased toxicity, but the results are usually consistent with additive cytotoxic effects. Important interactions are reviewed in Chap. 17, Sec. 17.3.4.

14.4.4 High-LET Radiation

The use of high-LET (linear energy transfer) radiations might contribute to improvements in the therapeutic ratio in two different ways. First, particle beams, because much of their energy is deposited in

Figure 14.21. In vivo studies to illustrate the sensitizing effect of misonidazole. Tumor control versus dose curves for murine mammary tumors treated with x-irradiation in the presence or absence of misonidazole (1 mg/g). (Modified from Sheldon et al., 1974.)

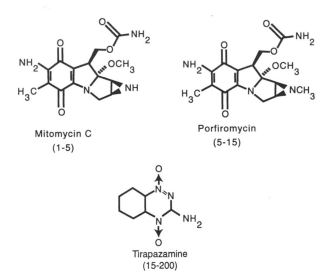

Mitomycin C
(1-5)

Porfiromycin
(5-15)

Tirapazamine
(15-200)

Figure 14.22. Structures of some of the bioreductive cytotoxic agents of current clinical interest. The numbers in parentheses associated with each drug show an approximate range of the ratios of drug concentrations to produce equal cell kill for aerobic and hypoxic cells for a variety of different tumor cell lines. (Modified from Brown and Siim, 1996.)

tissue at the end of particle tracks (i.e., in the region of the Bragg peak—see Chap. 13, Sec. 13.2.2), can be used to give improved depth-dose distributions for deep-seated tumors (Fig. 14.23). Neutron beams are not useful in this regard, since they do not demonstrate a Bragg peak and depth-dose distributions are similar to those for low-LET radiation. Second, the oxygen enhancement ratio is reduced at high LET (see Chap. 13, Sec. 13.5.2), so that hypoxic cells are protected to a lesser degree. Studies with fast neutron irradiation have indicated that the OER is in the range 1.5 to 2.0; for accelerated ion beams, it may be lower. Thus, high-LET radiation is potentially useful in the treatment of tumors that contain hypoxic cells.

The variation in radiosensitivity with position in the cell cycle is reduced for high-LET radiation and, in general, there is reduced variability in response between different cells. Cells also exhibit reduced capacity for repair following high-LET radiation relative to that following low-LET radiation. This property leads to an increased relative biological effectiveness (RBE; Chap. 13, Sec. 13.5.1), with the RBE increasing as the fraction size decreases. Because late-responding tissues demonstrate greater repair capacity than early-responding tissues (see Sec. 14.3.7), the reduction in repair capacity following high-LET irradiation will result in relatively higher

RBE values for late-responding tissues. In general, this will contribute to a decrease in therapeutic ratio.

A comparison of various different radiations in relation to their potential physical or biological therapeutic advantages is shown in Fig. 14.24. The vertical axis represents the potential gain due to improved depth-dose distribution, while the horizontal axis represents that due to the biological aspects of increased LET. The expected gains with protons are largely confined to improved dose distribution, while for neutrons any gains are likely to be related to the biological factors. Negative pions and accelerated ions can give both advantages, but it is likely that they will have only limited applicability because they are very expensive to produce and only a few places in the world have suitable facilities.

Clinical studies using high-LET radiation have been most extensive with fast neutrons. Clinical results with neutron therapy have, however, been associated with an increase in complications, and randomized trials have not demonstrated therapeutic gain (Fowler, 1988; Raju, 1996). Similarly, recent randomized results with pion therapy also failed to suggest any clinical advantage compared to photons (Pickles, 1995). The experience with heavy ions is not sufficient for an assessment of any clinical treatment advantage. Results with protons, however, have demonstrated a clear advantage for treatment

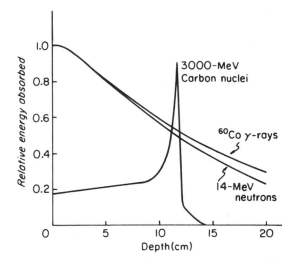

Figure 14.23. Depth-dose distributions for three different types of radiation. The energy deposited decreases as a function of depth into the body for both γ-rays and 14-MeV neutrons. For the 3000-MeV carbon nuclei, energy deposition increases to a peak (the Bragg peak) at a depth of about 12 cm. The vertical scale relates to the three types of radiation independently and does not provide an intercomparison. (Redrawn from Hall, 1988.)

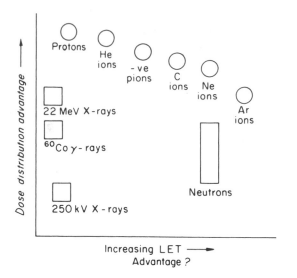

Figure 14.24. Schematic comparison of the possible therapeutic advantage from using different types of radiation. The vertical axis represents the advantage due to improved depth-dose distribution. The horizontal axis represents increasing LET, which may give an advantage for the treatment of some tumors but not others. (Adapted from Raju, 1980.)

of tumors such as choroidal melanomas and skull-base tumors that require precise treatment of a highly localized lesion (Suit and Urie, 1992; Slater et al., 1995).

Recently there has been renewed interest, particularly for treatment of brain tumors, in boron neutron capture therapy (BNCT), which is a two-component modality in which compounds enriched with ^{10}B are administered prior to irradiation with a thermal neutron beam. Neutrons are captured by ^{10}B atoms in the tumors (or tissues), and, a fission reaction produces high-energy charged particles (^{7}Li and ^{4}He). For an improved therapeutic ratio with BNCT, relatively high concentrations of ^{10}B must be achieved in the tumor, with low concentrations in normal tissues (Hatanaka and Nakagawa, 1994; Coderre et al., 1995). New boronated compounds and new strategies for delivering the compounds have improved the differential concentrations achievable in tumors and surrounding normal tissues, and rodent models have given encouraging results (Barth et al., 1997).

14.5 PREDICTIVE ASSAYS

Currently, the choice of treatment for a patient is based largely on clinical and histopathologic prognostic parameters; these include tumor- and host-related factors and knowledge of the dose-response relationships for control of tumors of a similar type

and for the normal tissues to be included in the treatment field. It would be desirable to predict the tumor and normal tissue response of an individual patient. The heterogeneity of radiobiological properties that govern tissue response to radiation treatment among individual patients suggests the need for predictive assays that focus on specific biological properties. This is particularly important in testing new treatment strategies, because if only a fraction of patients can benefit, the improvement in the response of their tumors will be obscured by that in the majority of patients who do not benefit from the particular strategy being tested. Predictive assays assessing radiobiological factors that may influence the response of tumors and normal tissues to treatment are focused largely in three areas: (1) intrinsic radiosensitivity of tumor and normal cells, (2) tumor-cell proliferation kinetics, and (3) tumor hypoxia.

14.5.1 Intrinsic Radiosensitivity of Tumor and Normal Cells

The concept that the radiosensitivity of tumor cells, particularly the survival following a small dose (2 Gy) of radiation, might be predictive for the outcome of fractionated treatment was discussed in Sec. 14.2.1. Studies have been undertaken to determine whether measurement of parameters defining the low-dose region of survival curves for tumor cells, taken directly from biopsies, would correlate with the outcome of the treatment of that particular tumor. Studies with experimental tumors and with xenografts of human tumors have supported such a correlation (Rofstad and Brustad, 1987; Bristow and Hill, 1990). In vitro radiosensitivity of tumor cells has been assayed using the cell-adhesive matrix (CAM) and a clonogenic assay. In the CAM assay (see also Chap. 13, Sec. 13.3.4), a suspension of cells from the tumor is plated into wells coated with CAM and the relative density of cells in control and irradiated wells after a period of growth, usually 2 to 3 weeks, is used to estimate surviving fraction. In the clonogenic assay, colony-forming efficiency of irradiated and control cells is determined after plating in soft agar. The CAM assay is more rapid, but nontumor cells may contribute to the growth density used as the endpoint. The clonogenic assay takes 5 to 6 weeks before results are available, but it is believed to give an estimate of the sensitivity of clonogenic cells in the tumor. Other limitations of such measurements are that (1) in vitro assays may not account for microenvironmental factors influencing radiosensitivity in vivo, (2) tumors may contain clonogenic subpopulations of different intrinsic radiosensitivity, (3) the assay may not be measuring the radiosensitivity of the stem cells in vivo, (4) assay-specific variations in radiosensitivity measures (e.g., SF2) are considerable, and (5) measurements may not be obtained in 25 to 30 percent of tumors.

Using the CAM assay, Girinsky et al. (1992) reported that an α value of < 0.07 Gy^{-1} was associated with decreased local control and survival in patients treated with radiation for head and neck cancer or cervical carcinoma, but SF2 values were not predictive of outcome. In another study of head and neck cancer treated by surgery and postoperative radiotherapy, SF2 values obtained from the CAM assay, did not discriminate patients who achieved local control versus those who failed locally (Brock et al., 1990). Intrinsic radiosensitivity was able to discriminate between outcomes for patients with cervical cancer treated with radiation therapy in a study from Manchester (Levine et al., 1995). In this study SF2 was measured using a clonogenic assay, and in a multivariate analysis that included clinical and histopathologic prognostic parameters, patients with radioresistant tumors (SF2 > median of 0.41) had significantly worse local control and survival than those with more radiosensitive tumors (SF2 < 0.41) (see Fig. 14.25).

Patients receiving identical radiation treatments may experience widely differing levels of normal tissue injury. Predictive assays for normal tissue radiosensitivity may be useful if variations in normal

tissue injury observed clinically are due largely to individual differences in radiosensitivity and not simply to random effects. The enhanced radiosensitivity of patients with ataxia telangiectasia who have a deficiency in DNA repair (see Chap. 4, Sec. 4.4) supports a genetic contribution to individual variability in radiosensitivity (Jorgensen and Shiloh, 1996). Clinical studies in breast cancer patients have also shown individual correlation of acute and late skin reactions in one treatment field with those in a different treatment field, again suggesting a genetic basis of individual differences in normal-tissue radiosensitivity (Tucker et al., 1992). A number of studies have examined in vitro radiosensitivity of fibroblasts as a potential predictive assay. These studies have suggested a correlation between the SF2 of fibroblasts and late clinical reactions but showed no correlation between SF2 of fibroblasts and early reactions (Johanson et al., 1994; Brock et al., 1995). The number of patients assayed in these studies was small, but these preliminary results support the validity of a predictive assay of normal tissue radiosensitivity. By identifying patients as being more or less radioresistant to normal tissue injury, such assays could lead to an improvement in therapeutic ratio by tailoring treatment regimens to individual patients (Bentzen, 1997.).

14.5.2 Tumor-Cell Kinetics and Cell Death

The demonstration by Withers et al. (1988) that rapid repopulation may occur in tumors during the course of fractionated radiation therapy (see Sec. 14.3.2) has reinforced interest in treatment using accelerated fractionation (see Sec. 14.4.1). Such treatments, however, are likely to result in more severe early tissue reactions. It is thus important to select tumors most likely to benefit from such treatment; in theory, these should be the most rapidly growing tumors. As discussed in Chap. 7 (Sec. 7.4 and 7.6), three parameters influence tumor growth rate, the cell-cycle time of the dividing cells, the fraction of cells in the tumor that are in the proliferation cycle (growth fraction), and the rate of cell loss. The cycle time and growth fraction combine to give a parameter, known as the *potential doubling time* (T_{pot}), that expresses the rate at which new tumor cells are added to the tumor-cell population. Values of T_{pot} for human tumors vary quite widely, but the median is in the range 4 to 5 days (Begg, 1995). The difference between values of T_{pot} and of the volume doubling time is due to cell loss.

Because radiation-damaged cells often divide once or twice before expressing their lethal damage,

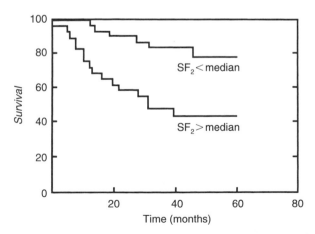

Figure 14.25. Actuarial survival in patients with cervical cancer treated by radical radiotherapy as a function of intrinsic radiosensitivity of tumors stratified as above or below the median SF$_2$ of 0.41. Survival and local control (*not shown*) are significantly worse for patients with SF$_2$ > 0.41; p = 0.003 and 0.002, respectively. (Redrawn from Levine et al., 1995.)

assessment of cell kinetics in irradiated tumors may not give information about the kinetics of the cells surviving the treatment. It is expected, however, that cell loss from the population of surviving cells may decline during treatment because radiation-killed cells are being lost and there is less demand on the nutrient supply. Thus the growth rate of the surviving tumor cells may be better characterized by the value of T_{pot} than by the volume doubling time (Trott and Kummermehr, 1985). This concept underlies the principle of using pretreatment T_{pot} as a predictive assay.

A technique for measuring T_{pot} for human tumors in vivo using a single biopsy is described in Chap. 7, Sec. 7.4.3. This method depends on taking a tumor biopsy a few hours after the injection of bromodeoxyuridine, which is taken up by S-phase cells and detected subsequently in the cells by flow cytometry (Wilson et al., 1988). Measurement of T_{pot} can be used as a predictive assay before a treatment decision, as has been demonstrated for tumors in animals (Trott, 1990). A trend for an adverse treatment outcome associated with short T_{pot} has been reported in patients with cancers of the head and neck or cervix, but this remains controversial (Begg, 1995). One problem with determining T_{pot} using flow cytometry is the difficulty of separating tumor cells from nontumor cells, particularly for tumors with diploid DNA content. This problem can be overcome by determining T_{pot} values from histologic sections of tumors, although this is more labor-intensive (Wilson et al., 1995).

Assays for tumor proliferation have been studied extensively, but until recently little attention has been devoted to cell death. The observation of radiation-induced apoptosis in many tumors as well as normal tissues, has ignited interest in the predictive role of spontaneous and radiation-induced apoptosis in human tumors treated by radiotherapy. Data from murine tumors suggest that the levels of pretreatment apoptosis correlate with radiation-induced apoptosis and predict tumor response (Stephens et al., 1991b; Meyn et al., 1993). The value of pretreatment apoptotic index (determined from characteristic morphologic features on histologic sections) as a predictive assay has been reported in patients with cervical and bladder carcinoma treated with radiotherapy (Levine et al., 1995; Wheeler et al., 1995; Chyle et al., 1996). It is uncertain whether larger studies will confirm the predictive value of the apoptotic index, given the limited correlation with cell death as assessed by a colony-forming assay (see Chap. 13, Sec. 13.3.3).

14.5.3 Hypoxia

Since hypoxia in tumors conveys resistance to radiation (see Chap. 13, Sec. 13.5.2), techniques to determine tumor oxygenation in individual tumors might allow for more rational selection of patients for new treatment modalities targeted at hypoxic cells. Commercially available polarographic oxygen electrodes (from Eppendorf) can measure microregional P_{O_2} directly in human tumors (Stone et al., 1993). Measurements of tumor P_{O_2} in individual patients using this technology have revealed wide differences from tumor to tumor (see Fig. 14.26). Preliminary results from clinical studies in cancers of the cervix and head and neck managed by radiotherapy or radiotherapy and chemotherapy suggest that hypoxic tumors (median P_{O_2} value < 10 mmHg) have poorer disease-free and overall survival (Hockel et al., 1996; Nordsmark et al., 1996). The study of Hockel et al. (1996) suggests that hypoxic tumors treated with surgery also have a poorer prognosis than better-oxygenated tumors, raising the possibility that hypoxia may be a marker for more aggressive disease as well as a specific marker for radiation resistance (see also Chap. 13, Sec. 13.5.2). This is consistent with the results of a small study of soft tissue sarcoma suggesting that hypoxic tumors were more likely to metastasize (Brizel et al., 1996).

The polarographic oxygen probe measures tissue oxygen directly, but it has the disadvantage that it is invasive, and it is difficult to distinguish between measurements made in viable versus nonviable tissue regions. Other techniques are currently at various stages of development for application in the clinical environment (Stone et al., 1993; Evans et al., 1996; Raleigh et al., 1996).

14.6 SUMMARY

Radiotherapy for cancer usually involves giving 25 to 35 individual dose fractions of about 2 Gy once daily, over a period of 5 to 7 weeks. These treatment schedules have been developed empirically and shown to have a better therapeutic ratio than single doses because they give greater tumor control at tolerable levels of normal-tissue damage. Experimental studies with cells in culture and with animal models have identified four factors (the "four R's") that influence response to fractionated treatment. These are repair of radiation damage, repopulation of damaged tissues by proliferation of surviving cells, redistribution of proliferating cells through the cell cycle, and reoxygenation of hypoxic cells. Repair and repopulation are the reasons why cells and tis-

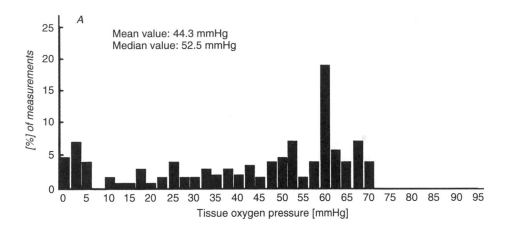

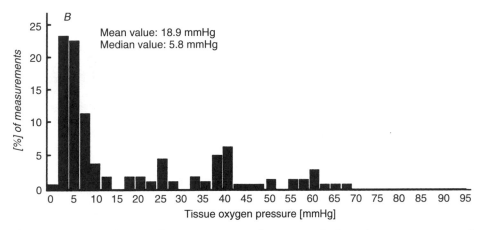

Figure 14.26. Distribution of tumor P_{O_2} in two human cervical carcinomas as measured by the Eppendorf polarographic oxygen electrode. Each distribution represents 160 individual measurement points in the tumor. The tumor in *A* is less hypoxic and shows fewer regions with low P_{O_2} measurements than the tumor in *B*. (Courtesy of Fyles et al., unpublished.)

sues can tolerate a larger total dose when it is fractionated. They occur both in tumors and normal tissues, although repopulation has a minor effect on the late radiation damage that occurs in slowly proliferating normal tissues and is often dose-limiting. Repopulation during the latter part of conventional (5 to 7 week) fractionated treatments may play an important role in increasing the dose required for tumor control. Reoxygenation in tumors also contributes to the improved therapeutic ratio obtained with fractionated treatment.

In clinical practice, different fractionated schedules that give an equal level of normal-tissue response or tumor control can be expressed in the form of an isoeffect relationships described by the parameters α and β of the linear-quadratic model. Late-responding tissues tend to have smaller α/β values than early-re-

sponding tissues, implying greater capacity for repair of damage that leads to late effects. The difference in the isoeffect relationships for early and late damage implies that reducing fraction size will reduce damage to late-responding tissues to a greater extent than to early-responding tissues or tumors. A therapeutic gain might therefore be achieved by using hyperfractionation, where treatment with smaller dose fractions is given several times per day. Giving treatments more than once per day with the aim of reducing overall treatment time might also lead to a therapeutic gain if repopulation occurs more rapidly in the tumors than in the dose-limiting normal tissues. Other approaches to improving the therapeutic ratio have included attempts to reduce the resistance due to hypoxic cells in tumors, such as strategies to increase oxygen delivery to hypoxic cells in tumor, or drugs capable of specific sensitization (and toxicity for) hypoxic cells.

The improved understanding of biological factors that influence the response of tissues and tumors to fractionated irradiation has led to renewed interest in the possibility of predicting treatment outcome for individual patients based on assays that assess relevant biological parameters. Parameters currently under investigation include intrinsic radiation sensitivity of tumor and normal cells, tumor-cell kinetics, and the extent of hypoxia. The next few years should see some conclusive information on the predictive role of these parameters for outcome after radiotherapy.

REFERENCES

Ang KK, Jiang GL, Guttenberger HD, et al: Impact of spinal cord repair kinetics on the practice of altered fractionation schedules. *Radiother Oncol* 1992; 25: 287–294.

Barth RF, Yang W, Rotaru JH, et al: Boron neutron capture therapy of brain tumors: Enhanced survival following intracarotid injection of either sodium borocaptate or borophenylalanine with or without blood-brain-barrier disruption. *Cancer Res* 1997; 57:1129–1136.

Begg AC: The clinical status of Tpot as a predictor? Or, why no tempest in the Tpot! *Int J Radiat Oncol Biol Phys* 1995; 32:1539–1541.

Begg AC, Hofland I, Moonen L, et al: The predictive value of cell kinetic measurements in a European trial of accelerated fractionation in advanced head and neck tumors: An interim report. *Int J Radiat Oncol Biol Phys* 1990; 19:1449–1453.

Bentzen SM: Potential clinical impact of normal tissue intrinsic radiosensitivity testing. Radiother Oncol 43: 121–131, 1997.

Bentzen SM, Ruifrok ACC, Thames HD: Repair capacity and kinetics for human mucosa and epithelial tumors in the head and neck: Clinical data on the effect of changing the time interval between multiple fractions per day in radiotherapy. *Radiother Oncol* 1996; 38: 89–101.

Bristow RG, Hill RP: Comparison between in vitro radiosensitivity and in vivo radioresponse in murine tumor cell lines: In vivo radioresponse following fractionated treatment and in vitro/in vivo correlations. *Int J Radiat Oncol Biol Phys* 1990; 18:331–345.

Brizel DM, Scully SP, Harrelson JM, et al: Tumor oxygenation predicts for the likelihood of distant metastases in human soft tissue sarcoma. *Cancer Res* 1996; 56: 941–943.

Brock WA, Baker FL, Wike J, et al: Cellular radiosensitivity of primary head and neck squamous cell carcinomas and local tumor control. *Int J Radiat Oncol Biol Phys* 1990; 18:1283–1286.

Brock WA, Tucker SL, Geara FB, et al: Fibroblast radiosensitivity versus acute and late normal skin responses in patients treated for breast cancer. *Int J Radiat Oncol Biol Phys* 1995; 32:1371–1379.

Browman GP, Wong G, Hodson I: Influence of cigarette smoking on the efficacy of radiation therapy in head and neck cancer. *N Engl J Med* 1993; 328:159–163.

Brown JM: SR4233 (tirapazamine): A new anticancer drug exploiting hypoxia in solid tumors. *Br J Cancer* 1993; 67:1163–1170.

Brown JM, Giaccia AJ: Tumor hypoxia: The picture has changed in the 1990s. *Int J Radiat Biol* 1994; 65: 95–102.

Brown JM, Siim BG: Hypoxia-specific cytotoxins in cancer therapy. *Semin Radiat Oncol* 1996; 6:22–36.

Bush RS: The significance of anemia in clinical radiation therapy. *Int J Radiat Oncol Biol Phys* 1986; 12:2047–2050.

Chaplin DJ, Horsman MR, Aoki D: Nicotinamide, fluosol DA and carbogen: A strategy to reoxygenate acutely and chronically hypoxic cells in vivo. *Br J Cancer* 1991; 63:109–113.

Chassagne D, Sancho-Garnier H, Charreau I, et al: Progress report of a phase II and a phase III trial with etanidazole (SR-2508): A multicentre European study. *Radiother Oncol* 1991; 20S:121–127.

Chyle V, Pollack A, Czerniak B, et al: Apoptosis and downstaging after preoperative radiotherapy for muscle-invasive bladder cancer. *Int J Radiat Oncol Biol Phys* 1996; 35:281–287.

Coderre JA, Morris GM, Micca PL, et al: Comparative assessment of single dose and fractionated beam neutron therapy. *Radiat Res* 1995; 144:310–317.

Deacon J, Peckham MJ, Steel GG: The radioresponsiveness of human tumors and the initial slope of the cell survival curve. *Radiother Oncol* 1984; 2:317–323.

del Regato JA: Our history and heritage: Claudius Regaud. *Int J Radiat Oncol Biol Phys* 1976; 1:993–1001.

Denekamp J: Changes in the rate of repopulation during multifraction irradiation of mouse skin. *Br J Radiol* 1973; 46:381–387.

Denekamp J: Cell kinetics and radiation biology. *Int J Radiat Biol* 1986; 49:357–380.

Dewey WC, Ling CC, Meyn RE: Radiation-induced apoptosis: Relevance to radiotherapy. *Int J Radiat Oncol Biol Phys* 1995; 33:781–796.

Dische S: Hypoxic cell sensitizers: Clinical developments. *Int J Radiat Oncol Biol Phys* 1989; 16:1057–1060.

Dische S, Saunders MI: Continuous, hyperfractionated, accelerated radiotherapy (CHART): An interim report upon late morbidity. *Radiother Oncol* 1989; 16:67–74.

Dische S, Saunders MI, Barrett A, et al: A randomised multicentre trial of CHART versus conventional radiotherapy in head and neck cancer. *Radiother Oncol* 1997; 44:123–136.

Ellis F: Dose, time and fractionation: A clinical hypothesis. *Clin Radiol* 1969; 20:1–7.

Ellis F: Is NSD-TDF useful to radiotherapy? *Int J Radiat Oncol Biol Phys* 1985; 11:1685–1697.

Evans SM, Jenkins WT, Joiner BJ, et al: 2-Nitroimidazole (EF5) binding predicts radiation resistance in individual 9L s.c tumors. *Cancer Res* 1996; 56:405–411.

Fertil B, Malaise EP: Inherent cellular radiosensitivity as a basic concept for human tumor radiotherapy. *Int J Radiat Oncol Biol Phys* 1981; 7:621–629.

Fertil B, Malaise EP: Radiosensitivity of human cell lines is correlated with radioresponsiveness of human tumors: Analysis of 101 published survival curves. *Int J Radiat Oncol Biol Phys* 1985; 11:1699–1708.

Fowler JF: Experimental animal results relating to time-dose relationships in radiotherapy and the "ret" concept. *Br J Radiol* 1971; 44:81–90.

Fowler JF: What next in fractionated radiotherapy? *Br J Cancer* 1984; 49(suppl VI):285–300.

Fowler JF: What to do with neutrons in radiotherapy. *Radiother Oncol* 1988; 13:233–235.

Fowler JF: The linear-quadratic formula and progress in fractionated radiotherapy. *Br J Radiol* 1989; 62:679–694.

Fowler JF, Lindstrom MJ: Loss of local control with prolongation in radiotherapy. *Int J Radiat Oncol Biol Phys* 1992; 23:457–467.

Fowler JF, Stern BE: Dose-time relationships in radiotherapy and the validity of cell survival curve models. *Br J Radiol* 1963; 36:163–173.

Fuks Z, Persaud RS, Alfieri A, et al: Basic fibroblast growth factor protects endothelial cells against radiation-induced programmed cell death in vitro and in vivo. *Cancer Res* 1994; 54:2582–2590.

Fuks Z, Weichselbaum RR: Radiation tolerance and the new biology: Growth factors in the radiation injury to the lung. *Int J Radiat Oncol Biol Phys* 1992; 24:183–184.

Fyles A, Keane TJ, Barton M, Simm J: The effect of treatment duration in the local control of cervix cancer. *Radiother Oncol* 1992; 25:273–279.

Girinsky T, Lubin R, Pignon JP, et al: Predictive value of in vitro radiosensitivity parameters in head and neck cancers and cervical carcinomas: Preliminary conclusions with local control and overall survival. *Int J Radiat Oncol Biol Phys* 1992; 25:3–7.

Haimovitz-Friedman A, Kolesnick RN, Fuks Z: Modulation of the apoptotic response: Potential for improving the outcome in clinical radiotherapy. *Semin Radiat Oncol* 1996; 6:273–283.

Hall EJ: *Radiobiology for the Radiologist,* 3d ed. Philadelphia: Lippincott; 1988.

Hallahan DE: Radiation-mediated gene expression in the pathogenesis of the clinical radiation response. *Sem Radiat Oncol* 1996; 6:250–267.

Hatanaka H, Nakagawa Y: Clinical results of long-surviving brain tumor patients who underwent boron neutron capture therapy. *Int J Radiat Oncol Biol Phys* 1994; 28:1061–1066.

Henk JM, Kunkler PB, Smith CW: Radiotherapy and hyperbaric oxygen in head and neck cancer: Final report of first controlled clinical trial. *Lancet* 1977; 313:104–105.

Hill RP: Sensitizers and radiation dose fractionation: Results and interpretations. *Int J Radiat Oncol Biol Phys* 1986; 12:1049–1054.

Hill RP, Milas L: The proportion of stem cells in murine tumors. *Int J Radiat Oncol Biol Phys* 1989; 16:513–518.

Hockel M, Schlenger K, Aral B, et al: Association between tumor hypoxia and malignant progression in advanced cancer of the uterine cervix. *Cancer Res* 1996; 56:4509–4515.

Hong JH, Chiang CS, Campbell IL, et al: Induction of acute phase gene expression by brain irradiation. *Int J Radiat Oncol Biol Phys* 1995; 33:619–626.

Horiot JC, Bontemps P, van den Bogeart W, et al: Accelerated fractionation (AF) compared to conventional fractionation (CF) improves locoregional control in the radiotherapy of advanced head and neck cancers: Results of the EORTC 22851 randomized trial. *Radiother Oncol* 1997; 44:111–122.

Horiot JC, LeFur R, N'Guyen T, et al: Hyperfractionation versus conventional fractionation in oropharyngeal carcinoma: Final analysis of a randomized trial of the EORTC cooperative group of radiotherapy. *Radiother Oncol* 1992; 25:231–241.

Horsman MR, Khalil AA, Nordsmark M, et al: Relationship between radiobiological hypoxia and direct estimates of tumor oxygenation in a mouse tumor model. *Radiother Oncol* 1993; 28:69–71.

Johansen J, Bentzen SM, Overgaard J, et al: Evidence for a positive correlation between in vitro radiosensitivity of normal human fibroblasts and the occurrence of subcutaneous fibrosis after radiotherapy. *Int J Radiat Biol* 1994; 66:407–412.

Jorgensen TJ, Shiloh Y: The ATM gene and the radiobiology of ataxia telangiectasia. *Int J Radiat Biol* 1996; 69:527–537.

Kallman RF: Reoxygenation and repopulation in irradiated tumors. *Front Radiat Ther Oncol* 1988; 22:30–49.

Kim JJ, Hao Y, Jang D, Wong CS: Lack of influence of sequence of top-up doses on repair kinetics in rat spinal cord. *Radiother Oncol* 1997; 43:211–217.

Kirk J, Gray WM, Watson ER: Cumulative radiation effect. Part I: fractionated treatment regimes. *Clin Radiol* 1971; 22:145–155.

Koh W, Bergmans KS, Rasey JS, et al: Evaluation of oxygenation status during fractionated radiotherapy in human nonsmall cell lung cancers using [F-18]fluoromisonidazole positron emission tomography. *Int J Radiat Oncol Biol Phys* 1995: 33:391–398.

Lavey RS, Dempsey WH: Erythropoietin increased hemoglobin in cancer patients during radiation therapy. *Int J Radiat Oncol Biol Phys* 1993; 27:1147–1152.

Lee D-J, Cosmatos D, Marcial VA, et al: Results of an RTOG phase III trial (RTOG 85-27) comparing radiotherapy plus etanidazole (SR-2508) with radiotherapy alone for locally advanced head and neck carcinomas. *Int J Radiat Oncol Biol Phys* 1995; 32:567–576.

Levine EL, Renehan AR, Gossiel R, et al: Apoptosis, intrinsic radiosensitivity and prediction of radiotherapy response in cervical carcinoma. *Radiother Oncol* 1995; 37:1–9.

Li YQ, Jay V, Wong CS: Oligodendrocytes in rat spinal cord undergo radiation-induced apoptosis. *Cancer Res* 1996; 56:5417–5422.

Marples B, Joiner MC: The elimination of low-dose hypersensitivity in Chinese hamster V79-379A cells by pretreatment with x-rays or hydrogen peroxide. *Radiat Res* 1995; 141:160–169.

Marshall RS, Rauth AM: Oxygen and exposure kinetics as factors influencing the cytotoxicity of porfiromycin, a mitomycin analogue in Chinese hamster ovary cells. *Cancer Res* 1988; 48:5655–5659.

Meyn RE, Stephens LC, Ang KK, et al: Heterogeneity in apoptosis development among irradiated murine tumors of different histologies. *Int J Radiat Oncol Biol* 1993; 64:583–591.

Meyn RE, Stephens LC, Milas L: Programmed cell death and radioresistance. *Cancer Metastasis Rev* 1996; 15: 119–131.

Mitchell JB, Bedford JS, Bailey SM: Dose-rate effects on the cell cycle and survival of S3-HeLa and V79 cells. *Radiat Res* 1979; 79:520–536.

Newcombe C, Van Dyk J, Hill RP: Evaluation of isoeffect formulae for predicting radiation-induced lung damage. *Radiother Oncol* 1993; 26:51–56.

Nordsmark M, Overgaard M, Overgaard J: Pretreatment oxygenation predicts radiation response in advanced squamous cell carcinoma of the head and neck. *Radiother Oncol* 1996; 41:31–39.

Orton CG, Ellis F: A simplification in the use of the NSD concept in practical radiotherapy. *Br J Radiol* 1973; 46:529–537.

Overgaard J: Clinical evaluation of nitroimidazoles as modifiers of hypoxia in solid tumor. *Oncol Res* 1995; 6:509–518.

Overgaard J, Horsman MR: Modification of hypoxia- induced radioresistance in tumors by the use of oxygen and sensitizers. *Semin Radiat Oncol* 1996; 6:10–21.

Overgaard J, Sand Hansen J, Overgaard M, et al: A randomized double-blind phase III study of nimorazole as a hypoxic radiosensitizer of primary radiotherapy in supraglottic larynx and pharynx carcinoma. Results of the Danish Head and Neck Cancer Study (DAHANKA) Protocol 5–85. *Radiother Oncol* 1998; 46:135–146.

Peters LJ, Brock WA, Travis EL: Radiation biology at clinically relevant fractions. In: Hellman S, DeVita V, eds. *Important Advances in Oncology*, Philadelphia: Lippincott; 1990:65–83.

Pickles T: Pion studies completed at TRIUMF, Vancouver Canada. *Particles News Letter* 1995; 16:11.

Potten CS: The significance of spontaneous and induced apoptosis in the gastrointestinal tract of mice. *Cancer Metastasis Rev* 1992; 11:179–195.

Raju MR: *Heavy Particle Radiotherapy*. New York: Academic Press; 1980.

Raju MR: Particle radiotherapy. *Radiat Res* 1996; 145: 391–407.

Raleigh JA, Dewhirst MW, Thrall DE: Measuring tumor hypoxia. *Semin Radiat Oncol* 1996; 6:37–45.

Rofstad EK: Human tumor xenografts in radiotherapeutic research. *Radiother Oncol* 1985; 3:35–46.

Rofstad EK, Brustad T: Radioresponsiveness of human melanoma xenografts given fractionated irradiation in vivo: Relationship to the initial slope of the cell survival curves in vitro. *Radiother Oncol* 1987; 9:45–56.

Rubin P, Johnston CJ, Williams JP, et al: A perpetual cascade of cytokines post-irradiation leads to pulmonary fibrosis. *Int J Radiat Oncol Biol Phys* 1995; 33:99–109.

Sheldon PW, Foster JL, Fowler JF: Radiosensitization of C_3H mouse mammary tumors by a 2-nitroimidazole drug. *Br J Cancer* 1974; 30:560–565.

Shinohara C, Gobbel GT, Lamborn KR, et al: Apoptosis in the subependyma of young adult rats after single and fractionated doses of x-rays. *Cancer Res* 1997; 57: 2694–2702.

Siemann DW, Hill RP, Bush RS: Smoking: The influence of carboxy-hemoglobin (HbCO) on tumor oxygenation and response to radiation. *Int J Radiat Oncol Biol Phys* 1978; 4:657–662.

Slater JM, Slater JD, Archambeau JO: Proton therapy for cranial base tumors. *J Craniofac Surg* 1995; 6:24–26.

Steel GG, Down JD, Peacock JH, Stephens TC: Dose-rate effects and the repair of radiation damage. *Radiother Oncol* 1986; 5:321–331.

Stephens LC, Schultheiss TE, Price RE, et al: Radiation apoptosis of serous acinar cells of salivary and lacrimal glands. *Cancer* 1991a; 67:1539–1543.

Stephens LC, Ang KK, Schultheiss TE, et al: Apoptosis in irradiated murine tumors. *Radiat Res* 1991b; 127: 308–316.

Stewart FA, Oussoren Y, Van Tinteren H, et al: Loss of re-irradiation tolerance in the kidney with increasing time after single and fractionated partial tolerance doses. *Int J Radiat Biol* 1994; 66:169–179.

Stone HB, Brown JM, Philips TL, et al: Oxygen in human tumors: Correlations between methods of measurement and response to therapy. *Radiat Res* 1993; 136: 422–434.

Strandqvist M: Studien uber die kumulative Wirkung der Rontgenstrahlen bei Fracktionierung. *Acta Radiol* 1944; 55:1–300.

Suit HD, Urie M: Proton beams in radiation therapy. *J Natl Cancer Inst* 1992; 84:155–164.

Suit HD, Howes AE, Hunter N: Dependence of response of a C_3H mammary carcinoma to fractionated irradiation on fractionation number and intertreatment interval. *Radiat Res* 1977; 72:440–454.

Tannock IF: Combined modality treatment with radiotherapy and chemotherapy. *Radiother Oncol* 1989; 16: 83–101.

Terry NHA, Tucker SL, Travis EL: Time course of loss of residual radiation damage in murine skin assessed by retreatment. *Int J Radiat Biol* 1989; 55:271–283.

Thames HD: Repair kinetics in tissues: alternative models. *Radiother Oncol* 1989; 14:321–327.

Thames HD, Withers HR, Peters LJ, Fletcher GH: Changes in early and late radiation responses with altered dose fractionation: Implications for dose-survival relationships. *Int J Radiat Oncol Biol Phys* 1982; 8: 219–226.

Thames HD, Bentzen SM, Turesson I, et al: Time-dose factors in radiotherapy: A review of the human data. *Radiother Oncol* 1990; 19:219–235.

Trott KR: Cell repopulation and overall treatment time. *Int J Radiat Oncol Biol Phys* 1990; 19:1071–1075.

Trott KR, Kummermehr J: What is known about tumor proliferation rates to choose between accelerated fractionation or hyperfractionation? *Radiother Oncol* 1985; 3:1–9.

Tucker SL, Turesson I, Thames HD: Evidence for individual differences in the radiosensitivity of human skin. *Eur J Cancer* 1992; 28A:1783–1791.

Watson ER, Halnan KE, Dische S, et al: Hyperbaric oxygen and radiotherapy: A Medical Research Council trial in carcinoma of the cervix. *Br J Radiol* 1978; 51: 879–887.

Wheeler JA, Stephens LC, Tomos C, et al: Apoptosis as a predictor of tumor response to radiation in stage 1B cervical carcinoma. *Int J Radiat Oncol Biol Phys* 1995; 32:1487–1493.

Wilson GD, Dische S, Saunders MI: Studies with bromo-deoxyuridine in head and neck cancer and accelerated radiotherapy. *Radiother Oncol* 1995; 36:189–197.

Wilson GD, McNally NJ, Dische S, et al: Measurement of cell kinetics in human tumors in vivo using bromo-deoxyuridine incorporation and flow cytometry. *Br J Cancer* 1988; 58:423–431.

Withers HR, Mason KA: The kinetics of recovery in irradiated colonic mucosa of the mouse. *Cancer* 1974; 34: 896–903.

Withers HR, Peters JL, Taylor JM, et al: Local control of carcinoma of the tonsil by radiation therapy: an analysis of patterns of fractionation in nine institutions. *Int J Radiat Oncol Biol Phys* 1995; 33:549–562.

Withers HR, Taylor JMG, Maciejewski B: The hazard of accelerated tumor clonogen repopulation during radiotherapy. *Acta Oncol* 1988; 27:131–146.

Wong CS, Hao Y: Long term recovery kinetics of radiation damage in rat spinal cord. *Int J Radiat Oncol Biol Phys* 1997; 33:171–179.

Wong CS, Minkin S, Hill RP: Linear-quadratic model underestimates sparing effect of small doses per fraction in rat spinal cord. *Radiother Oncol* 1992; 23:176–184.

Wouters BG, Brown JM: Cells at intermediate oxygen levels can be more important than the "hypoxic fraction" in determining the response to fractionated radiotherapy. *Radiat Res* 1997; 147:541–550.

Wyllie AH, Kerr JFR, Currie AR: Cell death: The significance of apoptosis. *Int Rev Cytol* 1980; 68:251–306.

Zackrisson B, Franzen L, Henriksson R, et al: Acute effects of accelerated radiotherapy in combination with carbogen breathing and nicotinamide (ARCON). *Acta Oncol* 1994; 33(4):377–381.

Zywietz F, Reeker W, Kochs E: Tumor oxygenation in a transplanted rat rhabdomyosarcoma during fractionated irradiation. *Int J Radiat Oncol Biol Phys* 1995; 32:1391–1400.

BIBLIOGRAPHY

Awwad HK: *Radiation Oncology: Radiobiological and Physiological Perspectives.* Dordrecht: Kluwer; 1990.

Hall EJ: *Radiobiology for the Radiologist,* 4th ed. Philadelphia: Lippincott; 1994.

Hallahan DE, ed. Molecular biology and its clinical implications. *Semin Radiat Oncol* 1996; 6:243–328.

Raleigh TA, ed. Hypoxia and its clinical significance. *Sem Radiat Oncol* 1996; 6:1–70.

Steel GG(ed): *Basic Clinical Radiobiology.* 2nd ed. London, England: Edward Arnold; 1997.

Thames HD, Hendry JH: *Fractionation in Radiotherapy.* London: Taylor and Francis; 1987.

15

Cellular and Molecular Basis of Chemotherapy

Michael J. Boyer and Ian F. Tannock

15.1 INTRODUCTION

15.2 CELLULAR EFFECTS OF DRUGS
    15.2.1 Types of Cell Damage
    15.2.2 Nonclonogenic Assays
    15.2.3 Colony-Forming Assays and Cell-Survival Curves
    15.2.4 Cell-Cycle Effects

15.3 EFFECTS OF DRUGS AGAINST TUMORS
    15.3.1 In Situ Assessment
    15.3.2 Xenografts
    15.3.3 Predictive Assays for Tumor Response
    15.3.4 Influence of Tumor Microenvironment

15.4 DRUG TOXICITY
    15.4.1 Bone Marrow

15.4.2 High-Dose Chemotherapy
    with Stem-Cell Transplantation
15.4.3 Toxicity to Other Proliferative Tissues
15.4.4 Determinants of Normal-Tissue Toxicity
15.4.5 Nausea and Vomiting
15.4.6 Drugs as Carcinogens

15.5 DISCOVERY AND DESIGN OF NEW ANTICANCER DRUGS
    15.5.1 Screening for Activity of New Compounds
    15.5.2 Rational Design of New Anticancer Drugs
    15.5.3 New Targets for Cancer Chemotherapy

15.6 SUMMARY

REFERENCES

15.1 INTRODUCTION

This chapter is the first of three dealing with the scientific basis for cancer chemotherapy. It introduces the more important anticancer drugs and their biologic properties, experimental methods used to determine their activity, and some of the methods used to discover and design new drugs; Chap. 16 describes the pharmacology of anticancer drugs, and Chap. 17 gives an overview of experimental chemotherapy, with particular emphasis on mechanisms of drug resistance.

The first documented clinical use of chemotherapy was in 1942, when the alkylating agent nitrogen mustard was used to obtain a brief clinical remission in a patient with lymphoma (Gilman, 1963). About 40 cytotoxic drugs (excluding hormonal agents) are currently (1997) licensed for use in North America

as anticancer drugs, and several new agents are undergoing clinical trials.

Anticancer drugs can be classified into a number of families (see Fig. 15.1) based on their biochemical activities or their origins. These families include the alkylating agents, antimetabolites, and several types of natural products and their derivatives. When a lead compound is shown to have activity as an anticancer drug, numerous drugs with related structures are synthesized and their biologic activities assessed. Following the initial use of nitrogen mustard, this study of structure-activity relationships produced several alkylating agents that are in current clinical use, such as cyclophosphamide and melphalan. Alkylating agents have one or two side chains that are electron-deficient and will bind to electron-rich groups of biologic molecules. Their major mechanism of lethal activity is thought to in-

Alkylating Agents

Nitrogen Mustard
Chlorambucil
Melphalan
Cyclophosphamide
Mitomycin C
Ifosfamide
Busulfan
Nitrosoureas
  BCNU
  CCNU
  Methyl CCNU

Antimetabolites

Methotrexate
5-Fluorouracil
Cytosine Arabinoside
6-Thioguanine
6-Mercaptopurine
Gemcitabine

Natural Products and their Derivatives

Anthracyclines
  Doxorubicin
  Daunorubicin
  Epirubicin
Mitoxantrone
Actinomycin D
Bleomycin

Vinca Alkaloids
  Vinblastine
  Vincristine
  Vindesine
  Vinorelbine
Etoposide (VP-16)
Camptothecins

Taxanes
  Paclitaxel
  Docetaxel

Miscellaneous Agents

Cisplatin
Carboplatin
Dacarbazine (DTIC)

Figure 15.1. Important drugs used in cancer chemotherapy.

volve interaction with bases in DNA (Chap. 16, Sec. 16.3).

The development of a second major class of compounds followed the unraveling of biochemical pathways in intermediate metabolism and represented the first example of rational drug design as applied to anticancer agents. Drugs that resembled normal metabolites and could compete as substrates for enzyme activity were synthesized (Chap. 16, Sec. 16.4). Examples of these antimetabolites (Fig. 15.1) are methotrexate (an analogue of the vitamin folic acid, which is essential for the transfer of methyl groups in several biosynthetic reactions) and 5-fluorouracil (which closely resembles the bases thymine and uracil, which are constituents of DNA and RNA, respectively). Most antimetabolites inhibit nucleic acid synthesis either directly or indirectly and tend to be active mainly against proliferating cells.

Other new drugs are heterogeneous and include derivatives of naturally occurring species (antibiotics) and synthesized chemicals (e.g., cisplatin). Several naturally occurring compounds have important antitumor activity. The anthracyclines, such as doxorubicin (Adriamycin), are planar multiring structures that are thought to intercalate between turns of the double helix in DNA; they and drugs

such as etoposide also bind to DNA and inhibit the enzyme topoisomerase II, which catalyzes the orderly breaking of DNA strands, unwinding of DNA, and religation during DNA synthesis or RNA transcription (Chap. 16, Sec. 16.5). Newer drugs (camptothecins) inhibit the action of the enzyme topoisomerase I. The vinca alkaloids (e.g., vincristine and vinblastine) are derived from the periwinkle plant; they bind to tubulin and disrupt the mitotic spindle. The taxanes (paclitaxel and docetaxel) are also naturally derived compounds that act by stabilizing microtubules. Platinum-based compounds (cisplatin, carboplatin, and others) are very active compounds derived by chemical synthesis; their activity is thought to be due to their alkylating properties. The pharmacology of each of these compounds is reviewed in Chap. 16.

15.2 CELLULAR EFFECTS OF DRUGS

15.2.1 Types of Cell Damage

The concept that tumors contain a population of cells, known as stem cells, which have a very large potential for cell proliferation, was introduced in Chap. 7, Sec. 7.6.2. Stem cells may constitute only a small proportion of the total cells in a human tumor; but since the aim of tumor treatment is cure or long-term remission, the critical test of drug effects against tumors is lethality for stem cells. In practice, the survival of such cells after treatment is assessed by their ability to produce colonies of progeny of a defined minimum size. Thus, measurement of cell survival after drug treatment is analogous to that for radiation, and involves the use of a clonogenic assay (see Chap. 13, Secs. 13.3.4 and 13.3.5). Other types of damage, leading to transient changes in cell metabolism and proliferation and loss of nonclonogenic cells, occur frequently after drug treatment. These effects, which can lead to normal-tissue toxicity (Sec. 15.4), may contribute to tumor remission (i.e., to transient changes in tumor volume) but not to cure.

15.2.2 Nonclonogenic Assays

Many investigators have sought to assess the cellular toxicity of anticancer drugs by a variety of methods that do not measure reproductive potential in a clonogenic assay (see Table 15.1).

Each of the end points in Table 15.1 has been proposed as a method for predicting the inhibition of reproductive potential by drugs without the need to do clonogenic assays. In general, these methods, as compared with clonogenic assays, have the advan-

Table 15.1. Nonclonogenic Assays Used to Assess
Drug Activity

- Microscopic evidence of cell damage
- Damage to cell membranes, as measured by failure to exclude dyes such as trypan blue, or loss of radioactivity (e.g., ^{51}Cr) from prelabeled cells
- Impairment of macromolecular synthesis, usually assessed by measuring the uptake of ^3H-thymidine into DNA, ^3H-uridine into RNA, or ^3H-amino acids into proteins
- Inhibition of cell growth under defined conditions, which may be assessed in multiple samples by automated methods (e.g., by the MTT assay; see text)
- Changes in proliferative parameters such as thymidine-labeling index or S-phase fraction assessed by flow cytometry
- Formation of micronuclei in cells
- Exchange of sister chromatids detected at mitosis as an assay of damage to DNA
- Assays of apoptosis (by morphologic criteria or by flow cytometry)

tage of providing results rapidly. Unfortunately, many of these end points correlate poorly with loss of reproductive integrity as measured by a clonogenic assay.

If the assessment of toxicity is delayed for a few hours to days after drug exposure, thereby allowing for the expression of lethal damage and/or the proliferation of surviving cells, then exclusion of dye from intact cells or assessment of metabolic activity can give reasonable correlations with a colony-forming assay (Weisenthal et al., 1983; Scheithauer et al., 1986). The MTT assay depends on the reduction of a tetrazolium-based compound to a blue formazan product by living but not dead cells (Carmichael et al., 1987). The amount of reduced product is quantitated in an automated system using multiple tissue-culture wells in which cells have been exposed to a range of doses of the drugs under test. Another dye that has been found to be useful in quantitating cell number is sulforhodamine B (SRB), a pink anionic dye that binds to basic amino acids of fixed cells such that dye intensity is linearly related to the number of cells (Rubinstein et al., 1990; Skehan et al., 1990). These methods are being used in the screening of new agents (Sec. 15.5.1). Technical factors must be optimized for each cell type studied, ideally by comparing with a clonogenic assay, because results have been shown to vary when applied to different types of cells.

Following treatment with drugs many cells undergo apoptosis (see Chap. 7, Sec. 7.3). Apoptosis

may be quantitated by morphologic criteria or by using flow cytometric methods to detect breaks in DNA leading to an "apoptotic index." While this measure of the proportion of cells undergoing apoptosis may give a broad indication of drug effectiveness, apoptosis is a dynamic process and results are very dependent on the time after treatment that observations are made (Potten, 1996).

A general problem with most of the nonclonogenic assays is that they lead to some measure of cell death or damage that is quantitated on a linear scale from 0 to 100 percent. Major effects of drugs against a tumor-cell population require reduction in cell survival by several orders of magnitude; this is measured most easily by observation of colony formation from serial dilutions of cells, as described in Sec. 15.2.3. Even when cell survival (assessed by colony formation) is less than 1 percent, many of the cells in the population appear to be "viable" by morphologic or metabolic criteria at short intervals after treatment.

15.2.3 Colony-Forming Assays and Cell-Survival Curves

Colony-forming assays and others that allow quantitation of stem cells were described in detail in Chap. 13, Secs. 13.3.4 and 13.3.5, as methods for assessment of the lethal effects of radiation. The same assays are often used for assessing the lethal effects of drugs (Table 15.2). The major modification for assessment of drug effects is that, whereas even high doses of radiation may be delivered over a few seconds or minutes, some drugs may require exposures of several hours to exert lethal effects on cells. Metabolism of the drug to active or inactive products during the exposure period may thus influence cell survival. The

Table 15.2. Assays Used to Quantitate Stem Cells after Drug Treatment

- Colony formation on plastic or glass in liquid medium
- Colony formation in semisolid medium such as dilute agar or methylcellulose
- Serial dilution of cells into multiwell plates to establish the minimum number of cells that will lead to growth
- Serial dilutions of cells implanted into syngeneic animals to establish the TD_{50} (i.e., the number of cells that lead to growth of tumors in 50 percent of animals)
- Formation of spleen colonies after intravenous injection of hematologic cells into irradiated mice
- Formation of metastatic lung colonies after intravenous injection of tumor cells

biologic effectiveness of a drug is dependent on both the concentration of the drug and the duration of exposure. Thus, it is usual to relate cell survival after drug treatment to both the drug concentration (for a constant exposure time) and to the duration of exposure (at a constant drug concentration).

The simplest assay for assessing drug-induced lethality is to treat cells that will grow in tissue culture with the drug to be tested, followed by plating of different dilutions of cells in Petri dishes. Colony-forming assays in culture may also be used to study drug effects in vivo by using tumors whose cells have the ability to generate colonies in vitro following removal and dissociation of the tumor. Assessment of colony formation after treatment of transplanted tumors in vivo allows for drug metabolism and other aspects of drug pharmacology to be assessed. Toxicity to colony-forming cells of bone marrow can also be determined by removal and culture of marrow in the same experiment.

For some drugs, the proportion of cells surviving treatment is found to be exponentially related to drug concentration. As in the analysis of radiation effects (Chap. 13, Sec. 13.4.1), cell survival curves are often plotted using a logarithmic axis for cell survival and a linear axis for either drug concentration (using a constant exposure time) or for exposure time to a constant drug concentration; exponential survival curves are then represented by a straight line (Fig. 15.2). Exponential cell survival

curves are expected if cell lethality is due to a simple chemical interaction between molecules of the drug and a molecular "target" in the cell. The relationship is then analogous to the interaction of ionizing events due to radiation with a molecular target (thought to be DNA).

Tumors and normal tissues may be expected to contain cells that are heterogeneous with respect to proliferative rate and intrinsic drug sensitivity, which depends on many factors including drug uptake and retention, and the proficiency for repair of drug-induced damage. In addition, limited diffusion of some drugs and changes in activity due to metabolism may lead to delivery of varying drug doses to cells within the population. Each of these factors may influence the shape of the cell-survival curve after drug treatment, so that departures from an exponential relationship between cell survival and dose occur commonly. As discussed in subsequent sections, the shape of the dose-survival relationship may give important clues to mechanisms underlying drug activity.

15.2.4 Cell-Cycle Effects

If bone marrow from a mouse is injected into an irradiated genetically identical animal, the stem cells will generate colonies in the spleen after a few days (Till and McCulloch, 1961). This spleen-colony assay has been used to compare the effects of drugs on the cell survival of slowly proliferating bone marrow precursors (CFU-S) with either rapidly proliferating murine lymphoma cells or with CFU-S that have been induced to proliferate (e.g., Bruce et al., 1966; Van Putten et al., 1972). Two basic types of survival curve were obtained. For some drugs, including most of the alkylating agents and 5-fluorouracil, cell survival was exponentially related to dose, and most drugs had greater activities against proliferating cells (Fig. 15.2A). For other drugs, survival decreased exponentially at low drug doses, but if the exposure time was short there was no further decrease in survival above a threshold drug concentration, leading to a plateau in the cell-survival curve (Fig. 15.2B). The plateau level of cell survival was always lower for rapidly proliferating cells. Drugs that show this pattern of survival are now known to act primarily at one phase of the cell cycle (see below); they include most of the antimetabolites and tubulin-binding agents such as methotrexate, cytosine arabinoside, 6-thioguanine, 6-mercaptopurine, vincristine, and vinblastine. (The taxanes, which also bind tubulin, appear to have relative but not absolute specificity for cycling cells.) An in-

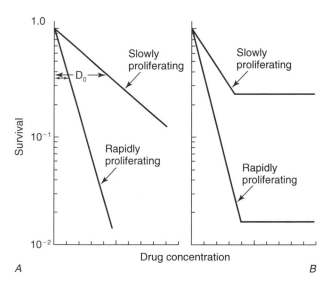

Figure 15.2. Model cell-survival curves for rapidly and slowly proliferating cells generated following a short duration of exposure to varying concentrations of drugs *(A)* for drugs that are not cell cycle–phase specific; *(B)* for drugs that are active in only certain phases of the cell cycle.

crease in concentration of cell cycle–specific drugs with a short exposure time gives no further cell kill once a threshold is exceeded, since all cells in the drug-sensitive phase of the cycle are killed and those in the other phases of the cell cycle are not affected. An increase in exposure time with constant drug concentration may allow more cells to enter the drug-sensitive phase, leading to an exponential relationship between cell survival and exposure time (Bruce et al., 1969). However, many drugs also inhibit the transit of surviving cells through the cell cycle (and hence their progression into the sensitive phase of the cycle).

Similar techniques can be applied in vitro to study drug effects on cells with different rates of proliferation. Most drugs have greater sensitivity for rapidly proliferating (exponentially growing) cells than for cells that are proliferating slowly (plateau phase). Exceptions to this include the nitrosoureas (BCNU, CCNU), bleomycin, and cisplatin, which show similar effects against proliferating and non-proliferating cells (Twentyman and Bleehan, 1975).

For drugs that show an exponential relationship between cell survival and dose, the relative sensitivity of rapidly and slowly proliferating cells may be expressed as the ratio of doses required to achieve the same level of cell kill (Fig. 15.2A). Values of this ratio generally lie between 1.0 and 2.0 for alkylating agents, but cyclophosphamide has greater specificity for cycling cells with values in the range of 2.0 to 5.0 when tested using the spleen colony assay. Doxorubicin, 5-fluorouracil, and bleomycin also show marked selectivity for proliferating cells (data reviewed in Tannock, 1978). Thus, the proliferative rate of the cell population being treated is a major determinant of drug activity.

Information about the activities of drugs at different phases of the cell cycle has been obtained by treatment of cells that have been synchronized in tissue culture (e.g., Donaldson et al., 1994; see also Chap. 13, Sec. 13.5.3). As cells progress in a cohort around the cell cycle, drug administration may be timed to treat a population that is enriched for cells in G1, S, G2, or mitotic phase. Alternative methods for studying drug effects involve separation of asynchronous cells on the basis of cell-cycle phase either before or immediately after drug treatment, followed by assessment of colony formation. Techniques that have been used for this purpose include separation of cells on the basis of DNA content (by flow cytometry; see Chap. 7, Sec. 7.4.3) or separation by size or density using centrifugation (Donaldson et al., 1994).

Most drugs show variations in lethal toxicity around the cell cycle (e.g., Mauro and Madoc-Jones, 1970; Donaldson et al., 1994; Hennequin et al., 1995; Fig. 15.3). Many of the antimetabolites exert lethal toxicity only for cells that are synthesizing DNA, whereas methotrexate and doxorubicin have maximum toxicity for S-phase cells but have some activity during other phases of the cycle. Studies using thymidine labeling or flow cytometry have demonstrated that many of these drugs also inhibit the onset or continuation of DNA synthesis in cells that survive treatment. Such studies of nonlethal progression delay are always subject to problems of interpretation because of difficulty in recognizing surviving cells as opposed to lethally damaged cells prior to their lysis. Vincristine and vinblastine are known to disrupt formation of the mitotic spindle, leading to arrest of cells in mitosis. Experiments with synchronized cells have shown, however, that lethal effects of these drugs occur when cells are in S phase, presumably when formation of the mitotic spindle is initiated. Docetaxel and paclitaxel, which act to stabilize tubulin, have somewhat different cell-cycle dependence: docetaxel is maximally toxic in S phase, whereas paclitaxel shows increasing toxicity for cells as they progress from S phase through G2 phase to mitosis (Donaldson et al., 1994; Hennequin et al., 1995). Many alkylating agents (e.g., nitrogen mustard, melphalan) have a phase activity

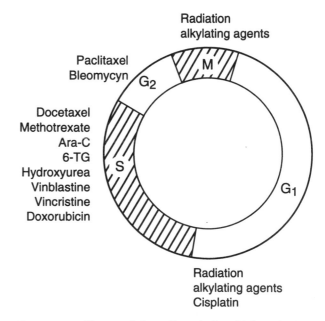

Figure 15.3. Phases of the cell cycle in which anticancer drugs show selective lethal toxicity. Ara-C = cytosine arabinoside; 6-TG = 6-thioguanine.

similar to that observed for radiation (see Chap. 13, Sec. 13.5.3), with two peaks of maximum lethal activity—one in G2/M phase and one near the G1-phase/S-phase boundary. Cisplatin also appears to exert maximum lethal activity in late G1 phase (Donaldson et al., 1994).

The relative specificity of most drugs for one or more phases of the cell cycle leaves a partly synchronized population of surviving cells after treatment. Several investigators have proposed that such synchrony may allow scheduling of anticancer drugs to maximize killing of tumor cells by giving subsequent treatments when a large number of survivors are again in a drug-sensitive phase. In practice, the wide variation of cell-cycle times observed in vivo leads to rapid loss of synchrony, and, together with heterogeneity of the tumor-cell population and of drug distribution, make optimal treatment scheduling difficult to apply (Tannock, 1978). Furthermore, any such scheduling would have to avoid increased toxicity to critical normal tissues.

15.3 EFFECTS OF DRUGS AGAINST TUMORS

15.3.1 In Situ Assessment

The clonogenic assays described in the preceding sections have the advantage that they seek to assess directly the reproductive death of cells after drug treatment. When used to study drug treatment in vivo, they require removal of tissue and production of a suspension of single cells, followed by study of colony formation in an environment that differs markedly from that in a tumor or normal tissue that is left in situ after treatment. These processes may (1) add to cellular damage caused by drugs, (2) rescue cells that would have died in situ but are "rescued" by removal into a tissue culture environment, and (3) bias the results by assessment only of cells that can proliferate in the new environment. In situ assays avoid such problems, but do not provide a direct assessment of cell survival after drug treatment (Kallman, 1987). In situ assays that have been used to assess the effects of drugs on tumors include the duration of animal survival after treatment or drug-induced delay in tumor growth.

The influence of a drug on survival of animals (usually mice) bearing syngeneic transplanted tumors has been used as a method for screening of new agents. In a typical experiment, a number of mice are implanted with identical numbers of tumor cells; they are randomly assigned to drug treatment and control groups and their survival time is recorded. The use of animal survival to predict cell lethality is complicated by nonlethal effects of drugs that can delay tumor growth and by toxic effects of drugs on normal tissues that tend to shorten animal survival. Assessment of relative effects of drugs on tumor and normal tissues in one experiment has been claimed to offer an advantage for drug screening. Revised attitudes to the ethics of animal experimentation, however, have resulted in the severe curtailing of such experiments and their replacement by more humane methods.

Comparison of tumor growth in treated and untreated animals is the preferred in situ method for assessing drug effects against solid tumors in animals (Fig. 15.4A). The determination of tumor shrinkage and delay in regrowth models the clinical assessment of tumor remission. It is more humane, since animals can be killed painlessly before their (regrowing) tumors are sufficiently large to cause discomfort. The effect of drugs to cause delay in tumor growth is usually studied in groups of animals that received different doses of drugs. A dose-response curve can then be generated to relate drug dose with some measure of growth delay (e.g., the time for the tumor to grow to a fixed volume; Fig. 15.4B). Experiments with many drugs and tumors lead to regrowth curves after treatment that are parallel to (but displaced from) the growth curve for untreated controls. Under these conditions, the shape of the dose-response curve is independent of the end point selected as a measure of growth delay. Treatment with other drugs may lead to tumor regrowth that is slower than in controls, perhaps because of damage to blood vessels. Growth delay may then be due not only to lethal effects against tumor stem cells but also to the effect of the drug on other cells that may be present in the tumor as well as nonlethal effects that may lead to slower proliferation of tumor cells. Likewise, partial remission of human tumors after drug treatment does not necessarily imply major lethal effects of the drugs for the tumor cells.

15.3.2 Xenografts

Human tumors may be implanted into immune-deficient mice to generate xenografts and study their responsiveness to drugs in vivo (Arnold et al., 1996). The most widely used host for xenografting of human tumors is the congenitally athymic nude mouse. The nude mouse is not a perfect host, since it may produce antibodies and also has large numbers of natural killer cells that may inhibit tumor growth. Alternative hosts include mice with severe

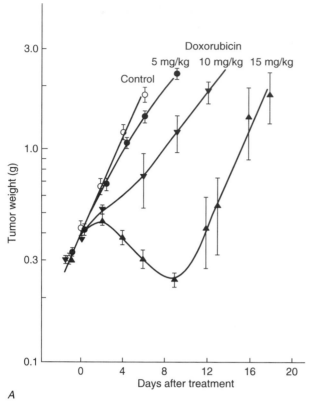

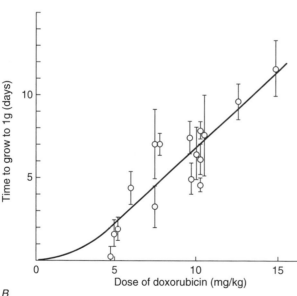

Figure 15.4. *A.* Illustration of tumor growth curves for treatment of an experimental tumor with doxorubicin. Tumor weight was estimated by prior calibration with measurements of tumor diameter. Note that growth curves after drug treatment are not always parallel to the growth curve for controls and that interanimal variation may lead to large standard errors. *B.* Dose-response curve relating drug dose to the time for tumors to grow from size at treatment (~0.4 g) to 1 g. The curve was obtained from multiple experiments similar to that shown in Fig. 15.4A. (Adapted from Tannock, 1982.)

combined immune deficiency (SCID). These mice may be better recipients for transplanted human tissues and have allowed the establishment of grafts of lymphoid and hematopoietic tissues, as well as of solid tumors (von Kalle et al., 1992).

Xenografts have the advantage that they may have characteristics similar to those of the human tumors from which they are derived (e.g., enzyme activities or levels of detoxifying molecules). They have been useful in assessing the activities of both new and established drugs against human tumors of varying origins and histologic types. Usually, drug effects are assessed by delay in tumor growth. There is a correlation between response to drugs of such xenografts and the clinical response of human tumors of the same histologic type to the same drugs. Xenografts grown using cell lines derived from common types of human tumor (e.g., breast, colon, lung) are used in the preclinical evaluation of new agents (Sec. 15.5.1).

15.3.3 Predictive Assays for Tumor Response

Anticancer drugs are toxic (Sec. 15.4) and many tumors do not respond to empirically chosen chemotherapy. Consequently, a reliable in vitro assay that could predict tumor responsiveness to drugs would be very valuable. Such predictive assays would be analogous to those used in selecting antibiotics to treat bacterial infections, where sensitivity of the bacteria to a range of antibiotics can be assessed in culture. Predictive assays employing a variety of the end points listed in Table 15.1 have been used to assess the effects of anticancer drugs against tumor biopsies since the early days of chemotherapy. Such tests have been quite successful in predicting clinical resistance (i.e., if a drug had no effect in the assay, it had no therapeutic effect in the patient donating the biopsy). Unfortunately the assays have had less success in predicting those tumors that were sensitive to drugs. For example, an assay based on the efficacies of drugs in inhibiting DNA synthesis did not lead to an improvement in survival of patients with ovarian or lung cancer when drugs selected by the in vitro assay were compared with empirical treatment (or to no adjuvant therapy) in randomized clinical trials (Nissen et al., 1978).

Courtenay et al. (1976) and Hamburger and Salmon (1977) have developed assays using semi-solid agar and enriched media that support colony growth from cell suspensions derived from a variety of human tumors (see also Chap. 7, Sec. 7.6.2). These assays have several limitations relating to the suitability of the growth conditions and to other factors such as preparing suspensions of single cells. The presence of even a small number of clumps of cells can cause artifacts, since it is difficult to distinguish residual clumps from colonies growing from single cells (Selby et al., 1983). Clonogenic assays have the advantage, however, that they assess directly the effects of drugs on colony-forming cells from human tumors, and, when optimized, might be expected to predict long-term benefit from treatment.

Several nonclonogenic assays have been re-evaluated for their ability to predict clinical response. One assay involves the plating of cells on a special matrix (cell adhesive matrix, or CAM), which appears to be optimal for the selection and growth of tumor cells (Ajani et al., 1987). Growth can then be assessed with and without drug exposure by staining multiwell plates and estimating cell number by automated densitometry. The assay does not require a suspension of single cells to initiate growth and gives a reasonable correlation with clonogenic assays in experimental systems.

The problems associated with the use of predictive assays are summarized in Table 15.3. At present,

Table 15.3. Problems Associated with the Use of In Vitro Assays to Predict the Response of Human Tumors to Chemotherapy

- Often only a low proportion of tumor cells will grow in culture. This limits the range of the assay and excludes some tumors from being assessed.

- The tissue culture environment may lead to selective growth of only some subpopulations of cells from a heterogeneous tumor.

- The assays must utilize a limited number of fixed concentration-×-time exposures, which do not necessarily match the time variation of drug exposure in vivo (often unknown).

- Patients are treated most often with drugs in combination. It is difficult to test drug combinations in vitro and difficult to relate sensitivity to individual drugs with clinical response to combination treatment.

- The predictive value of an assay depends on the prevalence of drug resistance or sensitivity among the patients tested. Thus assays are useful only if the predictive value for drug resistance (or sensitivity) exceeds its prevalence among the treated patients (probability of resistance is frequently > 80 percent).

- The ability of many assays to predict cell killing has not been validated by using a positive control, such as radiation, where the relationship between survival and dose may be predicted.

- There is potential for large errors in assessment of "response" in both the assay and in patients.

both the human tumor clonogenic assays and some nonclonogenic assays have demonstrated the following:

1. In vitro predictive assays can give information in up to 70 percent of tumors evaluated.
2. Cells from human tumors of differing histologic types and sites of origin have a range of responsiveness to in vitro assays that is similar to the range of clinical responsiveness to drug treatment.
3. An assay that predicts for drug resistance may be correct for at least 90 percent of tumors, whereas the prediction of clinical drug sensitivity is, at best, correct in about 70 percent of patients (Von Hoff, 1990). In vitro exposure to very high doses of drugs can give assays that are highly specific in predicting clinical resistance (Kern and Weisenthal, 1990), but there is a decrease in detection of clinical sensitivity.
4. The response rate of tumors in patients treated with drugs selected by predictive assays is higher than that in patients treated empirically (Von Hoff et al., 1991; Gazdar et al., 1990). As yet, however, there has been no evidence that the assays lead to improved survival of patients, and their use outside a research setting should await their validation in prospective, randomized clinical trials.

15.3.4 Influence of Tumor Microenvironment

Many tumors are known to have a poorly organized vascular system, so that some tumor cells are deficient in oxygen and other nutrients. Hypoxic cells are known to be resistant to radiation (Chap. 13, Sec. 13.5.2) and to the activity of several anticancer drugs. This protection may occur because of limited penetration of drugs from tumor blood vessels and because nutrient-deprived cells tend to proliferate slowly (Fig. 15.5; Chap. 7, Sec. 7.6.3). The nutritional state of the cells is also known to influence directly the cellular uptake, metabolism, and toxicity of some anticancer drugs (Teicher, 1994).

Penetration of drugs into tissue and toxicity of drugs for cells in different nutritional microenvironments has been studied in spheroids (Sutherland, 1988; Erlanson et al., 1992; Durand, 1994). Spheroids are spherical aggregates of tumor cells resembling tumor nodules that will grow in suspension culture (Chap. 7, Sec. 7.6.3). More recently, a simpler technique for studying drug penetration through tissue has been devised (Fig. 15.6; Cowan et al., 1996; Hicks et al., 1997). In this multicellular membrane method, tumor cells are grown as a solid

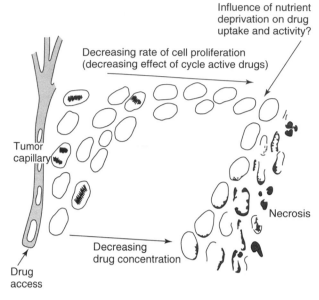

Figure 15.5. Influence of drug diffusion and nutrient environment on drug activity for cells within solid tumors.

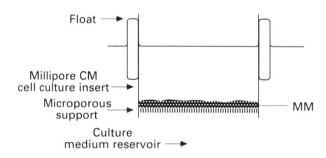

A

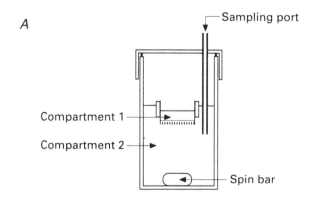

B

Figure 15.6. The multilayer-membrane (MM) method. *A.* Cells are grown as a solid layer on a semipermeable membrane. *B.* In studies of drug penetration, drug is added to medium in compartment 1; its appearance in compartment 2 is studied as a function of time. (Reproduced from Cowan et al., 1996, with permission.)

layer of tissue (~200 μm in thickness) on a semipermeable support membrane that separates two compartments containing tissue culture medium. Drug penetration is then measured by the rate of appearance of drug in the lower compartment (compartment 2 of Fig. 15.6). Drug penetration is compared with (1) diffusion across the semipermeable membrane in the absence of a layer of tissue, and (2) penetration of a control substance such as ^{14}C sucrose. There is evidence (at present largely from spheroids) that several drugs have poor penetration into tissue; these include doxorubicin, methotrexate, vinblastine, vincristine, and paclitaxel.

Factors that may influence drug delivery to cells within solid tumors include variability in blood flow (Chap. 9, Sec. 9.3.1), permeability of blood vessel walls to anticancer drugs, and the interstitial fluid pressure within solid tumors. Several investigators have established that the interstitial pressure in a variety of solid tumors in humans and animals is high (typically 4 to 50 mmHg in tumors, compared with ~2 mmHg in normal tissues), and this may provide an additional barrier to drug penetration (e.g., Less et al., 1992). Various agents that decrease interstitial pressure, such as dexamethasone (given often as an antiemetic drug to patients), or intermittent modulation of systemic blood pressure might improve drug delivery (Kristjansen et al., 1993; Netti et al., 1995).

The relationship between the toxicity of an anticancer drug and depth of penetration in tissue may be studied in spheroids or in experimental tumors by using a fluorescent dye that sets up a decreasing gradient of fluorescence with increasing distance from tumor capillaries or from the surface of the spheroid (Chaplin et al., 1985; Durand 1989, 1994; Fig. 15.7). For tumors, the method involves intravenous injection of a fluorescent dye (Hoechst 33342) at a dose that is not toxic to cells, followed by removal and disaggregation of the tumor. Spheroids are exposed to the dye in medium. Since the dye binds tightly to DNA, cells at different depths of penetration can be separated on the basis of their fluorescence using flow cytometry and assessed for colony-forming ability. If the tumor or spheroid has been treated previously with drugs or radiation, the method allows an estimate of cell survival at different distances from tumor capillaries or from the surface of the spheroid. The technique has been used to demonstrate that cells distant from blood vessels are resistant to radiation (because of hypoxia, Chap. 13, Sec. 13.5.2) and also to doxorubicin, presumably because of poor drug penetration (Fig. 15.8). For

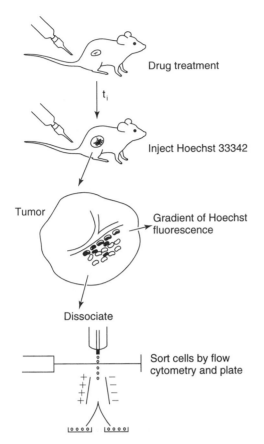

Figure 15.7. Use of the fluorescent vital dye Hoechst 33342 to separate cells at varying distances from tumor blood vessels. If the tumor has received prior treatment, the separated cells may be assessed for colony formation in order to determine the relationship between cell survival and distance of cells from blood vessels.

many agents, the relationship between cell survival and depth in tissue appears to be quite complex (Durand; 1989, 1994). Moreover, the net effect of drugs in solid tissue is often not predictable from their effects against single cells in culture, suggesting a limitation to the potential benefits of some of the in vitro assays that seek to predict clinical response to drugs (Sec. 15.3.3 and Chap. 17, Sec. 17.2.9).

Since nutrient-deprived cells in solid tumors may be spared from radiation and some anticancer drugs, there is potential for therapeutic benefit by combining these agents with other drugs that show selectivity for hypoxic or nutrient-deprived cells and distribute well in tissue. Drugs that require bioreductive activation, such as mitomycin C and tirapazamine, are selectively toxic under hypoxic conditions. Tirapazamine is a particularly promising agent, as it has been shown to kill hypoxic cells in several experimental tumors and to enhance the effects of fractionated radiation at tolerable doses (Brown, 1993). The availability of effective drugs that are specific for hypoxic cells could lead to a considerable therapeutic advantage, since hypoxic cells are not usually found in normal tissues; several other drugs that require reductive activation are in various phases of development (e.g., Siim et al., 1994). The effectiveness of drugs that are selectively toxic for hypoxic cells might be increased by coadministration of vasodilating drugs such as hydralazine, which redistribute blood flow from tumors to normal tissues, leading to a transient

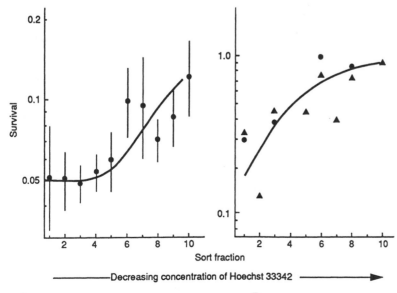

Figure 15.8. Survival of cells at varying distance from blood vessels in the murine Lewis lung tumor after treatment with *(A)* radiation or *(B)* doxorubicin. Cells close to the vessels contain a high concentration of Hoechst 33342 (sort fractions 1–2). As distance from the blood vessels increases, the concentration of Hoechst 33342 in the cells decreases so that sort fractions 9–10 represent cells furthest from the vessels. (Adapted from Chaplin et al., 1985).

A   *B*

increase in the proportion of tumor cells that is hypoxic (Chaplin, 1989).

It may be possible to select drugs that are active against nutrient-deprived cells for reasons other than hypoxia; for example, poorly nourished cells have reduced clearance of acidic products of metabolism, and the microenvironment of solid tumors is often found to be acidic. Within an acidic environment, cellular viability becomes dependent on membrane-based ion-exchange mechanisms that regulate intracellular pH (Tannock and Rotin, 1989). Drugs that become more effective at low extracellular pH and/or that cause cytoplasmic acidification by inhibiting regulatory mechanisms that control intracellular pH may exert selective toxicity for cells within the acidic microenvironment of tumors. Screening for activities of drugs that are selectively toxic for a subpopulation of nutrient-deprived cells in tumors will require the use of prior treatment with agents such as radiation or doxorubicin to reveal effects against this subpopulation.

15.4 DRUG TOXICITY

Toxicity to normal tissues limits both the dose and frequency of drug administration. Many drugs cause toxicity because of their preferential activity against rapidly proliferating cells. Adult tissues that maintain a high rate of cellular proliferation include the bone marrow, intestinal mucosa, hair follicles, and gonads (Chap. 7, Sec. 7.5). Nausea, vomiting, and carcinogenic effects are also common side effects of many drugs, while there are several drug-specific toxicities to other tissues of the body. Toxic damage to normal tissues that may occur through a common mechanism for several drugs is discussed below, whereas toxic effects specific for individual drugs are described in Chap. 16.

15.4.1 Bone Marrow

The pattern of cell proliferation and differentiation of hemopoietic cells in the bone marrow has been described in Chap. 7, Sec. 7.5.1. There is evidence for a pluripotent stem cell that under normal conditions proliferates slowly to replenish cells in the myelocytic, erythroid, and megakaryocytic lineages. Lineage-specific precursors proliferate more rapidly than stem cells, while the morphologically recognizable but immature precursor cells (e.g., myeloblasts) have a very rapid rate of cell proliferation. Beyond a certain stage of maturation, proliferation ceases and the cells mature into circulating blood cells.

The relationship between proliferation and maturation in bone-marrow precursor cells provides a plausible explanation for the observed fall and recovery of blood granulocytes that follows treatment with most anticancer drugs (Fig. 15.9). The effect of treatment will be to deplete the rapidly proliferating cells in the earlier part of the maturation series, with minimal effects against the more mature nonproliferating cells and against slowly proliferating stem cells. Blood counts may remain in the normal range while the more mature surviving cells continue to differentiate but will then fall rapidly at a time when the cells depleted earlier would normally have completed maturation. A decrease in the number of mature cells is common for granulocytes, since their lifetime is only 1 to 2 days, less common for platelets (lifetime of a few days), and rare for red blood cells (mean lifetime of about 120 days), but it may also be influenced by differences in the intrinsic sensitivities of their precursor cells for different drugs. The number of mature granulocytes usually decreases at 8 to 10 days after treatment with drugs such as cyclophosphamide or doxorubicin but

Figure 15.9. *A.* Fall and rapid recovery of the peripheral granulocyte count after chemotherapy (e.g., with cyclophosphamide and/or doxorubicin). For most drugs the count falls to a nadir at 10 to 14 days after treatment, with complete recovery by 3 to 4 weeks. *B.* Delayed and sometimes incomplete recovery is observed after treatment with wide-field radiation and some drugs (e.g., melphalan, mitomycin C, and nitrosoureas).

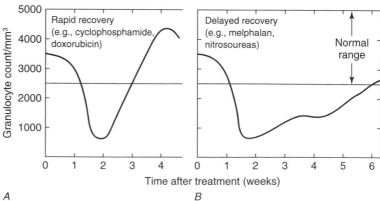

may do so earlier for other drugs (e.g., vinblastine). The variation in time from treatment to the fall in peripheral blood counts for different drugs probably reflects their different effects on the rate of cell maturation (Tannock, 1986).

When the peripheral granulocyte count falls, proliferation of stem cells is mediated by the production of growth factors (Chap. 7, Sec. 7.5.1), with subsequent recovery of the entire bone marrow population. Administration of growth factors (e.g., granulocyte colony-stimulating factor, or G-CSF) after chemotherapy has been shown to accelerate the reappearance of mature cells in the peripheral blood; this may decrease the possibility of infection that can occur in the absence of mature granulocytes.

For many drugs (e.g., cyclophosphamide, doxorubicin), recovery of peripheral blood counts is complete at 3 to 4 weeks after therapy (or at 2 to 3 weeks if growth factors are given), and further treatment may be given with little or no evidence of residual damage to bone marrow. For other drugs, such as melphalan and nitrosoureas, recovery of mature granulocytes and platelets to normal levels is slower, usually requiring about 6 weeks after treatment (Fig. 15.9). For such drugs, the bone marrow may be less tolerant of further treatment, indicating some latent damage. Drugs that produce prolonged myelosuppression tend to show small differential effects against slowly and rapidly proliferating cells and may cause direct damage to stem cells; thus recovery is delayed because of repopulation from a smaller number of bone marrow stem cells and some of this damage may be permanent because of incomplete repopulation of the stem-cell pool.

There is experimental evidence that some drugs may damage stem cells and limit their ability to repopulate the bone marrow (Morley et al., 1975). Botnick et al. (1978, 1981) studied the proliferative potential of treated bone marrow by transplanting it serially into irradiated mice; they also studied the ability of treated bone marrow to regenerate stem cells (CFU-S) by removing marrow at intervals after drug treatment and assessing its ability to form colonies in the spleens of irradiated mice following a single transplantation (Fig. 15.10). Busulfan and carmustine (BCNU) caused long-lasting defects in the ability of stem cells to repopulate; melphalan had an intermediate effect; while full and rapid recovery was observed after treatment with cyclophosphamide and 5-fluorouracil. These results agree with the clinical experience of bone marrow reserve following treatment of patients with the same drugs.

Recovery of blood counts after treatment with anticancer drugs is the usual determinant of the interval between courses of treatment. If myelosuppressive drugs are given when peripheral blood counts are low, they will not only delay recovery and increase the chance of infection and bleeding but will also have a higher chance of depleting the stem-cell population, since it is likely to be proliferating rapidly. Drug administration can be repeated up to 1 week after initial treatment, before the decrease in mature granulocytes and platelets is observed; this schedule has been incorporated into several drug regimens (e.g., the "MOPP" regimen for Hodgkin's disease, where nitrogen mustard is given on days 1 and 8 of a 28-day cycle). Some drugs cause only minimal toxicity to bone marrow (e.g., bleomycin and vincristine), probably because of intrinsic resistance of the precursor cells; they can be given when peripheral granulocyte and platelet counts are low following the use of myelosuppressive agents.

15.4.2 High-Dose Chemotherapy with Stem-Cell Transplantation

The dose of chemotherapy that can be administered to a patient is usually limited by toxicity to the bone marrow. A technique that can allow delivery of higher doses of chemotherapy involves replacement of bone marrow stem cells after drug treatment. Stem cells for transplantation may be derived from the bone marrow or peripheral blood of other individuals (allogeneic transplantation), when they are matched closely for histocompatibility (HLA) antigens with the recipient (Chap. 11, Sec. 11.3.2); or they may be the recipient's own stored stem cells that were harvested prior to chemotherapy (autologous transplantation).

The most successful use of allogeneic stem-cell transplantation has been in the treatment of acute leukemia (for reviews, see Bensinger, 1995; Gorin, 1995). Following initial chemotherapy to achieve a complete remission (when no leukemic cells can be detected), patients are subjected to high-dose chemotherapy and whole-body irradiation aimed at eradicating subclinical disease. Then they are injected with HLA-matched bone marrow, usually from a close relative. About 50 percent of recipients now survive long-term if there is a suitable donor. Limitations include regrowth of leukemia despite high-dose chemotherapy, nonhematologic toxicity of the intensive treatment (e.g., to lungs and other organs), failure of the implant to regenerate, and graft-versus-host disease. This last syndrome occurs

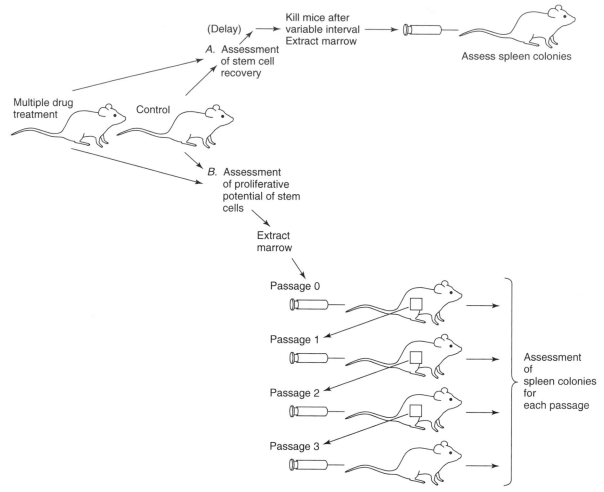

Figure 15.10. Experiments designed to study *(A)* recovery of stem-cell function after chemotherapy and *(B)* repopulating ability of stem cells after chemotherapy. (Methods were described by Botnick et al., 1978, 1981.)

because immunologically competent stem cells are implanted into the host. Unless the patient has an identical twin, immunologic matching is always imperfect and the transplanted marrow will try to "reject" the host. This can lead to damage in multiple organs and, despite the use of immunosuppressive agents such as cyclosporin A, occasionally ends in death.

Autologous stem-cell transplantation is being used for patients with lymphoma who have not responded to conventional therapy or for selected patients with metastatic solid tumors that respond to chemotherapy but cannot be cured by conventional doses. Autologous transplantation avoids graft-versus-host disease, since the patient receives his or her own marrow. There is considerable research into the role of high-dose chemotherapy with autol-

ogous stem-cell transplantation for patients with metastatic breast cancer or as adjuvant therapy in patients at high risk for recurrence. Although there are some encouraging results (Bezwoda et al., 1995), the value of this approach in comparison with conventional therapy must await the results of the large randomized trials in progress.

A major limitation of high-dose chemotherapy with stem-cell transplantation is the toxicity of chemotherapy to organs other than bone marrow, especially liver, heart, lungs, and nervous system. Although drugs are selected (e.g., alkylating agents, carboplatin) whose major toxicity is to bone marrow, dose-limiting toxicity to other organs occurs commonly at about three to five times the dose that could be given in the absence of stem-cell transplantation. For many solid tumors, this dose increment is unlikely to be sufficient to eradicate all of the tumor cells. Another problem may be the reimplantation of undetected tumor cells that had invaded the bone marrow prior to harvest from the patient. Methods using monoclonal antibodies and/or the polymerase chain reaction (Chap. 3, Sec. 3.3.7) applied to tumor-specific genes are being used to increase the sensitivity of detection of contaminating tumor cells in bone marrow. Techniques that allow the selective removal (purging) of such cells are also under investigation.

15.4.3 Toxicity to Other Proliferative Tissues

Ulceration of the intestinal mucosa is a common dose-limiting toxicity when rodents are treated with anticancer drugs. It is due to interruption of the production of new cells (in the crypts of Lieberkuhn) that normally replace the mature cells continually being sloughed into the intestinal lumen from the villi (Chap. 7, Sec. 7.5.2). Damage to bone marrow is more commonly dose-limiting in humans, but mucosal ulceration may occur after treatment with several drugs, including methotrexate, 5-fluorouracil, bleomycin, and cytosine arabinoside; other drugs—such as cyclophosphamide and doxorubicin—may increase the severity of ulceration when used in combination with these drugs. Mucosal damage, resulting in mouth soreness and/or diarrhea, usually begins about 5 days after treatment, and its duration increases with the severity. Full recovery is usually possible if the patient can be supported through this period; recovery is analogous to that in the bone marrow, with repopulation from slowly proliferating stem cells in the crypts.

Partial or complete hair loss is common after treatment with many anticancer drugs and is due to lethal effects of drugs against proliferating cells in hair follicles; this usually begins about 2 weeks after treatment. Full recovery occurs after cessation of treatment, suggesting the presence of drug-resistant, slowly proliferating precursor cells. In some patients, regrowth of hair is observed despite continued treatment with the agent that initially caused its loss. Regrowth of hair might reflect a compensating proliferative process that increases the number of stem cells or may represent the development of drug resistance in a normal tissue akin to that which occurs in tumors (See Chap. 17, Sec. 17.2).

Spermatogenesis in men and formation of ovarian follicles in women both involve rapid cellular proliferation and are susceptible to the toxic effects of many anticancer drugs. Men who receive chemotherapy often have decreased production of sperm and consequent infertility. Testicular biopsy usually demonstrates a loss of germinal cells within the seminiferous tubules, presumably because of drug effects against these rapidly proliferating cells. Antispermatogenic effects may be reversible after lower doses of chemotherapy (Schilsky et al., 1980), but some men remain permanently infertile; it is now usual to recommend sperm banking for young men who undergo intensive chemotherapy for potentially curable malignancies such as Hodgkin's disease.

Chemotherapy given to premenopausal women often leads to temporary or permanent cessation of menstrual periods and to menopausal symptoms. Reversibility of this effect depends on age, the types of drug used, and the duration and intensity of chemotherapy. Biopsies taken from the ovaries have shown failure of formation of ovarian follicles, sometimes with ovarian fibrosis. The pathologic findings are consistent with a primary effect of drugs against the proliferating germinal epithelium.

15.4.4 Determinants of Normal-Tissue Toxicity

When chemotherapy is given to a patient, a drug dose is selected on the basis of early-phase clinical trials that have determined the *average* dose (usually per unit of body surface area) that gives some toxicity, but at an acceptable level. At this dose, there will be no detectable effects on normal tissues in a few patients while severe, potentially lethal toxicity may be seen in others.

Multiple factors influence the distribution of drugs to tissues in the body (i.e., pharmacokinetics, see Chap. 16, Sec. 16.2) and the response of normal cells to these drugs. Some patients have genetically determined traits that change drug metabolism. For example, patients who lack the enzyme dihydropyrimidine dehydrogenase (DPD), which catabolizes 5-fluorouracil (Chap. 16, Sec. 16.4.2), show extreme sensitivity to this drug (Milano and Etienne, 1994). Changes in the activity of enzymes that metabolize other drugs, either genetically determined or induced by concomitant medications, may also have a profound effect on drug-induced toxicity.

Since lethal damage results most often from interaction of drugs with DNA, patients with deficiencies in DNA repair (see Chap. 4, Sec. 4.4) are very sensitive to anticancer drugs, as they are to radiation. Heterozygotes for these defects (e.g., patients with xeroderma pigmentosum) are usually asymptomatic but may be at high risk for severe toxicity if treated by chemotherapy. Unfortunately, at present, there is no simple and cost-effective test that allows for prediction of normal tissue toxicity prior to treatment.

15.4.5 Nausea and Vomiting

Nausea and vomiting are frequent during the first few hours after treatment with many anticancer drugs but are not due primarily to direct effects on intestinal mucosa. Drug-induced vomiting is thought to occur because of direct stimulation of chemoreceptors in the brainstem, which then emit signals via connecting nerves to the neighboring vomiting center, thus eliciting the vomiting reflex. Major evidence for this mechanism comes from studies in animals, where induction of vomiting by chemotherapy is prevented by removal of the chemoreceptor zone. In addition to a central mechanism, some chemotherapeutic agents exert direct effects on the gastrointestinal tract that may contribute to nausea and vomiting (Andrews et al., 1990). Several medications have been developed that inhibit nausea and vomiting after chemotherapy. The most effective of these are the serotonin antagonists, which block $5HT_3$ receptors. Examples of these drugs are ondansetron, tropisetron, and granisteron.

15.4.6 Drugs as Carcinogens

Many anticancer drugs cause toxic damage through effects on DNA; they can also cause mutations and chromosomal damage. These properties are shared with known carcinogens (see Chap. 8), and patients who are long-term survivors of chemotherapy may be at an increased risk for developing a second malignancy. This effect has become apparent only under conditions where chemotherapy has resulted in long-term survival for some patients with drug-sensitive diseases (e.g., lymphomas, myeloma, and carcinoma of the ovary) or where it is used as an adjuvant to decrease the probability of recurrence of disease following local treatment (e.g., breast cancer). Many of the second malignancies are acute leukemias, and their most common time of presentation is 2 to 6 years after initiation of chemotherapy. Increased incidence of solid tumors may also be observed after longer periods of follow-up.

Alkylating agents are the drugs most commonly implicated as the cause of second malignancy, and there is increased risk if patients also receive radiation. It is often difficult to separate an increase in the probability of second malignancy that may be associated with the primary neoplasm (e.g., in a patient with lymphoma) from that associated with its treatment. Comparisons of the incidence of leukemia and other malignancies in clinical trials that randomize patients to receive adjuvant chemotherapy or no chemotherapy after primary treatment have given conclusive evidence of the carcinogenic potential of some drugs. The relative risk of leukemia in drug-treated, as compared with control patients, may be substantial; for example, the relative risk of leukemia was about 12 for 2000 patients receiving methyl-CCNU as adjuvant therapy for gastrointestinal cancer (Boice et al., 1983) and also for 19,000 women receiving adjuvant therapy (which included alkylating agents) for breast cancer (Fisher et al., 1985; Curtis et al., 1990). Leukemia is more common after treatment with alkylating agents that are damaging to bone marrow stem cells (e.g., melphalan; Sec. 15.4.1) than for cyclophosphamide.

Recently, leukemia has been recognized as a complication of treatment with anthracyclines such as doxorubicin and epirubicin and podophyllotoxins such as etoposide. Leukemias that occur following treatment with these drugs have cytogenetic abnormalities distinguishing them from those that occur following alkylating agents (Pedersen-Bjergaad and Philip, 1991).

The absolute risk of second malignancy remains low and the risks of second malignancy are small compared with the potential benefits in treating patients with breast cancer or curable tumors such as Hodgkin's disease or testicular germ-cell tumors (Bajorin et al., 1993; Tallman et al., 1995). However, care is needed in using carcinogenic drugs as adjuvant chemotherapy for malignancies where benefit is minimal.

15.5 DISCOVERY AND DESIGN OF NEW ANTICANCER DRUGS

15.5.1 Screening for Activity of New Compounds

The synthesis and extraction of new compounds have led to a very large number of agents that might be considered for use as anticancer drugs. A major problem confronting cancer agencies and pharmaceutical companies is the selection for clinical testing of the compounds that have the highest probability of clinical activity. Ideally, the models chosen for screening should be rapid and simple (and hence inexpensive) and should have both a good chance of detecting clinically active agents (i.e., high sensitivity) and of excluding clinically inactive agents (i.e., high specificity).

Until recently, most screening assays were based on assessment of drug activity against rapidly growing transplanted tumors in mice, including ascites tumors (Driscoll, 1984). From a large number of potential anticancer drugs (~40,000 per year between 1975 and 1982), the screening programs have identified a few drugs active against rapidly growing human tumors (e.g., testicular cancer) but have met with little success in identifying new agents active against more common human tumors such as cancer of the colon or lung. This limited success may reflect major differences between the properties of slowly growing tumors in humans and those of the rapidly growing murine tumors used in screening.

The National Institutes of Health (NIH) in the United States has been searching for more economical screening methods that will detect a larger number of clinically active drugs, particularly those with activity against the more common human tumors. Current assays depend on the initial assessment of drugs against a panel of cell lines derived from human tumors, using automated staining with the dye sulforhodamine B (SRB) to assess the number of viable cells after drug-induced damage (Sec. 15.2.2; Skehan et al., 1990; Boyd and Paull, 1995). Other automated methods of drug screening include the MTT assay (described in Sec. 15.2.2; Carmichael et al., 1987). New agents that show activity in culture are then selected for further testing in mice, using the end point of growth delay to assess drug effects against a panel of human tumor cell lines that generate xenografts in nude mice. Promising drugs are tested against xenografts derived from common solid tumors, including those derived from colorectal and non-small-cell lung cancer, which demonstrate clinical resistance to most anticancer drugs currently available. This process may be more successful in identifying new agents with improved activity against a range of human tumors.

15.5.2 Rational Design of New Anticancer Drugs

The identification and characterization of some of the targets of existing anticancer agents have provided the opportunity for the rational design and subsequent development of new agents. This applies particularly to those drugs where the putative mechanism of action is the interaction of the drug with an enzyme. The technique of x-ray crystallography (of the target, either alone or complexed with a ligand) combined with molecular modeling has enabled the design of compounds with specific properties. For example, the use of this approach has resulted in the development of new inhibitors of the enzyme thymidylate synthase, the target for the drug 5-fluorouracil (Hardy et al., 1987; Webber et al., 1993; Varney et al., 1995). In addition, improved understanding of the interactions of thymidylate synthase with its cofactor, 5-10-methylenetetrahydrofolate, has allowed the development of inhibitors that are more specific. The new inhibitors are being evaluated in clinical trials.

If the crystal structures of potential targets for anticancer chemotherapy are not known, other techniques have been used to aid in the design of new drugs. Structure-activity studies examine systematically the effects of modification of a drug's structure on its properties and activity. This approach may be applied to lead compounds, which may have been discovered fortuitously or may themselves have been the product of a rational design process. For example, the approach has been used in the development of new topoisomerase inhibitors (Leteurtre et al., 1992).

15.5.3 New Targets for Cancer Chemotherapy

Many of the biochemical and molecular changes that occur in malignancy are becoming better defined. As these processes are elucidated, they become potential targets for new therapeutic strategies. In particular, knowledge of the products of oncogenes, and increased understanding of the processes of intracellular signaling, angiogenesis, and metastasis has provided the opportunity for novel therapeutic approaches. Some examples are given below.

The Ras Oncogene: The importance of the *ras* oncogene in malignancy has been described in Chap. 5, Sec. 5.4 and Chap. 6, Sec. 6.3.4. The existence of an oncogene that is mutated so commonly in human malignancy has prompted the search for methods of exploiting this abnormality therapeutically. The transforming activity of Ras proteins is dependent on their migration from the cytoplasm to the plasma membrane, an event that is facilitated by a series of posttranslational modifications. The first (and necessary) step in this process is the addition of a farnesyl group to a cysteine residue, which is catalyzed by the enzyme farnesyl transferase (Manne et al., 1990). Inhibitors of farnesyl transferase might thus act as anticancer agents. Several such compounds have been synthesized, using rational design techniques based on knowledge of the enzyme structure and its interaction with substrates (Patel et al., 1995). When tested in vivo, such compounds are able to suppress the growth of tumors derived from *ras*-transfected cell lines (Kohl et al., 1994). This effect is specific, with no effect on tumors derived from cell lines transformed by other oncogenes. It is not clear how effective such approaches will be in human malignancy, where multiple oncogenic abnormalities often occur. Nonetheless, encouraging preclinical results have prompted the further study of farnesylation inhibitors, and clinical trials of these compounds are now commencing.

Protein tyrosine kinases offer a potential target for novel anticancer strategies. As described in Chap. 6, these enzymes often play a central role in the generation of signals involved in proliferation and malignancy. The use of recombinant DNA techniques in vitro to inactivate kinase activity is associated with a loss of transforming potential (Snyder et al., 1985), suggesting that these enzymes may be a suitable target for anticancer drug development. Several inhibitors of protein tyrosine kinases have been identified, including erbstatin, the flavonoids quercetin and genistein, and tyrophostins (Workman et al., 1992). These agents have many effects, including the ability to slow or inhibit the growth of tumor cell lines in vitro, inhibit invasion (Scholar and Toews, 1994), and slow experimental tumor growth in vivo. Clinical trials of these compounds have not yet commenced.

Angiogenesis: Tumor growth is dependent on angiogenesis, and various inhibitors of angiogenesis are now in clinical trials. This approach is described in Chap. 9, Sec. 9.3.3.

Telomerase This is a ribonucleoprotein enzyme that maintains the length of the telomeres of chromosomes may play a role in the development and maintenance of the malignant phenotype (Chap. 7; Sec. 7.3.5). The presence of an enzyme, such as telomerase, which is active in many malignant tumors but few normal tissues (with the exception of germ cells and possibly hemopoietic stem cells) raises the possibility of its therapeutic exploitation. Several strategies may be used to develop inhibitors of telomerase. These include the search for inhibitors using a "screening" approach; the use of gene therapy, with antisense oligonucleotides targeting either the RNA or the protein component of the enzyme; and the rational development of specific inhibitors once telomerase structure and function are characterized further (Healy, 1995; Axelrod, 1996).

The cyclins are potential targets for therapeutic attack because they are responsible for control of the cell cycle. Details of the interactions between cyclins, the cyclin-dependent kinases (CDKs), and the retinoblastoma protein pRb are presented in Chap. 7; Sec. 7.2.2. Expression of D-type cyclins usually follows stimulation of the cell by growth factors. Constitutive expression may be perceived by the cell as a signal that growth factors are present continuously, and this may be a step in oncogenesis. Consequently, inhibitors of the expression of D-type cyclins or of their interaction with other molecules such as the CDKs could have anticancer properties. Compounds such as these are now under development.

Cellular Differentiation: In general, there is an inverse relationship between the degree of cellular differentiation and the rate of cell proliferation in tumors. Whether cells differentiate or proliferate depends on cell signaling pathways, described in Chap. 6. Although the precise mechanisms remain poorly understood, several agents have been shown to stimulate differentiation (and inhibit proliferation) of malignant cells in culture: these agents include retinoids, various cytokines, and analogues of vitamin D (Bollag, 1994). One agent that induces differentiation, all-trans retinoic acid, gives a high rate of complete clinical remission in the treatment of acute promyelocytic leukemia (APL). In this (rare) disease, the *retinoic acid receptor*–α gene is frequently rearranged and fused with another (*PML*) gene. Interaction of retinoic acid with this fusion product is the probable cause of differentiation and response in APL (Cornic et al., 1994). Unfortunately, retinoids have proven useful only in the management of APL, some skin cancers, and superficial bladder cancer, but research continues into agents that influence the balance between cell differentiation and proliferation in tumors.

Conventional cancer chemotherapy is based upon the concept of killing tumor stem cells in order to produce a cure (scc Sec. 15.2). For many of the newer approaches to cancer control, cell kill is a less relevant end point. Inhibition of intracellular signaling may act to interfere with transformation and uncontrolled cell growth but may produce little or no cell killing. Similarly, inhibitors of angiogenesis (Chap. 9, Sec. 9.3.3) and stimulators of differentiation are unlikely to produce cell killing that could be measured by using traditional in vitro assays of anticancer drug activity. The effect of these agents may be to inhibit proliferation of tumor cells while cell death continues leading to gradual involution of the tumor. Toxicities of these agents are also likely to differ from those of current cytotoxic agents, since a major goal is to achieve greater specificity for tumor cells by targeting molecular products that are specific to tumor cells. New assays, both in vitro and in vivo, may be required to fully assess the therapeutic potential of these agents. Likewise, novel approaches may be required to evaluate the role of new agents in clinical practice.

15.6 SUMMARY

Chemotherapy for cancer has evolved rapidly since the first patient was treated with nitrogen mustard in 1942, with about 40 drugs licensed for clinical use in North America. Major classes of drugs include alkylating agents, antimetabolites, and a variety of natural or semisynthetic compounds.

The most relevant end point for assessing lethal effects of drugs on cells is loss of reproductive potential as measured by a colony-forming assay. Survival curves that relate colony-forming ability to drug concentration may be exponential or may demonstrate no further killing above a certain concentration if the drugs are cell-cycle phase–specific. Most drugs are more toxic to rapidly proliferating cells.

In situ assays of tumor response following drug treatment in animals include assessment of delay in tumor growth. Growth delay has been applied to the study of drug response of human tumor xenografts in immune-deficient mice. Automated assays of drug toxicity in culture are used for screening the activity of new agents, and promising drugs are tested against xenografts derived from drug-resistant human tumors. Attempts have been made to apply in vitro assays following drug treatment of cells obtained by biopsy from human tumors with the aim of prediction of clinical response. At present, several problems exist that should limit the use of such assays to a research setting. The microenvironment in solid tumors may limit drug penetration and activity, and there is therapeutic potential for drugs that have activity against nutrient-deprived, slowly proliferating cells in solid tumors.

The toxicity of many drugs for bone marrow, intestine, hair follicles, and gonads is probably due to depletion of rapidly proliferating cells in these tissues, with subsequent recovery from slowly proliferating stem cells. However, some drugs may cause permanent damage to stem-cell function. High-dose chemotherapy with stem-cell transplantation provides a strategy to circumvent stem-cell toxicity, but the dose of anticancer drugs is still limited by toxicity to other organs. Nausea and vomiting may occur through stimulation of chemoreceptors in the brainstem, and several drugs cause specific damage to organs such as heart, lung, or kidney. Many drugs cause damage to DNA, which may occasionally result in the induction of a second malignancy. There is a need for simple assays that can identify patients with genetically based defects having unusual sensitivity to anticancer drugs.

The molecular characterization of events that occur in cellular transformation to malignancy and in tumor progression is being used to synthesize new types of anticancer drugs whose targets may be more specific to tumor cells. Such targets include the products of (mutated) oncogenes, other molecules involved in cell signaling or cell-cycle control; the enzyme telomerase, which inhibits cellular senescence; and growth factors or their receptors that are essential for angiogenesis in tumors.

REFERENCES

Ajani JA, Baker FL, Spitzer G, et al: Comparison between clinical response and in vitro drug sensitivity of primary human tumors in the adhesive tumor cell culture system. J Clin Oncol 1987; 5:1912–1921.

Andrews PLR, Davis CJ, Bingham S, et al: The abdominal visceral innervation and the emetic reflex: Pathways, pharmacology and plasticity. Can J Physiol Pharmacol 1990; 68:325–330.

Arnold W, Köpf-Maier P, Michael B (eds): Immunodeficient Animals: Models for Cancer Research. Contributions to Oncology: 51. Basel and New York: Carter; 1996; 1–229.

Axelrod N: Of telomeres and tumors. Nature Med 1996; 2:158–159.

Bajorin DF, Motzer RJ, Rodriguez E, et al: Acute nonlymphocytic leukemia in germ cell tumor patients treated with etoposide-containing chemotherapy. J Natl Cancer Inst 1993; 85:60–62.

Bensinger W: Peripheral blood stem cell transplantation. Cancer Treat Res 1995; 76:169–193.

Bezwoda WR, Seymour L, Dansey RD: High-dose chemotherapy with hematopoietic rescue as primary treatment for metastatic breast cancer: A randomized trial. J Clin Oncol 1995; 13:2483–2489.

Boice JD Jr, Greene MH, Killen JY Jr, et al: Leukemia and preleukemia after adjuvant treatment of gastrointestinal cancer with semustine (methyl-CCNU). N Engl J Med 1983; 309:1079–1084.

Bollag W: Experimental basis of cancer combination chemotherapy with retinoids, cytokines, 1,25-dihydroxyvitamin D3, and analogs. J Cell Biochem 1994; 56:427–435.

Botnick LE, Hannon EC, Hellman S: Multisystem stem cell failure after apparent recovery from alkylating agents. Cancer Res 1978; 38:1942–1947.

Botnick LE, Hannon EC, Vigneulle R, Hellman S: Differential effects of cytotoxic agents on hematopoietic progenitors. Cancer Res 1981; 41:2338–2342.

Boyd MR, Paull KD: Some practical considerations and applications of the National Cancer Institute in vitro anticancer drug discovery screen. *Drug Dev Res* 1995; 34:91–109.

Brown JM: SR4233 (Tirapazamine): A new anticancer drug exploiting hypoxia in solid tumor. *Br J Cancer* 1993; 67:1163–1170.

Bruce WR, Meeker BE, Valeriote FA: Comparison of the sensitivity of normal hematopoietic and transplanted lymphoma colony-forming cells to chemotherapeutic agents administered *in vivo. J Natl Cancer Inst* 1966; 37:233–245.

Bruce WR, Meeker BE, Powers WE, Valeriote FA: Comparison of the dose and time-survival curves for normal hematopoietic and lymphoma colony-forming cells exposed to vinblastine, vincristine, arabinosylcytosine, and amethopterin. *J Natl Cancer Inst* 1969; 42:1015–1023.

Carmichael J, DeGraff WG, Gazdar AF: Evaluation of a tetrazolium-based semiautomated colorimetric assay: Assessment of chemosensitivity testing. *Cancer Res* 1987; 47:936–942.

Chaplin DJ: Hydralazine-induced tumor hypoxia: a potential target for cancer chemotherapy. *J Natl Cancer Inst* 1989; 81:618–622.

Chaplin DJ, Durand RE, Olive PL: Cell selection from a murine tumour using the fluorescent probe Hoechst 33342. *Br J Cancer* 1985; 51:569–572.

Cornic M, Agadir A, Degos L, Chomienne C: Retinoids and differentiation treatment: A strategy for treatment in cancer. *Anticancer Res* 1994; 14:2339–2346.

Courtenay VD, Smith IE, Peckham MJ, Steel GG: In vitro and in vivo radiosensitivity of human tumour cells obtained from a pancreatic carcinoma xenograft. *Nature* 1976; 263:771–772.

Cowan DSM, Hicks KO, Wilson WR: Multicellular membranes as an *in vitro* model for extravascular diffusion in tumours. *Br J Cancer* 1996; 74(suppl 27):S28–S31.

Curtis RE, Boice JD Jr, Moloney WC, et al: Leukemia following chemotherapy for breast cancer. *Cancer Res* 1990; 50:2741–2746.

Donaldson KL, Goolsby GL, Wahl AF: Cytotoxicity of the anticancer agents cisplatin and taxol during cell proliferation and the cell cycle. *Int J Cancer* 1994; 57:847–855.

Driscoll JS: The preclinical new drug research program of the National Cancer Institute. *Cancer Treat Rep* 1984; 68:63–76.

Durand RE: Distribution and activity of anti-neoplastic drugs in a tumor model. *J Natl Cancer Inst* 1989, 81:146–152.

Durand RE: The influence of microenvironmental factors during cancer therapy. *In Vivo* 1994; 8:691–702.

Erlanson M, Daniel-Szolgay E, Carlsson J: Relations between the penetration, binding and average concentration of cytostatic drugs in human tumour spheroids. *Cancer Chemother Pharmacol* 1992; 29:343–353.

Fisher B, Rockette H, Fisher ER, et al: Leukemia in breast cancer patients following adjuvant chemotherapy or postoperative radiation: The NSABP experience. *J Clin Oncol* 1985; 3:1640–1658.

Gazdar AF, Steinberg SM, Russell EK, et al: Correlation of in vitro drug sensitivity testing results with response to chemotherapy and survival in extensive stage small-cell lung cancer: A prospective clinical trial. *J Natl Cancer Inst* 1990; 82:117–124.

Gilman A: The initial clinical trial of nitrogen mustard. *Am J Surg* 1963; 105:574–578.

Gorin NC: Stem cell transplantation in acute leukemia. *Ann NY Acad Sci* 1995; 770:262–287.

Hamburger AW, Salmon SE: Primary bioassay of human tumor stem cells. *Science* 1977; 197:461–463.

Hardy LW, Finer-Moore JS, Montfort WR, et al: Atomic structure of thymidylate synthase: Target for rational drug design. *Science* 1987; 235:448–455.

Healy KC: Telomere dynamics and telomerase activation in tumor progression: Prospects for prognosis and therapy. *Oncology Res* 1995; 7:121–130.

Hennequin C, Giocanti N, Favaudon V: S-phase specificity of cell killing by docetaxel (Taxotere) in synchronized HeLa cells. *Br J Cancer* 1995; 71:1194–1198.

Hicks KO, Ohms SJ, van Zijl PL, et al: An experimental and mathematical model for the extravasular transport of a DNA intercalator in tumours. *Br J Cancer* 1997; 76:894–903.

Kallman RF, ed: *Rodent Tumor Models in Experimental Cancer Therapy.* Elmsford; NY: Pergamon Press; 1987.

Kern DH, Weisenthal LM: Highly specific prediction of antineoplastic drug resistance with an in vitro assay using suprapharmacologic drug exposures. *J Natl Cancer Inst* 1990; 82:582–588.

Kohl NE, Wilson FR, Mosser SD, et al: Protein farnesyltransferase inhibitors block the growth of ras-dependent tumors in nude mice. *Proc Natl Acad Sci USA* 1994; 91:9141–9145.

Kristjansen PEG, Boucher Y, Jain RK: Dexamethasone reduces the interstitial fluid pressure in a human colon adenocarcinoma xenograft. *Cancer Res* 1993; 53: 4764–4766.

Less JR, Posner MC, Boucher Y, et al: Interstitial hypertension in human breast and colorectal tumors. *Cancer Res* 1992; 52:6371–6374.

Leteurtre F, Madalengoitia J, Orr A, et al: Rational design and molecular effects of a new topoisomerase II inhibitor, azatoxin. *Cancer Res* 1992; 52:4478–4483.

Manne V, Roberts D, Tobin A, et al: Identification and preliminary characterisation of protein-cysteine farnesyltransferase. *Proc Natl Acad Sci USA* 1990; 87:7541–7545.

Mauro F, Madoc-Jones H: Age response of cultured mammalian cells to cytotoxic drugs. *Cancer Res* 1970; 30:1397–1408.

Milano G, Etienne MC: Dihydropyrimidine dehydrogenase (DPD) and clinical pharmacology of 5-fluorouracil (review). *Anticancer Res* 1994; 14:2295–2297.

Morley A, Trainor K, Blake J: A primary stem cell lesion in experimental chronic hypoplastic marrow failure. *Blood* 1975; 45:681–688.

Netti PA, Baxter LT, Boucher Y, et al: Time-dependent behaviour of interstitial fluid pressure in solid tumors:

Implications for drug delivery. *Cancer Res* 1995; 55:5451–5458.

Nissen E, Tanneberger S, Projan A, et al: Recent results of *in vitro* drug prediction in human tumour chemotherapy. *Arch Geschwulstforsch* 1978; 48:667–672.

Patel DV, Schmidt RJ, Biller SA, et al: Farnesyl diphosphate-based inhibitors of ras farnesyl protein transferase. *J Med Chem* 1995; 38:2906–2921.

Pedersen-Bjergaad J, Philip P: Balanced translocations involving chromosome bands 11q23 and 21q22 are highly characteristic of myelodysplasia and leukemia following therapy with cytostatic agents targeting DNA topoisomerase II. *Blood* 1991; 78:1147–1148.

Potten CS: What is an apoptotic index measuring? A commentary. *Br J Cancer* 1996, 74:1743–1748.

Rubinstein LV, Shoemaker RH, Paull KD, et al: Comparison of in vitro anticancer-drug-screening data generated with a tetrazolium assay versus a protein assay against a diverse panel of human tumor cell lines. *J Natl Cancer Inst* 1990; 82:113–118.

Scheithauer W, Clark GM, Moyer MP, von Hoff DD: New screening system for selection of anticancer drugs for treatment of human colorectal cancer. *Cancer Res* 1986; 46:2703–2708.

Schilsky RL, Lewis BJ, Sherins RJ, Young RC: Gonadal dysfunction in patients receiving chemotherapy for cancer. *Ann Intern Med* 1980; 93:109–114.

Scholar EM, Toews ML. Inhibition of invasion of murine mammary carcinoma cells by the tyrosine kinase inhibitor genistein. *Cancer Lett* 1994; 87: 159–162.

Selby P, Buick RN, Tannock I: A critical appraisal of the "human tumor stem cell assay." *N Engl J Med* 1983; 308:129–134.

Siim BG, Atwell GJ, Wilson WR: Oxygen dependence of the cytotoxicity and metabolic activation of 4-alkylamino-5-nitroquinidine bioreductive drugs. *Br J Cancer* 1994; 70:596–603.

Skehan P, Storeng R, Scudiero D, et al: New colorimetric cytotoxicity assay for anticancer-drug screening. *J Natl Cancer Inst* 1990; 82:1107–1112.

Snyder MA, Bishop JM, McGrath JP, Levinson AD. A mutation of the ATP binding site of pp60v-src abolishes kinase activity, transformation, and tumorigenicity. *Mol Cell Biol* 1985; 5:1772–1779.

Sutherland RM: Cell and environment interactions in tumor microregions: The multicell spheroid model. *Science* 1988; 240:177–184.

Tallman MS, Gray R, Bennett JM, et al: Leukemogenic potential of adjuvant chemotherapy for early-stage breast cancer: The Eastern Cooperative Oncology Group experience. *J Clin Oncol* 1995; 13:1557–1563.

Tannock IF: Cell kinetics and chemotherapy: A critical review. *Cancer Treat Rep* 1978; 62:1117–1133.

Tannock IF: Response of aerobic and hypoxic cells in a solid tumor to Adriamycin and cyclophosphamide and interaction of the drugs with radiation. *Cancer Res* 1982; 42:4921–4926.

Tannock IF: Experimental chemotherapy and concepts related to the cell cycle. *Int J Radiat Biol* 1986; 49:335–355.

Tannock IF, Rotin D: Acid pH in tumors and its potential for therapeutic exploitation. *Cancer Res* 1989; 49:4373–4384.

Teicher BA: Hypoxia and drug resistance. *Cancer Metastasis Rev* 1994; 13:139–168.

Till JE, McCulloch EA: A direct measurement of the radiation sensitivity of normal mouse bone marrow cells. *Radiat Res* 1961; 14:213–222.

Twentyman PR, Bleehen NM: Changes in sensitivity to cytotoxic agents occurring during the life history of monolayer cultures of a mouse tumour cell line. *Br J Cancer* 1975; 31:417–423.

Van Putten LM, Lelieveld P, Kram-Idsenga LKJ: Cell cycle specificity and therapeutic effectiveness of cytostatic agents. *Cancer Chemother Rep* 1972; 56:691–700.

Varney MD, Palmer CL, Deal JG, et al: Synthesis and biological evaluation of novel 2,6-diaminobenzindole inhibitors of thymidylate synthase using the protein structure as a guide. *J Med Chem* 1995; 38:1892–1903

Von Hoff DD: He's not going to talk about in vitro predictive assays again, is he? *J Natl Cancer Inst* 1990; 82:96–101.

Von Hoff DD, Kronmal R, Salmon SE, et al: A Southwest Oncology Group study on the use of a human tumor cloning assay for predicting response in patients with ovarian cancer. *Cancer* 1991; 67:20–27.

von Kalle C, Wolf J, Becker A, et al: Growth of Hodgkin cell lines in severely combined immunodeficient mice. *Int J Cancer* 1992; 52:887–891.

Webber SE, Bleckman TM, Deal JG, et al: Design of thymidylate synthase inhibitors using protein crystal structures: The synthesis and biological evaluation of a novel class of 5-substituted quinazolinones. *J Med Chem* 1993; 36:733–746.

Weisenthal LM, Dill PL, Kurnick NB, Lipman ME: Comparison of dye exclusion assays with a clonogenic assay in the determination of drug-induced cytotoxicity. *Cancer Res* 1983; 43:258–264.

Workman P, Brunton VG, Robins DJ. Tyrosine kinase inhibitors. *Semin Cancer Biol* 1992; 3:369–381.

16

Pharmacology of Anticancer Drugs

Malcolm J. Moore and Charles Erlichman

16.1 INTRODUCTION

16.2 PHARMACOKINETICS AND PHARMACODYNAMICS
    16.2.1 General Principles
    16.2.2 Regional Chemotherapy

16.3 ALKYLATING AGENTS
    16.3.1 General Properties
    16.3.2 Nitrogen Mustards
    16.3.3 Nitrosoureas
    16.3.4 Other Alkylating Agents

16.4 ANTIMETABOLITES
    16.4.1 Methotrexate
    16.4.2 5-Fluorouracil
    16.4.3 Cytidine Analogues
    16.4.4 Purine Antimetabolites
    16.4.5 Thymidylate Synthase Inhibitors

16.5 NATURAL PRODUCTS
    16.5.1 Anthracyclines and Anthracenediones
    16.5.2 Bleomycin
    16.5.3 Vinca Alkaloids
    16.5.4 Taxanes
    16.5.5 Epipodophyllotoxins
    16.5.6 Camptothecin Derivatives
    16.5.7 Mitomycin C

16.6 MISCELLANEOUS DRUGS
    16.6.1 Cisplatin and Carboplatin
    16.6.2 Other Drugs

16.7 SUMMARY

REFERENCES

16.1 INTRODUCTION

In this chapter some general principles of pharmacology relevant to anticancer drug treatment are presented. The specific properties of the most important anticancer drugs in clinical use are then reviewed, with particular emphasis on their structure, mechanism of action, pharmacokinetics, and host toxicity.

16.2 PHARMACOKINETICS AND PHARMACODYNAMICS

16.2.1 General Principles

Pharmacokinetics is the study of the time course of drug and metabolite levels in different body fluids and tissues; it includes drug absorption, distribution, metabolism, and elimination, while the study of drug effects at the cellular level is known as *phar-*

macodynamics. Alterations in drug pharmacokinetics may account for subsequent differences in drug effect or response.

A variable proportion of an orally administered drug may be delivered into the circulation and become available for a potential therapeutic effect (bioavailability). Factors influencing the bioavailability of a drug include patient compliance, dissolution of the capsule or tablet, absorption through the gastrointestinal mucosa, and "first-pass" metabolism in the liver. Absorption of an oral anticancer agent (e.g., melphalan, etoposide) may vary among patients receiving similar treatments or within one patient from one course of treatment to another. This can account for some differences in the toxicity, and possibly tumor response, when such agents are used.

Distribution of a drug or its metabolites in the body is governed by factors such as blood flow to different organs and diffusion of the drug from blood vessels, protein binding in plasma or elsewhere, and lipid solubility. In general, drugs with extensive binding to tissues (e.g., doxorubicin) or with high lipid solubility will tend to exhibit prolonged elimination phases because there is slow release of drug from these sites. However, this also depends on the rate of drug inactivation. For example, BCNU (bis-chloroethylnitrosourea) is a lipid-soluble drug and penetrates well into the central nervous system, but it is rapidly inactivated, resulting in a short duration of exposure to body tissues.

Metabolism of a drug in any organ (most commonly in the liver) will contribute to elimination of the parent compound from the plasma. For some drugs, metabolites retain therapeutic activity; for others (e.g., cyclophosphamide), metabolism is required for activation. Many anticancer drugs have active metabolites; this introduces an additional complexity into understanding the relationship between drug pharmacokinetics and antitumor effects. Many drugs and their metabolites are eliminated from the body by excretion into the urine. For drugs that are potentially toxic to the kidney (e.g., high-dose methotrexate and cisplatin), it may be important to stimulate drug elimination by maintaining the urine at an alkaline pH (methotrexate) or by maintaining a rapid urinary flow (cisplatin). If a patient has abnormalities in renal function, a dosage reduction of drugs that are eliminated unchanged by the kidney (e.g., methotrexate, carboplatin) may be necessary. Some anticancer drugs (e.g., doxorubicin) are excreted predominantly via hepatic metabolism and biliary tract excretion and are eliminated in the feces. Therefore, the tolerated dose of doxorubicin is lower in patients with elevated levels of bilirubin secondary to liver disease because in this case the elevated bilirubin indicates impairment of hepatic metabolism.

Once a drug is delivered to the tumor, the important processes include uptake of the drug into cells, intracellular metabolism, binding to molecular targets, and cellular mechanisms for overcoming drug-induced damage. Anticancer drugs may enter cells by passive diffusion, facilitated diffusion, or active transport. Passive diffusion is energy-independent but concentration-dependent and is influenced by physicochemical characteristics of the drug such as lipid solubility and degree of ionization. Active transport is an energy-dependent process involving a receptor molecule to which the drug is bound as it is transported across the cell membrane. This process is saturable, may be blocked by metabolic inhibitors, and allows transport of drug against a concentration gradient. Active transport systems have been demonstrated for methotrexate, doxorubicin, vinca alkaloids, and several other drugs. Facilitated diffusion is also thought to involve a carrier molecule; thus drugs can enter the cell more rapidly than by passive diffusion but can only be transported down a concentration gradient. Some drugs are transported into cells by more than one mechanism, and the dominant process then depends on the concentration gradient across the cell membrane and the degree of saturation of available carrier sites. Drug effects inside cells, and the mechanisms that cells use to try to circumvent or repair damage caused by them, vary widely among the different types of drugs; these factors are described for individual drugs in subsequent sections.

Most anticancer drugs can be measured in plasma or in the tissues of a patient. Measurement of drug concentrations is an important research tool that aids in the understanding of drug pharmacology and response. If a drug is measured in plasma, then a curve relating drug concentration to time can be defined. From these concentration–time profiles models can be defined to characterize drug pharmacokinetics. Some of the important terms that can be derived from such models are listed in Table 16.1 (Allen et al., 1982). These terms and models are tools that can be used to predict a drug's behavior in the body. The volume of distribution (V_d) represents a *hypothetical* volume of body fluid that would be required to dissolve the total amount of drug at

Table 16.1. Glossary of Terms Used Commonly in Pharmacokinetics

AUC	Area under the plasma concentration–time curve from zero to infinity (also referred to as $C \times T$); determined by integrating drug concentration in plasma over time.
$C(t)$	Drug concentration in plasma at time t.
$t_{1/2}$	Half-life. The time required for the drug concentration in plasma to decrease by half. $t_{1/2}\alpha$ = distribution half-life; $t_{1/2}\beta$ = elimination half-life.
V_d	Apparent volume of distribution. A hypothetical volume required to dissolve the total amount of drug at the same concentration as is found in blood immediately after injection.
Cl	Clearance. This is an indicator of the rate of elimination of the drug from the body.

the same concentration as that found in plasma immediately after injection. The calculation of a value of V_d that is larger than the total volume of the body is possible and usually represents extensive binding of drug in tissue. The area under the concentration–time curve (AUC) is a commonly used measure of total drug exposure; for drugs such as alkylating agents, the effect is generally proportional to the AUC. For other drugs, such as antimetabolites or topoisomerase I inhibitors, the duration of exposure may be relatively more important than concentration, and weaker relationships between AUC and response are seen.

The half-life of a drug represents the time required for the drug concentration to decrease by half. This is dependent upon both the rate of elimination of the drug (the clearance) and the volume of distribution. Most drugs undergo both distribution to tissues and subsequent elimination from the body. Separate half-lives that reflect the rate of distribution into other tissues ($t_{1/2}\alpha$) and the rate of removal from the body ($t_{1/2}\beta$) can thus be determined (Fig. 16.1). For some drugs there may also be a slow, delayed elimination (e.g., removal of cisplatin bound to plasma proteins) that may be apparent if plasma drug concentrations are measured for several days. The half-life of this third component of the plasma clearance curve is referred to as $t_{1/2}\gamma$.

Pharmacokinetic models can have practical applications in the use of chemotherapeutic agents. Organ dysfunction (e.g., renal or hepatic disease) may alter drug disposition in the body. Recommendations regarding drug dose in patients with such disease are one practical application of pharmacokinetic analysis of drug behavior. This has been most commonly applied in the dosing of carboplatin in the setting of renal dysfunction (Egorin et al., 1984). Pharmacokinetic/pharmacodynamic modeling attempts to define a relationship between a clinical endpoint such as toxicity or antitumor effect of a drug to its pharmacokinetic parameters (Mick and Ratain, 1993; Newell, 1994; Evans et al., 1998). This approach has the potential for identifying parameters that are important in clinical toxicity or efficacy and may lead to incorporation of blood sampling into patient management. However, for most anticancer drugs, the lack of simple and rapid assays and the absence of a direct relationship between drug concentration in blood and tumor response or normal-tissue toxicity has limited the practical utility of routine therapeutic drug monitoring (Moore and Erlichman, 1987).

Cancer therapy often involves the administration of several anticancer drugs to patients during a

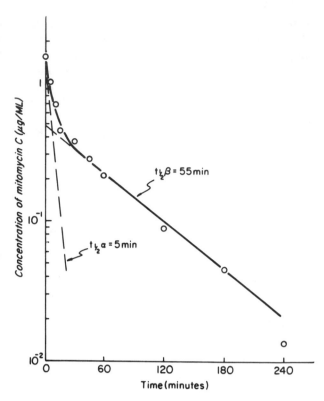

Figure 16.1. Plasma clearance curve for the drug mitomycin C. Initial and final plasma half-lives are referred to as $t_{1/2}\alpha$ and $t_{1/2}\beta$, respectively (Modified from Erlichman et al., 1987.)

short interval of time, in addition to medications for relief of pain, nausea, and other symptoms. Interactions between drugs may influence each of the processes of absorption, metabolism, distribution, and excretion. Although there are documented examples where administration of one drug has been found to influence the disposition of another (e.g., excretion of methotrexate is inhibited by aspirin, since both compete for transporters of weak acids in kidney tubules), the clinical significance of interactions between anticancer drugs has not been investigated extensively.

16.2.2 Regional Chemotherapy

Regional chemotherapy has been used in attempts to achieve high local concentration of a drug and hence to obtain a therapeutic advantage when treating malignant disease localized to one region of the body. Many anticancer drugs have limited access to the central nervous system (CNS), and one form of regional chemotherapy has involved injection of drugs into the cerebrospinal fluid (CSF), which flows around and through the CNS. Such intrathecal administration can be achieved by lumbar puncture (injection into the CSF in the space below the spinal cord in the lower back), or into an Ommaya reservoir, a small device that is implanted surgically just under the skin of the head, through which CSF circulates via a catheter in contact with one of the ventricles (spaces containing CSF) of the brain. Other uses of regional chemotherapy involve instillation of drugs into the bladder for treatment of superficial bladder cancer, injection of drugs into the peritoneal cavity in patients with peritoneal seeding of malignant disease, or arterial infusion into limbs, liver, or other organs of the body.

Regional administration of chemotherapy offers a therapeutic advantage only if the initial exposure due to regional administration is much higher than subsequent exposure due to recirculation of drug through the systemic circulation (Collins, 1984). One favorable circumstance for regional delivery is the administration of drug that will be removed rapidly from plasma by the region being perfused. Systemic exposure to drug will subsequently be low. A low rate of drug exchange between the site of perfusion and the systemic circulation is responsible for the therapeutic advantage of intrathecal treatment for meningeal disease and for intravesical therapy of bladder cancer as compared with systemic administration of drug. However, clear evidence for benefit of intra-arterial chemotherapy has yet to be established. It will depend on the use of drugs that are removed rapidly and effectively from blood and have a low regional rate of exchange; e.g., intrahepatic administration of drugs such as methotrexate and doxorubicin is unlikely to result in a major therapeutic benefit, since these drugs have low plasma clearance and a ready access to other organs when injected into the hepatic artery. The use of 5-fluorodeoxyuridine (5-FUdR) by intrahepatic infusion is based on the rapid removal of this drug from blood by the liver, resulting in a high exposure of the liver as compared with organs supplied by the systemic circulation. This treatment is more effective than systemic therapy in shrinking hepatic metastases, but it has not been shown to increase the overall survival of patients who have liver metastases (Kemeny et al., 1987).

16.3 ALKYLATING AGENTS

16.3.1 General Properties

Alkylating agents are chemically diverse drugs that act through the covalent bonding of alkyl groups (e.g., $-CH_2Cl$) to intracellular macromolecules. In general they act through the generation of highly reactive, positively charged intermediates, which then combine with an electron-rich "nucleophilic" group such as an amino, phosphate, sulfhydryl, or hydroxyl moiety. Alkylating agents may contain either one or two reactive groups and are thus classified as monofunctional or bifunctional, respectively. Bifunctional alkylating agents have the ability to form cross-links between biological molecules and are the most clinically useful of these agents.

Nucleophilic groups that are potential sites of alkylation occur on almost all biological molecules. Alkylation of bases in DNA appears to be the major cause of lethal toxicity. This is supported by a quantitative relationship between the concentration of drug that causes toxicity to cells and the production of lesions in DNA, such as single-strand breaks and cross-links (Kohn, 1979). Also, increased toxicity of alkylating agents has been found in mutant cells that are deficient in the enzymes required for repair of DNA (see Chap. 4, Sec. 4.4). Cross-linking of DNA strands seems to be the major mechanism of damage for bifunctional alkylating agents (Garcia et al., 1988). The cytotoxicity of monofunctional alkylating agents is probably related to single-strand breaks in DNA or to damaged bases. Identified mechanisms of resistance to alkylating agents include decreased transport across the cell membrane, increased intracellular thiol (e.g., glutathione) concentration, increased enzymatic detoxification of reactive intermediates, and alterations in DNA repair enzymes such as guanine-O^6-alkyltransferase (Chap. 17, Sec. 17.2). While the nitrogen mustards are the most clinically useful alkylating agents, many of other alkylating compounds have been synthesized, and several of them are used clinically.

As alkylating agents bind directly to DNA, they have limited cell-cycle specificity. The sensitivity to these drugs is dependent upon the area under the concentration curve and is relatively independent of the schedule of administration used. They do have longer-term effects, such as infertility and carcinogenesis, that reflect their ability to cause DNA damage (Erlichman and Moore, 1996; Chap. 15, Sec. 15.4). Mechlorethamine, melphalan, and the nitrosoureas have been associated with an increased incidence of acute myelogenous leukemia. The development of infertility and carcinogenesis depend both upon which alkylating agent is used and the cumulative dose given.

16.3.2 Nitrogen Mustards

This family of drugs, derived from the prototype alkylating agent nitrogen mustard (or mechlorethamine), contains several drugs in common clinical use, including cyclophosphamide, ifosfamide, melphalan, and chlorambucil. The structures of these drugs are shown in Fig. 16.2: Each of them is bifunctional, with two chloroethyl groups that form the reactive electron-deficient groups responsible for alkylation of DNA.

The most common site of alkylation of DNA by the nitrogen mustards is the N-7 position on the base guanine (Fig. 16.3). First, one of the chloroethyl side chains of nitrogen mustard undergoes a first-order reaction, leading to release of a chloride ion and to formation of a highly reactive, positively charged intermediate. This intermediate may then bind covalently with the electronegative N-7 group on a guanine base, resulting in alkylation. Alkylation of guanine may lead to mispairing with thymine or to strand breakage. The second chloroethyl side chain of nitrogen mustard may undergo a similar reaction, leading to covalent binding with another base on the opposite strand of DNA and thus to formation of an interstrand cross-link.

In the 1940s mechlorethamine was the first nonhormonal anticancer agent to be used clinically. The original studies in malignant lymphoma were instituted based on observations of lymphoid aplasia in men exposed during war to the more reactive but chemically similar sulfur mustard gas. Following in-

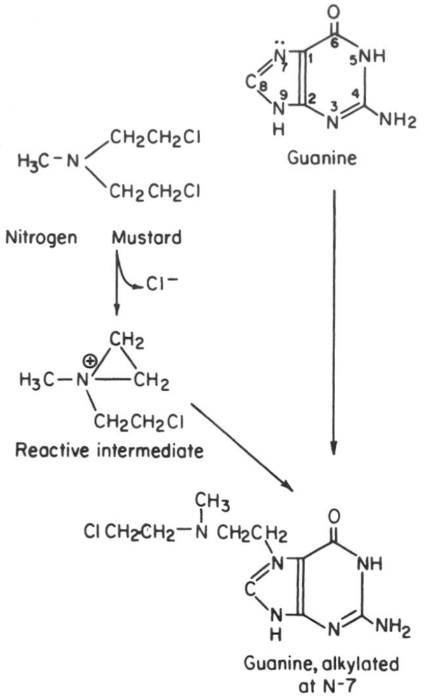

Figure 16.3. Reactions leading to alkylation at the N-7 position of guanine by nitrogen mustard.

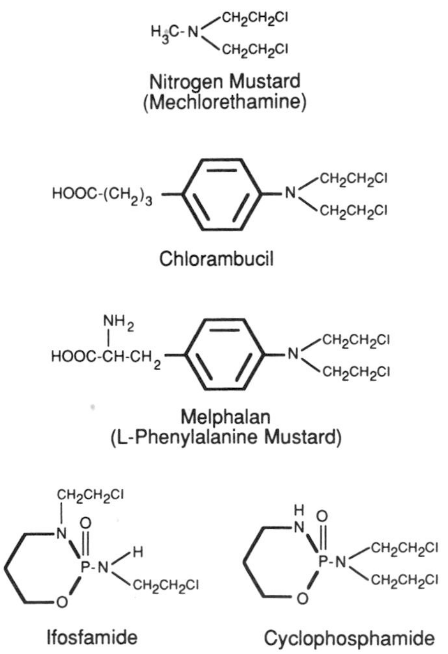

troduction of mechlorethamine, a large number of analogues were produced in an attempt to reduce the reactivity and improve the therapeutic ratio. These studies identified what are still (in the 1990s) the four most commonly used alkylating agents, cyclophosphamide, ifosfamide, melphalan, and chlorambucil (Fig 16.2).

Although mechlorethamine is still used clinically as part of the four-drug "MOPP" protocol for Hodgkin's disease, it has been replaced by the other nitrogen mustards for the treatment of other tumors. The addition of ring structures to the nitrogen mustard molecule conveys increased stability, such that oral preparations of chlorambucil, melphalan, and cyclophosphamide are available.

Chlorambucil is a well-absorbed drug with a narrow spectrum of activity that is used mainly in slowly progressive neoplasms such as low-grade lymphomas and chronic lymphocytic leukemia. Melphalan is used for treatment of multiple myeloma and in some high-dose bone marrow transplantation protocols. It was used previously for ovarian and breast cancer but has largely been replaced by cyclophosphamide and other newer drugs. Absorption of melphalan is low and variable after oral administration; some patients with poor bioavailability after oral dosage have responded to the drug given intra-

Figure 16.2. Structures of clinically used alkylating agents of the nitrogen mustard family.

venously. Detoxification is primarily through spontaneous hydrolysis, although increased toxicity is seen in patients with renal dysfunction, suggesting that elimination by the kidney also plays a role. Uptake of melphalan into cells is mediated by an amino acid active transport system, and resistance may occur because of changes in this transport system. Both chlorambucil and melphalan are almost equally toxic to cycling and noncycling cells and may lead to delayed and/or cumulative effects on bone marrow because of their toxicity to hemopoeitic stem cells (Chap. 15, Sec. 15.4.1).

Cyclophosphamide is the alkylating agent in widest clinical use and is part of treatment protocols for many types of cancer. The parent compound is inactive, requiring metabolism by hepatic mixed-function oxidases to form the alkylating intermediate phosphoramide mustard (Fig. 16.4). Cyclophosphamide was synthesized originally because tumor cells were known to contain phosphoramidase and phosphatase enzymes at high activity. It was thought that these enzymes might lead to selective activation of alkylating activity by cleavage of the ring structure within tumor cells. However, it is now apparent that primary activation takes place in the liver rather than within tumors. Hepatic microsomal enzymes metabolize cyclophosphamide to 4-hydroxycyclophosphamide, which exists in equilibrium with its acyclic isomer aldophosphamide (Fig. 16.4). The 4-hydroxycyclophosphamide enters cells and spontaneously decomposes to form phosphoramide mustard plus acrolein, or it is detoxified by aldehyde dehydrogenase to form inactive metabolites. The metabolites 4-ketocyclophosphamide and car-

boxyphosphamide account for most of the urinary excretion of cyclophosphamide. Acrolein appears to be the major cause of the bladder toxicity (hemorrhagic cystitis) that may occur with chronic usage or higher dosage, particularly if a high urine output is not maintained (Cox, 1979).

Study of the pharmacokinetics of cyclophosphamide is complicated by the number of unstable metabolites formed. The drug is well absorbed after oral administration. Elimination of the parent drug is initially by hepatic transformation to the active metabolites, and then most of the drug is eventually eliminated via renal excretion of inactive metabolites (Moore, 1991). The use of cyclophosphamide in patients with renal failure has not been associated with increased toxicity, as renal clearance of the parent compound and active metabolites is quite low. Cyclophosphamide induces cytochrome P-450 enzymes and will induce its own metabolism with repeated administration (Moore et al., 1988). This alters the rate but not the absolute amount of phosphoramide mustard formation, so no alteration in therapeutic ratio is likely to occur.

The dose-limiting toxicity of cyclophosphamide is myelosuppression, and the drug causes a fall in granulocyte count, with rapid recovery by 3 to 4 weeks after administration (Chap. 15, Sec. 15.4.1). There is relative sparing of stem cells and platelets owing partly to the higher concentrations of aldehyde dehydrogenase (which inactivates the drug intracellularly) in early progenitor cells (Kastan et al., 1990). Cumulative toxicity to bone marrow is not commonly seen. Toxicities of cyclophosphamide common to many alkylating agents include nausea,

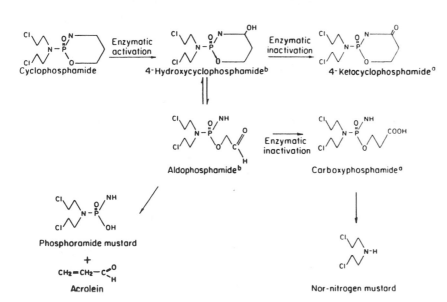

Figure 16.4. The metabolism of cyclophosphamide. *a,* Major urinary metabolites; *b,* transport forms. Phosphoramide mustard is an active alkylating agent, and acrolein is the probable cause of toxicity to the bladder.

vomiting, hair loss, gonadal damage, and potential carcinogenicity. Very high doses are commonly used in preparation for bone marrow transplantation. The dose in this setting is limited by irreversible myocardial necrosis, which occurs with single dosages greater than 60 mg/kg.

Ifosfamide is an analogue of cyclophosphamide that differs in the presence of one chloroethyl group on the oxazaphosphorine ring (Fig 16.2). It is used in the treatment of testicular cancer, sarcoma, and lung cancer. In animals, ifosfamide has a therapeutic ratio equivalent or superior to that of cyclophosphamide, particularly when repeated daily doses are used. Although the metabolism of ifosfamide is similar to that of cyclophosphamide, there is less affinity for the microsomal mixed-function oxidases and more drug undergoes transformation by other pathways, including dechloroethylation. This alteration in metabolism is the reason why higher doses of ifosfamide are used and some differences in toxicity are seen. Hemorrhagic cystitis due to increased production of acrolein is more common with ifosfamide, such that all patients receiving the drug require coadministration of a sulfhydryl-containing compound such as 2-mercaptoethane sulfonate (Mesna), which conjugates with acrolein in the urinary tract and protects the bladder from damage. As Mesna is inactive in plasma and is converted to its active form only in urine, it does not influence the cytotoxicity of cyclophosphamide or ifosfamide at other sites (Benvenuto et al., 1992). Neurotoxicity, manifesting as changes in mental status, may occur with higher doses of ifosfamide. This is not seen with cyclophosphamide and is probably related to the differences in metabolism and the formation of chlorethylacetaldehyde from ifosfamide. Other toxicities are similar to those observed with cyclophosphamide.

16.3.3 Nitrosoureas

The chloroethylnitrosoureas—BCNU (carmustine), CCNU (lomustine), and methyl-CCNU (Fig. 16.5)—are lipid-soluble drugs that can penetrate into the CNS for treatment of intracranial tumors. The drugs are effective for treatment of experimental tumors but have found only limited clinical application. This is partially because normal tissue toxicity has limited the ability to achieve a cytotoxic concentration in vivo. They tend to cause prolonged myelosuppression and are highly leukemogenic, probably because of direct effects on bone marrow stem cells.

BCNU resembles the nitrogen mustards in having two chloroethyl groups, whereas CCNU and methyl-

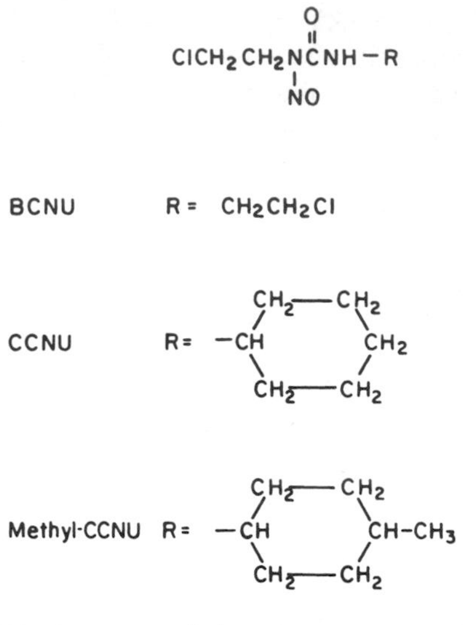

Figure 16.5. Structure of the nitrosoureas: BCNU = bis-chloroethylnitrosourea; CCNU = cyclohexyl-chloroethylnitrosourea; methyl-CCNU = methylcyclohexyl-chloroethylnitrosourea.

CCNU are monofunctional agents with a single chloroethyl group. BCNU forms DNA interstrand cross-links by chloroethylation of two nucleophilic sites on opposite DNA strands (Prestayko et al., 1981). Both CCNU and methyl-CCNU are rapidly and completely absorbed after oral administration, but BCNU must be given intravenously. The parent drugs undergo rapid tissue uptake and metabolism and have not been identified in plasma or urine. The extent to which metabolites contribute to the toxicity of these agents is unknown.

Many other nitrosoureas have been synthesized, but only streptozotocin, a methylnitrosourea that has a direct toxic effect on pancreatic islet cells, has proven to be useful clinically. It is a component of first-line treatment regimens for pancreatic islet-cell tumors and other gastrointestinal endocrine tumors (Moertel et al., 1992).

16.3.4 Other Alkylating Agents

Busulfan is an alkyl alkane sulfonate (Fig 16.6). It has a different mechanism of alkylation to the nitrogen mustards and has selective effects on blood-forming cells. It is used for the treatment of chronic myelogenous leukemia as well as in high-dose bone marrow transplantation regimens. Busulfan is eliminated via hepatic metabolism, and clearance is dependent on age and hepatic function. The higher doses of busulfan used in marrow transplantation may cause hepatic veno-occlusive disease in patients who metabolize the drug slowly (Grochow et al.,

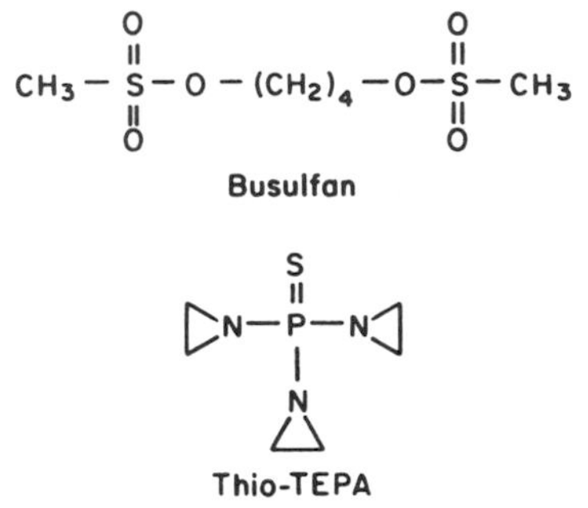

$$CH_3 - \overset{\overset{O}{\|}}{\underset{\underset{O}{\|}}{S}} - O - (CH_2)_4 - O - \overset{\overset{O}{\|}}{\underset{\underset{O}{\|}}{S}} - CH_3$$

Busulfan

Thio-TEPA

Figure 16.6. Structure of the alkylating agents busulfan and thio-TEPA (triethylenethiophosphoramide).

1992). Prolonged administration of busulfan may cause marrow aplasia and pulmonary fibrosis.

Aziridines such as thio-TEPA are structurally similar to intermediate alkylating species of the nitrogen mustards but are less reactive (Fig. 16.6) They have no unique advantages, but thio-TEPA has been used for intravesical treatment of superficial bladder cancer and is occasionally used in the treatment of breast cancer and as intrathecal therapy of meningeal carcinomatosis.

Procarbazine is a synthetic derivative of hydrazine that is used in combination to treat lymphomas, including Hodgkin's disease. The drug undergoes extensive metabolism to produce alkylating species, although details of its metabolism and mechanism of action remain unclear.

Dacarbazine (DTIC) was synthesized originally as an antimetabolite to inhibit purine biosynthesis. It is believed to function through formation of a metabolite with alkylating properties. The drug is used mainly for treatment of sarcomas, Hodgkin's disease, and melanoma. It causes severe nausea and vomiting and the dose-limiting toxicity is myelosuppression. Temozolomide is an oral agent that contains a triazine that is thought to be the active component of dacarbazine. It has a simpler metabolism and undergoes spontaneous decomposition to an alkylating intermediate. This drug is still in clinical testing and has promising activity against malignant glioma and possibly also against melanoma. Hexamethylmelamine is another oral triazine derivative that requires activation to an alkylating intermediate. It has demonstrated activity against ovarian cancer but has largely been replaced by cisplatin, cyclophosphamide, and paclitaxel.

16.4 ANTIMETABOLITES

Antimetabolites are drugs that interfere with normal cellular function, particularly the synthesis of DNA that is required for replication. Many of the clinically useful agents are purine (e.g., 6-thioguanine, 2-chlorodeoxyadenosine) or pyrimidine (e.g., 5-fluorouracil, cytosine arabinoside) analogues that either inhibit the formation of the normal nucleotides or interact with DNA and prevent normal cell division from occurring. The antifolates (e.g., methotrexate) are not nucleoside analogues, and prevent the formation of reduced folates, which are required for the synthesis of DNA. Recently, specific inhibitors of critical enzymes required for DNA synthesis (e.g., thymidylate synthase) have been brought into clinical practice and a number of others are undergoing early clinical studies.

Most antimetabolites are cell cycle–specific; their toxicity reflects effects on proliferating cells and is primarily seen in bone marrow cells and gastrointestinal mucosa (see Chap. 15, Sec. 15.4). As they do not interact directly with DNA, they do not cause the later problems of carcinogenesis seen with DNA-binding drugs like the alkylating agents. The effects of these drugs are dependent upon the schedule of administration. In many cases the duration of exposure above a critical threshold required to inhibit an enzyme is more important than the peak concentration. Therefore, while large doses may be tolerated if the drug is given as a single intravenous injection, a much lower dose is required if the drug is given repeatedly or by a continuous infusion.

16.4.1 Methotrexate

Methotrexate is an analogue of the vitamin folic acid (Fig. 16.7). Reduced folate is required for transfer of methyl groups in the biosynthesis of purines and in the conversion of deoxyuridine monophosphate (dUMP) to thymidine monophosphate (dTMP), a reaction catalyzed by thymidylate synthase. Reduced folate becomes oxidized in the latter reaction; its regeneration is dependent on the enzyme dihydrofolate reductase (DHFR) for further reduction to its active form. Methotrexate is a competitive inhibitor of DHFR and thus prevents the formation of reduced folate (Fig. 16.8). The result of this inhibition may be cessation of DNA synthesis due to nonavailability of dTMP and/or purines, leading to cell death.

Methotrexate enters the cell primarily by active transport. However, drug uptake may be by passive diffusion at high drug concentration (> 20 μM). Intracellular metabolism of methotrexate may lead to addition of glutamic acid residues to the initial glutamate residue of the drug (Fig. 16.7), a process

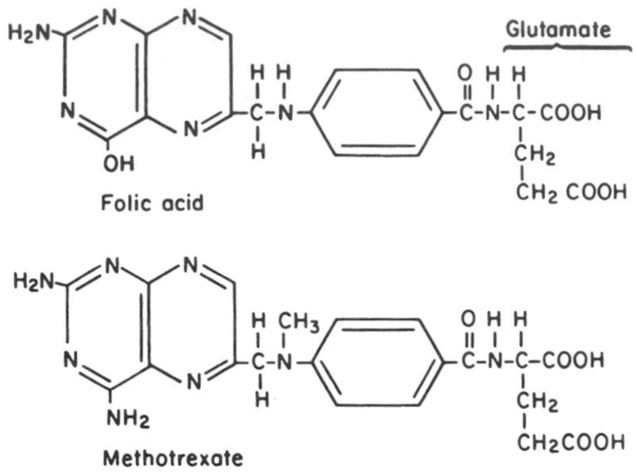

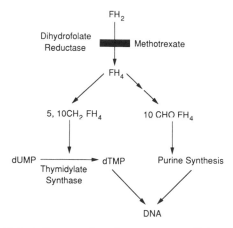

Figure 16.7. The structure of folic acid and its analogue methotrexate. Note that glutamate forms one end of these molecules and further glutamic acid molecules may be added to methotrexate within the cell.

known as *polyglutamation*. Methotrexate polyglutamates cannot be transported across the cell membrane, so their formation prevents efflux of the drug, and they appear to be more effective than methotrexate in inhibiting the activity of DHFR. The cytotoxic action of methotrexate depends critically on the duration of exposure of tissue to levels of drug above a certain threshold rather than on the peak levels of drug in the tissue. Methotrexate has selective toxicity for cells synthesizing DNA, and prolonged treatment with the drug may expose more cells that enter this drug-sensitive phase of the cell cycle. For many tissues, the threshold concentration for cytotoxicity appears to be in the range of 10^{-8} to 10^{-7} M.

The toxicity of methotrexate may be reversed by administration of thymidine and exogenous purines or by a source of reduced folate (FH_4). These agents circumvent the effects of methotrexate by providing products of the interrupted metabolism (Fig. 16.8); they have been used clinically to reverse the activity of methotrexate following a defined period of exposure (usually 24 to 36 h) to methotrexate at high doses. Reduced folate in the form of 5-formyltetrahydrofolate (also known as leucovorin or folinic acid) has been used in many clinical protocols and has allowed the administration of doses of methotrexate that are increased by factors of 10 to 100 over conventional doses. The arguments put forward for such high-dose methotrexate treatment include (1) selective uptake by tumor cells, (2) better CNS penetration, and (3) lack of myelosuppression. This type of protocol may allow for frequent administration of methotrexate and retained therapeutic efficacy with little or no toxicity in many patients. However, responses to treatment are ob-

served only rarely in patients who are refractory to conventional doses of methotrexate given without leucovorin rescue. Although toxicity is often lower with the use of high doses of methotrexate and leucovorin, an occasional patient may experience life-threatening toxicity, usually due to damage to the kidney or sequestration in fluid-filled spaces (e.g., ascites, pleural effusions) and consequent delayed clearance of drug.

Methotrexate can be given orally, intramuscularly, intravenously, and intrathecally. It crosses the blood-brain barrier but achieves cytotoxic concentrations in the central nervous system only with intrathecal or high-dose intravenous administration. It accumulates in fluid-filled spaces such as pleural effusions, from which it is released slowly. The parent compound and hepatic metabolites such as 7-hydroxymethotrexate are excreted by the kidney. This excretion can be inhibited by the presence of weak organic acids such as aspirin or penicillin. Aspirin may also displace methotrexate from its binding site on plasma albumin, and these two effects of aspirin can increase the toxicity of methotrexate. Most reports indicate that the pharmacokinetics of methotrexate can be described by an initial phase of drug disappearance from plasma, which has a half-life of 2 to 3 h, and a final phase with a half-life of 8 to 10 h. This terminal half-life may be prolonged in patients with poor kidney function. Enterohepatic circulation of methotrexate (i.e., circulation from liver to intestine to liver via the biliary tract and por-

Figure 16.8. Influence of methotrexate on cellular metabolism. Through competitive inhibition of the enzyme dihydrofolate reductase, the drug depletes the pools of reduced folates (FH_4):5,10-methylene tetrahydrofolate ($5,10CH_2FH_4$) and 10 formyltetrahydrofolate ($10CHOFH_4$). These reduced folates are required in the conversion of deoxyuridine monophosphate (dUMP) to thymidine monophosphate (dTMP) and for purine synthesis, respectively. Interruption of these processes leads to inhibition of DNA synthesis.

tal veins), which has been reported in some studies, may contribute to a slow third phase of elimination from plasma. Mechanisms which cause resistance to methotrexate include decreased uptake into cells, variant forms of DHFR, and increased production of DHFR because of gene amplification (Chap. 17, Sec. 17.2.2).

Methotrexate has a wide spectrum of clinical activity and may be curative for women with choriocarcinoma, a tumor derived from fetal elements. Its major toxicities are myelosuppression and inflammation of the oral and gastrointestinal mucosa; these toxicities are usually observed within 5 to 7 days of administration, earlier than for many other drugs. Damage to kidneys may occur after high doses of methotrexate due to precipitation of the drug in renal tubules; the risk of such toxicity may be minimized by maintaining a high output of alkaline urine to prevent precipitation. Rarer toxicities include damage to liver, lung, and brain—the latter occurring most frequently after intrathecal administration. In general, the drug is well tolerated compared with many other anticancer drugs.

16.4.2 5-Fluorouracil

5-Fluorouracil (5-FU or FURa) is a drug that resembles the pyrimidine bases uracil and thymine (Fig. 16.9), which are components of RNA and DNA, respectively. The drug penetrates rapidly into cells, where it is metabolized to nucleoside forms by the

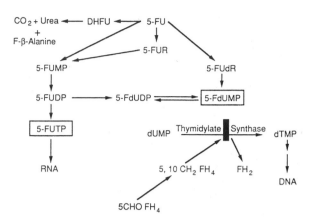

Figure 16.10. Metabolic activation of 5-fluorouracil (5-FU) leads to formation of 5-fluorodeoxyuridine monophosphate (5-FdUMP), which inhibits the enzyme thymidylate synthase, and 5-fluorouridine triphosphate (5-FUTP), which may be incorporated into RNA. Folinic acid (5-CHOFH$_4$) is metabolized to 5,10-methylene tetrahydrofolate (5,10CH$_2$FH$_4$), the cofactor that forms a ternary complex with 5-FdUMP and enzyme. 5-FU is catabolized to dihydrofluorouracil (DHFU) and excreted as CO$_2$, urea, and α-fluoro-β-alanine.

addition of the sugars ribose or deoxyribose; these reactions are catalyzed by enzymes that normally act on uracil and thymine. Phosphorylation then leads to the active fluorinated nucleotides 5-FUTP and 5-FdUMP (Fig. 16.10). 5-FUTP can be incorporated into RNA in place of UTP (uridine triphosphate); this leads to inhibition of the nuclear processing of ribosomal and messenger RNA and may cause other errors of base pairing during transcription of RNA. 5-FdUMP inhibits irreversibly the enzyme thymidylate synthase, leading to depletion of dTMP (thymidine monophosphate), which is required for DNA synthesis.

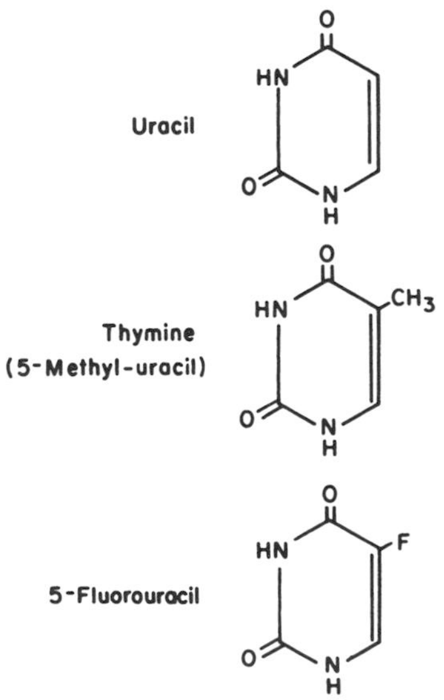

The relative importance of the above mechanisms for toxicity of 5-FU are disputed. Separation of these effects may be achieved by administration of (1) 5-fluorodeoxyuridine (5-FUdR), another agent that is available for clinical use and that seems to act solely (after phosphorylation) to inhibit thymidylate synthase (Fig. 16.10), or (2) 5-FU together with thymidine, which should prevent any toxic effects from inhibition of thymidylate synthase. Both of these measures lead to toxicity for various types of cells. The relative importance of the two mechanisms underlying cytotoxicity of 5-FU probably varies for treatment of different tumors and normal tissues. In cells where toxicity is due to interruption of DNA synthesis through inhibition of thymidylate syn-

Uracil

Thymine (5-Methyl-uracil)

5-Fluorouracil

Figure 16.9. Structures of uracil, thymine, and the analogue 5-fluorouracil.

thase, the drug should have specificity for cells in the S phase of the cycle; when the major mechanism is incorporation of 5-FUTP into RNA, the effects may be independent of cell-cycle phase. Approximately 80 percent of 5-FU administered clinically is catabolized to the end products of CO_2, urea, and α-fluoro-β-alanine, mainly in the liver. The catabolism of 5-FU appears to be an important determinant of normal-tissue toxicity. If 5-FU is catabolized rapidly, then the exposure of both tumor and normal tissues to active metabolites of the drug will be decreased. About 3 percent of patients have a partial deficiency of the rate-limiting enzyme for elimination of 5-FU, dihydropyrimidine dehydrogenase (DPD), and are at risk for severe toxicity from the drug (Milano and Etienne, 1994). An experimental approach to therapy involves very low dose oral 5-FU given with an inhibitor of DPD; this gives relatively constant plasma levels of 5-FU.

Inhibition of thymidylate synthase by FdUMP is dependent on the presence of the cofactor 5,10-methylenetetrahydrofolate, which combines with thymidylate synthase and FdUMP to form a covalent ternary complex (Fig. 16.10). The dissociation rate of this complex is decreased in the presence of excess cofactor (Moran and Keyomarsi, 1987). This led to experiments indicating that addition of the prodrug 5-formyltetrahydrofolate (folinic acid or leucovorin) increased the cytotoxicity of 5-FU (Fig. 16.10; Keyomarsi and Moran, 1986). Clinical studies have demonstrated that this combination has greater activity in the treatment of patients with metastatic colorectal cancer than 5-FU alone (Erlichman et al., 1988).

5-Fluorouracil is most commonly used for treatment of breast and gastrointestinal cancer. The drug is usually given intravenously, because bioavailability after oral administration is variable. It is eliminated rapidly from plasma with a half-life of a few minutes. This agent demonstrates nonlinear pharmacokinetics due to a saturation of metabolism at higher peak concentrations, which may be seen when it is given by bolus injection but not when given by infusion. This difference in pharmacokinetic behavior under the two conditions of administration may explain why the dose-limiting toxicity differs for bolus and infusion. Major toxicity is to bone marrow and mucous membranes; the latter becomes dominant if the drug is given over 4 to 5 days by continuous infusion. Rarer toxicity includes skin rashes, conjunctivitis, ataxia (loss of balance) due to effects on the cerebellum, and cardiotoxicity. Prolonged low-dose infusions of 5-FU can be administered with a decrease in some of the above forms of systemic toxicity, but they are associated with changes in sensation as well as with redness and peeling of the skin on the palms of the hands and the soles of the feet, referred to as the *hand–foot syndrome*. There is limited evidence that this method of 5-FU administration results in improvement of antitumor effects when compared with 5-FU given by bolus schedules (Lokich et al., 1989).

Several investigators have studied the interaction between 5-FU and methotrexate because they both inhibit DNA synthesis by influencing the reaction catalyzed by thymidylate synthase, which converts dUMP to dTMP. Mechanisms that suggest a sequence dependency for the combined activity of methotrexate and 5-FU include the following: (1) methotrexate given first might block purine synthesis, leading to elevation of phosphoribosyl-pyrophosphate (PRPP), which is necessary for activation of 5-FU, (2) 5-FU given first might block thymidylate synthesis, thus preventing consumption of reduced folates, and antagonize the antipurine effects of methotrexate. Increased toxicity has been observed in tissue culture when methotrexate is given from 1 to 24 h prior to 5-FU (Cadman et al., 1979). When studied in clinical trials, however, this sequence led to little or no therapeutic advantage in comparison with simultaneous administration.

16.4.3 Cytidine Analogues

Cytosine arabinoside (ara-C) differs from the nucleoside deoxycytidine only by the presence of a β-hydroxyl group on the 2-position of the sugar, so that the sugar moiety is arabinose instead of deoxyribose (Fig. 16.11). Ara-C penetrates cells rapidly by a carrier-mediated process shared with deoxycytidine and is phosphorylated to ara-CTP (Fig. 16.12). Ara-CTP is a competitive inhibitor of DNA polymerase, an enzyme necessary for DNA synthesis, and has similar affinity for this enzyme to the normal substrate dCTP. When ara-CTP binds to this enzyme, DNA synthesis is arrested and S-phase cells may die. Incorporation of ara-C into DNA also occurs and may contribute to its cytotoxic effects, possibly because of defective ligation or incomplete synthesis of DNA fragments.

The availability of ara-CTP for cytotoxic activity depends critically on the balance between the kinases that activate the drug and the deaminases that degrade it (Fig. 16.11). The activity of these enzymes varies greatly among different types of cells, leading to different rates of generation of ara-CTP. Resistance to the action of ara-C may occur by mutations that lead to deficiency in deoxycytidine kinase

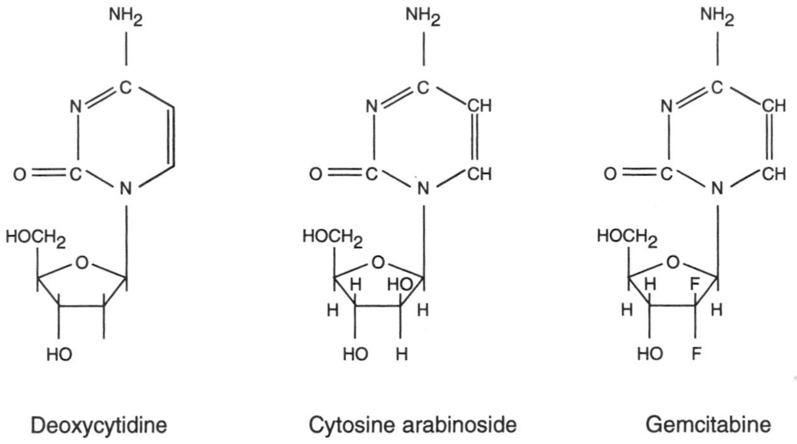

Figure 16.11. Structure of deoxycytidine and its analogues cytosine arabinoside and gemcitabine.

Deoxycytidine   Cytosine arabinoside   Gemcitabine

or to cells with an expanded pool of dCTP that competes with the active metabolite ara-CTP and regulates enzymes involved in activation and degradation of the drug. Ara-C is specific in its activity for cells synthesizing DNA. Since it is rapidly degraded in plasma with a half-life of 7 to 20 min, it must be given intravenously by frequent injections or by continuous infusion to kill cells as they pass from G1 to S phase of the cycle. The drug is used primarily for treatment of acute leukemia. Myelosuppression and gastrointestinal toxicity are the major side effects, but abnormal behavior and thought processes may also occur following high doses.

Gemcitabine (2'2'-difluorodeoxycytidine) is a cytosine analogue with structural similarities to ara-C (Fig 16.11). Unlike ara-C, gemcitabine has antitumor activity against a variety of solid tumors. Like ara-C, gemcitabine requires intracellular activation to its triphosphate derivative dFdCTP, which is incorporated into DNA and then inhibits DNA synthesis. Gemcitabine has other intracellular effects that may contribute to its cytotoxic activity; these include inhibition of ribonucleotide reductase; stimulation of deoxycytidine kinase, the enzyme responsible for its activation; and inhibition of cytidine deaminase, the primary enzyme responsible for its degradation (Huang et al., 1991). The intracellular half-life of the nucleotide triphosphate of gemcitabine is much longer than that formed from ara-C. The drug is schedule-dependent, with once-weekly administration providing a good therapeutic ratio. In clinical studies, gemcitabine has activity against non-small-cell lung cancer, pancreatic cancer, breast cancer, and bladder cancer. Toxicity is primarily myelosuppression.

16.4.4 Purine Antimetabolites

Many purine analogues have been synthesized, and a few of these have found application as antiviral agents (e.g., adenosine arabinoside, ara-A), immunosuppressive agents used in preservation of kidney and other organ grafts (e.g., azathioprine), and as anticancer drugs [e.g., 6-mercaptopurine (6-MP) and 6-thioguanine (6-TG); Fig. 16.13]. Use of the last two of these drugs is limited to treatment of leukemia.

Like guanine, 6-MP and 6-TG are metabolized to deoxynucleotides by addition of the sugar-phosphate moiety and are incorporated into DNA. This mechanism presumably accounts for their selective toxicity for cells in DNA synthesis. Metabolites of the drugs may also inhibit purine and RNA synthesis; the relative importance of these mechanisms is unclear. Cross-resistance is usually observed between

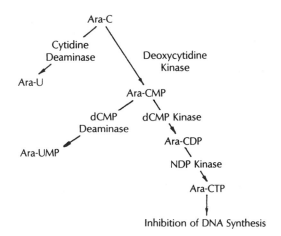

Figure 16.12. Metabolic activation and degradation of cytosine arabinoside (ara-C). Formation of the active metabolite ara-CTP depends on the balance between kinases that activate the drug and deaminases that degrade it.

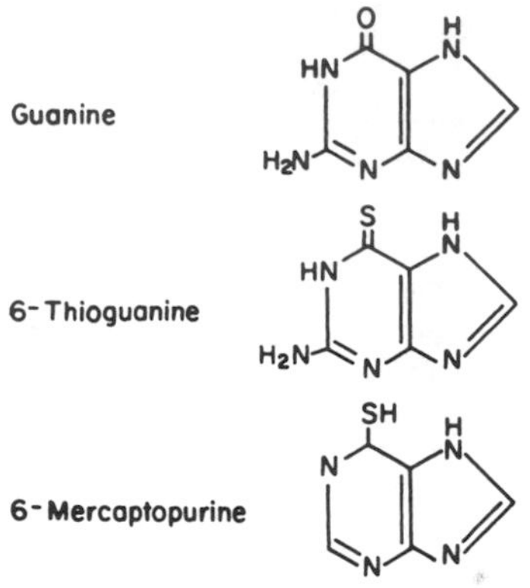

Guanine

6-Thioguanine

6-Mercaptopurine

Figure 16.13. Structures of guanine and the analogues 6-thioguanine and 6-mercaptopurine.

6-MP and 6-TG, and drug-resistant mutant cells may have decreased activity of the enzyme HGPRT (hypoxanthine–guanine phosphoribosyltransferase), which is necessary for their activation. Alternative mechanisms that convey resistance probably involve increased degradation of the drugs and their metabolites.

Recent studies of the clinical pharmacology of 6-MP have revealed a low bioavailability of drug when administered orally because of first-pass hepatic metabolism and wide patient-to-patient variability. The clinical toxicities of 6-MP include myelosuppression, mucositis, diarrhea, nausea, and vomiting.

Analogues of adenine and its nucleoside derivative adenosine (Fig. 16.14) are the most recent of the DNA base analogues to be introduced into clinical practice. Early analogues were limited by their rapid deamination by adenosine deaminase (ADA). Fludarabine (9-β-arabinofuranosyl-2-fluoroadenine monophosphate) is a derivative that is resistant to deamination and has activity against low-grade lymphomas, chronic lymphocytic leukemia, and hairy cell leukemia (Keating et al., 1994). After administration, fludarabine is rapidly dephosphorylated to 2-flu-

oro–ara-A, which then is transported into cells and converted to the active triphosphate derivative. Since 2-fluoro–ara-A is excreted primarily unchanged in the urine, dose reduction is necessary in the setting of renal insufficiency. The major toxicity of fludarabine is myelosuppression and immunosuppression.

2-chlorodeoxyadenosine (2CdA) is a potent chlorinated adenosine derivative (Fig. 16.14) that is resistant to deamination. It has a similar spectrum of clinical activity and toxicity to fludarabine. It is transported directly into cells, where the triphosphate 2-CdATP is formed by deoxycytidine kinase. While 2-CdATP can induce DNA breaks and inhibit replication, its mechanism of cytotoxicity in slowly proliferating cells is not well understood.

Deoxycoformycin (Fig. 16.14) is an inhibitor of adenosine deaminase (ADA) that has demonstrated activity against hairy cell leukemia and some indolent lymphomas. Why inhibition of the ability of cells to break down normal nucleosides should be cytotoxic is not understood, but accumulation of adenine nucleosides might lead to secondary inhibition of DNA synthesis. Most of the drug is excreted unchanged in urine and, as with fludarabine, dose reduction is necessary in the setting of renal insufficiency. The dose of deoxycoformycin required to maximally inhibit ADA leads to substantial toxicity. However hairy cell leukemias have low ADA activity, and the lower dose of deoxycoformycin required to treat this disease has minimal toxicity.

16.4.5 Thymidylate Synthase Inhibitors

New compounds designed specifically to inhibit thymidylate synthase (TS), by binding to the site for 5,10-methylene tetrahydrofolate, have been developed (Tourtoutoglou and Pazdur, 1996). These compounds are intended to bind to TS and deplete dTMP required for DNA synthesis. Two compounds are undergoing clinical development (Fig. 16.15). Tomudex and LY231514 are folate-based TS in-

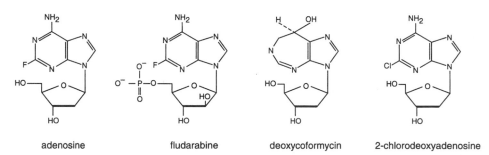

adenosine   fludarabine   deoxycoformycin   2-chlorodeoxyadenosine

Figure 16.14. Structures of adenosine and the analogues fludarabine, deoxycoformycin, and 2-chlorodeoxyadenosine.

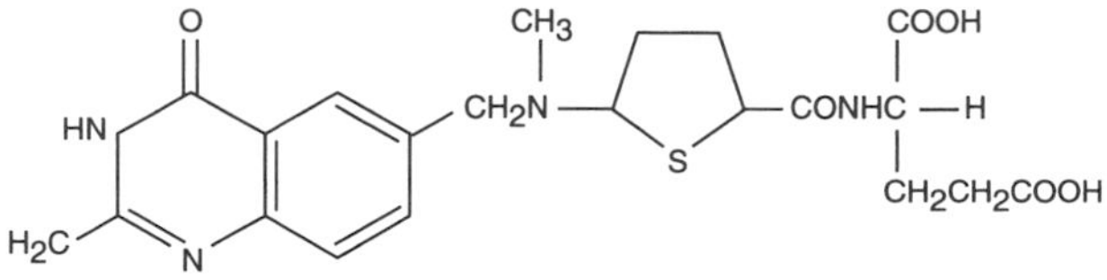

Tomudex
(ZD1694)

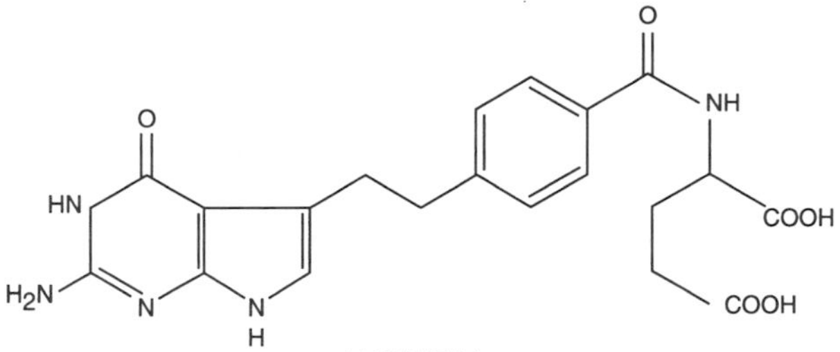

LY231514

Figure 16.15. Structure of the thymidylate synthase inhibitors Tomudex and LY231514.

hibitors with glutamic acid at one end of the molecule (similar to methotrexate) and can be polyglutamated for increased retention in cells and increased potency of TS inhibition. These agents require transport via the reduced folate carrier and are potent inhibitors of TS.

Both Tomudex and LY231514 are administered intravenously. Renal excretion appears to be the major route of elimination for both agents. The clinical activity of Tomudex appears comparable to that of 5-FU combined with leucovorin in metastatic colorectal cancer, and activity has also been seen in breast cancer (Cunningham et al., 1995). LY231514 has demonstrated clinical activity in colon cancer. The main clinical toxicities are myelosuppression, inflammation of the oral and gastrointestinal mucosa, and skin rash. Tomudex has been associated with transient elevations in some liver-function tests. The ultimate clinical utility of these compounds is yet to be defined.

16.5 NATURAL PRODUCTS

No satisfactory classification of cytotoxic agents currently exists. The classification presented in this chapter is the one usually used in discussing these drugs. However, while the previous categories are based on mechanism of action, the natural products include a variety of agents with a variety of mechanisms of action. They are either compounds isolated from plants, fungi, or bacteria or derivatives of products isolated in this manner. Within this category are drugs that interfere with topoisomerase I

(e.g., camptothecins) or topoisomerase II (e.g., doxorubicin, etoposide), that bind directly with DNA (e.g., bleomycin), and that interfere with microtubules (e.g., paclitaxel, vincristine).

16.5.1 Anthracyclines and Anthracenediones

The original anthracycline, daunorubicin, is a product of a *Streptomyces* species isolated from an Italian soil sample in 1958. The drug had high activity against acute leukemia and remains a component of many current protocols for acute myelogenous leukemia. Modifications of the structure of daunorubicin led to the identification of doxorubicin, an analogue with greater activity against many solid tumors and one of the most active anticancer drugs in current clinical practice (Fig. 16.16). The success of doxorubicin led to a major effort to synthesize other analogues, but of the hundreds developed and tested, only two are used currently; both have only marginal advantages. Idarubicin is an orally absorbed daunorubicin analogue with similar activity against acute leukemia. Epirubicin differs from doxorubicin only in its three-dimensional configuration; it has equivalent activity and possibly less toxicity.

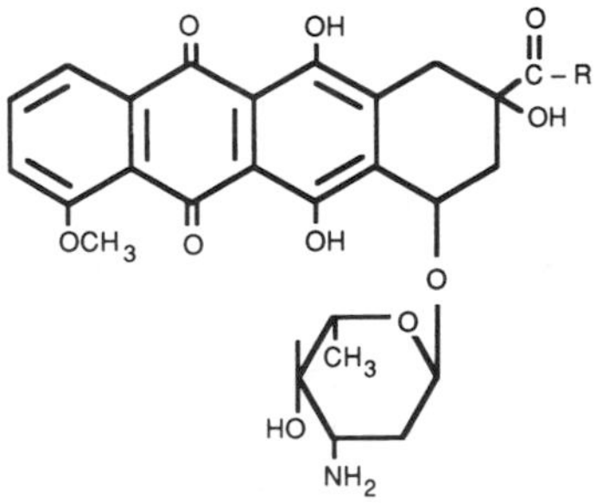

R = CH₂ OH, doxorubicin

= CH₃ daunorubicin

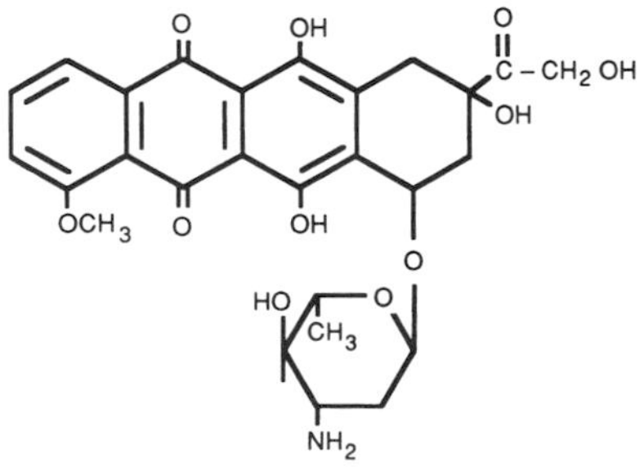

Epirubicin

Figure 16.16. Structure of doxorubicin (Adriamycin), daunorubicin, and epirubicin.

Several mechanisms may contribute to the cytocidal effect of doxorubicin and related drugs. These include DNA intercalation, interaction with topoisomerase II, formation of free radicals, and effects on the cell membrane. Doxorubicin can intercalate between base pairs perpendicular to the long axis of the double helix, leading to partial unwinding of the DNA helix. However, much of the DNA is organized and folded into chromatin and may be protected from this type of drug interaction. Also, the concentration of doxorubicin required to intercalate into DNA and to cause inhibition of DNA and RNA polymerase cannot be achieved in vivo without excessive toxicity.

Doxorubicin may also cause single- and double-strand breaks in DNA, which are probably mediated through binding to topoisomerase II. The enzyme topoisomerase II is involved in the cleavage, unwinding, and rejoining of segments of DNA—processes that are required during DNA and RNA synthesis (see Chap. 17, Sec. 17.2.5). Doxorubicin can interact with topoisomerase II by binding directly with the enzyme and preventing resealing of topoisomerase II–induced DNA cleavage. It can also indirectly produce topoisomerase II–mediated cleavage of DNA.

Doxorubicin may undergo metabolism of its quinone ring to a semiquinone radical (i.e., a group containing an unpaired electron) that, in turn, reacts rapidly with oxygen to yield superoxide, O_2^- (Bachur et al., 1977). The superoxide radical is known to undergo several reactions that can lead to cell death, including oxidative damage of cell membranes and DNA. There is evidence that free radical formation accounts for the cardiac toxicity of anthracyclines, but the contribution of free radicals to the killing of cancer cells is uncertain. Resistance to anthracyclines has been associated with an increase in the free radical scavenger system (glutathione and related compounds), but doxorubicin retains toxicity under hypoxic conditions, when superoxide radicals cannot be formed (Tannock and Guttman, 1981).

Doxorubicin and related drugs also bind to cell membranes and may kill cells through membrane-related effects. Tritton and Yee (1982) studied the effects of doxorubicin in vitro, when it was linked to beads, and demonstrated that the drug could cause cell death without being transported into the cell.

With the exception of idarubicin, all anthracyclines are administered intravenously, because oral absorption is poor. They are widely distributed in the body, with significant binding to plasma proteins and tissue. Plasma clearance after intravenous administration may be described by three exponential components with half-lives in the ranges of 8 to 25 min, 1.5 to 10 h, and 24 to 48 h (Robert and Gianni, 1993). The second phase is attributed to metabolism of the drug in liver and the final phase to release of drug from tissue-binding sites. Doxorubicin is metabolized in the liver to doxorubicinol, which retains some cytotoxic activity, and to several other metabolites; the drug and its metabolites are excreted via the bile. Thus, dosage reduction is required for patients with hepatic dysfunction or biliary obstruction.

The acute toxicities of doxorubicin include myelosuppression, total loss of hair, nausea, vomiting, mucositis, and local tissue necrosis following leakage of drug at the injection site. Repeated administration is limited by a chronic irreversible cardiomyopathy that occurs with increasing frequency once a total dose of 450 mg/m^2 has been given. The mechanism of cardiotoxicity is probably related to damage to sarcoplasmic reticulum mediated by the formation of free radicals within cardiac muscle. Patients with pre-existing cardiac disease or those who have received mediastinal radiation are more likely to develop this problem. Cardiac toxicity appears to be more related to peak concentration of drug than to overall exposure, so that infusional or repeated lower-dose administration will reduce the chances of its occurrence. Dexrazoxane, an iron-chelating agent, has been demonstrated to reduce cardiac toxicity without compromising efficacy when given concurrently with doxorubicin.

Mitoxantrone is an anthracenedione that differs from the anthracyclines in lacking the sugar and the tetracyclic ring. It is a synthetic drug with three planar rings that intercalates into DNA, with a preference for guanine-cytosine base pairs. It may also function as an inhibitor of topoisomerase II. This drug is used as an alternative to anthracyclines in the treatment of acute myelogenous leukemia and breast cancer. While generally less active than doxorubicin, it causes less nausea, vomiting, mucositis, and hair loss and has found a role in the palliative treatment of cancers of the breast and prostate.

Multiple mechanisms which can lead to resistance to anthracyclines and anthracenediones are summarized in Chap. 17, Tables 17.2 and 17.3.

16.5.2 Bleomycin

Bleomycin consists of a family of molecules with a complex structure; it is derived from fungal culture, the dominant active component being known as bleomycin A2 (Lazo and Chabner, 1996).

Bleomycin causes DNA double-strand breaks through a complex sequence of reactions involving the binding of a bleomycin–ferrous iron complex to DNA. This binding leads to insertion of the drug between base pairs (intercalation) and unwinding of the double helix. A second step in the formation of DNA strand breaks may involve the reduction of molecular oxygen to superoxide or hydroxyl radicals, catalyzed by the bleomycin–ferrous iron complex. However, like doxorubicin, bleomycin retains some of its lethal activity under hypoxic conditions. Bleomycin may exert preferential toxicity in the G2 phase of the cell cycle, but it also has toxicity for slowly proliferating cells in plateau-phase cell culture. Bleomycin is a large molecule that crosses cell membranes slowly. Once within the cell, it can be activated or broken down by bleomycin hydrolase; cellular sensitivity to bleomycin has been found to correlate inversely with the concentration of this enzyme.

After intravenous injection, most of the administered drug is eliminated unchanged in the urine. Plasma clearance curves have two components with half-lives of about 0.5 h and 4 to 8 h, respectively. The major use of bleomycin is in combination with other drugs for the curative therapy of testicular cancer and lymphomas. Bleomycin has little toxicity to bone marrow but may cause fever, chills, and damage to skin and mucous membranes. The most serious toxicity is interstitial fibrosis of the lung; its incidence is related to cumulative dose, age, renal function, and the use of other agents that may damage the lung, such as high oxygen concentrations or radiation therapy.

16.5.3 Vinca Alkaloids

The vinca alkaloids—vinblastine, vincristine, and vinorelbine—are naturally occurring or semisynthetic derivatives from the periwinkle plant. These compounds bind to the protein tubulin and inhibit its polymerization to form microtubules (Rowinsky and Donehower, 1996). Microtubules have several important cellular functions, including formation of the mitotic spindle responsible for separation of chromosomes, and structural and transport functions in axons of nerves. Microtubules are in a state of dynamic equilibrium, with continuous formation and degradation from cytoplasmic tubulin. This process is interrupted by treatment with vinca alkaloids, and lethally damaged cells may be observed to enter an abortive metaphase and then lyse. However, experiments with synchronized cells have

demonstrated that maximum lethal toxicity for vinblastine and vincristine occurs when cells are exposed during the period of DNA synthesis; presumably the morphologic expression of that damage is observed in the attempted mitosis.

Vincristine and vinblastine are structurally similar, differing only in a substitution on the central rings (Fig. 16.17; Chabner and Chabner, 1994). Vinca alkaloids have large volumes of distribution, indicating a high degree of tissue binding, and are eliminated mainly by hepatic metabolism and biliary excretion. Their plasma clearance is described by a triexponential curve, with terminal half-lives of about 20 to 40 h.

Despite similarities in their structures, these drugs differ in both their clinical spectra of activity and their toxicities. Vinblastine is an important drug in combination chemotherapy of testicular cancer, while vincristine is a mainstay of treatment for childhood leukemia. Both drugs have been combined with other cytotoxic agents to treat lymphomas or various solid tumors. Vinorelbine has been introduced more recently and has activity as a single agent against lung and breast cancers. Vinblastine causes major toxicity to bone marrow, with some risk of autonomic neuropathy, leading to constipation. The dose of vincristine is limited by its toxicity to peripheral nerves, and this damage relates to the duration of treatment as well as the total dose of vincristine used. This neurotoxicity probably occurs because of damage to the microtubules in axons. The dose-limiting toxicity of vinorelbine is myelosuppression. Neurotoxicity can occur but is less common than with vincristine, possibly due to a lower affinity for axonal microtubules.

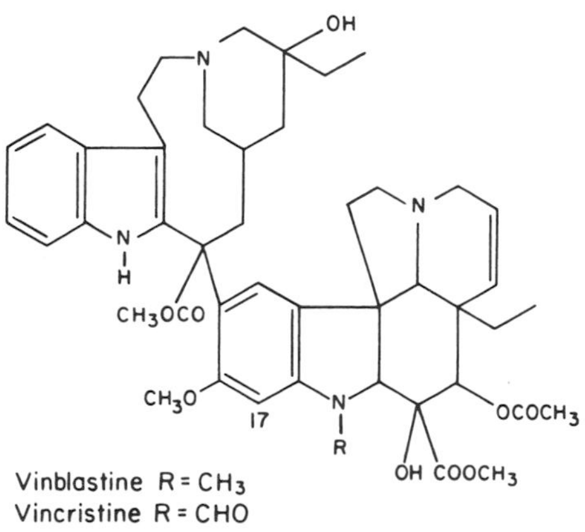

Vinblastine R = CH₃
Vincristine R = CHO

Figure 16.17. Structures of vinblastine and vincristine.

16.5.4 Taxanes

The taxanes paclitaxel (Taxol) and docetaxel (Taxotere) are plant alkaloids extracted from the bark and needles of the western yew tree *Taxus brevifolia* (Fig. 16.18). Paclitaxel was identified originally as an anticancer drug more than 25 years ago, but its clinical development was hampered by a limited drug supply, which depended on the bark of the relatively rare yew tree. Interest increased once it became apparent that the mechanism of action was unique and that there was evidence of activity in ovarian cancer. Docetaxel is a semisynthetic derivative of the needles of the yew tree and is a more potent tubulin inhibitor in vitro.

Taxanes are antimicrotubular agents and bind to tubulin at a site different to that of the vinca alkaloids. In contrast to the vinca alkaloids, which inhibit the polymerization of tubulin into microtubules, taxanes inhibit microtubular disassembly, which then prevents the normal growth and breakdown of microtubules that is required for cell division (Rowinsky and Donehower, 1995).

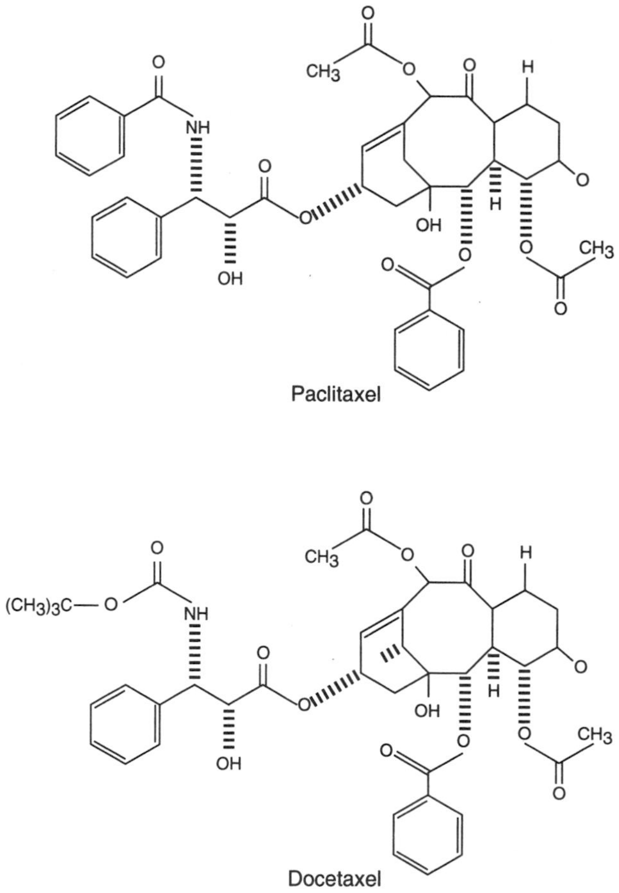

The pharmacokinetics of paclitaxel and docetaxel are characterized by a large volume of distribution with extensive tissue binding, elimination by hepatic metabolism, and elimination half-lives of 10 to 12 h (Sonnichsen and Relling, 1994). As hepatic elimination to inactive metabolites is mediated through cytochrome P-450 enzymes, agents that influence cytochrome P-450 can influence the clearance and toxicity of the taxanes; thus patients on anticonvulsants have demonstrated increased clearance and reduced toxicity. The ideal schedule of administration for taxanes remains to be determined. Paclitaxel is generally given as a 3-h infusion, although longer infusion schedules have better activity in vitro and are undergoing clinical testing.

Paclitaxel and docetaxel share many common toxicities. The dose-limiting toxicity is a noncumulative myelosuppression, mainly neutropenia. Both can cause hypersensitivity reactions with bronchial constriction, urticaria, and hypotension. This problem has been reduced substantially by prophylactic treatment with steroids and histamine blockers. A sensory peripheral neuropathy can occur with repeated or high-dose administration. Docetaxel can also cause fluid retention and skin and nail changes with repeated usage. These drugs have activity against ovarian, breast, and lung cancer and are undergoing more detailed evaluation in patients with a number of other tumors.

16.5.5 Epipodophyllotoxins

VP-16 (etoposide) and VM-26 (teniposide) are semisynthetic glycoside derivatives of podophyllotoxin, an antimitotic agent derived from the mandrake plant. Although podophyllotoxin binds to tubulin and inhibits its polymerization, VP-16 and VM-26 act through inhibition of DNA topoisomerase II (Van Mannen et al., 1988). VP-16 is a widely used drug and is a component of first-line treatment regimens in small-cell lung cancer, testicular cancer, pediatric tumors, and malignant lymphomas. It also has activity against gastric cancer, non-small-cell lung cancer, and acute leukemia. VM-26 has a more limited role in childhood hematologic cancer. VP-16 is markedly schedule-dependent, with repeated daily doses providing greater activity than a single intravenous injection. Synergy between cisplatin and etoposide has been demonstrated in vitro, and these two drugs are commonly given together to patients with lung or testicular tumors (Eder et al., 1990).

VP-16 and VM-26 form a complex with topoisomerase II after cleavage of DNA and inhibit religa-

Figure 16.18. Structures of paclitaxel and docetaxel.

tion of the DNA strands (Pommier, 1993). This leads to inhibition of DNA replication and to single- and double-strand breaks in DNA. Cells with higher concentration of topoisomerase II are more sensitive to the effects of the epipodophyllotoxins (see also Chap. 17, Sec. 17.2.5).

Etoposide is usually given intravenously but can be given orally, with a bioavailability of approximately 50 percent and considerable interindividual variability. Following intravenous administration, etoposide is eliminated by hepatic glucuronidation and approximately 40 percent of the drug is excreted unchanged in the urine.

The toxicity of VP-16 at standard doses is myelosuppression and hair loss, with other effects being uncommon. This toxicity profile makes etoposide ideal for high-dose transplantation regimens, and at these higher doses (1.0 to 1.5 g/m^2), mucositis becomes dose-limiting. An association between the use of etoposide and a secondary leukemia with a characteristic 11q23 translocation has been described (Winick et al., 1993).

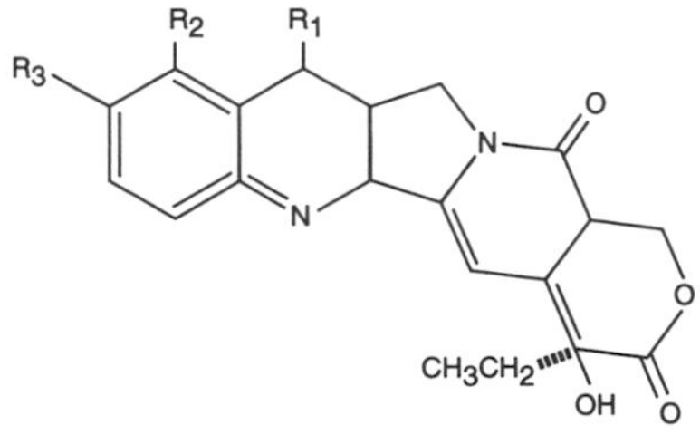

16.5.6 Camptothecin Derivatives

Camptothecin is an extract from the wood of the Chinese tree *Camptotheca acuminata* (Fig. 16.19). Camptothecin was found to be active in vivo against a murine leukemia, but phase I studies conducted in the early 1970s were terminated because of severe and unpredictable toxicity. This class of agents is unique in affecting topoisomerase I activity. Topoisomerase I is a ubiquitous nuclear enzyme that relaxes torsionally strained DNA by the formation of a single-strand nick in the backbone. The opposite DNA strand then passes through the nick and the DNA backbone is rejoined (Chap. 17, Sec. 17.2.5). Camptothecin and its analogues act by binding to and stabilizing DNA/topoisomerase I adducts, which leads to an inhibition of the religation of the DNA and to DNA single-strand breaks. Cells in S phase are very sensitive to camptothecin and its analogues, possibly because the process of DNA replication requires topoisomerase I activity and because the topoisomerase-associated single-strand breaks are converted into double-strand breaks (Pommier, 1993). However, cytotoxicity is not restricted to cells in S phase, and the proportion of cells killed following an exposure to camptothecin has been demonstrated in vitro to exceed the S-phase fraction.

Several analogues of camptothecin have been synthesized. Those under clinical development have either substitutions on the "A" ring, which increase

	R$_3$	R$_2$	R$_1$
Camptothecin	H	H	H
CPT-11	(piperidine-N-C(=O)-O)	H	CH$_3$CH$_2$
Topotecan	OH	(CH$_3$)$_2$NCH$_2$	H
9-Aminocamptothecin	H	NH$_2$	H

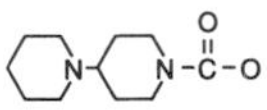

Figure 16.19. Structures of camptothecin and analogues topotecan, CPT-11, and 9-aminocamptothecin.

the aqueous solubility while retaining cytotoxicity (topotecan and CPT-11), or addition of an amino group to the "B" ring, which leads to increased potency, but the problems with solubility remain (9-aminocamptothecin) (Fig. 16.19).

Topotecan has activity in vitro and in vivo that is similar to that of camptothecin. It does not undergo any appreciable metabolism and is primarily eliminated unchanged by the kidneys. Therefore dose reduction in the setting of renal dysfunction is required. Topotecan can be given either intravenously or orally. Interest in the oral formulation has been stimulated by preclinical evidence of a better cell kill when this drug is given continuously. The dose-limiting toxicity in most clinical studies is myelosuppression. Topotecan has promise as a treatment for ovarian cancer and some types of lung cancer.

CPT-11 requires esterification to an active metabolite SN-38 before becoming cytotoxic. It has activity in vivo that is greater than or equal to that seen with camptothecin. Dose-limiting toxicity has consisted of both myelosuppression and diarrhea. In phase II studies using a once-weekly schedule, activity was seen in small-cell lung cancer, non-small-cell lung cancer, ovarian cancer, and most notably colon cancer refractory to 5-FU.

While 9-aminocamptothecin is a more potent agent, its clinical development has lagged behind that of the others because of problems with solubility and formulation. These have now been solved and it is undergoing broad phase II testing.

16.5.7 Mitomycin C

Mitomycin C is derived from a *Streptomyces* species and is a quinone-containing compound that requires activation to an alkylating metabolite by reductive metabolism. The drug is more active against hypoxic than aerobic cells in tissue culture, but it has not been shown to have preferential toxicity for hypoxic cells in vivo, perhaps because of limited penetration from tumor blood vessels (Rauth et al., 1983). Mitomycin C causes delayed and rather unpredictable myelosuppression. More seriously, the drug can produce a hemolytic-uremic syndrome, which is usually fatal and is probably due to small-vessel endothelial damage. Another potentially lethal effect is interstitial lung disease with progression to pulmonary fibrosis. The availability of equally active drugs with lower toxicities limits the clinical utility of mitomycin C. It is sometimes used intravesically to treat superficial bladder cancer and is also used with radiation therapy in cancer of the anal canal, head and neck, and esophagus. Analogues of the drug that are less toxic or better hypoxic cell cytotoxins are undergoing clinical testing.

16.6 MISCELLANEOUS DRUGS

16.6.1 Cisplatin and Carboplatin

Cisplatin (*cis*-diamminedichloroplatinum II; Fig. 16.20) is an important anticancer drug whose discovery followed an observation that an electric current delivered to bacterial culture via platinum electrodes led to inhibition of bacterial growth. The active compound was found to be cisplatin, and this compound was shown subsequently to exert major activity against several tumors in mice.

Cisplatin acts by a mechanism that is similar to that of classical alkylating agents (Roberts et al., 1988). The chlorine atoms are leaving groups that may be compared to those of nitrogen mustards (Fig. 16.2); these atoms may be displaced directly by nucleophilic groups of DNA or indirectly after chloride ions are replaced by hydroxyl groups through reaction of the drug with water. The preferred sites for binding of cisplatin to DNA are the N-7 positions of guanine and adenine bases. Cisplatin binds to two sites on DNA with the production of interstrand cross-links and interstrand adducts (Fichtinger-Schepman et al., 1987). Lethal effects against cells seem to correlate with the number of cross-links formed between the DNA strands. Studies of the kinetics of formation and removal of cross-links (Kohn, 1979) have shown that both cisplatin and its trans isomer lead to formation of DNA protein cross-links, but only cisplatin pro-

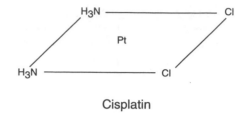

Cisplatin

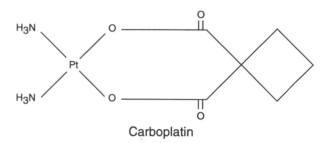

Carboplatin

Oxaliplatin

Figure 16.20. Structures of cisplatin, carboplatin, and oxaliplatin.

duces DNA interstrand cross-links at clinically achievable concentration. These cross-links continue to be formed for several hours after removal of the drug and are then repaired.

Following administration, cisplatin is rapidly and tightly bound to plasma proteins, with greater than 90 percent of free cisplatin lost in the first 2 h. Total cisplatin (free and bound drug) disappears more slowly from plasma, with a prolonged half-life of 2 to 3 days. Cisplatin is excreted mainly via the urine, and 15 to 30 percent of the administered dose is excreted during the first 24 h.

Cisplatin is used as part of drug combinations that can cure testicular cancer and, in combination with other drugs, for palliation of a variety of solid tumors. It causes little toxicity to bone marrow by itself but can add to the toxic effects of other drugs and may lead to anemia. Its major dose-limiting toxicities are severe nausea and vomiting, damage to the kidneys, and loss of hearing and neurotoxicity after prolonged use. The effects on the kidneys may be minimized by maintaining a rapid urine output during and after drug administration. A large number of analogues of cisplatin have been synthesized and are being tested in experimental animals and in humans. Resistance to cisplatin may develop by multiple mechanisms (see Chap. 17, Table 17.2).

Carboplatin is an analogue of cisplatin that has a similar spectrum of activity (Fig. 16.20). Carboplatin is less nephrotoxic and causes less nausea and vomiting than cisplatin, but it causes thrombocytopenia. Carboplatin also binds avidly to plasma proteins and is excreted primarily by the kidney. The relationship between dose and renal function has been determined, leading to the definition of a model that can be used to predict the dose of carboplatin required to achieve a predetermined level of toxicity, such as the nadir platelet count (Egorin et al., 1984).

Oxaliplatin (Fig. 16.20) is an analogue of cisplatin that differs from cisplatin in that it has mild renal toxicity. Its dose-limiting toxicity is peripheral neuropathy, which is cumulative. There is no apparent relationship between oxaliplatin's pharmacokinetics and neurotoxicity (Weiss and Christian, 1993). Oxaliplatin has shown antitumor activity in colorectal cancer, melanoma, glioma, lung cancer, ovarian cancer, and breast cancer.

16.6.2 Other Drugs

Drugs with limited clinical use that are not described in the preceding sections include hydroxyurea and L-asparaginase. Hydroxyurea is a simple structural analogue of urea that was synthesized more than a century ago. The drug inhibits ribonucleotide reductase enzymes, which catalyze the conversion of ribonucleotides (e.g., CDP) to the deoxyribonucleotides (dCDP) necessary for DNA synthesis. It is used as an alternative to busulfan in the treatment of chronic myelocytic leukemia. Hydroxyurea is used experimentally to cause cell synchronization, since it kills cells in S phase and blocks them reversibly at the G1/S border.

L-Asparaginase is an enzyme purified from bacterial sources, which causes degradation of the amino acid L-asparagine. Asparagine is synthesized from aspartic acid and glutamine through the enzyme L-asparagine synthase. However, this enzyme appears to be lacking in some tumors, particularly acute leukemia in children. L-Asparaginase may then lead to death of these leukemic cells, since their viability depends on the availability of asparagine in the circulation. The major toxicity of the drug is due to hypersensitivity reactions and to inhibition of synthesis of important proteins such as clotting factors.

16.7 SUMMARY

Anticancer drugs are grouped for convenience into categories based on their mechanism of action or derivation. The intracellular effects that lead to cell death following administration of these drugs are varied and complex, but most of them cause damage to DNA, either directly or indirectly. Several anticancer drugs have been introduced recently. These include not only analogues of previously existing drugs, such as vinorelbine or gemcitabine, but also new categories of agents with different cellular targets and novel mechanisms of action, such as the taxanes and the camptothecin derivatives.

The efficacy of anticancer drugs depends on drug concentration and time of exposure, which in turn depend on absorption, metabolism, distribution, and excretion. An understanding of the basic components of the pharmacology of these drugs is essential if we are to use them effectively and safely.

REFERENCES

Allen L, Kimura K, MacKichan J, Ritschel WA: Manual of symbols, equations and definitions in pharmacokinetics. *J Clin Pharmacol* 1982; 22:1S–23S.

Bachur NR, Gordon SL, Gee MV: Anthracycline antibiotic augmentation of microsomal electron transport and free radical formation. *Mol Pharmacol* 1977; 13: 901–910.

Benvenuto JA, Ayele W, Legha SS, et al: Clinical pharmacokinetics of ifosfamide in combination with *N*-acetylcysteine. *Anticancer Drugs* 1992; 3:19–23.

Cadman E, Heimer R, Davis L: Enhanced 5-fluorouracil nucleotide formation after methotrexate administration: Explanation for drug synergism. *Science* 1979; 205:1135–1137.

Chabner BA, Chabner AS. Mitotic inhibitors. *Cancer Chemother Biol Response Modi* 1994; 15:58–66.

Collins JM: Pharmacologic rationale for regional drug delivery. *J Clin Oncol* 1984; 2:498–504.

Cox PJ: Cyclophosphamide cystitis—Identification of acrolein as the causative agent. *Biochem Pharmacol* 1979; 28:2045–2049.

Cunningham D, Zalcberg JR, Rath U, el al: Tomudex (ZD1694)—Results of a randomized trial in advanced colorectal cancer demonstrate efficacy and reduced mucositis and leucopenia. *Eur J Cancer* 1995; 31A: 1945–1954.

Eder JP, Teicher BA, Holder SA, et al: Ability of 4 potential topoisomerase II inhibitors to enhance the cytotoxicity of cis-platin in Chinese hamster ovary cells and in epipodophyllotoxin-resistant subline. *Cancer Chemother Pharmacol* 1990; 26:423–428.

Egorin MJ, Van Echo DA, Tipping SJ: Pharmacokinetics and dosage reduction of cis-diammine (1.1-cyclobutane-dicarboxylato) platinum in patients with impaired renal function. *Cancer Res* 1984; 44:5432–5438.

Erlichman C, Fine S, Wong A, Elhakim T: A randomized trial of fluorouracil and folinic acid in patients with metastatic colorectal carcinoma. *J Clin Oncol* 1988; 6:469–475.

Erlichman C, Moore M: Carcinogenesis: A late complication of cancer chemotherapy. In: Chabner BA, Longo DL, eds. *Cancer Chemotherapy and Biotherapy.* Philadelphia: Lippincott; 1996:45–58.

Erlichman C, Rauth AM, Battistella R, et al: Mitomycin C pharmacokinetics in patients with recurrent or metastatic colorectal carcinoma. *Can J Physiol Pharmacol* 1987; 65:404–411.

Evans WE, Relling MV, Rodman JH, et al: Conventional compared with individualized chemotherapy for childhood acute lymphoblastic leukemia. *N Engl J Med* 1998; 338:499–505.

Fichtinger-Shepman AMJ, van Oosterom AT, et al: *Cis*-diamminechloroplatinum (II)-induced DNA adducts in peripheral leukocytes from seven cancer patients: Quantitative immunochemical detection of the adduct induction and removal after a single dose of *cis*-diamminechloroplatinum (II). *Cancer Res* 1987; 47:3000–3004.

Garcia ST, McQuillan A, Panasci I. Correlation between the cytotoxicity of melphalan and DNA crosslinks as detected by the ethidium bromide fluorescence assay. *Biochem Pharmacol* 1988; 37:3189–3196.

Grochow LLB, Piantadosi S, Santos G, et al: Busulfan dose adjustment decreases the risk of hepatic veno-occlusive disease in patients undergoing bone marrow transplantation. *Proc Am Assoc Cancer Res* 1992; 33:200.

Huang P, Chubb S, Hertel LW, et al: Action of gemcitabine on DNA synthesis. *Cancer Res* 1991; 51:6110–6117.

Kastan MB, Schlaffer E, Russo JE, et al: Direct demonstration of elevated aldehyde dehydrogenase in human hematopoietic progenitor cells. *Blood* 1990; 75:1947–1950.

Keating MJ, O'Brien S, Plunkett W, et al: Fludarabine phosphate: A new active agent in hematogic malignancies. *Semin Hematol* 1994; 31:28–39.

Kemeny N, Daly J, Reichman B, et al: Intrahepatic or systemic infusion of fluorodeoxyuridine in patients with liver metastases from colorectal carcinoma. *Ann Intern Med* 1987; 107:459–465.

Keyomarsi K, Moran RG: Folinic acid augmentation of the effects of fluoropyrimidines on murine and human leukemic cells. *Cancer Res* 1986; 46:5229–5235.

Kohn KW: DNA as a target in cancer chemotherapy: Measurement of macromolecular DNA damage produced in mammalian cells by anticancer agents and carcinogens. *Methods Cancer Res* 1979; 16:291–345.

Lazo JS, Chabner BA: Bleomycin. In: Chabner BA, Longo DL, eds. *Cancer Chemotherapy and Biotherapy.* Philadelphia: Lippincott; 1996:263–275.

Lokich JJ, Ahlgren JD, Gullo JJ, et al: A prospective randomized trial of continuous infusion fluorouracil with a conventional bolus schedule in metastatic colorectal carcinoma: A mid-Atlantic oncology program study. *J Clin Oncol* 1989; 7:425–432.

Mick R, Ratain MJ: Statistical approaches to pharmacodynamic modelling: Motivations, methods, and misconceptions. *Cancer Chemother Pharmacol* 1993; 33:1–9.

Milano G, Etienne MC: Dihydropyrimidine dehydrogenase (DPD) and clinical pharmacology of 5-fluorouracil (review). *Anticancer Res* 1994; 14:2295–2297.

Moertel CG, Lefkopoulo M, Lipsitz S, et al: Streptozocin-doxorubicin, streptozocin-fluorouracil, or chlorozotocin in the treatment of advanced islet cell carcinoma. *N Engl J Med* 1992; 326:519–523.

Moore MJ: Clinical pharmacokinetics of cyclophosphamide. *Clin Pharmacokinet* 1991; 20:194–208.

Moore MJ, Erlichman C: Therapeutic drug monitoring in oncology. *Clin Pharmacokinet* 1987; 13:205–227.

Moore MJ, Hardy RW, Soldin SJ, et al: Rapid development of enhanced clearance following high dose cyclophosphamide. *Clin Pharmacol and Ther* 1988; 44:622–628.

Moran RG, Keyomarsi K: Biochemical rationale for the synergism of 5-fluorouracil and folinic acid. *Natl Cancer Inst Monogr* 1987; 5:159–163.

Newell DR: Can pharmacokinetic and pharmacodynamic studies improve cancer chemotherapy? *Ann Oncol* 1994; 5(suppl 4):9–14.

Pommier Y: DNA topoisomerases I & II in cancer chemotherapy. *Cancer Chemother Pharmacol* 1993; 32:103–112.

Prestayko AW, Crooke ST, Baker LM, et al: *Nitrosoureas: Current Status and New Developments.* New York: Academic Press; 1981.

Rauth AM, Mohindra JK, Tannock IF: Activity of mitomycin C for aerobic and hypoxic cells in vitro and in vivo. *Cancer Res* 1983; 43:4154–4158.

Robert J, Gianni L: Pharmacokinetics and metabolism of anthracyclines. *Cancer Surv* 1993; 17:219–252.

Roberts JJ, Know RJ, Rera MF, et al: The role of platinum-DNA interactions in the cellular toxicity and the antitumor effect of platinum coordinated compounds. *Dev Oncol* 1988; 54:16–31.

Rowinsky EK, Donehower RD. Paclitaxel. *N Engl J Med* 1995; 332:1004–1014.

Rowinsky E, Donehower R: In: Chabner BA, Longo DL (eds). *Cancer Chemotherapy and Biotherapy.* Philadelphia: Lippincott; 1996:379–393.

Sonnichsen DS, Relling MV: Clinical pharmacokinetics of paclitaxel. *Clin Pharmacokinet* 1994; 27:256–269.

Tannock I, Guttman P: Response of chinese hamster ovary cells to anticancer drugs under aerobic and hypoxic conditions. *Br J Cancer* 1981; 43:245–248.

Touroutoglou N, Pazdur R: Thymidylate synthase inhibitors (review). *Clin Cancer Res* 1996; 2:227–243.

Tritton TR, Yee G: The anticancer agent Adriamycin can be actively cytotoxic without entering cells. *Science* 1982; 217:248–250.

Van Mannen JM, Retel J, de Vries J, Pinedo HM: Mechanism of action of antitumor drug etoposide: A review. *J Natl Cancer Inst* 1988; 80:1526–1533.

Weiss RB, Christian MC: New cisplatin analogues in development. *Drugs* 1993; 46:360–377.

Winick NJ, McKenna RW, Shuster JJ, et al: Secondary acute myeloid leukemia in children with acute lymphoblastic leukemia treated with etoposide. *J Clin Oncol* 1993; 11:29–214.

17

Drug Resistance and Experimental Chemotherapy

Ian F. Tannock and Gerald J. Goldenberg

17.1 PRINCIPLES OF CHEMOTHERAPY
    17.1.1 Therapeutic Index
    17.1.2 Relationship between Tumor Remission and Cure
    17.1.3 Adjuvant Chemotherapy
    17.1.4 Directed Drug Delivery

17.2 DRUG RESISTANCE
    17.2.1 Mechanisms of Drug Resistance
    17.2.2 Resistance to Methotrexate and Other Antimetabolite Drugs
    17.2.3 Drug Resistance due to Impaired Drug Influx
    17.2.4 Multiple Drug Resistance: P-Glycoprotein, MRP, and LRP
    17.2.5 Topoisomerases and Drug Resistance

17.2.6 Glutathione and Drug Resistance
17.2.7 Drug Resistance and DNA Repair
17.2.8 Resistance to Apoptosis
17.2.9 Drug Resistance In Vivo

17.3 TREATMENT WITH MULTIPLE AGENTS
    17.3.1 Influence on Therapeutic Index
    17.3.2 Synergy and Additivity: Isobologram Analysis
    17.3.3 Modifiers of Drug Activity
    17.3.4 Drugs and Radiation

17.4 SUMMARY

REFERENCES

17.1 PRINCIPLES OF CHEMOTHERAPY

In current clinical practice, chemotherapy is used primarily (1) as the major curative modality for a few types of malignancies, such as Hodgkin's disease and other lymphomas, acute leukemia in children, and testicular cancer in men; (2) as palliative treatment for many types of advanced cancers; and (3) as adjuvant treatment before, during, or after local treatment (surgery and/or radiotherapy) with the aim of both eradicating occult micrometastases and of improving local control of the primary tumor. Such treatments usually involve a combination of drugs. The most important factors underlying the successful use of drugs in combination are (1) the ability to combine drugs at close to full tolerated doses with additive effects against tumors and less than additive toxicities to normal tissues and (2) the expectation that drug combinations will include at least one drug to which the tumor is sensitive. Some drugs are also combined because there is a theoretical or experimental basis for expecting synergistic interaction. This is either through their known mechanisms of action at the molecular level or because of their complementary effects on cell-cycle kinetics. Synergy does not lead to therapeutic benefit, however, unless the interaction between drugs leads to greater effects against tumor cells than against dose-limiting normal tissues.

17.1.1 Therapeutic Index

In addition to their antitumor effects, all anticancer drugs are toxic to normal tissues. It is this toxicity that limits the dose of drugs which can be given to patients. The relationship between the probability of a biologic effect of a drug and the administered dose is usually described by a sigmoid curve (Fig. 17.1). If the drug is to be useful, the curve describing the probability of antitumor effect (e.g., com-

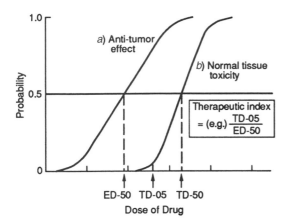

Figure 17.1. Schematic relationships between dose of a drug and (curve *a*) the probability of a given measure of antitumor effect, and (curve *b*) the probability of a given measure of normal-tissue toxicity. The therapeutic index might be defined as the ratio of doses to give 50 percent probabilities of normal-tissue damage and antitumor effects. However, if the endpoint for toxicity is severe (e.g., sepsis due to bone marrow suppression), it would be more appropriate to define the therapeutic index at a lower probability of toxicity (e.g., TD-05/ED-50).

plete clinical remission) must be displaced toward lower doses as compared with the curve describing the probability of major toxicity to normal tissues (e.g., myelosuppression leading to infection). Therapeutic index (or therapeutic ratio) may be defined from such curves as the ratio of the dose required to produce a given probability of toxicity and the dose required to give a defined effect against the tumor (see Chap. 14; Sec. 14.2.3). Therapeutic index in Fig. 17.1 might be represented by the ratio of the drug dose required for a 5 percent level of probability of severe toxicity (sometimes referred to as toxic dose-05 or TD-05) to that required for 50 percent probability of antitumor effect (i.e., effective dose 50 or ED-50). Any stated levels of probability might be used. The appropriate endpoints of tumor response and toxicity will depend on the limiting toxicity of the drug and the intent of treatment (i.e., cure versus palliation).

Improvement in the therapeutic index is the goal of experimental chemotherapy. However, although dose-response curves similar to those of Fig. 17.1 have been defined in animals, they have rarely been obtained for drug effects in humans. They emphasize the important concept that any modification in treatment that leads to increased killing of tumor cells in tissue culture or animals must be assessed for its effects on critical normal tissues prior to therapeutic trials.

17.1.2 Relationship between Tumor Remission and Cure

For most solid tumors the limit of clinical and/or radiologic detection is about 1 g of tissue ($\sim 10^9$ cells). If therapy can reduce the number of malignant cells below this limit of detection, the patient will be described as being in complete clinical remission. Surgical biopsy of sites that were known to be involved with tumor previously may lower the limit of detection, but a pathologist is unlikely to detect sporadic tumor cells present at a frequency of less than 1 in 1000 normal cells. Therefore, even a "surgically confirmed complete remission" may be compatible with the presence of a large number of tumor cells (up to $\sim 10^6$/g tissue). Tumor cure requires eradication of all tumor cells that have the capacity for tumor regeneration. The proportion of such stem cells among those of the tumor population is unknown (see Chap. 7, Sec. 7.6.2), but clinical and even surgically confirmed complete remissions are compatible with the presence of a substantial residual population of tumor stem cells.

For some drugs the relationship between cell survival and dose is close to exponential, so that a constant *fraction* of the cells (rather than a constant *number*) is killed by a given dose of drug (Chap. 15, Sec. 15.2.3). Drugs are usually given in sequential courses, with dosage and schedule limited by normal-tissue tolerance. Some repopulation of tumor cells may take place between courses, so that the number of tumor cells in a drug-sensitive tumor may change with time during a course of chemotherapy, as illustrated in Fig. 17.2. In this example, each course of drug kills 90 percent of the tumor cells, and starting from a large (~ 100 g) tumor, complete clinical remission is achieved after three courses. Note that a further 6 to 10 courses (depending on the prevalence of tumor stem cells) would be required to achieve cure, even if all cells in the population were equally sensitive. Realization of the need to continue aggressive treatment during complete remission led to success in the treatment of acute lymphoblastic leukemia in children and subsequently to cures in other tumors, such as lymphomas. Unfortunately, for most solid tumors, a drug-resistant subpopulation emerges and leads to relapse, as shown in Fig. 17.2.

17.1.3 Adjuvant Chemotherapy

Chemotherapy is often given to patients who have no overt evidence of residual cancer after local treatment with surgery or radiation. This strategy

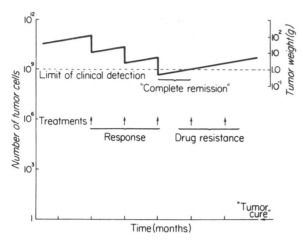

Figure 17.2. Illustration of the relationship between tumor remission and cure. In this hypothetical example, treatment of a human tumor starts when it has 10^{11} cells (at about 100 g), and each treatment, given at monthly intervals, kills 90 percent of the cells present. This course of therapy leads to complete disappearance of clinical tumor. Drug resistance then develops, and the tumor grows despite continued treatment. Note that despite the attainment of a complete clinical response, there are always at least 10^8 viable cells present, and that the reduction in cell number is small compared with that required for cure.

derives from past experience with similar patients who have shown a high rate of relapse from the presence of undetectable micrometastatic disease. Adjuvant chemotherapy is used widely in the clinic and has demonstrated a small but important effect to increase the probability of cure for some types of malignancy, including breast and colorectal cancer.

Several mechanisms may allow for increased curability of micrometastatic disease. Eradication of a smaller number of cells is more likely with a given dose of drug (see Fig. 17.3). Smaller tumors may have better perfusion of blood than larger tumors, allowing better access of drug to the tumor cells. A higher rate of cell proliferation due to better nutrition may also be important, since rapidly proliferating cells are more sensitive to most anticancer drugs (Chap. 15, Sec. 15.2.4). Finally, drug-resistant cells may be present in larger tumors, thus reducing the chance of cure (Sec. 17.2.1).

Despite the multiple mechanisms supporting the use of adjuvant treatment, as well as the definitive evidence of benefit for transplanted tumors in mice (Schabel, 1975), it is disappointing that adjuvant chemotherapy has not been more beneficial to patients. This may be because transplanted tumors in mice are poor models for slowly growing and heterogeneous tumors in humans. A model to estimate the reduction in survival of tumor cells due to adjuvant chemotherapy for breast cancer has been proposed by Withers (1991). In this model (Fig. 17.4), it is assumed that in a large population of patients who are destined to develop disease recurrence, the distribution of cells after surgery (plus or minus adjuvant chemotherapy) ranges from 1 cell to 10^9 cells (the limit of *clinical detection*). If adjuvant chemotherapy leads to an increase in 10-year recurrence-free survival for node-positive women from about 30 percent to about 40 to 45 percent, as suggested by various clinical trials, this model suggests a fractional reduction in cell survival due to chemotherapy of only 10^{-1} to 10^{-2} (Fig. 17.4). Further improvements in the probability of cure due to adjuvant chemotherapy will require either more active drugs or the use of higher doses in order to increase the fractional cell kill. Clinical trials of high-dose chemotherapy

Figure 17.3. Result of an experiment in which mice were treated at different times after intravenous injection of Lewis lung tumor cells. Therapy is curative only if it is started early, when the number of tumor cells is low. (Adapted from Hill and Stanley, 1977.)

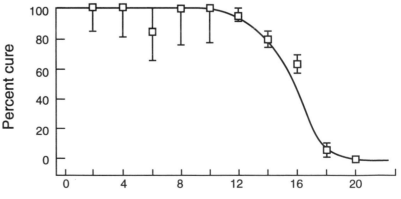

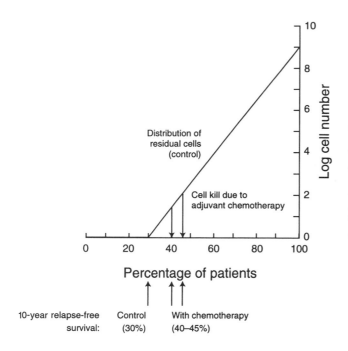

Figure 17.4. A model for the distribution of number of cells that remain after local treatment of patients with node-positive breast cancer, about 70 percent of whom will relapse within 10 years. The distribution is assumed to be exponential from 1 cell to 10^9 cells (lower limit of clinical detection). If adjuvant chemotherapy increases 10-year relapse-free survival by 10 to 15 percent, as found in various clinical trials, the fractional cell survival due to this treatment is about 10^{-1} to 10^{-2}. (Adapted from Withers, 1991).

with stem-cell rescue (Chap. 15, Sec. 15.4.2) are in progress for patients with breast cancer who are at high risk for recurrence.

Adjuvant chemotherapy is sometimes started in patients before treatment of the primary tumor with surgery or radiation—a strategy that has been termed *neoadjuvant chemotherapy*. This approach is attractive because observation of the primary tumor during initial therapy may give an indication of responsiveness to the drugs used. Also, it has been shown that cancer cells may be spread into the bloodstream during surgery (see also Chap. 10, Sec. 10.2), so that chemotherapy given immediately prior to surgery might kill circulating cells and prevent seeding of metastases. However, experiments in animals suggest that neoadjuvant chemotherapy should be used with caution, since many drugs have been found to increase the chance of metastasis to the lungs from circulating tumor cells (e.g., Van Putten et al., 1975; Iwamoto et al., 1992). This effect is largest after treatment with cyclophosphamide, when the frequency of metastasis after intravenous injection of tumor cells may be increased by a factor of 100 to 1000; but smaller effects have been observed following treatment with several other anticancer drugs. There is also some evidence that drug treatment may increase spontaneous metastasis from transplanted tumors, although this is not a universal finding. The mechanisms underlying these effects appear to include drug-induced damage to endothelial cells, which may facilitate the trapping of tumor cells in small blood vessels (Nicolson and Custead, 1985; Orr et al., 1986), and drug-induced changes in malignant cells, which may increase their ability to metastasize (McMillan and Hart, 1986).

Neoadjuvant chemotherapy given before radiation therapy has been observed to cause initial shrinkage of tumors in some sites (e.g., head and neck cancer) without improvement in survival as compared with radiation treatment alone. It has been pointed out by Withers et al. (1988) that tumor shrinkage induced by drug therapy may stimulate proliferation of the surviving tumor cells. If this increased proliferation occurs during the subsequent radiation therapy, it could increase the effective number of target tumor cells that must be sterilized by radiation and decrease the probability of tumor control (see Chap. 14, Fig. 14.13).

17.1.4 Directed Drug Delivery

A major limitation to the use of chemotherapy is lack of selectivity of most anticancer drugs for tumor cells. A potential method for increasing the therapeutic index is to direct drugs to tumor cells by linking them to a carrier. Among these approaches are (1) linkage of drugs or toxins to antibodies or growth factors that recognize antigens or receptors on tumor cells and (2) entrapment of drugs in lipid vesicles known as *liposomes*. Each of these methods has led to improvement in the therapeutic index for selected tumors in animals and to products being tested in clinical trials.

Several anticancer drugs have been linked to monoclonal antibodies directed against tumor-associated antigens, with occasional evidence of substantial therapeutic effects in animal models, including human xenografts (e.g., Trail et al., 1993). Monoclonal antibodies or growth factors have also been linked to potent toxins such as *Pseudomonas* exotoxin, diphtheria toxin, and ricin (Wawrzynczak, 1991; Pastan and Fitzgerald, 1992). The genes encoding these toxins have been cloned, and the DNA sequences encoding the different parts of the molecules that cause toxicity and binding to cells are known. This has made it possible to engineer chimeric molecules in which a tumor-binding ligand is conjugated to the toxic part of the molecule. The therapeutic potential and problems associated with the use of these strategies are described in Chap. 18, Sec. 18.3.4.

Another novel strategy is to conjugate antibody and drug with an acid-labile linker region, so that the drug is released preferentially in the acidic microenvironment that is often present in solid tumors (Lavie et al., 1991). An antibody that recognizes a tumor antigen may also be linked to an enzyme that activates a nontoxic prodrug within a tumor (Bagshawe, 1989). This strategy (ADEPT, or *antibody-dependent enzyme-activated prodrug therapy*) overcomes the problem of limited delivery of conjugated drugs, since a single enzyme molecule can activate many prodrug molecules. For example, a conjugate between a monoclonal antibody (MAb) directed against carcinoembryonic antigen and alkaline phosphatase has been used to release the active drug etoposide from the inactive prodrug etoposide phosphate in model systems (Haisma et al., 1992). Whether these approaches will be useful for treatment of human cancer remains uncertain.

A large body of research relates to the entrapment of anticancer drugs in liposomes (Brenner, 1989; Gabizon, 1994). Liposomes may be constructed of varying size and with positive, neutral, or negative charge; they may be single or multilayered; and the lipid composition may be varied to provide solid or fluid forms of the lipid membrane. In general, liposomes are taken up by reticuloendothelial cells in liver, spleen, and lungs, but they may also deliver relatively high concentrations of drug in tumors; their site of localization depends on the size of the liposomes and their membrane composition. There is particular interest in liposomes that contain polyethylene glycol–derived phospholipids, which are sterically stabilized and may escape up-

take by the reticuloendothelial system, leading to long circulation times. There is evidence that these "stealth" liposomes may localize in tumors (Gabizon, 1994; Sakakibara et al., 1996).

There are several mechanisms whereby drugs encapsulated in liposomes might lead to improvement in therapeutic index relative to free drug: (1) Slow, continuous release of the anticancer drug into the circulation; this may protect against organ-specific toxicity (e.g., cardiotoxicity due to doxorubicin) and/or lead to improvement in anti-tumor effects. (2) Fusion of liposomes with cell membranes, leading to efficient internal delivery of drugs; this may overcome drug resistance due to impaired uptake of free drug. (3) Selective localization of liposomes (especially small, sterically stabilized liposomes) in tumor tissue. Indeed, superior therapeutic effects of drugs encapsulated in liposomes, as compared with use of free drug, have been demonstrated in several animal models, including human tumor xenografts (e.g., Sakakibara et al., 1996). Clinical trials are in progress with doxorubicin-containing sterically stabilized liposomes.

The above approaches have been combined in a strategy to conjugate doxorubicin-containing liposomes with Fab fragments of a monoclonal antibody that recognizes the *erbB-2/HER2/neu* oncogene product on the surface of many breast cancer cells (see Chap. 6, Sec. 6.7.2). This strategy is effective in delivering doxorubicin to *HER2*-expressing xenografts of human breast cancer (Park et al., 1995), and the use of these immunoliposomes is being evaluated in clinical trials.

All carrier-mediated drug delivery systems involve large molecules, and there may be problems in delivering such large molecules to cells within a solid tumor. Even some free drugs may have difficulty in diffusing from blood vessels to tumor cells (see Chap. 15, Sec. 15.3.4). For this reason, the clinical use of these approaches might be more successful against leukemias or as adjuvant treatment of micrometatases.

17.2 DRUG RESISTANCE

Many types of cancer that occur commonly in humans (e.g., colon cancer, lung cancer other than the small-cell type) have a relatively low probability of response to treatment with anticancer drugs. Other human tumors (e.g., breast cancer, ovarian cancer, or small-cell cancer of the lung) often respond to initial treatment, but acquired resistance to further therapy usually prevents drug treatment from being curative. This resistance to chemotherapy may be influenced by such factors as the proliferative state of the cells (Chap. 15, Sec. 15.2.4) and by factors related to the solid-tumor environment, such as limited vascular access and penetration of drugs into tissue (Chap. 15, Sec. 15.3.4). The most important factor is the intrinsic resistance of the tumor cells to available anticancer drugs. Intrinsic sensitivity to drugs may differ widely among cell populations from tumors and normal tissues and also among the cells of a single tumor. The selection or induction of a drug-resistant subpopulation in human tumors is probably the major factor limiting the efficacy of clinical chemotherapy. Even if drug-resistant cells are present initially only at low frequency (e.g., one drug-resistant cell per 10^5 drug-sensitive cells), their selective advantage during drug treatment will lead to their rapid emergence as the dominant cell population, giving the clinical impression of "acquired resistance."

The presence of drug-resistant cells in a population may be disclosed by a drug-resistant "tail" on the cell-survival curve. Survival curves with a terminal part of shallow slope may indicate a population that is drug-resistant for many reasons, including a population that is spared in a drug-resistant phase of the cell cycle (see Chap. 15, Sec. 15.2.4). If a population of cells with stable drug resistance has been selected, the survival curve will demonstrate resistance when the initial surviving cells are expanded and again treated with the same agent.

Table 17.1. General Mechanisms Associated with Resistance to Anticancer Drugs[a]

Mechanism	Drugs
Decreased uptake	Methotrexate, nitrogen mustard, melphalan, cisplatin
Increased efflux[b]	Anthracyclines, vinca alkaloids, etoposide, taxanes[b]
Decrease in drug activation	Many antimetabolites
Increase in drug catabolism	Many antimetabolites
Increase or decrease in levels of target enzyme	Methotrexate, topoisomerase inhibitors[b]
Alterations in target enzyme	Methotrexate, other antimetabolites, topoisomerase inhibitors
Inactivation by binding to sulfhydryls (e.g., glutathione)	Alkylating agents, cisplatin, anthracyclines
Increased DNA repair	Alkylating agents, cisplatin, anthracyclines, etoposide
Decreased ability to undergo apoptosis	Alkylating agents, cisplatin, anthracyclines, etoposide

[a]Additional mechanisms remain to be elucidated, including those which lead to drug resistance that is expressed selectively in a solid-tumor environment (see Sec. 17.2.9).

[b]See Table 17.3 for specificity of these mechanisms.

17.2.1 Mechanisms of Drug Resistance

A wide range of metabolic or structural properties of cells may lead to drug resistance; some of the underlying mechanisms are summarized in Table 17.1. Alkylating agents and cisplatin cause cellular damage by binding with DNA, leading to cross-linkages and breaks in DNA strands (Chap. 16, Secs. 16.3 and 16.6.1). Cells may be resistant to these drugs through a number of mechanisms, including decreased cellular uptake, reduced drug activation, binding of alkylating species by sulfhydryl compounds such as glutathione followed by transport out of cells (Sec. 17.2.6), increased removal of drug adducts from DNA, and increased repair of DNA damage (Sec. 17.2.7). Cross-resistance to chemically unrelated drugs has been observed for naturally occurring and semisynthetic compounds such as doxorubicin and etoposide, owing to common mechanisms of stimulated drug efflux from cells (Sec. 17.2.4) or to decreased activity of the enzyme topoisomerase II, which allows conformational changes in DNA (Sec. 17.2.5). A number of mechanisms may also lead to resistance to antimetabolite drugs (Sec. 17.2.2). These mechanisms include impaired drug transport into cells, overproduction or reduced affinity of the molecular target, stimulation of alternative biochemical pathways, and impaired activation or increased catabolism of the drug. Table 17.2 illustrates the multiple mechanisms that can lead to resistance to doxorubicin and cisplatin, which are commonly used in the clinic. Since multiple mechanisms may contribute to resistance to every anticancer drug, it is not surprising that initial or acquired drug resistance is observed after treatment of most cell populations.

The following evidence suggests that many types of drug resistance are genetic in origin:

Table 17.2. Mechanisms Known or Suspected to Cause Resistance to the Commonly Used Anticancer Drugs Doxorubicin and Cisplatin

Doxorubicin	Cisplatin
↑ Export from cells by P-glycoprotein or by multidrug-resistance protein (MRP)	↓ Net uptake into cells
↑ Lung-resistance protein (LRP)	↑ LRP
↓ Topoisomerase II activity	↑ Metallothionein
↑ Conjugation by glutathione (↑glutathione S-transferases)	↑ Conjugation by glutathione (↑ glutathione S-transferases)
↑ DNA repair	↑ DNA repair (↑ removal of cisplatin-DNA adducts)
↓ Apoptosis	↓ Apoptosis

1. Characteristics of drug-resistant cells (i.e., their phenotypes) are often stably inherited in the absence of the selecting drug.
2. Drug-resistant cells are generated spontaneously at a rate that is consistent with known rates of genetic mutation. A fluctuation test (Luria and Delbruck, 1943) has provided strong evidence for mutation and selection as a mechanism leading to resistance to a few anticancer drugs, including paclitaxel (Dumontet et al, 1996).
3. Generation of drug-resistant cells is increased by exposure to compounds that induce either mutation or amplification of genes. This property has been used to generate and select a large number of drug-resistant variant cells that have been used to study drug-resistant phenotypes (Fig. 17.5). Several anticancer drugs may themselves stimulate mutation or gene amplification, so that treatment may be expected to accelerate the development of drug resistance.
4. Altered gene products have been identified in some drug-resistant cells, and some of the genes have been cloned and sequenced.
5. Some drug-resistant phenotypes have been transferred to drug-sensitive cells by transfer of genes, using techniques described in Chap. 3, Sec. 3.3.10.

The presence of drug-resistant cells among the cells in human tumors has implications for planning optimal chemotherapy. Goldie and Coldman (1984)

have demonstrated that the probability of there being at least one drug-resistant cell in a tumor population is dependent on tumor size (Fig. 17.6). This probability increases from near zero to near unity over a small range of tumor sizes (six doublings), with the critical size depending on the rate of mutation to drug resistance. This effect implies a greater chance of cure if therapy is begun early, when only microscopic foci of tumor cells are present, although additional mechanisms contribute to the increased probability of eradication of very small tumors (see Sec. 17.1.3). The Goldie-Coldman model also predicts a better therapeutic effect when two equally effective and non-cross-resistant drugs are alternated rather than given sequentially, since this minimizes the emergence of cell populations that are resistant to both drugs. However, it has been difficult to demonstrate the validity of this prediction in clinical trials.

Although drug-resistant phenotypes in many types of cell have been shown to be due to mutation or amplification of genes, there is a concern that this may be of limited relevance to clinical drug treatments. The methods used for selection of drug-resistant cells, i.e., exposure of cells to mutagens, followed by selection in high concentrations of drug (Fig. 17.5), may predispose to selection of cells with genetically based drug resistance. Exposure of cells to lower concentrations of drugs, without prior exposure to mutagens, often leads to cells that show transient resistance to drugs; indeed, transient resistance of some cells in the population may occur spontaneously, without prior drug exposure (Cillo et al., 1989). Mechanisms underlying drug resistance that is unstable may include transient amplification of genes, changes in patterns of DNA methylation, and other factors that influence gene expression (these mechanisms are sometimes referred to as *epigenetic*). Such changes in drug sensitivity might be expected to occur in vivo, since the cells are exposed to relatively low concentrations of drugs during cancer treatment. Clinically important drug resistance is probably due to both genetic and epigenetic mechanisms.

17.2.2 Resistance to Methotrexate and Other Antimetabolite Drugs

Resistance to antimetabolites may arise from several mechanisms, including (1) downregulation or mutation of genes encoding drug-activating enzymes, (2) upregulation of drug-inactivating enzymes, (3) upregulation of the target enzyme, and/or (4) modification of the target enzyme, resulting in reduced

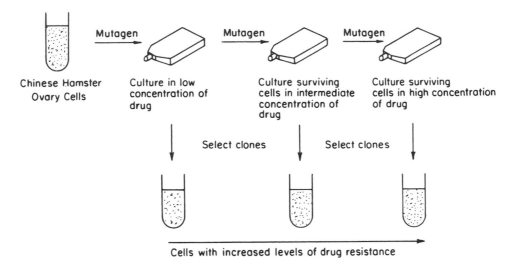

Figure 17.5. General method used for stepwise selection of drug-resistant mutant cells.

binding affinity for the drug. For example, resistance to the purine analogues 6-mercaptopurine and 6-thioguanine may arise as a result of decreased drug activation by the enzyme hypoxanthine-guanine-phosphoribosyltransferase and/or increased inactivation of thionucleotides by alkaline phosphatase. Resistance to the pyrimidine analogue cytosine arabinoside may occur as a result of decreased uptake into cells, decreased activation by kinases, and/or enhanced inactivation by deaminases (see also Chap. 16, Sec. 16.4).

Several mechanisms of resistance have been reported for 5-fluorouracil (5-FU); these include upregulation or alteration of the target enzyme thymidylate synthase (Peters et al., 1995), downregulation of enzymes that activate the drug to nucleotides, increase in the rate of breakdown of 5-FU, and increase in the pool size of deoxyuridine monophosphate (dUMP), the native substrate for thymidylate synthase (see also Chap. 16, Sec. 16.4.2).

Resistance to methotrexate may occur by several mechanisms (Gorlick et al., 1996; Fig. 17.7). Methotrexate is transported across cell membranes both by passive diffusion and by an energy-dependent active transport system, the reduced folate carrier; glutamic acid residues are then added to the drug inside cells (see Chap. 16, Sec. 16.4.1). Drug-resistant cells may arise that have impaired transport of methotrexate into the cell, due to mutation in the reduced folate carrier (Williams and Flintoff, 1995; Wong et al., 1995); this is a common mechanism of acquired resistance in patients with acute leukemia

(Gorlick et al., 1996). Other drug-resistant cells, including those from untreated human leukemia, may show a decrease in polyglutamation of intracellular methotrexate due to either decreased activity of the synthetic enzyme folylpolyglutamate synthase or increased activity of the catabolic enzyme folylpolyglutamate hydrolase (Lin et al., 1991; Rhee et al., 1993).

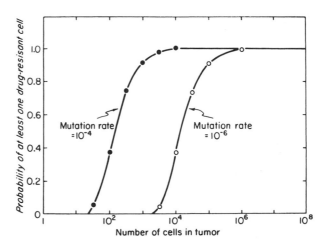

Figure 17.6. Probability that there will be at least one drug-resistant cell in a tumor containing varying numbers of cells, based on rates of mutation of 10^{-6} *(open symbols)* and 10^{-4} *(closed symbols)* per cell per generation. Note that this probability increases from low to high values over a relatively short period in the life history of the tumor and that drug-resistant cells are likely to be established prior to clinical detection. (Adapted from Goldie and Coldman, 1984.)

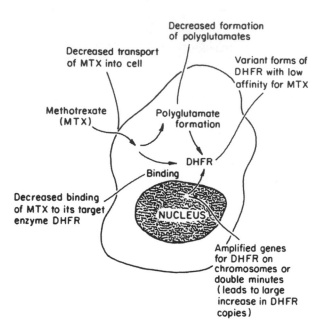

Figure 17.7. Probable mechanisms underlying cellular resistance to methotrexate.

Other mutations may lead to production of variant forms of dihydrofolate reductase (DHFR), the target enzyme for methotrexate (Goldie et al., 1980; Dicker et al., 1993). Variant enzymes have been found that retain adequate function for reduction of their normal substrate (dihydrofolate) but have decreased affinity for methotrexate. Primary defects in polyglutamation or in intracellular binding to the target enzyme will lead to a relative increase in free drug in the cytoplasm of cells and to a consequent decrease in uptake of methotrexate because of a reduced gradient in free-drug concentration across the cell membrane.

A common mechanism leading to methotrexate resistance in cell lines and experimental tumors exposed to increasing concentrations of the drug is overproduction of DHFR from amplified genes (Schimke, 1984; Stark et al., 1989). This process has also been observed in human tumors treated with methotrexate. It has been characterized as follows (e.g., Schimke, 1984):

1. High levels of resistance to methotrexate can be obtained only by a stepwise increase in drug concentration in the medium, and this may lead to as many as 100 to 1000 copies of the *DHFR* gene.
2. Resistance occurs from overproduction of the normal enzyme (although overproduction of variant forms of DHFR has also been observed).
3. Drug resistance due to gene amplification may be either stable or unstable when cells are grown

in the absence of the drug. Stable amplification is usually associated with a chromosomal location of the amplified genes, seen as homogeneously staining regions in stained chromosome preparations (Chap. 4, Sec. 4.3.3). Unstable amplification is usually associated with location of the genes in extrachromosomal chromatin structures known as *double minutes*. Both locations may be evident during selection for drug resistance.

4. Gene amplification appears to take place by multiple replication of the *DHFR* gene (and flanking sequences) during the S phase of the cell cycle. Interruption of DNA synthesis in synchronized cells by drugs such as hydroxyurea or by transient exposure to hypoxic conditions (Rice et al., 1986) leads to an increase in the extent of gene amplification. Other anticancer drugs may stimulate increased resistance to methotrexate by the mechanism of gene amplification.

Although gene amplification has been studied most extensively in relation to methotrexate, there is increasing evidence for the importance of this mechanism in determining resistance to several other drugs, including upregulation of the target enzymes for 5-FU and other antimetabolites and of membrane-based drug-export proteins, which lead to multiple drug–resistance phenotypes (Sec. 17.2.4).

17.2.3 Drug Resistance due to Impaired Drug Influx

Drug uptake occurs by one of three mechanisms: (1) passive diffusion, in which the drug enters the cell through the cell membrane by an energy- and temperature-independent process without interacting with specific sites on the membrane; (2) facilitated diffusion, in which the drug interacts in a chemically specific manner with a transport carrier on the cell membrane and is translocated into the cell in an energy- and temperature-independent process; and (3) active transport, in which the drug is actively transported by a carrier-mediated process that is both temperature- and energy-dependent (Goldenberg and Begleiter, 1984). All three mechanisms allow for drug entry into cells down a concentration gradient, but the third mechanism can also lead to transport "uphill" against a concentration gradient. One of the mechanisms of resistance to the antimetabolite methotrexate, described in the preceding section, is impaired unidirectional drug influx. Impaired drug influx is also a mechanism of resistance for other drugs, including several alkylating agents and cisplatin.

Uptake of nitrogen mustard by mammalian cells is an active process mediated by the transport carrier for choline. Resistance to nitrogen mustard is multifactorial, but one of the mechanisms leading to resistance is reduced binding affinity of the transport carrier for drug and either a reduced number of transport sites and/or slower carrier mobility. Uptake of melphalan is mediated by active transport using two independent amino acid transport systems: (1) system ASC, which transports preferentially the amino acids alanine, serine, and cysteine, and (2) system L, the leucine-preferring carrier (Goldenberg and Begleiter, 1984). Resistance to melphalan has been attributed to a specific mutation in the system L carrier leading to reduced binding affinity between the drug and this transport carrier. Uptake of cyclophosphamide is mediated by facilitated diffusion, while uptake of chlorambucil, BCNU (carmustine), CCNU (lomustine), busulfan, procarbazine, and hexamethylmelamine occurs by passive diffusion (Goldenberg and Begleiter, 1984). Drug uptake has not been invoked as a mechanism of resistance to these alkylating agents.

Variant cells have been isolated that are resistant to cisplatin because of decreased net uptake, and that express a 200-kDa surface glycoprotein (Kawai et al., 1990), but more common causes of resistance to this drug relate to binding to sulfhydryl compounds or to removal of DNA-platinum adducts and other mechanisms of DNA repair (see Table 17.2; Secs. 17.2.6 and 17.2.7).

17.2.4 Multiple Drug Resistance: P-Glycoprotein, MRP, and LRP

Many drugs that are either natural products or their derivatives (e.g., anthracyclines such as doxorubicin, vinca alkaloids, etoposide, and taxanes) share common mechanisms of resistance. Many of these drugs are substrates for membrane-based proteins that act to pump the drugs out of cells. The best characterized of these is P-glycoprotein (P = *pleiotropic*), which is encoded by the multiple drug–resistance (*mdr*) genes (for reviews see Endicott and Ling, 1989; Shustik et al., 1995). P-glycoprotein is now known to be one of a family of molecules (Childs and Ling, 1994; Fig. 17.8), referred to ATP-binding cassette (ABC) molecules. This family includes the cystic fibrosis transmembrane conductance regulator and at least one other molecule, the multidrug-

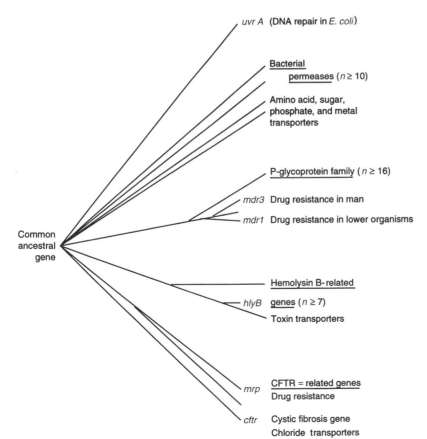

Figure 17.8. Selected members of the ATP-binding cassette (ABC) family of transport molecules, arranged according to homology in amino acid sequence. (Adapted from Childs and Ling, 1994.)

resistance protein (MRP), whose expression causes resistance to multiple anticancer drugs (Cole et al., 1992; Lautier et al., 1996). A molecule of a different family, known as the lung-resistance protein (LRP) is also associated with resistance to multiple drugs and probably causes export of drugs from cells by first sequestering them into intracellular organelles (Izquierdo et al., 1996a). These mechanisms of drug resistance are described in the current section. Alternative mechanisms that cause resistance to multiple drugs include changes in the activity of the enzyme topoisomerase II, changes in glutathione and other sulfhydryls, and increased DNA repair; these mechanisms are described in subsequent sections. Selected drugs whose resistance may be mediated by some of these mechanisms are indicated in Table 17.3.

P-Glycoprotein The genes responsible for the MDR phenotype have been cloned and sequenced from human, hamster, and murine cells (Gottesman and Pastan, 1988; Raymond and Gros, 1989; Endicott and Ling, 1989). In humans, two homologous linked genes, *mdr1* and *mdr2*, have been mapped to chromosome 7, but only *mdr1* is associated with drug resistance. *Mdr1* encodes a membrane glycoprotein of molecular weight 170 kDa, which is overexpressed in drug-resistant cells and has been called P-glycoprotein (Fig. 17.9) Three *mdr* genes have been identified in mouse and hamster cells, two of which appear to encode a functional P-glycoprotein.

The sequences of the human and rodent genes show about 80 percent identity, and each gene contains two homologous halves, suggesting that they were produced originally by duplication of a smaller gene. Activity of P-glycoprotein and its relative specificity for different drugs are influenced by phosphorylation; the major sites of phosphorylation are clustered within the linker region connecting the two homologous halves (Germann et al., 1995). Sequencing of the genes has allowed determination of the amino acid composition of the corresponding proteins, and the location of hydrophilic and hydrophobic regions has allowed modeling of the configuration and orientation of P-glycoprotein in the cell membrane (Fig. 17.10). This model suggests that there are 12 transmembrane domains with two internal ATP-binding sites.

Transfection studies have provided direct evidence that P-glycoprotein causes drug resistance. Transfection of the cDNA for *mdr* into drug-sensitive cells converts the transfectants from a negative to a positive multidrug-resistant phenotype with overexpression of P-glycoprotein and a decrease in chemosensitivity. Definitive evidence that P-glycoprotein functions as a drug export pump has been obtained by expressing the molecule in the surface of liposomes in an "inside-out" configuration and showing that a substrate would then accumulate in the liposomes (Shapiro and Ling, 1995).

Northern and Western blotting (see Chap. 3, Sec. 3.3.4) has been used to show that P-glycoprotein is

Table 17.3. Causes of Multiple Drug Resistance and Their Specificity for Individual Anticancer Drugs

P-Glycoprotein	Multidrug-Resistance Protein (MRP)	Lung-Resistance Protein (LRP)	Decreased Topoisomerase II Activity
Anthracyclines Doxorubicin Daunorubicin Epirubicin Mitoxantrone	Anthracyclines Doxorubicin Daunorubicin Epirubicin	Anthracyclines Doxorubicin Daunorubicin Mitoxantrone	Anthracyclines Doxorubicin Daunorubicin Epirubicin
Vinca alkaloids Vinblastine Vincristine	Vinca alkaloids Vinblastine (low level of resistance) Vincristine	? Cisplatin	Etoposide
Etoposide	Etoposide	? Alkylating agents	
Taxanes Paclitaxel Docetaxel			
Actinomycin D			

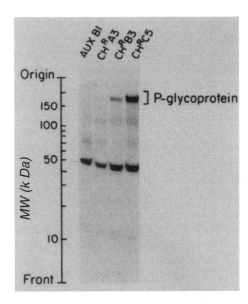

Figure 17.9. Increased levels of P-glycoprotein in increasingly drug-resistant mutant Chinese hamster ovary cells derived from wild-type (Aux B1 cells) by stepwise selection (as indicated in Fig. 17.5). Membrane components were separated by SDS polyacrilamide gel electrophoresis, transferred to nitrocellulose paper, and stained using a radiolabeled hetero-antiserum. (From Ling, 1982, with permission).

present at high levels in the normal human kidney and adrenal gland; at intermediate levels in lung, liver, colon, and rectum; and at low levels in most other tissues. Immunohistochemical techniques have shown that P-glycoprotein is localized to the surface of cells that line tubules or ducts in these organs, suggesting that the protein provides a mechanism for the excretion of xenobiotic molecules from such cells. P-glycoprotein is also expressed in a polarized way on endothelial cells lining the blood-brain barrier and probably performs a related function in excluding toxic natural products from the central nervous system.

Many investigators have measured levels of P-glycoprotein in human tumors, both before and after treatment with anticancer drugs. Elevated levels of P-glycoprotein have been found in untreated sarcomas and in cancers of the colon, adrenal, kidney, liver, and pancreas. All these tumors tend to be resistant to chemotherapy. Elevated levels of P-glycoprotein have also been detected following relapse after chemotherapy in more drug-sensitive tumors, including multiple myeloma and cancers of the breast and ovary. These findings suggest that multidrug resistance may contribute to clinical drug resistance. Increased expression of P-glycoprotein has

been reported to correlate with a poor prognosis in children with neuroblastoma, rhabdomyosarcoma, and osteogenic sarcoma (Chan et al., 1991).

A variety of agents are known to inhibit the function of P-glycoprotein and to increase the sensitivity of drug-resistant cells in culture (Bradley et al., 1988; Shustik et al., 1995). Compounds with this property include (1) nontoxic analogues of anticancer drugs whose resistance is determined by the multidrug-resistant phenotype; (2) calcium channel blockers such as verapamil; (3) calmodulin inhibitors such as quinidine, chloroquine, and trifluoperazine; and (4) the immunosuppressive agent cyclosporin A and its analogues. Some of these agents appear themselves to be substrates for the P-glycoprotein efflux pump and competitively inhibit the efflux of anticancer drugs, but noncompetitive mechanisms have also been implicated. Several clinical trials have assessed the potential of P-glycoprotein antagonists to increase the sensitivity of hu-

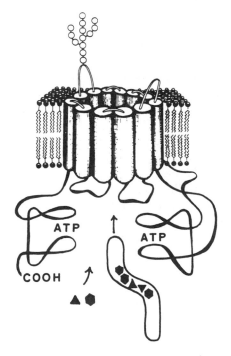

Figure 17.10. Model of P-glycoprotein as a channel-forming energy-dependent export pump. Analysis of DNA sequence has suggested the presence of 12 transmembrane domains (here drawn as cylinders); it is postulated that these are arranged to form a pore. ATP-binding domains have been localized to the cytoplasmic side using monoclonal antibodies. Drugs *(triangles and hexagons)*, which enter the cell by diffusion, are exported from the cell either directly through the pore or indirectly following binding to a carrier molecule. (From Bradley et al., 1988, with permission.)

man tumors to anticancer drugs such as doxorubicin. In a few of these studies, some patients with hematologic malignancies which were drug-resistant responded to the same anticancer drugs when an inhibitor of P-glycoprotein was added to the drug regimen (e.g., Miller et al., 1991). In general, however, the results of studies with solid tumors have been disappointing (Shustik et al., 1995). There are several possible reasons for the failure of these clinical trials. These include resistance due to mechanisms in addition to P-glycoprotein and achievement of inadequate levels of the reversing agent in tissue. In vitro studies suggest that these agents have decreased activity at the high cell concentration that exists in solid tumors. Several new reversal agents with higher affinity and greater specificity than previously available antagonists are under investigation in clinical trials.

Multidrug-Resistance Protein Cole et al., (1992) described a human lung cancer cell line that, although resistant to many drugs, did not overexpress P-glycoprotein. A novel cDNA was isolated from these resistant cells that encoded a gene product of molecular weight 190,000. The protein, which is now called the multidrug-resistance (associated) protein (MRP), is a member of the ATP-binding cassette (ABC) superfamily of transmembrane transporter proteins but shares only 15 percent amino acid sequence identity with P-glycoprotein (Fig. 17.8; Lautier et al., 1996; Loe et al., 1996). Like P-glycoprotein, MRP leads to a net decrease in cellular accumulation of a variety of anticancer drugs (Table 17.3). The spectrum of substrates is, however, slightly different in that MRP conveys at most low levels of resistance to paclitaxel and mitoxantrone. Transport across membranes of some drugs (e.g., vincristine) by MRP depends on the presence of reduced glutathione (Zaman et al., 1995; Loe et al., 1996), suggesting that MRP may act as a carrier for glutathione-conjugated drugs (see also Sec. 17.2.6). The gene encoding MRP has been located to chromosome 16 and analysis of its amino acid sequence suggests that the molecule has several membrane-spanning sequences. Studies with monoclonal antibodies have demonstrated that MRP is expressed in the cell membrane but also in internal cellular membranes of the endoplasmic reticulum.

MRP has been detected in a wide variety of human tumors and normal tissues, where it is usually expressed at low levels (Kruh et al., 1995; Nooter et al., 1995). Increased expression has been observed in several human tumors, such as lung cancer and some leukemias, and in many cell lines derived from human tumors. In children with neuroblastoma, expression of MRP was correlated with expression of the N-*myc* oncogene and predicted poor survival (Norris et al., 1996). Agents such as verapamil and cyclosporin A, which may reverse drug resistance due to P-glycoprotein in cell culture, have no effect on drug resistance due to MRP. A number of agents that antagonize the effects of MRP are under development, including drugs leading to depletion of glutathione (Zaman et al., 1995; Gonzalez Manzano et al., 1996; Vanhoefer et al., 1996).

Lung-Resistance Protein A third protein that causes resistance to a related spectrum of multiple drugs, called lung-resistance protein (LRP), is expressed by a gene on chromosome 16, close to the gene for MRP. LRP is a 100-kDa protein that has been identified as the major protein expressed on intracellular organelles known as *vaults,* which are multisubunit structures involved in nucleocytoplasmic transport (Scheffer et al., 1995). It is hypothesized that LRP causes drug resistance by pumping drugs into vaults and subsequently exporting them from the cell (Izquierdo et al., 1996a; Fig. 17.11).

The expression of P-glycoprotein, MRP, and LRP has been quantitated in a panel of 61 human tumor cell lines. These cell lines were ranked in terms of their in vitro sensitivity to drugs in the MDR family (e.g., doxorubicin, vinblastine, and etoposide) and to drugs not in the MDR family (e.g., 5-FU, alkylating agents, and cisplatin). High rates of expression

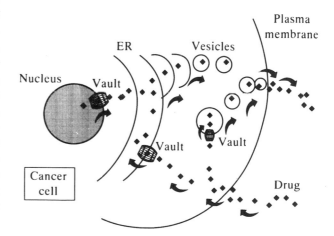

Figure 17.11. Proposed function of the lung resistance protein (LRP), which is the human vault protein: it probably mediates drug transport into vesicles that are then exocytosed. (Reproduced from Izquierdo et al., 1996a, with permission.)

of MRP and LRP (but not P-glycoprotein) were observed. Each marker of drug resistance correlated with resistance to MDR drugs, with increasing resistance if more than one of the molecules was expressed (Izquierdo et al., 1996b). Expression of LRP showed the greatest predictive value and was also correlated with resistance to non-MDR drugs. Staining for these markers was also carried out on tissue blocks from 57 patients who had undergone chemotherapy for ovarian cancer: MRP and LRP were expressed at higher levels (68 and 77 percent, respectively) than P-glycoprotein (16 percent), and only LRP expression correlated with poorer response to chemotherapy and shorter survival (Izquierdo et al., 1995). The relative importance of these molecules in contributing to drug resistance is currently not well established but seems likely to differ among tumors of different histologic types.

There are isolated reports of cell lines selected for resistance to drugs that express membrane-based proteins that are distinct from P-glycoprotein, MRP, or LRP (e.g., Doyle et al., 1996). It is likely that several drug-transport molecules may contribute to

drug resistance. Techniques for their detection and characterization are likely to increase rapidly, but overcoming resistance due to these multiple mechanisms will be a daunting task.

17.2.5 Topoisomerases and Drug Resistance

DNA topoisomerases are widespread nuclear enzymes that catalyze topologic changes of DNA structure required for recombination and replication of DNA and for transcription of RNA. These enzymes play a central role in chromosome structure, condensation/decondensation, and segregation (Froelich-Ammon and Osheroff, 1995). There are two highly conserved classes of topoisomerases: type I enzymes facilitate DNA strand unwinding by the passage of single-stranded DNA through a transient single-strand break in the complementary strand, whereas type II enzymes facilitate untwisting of the DNA by catalyzing passage of double-stranded DNA through double-strand breaks (Fig. 17.12). Under physiologic conditions, these covalent enzyme-DNA cleavage complexes are short-lived intermediates

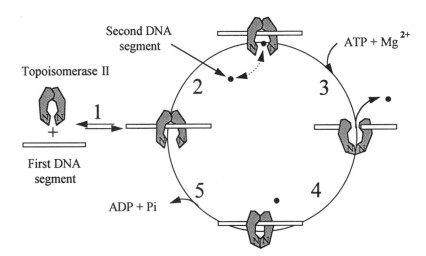

Figure 17.12. The catalytic cycle of topoisomerase II: the two-gate model. 1, DNA binding. In the absence of bound ATP, the enzyme is in the form of an open clamp and can bind to or dissociate from a segment of double-stranded DNA. The enzyme bound to the DNA creates a potential DNA gate. 2, Second DNA strand. A second DNA segment can enter and leave the DNA-bound enzyme as long as the gate remains open. 3, DNA cleavage and double-strand DNA passage. Binding of ATP to the enzyme closes the protein gate consisting of the N-terminal domain of each polypeptide in the homodimeric enzyme. A second gate on the opposite side to the N gate opens to allow exit to the second DNA segment from the interior of the enzyme. The opening of the second gate creates a transient double-stranded break in the DNA backbone. 4, Religation. The second gate closes, and the cleaved DNA is religated. 5, ATP hydrolysis and enzyme turnover. The enzyme returns to the open-clamp form bound to DNA following ATP hydrolysis. (Modified from Roca and Wang, 1994.)

present in low concentration that are well tolerated by the cell. Topoisomerases serve as cellular targets for several antineoplastic agents, which appear to stabilize the DNA-enzyme complex, leading to increased DNA strand cleavage and thereby mediating, at least in part, the cytocidal activity of these compounds (e.g., Fig. 17.13).

The gene for human topoisomerase I is located on chromosome 20 and encodes a 100-kDa monomeric protein. Camptothecin and its close structural analogues topotecan and CPT-11 exert their antitumor activity by inhibiting the enzyme DNA topoisomerase I (see Chap. 16, Sec. 16.5.6). Under physiologic conditions, the enzyme produces transient single-strand breaks in DNA, binds covalently to the 3'-phosphoryl end of DNA at the break site, facilitates passage of an intact DNA strand through the break site, and religates the cleaved DNA. In the presence of camptothecin or its analogues, the drug forms a complex with the enzyme and DNA, shifting the equilibrium reaction markedly in the direction of cleavage, and resulting in increased DNA damage and ultimately cell death. Downregulation and production of mutant forms of

DNA topoisomerase I, the target of these drugs, have been reported in drug-resistant cells (Schlichenmeyer et al., 1993).

Two isoforms have been described for human topoisomerase II: α and β. The gene for topoisomerase IIα encodes a 170-kDa protein and maps to chromosome 17 (Tsai-Pflugfelder et al., 1988), while that for topoisomerase II β forms a 180-kDa product and is located on chromosome 3 (Tan, et al., 1992). Although the two isozymes are closely related in sequence homology, they differ in biochemical and biophysical characteristics as well as in subcellular localization, cell-cycle specificity, and sensitivity to antineoplastic agents (Drake et al., 1989). The multiple steps in the catalytic cycle of topoisomerase II are illustrated schematically in Fig. 17.12. The DNA intercalating drugs doxorubicin, mitoxantrone, and amsacrine (Chap. 16, Sec. 16.5.1) as well as etoposide (VP-16) and teniposide (VM-26) (Chap. 16, Sec. 16.5.5) exert their cytocidal activity, at least in part, by interacting with topoisomerase II leading to double-strand breaks in DNA, as shown in Fig. 17.13.

Several laboratories have described downregulation of topoisomerase II in mammalian cells as a mechanism of resistance to topoisomerase II interactive agents (e.g., Harker et al., 1995). Induction of resistance by topoisomerase II−derived genetic suppressor elements and reversion of drug resistance by transfecting drug-resistant cells with the gene for topoisomerase IIα have provided direct functional evidence that resistance can be mediated by changes in topoisomerase II expression (Eder et al., 1993). A recent study suggested that in some leukemic cell lines the β, but not the α isoform may mediate the cytocidal activity of doxorubicin and etoposide (Brown et al., 1995); however, there have been relatively few studies of the β isoform, and the relative contribution of each isoform to total cellular topoisomerase II activity and sensitivity to antineoplastic agents is uncertain.

Drug-resistance has been attributed to qualitative as well as quantitative alteration in expression of topoisomerase IIα. Phosphorylation appears to alter the susceptibility of topoisomerase II to inhibition by antitumor drugs. It has been suggested that hyperphosphorylation of topoisomerase II might compensate for a decrease in the topoisomerase II protein level observed in drug-resistant cell lines and allow their proliferation and survival. Point mutations and other gene rearrangements have also been reported in the topoisomerase IIα gene in drug-resistant cell lines (McPherson et al., 1993).

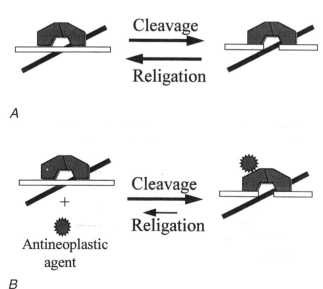

Figure 17.13. Interaction of antineoplastic agents with DNA topoisomerase II. *A.* In the absence of drug, topo II binds to the DNA and establishes a DNA cleavage/religation equilibrium. *B.* In the presence of drug, the antineoplastic agent binds to topo II, stabilizes the DNA-enzyme complex, and shifts the equilibrium markedly in the direction of DNA strand cleavage.

17.2.6 Glutathione and Drug Resistance

Glutathione (GSH)-mediated detoxification pathways play a central role in the inactivation and elimination of antineoplastic agents and chemical carcinogens. Many of these compounds cause cellular damage by the production of reactive charged intermediates. Similar processes are involved during the interaction of ionizing radiation with tissue (Chap. 13, Sec. 13.2.3). One mechanism by which cells can protect themselves from damage caused by reactive agents is the synthesis of a high concentration of sulfhydryl compounds, especially the tripeptide glutathione, which can react with such radicals and render them nontoxic (Fig. 17.14). The importance of glutathione in the protection of normal tissue is reflected in its widespread distribution. Reduced glutathione can inactivate peroxides and free radicals, which may be produced by drugs such as doxorubicin. It can also bind to positively charged electrophilic molecules, such as the active groups of alkylating agents (Chap. 16, Sec. 16.3), rendering them less toxic and more easily excreted. These reactions are catalyzed, respectively, by the enzymes glutathione peroxidase and glutathione S-transferase (Fig. 17.14).

Drugs conjugated to GSH must be extruded from cells by glutathione-conjugate export carriers known variably as the GS-X pump, the multispecific organic anion transporter, or the leukotriene C4 transporter. The GS-X pumps have broad specificity for substrates, including several anticancer drugs. This function is undertaken in part by the multidrug re-

sistance protein (MRP), so that c[...] to increased expression of MRP [...] on glutathione-mediated conjugatio[...] drugs (Loe et al., 1996, Sec. 17.2.4). [...] appear to transport cisplatin-GSH co[...] though both increased expression of M[...] creased synthesis of glutathione have been [...] in cisplatin-resistant cells (Chuman et al., 19[...] et al., 1996). MRP appears to be one of a family of carriers that facilitate the export from cells of glutathione-conjugated drugs.

Glutathione S-transferases (GSTs) represent a multigene family of enzymes that catalyze the conjugation of glutathione to a broad range of electrophilic compounds, including anticancer drugs and carcinogens. By conjugating glutathione (GSH) to various drugs, GSTs appear to play a role in the development of cellular resistance to antineoplastic agents (Waxman et al., 1992). Five distinct GST classes or gene families have been identified. The cytosolic GSTs are abundant and are classified by their isoelectric point as basic (α class), neutral (μ class), and acidic (π class); the other two GST classes are the microsomal isoform and the more recently described θ class. The π, θ, and microsomal classes each consist of a single gene product, whereas the α and μ classes contain more than one gene product. Each functional GST enzyme is a homo- or heterodimer made up of subunits encoded by gene loci from within a given class.

Several lines of evidence support a role for GSTs in resistance to alkylating agents (Tew, 1994): (1) nitrogen mustards can form GSH conjugates in reactions catalyzed by GSTs; (2) human tumors and cell lines often overexpress GST isozymes; (3) GST inhibitors cause sensitization of cultured cells to alkylating agents; (4) cell cycle–dependent sensitivity to melphalan correlates with the cell cycle–dependent expression of GSTs; and (5) elevation of GSTα occurs within several days of exposure to chlorambucil as part of the normal cellular response. In contrast, some cell lines selected for resistance to alkylating agents have shown no increase in GST protein or function. Also, in studies of melphalan-glutathione conjugate formation in tumor cells, GST-catalyzed conjugation made only a minimal contribution to the overall rate of conjugation.

Transfection of the human gene for GSTπ has been reported to increase resistance of Chinese hamster ovary cells, but not that of NIH-3T3 cells, to cisplatin. More consistently, transfection and expression of GSTπ has been associated with resistance to doxorubicin, GSTμ with resistance to cisplatin, and

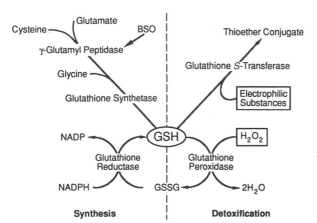

Figure 17.14. The metabolism of glutathione. Reduced glutathione (GSH) can inactivate peroxides and free radicals through reactions catalyzed by glutathione peroxidase and a family of glutathione S-transferases (GSTs). Synthesis of GSH is inhibited by buthionine sulfoximine (BSO).

GSTα with resistance to alkylating agents (e.g., Puchalski and Fahl, 1990). In contrast to the above results, several attempts to transfect MCF-7 human breast cancer cells with genes encoding class π, α, or μ GST have resulted in overexpression of the gene product but not in resistance to antineoplastic agents. One explanation for the contradictory results of the transfection experiments is that appropriate concentrations of cofactors, such as GSH and/or of carrier molecules required for export of glutathione-drug conjugates from the cell might be required for GST isozymes to confer resistance, and these may not be available (Tew, 1994). Overall, there is substantial evidence that high levels of GST isozymes are associated with resistance to alkylating agents.

There are several inhibitors of GST activity and some have been tested for their ability to alter the cytotoxicity of alkylating agents. In a chlorambucil-resistant cell line with elevated GSH and GST, cytotoxicity was increased with the use of buthionine sulfoximine (BSO), which causes reduced synthesis of glutathione, and/or with the GST inhibitors ethacrynic acid or indomethacin (Yang et al., 1992). Sensitivity to chlorambucil could be restored to that of the parental line by a combination of both inhibitors. Ethacrynic acid has been reported to potentiate the cytotoxicity of melphalan against MCF-7 breast cancer cells when given in combination with BSO. When given at concentrations sufficient to inhibit GST π, μ, and α by at least 50 percent in a melanoma cell line, a twofold increase in chemosensitivity to melphalan was observed. Phase I clinical testing of alkylating agents with the GST inhibitor ethacrynic acid has been initiated. Administration of BSO has also led to the reversal of drug resistance mediated by MRP, providing further evidence that substrates for MRP may require conjugation with GSH (Zaman et al., 1995).

Increased levels of metallothioneins, proteins rich in sulfhydryl-containing cysteine residues, are associated with resistance to cisplatin and alkylating agents. The presumed mechanism is interaction with toxic electrophilic drugs or their metabolites. A cause-and-effect relationship has been suggested by development of resistance to cisplatin and alkylating agents in cells that were transfected with a human metallothionein gene (Kelley et al., 1988) and by increased sensitivity of cells that do not produce metallothionein (Kondo et al., 1995). However, studies of cisplatin-resistant cells derived from human ovarian cancer did not show a correlation between resistance and metallothionein levels (Schilder et al., 1990), and multiple mechanisms are known to be involved in resistance to this drug (Table 17.2).

17.2.7 Drug Resistance and DNA Repair

The involvement of DNA repair in the development of resistance to alkylating agents and to cisplatin is suggested by the enhanced removal of DNA adducts and/or cross-links from resistant cells (Zamble et al., 1996). DNA lesions produced by alkylating agents may be repaired by at least three mechanisms: (1) damage reversal, (2) nucleotide-excision repair (NER), and (3) recombination or complementation (Chap. 4, Sec. 4.4). Two enzymes involved in repair are O^6-alkylguanine DNA alkyltransferase (AGAT; also known as MGMT where M = melthyl) and 3-methyladenine DNA glycosylase (GLY). The DNA repair enzyme AGAT removes adducts from the O^6 position of the base guanine and is a major contributor to resistance against nitrosoureas such as BCNU and to some other alkylating agents (Gerson and Willson, 1995). The enzyme GLY has been reported to be increased in lymphocytes from patients with chronic lymphocytic leukemia resistant to alkylating agents. Increased expression of the enzyme ERCC-2, which is a DNA helicase involved in the first step of nucleotide excision repair (see Chap. 4, Sec. 4.4.5), has been demonstrated recently by the polymerase chain reaction (see Chap. 3, Sec. 3.3.7) in human tumor cell lines resistant to the nitrosoureas BCNU and SarCNU (Chen et al., 1996).

Theoretical opportunities exist to circumvent drug resistance by inhibition of DNA repair enzymes. For example, O^6-benzylguanine acts as a substrate for AGAT, resulting in the transfer of the benzyl group to the active site of the enzyme and leading to the irreversible inactivation of the enzyme (Gerson and Willson, 1995). Completion of DNA repair requires unscheduled DNA synthesis to bridge the gap appearing in DNA as a result of base or nucleotide excision. In preclinical studies, inhibitors of DNA synthesis—such as aphidicolin, cytosine arabinoside, and hydroxyurea—have been reported to potentiate the toxicity of cross-linking agents such as nitrogen mustards and cisplatin by inhibiting DNA repair (Gosland et al., 1996). Inhibitors of DNA repair would have to be used with caution, however, since they are likely to increase the sensitivity of dose-limiting normal tissues.

17.2.8 Resistance to Apoptosis

Apoptosis was described in Chap. 7, Sec. 7.3 as an active process whereby intracellular signals trigger a sequence of events leading to cell death and lysis. Apoptotic death is observed frequently after treatment with anticancer drugs and occurs, therefore, in response to damage caused by them. Apoptosis may play a primary role in cell death following drug treatment or it may occur as a late event leading to lysis of cells secondary to irreversible damage that has caused loss of reproductive integrity (Smets, 1994). There is evidence for some drugs and cell lines that apoptotic pathways activated by anticancer drugs play a primary role in cell death. Decreased ability to undergo apoptosis may then cause drug resistance (Hickman, 1996).

Apoptosis is inhibited by expression of the *bcl-2* gene and stimulated by homologous members of the same gene family, such as *bax* and *bcl-X_S* (Yin et al, 1994; Chapter 7, Section 7.3.3). In some cell lines and human tumors, there is a correlation between increased expression of *bcl-2* or decreased expression of *bax* and resistance to anticancer drugs (e.g., Krajewski et al., 1995), but other studies have failed to reveal a correlation. In a human leukemia cell line, transfection of the *bcl-2* gene led to increased resistance to the anticancer drug cytosine arabinoside (Hu et al., 1995) but transfection of *bcl-2* into some other cell lines led to reduction or delay in apoptosis without influencing drug sensitivity as determined in clonogenic assays (Yin and Schimke, 1995; Lock and Strabinskiene, 1996). These observations presumably reflect the varying role of apoptosis as a primary cause of cell death versus its secondary role in the lysis of irreversibly damaged cells.

Independent evidence of the importance of apoptotic pathways in cellular sensitivity to anti-cancer drugs has been reported by Zanke et al. (1996). They found that thermoresistant murine TR-4 cells were unable to activate p54 stress-activated protein kinase (SAPK; Chap. 6, Sec. 6.4.1) in response to heat, whereas the heat-sensitive parental RIF-1 cells readily activated SAPK. Moreover, the TR-4 cells were resistant to several anticancer drugs, including cisplatin and doxorubicin, which also activated SAPK in the parental cell line but not in TR-4 cells. Introduction of a dominant mutation into sensitive RIF-1 cells that prevented upregulation of SAPK in response to stress caused resistance to heat and to several anticancer drugs, including cisplatin and doxorubicin, as determined by clonogenic assays (Zanke et al., 1996). The ability to activate SAPK in response to drug treatment appears to be an upstream event that allows a cell to undergo apoptosis, and downregulation of this signaling pathway by genetic or other events can cause cellular resistance to a variety of agents.

The *p53* gene also plays a role in apoptosis, and normal *p53* can stimulate apoptosis of cells that have sustained damage to DNA (Chap. 5, Sec. 5.5.2). A mutant *p53* gene, present in a substantial proportion of human cancers, may inhibit apoptosis. There is substantial evidence that the p53 protein may influence response to anticancer drugs, and several mechanisms of drug resistance are probably influenced by it (Lowe et al., 1994; Harris, 1996). For example, in one study, transfected wild-type *p53* could be induced in colon cancer cells that had an endogenous mutant p53 protein: induction of the wild-type p53 protein was found to increase sensitivity to 5-FU, camptothecin, and radiation (Yang et al., 1996).

Apoptosis is a complex pathway that is regulated by many cellular proteins (Park et al., 1996). Recent evidence suggests that drug resistance, mediated by inhibition of apoptosis, can arise through transfection of cytokeratin genes (Anderson et al., 1996) and by upregulation of the transcription factor NF-κB (Wang et al., 1996). A better understanding of the signaling pathways that lead to cell death in response to damaging agents such as anticancer drugs is likely to provide insight into other mechanisms of drug resistance and potential strategies for their reversal.

17.2.9 Drug Resistance In Vivo

Most studies of the mechanisms that underlie drug resistance have exposed cells at low density in tissue culture to various mutagens, followed by repeated selection in increasing concentration of the anticancer drug (Fig. 17.5). These studies have led to the characterization of mechanisms of drug resistance, described in previous sections, at least some of which appear to be relevant to human cancer. The clinical situation, especially for solid tumors, is rather different. Drug resistance may be present without prior drug exposure or may emerge after brief exposure of solid tissue at high cell density to a relatively low concentrations of drug or drugs achievable in plasma.

Two groups of investigators have shown that repeated treatment with alkylating agents of solid tissue, either in the form of spheroids (Chap. 7, Sec. 7.6.3) or tumor-bearing mice, may lead to drug resistance that is expressed only when the cells are regrown in contact as spheroids or tumors. The cells did not express drug resistance when grown in dilute cell culture (Teicher et al., 1990; Kerbel et al., 1994). Further work has suggested that drug resistance is correlated with the density of cell packing in spheroids and may be reversed by agents which inhibit adhesion between the cells (St. Croix et al., 1996). Adherent drug-resistant cells in spheroids over-express the cell cycle–inhibitory protein p27^{KIP1} (Chap. 7, Sec. 7.2.3), so that these effects may be mediated in part by a low rate of cell proliferation in the solid-tissue environment.

The above findings emphasize the importance of model systems to study drug resistance, which include those relevant to drug exposure of tumors in patients undergoing chemotherapy. Such experiments are likely to detect mechanisms of drug resistance that depend on the cellular environment, including tight junctions between cells in epithelial tumors, the presence of an extracellular matrix and cell-adhesion molecules (see Chap. 9, Sec. 9.2), and metabolic factors such as hypoxia and acidity (see Chap. 15, Sec. 15.3.4). These mechanisms may differ from those that have been characterized in more simple cell systems.

17.3 TREATMENT WITH MULTIPLE AGENTS

17.3.1 Influence on Therapeutic Index

Patients are frequently treated with combination chemotherapy or with drugs in combination with radiation therapy. When two or more agents are combined to give an improvement in the therapeutic index, this implies that the increase in toxicity to critical normal tissues is less than the increase in damage to tumor cells (Sec. 17.1.1). Since the dose-limiting toxicity to normal tissues may vary for different drugs and for radiation, two agents may often be combined with only minimal reduction in doses as compared with those that would be used if either agent were given alone. Additive effects against a tumor with less than additive toxicity for normal tissue may then lead to a therapeutic advantage.

Mechanisms by which different agents may give therapeutic benefit when used in combination have been classified by Steel and Peckham (1979) as follows: (1) independent toxicity, which may, for example, allow combined use of anticancer drugs at full dosage; (2) spatial cooperation, whereby disease that is missed by one agent (e.g., local radiotherapy) may be treated by another (e.g., chemotherapy); (3) protection of normal tissues; and (4) enhancement of tumor response.

The above mechanisms suggest guidelines for choosing drugs that might be given in combination. Most drugs exert dose-limiting toxicity for the bone marrow, but this is not the case for vincristine (dose-

limiting neurotoxicity), cisplatin (nephrotoxicity), or bleomycin (mucositis and lung toxicity). These and some other drugs can be combined with myelo-suppressive agents at close to full dosage and have contributed to the therapeutic success of drug combinations used to treat lymphoma and testicular cancer. Research on drug resistance (Sec. 17.2) has defined drugs that commonly (e.g., doxorubicin and vincristine) or rarely (e.g., doxorubicin and cyclophosphamide) demonstrate cross-resistance. Combination of non-cross-resistant drugs may contribute to therapeutic benefit, as, for example, in the combined use of doxorubicin and cyclophosphamide to treat many types of tumors. Nevertheless, most drug combinations in clinical use have evolved empirically through the combination of drugs that demonstrate some antitumor effects when used singly.

17.3.2 Synergy and Additivity: Isobologram Analysis

Claims are made frequently that two agents are "synergistic," implying that the two agents given together are more effective than would be expected from their individual activities. Confusion has arisen because of disagreement as to what constitutes an "expected" level of effect when two noninteracting agents are combined (Berenbaum, 1981; Merlin, 1994). An appropriate definition must take into account the dose-effect relationship for each agent used alone rather than a simple summation or multiplication of individual effects. The use of multiple agents may lead to an increase in the therapeutic index, but it is rare that a claim for synergy of effects against a single population of cells can be substantiated.

The concepts of synergy and additivity between two agents can be understood by considering the level of cell survival after treatment of a single population of cells, either in a tumor or in a normal tissue. Suppose a given dose of agent A gives a surviving fraction of cells (S_A), that a surviving fraction (S_B) follows treatment with a given dose of agent B, and a combination of the agents gives a surviving fraction (S_{A+B}) (Fig. 17.15). Claims for synergy are often made if S_{A+B} is less than the product $S_A \times S_B$. This conclusion is correct only if cell survival is exponentially related to dose for both agents. However, if the survival curves have an initial "shoulder" (Fig. 17.15), then the combined effects of the two agents may be expected to lead to an upper limit of survival equal to $S_A \times S_B$ if they act independently of each other, so that the shoulder of the survival curve

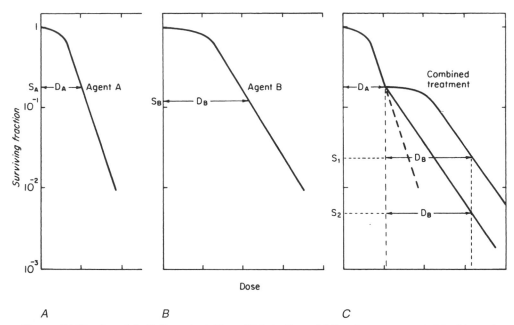

Figure 17.15. *A* and *B.* Cell survival (S_A or S_B) is indicated following treatment with either of two agents, A and B, each of which has a survival curve characterized by an initial shoulder followed by an exponential fall with increasing dose. *C.* Survival (S_{A+B}) after combined use of dose D_A of agent A and dose D_B of agent B will be equal to S_1 ($= S_A \times S_B$) if there is no overlap of damage, and the "shoulder" representing accumulation of sublethal damage is retained for the second agent. Survival after combined treatment (S_{A+B}) will be equal to S_2 if cells have accumulated maximum sublethal damage from the first agent, A, and the "shoulder" of the curve is lost for the second agent, B.

is retained for both agents. Combined treatment will lead to a lower level of survival if, after treatment with the first agent, A, the survival falls exponentially with dose (in the absence of a shoulder effect) for the second agent, B (Fig. 17.15C). The fallacy of defining this lower level of survival as a synergistic effect can be illustrated by replacing agent B with a second, equivalent dose of agent A given immediately after the first dose. The "combined" survival curve then follows that for agent A, with a survival level corresponding to a dose $2 \times D_A$ in Fig. 17.15A. If agent A has a survival curve with an initial shoulder, one would then conclude erroneously that the second dose of agent A was synergistic with the first (i.e., that agent A was synergistic with itself).

The above discussion implies that there is a range over which two agents can produce additive effects. Isobologram analysis provides a method for defining this range of additivity (Steel and Peckham, 1979). Dose-response curves are first generated for each agent used alone. These dose-response curves are then used to generate isoeffect plots (known as *isobolograms*). These curves relate the dose of agent A to the dose of agent B that would be predicted,

when used in combination, to give a constant level of biological effect (e.g., cell survival) for the assumptions of (1) independent damage and (2) overlapping damage (Fig. 17.15). These curves define an envelope of additivity (Fig. 17.16). If, when the two agents are given together, the doses required to give the same level of biological effect lie within the envelope, the interaction is said to be *additive.* If they lie between the lower isobologram and the axes (i.e., the combined effect is caused by lower doses of the two agents than predicted) the interaction is *supra-additive* or synergistic. If the required doses of the two agents in combination lie above the envelope of additivity (i.e., the effect is caused by higher doses than predicted), the interaction is *sub-additive* or antagonistic (Fig. 17.16).

Demonstration that two or more agents have a supra-additive or synergistic interaction has been used as a rationale for their inclusion in clinical protocols. This rationale is valid only if the interaction leads to a greater effect against the tumor as compared with that against limiting normal tissues (i.e., if it leads to an improvement in therapeutic index; Sec. 17.1.1). It is theoretically possible that antagonistic agents (subadditive interaction) could im-

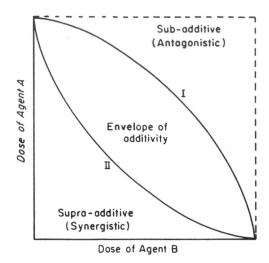

Figure 17.16. Isobologram relating the doses of two agents that would be expected to give a constant level of biologic effect when used together. It was generated from dose-response curves for each agent separately. Assumptions about overlap or nonoverlap of damage (Fig. 17.15) lead to the generation of two isobologram curves (I and II) that describe an envelope of additive interaction. Experimental data falling outside this envelope may indicate synergistic or antagonistic interactions, as shown. (Adapted from Steel and Peckham, 1979.)

prove therapeutic index provided that there was greater antagonism of toxic effects for normal tissue as compared with tumor.

17.3.3 Modifiers of Drug Activity

Some drugs with little or no toxicity for tumor cells may modify the action of anticancer drugs to produce increased antitumor effect or protection of normal tissue. Examples of interactions that might lead to therapeutic benefit through increased antitumor effects include (1) the use of doxorubicin with agents such as verapamil, cyclosporin A, or their analogues (which inhibit multidrug resistance; Sec. 17.2.4); (2) use of BSO (which inhibits the synthesis of glutathione; Sec. 17.2.6), or (3) use of folinic acid with 5-FU, which may provide a necessary cofactor for inhibition of the target enzyme thymidilate synthase (Chap. 16, Sec. 16.4.2).

Alternatively, reduction of the toxic effects of chemotherapy against bone marrow may be achieved by coadministration of growth factors such as granulocyte colony-stimulating factor (G-CSF) or granulocyte-macrophage colony-stimulating factor (GM-CSF), which are produced by recombinant DNA technology (Chap. 7, Sec. 7.5.1). It has been shown that these growth factors can stimulate earlier recov-

ery of mature granulocytes after bone-marrow suppression by chemotherapy, or after stem-cell transplantation (Chap. 15, Sec. 15.4). G-CSF is commonly used in situations where reduction in dosage of chemotherapy might lead to a decrease in the probability of cure or long-term survival of patients.

Two other agents that protect normal tissues from damage due to chemotherapy have been licensed for use in the United States. Dexrazoxane is a prodrug whose active form chelates iron. Since complexes between iron and anthracyclines such as doxorubicin (and the consequent formation of free radicals) appear to mediate cardiac toxicity but not antitumor effects, dexrazoxane may decrease cardiac toxicity of these drugs and increase their therapeutic index (Speyer et al., 1988, Venturini et al., 1996). Amifostine is also a prodrug that is converted to a sulfhydryl-containing active form. Amifostine is localized selectively in normal tissues, probably because of increased activity of the activating enzyme alkaline phosphatase on the membranes of normal cells. Therefore it may offer selective protection against a variety of drugs (and radiation) that damage cells by producing reactive intermediates which bind to sulfhydryl groups (Kemp et al., 1996).

17.3.4 Drugs and Radiation

Many patients receive treatment with both drugs and radiation (Tannock, 1996). Study of mechanisms of interaction between drugs and radiation at the cellular level may be evaluated from cell-survival curves for radiation obtained in the presence or absence of the drug (Fig. 17.17). Drugs may influence the survival curve in at least three ways: (1) the curve may be displaced downward by the amount of cell kill caused by the drug alone; (2) the "shoulder" on the survival curve may be lost, suggesting an inability to repair radiation damage in the presence of the drug; and (3) the slope of the exponential part of the survival curve may be changed, indicating sensitization or protection by the drug. Most drugs influence survival curves according to the first two patterns described above; this corresponds to the limits of additivity defined in Sec. 17.3.2, where sublethal damage may be independent or overlapping. The third pattern, leading to a change in slope of the dose-response curve, defines agents that are radiation sensitizers or protectors (Chap. 14, Sec. 14.4.3). Sensitization of this type has been reported inconsistently for cisplatin and for prolonged exposure to 5-FU after radiation.

The most common mechanism by which combined treatment with radiation and drugs leads to

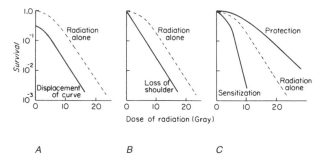

Figure 17.17. Possible influences of drug treatment on the relationship between radiation dose and cell survival: (*A*) displacement of curve; (*B*) loss of shoulder, indicating effects of drug on the repair of sublethal radiation damage; (*C*) change in the slope of the curve, indicating sensitization or protection.

therapeutic advantage arises when radiation is used to provide effective treatment for sites of bulk disease (usually the primary tumor) and drugs are used to treat metastatic sites containing smaller numbers of cells. This spatial co-operation (Sec. 17.3.1) requires no interaction of the two modalities but involves different dose-limiting toxicities. It is limited by the lack of availability of effective chemotherapy for many types of malignancy. There are also mechanisms whereby the combined use of radiation and drugs might be used to obtain therapeutic advantage for treatment of a primary tumor, although there are as yet few examples of unequivocal benefit in clinical trials (Tannock, 1996). Three properties of cells that might be exploited to give therapeutic advantage for the combined use of radiation and drugs are listed in Table 17.4.

Evidence was presented in Chap. 10, Sec. 10.1,

that tumors undergo both genetic and corresponding phenotypic changes that lead to heterogeneity among the cells of the population. Genetic instability implies progression to a state where many subclones will coexist in the tumor with different levels of sensitivity to drugs (see Sec. 17.2). When therapy is applied, any resistant cells that are present will have a selective survival advantage and will determine tumor response: thus, heterogeneity in therapeutic response will tend to make tumors more resistant to treatment than normal tissues. Combined treatment with radiation and drugs might then lead to improved therapeutic index if radiation can eradicate small populations of drug-resistant cells. This cooperative effect requires that mechanisms of resistance to the two therapeutic agents are independent.

There is quite marked variability in the surviving fraction of cells following a low radiation dose of 2 Gy, which is representative of the typical fraction size used in fractionated daily irradiation. The net effect after a 5- to 7-week course of such treatment will be a probability of cell survival that may differ by several orders of magnitude for different cell populations (Chap. 14, Sec. 14.5.1). Mechanisms (other than hypoxia) that convey clinical resistance to radiotherapy remain poorly understood but probably include enhanced ability to repair damage to DNA, increased levels of SH compounds such as glutathione (or of associated GST enzymes) that scavenge free radicals (especially in hypoxic cells), and decreased ability to undergo apoptosis. These mechanisms may also convey resistance to some anticancer drugs, whereas many other mechanisms of drug resistance (Sec. 17.2) are unlikely to cause re-

Table 17.4. Properties of Tumor Cells That Could Be Exploited to Provide Therapeutic Advantage from the Combined Use of Radiation and Drugs

Property	Effect of Combined Treatment
Genetic instability of tumors, leading to drug and radiation resistance for different clones	Killing of drug-resistant cells by radiation, and radiation-resistant cells by drugs *if* mechanisms of resistance are independent.
Differences in cell proliferation and especially in repopulation during radiation treatment for tumor and normal tissue	Inhibition of repopulation by drugs or selective uptake of radiosensitizing nucleosides (e.g., IUdR) could lead to therapeutic advantage *if* repopulation were faster in the tumor.
Environmental factors such as hypoxia and acidity, which are usually confined to tumors	Beneficial effects from drugs with selective toxicity for hypoxic and/or acidic cells.

sistance to radiation. Resistance to any given drug may be caused by multiple mechanisms (Table 17.2), so that a radiation-drug combination that provides therapeutic advantage for one tumor may not do so for another if different mechanisms of drug resistance are dominant. Effective use of combined treatment would be facilitated by rapid pretreatment assays that give insight into mechanisms of resistance prior to initiation of therapy.

Proliferation of surviving cells during a course of fractionated radiation (i.e., repopulation, Chap. 14, Sec. 14.3.2) acts to increase the total number of cells that must be killed. Anticancer drugs given *during* the course of fractionated radiation might be expected to inhibit repopulation, while agents such as iodo-deoxyuridine might be taken up selectively into proliferating cells (during S phase) and might sensitize them to radiation (McGinn et al., 1996). Combined treatment may then convey therapeutic advantage if the rate of repopulation is greater for the tumor cells than it is for normal tissues within the radiation field; this might apply to tumors growing in slowly proliferating or nonproliferating tissues such as lung or brain. In contrast, the same effect could lead to a therapeutic disadvantage, at least for acute normal-tissue reactions, if repopulation were faster in normal tissues; this effect might occur for tumors adjacent to rapidly proliferating normal tissues such as the mucous membranes in the head and neck. Greater specificity would be expected for agents that specifically inhibit the proliferation of tumor cells; this might be achieved through use of hormonal agents (tamoxifen, antiandrogens) used concurrently with radiation for treatment of breast or prostate cancer (Chap. 12; Sec. 12.4). Another possible strategy is to administer inhibitory growth factors (e.g., members of the TGF-β family) or agents that block receptors for stimulatory growth factors if they are expressed selectively on tumor cells.

As noted earlier, repopulation during fractionated radiation therapy might also be influenced by prior treatment with neoadjuvant chemotherapy (Sec. 17.1.3). Such chemotherapy may cause tumor shrinkage, followed by improved nutrition of surviving cells, with consequent stimulation of cell proliferation (Withers et al., 1988). If there is increased repopulation of surviving cells during the subsequent course of fractionated radiation therapy, any advantage from initial shrinkage of the tumor caused by chemotherapy may be lost or reversed because of the decreased net effectiveness of subsequent radiation treatment (see Chap. 14, Fig. 14.13).

A third mechanism that has potential for exploitation through combined use of radiation and drugs depends on the presence of a hypoxic microenvironment within solid tumors (see Chap. 7; Sec. 7.6.3, and Chap. 13, Sec. 13.5.2). A hypoxic environment conveys resistance to radiation because cell killing is dependent in part on the presence of oxygen. Drugs that have selective toxicity for hypoxic cells, such as tirapazamine, which requires bioreduction for activity, might therefore improve therapeutic index when used with radiation (see Chap. 15, Sec. 15.3.4). Drugs that are activated under hypoxic conditions may also kill tumor cells in neighboring aerobic regions (Brown et al., 1995). Such drugs should have minimal effects against normal tissues, where adequate vasculature usually prevents development of a hypoxic microenvironment.

Whenever radiation and drugs are used together or in sequence, there is potential for increased damage to normal tissues in the radiation field. Some of the effects of combined treatment may lead to changes in function that occur months to years after treatment. Both clinical experience and studies in animals have shown that most anticancer drugs can increase the incidence of toxicity from radiation, sometimes in organs (e.g., the kidney) where the drugs alone rarely cause overt toxicity (Phillips and Fu, 1976; von der Maase, 1986). There is rather minimal information about the ability of drugs to increase the late effects of radiation on normal tissue in animal systems, even though these late effects are most often dose-limiting (Chap. 14, Sec. 14.2.2). Some of the tissues in which important interactions of drugs and radiation have been documented in clinical experience are indicated in Table 17.5. These interactions may lead to a reduction in the maximally tolerated dose of radiation by factors of 10 to 50 percent as compared with treatment by radiation alone.

The effect of a drug on radiation toxicity to any organ may be expressed as the dose-enhancement ratio (DER), which is the dose of radiation to produce a given effect when used alone divided by the dose of radiation that gives the same effect when combined with the drug. For acute effects of radiation on normal tissues of mice, typical values of DER range from 1.0 to 1.5, depending on the drug and normal tissue; maximum interaction occurs when drug and radiation are administered within a short time span (von der Maase, 1986). The therapeutic gain factor equals the ratio of DER for the tumor to the DER for the dose-limiting normal tissue in the radiation field. In experimental systems, this may vary widely depending on the drug used, the doses

Table 17.5. Combined Effects of Radiation and Anticancer Drugs That Have Led to Increased Toxicity for Normal Tissues of Patients

Tissue	Drugs Used with Radiation
Lung	Actinomycin D Doxorubicin Bleomycin
Heart	Doxorubicin
Kidney	Actinomycin D Doxorubicin
Esophagus	Actinomycin D Doxorubicin Bleomycin
Lower gastrointestinal tract	Actinomycin D 5-Fluorouracil
Bladder	Cyclophosphamide
Central nervous system	Methotrexate
Peripheral nerves	Vincristine
Skin and mucous membranes	Actinomycin D Doxorubicin Bleomycin 5-Fluorouracil Cisplatin Methotrexate

of drug and radiation, and the sequence. It is difficult to predict the dose schedules that are likely to lead to therapeutic gain in patients.

17.4 SUMMARY

Experimental chemotherapy is directed toward improvement of the therapeutic index, which requires greater selectivity of drugs for tumors as compared to critical normal tissues. Experiments in animals have demonstrated that drug administration may lead to cure of microscopic tumors but not larger tumors; these experiments provide a model for adjuvant chemotherapy. Attempts have been made to improve therapeutic index through selective delivery of drugs to tumor cells by the use of carriers such as antibodies or liposomes. These methods have shown benefit in some animal models and are being investigated in clinical trials. A major problem may be presented by the limited penetration of these complexes into tumor tissue.

The most important limitation to the therapeutic effects of chemotherapy is the presence of intrinsic or acquired resistance to drugs by tumor-cell populations. Drug resistance occurs through a variety of mechanisms and usually results from mutation or altered expression of genes. Mechanisms such as an increase in extrusion of drugs from cells by P-glycoprotein, MRP or LRP, increased synthesis of glutathione and its associated enzymes, or an increase in potential for DNA repair may lead to cross-resistance between chemically unrelated drugs. These and other mechanisms provide a plausible explanation for the common observation of clinical resistance to multiple agents. Increased understanding of mechanisms that cause drug resistance may lead to the development of new agents or therapeutic strategies that circumvent drug resistance.

Anticancer drugs are frequently used in combination with each other and with radiation. Agents that modify the toxicity of anticancer drugs are leading to therapeutic benefit in selected situations. Mechanisms that may lead to therapeutic advantage from combined use of radiation and drugs include (1) spatial cooperation, whereby radiation is used to treat bulk disease and chemotherapy to treat metastases; (2) use of each modality to kill tumor cells that have developed resistance to the other, (3) inhibition by drugs of repopulation of surviving cells during fractionated radiotherapy, and (4) use of drugs that are selective for hypoxic cells that are resistant to radiation.

REFERENCES

Anderson JM, Heindl LM, Bauman PA, et al: Cytokeratin expression results in a drug resistant phenotype to six different chemotherapeutic agents. *Clin Cancer Res* 1996; 2:97–105.

Bagshawe KD: Towards generating cytotoxic agents at cancer sites. *Br J Cancer* 1989; 60:275–281.

Berenbaum MC: Criteria for analyzing interactions between biologically active agents. *Adv Cancer Res* 1981; 35:269–335.

Bradley G, Juranka P, Ling V: Mechanisms of multidrug resistance. *Biochim Biophys Acta* 1988; 948:87–128.

Brenner DE: Liposomal encapsulation: Making old and new drugs do new tricks. *J Natl Cancer Inst* 1989; 81:1436–1438.

Brown GA, McPherson JP, Liu G, et al: Relationship of DNA topoisomerase IIα and β expression to cytotoxicity of antineoplastic agents in human acute lymphoblastic leukemia cell lines. *Cancer Res* 1995; 55:78–82.

Chan HSL, Haddad G, Thorner PS, et al: P-glycoprotein expression as a predictor of the outcome of therapy for neuroblastoma. *N Engl J Med* 1991; 325:1608–1616.

Chen ZP, Malpetsa A, Marcantonio D, et al: correlation of chloroethylnitrosourea resistance with ERCC-2 expression in human tumor cell lines as determined by quantitative competitive polymerase chain reaction. *Cancer Res* 1996; 56:2475–2478.

Childs S, Ling V: The MDR superfamily of genes and its biological implications. In: DeVita VT, Hellman S,

Rosenberg S, eds. *Important Advances in Oncology.* Philadelphia: Lippincott; 1994; 21–36.

Chuman Y, Chen ZS, Sumizawa T, et al: Characterization of the ATP-dependent LTC-4 transporter in cisplatin-resistant human KB cells. *Biochem Biophys Res Commun* 1996; 226:158–165.

Cillo C, Ling V, Hill RP: Drug resistance to KHT fibrosarcoma cell lines with different metastatic ability. *Int J Cancer* 1989; 43:107–111.

Cole SPC, Ghardwaj G, Gerlach JH, et al: Overexpression of a transporter gene in a multidrug-resistant human lung cancer cell line. *Science* 1992; 258:1650–1654.

Dicker AP, Waltham MC, Volkenandt M, et al: Methotrexate resistance in an in vivo mouse tumor due to a non-active site dihydrofolate reductase mutation. *Proc Natl Acad Sci USA* 1993: 90:11797–11801.

Doyle LA, Yang W, Rishi AK, et al: H19 gene overexpression in atypical multidrug-resistant cells associated with expression of a 95 kilodalton membrane glycoprotein. *Cancer Res* 1996; 56:2904–2907.

Drake FH, Hofmann GA, Bartus HF, et al: Biochemical and pharmacological properties of p170 and p180 forms of topoisomerase II. *Biochemistry* 1989; 28:8154–8160.

Dumontet C, Duran GE, Steger KA, et al: Resistance mechanisms in human sarcoma mutants derived by single-step exposure to paclitaxel (Taxol). *Cancer Res* 1996; 56:1091–1097.

Eder JP Jr, Chan VT-W, Neimierko E, et al: Conditional expression of wild-type topoisomerase II complements a mutant enzyme in mammalian cells. *J Biol Chem* 1993; 268:13844–13849.

Endicott JA, Ling V: The biochemistry of P-glycoprotein-mediated multidrug resistance. *Annu Rev Biochem* 1989; 58:137–171.

Evans CD, Mirsky SEL, Danks MK and Cole SPC: Reduced levels of topoisomerase IIα and IIβ in a multidrug-resistant lung-cancer cell line. *Cancer Chemother Pharmacol* 1994; 34:242–248.

Fine RL, Patell J, Chabner BA: Phorbol esters induce multidrug resistance in human breast cancer cells. *Proc Natl Acad Sci USA* 1988; 85:582–586.

Froelich-Ammon SJ, Osheroff N: Topoisomerase poisons: Harnessing the dark side of enzyme mechanism. *J Biol Chem* 1995; 270:21429–21432.

Gabizon AA: Liposomal anthracyclines. *Hematol Oncol Clin North Am* 1994; 8:431–450.

Germann UA, Chambers TC, Ambudkar SV, et al: Effects of phosphorylation of P-glycoprotein on multidrug resistance. *J Bioenerg Biomembr* 1995; 27:53–61.

Gerson SL, Willson JK: O^6-alkylguanine-DNA alkyltransferase: A target for the modulation of drug resistance. *Hematol Oncol Clin North Am* 1995; 9:431–450.

Glisson BS, Ross WE: DNA Topoisomerase II: A primer on the enzyme and its unique role as a multidrug target in cancer chemotherapy. *Pharmacol Ther* 1987; 32:89–106.

Goldenberg GJ: Properties of L5178Y lymphoblasts highly resistant to nitrogen mustard. *Ann NY Acad Sci USA* 1969; 163:936–953.

Goldenberg GJ: The role of drug transport in resistance to nitrogen mustard and other alkylating agents in L5178Y lymphoblasts. *Cancer Res* 1975; 35:1687–1692.

Goldenberg GJ, Begleiter A: Alternations of drug transport. In: Fox BW, Fox M, eds. *Handbook of Experimental Pharmacology.* Berlin: Springer-Verlag; 1984: 72: 241–298.

Goldie JH, Coldman AJ: The genetic origin of drug resistance in neoplasms: Implications for systemic therapy. *Cancer Res* 1984; 44:3643–3653.

Goldie JH, Krystal G, Hartley D, et al: A methotrexate insensitive variant of folate reductase present in two lines of methotrexate-resistant L5178Y cells. *Eur J Cancer* 1980; 16:1539–1546.

Goldstein LJ, Galski H, Fojo A, et al: Expression of a multidrug resistance gene in human cancers. *J Natl Cancer Inst* 1989; 81:116–124.

Gonzalez MR, Wright KA, Twentyman PR: Modulation by acrolein and chloroacetaldehyde of multidrug resistance mediated by the multidrug resistance–associated protein (MRP). *Clin Cancer Res* 1996; 2:1321–1326.

Gorlick R, Goker E, Trippett T, et al: Intrinsic and acquired resistance to methotrexate in acute leukemia. *N Engl J Med* 1996; 335:1041–1048.

Gosland M, Lum B, Schimmelpfennig L, et al: Insights into mechanisms of cisplatin resistance and potential for its clinical reversal. *Pharmacotherapy* 1996; 16:16–39.

Gottesman MM, Pastan I: The multidrug transporter, a double-edged sword. *J Biol Chem* 1988; 263: 12163–12166.

Haisma HJ, Boven E, van Muijen M, et al: Analysis of a conjugate between anti-carcinoembryonic antigen monoclonal antibody and alkaline phosphatase for specific activation of the prodrug etoposide phosphate. *Cancer Immunol Immunother* 1992; 34:343–348.

Harker WG, Slade DL, Parr RL, et al: Alterations in the topoisomerase IIα gene, messenger RNA, and subcellular protein distribution as well as reduced expression of the DNA topoisomerase IIβ enzyme in a mitoxantrone-resistant HL-60 human leukemia cell line. *Cancer Res* 1995; 55:1707–1716.

Harris CC: Structure and function of the p53 tumor suppressor gene: Clues for rational cancer therapeutic strategies. *J Natl Cancer Inst* 1996; 88:1442–1455.

Heppner GH: Tumor heterogeneity. *Cancer Res* 1984; 44:2259–2265.

Hickman JA: Apoptosis and chemotherapy resistance. *Eur J Cancer* 1996; 32A:921–926.

Hill RP, Stanley JA: Pulmonary metastases of the Lewis lung tumor-cell kinetics and response to cyclophosphamide at different sizes. *Cancer Treat Rep* 1977; 61:29–36.

Hu Z-B, Minden MD, McCulloch EA: Direct evidence for the participation of bcl-2 in the regulation of retinoic acid of the Ara-C sensitivity of leukemic stem cells. *Leukemia* 1995; 9:1667–1673.

Iwamato Y, Fujita Y, Sugioka Y: VIGSR, a synthetic laminin peptide, inhibits the enhancement by cyclophosphamide of experimental lung metastasis of human fibrosarcoma cells. *Clin Exp Metastasis* 1992; 10:183–189.

Izquierdo MA, Scheffer GL, Flens MJ, et al: Major vault protein LRP-related multidrug resistance. *Eur J Cancer* 1996a; 32A:979–984.

Izquierdo MA, Shoemaker RH, Flens MJ, et al: Overlapping phenotypes of multi-drug resistance among panels of human cancer-cell lines. *Int J Cancer* 1996b; 65:230–237.

Izquierdo MA, van der Zee AGJ, Vermuken JB, et al: Drug resistant-associated marker Lrp for prediction of response to chemotherapy and prognoses in advanced ovarian carcinoma. *J Natl Cancer Inst* 1995; 87:1230–1237.

Kawai K, Kamatari N, Georges E, Ling V: Identification of a membrane glycoprotein overexpressed in murine lymphoma sublines resistant to cis-diamminedichloroplatinum (II). *J Biol Chem* 1990; 265:13137–13132.

Kelley SL, Basu A, Teicher BA, et al: Overexpression of metallothionein confers resistance to anticancer drugs. *Science* 1988; 241:1813–1815.

Kemp G, Rose P, Lurain J, et al: Amifostine pretreatment for protection against cyclophosphamide-induced and cisplatin-induced toxicities: Results of a randomized control trial in patients with advanced ovarian cancer. *J Clin Oncol* 1996; 14:2101–2112.

Kerbel RS, Rak J, Kobayashi H, et al: Multicellular resistance: A new paradigm to explain aspects of acquired drug resistance of solid tumors. *Cold Spring Harbor Symp Quant Biol* 1994; 59:661–672.

Kondo Y, Woo ES, Michalska AE, et al: Metallothionein null cells have increased sensitivity to anticancer drugs. *Cancer Res* 1995; 55:2021–2023.

Krajewski S, Blomqvist C, Franssila K, et al: Reduced expression of proapoptotic gene *BAX* is associated with poor response rates to combination chemotherapy and shorter survival in women with metastatic breast adenocarcinoma. *Cancer Res* 1995; 55:4471–4478.

Kruh GD, Gaughan KT, Goodwin A, Chan A: Expression pattern of MRP in human tissues and adult solid tumor cell lines. *J Natl Cancer Inst* 1995; 87:1256–1258.

Kuo MT, Bao JJ, Curley SA, et al: Frequent coordinated overexpression of the MRP/GS-X pump and gamma-glutamylcysteine synthetase genes in human colorectal cancer. *Cancer Res* 1996; 56:3642–3644.

Lautier D, Canitrot Y, Deeley RG, Cole SPC: Multidrug resistance mediated by the multidrug resistance protein (MRP) gene. *Biochem Pharmacol* 1996; 52:967–977.

Lavie E, Hirschberg DL, Schreiber G, et al: Monoclonal antibody L6-daunomycin conjugates constructed to release free drug at the lower pH of tumor tissue. *Cancer Immunol Immunother* 1991; 33:223–230.

Lin JT, Tong WP, Trippett TM, et al: Basis for natural resistance to methotrexate in human acute non-lymphocytic leukemia. *Leuk Res* 1991; 15:1191–1196.

Ling V: Genetic basis of drug resistance in mammalian cells. In: Bruchovsky N, Goldie JH, eds. *Drug and Hormone Resistance in Neoplasia.* Boca Raton, FL: CRC Press; 1982: 1–19.

Lock RB, Strabinskiene L: Dual modes of cell death induced by etoposide in human epithelial tumor cells allow Bcl-2 to inhibit apoptosis without affecting clonogenic survival. *Cancer Res* 1996; 56:4006–4012.

Loe DW, Deeley RG, Cole SPC: Biology of the multidrug resistance-associated protein, MPR. *Eur J Cancer* 1996; 32A:945–957.

Lowe SW, Bodis S, McClatchey A, et al: p53 status and the efficacy of cancer therapy in vivo. *Science* 1994; 266:807–810.

Luria SE, Delbruck M: Mutations of bacteria from virus sensitivity to virus resistance. *Genetics* 1943; 28:491–511.

McGinn CJ, Shewach DS, Lawrence TS: Radiosensitizing nucleosides. *J Natl Cancer Inst* 1996; 88:1193–1203.

McMillan TJ, Hart IR: Enhanced experimental metastatic capacity of a murine melanoma following pretreatment with anticancer drugs. *Clin Exp Metastasis* 1986; 4:285–292.

McPherson JP, Brown GA, Goldenberg GJ: Characterization of a DNA topoisomerase IIα gene rearrangement in Adriamycin-resistant P388 murine leukemia: Expression of a fusion mRNA transcript encoding topoisomerase IIα and the retinoic acid receptor α locus. *Cancer Res* 1993; 53:5885–5889.

Merlin J-L: Concepts of synergism and antagonism. *Anticancer Res* 1994; 14:2315–2320.

Miller TP, Grogan TM, Dalton WS, et al: P-Glycoprotein expression in malignant lymphoma and reversal of clinical drug resistance with chemotherapy plus high-dose verapamil. *J Natl Cancer Inst* 1991; 9:17–24.

Nicolson GL, Custead SE: Effects of chemotherapeutic drugs on platelet and metastatic tumor cell–endothelial cell interactions as a model for assessing vascular endothelial integrity. *Cancer Res* 1985; 45:331–336.

Nooter K, Westerman AM, Flens MJ, et al: Expression of the multidrug resistance-associate protein (MRP) gene in human cancers. *Clin Cancer Res* 1995; 1:1301–1310.

Norris MD, Bordow SB, Marshall GM, et al: Expression of the gene for multidrug-resistance-associated protein and outcome in patients with neuroblastoma. *N Engl J Med* 1996; 334:231–238.

Orr FW, Adamson IYR, Young L: Promotion of pulmonary metastasis in mice by bleomycin-induced endothelial injury. *Cancer Res* 1986; 46:891–897.

Park DS, Stefanis L, Yan CYI, et al: Ordering the cell death pathway. *J Biol Chem* 1996; 271:21898–21905.

Park JW, Hong K, Carter P, et al: Development of anti-p185[HER2] immunoliposomes for cancer therapy. *Proc Natl Acad Sci USA* 1995; 92:1327–1331.

Pastan I, Fitzgerald D: Recombinant toxins for cancer treatment. *Science* 1992; 254:1173–1177.

Peters GJ, van der Wilt CL, van Triest B, et al: Thymidilate synthase and drug resistance (review). *Eur J Cancer* 1995; 31A:1299–1305.

Phillips TL, Fu KK: Quantification of combined radiation therapy and chemotherapy effects on critical normal tissues. *Cancer* 1976; 37:1186–1200.

Puchalski RB, Fahl WE: Expression of recombinant glutathione *S*-transferase π, Ya or Yb confers resistance to alkylating agents. *Proc Natl Acad Sci USA* 1990; 87:2443–2447.

Raymond M, Gros P: Mammalian multidrug resistance gene: Correlation of exon organization with structural domains and duplication of an ancestral gene. *Proc Natl Acad Sci USA* 1989; 86:6488–6492.

Redmond SMS, Joncourt F, Buser K, et al: Assessment of P-glycoprotein, glutathione-based detoxifying enzymes and O^6-alkylguanine-DNA alkyltransferase as potential indicators of constitutive drug resistance in human colorectal tumors. *Cancer Res* 1991; 51:2092–2097.

Rhee MS, Wang Y, Nair GM, Galivan J: Acquisition of resistance to antifolates caused by enhanced gamma-glutamyl hydrolase activity. *Cancer Res* 1993; 53: (suppl):2227–2230.

Rice GC, Hoy C, Schimke RT: Transient hypoxia enhances the frequency of dihydrofolate reductase gene amplification in Chinese hamster ovary cells. *Proc Natl Acad Sci USA* 1986; 83:5978–5982.

Roca J, Wang JC: DNA transport by a type II DNA topoisomerase: Evidence in favor of a two-gate mechanism. *Cell* 1994; 77:609–616.

Sakakibara T, Chen FA, Kida H, et al: Doxorubicin encapsulated in sterically stabilized liposomes is superior to free drug or drug-containing conventional liposomes at suppressing growth and metastases of human lung tumor xenografts. *Cancer Res* 1996; 56:3743–3746.

Schabel FM Jr: Concepts for systemic treatment of micrometastases. *Cancer* 1975; 35:15–24.

Scheffer GL, Wijngaard PLJ, Flens MJ, et al: The drug resistance-related protein LRP is the human major vault protein. *Nature Med* 1995; 1:578–582.

Schilder RJ, Hall L, Monks A: Metallothionein gene expression and resistance to cisplatin in human ovarian cancer. *Int J Cancer* 1990; 45:416–422.

Schimke RT: Gene amplification, drug resistance, and cancer. *Cancer Res* 1984; 44:1735–1742.

Schlichenmeyer WJ, Rowinsky EK, Donehower RC, Kaufman SH: The current status of camptothecin analogues as antitumor agents. *J Natl Cancer Inst* 1993; 85: 271–291.

Shapiro AB, Ling V: Reconstitution of drug transport by purified P-glycoprotein. *J Biol Chem* 1995; 270: 16167–16175.

Shustik C, Dalton W, Gros P: P-glycoprotein-mediated multidrug resistance in tumor cells: Biochemistry, clinical relevance and modulation. *Mol Aspects Med* 1995; 16:1–78.

Smets L: Programmed cell death (apoptosis) and response to anti-cancer drugs. *Anticancer Drugs* 1994; 5:3–9.

Speyer JL, Green MD, Kramer E, et al: Protective effect of the bispiperazinedione ICRF-187 against doxorubicin-induced cardiac toxicity in women with advanced breast cancer. *N Engl J Med* 1988; 319:745–752.

St. Croix B, Rak JS, Kapitain S, et al: Reversal by hyaluronidase of adhesion-dependent multicellular drug resistance in mammary carcinoma cells. *J Natl Cancer Inst* 1996; 88:1285–1296.

Stark GR, Debatisse M, Giulotto E, Wahl GM: Recent progress in understanding mechanisms of mammalian DNA amplification. *Cell* 1989; 57:901–908.

Steel GG, Peckham MJ: Exploitable mechanisms in combined radiotherapy-chemotherapy: The concept of additivity. *Int J Radiat Oncol Biol Phys* 1979; 5:85–91.

Stelmack GL, Goldenberg GJ: Increased expression of cytosolic glutathione S-transferases in drug-resistant L5178Y murine lymphoblasts: Chemical selectivity and molecular mechanisms. *Cancer Res* 1993; 53: 3530–3535.

Tan KB, Dorman TE, Falls KM, et al: Topoisomerase IIα and topoisomerase IIβ genes: Characterization and mapping to human chromosomes 17 and 3, respectively. *Cancer Res* 1992; 52:231–234.

Tannock IF: Treatment of cancer with radiation and drugs. *J Clin Oncol* 1996; 14:3156–3174.

Teicher BA, Herman TS, Holden SA, et al: Tumor resistance to alkylating agents conferred by mechanisms operative only in vivo. *Science* 1990; 247:1457–1461.

Tew KD: Glutathione-associated enzymes in anticancer drug resistance. *Cancer Res* 1994; 54:4313–4320.

Thiebaut, F, Tsuruo T, Hamada H, et al: Cellular localization of the multidrug-resistance gene product P-glycoprotein in normal human tissues. *Proc Natl Acad Sci USA* 1987; 84:7735–7738.

Trail PA, Willner D, Lasch SJ, et al: Cure of xenografted human carcinomas by BR96-doxorubicin conjugates. *Science* 1993; 261:212–215.

Tsai-Pflugfelder M, Liu LF, Liu AA, et al: Cloning and sequencing of cDNA encoding human DNA topoisomerase II and localization of the gene to chromosome region 17q21-22. *Proc Natl Acad Sci USA* 1988; 85: 7177–7181.

Vanhoefer V, Cao S, Minderman H, et al: PAK-104P, a pyridine analogue, reverses paclitaxel and doxorubicin resistance in cell lines and nude mice bearing xenografts that overexpress the multidrug resistance protein. *Clin Cancer Res* 1996; 2:369–377.

Van Putten LM, Kram LKJ, Van Dierendenck HHC, et al: Enhancement by drugs of metastatic lung nodule formation after intravenous tumor cell injection. *Int J Cancer* 1975; 15:588–595.

Venturini M, Michelotti A, Del Mastro L, et al: Multicenter randomized controlled clinical trial to evaluate cardioprotection of dexrazoxane versus no cardioprotection in women receiving epirubicin chemotherapy for advanced breast cancer. *J Clin Oncol* 1996; 14: 3112–3120.

von der Maase H: Experimental studies on interactions of radiation and cancer chemotherapeutic drugs in normal tissues and a solid tumour. *Radiother Oncol* 1986; 7:47–68.

Wang C-Y, Mayo MW, Baldwin AS Jr: TNF- and cancer therapy-induced apoptosis: Potentiation by inhibition of NF-κB. *Science* 1996; 274:784–787.

Wawrzynczak EJ: Systemic immunotoxic therapy of cancer: advances and prospects. *Br J Cancer* 1991; 64:624–630.

Waxman DJ, Sundseth SS, Srivastava PK, Lapenson DP: Gene-specific oligonucleotide probes for α, μ, π and microsomal rat glutathione S-transferases: Analysis of liver transferase expression and its modulation by hepatic enzyme inducers and platinum and anticancer drugs. *Cancer Res* 1992; 52:5797–5802.

Williams FM, Flintoff WF: Isolation of a human cDNA that complements a mutant hamster cell defective in methotrexate uptake. *J Biol Chem* 1995; 270: 2987–2982.

Withers HR: From bedside to bench and back. In: Dewey WC, et al., eds. *Radiation Research: A Twentieth Century Perspective:* Vol II. *Congress Proceedings.* New York: Academic Press; 1991: 26–31.

Withers HR, Taylor JMF, Maciejewski B: The hazard of accelerated tumor clonogen repopulation during radiotherapy. *Acta Oncol* 1988; 27:131–146.

Wong SC, Proefke SA, Bhushan A, Matherly LH: Isolation of human cDNAs that restore methotrexate sensitivity and reduced folate carrier activity in methotrexate transport-defective Chinese hamster ovary cells. *J Biol Chem* 1995; 270:17468–17475.

Yang B, Eshlemen JR, Berger NA, et al: Wild-type p53 protein potentiates cytotoxicity of therapeutic agents in human colon cancer cells. *Clin Cancer Res* 1996; 2:1649–1657.

Yang WZ, Begleiter A, Johnston JB, et al: Role of glutathione and glutathione S-transferase in chlorambucil resistance. *Mol Pharmacol* 1992; 41:625–630.

Yin XM, Oltvai ZN, Veis-Novack DJ, et al: Bcl-2 gene family and the regulation of programmed cell death. *Cold Spring Harbor Symp Quant Biol* 1994; 59:387–394.

Ying DX, Schimke RT: BCL-2 expression delays drug-induced apoptosis but does not increase clonogenic survival after drug treatment in HeLa cells. *Cancer Res* 1995; 55:4922–4928.

Zaman GJR, Lankelma J, van Tellingen O, et al: Role of glutathione in the export of compounds from cells by the multidrug-resistance-associated protein. *Proc Natl Acad Sci USA* 1995; 92:7690–7694.

Zamble DB, Mu D, Reardon JT, et al: Repair of cisplatin-DNA adducts by the mammalian excision nuclease. *Biochemistry* 1996; 35:10004–10013.

Zanke BW, Boudreau K, Rubie E, et al: The stress-activated protein kinase (SAPK/JNK) pathway mediates cell death following cis-platinum or heat-induced injury. *Curr Biol* 1996; 6:606–613.

18

Biological Therapy of Cancer

Neil L. Berinstein

18.1. INTRODUCTION
    18.1.1 Tumor-Rejection Antigens
    18.1.2 Molecular and Cellular Requirements
        for Immune Activation

18.2. GENE THERAPY
    18.2.1 Approaches to Gene Therapy
    18.2.2 Viral Methods for Gene Transfer
    18.2.3 Physical Methods for Gene Transfer
    18.2.4 Clinical Studies of Gene Therapy

18.3. PASSIVE IMMUNOTHERAPY
    18.3.1 Cytokines

18.3.2 Adoptive Cellular Therapy
18.3.3 Production of Monoclonal Antibodies
18.3.4 Immunotherapy with Monoclonal Antibodies

18.4. ACTIVE IMMUNOTHERAPY
    18.4.1 Protein Immunogens
    18.4.2 DNA Immunogens
    18.4.3 Immunization with Tumor Cells
    18.4.4 Genetically Modified Tumor Cells
    18.4.5 Antigen-Pulsed Dendritic Cells

18.5. SUMMARY

REFERENCES

18.1 INTRODUCTION

Recent advances in understanding of both the genetic alterations that contribute to the pathogenesis of cancers and of the immune response to cancer have led to the development of biologically based approaches to anticancer treatment. These new strategies exploit expanding insights into the nature of tumor antigens, the molecular and cellular requirements for immune activation, the role of cytokines in amplifying the immune response, and the evolution of recombinant DNA approaches to introduce genetic material into eukaryotic cells.

18.1.1 Tumor-Rejection Antigens

The existence of tumor antigens that can be recognized by the immune system is critical for the generation of an immune response against the tumor. Such antigens may either be expressed on the cell surface, where they are available for recognition by antibodies, or they may be intracellular antigens, which can be presented by molecules of the major histocompatibility complex (MHC) to T cells (see

Chap. 11, Sec. 11.3.2). These antigens may be tumor specific, such as unique products of mutated or activated oncogenes, or they may be tumor associated antigens such as oncofetal or differentiation proteins, which are not normally expressed in normal tissues of the adult.

The existence of tumor rejection antigens (TRAs) was suggested about 40 years ago by the demonstration that mice injected with syngeneic tumor cells (i.e., those derived from the same inbred strain of mice) induced by the carcinogen methylcholanthrene developed a cellular immune response that could protect against subsequent challenge with the same tumor cells but not with other tumor cells. Numerous experiments have since demonstrated TRAs expressed by a variety of murine tumors induced by chemicals, ultraviolet (UV) radiation, and several oncogenic viruses. These TRAs can stimulate cytotoxic T-lymphocytes (CTLs) which express CD8 on their cell surface. In contrast to the TRAs of chemically-induced tumors, which are usually unique, the TRAs of tumors induced by viruses such as polyomavirus were often found to be cross-reactive.

More recently, the protein products of a number of altered oncogenes and tumor suppressor genes have been shown to be the targets of CTLs (Pardoll, 1994). Such oncogene products include mutated p53, *Ras* proteins, and the fusion product of the *bcr/abl* translocation in chronic myelogenous leukemia (Table 18.1). These alterations are usually obligatory events in the pathogenesis of the cancer and hence are retained in the tumor cells; they are not found in most normal tissues and hence may be considered tumor-specific. These observations emphasize that even intracellular proteins may be processed, presented by class I major histocompatibility complex (MHC) molecules on the cell surface, and serve as targets for T cell recognition (see Chap. 11, Sec. 11.3.2).

Tumor-specific CTLs have been a powerful tool for the identification of TRAs. For example, the methylcholanthrene-induced P815 mastocytoma cell line was mutagenized to obtain variant subclones that, unlike the parental cell clone, were unable to form tumors in syngeneic mice and were recognized by specific CTLs (Boon et al., 1980, 1994). These variants, called tum-, were used to prepare a library of total genomic DNA cloned into cosmid expression vectors, which was introduced into the parental clone (Chap. 3, Sec. 3.3.3). Parental clones activating CTLs that recognized the tum- variant were isolated, the cosmids recovered, and the re-

sponsible genes sequenced. A single point mutation in a protein known as P91A was found to be responsible for the ability of the tum- variants to activate the CTL clone, thus demonstrating the power of this approach to isolate TRAs. Subsequently, Boon and others have employed similar approaches to isolate a number of TRAs from human tumors, including the MAGE series of antigens and tyrosinase from human melanoma (Boon et al, 1994). These antigens all correspond to nonmutated nononcogenic proteins that either are developmental antigens re-expressed as a result of transformation (e.g., MAGE) or differentiation antigens that are lineage specific (e.g., tyrosinase) (Table 18.1).

An alternative method for detection and isolation of TRAs is to acid-elute peptides from MHC molecules and then separate them into fractions by reverse phase high performance liquid chromatography (Pardoll, 1994). Tumor-specific CTLs are used subsequently to detect bioactive fractions by adding the protein fractions to antigen-processing mutant cells that express MHC class I molecules alone. With this approach, a glycoprotein, gp100, was identified as a human melanoma TRA. Antimelanoma CTLs from four different patients recognized gp100, thus illustrating the potential of this approach to identify and isolate common shared antigens. The gp100 antigen is also expressed on normal melanocytes but not on other normal tissues.

Table 18.1. Human Tumor-Rejection Antigens

Tumor Rejection Antigen	Cancer	Normal Tissue Expression	Genetic Alteration	Immune system Recognition
Bcr/Abl	Chronic myelogenous leukemia	Tumor-specific	Translocation	T cells
Mutated p53	Many cancers	Tumor-specific	Mutation	T cells
Immunoglobulin idiotype	B cell lymphoma	Tumor-specific	None	Antibodies and T cells
Mutated Ras	Adeno-carcinomas	Tumor-specific	Mutation	T cells
MAGE 1	Melanoma	Testis	None	T cells
MAGE 3	Melanoma	Testis	None	T cells
MART 1	Melanoma	Melanocytes	None	T cells
Tyrosinase	Melanoma	Melanocytes	None	T cells
Gp100	Melanoma	Melanocytes	None	T cells
MUC 1	Pancreas, breast	Epithelium	None	T cells

18.1.2 Molecular and Cellular Requirements for Immune Activation

The existence of TRAs has fundamental importance for therapeutic strategies to augment the immune response against tumors. As reviewed in Chap. 11, Sec. 11.2.2 the first step in lymphocyte activation is recognition of antigen. Unfortunately, the failure of CTLs to eradicate the cancers toward which they are sensitized indicates that tolerance or anergy to these TRAs has developed, just as tolerance/anergy may develop to other self antigens. Consequently, many biological approaches to cancer therapy are directed at strategies to augment T-cell activation by TRAs and to reverse this tolerance. Such strategies must take into account the following factors which were discussed in detail in Chap. 11, Sec. 11.3: (1) the existence and nature of TRAs; (2) the properties of CTLs that can recognize these antigens; (3) the complexity of T-cell activation, which requires accessory signals in addition to those generated through the T-cell receptor; and (4) the pattern of lymphokine release, which further amplifies the immune response (Fig. 18.1).

18.2. GENE THERAPY

18.2.1 Approaches to Gene Therapy

Numerous strategies for gene therapy have been investigated. These include (1) reversing the genetic alteration associated with the cancer cell by gene transfer of oncogene antisense or wild-type tumor suppressor genes such as *p53*, (2) enhancing the chemosensitivity of cancer cells by the transfer of genes that cause death of the cell, (3) enhancing the activity of immune effector cells by the transfer of genes encoding cytokines such as interferon or interleukin 2 (IL-2), (4) increasing the drug resistance of hemopoietic stem cells by transfer of genes that encode drug resistance (see Chap. 17, Sec. 17.2), and (5) enhancing the immunogenicity of the cancer cell itself by the transfer of genes encoding cytokines or costimulatory molecules (Fig. 18.2).

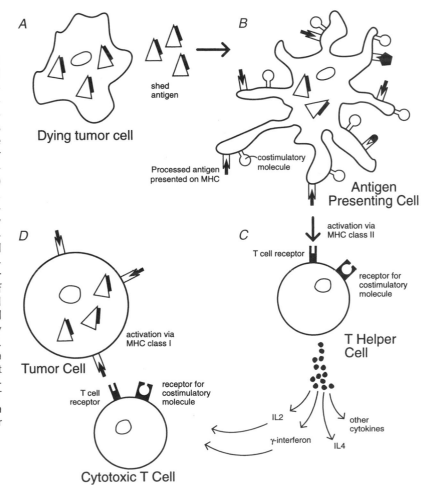

Figure 18.1. Features of the normal immune response that have guided biological antitumor strategies. Activation of T cells is central to the generation of an effective immune response. Four important features of this activation that have influenced the development of biological anticancer approaches are as follows: *A.* intracellular tumor rejection antigens (TRAs) may be shed from dying tumor cells. *B.* TRAs may be presented by molecules of the major histocompatibility complex (MHC) on antigen-presenting cells such as dendritic cells and provide the first signal for T-cell activation and an immunologic antitumor response. *C.* Effective activation of specific T cells requires both a signal through the T-cell receptor and through receptors for costimulatory molecules such as B7-1 or B7-2. *D.* Activation of T-helper cells results in the secretion of various cytokines that help activate other immunologic effector cells, including cytotoxic T cells, which do not require interaction through their costimulating receptor in order to mediate cell kill.

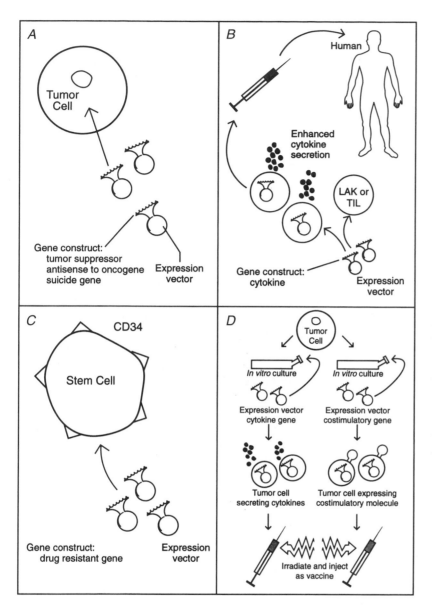

Figure 18.2. Approaches to gene therapy for cancer: *A.* Expression vectors containing gene constructs for tumor suppressor genes, antisense to oncogenes, or suicide genes can be introduced in vivo into tumor cells. *B.* Expression vectors containing genes for various cytokines can be introduced into tumor-infiltrating lymphocytes (TIL) or lymphokine-activated killer (LAK) cells that have been expanded in vitro. *C.* Expression vectors containing genes for drug-resistance proteins can be introduced into stem cells that have been cultured in vitro. *D.* Expression vectors containing genes for cytokines or costimulatory molecules can be introduced either in vitro or in vivo into tumor cells. In vitro gene-modified tumor cells (shown in figure) are irradiated and then injected with an immune adjuvant back into the patient.

Promising results in animal models have been obtained using several of these strategies, and a number of clinical trials of gene therapy are evaluating the safety and efficacy of these approaches in patients with cancer (see Sec. 18.2.4).

Gene transfer may be performed in vitro (e.g., enhancing immune effector cells with cytokine genes or increasing drug resistance of hemopoietic stem cells) or in vivo (e.g. reversing the genetic alteration of cancer cells or transfer of suicide genes). Because current gene transfer technologies do not permit transfer of the therapeutic gene to every cancer cell, strategies for in vivo gene therapy generally aim to augment other therapies.

Genetic material can be introduced into cells by physical methods or by infection with viruses. Because physical methods are characterized by a 100- to 1000-fold lower efficiency of gene transfer and because some cell types are fragile or resistant to these methods, most investigators have focused on viral approaches for gene transfer, referred to as *transduction* (for review, see Miller, 1992; Crystal, 1995).

18.2.2 Viral Methods for Gene Transfer

Retroviruses: Retroviruses contain a diploid RNA genome that is converted into a DNA intermediate by the retrovirally encoded enzyme reverse transcriptase upon entry into the cytoplasm of a cell. The DNA is then transported to the nucleus, where it integrates randomly into the genome. The viral genetic material contains information for the three protein regions of the virus: *gag* (structural proteins), *pol* (RNA-dependent DNA polymerase–reverse transcriptase), and *env* (surface or envelope proteins). The linear double-stranded viral DNA is flanked by long terminal repeats (LTR) and has an RNA polymerase II promoter in the 5'LTR. In addition, the DNA contains motifs to allow efficient encapsidation and DNA priming. Once the DNA has integrated into the cellular genome, it is transcribed, processed, and translated into proteins. These proteins subsequently assemble into virions, which encapsidate two copies of viral RNA, leave the cell, and infect other cells to complete the viral life cycle (see Chap. 5, Sec. 5.3.1).

The use of retroviruses for gene transfer requires a two-component approach. The first involves the replacement of the genetic material encoding the gag, pol, and env proteins with the DNA to be transferred. This DNA is expressed under the control of the promoter elements in the 5'LTR. Strategies have been developed to insert more than one gene into this region and can include alternative splicing of LTR-initiated transcripts, the use of multiple internal promoters, or the use of specific regions of DNA that can initiate internal translation of the tandemly linked mRNA (Hawley et al., 1994). The second component involves the introduction of this DNA into a retroviral packaging cell line to produce virus able to infect the appropriate host species. This cell line contains a replication-defective helper retrovirus that will provide the gag, pol, and env proteins and an encapsidation signal for efficient viral packaging. Several generations of such packaging lines/helper viruses have been developed to reduce the likelihood of replication-competent retroviruses being generated through random recombination events between the genetically modified retrovirus and the helper virus. Most recently the envelope proteins of such helper viruses have been modified to alter the host range of infectivity of the virus and to target retroviruses specifically to a cell of interest for the purposes of gene therapy (Kasahara et al., 1995; Miller and Vile, 1995).

Although retroviruses can infect cells and transfer the gene of interest at a relatively high efficiency (usually greater than 10 percent), there are some disadvantages associated with their use (Table 18.2). First retroviruses transfer the gene of interest permanently into the genome of the target cell, which could result in chronic overexpression of the inserted gene or to insertional mutagenesis. In addition, retroviruses can infect proliferating cells only. This may decrease their usefulness for gene transfer into stem cells, which are largely noncycling. Retroviruses can only accommodate less than 9 kb of foreign genetic information. Finally, retroviruses are associated with numerous technical problems related to recombination, rearrangement, and low viral titers.

Adenoviral Vectors: Adenoviruses are DNA viruses with a 36-kb genome that encode four early proteins (E1 to E4) and five late proteins (L1 to L5). Because replication is controlled by E1, it is usually deleted in adenoviral vectors used for gene therapy and replaced by the gene to be transferred. The resultant recombinant adenovirus is replication-incompetent. This recombinant adenoviral DNA is then transferred into a complementing cell line containing E1 sequences in its genome (but lacking other sequences required for replication) to generate viral particles that are infectious but replication-defective.

Adenoviruses enter a cell by means of two receptors that interact with the adenovirus fiber and penton proteins. After binding, the virus is internalized into a cytoplasmic endosome; it then enters the cytoplasm and subsequently the nucleus, where its double-stranded DNA is transcribed episomally without integrating into the cell's genome.

Adenoviruses have certain advantages over retroviruses for gene therapy (Table 18.2). They can be produced in high titer ($>10^{13}$ viral particles/per milliliter) and can transfer genes efficiently into both replicating and nonreplicating cells. As the transferred genetic material exists episomally, the risks of permanently altering the genetic material of the cell and of insertional mutagenesis are avoided. A disadvantage of adenoviral vectors is that the viral proteins are immunogenic and can induce nonspecific inflammation and specific cellular responses to viral proteins. Only approximately 7 kb of foreign DNA can be accommodated. Also, episomes tend to be lost from infected cells within 2 to 4 weeks, so that repeated administration may be necessary. Immune responses may, however, limit this possibility.

Adeno-Associated Viruses Adeno-associated viruses (AAV) are parvoviruses that are not pathogenic in humans. Unlike adenoviruses, AAV may integrate into the host genome and do so at preferred locations—in particular, at one site on chromosome 19. Thus, long term expression is more stable than with

Table 18.2. Advantages and Disadvatages of Vectors for Gene Therapy

	Advantages	Disadvantages
Retroviruses	Moderate gene transfer efficiency Long-term expression	Recombination Low titer Insertional mutagenesis Infect replicating cells only Accomodate less than 9 kb of foreign DNA
Adenoviruses	High gene-transfer efficiency Infect replicating and non-replicating cells High titer	Transient expression Immunogenic Accomodate less than 7 kb of foreign DNA
Adeno-associated viruses	High gene-transfer efficiency Infect replicating and non-replicating cells	Insertional mutagensis Often low titer Contamination with helper virus Long-term expression
Plasmid liposomes	Nonreplicating	Low gene-transfer efficiency
DNA complexes or naked DNA	Accomodate large therapeutic genes	No specific target-cell population

adenoviruses. Recombinant AAV vectors used for gene transfer contain a 145-bp terminal repeat sequence, and a polyadenylation site; they have had most of the viral genome deleted and replaced with DNA encoding the therapeutic gene. Because few viral proteins are expressed, these viruses induce less of an immune response than adenoviruses. Like adenoviruses, AAV vectors do not require cell replication for integration, but high AAV titers are often difficult to obtain. Also, because the production of infectious AAV requires the use of an adenoviral helper virus, contamination of the AAV with adenovirus is a concern.

Other Viral Vectors: A number of other viruses have been studied as vectors for introducing genes into cells. Several different members of the herpesvirus family are of interest because they infect specific cell types. Herpes simplex virus is specific for neurons, while human herpes virus 7 infects T lymphocytes. Recombinant vaccinia and poxviruses can accommodate large foreign therapeutic genes, do not induce significant immune response against viral proteins, and do not integrate into the genome (Perkus et al., 1995). Expression is thus transient

and decreases over weeks. These viral vectors have proven to be safe in initial phase I and II clinical studies.

18.2.3 Physical Methods for Gene Transfer

DNA on a plasmid can be introduced into cells by a number of physical strategies. It can be injected directly into smooth muscle or a "gene gun" can be used to bombard skin or subcutaneous tissue with microparticles coated with DNA (see Sec. 18.4.2).

Another promising approach involves encapsulation of plasmid DNA containing the therapeutic gene into lipid complexes called *liposomes* (Farhood et al., 1994). These complexes fuse with the plasma membrane, their contents enter the cell, and the plasmid DNA is expressed extrachromosomally.

There are many potential advantages of using physical methods for gene transfer; (1) expression cassettes containing the therapeutic foreign DNA can be of almost any size; (2) liposomes and naked plasmid DNA are noninfectious and cannot replicate, and (3) liposomes do not express foreign proteins and hence will not elicit an inflammatory response. The disadvantages of plasmid-liposome vectors are primarily related to their inefficiency of gene transfer and to inability to target specifically.

18.2.4 Clinical Studies of Gene Therapy

At present there are over a hundred clinical studies worldwide evaluating gene therapy approaches for cancer (for review, see Roth and Cristiano, 1997). These are all either phase I clinical studies evaluating safety and toxicity issues or early phase II studies of efficacy. Both in vitro and in vivo approaches are being studied, and most studies have used retroviral vectors. Expression of transferred genes has been documented with viral and nonviral vectors. For the most part, unexpected serious toxicities have not occurred, and retroviruses have been shown to be safe. Some investigators have documented tumor regression, but these results must be interpreted cautiously. Advances in vector technology and in our understanding of tumor biology and immunology make this a promising area for cancer therapeutics.

Many strategies of gene therapy seek to induce or augment an immune rejection response against tumor cells; these methods are described below, in Secs. 18.3 and 18.4. Strategies for gene therapy that do not depend on immunologic mechanisms and will be or are being tested clinically include the following:

1. *Tumor Suppressor/Antisense:* In this approach, expression vectors containing tumor suppressor genes such as *p53* or antisense constructs for oncogenes such as *bcr-abl* (in chronic myelogenous leukemia), c-*myb* (in acute and chronic myelogeneous leukemia), or c-*fos* (in breast cancer) are introduced in vivo. Antisense constructs have been delivered as retroviruses, adenoviruses, or oligonucleotides. Recently, antisense oligonucleotides to the *bcl*-2 proto-oncogene were administered subcutaneously to nine patients with non-Hodgkin's lymphoma. Objective improvement in symptoms, in biochemical and radiologic measurements of disease, as well as in reduction in the expression of the bcl-2 protein in lymphoma cells were documented (Webb et al., 1997).
2. *Drug Sensitivity:* A number of clinical trials are testing the efficacy of gene transfer of the herpes simplex virus thymidine kinase (HSV-TK) gene in sensitizing various cancer cells to the drug gancyclovir. Gancyclovir, which is nontoxic in eukaryotic cells, is metabolized to the cytotoxic gancyclovir triphosphate in cells expressing HSV-TK. In animal models, a "bystander" effect occurs where neighboring cells that have not been trans-

duced are also lysed. This may be mediated by transfer of toxic metabolites through gap junctions or phagocytosis by live tumor cells. The clinical trials for the most part involve in vivo gene transfer, usually by retroviruses, and are directed at glioblastomas, ovarian cancers, and melanomas.
3. *Drug Resistance:* These studies have involved transferring genes that mediate drug resistance, such as multidrug resistance-1 (*mdr-1*), into hemopoietic stem cells ex vivo to enhance bone marrow protection during chemotherapy. Most of these studies use retroviruses to mediate gene transfer. It remains to be determined whether the degree of bone marrow protection will be sufficient to allow high enough increases in the intensity of chemotherapy to enhance therapeutic outcome.

18.3. PASSIVE IMMUNOTHERAPY

The biological treatment of cancer includes both active and passive immunotherapy. Passive immunotherapy includes the use of antitumor reagents that have been generated in vitro, such as monoclonal antibodies (MAbs) or cytokines or the use of expanded effector cells such as lymphokine-activated killer (LAK) cells or tumor-infiltrating lymphocytes (TILs) in adoptive cellular therapy.

18.3.1 Cytokines

Many cytokines have been evaluated in animal models and clinical trials for their antitumor activity. These molecules have been chosen because they are known to regulate various aspects of the immune response and hence are also referred to as *biological response modifiers*. Most of these molecules are produced by recombinant genetic techniques and hence are available in large quantities as highly purified products. Several of these cytokines mediate antitumor activity against specific types of cancer (for review, see Takaku, 1994).

The *interferons* (IFN) have been studied most extensively. Interferons inhibit cell proliferation, increase gene expression, and augment the proliferation and cytotoxicity of cytotoxic T cells (CTL) and natural killer (NK) cells (see Chap. 11, Sec. 11.3.7). IFN-α induces responses in over 90 percent of patients with hairy cell leukemia, although most patients will relapse within 2 years. IFN-α may also prolong remissions obtained with chemotherapy in patients with chronic myelogeneous leukemia, and it has some antitumor activity against myeloma, low-grade non-Hodgkin's lymphoma, metastatic renal carcinoma, and Kaposi's sarcoma related to acquired immunodeficiency syndrome (AIDS).

Interleukin 2 (IL-2) stimulates the proliferation of T lymphocytes, NK cells, LAK cells, and TILs. IL-2 has been used alone or with LAK cells or TILs (see Sec. 18.3.2). It has been approved by the U.S. Food and Drug Administration (FDA) for the treatment of renal cell carcinoma and malignant melanoma based on an approximate 20 percent partial response rate for these cancers. A major limiting feature of IL-2 treatment is toxicity, and particularly the "capillary-leak syndrome" which results in hypotension, weight gain, and peripheral and pulmonary edema.

Interleukin 4 (IL-4) enhances proliferation of B and T lymphocytes, facilitates immunoglobulin class switching to IgG and IgE from IgM, and has multiple other pleiotrophic effects on the immune system (Puri and Siegel, 1993). IL-4 along with IL-2 can increase the expansion of TILs. Infusion of IL-4 has been ineffective against solid tumors but has induced antitumor responses in several hematologic malignancies.

Tumor necrosis factor (TNF) is produced by macrophages and is available by recombinant technologies. TNF is cytostatic or cytolytic for many human tumor cells in culture and has been shown to induce necrosis of transplanted tumors (including human xenografts) in mice. Unfortunately, TNF has proven to be toxic with only minimal activity in the clinic.

Interleukin 12 (IL-12) has been shown to mediate promising antitumor activity in animal models (for review, see Banks et al., 1995). This cytokine—secreted primarily by macrophages, monocytes, and B lymphocytes—is a heterodimer consisting of 35- and 40-kDa subunits; it can be synthesized by recombinant DNA technologies. IL-12 is an essential factor for the generation of helper T (T_h1) cells, which express CD4 (see Chap. 11, Sec. 11.3.3). It causes the proliferation of activated T lymphocytes and NK cells. It synergizes with the costimulatory molecule B7-1 in the activation of T-cell proliferation and cytokine secretion and produces dramatic increases in IFN-γ from T and NK cells. In a number of animal models, IL-12 injected systemically or locally into tumors or secreted locally by fibroblasts results in marked antitumor activity. Both T and NK cells may play important roles in this antitumor activity.

18.3.2 Adoptive Cellular Therapy

The immune rejection of cancers in animal models can be mediated by the *adoptive transfer* of sensitized lymphocytes. Studies of adoptive cellular therapy in murine models have established that (1) efficacy is dependent on the number of immune cells infused, (2) both fresh and cultured immune lymphocytes can mediate the effect, and (3) concomitant administration of IL-2 can enhance the in vivo activity of adoptive cellular therapy (for review, see Ettinghausen and Rosenberg, 1995).

Grimm et al. (1982) performed experiments in which they cultured lymphocytes in IL-2 to generate *lymphokine-activated killer* (LAK) cells. These cells did not express B- or T-cell markers and were able to lyse nonspecifically autologous and allogeneic tumor cells but not normal untransformed cells. In vivo administration of LAK cells with IL-2 reduced micrometastatic tumor burden in a murine model of pulmonary metastases. The above results prompted the assessment of adoptive immunotherapy with LAK cells and IL-2 in patients with cancer. Responses have been observed in patients with renal cell cancer or melanoma, and the overall results of studies involving almost 400 highly selected patients show a response rate of about 15 to 20 percent in patients with these tumors. Although the infusions of LAK cells were well tolerated, the systemic administration of high doses of IL-2 produced major toxicity, predominantly related to the development of a capillary leak syndrome. Subsequent studies comparing treatment with IL-2 alone to that with IL-2 and LAK cells together suggested that IL-2 treatment alone produces response rates equivalent to those seen with combined treatment (Rosenberg et al., 1993).

Lymphocytes from tumors can be isolated by culturing dissociated tumor biopsies in IL-2. These *tumor-infiltrating lymphocytes* (TILs) are CD3- and CD8-positive and lyse specifically cells in the tumor from which they are derived in an MHC-restricted fashion. They do not lyse tumors from other patients. Studies in mice showed that TILs were approximately 50 to 100 times more effective than LAK cells in treating pulmonary micrometastases, and the combination of cyclophosphamide, TILs, and IL-2 could effectively treat macroscopic pulmonary metastases. Based on these results, TILs and IL-2 have been evaluated in patients with metastases from various cancers. The treatment may cause tumor regression, especially in patients with melanoma or renal cancer, and current studies are comparing such treatment to that with IL-2 alone.

Some of the earliest gene therapy studies in humans involved transfer of either marker genes, such as that conferring neomycin drug resistance (*neo*), or cDNAs encoding cytokines, such as tumour necrosis factor (TNF), into TILs (Hwu and Rosen-berg, 1994). The objectives were to mark TIL survival and trafficking in the patient or to enhance cytolytic capabilities of TILs. The *neo* gene was introduced into expanded TILs using the Moloney MuLV–derived retroviral vector N2 and the LNL6 helper packaging retrovirus and infused into patients with metastatic melanoma (Rosenberg et al., 1990). This study demonstrated that (1) 1 to 10 percent of cells were transduced with this vector; (2) circulating mononuclear cells containing the *neo* gene were consistently present for 20 days postinfusion and could be found in the peripheral blood about 2 months postinfusion in some patients, and (3) modified TILs could be found in skin lesions biopsied 2 months postinfusion. Therapeutic studies are in progress.

18.3.3 Production of Monoclonal Antibodies

Kohler et al. (1977) showed that it was possible to stimulate hybridization between malignant plasma cells maintained in continuous culture and immune lymphoid cells. Hybrid cells that grew in culture and produced antibodies with the single defined specificity of the immune lymphoid cell could then be selected by cloning. The basic technique for production of such monoclonal antibodies (MAbs) is shown in Fig. 18.3. Spleen cells from an animal that has been immunized with foreign antigens are placed in culture with a continuously growing myeloma cell line in the presence of polyethylene glycol to stimulate cell fusion. The myeloma line used in the experiments is a mutant that does not secrete immunoglobulin and has been selected for an enzyme deficiency that prevents its growth in medium containing hypoxanthine, aminopterin, and thymidine (HAT medium). The normal spleen cells cannot grow in culture; thus only hybrid cells, formed by fusion, will grow in HAT medium, since the missing enzyme is provided by the fused lymphoid spleen cell.

After selection in HAT medium, hybrid cells are cloned by placing individual cells into single wells of a multiwell tissue-culture plate. Antibodies secreted by each clone of hybrid cells (known as a *hybridoma*) can then be tested for specificity—for example, by reactivity to tumor cells but not to normal cells. Large quantities of MAbs may be obtained from supernatants of "hybridoma" cell cultures or by growing the hybridoma as an ascites tumor in mice. Hybrid cells can also be frozen and stored.

MAbs that recognize antigenic determinants on cells of human tumors of a given histologic type

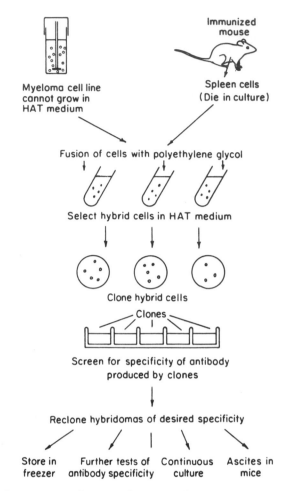

Figure 18.3. Schematic diagram indicating major steps in the production of monoclonal antibodies.

(e.g., melanoma-associated antigens) are now available for many types of tumors. Most of these antibodies show some cross-reactivity with the cells of a few normal tissues. Many of these MAbs probably recognize antigens that are related to cell differentiation, such as carcinoembryonic antigen (CEA), which is expressed at high frequency on cells from tumors of the colon.

Most MAbs have been made using rodent cell lines. This is a problem when they are to be used for treatment of human cancer, because they are recognized as foreign proteins and elicit an immune response that leads to their rapid clearance and loss of activity or to anaphylactic reactions. This response is due to human antimouse antibodies (HAMA) and is referred to as the *HAMA response.* The strength of such a reaction might be decreased or even eliminated by using MAbs of human origin, and if a patient's own lymphoid cells were used as a fusion partner, syngeneic MAbs could be obtained.

Attempts to obtain stable hybridoma cultures by fusion of human lymphoid and mouse myeloma cells have been frustrated by selective loss of human chromosomes from the hybrid cells, with consequent failure to continue secretion of antibody. Problems have also been encountered in attempts to fuse human lymphoid cells with human myeloma cell lines. This is primarily because there are few established human myeloma cell lines. In addition, the human myeloma cell lines often continue to secrete antibody or heavy or light immunoglobulin chains.

Strategies which utilize molecular genetic techniques have been developed to produce human MAbs (Figure 18.4). The first such approach involved generation of *chimeric antibodies* that have a constant region of human origin and a variable region of murine origin (Morrison et al., 1984). These can be generated by molecular cloning of the hybridoma's heavy- and light-chain immunoglobulin genes and linking the variable region components to human heavy- and light-chain constant regions. Alternatively, utilizing the process of homologous recombination, the human heavy- and light-chain constant regions can be introduced into the hybridoma cells to replace the murine constant region. Another approach, termed *CDR engraftment*, involves cloning only the variable regions of the murine heavy and light chains that bind to antigen (the CDR 1, 2, and 3 regions) and replacing the corresponding human regions with these (Verhoeyen et al., 1988). A third strategy for producing human MAbs involves *phage display* (McCafferty et al., 1990). This approach is based upon the random recombi-

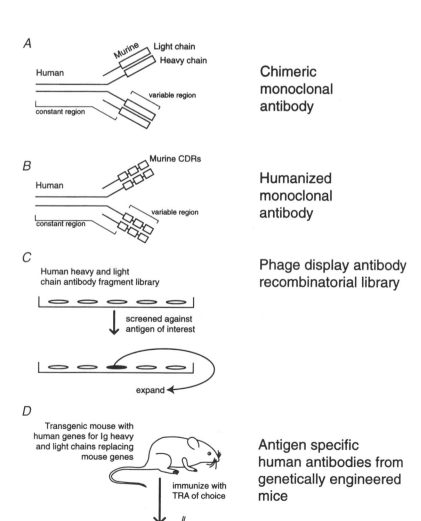

Chimeric monoclonal antibody

Humanized monoclonal antibody

Phage display antibody recombinatorial library

Antigen specific human antibodies from genetically engineered mice

Figure 18.4. Strategies to generate human monoclonal antibodies. *A.* Chimeric antibodies can be generated by recombinant genetic techniques where the gene fragments for the murine heavy- and light-chain immunoglobulin constant regions are replaced by the equivalent human gene fragments. *B.* Humanized monoclonal antibodies can be generated by using recombinant genetic techniques to replace the regions for the human heavy- and light-chain CDR regions (which bind to antigen) with the corresponding murine CDR regions specific for a particular monoclonal antibody. *C.* Recombinatorial phage display libraries for human heavy- and light-chain immunoglobulin proteins can be generated and screened for reactivity to a particular antigen. *D.* Transgenic mice generated by deleting the endogenous heavy- and light-chain genes, and by introducing genomic material for human immunoglobulin heavy- and light-chain genes can be immunized to a particular antigen. Hybridomas can be generated by standard techniques and screened for reactivity to the antigen used for immunization.

nation of independently cloned heavy- and light-chain human immunoglobulin genes, which are expressed in λ or filamentous phage systems.

Most recently, mice that contain large regions of unrearranged human immunoglobulin genes have been generated by transgenic technology. In addition, the endogenous murine heavy- and light-chain immunoglobulin loci were disrupted. Immunization and subsequent hybridoma generation produce hybridomas secreting human immunoglobulin genes of the desired specificity (for review see Morrison, 1994).

18.3.4 Immunotherapy with Monoclonal Antibodies

Monoclonal antibodies (MAbs) against tumor antigens can bind to their specific targets and mediate lysis of tumor cells either through complement-mediated lysis or antibody-dependent cellular cytotoxicity (ADCC). In ADCC, Fc receptor–bearing effector cells such as NK cells, macrophages, or polymorphonuclear cells bind to the Fc part of the targeting MAb and lyse the tumor cell to which the antibody is bound. MAbs may also elicit antitumor activity by blocking a receptor for a growth factor that the cell depends upon for proliferation or by inducing apoptosis through direct intracellular signaling (Fig. 18.5).

MAbs recognizing surface determinants expressed on human cancer cells have been tested for their therapeutic value in patients (Matthews et al., 1992; Dillman, 1994). Although objective and occasionally even complete responses have been documented, the overall response rates and duration of responses have been disappointing. A number of factors limit the therapeutic effectiveness of MAbs in patients. These include the following (See Table 18.3).

Tumor Cell Heterogeneity: The effectiveness of MAb immunotherapy depends on the antigenic target being present in relatively high levels on all tumor cells. Some antigenic targets are subject to normal physiologic alterations in their identity or levels of expression. In addition, ongoing mutagenesis may alter antigenic targets, so that antigenic targets are expressed on only a subpopulation of tumor cells. For example, the process of somatic hypermutation that occurs normally in germinal-center B cells produces idiotypic variants in follicular lymphoma B cells. The results of clinical trials with monoclonal anti-idiotype MAbs demonstrated that these antibodies could eliminate B lymphoma cells expressing the idiotype but that variant cells that ex-

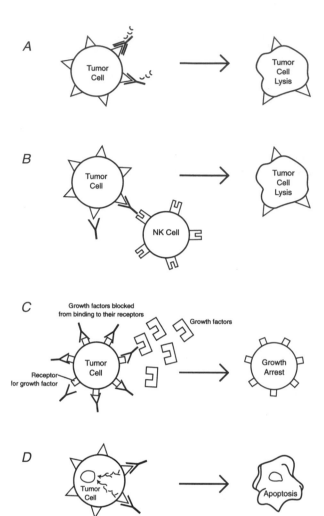

Figure 18.5. Mechanisms of tumor-cell lysis by monoclonal antibodies. Monoclonal antibodies can mediate tumor cell lysis by binding to their tumor target through the Fab part of the molecule and (*A*) activating the complement cascade through interactions mediated by the Fc regions of certain antibody isotypes, (*B*) interacting with the Fc receptors expressed on certain host effector cells (macrophages, natural killer cells and polymorphonuclear leukocytes), (*C*) blocking the binding of certain important growth factors to their receptors expressed on some tumor types, (*D*) generating an intracellular signal that activates a pathway to programmed cell death.

pressed altered idiotypes were not killed and repopulated the tumor (Meeker et al., 1985).

Antigenic Cross-Reactivity: Because most tumor antigens are not tumor-specific, MAbs may react with some normal tissues. Important toxicities may occur due to this cross-reactivity: for example, although the CDw52 antigen recognized by a MAb is expressed only on B and T lymphocytes, the conse-

Table 18.3. Strategies to Enhance the Efficacy of Monoclonal Antibody Therapy

Factors Limiting the Efficacy of Monoclonal Antibody Therapy	Approach to Enhance Efficacy
Specificity of tumor antigen	Identification of tumor-specific antigens
Tumor-cell heterogenicity	Radiolabeled MAb
Antigenic cross-reactivity	Antibody specificity
Antigenic modulation and shedding	Antibody specificity
Tumor penetration	Radiolabeled MAb Cytokine enhancement
Immune response (HAMA) to rodent antibody	Chimeric/humanized MAb
Defects in the host immune system	Chimeric/humanized MAb Radiolabeled MAb Immunotoxins Cytokine enhancement Bispecific MAb

quences of treatment of lymphoma with this MAb are lymphopenia with immunosuppression and susceptibility to opportunistic infections (Tang et al., 1996).

Antigenic Modulation and Shedding: Many cell surface antigens become internalized after binding to a MAb, a process known as *antigenic modulation.* As a result, the antigen is no longer available to bind further antibodies or to attract complement or Fc receptor–bearing effector cells to mediate lysis. Conversely, some antigens are shed into the surrounding tissues and may even accumulate in the circulation. This shed antigen may bind to the MAb and prevent it from reaching its tumor target.

Tumor Penetration: The effectiveness of immunotherapy with MAbs is dependent upon the ability of the MAb to reach all of the tumor cells. Biopsies of solid tumors, taken after the therapeutic injection of antitumor antibodies, have revealed uneven binding of antibody to tumor cells. This may be related to uneven expression of the antibody target and also to physical factors such as irregular blood flow and slow penetration of large antibody molecules from tumor blood vessels, often confounded by elevated interstitial pressure in the tumor (Jain, 1990).

Immune Response to Rodent Antibody: Because most MAbs are of murine or rat origin, the human immune system may recognize them as foreign proteins. Treated patients may, therefore, develop human antimouse antibodies (HAMA). This immune response can be directed at either the constant or the variable (idiotype) regions of the antibody, neutralizing its effect. Additionally, serum sickness may develop, with deposition of immune complexes in various organs.

Defects in the Host Immune System: The therapeutic activity of MAbs is dependent upon the activity of the host immune system. Either complement or Fc receptor–bearing effector cells must be available to mediate tumor lysis. The immune system of patients with cancer may be defective. The cancer itself may produce immunosuppression through various mechanisms discussed in Chap. 11, Sec. 11.4.3. In addition, most clinical trials of new agents such as MAbs have been performed in patients who have failed multiple anticancer treatments such as combination chemotherapy and irradiation. These treatments are also immunosuppressive and may limit the effectiveness of MAbs.

The following approaches have been proposed to address some of the problems discussed above and to enhance the therapeutic effectiveness of MAbs (see Table 18.3).

Chimeric or Humanized Monoclonal Antibodies: Rodent-derived MAbs are less efficient than human MAbs in interacting with human effector cells and human complement. Also, rodent MAbs can trigger a HAMA response. To circumvent these problems, MAbs have been genetically engineered to contain either human constant regions (chimeric antibodies) or to be almost entirely human, containing only the murine variable region that recognizes the tumor antigen, as described in Sec. 18.3.3. Some of these chimeric or humanized antibodies have been tested in phase I and II clinical studies. For example, a study of the chimeric antimelanoma MAb ch14.18 in patients with melanoma showed a prolonged half-life in serum compared to rodent antibodies, but a HAMA response directed at the variable region still developed in half of the patients. The most promising results have been obtained using the CDR-engrafted humanized MAb C2B8, which is specific for the CD20 antigen expressed on normal and malignant B cells. Approximately 50 percent of 164 patients with low-grade lymphoma achieved objective responses, with a median response duration of 9 months (McLaughlin et al., 1996). Other humanized MAbs are being assessed in clinical trials.

Radiolabeled Monoclonal Antibodies: Radioisotopes have been attached to MAbs for the targeted delivery of radiation to cancer cells (Larson et al., 1993; Wilder et al., 1996). Antibody coupling has most frequently involved the use of long-range β-emitting radioisotopes, such as iodine 131 (^{131}I), yttrium 90 (^{90}Y), and rhenium 186 (^{186}Re). With this approach, the problems of tumor penetration, uneven tumor-cell binding, and host effector cell dysfunction are circumvented, as cancer cells are killed by the radiation and not by the immune system. However, normal cells adjacent to tumor cells that have bound the antibody may be killed as well as cells in sites of nonspecific MAb uptake (e.g., liver, bone marrow). Animal studies have shown that the doses of radiation delivered by a specific radiolabeled MAb are more effective than those delivered by a nonspecific MAb.

Radiolabeled MAbs have induced regression of some hematologic malignancies. For example, complete remissions were seen in low-grade B-cell lymphoma using ^{131}I-anti-MB1 and ^{131}I-anti-B1 antibodies (Press et al., 1989; Kaminsky et al., 1993). In the former study, relatively high doses of radiation were delivered and support with autologous bone marrow grafts was required. Another study used ^{90}Y-anti-CD20 (C2B8) MAbs in 18 patients with recurrent B- cell lymphoma and obtained responses in 50 percent of these patients. Although myelotoxicity occurred, stem-cell infusions were not required

(Knox et al., 1995). The radiolabeled ^{131}I-anti-CD33 MAb, which targets leukemic blasts and myeloid progenitors, has been used for marrow ablation prior to stem cell transplantation for acute and chronic myelogeneous leukemia (Jurcic et al., 1995). Responses to radiolabeled MAbs have also been observed in a variety of solid tumors, although the response rate and duration of response is less than that seen with treatment for hematologic malignancies (for review, see Wilder et al., 1996).

Immunotoxins: The conjugation of a toxin to a MAb overcomes the requirement for a functioning immune system to effect cell killing, but the problem of targeting each and every tumor cell remains. Although only a few toxin molecules may be needed to effect killing, absence of antigenic expression on a cancer cell will be protective. The three toxin molecules that have been most studied are ricin, *Pseudomonas* exotoxin A, and diphtheria toxin (for reviews, see Vitetta et al., 1993; Pai and Pastan, 1994). The first generation of immunotoxins employed chemical coupling, but because the genes for the toxin molecules have now been cloned, the newer immunotoxins are made by recombinant genetic techniques and can be produced in bulk in *Escherichia coli* bacteria for clinical trials.

Pseudomonas exotoxin is a single-chain protein that inhibits protein synthesis irreversibly. It binds to a high-molecular-weight cell-surface glycoprotein, the α2-macroglobulin receptor. An immunotoxin in which the toxin was linked chemically to a monoclonal antibody that binds to almost all ovarian carcinomas was shown to kill ovarian cancer cells in cell culture and in nude mouse models. In patients with ovarian carcinoma, the clinical activity of this immunotoxin was limited by hepatic and neural toxicities due to nonspecific uptake of the *Pseudomonas* toxin in liver and by cross-reactivity of the antibody with neural tissue. More recently, the toxin has been modified by genetic techniques to delete the region of the molecule that binds to hepatic tissue and newer immunotoxins have been generated by linkage to other MAbs. The toxin has also been linked to growth-factor receptors by recombinant genetic techniques.

Ricin toxin is a 65 kDa glycoprotein consisting of A and B subunits. The A subunit kills cells by inactivating ribosomes, while the B subunit is responsible for nonspecific cell binding. Immunotoxins were generated that contained only the A chain, but clinical studies with this approach demonstrated toxicities including a vascular leak syndrome, flulike illness and the development of antimouse and antiricin antibodies. In addition, the half-lives of the immunotoxins were very short, owing to clearance by the liver following the binding of mannose and fucose residues on ricin to receptors present on reticuloendothelial cells. Deglycosylated ricin A-chain immunotoxins were generated subsequently to abrogate this problem and were tested in patients with refractory non-Hodgkin's lymphoma. Although vascular leak syndrome remained a problem, objective clinical responses were seen (Amlot et al., 1993) .

Diptheria toxin is a single-chain polypeptide that arrests cellular protein synthesis. Diptheria toxin with the cell-binding domain replaced with IL-2 has been tested in patients with refractory T-cell malignancies whose cells express IL-2 receptors. Toxicities included fevers and elevation of hepatic transaminases, but objective responses have been seen.

In a strategy that avoids unwanted toxicities, immunotoxins are being assessed for ex vivo purging of cancer cells from bone marrow for autologous transplantation.

Cytokine Enhancement of Effector Function: Studies in animal models have shown that concomitant infusions of cytokines such as IFN-γ, IL-2, or GM-CSF can increase the effectiveness of MAb treatment. These cytokines increase the number and activity of Fc receptor–bearing effector cells and enhance their ability to mediate antibody-dependent cellular cytotoxicity. Initial clinical studies suggest that these approaches may have some value in patients. For example, monoclonal anti-idiotype therapy was enhanced in patients with follicular lymphoma by concomitant treatment with interferon (Brown et al., 1989). These cytokines may also increase MAb uptake in tumors by increasing vascular permeability (LeBerthon et al., 1991).

Bispecific Monoclonal Antibodies: Two antibodies that recognize different specificities can be linked together by chemical or recombinant genetic techniques (Renner and Pfreundschuh, 1995). Thus it is possible to link an antibody recognizing a tumor rejection antigen (TRA) to an antibody that can target or activate a particular subset of effector cells. This approach may help to overcome cancer-related immunosuppression. Such approaches have been shown to be effective and specific in experiments in vitro and in mice. For example, bispecific antibodies made up of an anti-IL-2 receptor MAb linked to an anti-CD3 antibody can conjugate to peripheral blood mononuclear T cells and lyse specifically tumor cells expressing the IL-2 receptor. Bispecific antibodies are being tested in clinical trials.

18.4. ACTIVE IMMUNOTHERAPY

Active immunotherapy involves strategies that attempt to generate an anti-tumor response in vivo. The earliest approaches included immunization with lethally damaged tumor cells or with protein TRAs. More recently, DNA encoding TRAs has been incorporated into plasmid vectors for direct immunization. Other approaches have included gene therapy to enhance the immunogenicity of the tumor or the use of antigen-presenting cells such as dendritic cells to present TRAs to the host immune system.

18.4.1 Protein Immunogens

Tumor rejection antigens (TRAs) may be used as relatively specific protein immunogens for antitumor vaccines. Such approaches can induce effective and specific antitumor responses in animals. For example, injection of the purified immunoglobulin idiotype protein expressed on murine B-cell lymphomas was able to induce protection of animals from subsequent challenge with tumor and some animals with pre-existing tumors could be cured (Campbell et al., 1989; George and Stevenson, 1989). The activity of these vaccines has been associated with the development of high titers of anti-idiotype antibodies, and idiotype-specific CD4-positive T cells have also been detected. In these experiments, the idiotype protein was administered with an immune adjuvant (see Chap. 11, Sec. 11.2.1) and was often coupled to a carrier protein to enhance its immunogenicity.

Protein TRAs can be prepared in several ways for use in patients (Figure 18.6). Supernatants containing antigen shed from the tumor cells have been used in patients with melanoma and have resulted in the induction of both cellular and humoral responses. Tumor-cell lysates, purified proteins, or glycoproteins have been used as immunogens. Often, as with the polyvalent ganglioside vaccines for melanoma, multiple TRAs are included in the vaccine preparation. Conjugation to a carrier such as keyhole limpet hemocyanin or addition of an adjuvant such as bacillus Calmette-Guérin (BCG) may enhance the activity of the vaccine (Barth et al., 1994). Recombinant genetic techniques have been used to synthesize TRA immunogens. For example, a fusion protein between the idiotype protein of B-cell lymphomas and granulocyte-macrophage colony-stimulating factor (GM-CSF) generated an anti-idiotype humoral response and protection against tumor challenge without the need for carrier proteins or adjuvant (Tao and Levy, 1993).

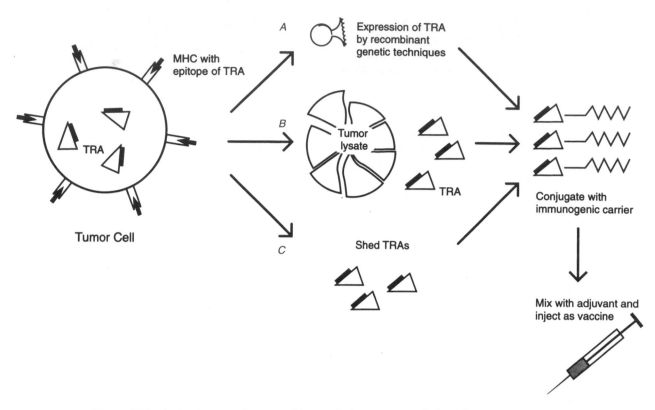

Figure 18.6. Active immunotherapy with protein immunogens derived from tumor rejection antigens. Protein immunogens of intracellular tumor rejection antigens (TRAs) may be generated by (A) cloning the cDNA for the TRA and expressing the TRA protein in vitro, (B) purifying the TRA of interest from tumor cell lysates, or (C) purifying the TRA of interest from protein shed or secreted from the tumor cells after in vitro culture. The purified TRA is then conjugated to an immunogenic carrier and injected with an adjuvant as a vaccine.

In a novel approach, antibodies called Ab1 generated to a particular antigen can induce the generation of another set of antibodies (Ab2) that may structurally resemble the antibody-binding component of the original antigen (Chatterjee et al., 1994). These "anti-idiotype" antibodies, in turn, can induce a third set of antibodies, called Ab3, which may bind to the original antigen and mediate an antitumor response. Thus, Ab2 antibodies can be used for vaccination purposes. In mice, humoral and cellular antitumor activity has been induced by this technique against established sarcomas and L1210 murine leukemia cells. Early studies have demonstrated specificity and immunogenicity using Ab2s to gp37 on acute lymphoblastic leukemias/cutaneous T-cell lymphomas, CEA on colon carcinomas, melanoma associated proteoglycan (MPG), as well as several other TRAs expressed on solid tumors. Phase I clinical trials are in progress, but preliminary results have already demonstrated the induction of antitumor Ab3 and proliferative T cell responses.

Another novel approach to tumor vaccination makes use of the observation that tumor-derived heat-shock proteins (HSPs) could induce specific immunity directed at the tumor from which they were isolated (Srivastava and Udono, 1994). HSPs such as HSPgp96 or HSP70 bind a broad array of peptides derived from several hundred cellular proteins, and antitumor immunity elicited by HSPs is lost when these peptides are eluted from the HSP. The mechanism of the antitumor response involves macrophages and CD8-positive CTLs, because depletion of these subsets in the priming phase abrogates the antitumor response elicited by HSPgp96. T cells may recognize the peptide fragments of TRAs presented on surface-expressed HSPs. Approaches using HSPs to elicit antitumor immunity might involve immunization with tumor-derived HSPs or immunization with an HSP mixed with peptides generated from a common TRA such as MAGE1.

18.4.2 DNA Immunogens

The ability to introduce DNA into cells by various physical techniques in vivo has prompted the development of immunization approaches using purified plasmid DNA (for review, see Donnelly et al., 1997). DNA can be introduced into cardiac or skeletal muscle and into epithelial or other cells by a number of strategies including injection or bombardment with microparticles, often gold, coated with DNA (Fig. 18.7). The particles and DNA enter the cytosol through the cell membrane and cells that have taken up these microparticles express the genetic material encoded on the plasmid. DNA not taken up is degraded by nucleases present in serum and tissue fluids. In muscle cells, expression of the plasmid DNA has been documented for up to 1 year after introduction. In studies using DNA encoding for influenza A hemagglutinin, both humoral and cell mediated responses comparable to the responses seen after influenza A virus infection can be generated (Ulmer et al, 1993).

The direct injection of plasmid DNA encoding CD4 or HIV gp160 has induced protective antitumor responses against a murine myeloma cell line that had been transfected with these antigens (Wang et al., 1993). Humoral responses were generated and were thought to mediate the antitumor response. In vivo immunization with plasmids encoding the immunoglobulin idiotype protein elicited anti-idiotype antibody responses that recognized the idiotype expressed on the Bcl1 murine B-cell lymphoma (Winter and Harris, 1993). Recently, anti-tumor responses against established adenocarcinomas

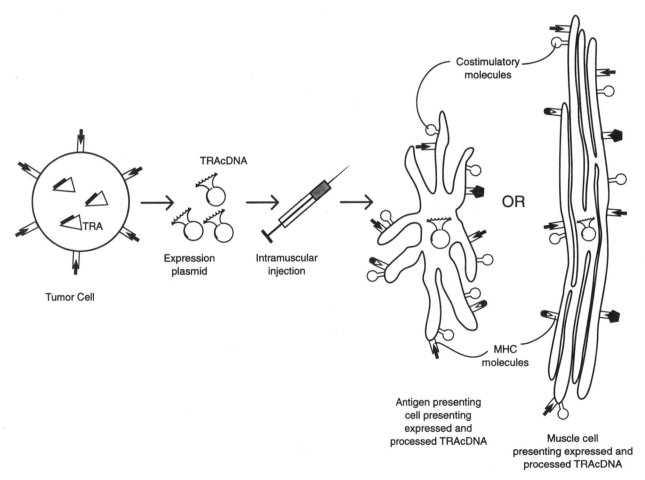

Figure 18.7. Active immunotherapy with DNA immunogens derived from tumor-rejection antigens. The cDNA encoding a particular TRA, isolated by recombinant techniques, or the cDNA encoding a known common TRA, is cloned into an expression plasmid. This is then injected intramuscularly or subcutaneously into the patient without the requirement for an adjuvant. The cDNA is taken up by muscle or antigen-presenting cells and the encoded protein is processed and presented on MHC molecules for T- cell activation.

expressing the β-gal TRA were elicited by gold-coated plasmid DNA encoding β-gal administered intradermally using a helium-powered "gene gun." Splenocytes from immunized mice were able to produce an antitumor effect after adoptive transfer (Irvine et al., 1996). Coadministration of cytokines (particularly IL-12) enhanced the antitumor activity. In preliminary studies of six patients with melanoma, CTLs were generated against autologous tumor cells after in vivo intratumoral inoculation with plasmids encoding HLA-B7 DNA complexed to liposomes to enhance gene delivery (Nabel et al., 1993). DNA was injected multiple times without complications, and plasmid DNA could be found in biopsies for up to 1 week after treatment. Patients did not make antibodies to DNA. Antitumor responses occurred within the inoculated tumors, and one patient responded at distant sites.

18.4.3 Immunization with Tumor Cells

Immunization with autologous or allogeneic tumor cells (which have usually received a lethal dose of radiation) either with or without a nonspecific adjuvant have been used to elicit an enhanced immune response against tumors. Many such experiments have been performed in animal models and clinical trials have been conducted in cancer patients, especially those with melanoma and renal cancer. Two mechanisms could explain T-cell activation by these allogeneic tumor cells. First, tumor cells might activate T cells by behaving as antigen-presenting cells and present TRAs on shared MHC molecules. Second, the allogeneic cells could be broken down *in vivo* and TRAs could be presented on self MHC molecules by host antigen-presenting cells.

The use of a common allogeneic vaccine (e.g., pooled melanoma cells) has the advantage that it can be mass produced and made easily available. A major disadvantage is that the vaccine may not contain TRAs expressed on the recipient patient's melanoma or may not express similar MHC molecules. Morton et al. treated 186 patients with stage III or IV melanoma using an irradiated melanoma cell vaccine from three melanoma cell lines that express six known TRAs (Morton et al., 1993). The vaccine was injected intradermally (and initially with BCG). In addition, some patients received cimetidine, indomethacin, or cyclophosphamide as immunomodulators. Delayed-type hypersensitivity and IgM responses were measured in some patients and correlated with clinical response. Of 40 patients with measurable disease, 3 had a complete response and 6 had a partial response; a randomized phase III study is in progress.

Active immunotherapy has led to tumor responses in many transplantable animal tumors, usually when immunization is applied either before tumor transplantation or when the tumor burden is low. Although some responses have been seen in patients, for the most part these are inconsistent and the overall clinical experience is much less encouraging. The animal tumors may not be ideal models for human cancer for the following reasons: (1) genetic drift of the cell lines, and of the animals into which they are implanted, may lead to effects that are due to transplantation antigens rather than to TRAs; (2) prevention of tumor outgrowth by vaccination in an animal model is not analogous to inducing regression of established tumors in patients; and (3) the immune system of a patient with an extensive and progressive cancer (and after immunosuppressive chemo- and radiation therapies) may not be as responsive to active immunotherapeutic approaches as that of a healthy murine immune system. Active immunotherapy with tumor cells has not been adopted as part of routine clinical practice.

18.4.4 Genetically Modified Tumor Cells

The introduction of cytokine genes into tumor cells that possess TRAs will result in the local secretion of specific cytokines; this should enhance the activation of immunoreactive lymphocytes, and this activation might be sufficient to eliminate unmodified tumor cells (Fig. 18.8). Moreover the local delivery of a cytokine should eliminate the common major toxicities associated with the high systemic doses of cytokines that are often required to mediate immune activation.

Many experimental studies have evaluated the antitumor effects of various cytokines introduced into tumor cells (Colombo and Forni, 1994; Fujiwara et al., 1994; Miller et al., 1994). Genetically modified tumor cells, often irradiated, are introduced into syngeneic mice to determine whether the expressed cytokine gene can induce an antitumor immune response against the unmodified tumor cells. Experiments to identify the cell types that mediate the antitumor response may include deletion of various host effector-cell subsets to test their importance or in vitro assessments of lymphocyte proliferation or cytotoxic T lymphocyte activity. Some of the results obtained in such studies are discussed below.

Interleukin 2 (IL-2) Tumor cells engineered to express high levels of interleukin 2 (IL-2) usually mediate regression of even large inocula of parental, unmodified tumor cells (Miller et al., 1994). The

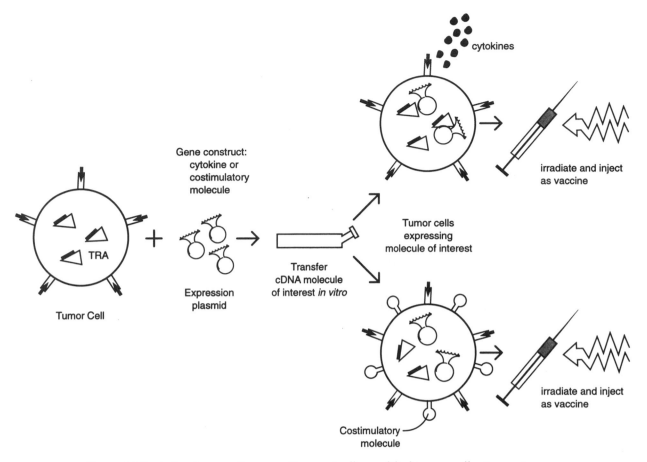

Figure 18.8. Active immunotherapy with genetically modified tumor cells. Expression vectors containing genes for costimulatory molecules or cytokines are introduced in vitro into cells obtained from a tumor biopsy. The tumor cells, now expressing the introduced gene, are irradiated and injected subcutaneously or intramuscularly into the patient in an attempt to enhance the activation of tumor- specific T cells.

site of tumor rejection is usually infiltrated massively with lymphocytes. Often a systemic immune response against the unmodified parental cells can be demonstrated. Depletion studies have shown that tumor rejection is mediated by CD8-positive T cells, although NK cells may also play a role. A strong correlation between the amount of cytokine secreted and the degree of local and systemic antitumor response has been documented.

Interleukin 4 (IL-4) Transduction of murine renal cell tumors with interleukin 4 (IL-4) has induced an antitumor response that was active against established and remote tumor cells. This response was completely abrogated by depletion of CD8-positive T cells (CTLs) and partially abrogated by depletion of CD4-positive helper T cells. Macrophages were also found to infiltrate the regressing tumor. Tu-

mor inhibition in syngeneic mice by IL-4 transduced tumor cells has also been seen with J558 plasmacytoma and K485 mammary adenocarcinoma.

Interferon-γ Several experiments using a variety of tumors have shown that tumor cell transduction with interferon-γ (IFN-γ) can generate antitumor responses mediated by CD8-positive T cells. For example, retroviral transduction of IFN-γ into murine sarcoma cells that express low levels of MHC class I molecules resulted in upregulation of class I expression and an antitumor effect.

Tumor Necrosis Factor α Sarcoma cells transfected with tumor necrosis factor α (TNF-α) were rejected after an initial phase of slow growth. This inhibition was blocked by depletion of CD4-positive or CD8-positive T cells and with antibodies to TNF-α. Nontransduced parental cells at the same site were also inhibited. Similar results have been reported using J558 plasmacytoma and UV light-induced skin-tumor cells.

Interleukin 6   IL-6 enhances the activity of cytotoxic T lymphocytes in vitro. In vivo administration of tumor cells transfected with IL-6 decreases the growth of some but not all tumors in mice. This effect is lost by sublethal irradiation of the animals, suggesting the need for the cellular immune system in mediating the response. Where growth inhibition was seen, it was correlated with the levels of IL-6 secreted; protection against tumor rechallenge was also observed.

Interleukin 7   IL-7 cooperates in the growth and differentiation of lymphocytes. IL-7 may also increase the expression of IL-6 and decrease the expression of TGF-β. Systemic administration of IL-7 may decrease tumor growth and induce protection against subsequent tumor challenge. Tumor cells transduced with IL-7 are less tumorigenic and induce immunity against subsequent rechallenge. In one study, the antitumor effect was found to be dependent on CD4-positive T cells and to some extent on macrophages but not on CD8-positive cells. Lymphocytes isolated from tumor infiltrates were cytotoxic against unmodified tumor cells.

Interleukin 12   IL-12 promotes the differentiation and activation of lymphocytes and natural killer (NK) cells. IL-12 stimulates T_h1 cells and enhances the secretion of INF-γ by both resting and activated T cells. The systemic or peritumoral administration of IL-12 can inhibit the growth of subcutaneous, hepatic or pulmonary tumors (see Sec. 18.3.1). CD8-positive T cells are critical in this antitumor activity, and NK cell deletion does not reduce the antitumor effect. When injected into murine sarcomas, fibroblasts transduced to express IL-12 have eliminated established tumors (Zitvogel et al., 1995). Intradermal injections of these modified fibroblasts effectively treated remote tumor deposits, and protective antitumor immunity against later challenges was generated. Infiltrates of CD4- and CD8-positive T cells were seen in regressing tumor sites.

Granulocyte Colony-Stimulating Factor and Granulocyte-Macrophage Colony-Stimulating Factor   G-CSF promotes differentiation of the myeloid lineage (see Chap. 7, Sec. 7.5.1). Transduction of a murine adenocarcinoma cell line with a G-CSF cDNA decreased the ability of that cell line to produce tumors even in mice that lacked T cells or NK cells, suggesting

that antitumor enhancement was being mediated by granulocytes or macrophages. GM-CSF is important for the differentiation of cells of the myeloid lineage, including macrophages and dendritic cells. Macrophages treated with GM-CSF demonstrate enhanced antibody-dependent cellular cytotoxicity as well as enhanced phagocytosis and antigen presentation. Dranoff et al, (1993) showed that irradiated B16 murine melanoma cells expressing GM-CSF induced long-lasting and specific anti-tumor immunity that was dependent on both CD4- and CD8-positive T cells. These authors also compared the relative efficacy of 10 different cytokines used for tumor-cell transduction and antitumor immunity using the same syngeneic tumor model. Live and irradiated transduced tumor cells were assessed. This group found that (1) irradiation of tumor cells appeared to enhance their immunogenicity, (2) IL-2 transduced cells could produce local but not systemic protection, and (3) GM-CSF was the most effective of the cytokines in inducing specific and systemic antitumor protection. Clinical studies to evaluate active immunotherapy with GM-CSF transduced melanoma cells are under way.

Introduction of Genes for Costimulatory Molecules: B7-1 and B7-2 costimulatory molecules provide the second signal required to activate T lymphocytes after engagement of their antigen receptor (Guinan et al., 1994). The immune response to autologous or syngeneic tumors can be modulated by manipulation of B7-1 expression. Townsend and Allison (1993) transferred a B7 expression vector into the murine melanoma cell line K1735 and showed that immunization with this B7-1–expressing cell line protected against subsequent challenge with modified or unmodified tumor cells. Rejection was mediated by CD8-positive T cells. Similar results were obtained by Chen et al. (1992), who introduced both B7-1 and a viral tumor antigen into melanoma cells and showed that established unmodified tumor cells were eliminated by immunization with the genetically altered tumor variants. Coexpression of B7-1 and MHC class II molecules in class II–expressing tumor cell lines has resulted in enhanced immunogenicity that was mediated primarily by CD8-positive T lymphocytes (Baskar et al., 1995). Studies are in progress to test the role of gene therapy with costimulatory molecules in patients with cancer.

18.4.5 Antigen-Pulsed Dendritic Cells

Dendritic cells are bone marrow–derived antigen-presenting cells that express relatively high cell-surface levels of critical costimulatory and adhesive molecules such as B7-1, B7-2, ICAM-1, and ICAM-3 as well as MHC class I and class II molecules (Inaba et al., 1990; Young and Inaba, 1996). They are able to internalize, process, and present soluble antigen and have been shown to prime class I and class II restricted T cells in vivo. Dendritic cells can be purified from mouse bone marrow or from the peripheral blood of humans using a variety of techniques. A number of cytokines, including GM-CSF, IL-4, steel factor, CD40 ligand, TNF-α and Flt-3 ligand have been shown to induce proliferation of dendritic cells, thus providing adequate numbers of dendritic cells for antitumor therapy.

Small numbers of dendritic cells incubated or "pulsed" with an ovalbumin peptide protected mice against challenge with thymoma or melanoma tumor cells transfected with the peptide (Fig. 18.9; Celluzzi et al., 1996). This protection was mediated by CD8-positive T cells. Mice that were protected against transfected tumor cells were also protected against subsequent challenge with the nontransfected tumor cells. A major limiting factor with this

approach was that a purified known TRA was added to the dendritic cells. This drawback may have been eliminated by a recent study, in which peptides were acid-eluted from MHC molecules on various tumor cells. When incubated with dendritic cells, these peptides were able to induce immunity against subsequent challenge with the tumor cells from which they had been eluted (Zitvogel et al., 1996). Furthermore, this immunization mediated regression of established tumors. The antitumor response was dependent on both CD4- and CD8-positive T cells, while neutralizing antibodies to IL-12, TNF-α, IFN-γ, and the B7 pathway blocked the response.

Recently, dendritic cells were obtained from the peripheral blood of patients with B-cell lymphoma and pulsed with purified immunoglobulin idiotype proteins expressed on the surface of the patient's lymphoma cells (Hsu et al., 1996). Subsequently the dendritic cells were infused into four patients, and two of them responded to this treatment. Cellular proliferative responses specific for the patient's idiotype protein were induced in all patients. Cytotoxic T-cell lytic activity against the patients' tumor cells

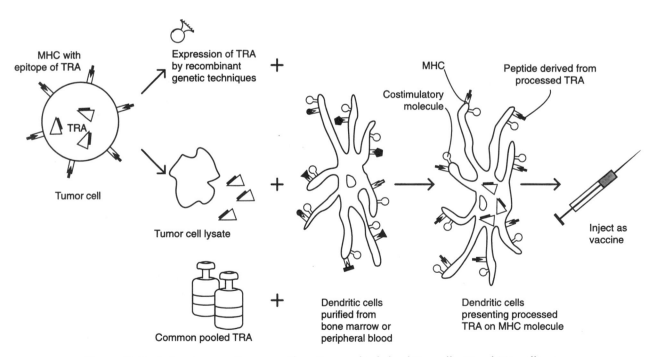

Figure 18.9. Active immunotherapy with antigen pulsed dendritic cells. Dendritic cells are purified from the peripheral blood of a patient and may be expanded in vitro by culture with various growth factors. These dendritic cells are incubated with a source of TRA extracted from lysis of the patient's tumor cells or generated by recombinant genetic techniques. Protein formulations of common TRAs may also be commercially available. The dendritic cells will process and present the TRA on MHC molecules and, in the context of other costimulatory molecules endogenously expressed on dendritic cells, will activate tumor-specific T cells.

could also be demonstrated in vitro. The use of acid eluted peptides to pulse the dendritic cells is advantageous in that the identity of the TRAs does not need to be known.

18.5. SUMMARY

The generation of a specific antitumor immune response requires that tumor cells present tumor rejection antigens with major histocompatibility molecules for recognition by T lymphocytes. Through a variety of experimental techniques, many tumor-rejection antigens have been identified, including the intracellular protein products of altered oncogenes or tumor suppressor genes as well as differentiation or developmental proteins. These tumor-rejection antigens may serve as the target for mobilization of the immune response by gene therapy or by passive or active immunotherapy. Approaches to gene therapy for cancer treatment exploit any of a number of gene-transfer techniques utilizing viral vectors or physical methods to introduce therapeutic genes into either the tumor cell, bone marrow stem cell, or immune effector cell. Nonimmunologic strategies involve transferring tumor suppressor genes, antisense oncogenes, genes to increase sensitivity of tumor cells to cytotoxic agents, or genes to enhance the resistance of stem cells to chemotherapy. Approaches using passive immunotherapy include the use of cytokines to enhance effector cell function or infusion of effector cell subsets expanded in vitro.

Monoclonal antibodies to tumor-rejection antigens expressed on the surface of tumor cells can be generated by cellular or molecular techniques and modified to closely resemble human proteins. These have been tested extensively in the clinic, and a number of strategies have been employed to overcome factors that limit their effectiveness. Approaches to active immunotherapy initially involved attempts at vaccination using tumor-rejection antigens isolated from tumor cells, or whole tumor cells themselves, and usually required some form of immunologic adjuvant. More recently, vaccines using naked DNA encoding tumor-rejection antigens or tumor cells genetically modified with cytokine or costimulatory molecules have been effective in animal models of cancer and are being tested in clinical trials. Professional antigen-presenting cells such as dendritic cells incubated or pulsed with preparations of proteins containing tumor rejection antigens have shown great promise for animal models in inducing specific antitumor immune responses and tumor regression.

ACKNOWLEDGMENT

The author acknowledges the critical review of this chapter by Dr. Andre Schuh.

REFERENCES

Amlot PL, Stone MJ, Cunningham D, et al: A phase I study of an anti-CD22-deglycosylated ricin A chain immunotoxin in the treatment of B cell lymphomas resistant to conventional therapy. *Blood* 1993; 82: 2624–2633.

Banks RE, Patel PM, Selby PJ: Interleukin12: A new clinical player in cytokine therapy. *Br J Cancer* 1995; 71: 655–659.

Barth AM, Reiko FI, Morton DL: Update on immunotherapy of advanced melanoma. *Contemp Oncol* 1994; 4: 52–60.

Baskar S, Glimcher L, Nabavi N, et al: Major histocompatibility complex class II+ B7–1+ tumor cells are potent vaccines for stimulating tumor rejection in tumor-bearing mice. *J Exp Med* 1995; 181:619–629.

Boon T, Cerottini J-C, Van den Eynde B, et al: Tumor antigens recognized by T lymphocytes. *Annu Rev Immunol* 1994; 12:337–365.

Boon T, Van Snick J, Van Pel A, et al: Immunogneic variants obtained by mutagenesis of mouse mastocytoma P815:II.T lymphocyte-mediated cytolysis. *J Exp Med* 1980; 152:1184–1193.

Brown SL, Miller RA, Horning SJ, et al: Treatment of B cell lymphomas with anti-idiotype antibodies alone and in combination with alpha interferon. *Blood* 1989; 73:651–661.

Campbell MJ, Esserman L, Byars NE, et al: Development of new therapuetic approach to B cell malignancy: The induction of immunity by the host against cell surface receptor on the tumor. *Int Rev Immunol* 1989; 4:251–270.

Celluzzi CM, Mayordomo JI, Storkus WJ, et al: Peptide-pulsed dendritic cells induced antigen-specific, CTL-mediated protective tumor immunity. *J Exp Med* 1996; 183:283–287.

Chatterjee MB, Foon KA, Kohler H: Idiotypic antibody immunotherapy of cancer. *Cancer Immunol Immunother* 1994; 38:75–82.

Chen L, Ashe S, Brady WA, et al: Costimulation of anti-tumor immunity by the B7 counterreceptor for T lymphocyte molecules CD28 and CTLA-4. *Cell* 1992; 71:1093–1102.

Colombo MP, Forni G: Cytokine gene transfer in tumor inhibition and tumor therapy: Where are we now? *Immunol Today* 1994; 15:48–51.

Crystal RG: Transfer of genes to humans: Early lessons and obstacles to success. *Science* 1995; 270:404–410.

Dillman RO: Antibodies as cytotoxic therapy. *J Clin Oncol* 1994; 12:1497–1515.

Donnelly JJ, Ulmer JB, Liu MA: DNA vaccines. *Life Sci* 1997; 60:163–172.

Dranoff G, Jaffee E, Lazenby A, et al: Vaccination with irradiated tumor cells engineered to secrete murine granulocyte-macrophage colony-stimulating factor stimulates potent, specific, and long-lasting anti-tumor immunity. *Proc Natl Acad Sci USA* 1993; 90: 3539–3543.

Ettinghausen SE, Rosenberg SA: Immunotherapy and gene therapy of cancer. *Adv Surg* 1995; 28:223–254.

Farhood H, Gao X, Son K, et al: Cationic liposomes for direct gene transfer in therapy of cancer and other diseases. *Ann NY Acad Sci* 1994; 716:23–34.

Fujiwara T, Grimm AE, Roth JA: Gene therapeutics and gene therapy for cancer. *Curr Opin Oncol* 1994; 6:96–105.

George AJT, Stevenson FK: Prospects for the treatment of B cell tumors using idiotypic vaccination. *Int Rev Immunol* 1989; 4:271–310.

Grimm EA, Mazumder A, Zhang HZ, Rosenberg SA: Lymphokine activated killer cell phenomenon. Lysis of natural killer–resistant fresh solid tumor cells by interleukin-2-activated autologous human peripheral blood lymphocytes. *J Exp Med* 1982; 155:1823–1841.

Guinan EC, Gribben JG, Boussiotis VA, et al: Pivotal role of the B7:CD28 pathway in transplantation tolerance and tumour immunity. *Blood* 1994; 84:3261–3282.

Hawley RG, Lieu FHL, Fong AZC, Hawley TS: Versatile retroviral vetors for potential use in gene therapy. *Gene Ther* 1994; 1:136–138.

Hsu FJ, Benike C, Fagnoni F, et al: Vaccination of patients with B-cell lymphoma using autologous antigen-pulsed dendritic cells. *Nature Med* 1996; 2:52–58.

Hwu P, Rosenberg SA: The genetic modification of T cells for cancer therapy: An overview of laboratory and clinical trials. *Cancer Detect Prev* 1994; 18:43–50.

Inaba K, Metlay MT, Crowley M, et al: Dendritic cells as antigen presenting cells in vivo. *Int Rev Immunol* 1990; 6:197–206.

Irvine, KR Rao JB, Rosenberg SA, Restifo NP: Cytokine enhancement of DNA immunization leads to effective treatment of established pulmonary metastases. *J Immunol* 1996; 156:238–245.

Jain RK: Physiologic barriers to delivery of monoclonal antibodies and other macromolecules in tumors. *Cancer Res* 1990; 50 (suppl):814s–818s.

Jurcic JG, Caron PC, Miller WH Jr, et al: Sequential targeted therapy for relapsed acute promyelocytic leukemia with all trans-retinoic acid and anti-CD33 monoclonal antibody, M195. *Leukemia* 1995; 9:244–248.

Kaminski MS, Zasadny KR, Francis IR, et al: Radioimmunotherapy of B-cell lymphoma with [^{131}I] anti-B1 (anti-CD20) antibody. *N Engl J Med* 1993; 329:459–465.

Kasahara N, Dozy A, and Kan Y-W. Targeting retroviral vectors to specific cells. *Science* 1995; 269:417.

Knox SJ, Goris ML, Trisler KD: 90Y-Anti- CD20 monoclonal antibody therapy for recurrent B cell lymphoma (abstr). *Int J Radiat Oncol Biophys* 1995; 32 (suppl1): 215.

Kohler G, Howe SC, Milstein C: Fusion between immunoglobulin-secreting and non-secreting myeloma cell lines. *Eur J Immunol* 1976; 6:292–295.

Larson SM, Macapinlac HA, Scott AM, Divgi CR: Recent achievments in the development of radiolabeled monoclonal antiboides for diagnosis, therapy and biologic characterization of human tumors. *Acta Oncol* 1993; 32:709–715.

LeBerthon B, Khali LA, Alauddin M, et al: Enhanced tumor uptake of macromolecules induced by a novel vasoactive interleukin 2 immunoconjugate. *Cancer Res* 1991; 51:2694–2698.

Matthews DC, Smith FO, Bernstein ID: Monoclonal antibodies in the study and therapy of hematopoietic cancers. *Curr Opin Immunol* 1992; 4:641–646.

McCafferty J, Grifffiths AD, Winter G, Chiswell DJ: Phage antibodies: Filamentous phage displaying antibody variable domains. *Nature* 1990; 348:552–554.

McLaughlin P, Cabinallas F, Grillo-Lopez AJ, et al: IDED C2B8 anti-CD20 antibody: Final report on a phase III pivotal trial in patients with relapsed low grade or follicular lymphoma (abstr). *Blood* 1996; 88:A349.

Meeker T, Lowder JN, Cleary ML, et al: Emergence of idiotype variants during treatment of B-cell lymphoma with anti-idiotype antibodies. *N Engl J Med* 1985; 312:1658–1665.

Miller AD: Retroviral vectors. *Curr Top Microbiol Immunol* 1992; 158:1–24.

Miller AR, McBride WH, Hunt K, Economou JS: Cytokine-mediated gene therapy for cancer. *Ann Surg Oncol* 1994; 1:436–450.

Miller N, Vile R: Targeted vectors for gene therapy. *FASEB J* 1995; 9:190–199.

Morrison SL: Success in specification. *Nature* 1994; 368:812–813.

Morrison SL, Johnson MJ, Herzenberg LA, Oi VT: Chimeric human antibody molecules: Mouse antigen-binding domains with human constant region domains. *Proc Natl Acad Sci USA* 1984; 81:6851–6855.

Morton DL, Foshag LJ, Hoon DS, et al: Prolongation of survival in metastatic melanoma after active specific immunotherapy with a new polyvalent melanoma vaccine. *Ann Surg* 1992; 216:463–482.

Nabel GJ, Nabel EG, Yang ZY, et al: Direct gene transfer with DNA-liposome complexes in melanoma: Expression, biologic activity, and lack of toxicity in humans. *Proc Natl Acad Sci USA* 1993; 90:11307–11311.

Pai LH, Pastan I: Immunotoxins and recombinant toxins for cancer treatment. In: eds. De Vita, VT, Hellman S, and Rosenberg SA. *Important Advances in Oncology.* Philadelphia: Lippincott; 1994:3–19.

Pardoll DM: Tumor antigens: A new look for the 1990s. *Nature* 1994; 369:357–358.

Perkus ME, Tartaglia J, Paoletti E: Pox virus–based vaccine candidates for cancer, AIDS, and other infectious diseases. *J Leuk Biol* 1995; 58:1–13.

Press OW, Eary JF, Badger CC, et al: Treatment of refractory non-Hodgkin's lymphoma with radiolabelled MB-1 (anti-CD37) antibody. *J Clin Oncol* 1989; 7:1027–1038.

Puri RK, Siegel JP: Interleukin-4 and cancer therapy. *Cancer Invest* 1993; 11:473–486.

Renner C, Pfreundschuh M: Tumor therapy by immune recruitement with bispecific antibodies. *Immunol Rev* 1995; 145:179–209.

Rosenberg, SA, Aebersold, P, Cornetta, K, et al: Gene transfer into humans immunotherapy of patients with advanced melanoma using tumor infiltrating lymphocytes modified by retroviral gene transduction. *N Engl J Med* 1990; 323:570–578.

Rosenberg SA, Lotze MT, Yang JC, et al: Prospective randomized trial of high dose interleukin-2 alone or in combination with lymphokine-acitivated killer cells for the treatment of patients with advanced cancer. *J Natl Cancer Inst* 1993; 85:622–632.

Roth JA, Cristiano RJ: Gene therapy for cancer: What have we done and where are we going? *J Natl Cancer Inst* 1997; 89:21–39.

Srivastava PK, Udono H: Heat shock protein-peptide complexes in cancer immunotherapy. *Curr Opin Immunol* 1994; 6:728–732.

Takaku F: Clinical application of cytokines for cancer treatment. *Oncology* 1994; 51:123–128.

Tang SC, Hewitt K, Reis MD, Berinstein NL: Immunosuppressive toxicity of CAMPATH 1H monoclonal antibody in the treatment of patients with recurrent low grade lymphoma. *Leuk Lymphoma* 1994; 24:93–101.

Tao MH, Levy R: Idiotype/granulocyte-macrophage colony-stimulating factor fusion protein as a vaccine for B cell lymphoma. *Nature* 1993; 362:755–758.

Townsend SE, Allison JP: Tumor rejection after direct costimulation of CD8+ T cells by B7-transfected melanoma cells. *Science* 1993; 259:368–370.

Ulmer JB, Donnelly JJ, Parker SE, et al: Heterologous protection against influenza by injection of DNA encoding a viral protein. *Science* 1993; 259:1745–1749.

Verhoeyen M, Milstein C, Winter G: Reshaping human antibodies: Grafting an antilysozyme activity. *Science* 1988; 239:1534–1536.

Vitetta ES, Thorpe PE, Uhr JW: Immunotoxins: Magic bullets or misguided missiles. *Trends Pharmacol Sci* 1993; 14:148–154.

Wang B, Ugen KE, Srikantan V, et al: Gene inoculation generates immune responses against human immunodeficiency virus type I. *Proc Natl Acad Sci USA* 1993; 90:4156–4160.

Webb A, Cunningham D, Cotter F, et al. BCL-2 antisense therapy in patients with non-Hodgkin's lymphoma. *Lancet* 1977; 349:1137–1141.

Wilder RB, DeNardo GL, DeNardo SJ: Radioimmunotherapy: Recent results and future directions. *J Clin Oncol* 1996; 14:1383–1400.

Winter G, Harris WJ: Humanized antibodies. *Immunol Today* 1993; 14:243–246.

Young JW, Inaba K: Dendritic cells as adjuvants for class I major histocompatibility complex–restricted antitumor immunity. *J Exp Med* 1996; 183:7–11.

Zitvogel L, Mayordomo JI, Tjandrawan T, et al: Therapy of murine tumors with tumor peptide-pulsed dendritic cells: Dependence on T-cells, B7 costimulation, and T helper cell 1-associated cytokines. *J Exp Med* 1996; 183:87–97.

Zitvogel L, Tahara H, Robbins PD, et al: Cancer immunotherapy of established tumors with IL-12. Effective delivery by genetically engineered fibroblasts. *J Immunol* 1995; 155:1393–1403.

19

Hyperthermia and Photodynamic Therapy

Fei-Fei Liu and Brian C. Wilson

19.1 HYPERTHERMIA
    19.1.1 Introduction
    19.1.2 Cell Survival
    19.1.3 Fractionation of Heat Treatment, Thermotolerance, and Step-Down Heating
    19.1.4 Mechanisms of Heat-Induced Cell Death
    19.1.5 Influence of Time and Temperature
    19.1.6 Blood Flow
    19.1.7 Hyperthermia and Radiation
    19.1.8 Hyperthermia and Drugs

19.2 PHOTODYNAMIC THERAPY
    19.2.1 Introduction
    19.2.2 Photophysics and Photochemistry
    19.2.3 Properties of Photosensitizers
    19.2.4 Mechanisms of Action
    19.2.5 Technologies
    19.2.6 Detection of Tumors with Fluorescence

19.3 SUMMARY

REFERENCES

19.1 HYPERTHERMIA

19.1.1 Introduction

Hyperthermia as a treatment for cancer extends back to antiquity (see Hornback, 1984, for historical review), but renewed interest over recent decades has been stimulated by biological studies that have defined a rationale for hyperthermia treatment based on cellular and tissue responses to heat alone and to the combination of heat with radiation or chemotherapy. Hyperthermia treatments alone produce regression in about 50 percent of spontaneous human and domestic animal tumors with minimal acute normal tissue complications (reviewed by Mayer, 1984). However, the responses are often transient, which has led to the investigation of treatment with heat combined with radiation or chemotherapy. Results of these studies are discussed in Secs. 19.1.7 and 19.1.8.

There are major difficulties in the application of hyperthermia, particularly regional hyperthermia, since, despite advances in the technology of heat-ing, it is almost impossible to obtain a uniform regional rise in temperature that is reproducible from treatment to treatment or from tumor to tumor. Whole-body heating or regional perfusion with heated blood can provide greater temperature uniformity, but these procedures are limited in their applicability. Further improvements in the technology of heating and in methods of thermal dosimetry are urgently needed, but a detailed discussion of methods for delivering heat and of techniques for measuring tissue temperatures are beyond the scope of this chapter (see Field and Hand, 1990, for comprehensive review). Emerging technologies include magnetic resonance imaging for real-time thermometry (Clegg et al., 1995) and high-intensity focused ultrasound techniques to heat human tumors (Hill and ter Haar, 1995).

19.1.2 Cell Survival

Cells in tissue culture can be easily maintained at a uniform temperature, and it has been shown that raising the temperature above normal influences a wide range of metabolic functions. For treatment of cancer, the most important property of cells is their reproductive integrity, as measured by a colony-forming assay (cell survival), since this parameter relates directly to the ability of a cancer to maintain growth (Chap. 13, Sec. 13.3). Results from experiments in which cell survival was measured for Chinese hamster ovary cells exposed to varying heat treatments are illustrated by the survival curves shown schematically in Fig 19.1. These and other studies of cells in culture have identified a number of important characteristics of cellular response to heat treatment.

1. Significant cytotoxicity occurs at temperatures above 41°C, but both duration of heating and temperature are important in determining heat dose.

2. At higher temperatures, cell survival decreases exponentially with heating time after an initial shoulder, as is observed following radiation treatment (Chap. 13, Sec. 13.4.1). At lower temperatures, there is a resistant tail to the curve. This resistance is due to the development of thermo-tolerance (Sec. 19.1.3) and does not reflect the presence of a subpopulation of cells that is intrinsically resistant.

3. Small changes in time or temperature can result in large differences in cell survival. This observation has major implications for the use of hyper-

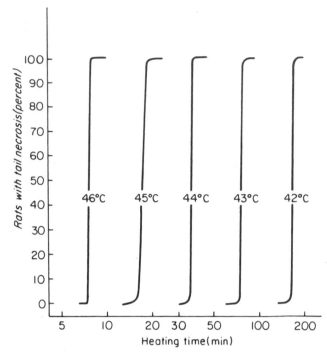

Figure 19.2. Percentage of baby rats developing tail necrosis following heating of the distal part of the tail for various times at different temperatures. (Adapted from Morris et al., 1977.)

thermia in cancer treatment. Its importance is illustrated by in vivo studies of heat treatments required to produce tissue damage. An example is shown in Fig. 19.2, where the sensitivity of the tissue (rat tail) to small increases in heating time or temperature is readily apparent.

4. Morphologic studies of heat-treated tissues, particularly tumors, have found that heat damage to cells is often observable within a few hours of treatment. This observation is consistent with in vitro cell studies demonstrating that heat-killed cells often express their damage and die during interphase. After low-temperature heating, apoptosis (see Chap. 7, Sec. 7.3) can be identified; but at higher temperatures (> 46°C), necrosis develops (Fairbairn et al., 1995). This response is in contrast to that of cells killed by ionizing radiation, which usually undergo one or more cell divisions before expressing their damage (see Chap. 13, Sec. 13.3.3).

5. Different cell types vary widely in their intrinsic sensitivities to heat (see Fig. 19.3). There is no consistent difference in sensitivity between tumor and normal cells, but there may be a difference in sensitivity between rodent and human cells, particularly for prolonged heating at low temper-

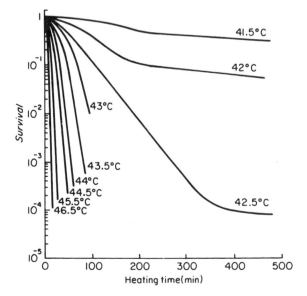

Figure 19.1. Survival of Chinese hamster ovary cells plotted as a function of duration of heating at a number of different temperatures. (Adapted from Dewey et al., 1977.)

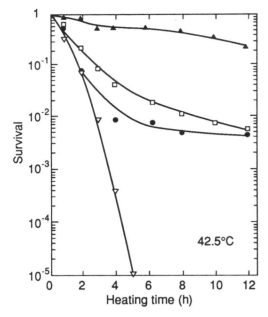

Figure 19.3. Survival curves for four different types of cells heated for various lengths of time at 42.5°C. The cells were all treated under identical conditions. (Data derived from Raaphorst et al., 1979.)

atures (~ 41°C). Recent data for various human cell lines and a rat brain tumor cell line are illustrated in Fig. 19.4 (cf. Fig. 19.1). The reason for this apparent difference is not known (Armour et al., 1993).

6. The sensitivity of cells to heat varies with position in the cell cycle, and cells in S phase and mitosis seem to be the most sensitive, which theoretically complements the pattern observed for radiation therapy (Chap. 13, Sec. 13.5.3). Cells in different phases of the cycle respond to heat differently (Fig 19.5); cells heated during G_1 usually die in interphase a few hours to a few days after heating. For cells heated in the S and G_2 phases (at a heat dose that will give 90 to 99% killing), there is a long delay before the cells divide. They can often complete this division but die attempting further divisions, similar to cell killing due to ionizing radiation (Dewey, 1989).

7. Cells exposed acutely to acid pH during heating have been found to be much more sensitive to heat treatment (see Fig. 19.6). The critical determinant of survival under different external con-

Figure 19.4. Survival of rodent and various human tumor cell lines following mild-temperature long-duration heating (41°C). (Adapted from Armour et al., 1993.)

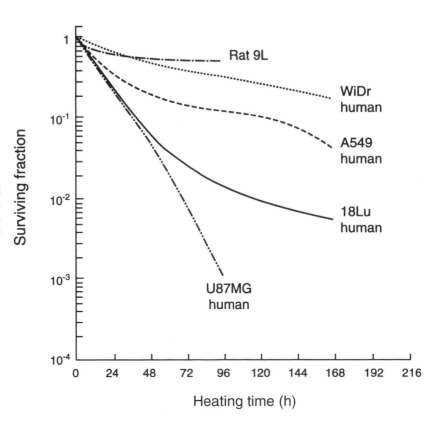

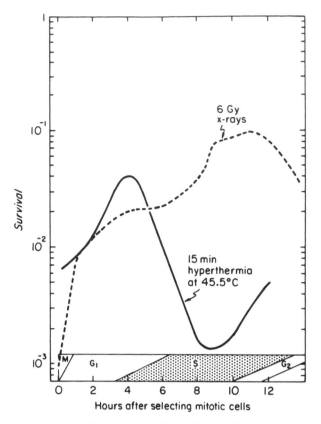

Figure 19.5. Survival of cells following heat treatment (15 min at 45.5.°C) or x-irradiation (6 Gy) delivered at various times after the selection of cells synchronized at mitosis. (Adapted from Dewey et al., 1977.)

due to concomitant changes in pH_i, since acute exposure to hypoxia does not affect sensitivity to heat if other conditions are normal. Chronic exposure of cells to hypoxia increases heat sensitivity, but again, this is unlikely to be due to hypoxia alone. Changes in the cell population (e.g., cell-cycle distribution and/or changes in nutrient status) induced by prolonged hypoxic exposure are the likely explanations.

Some of these results, obtained using cells in culture, provide a rationale for hyperthermic therapy. Tumors, because of their poorly organized vasculature, often have regions where the cells are poorly supplied with nutrients, including glucose, and where the pH is acid due to anaerobic glycolysis (Wike-Hooley et al., 1984; Engin et al., 1995). Cells in these regions of tumors should be more sensitive to heat treatment than those in normal tissues, which usually have better nutrition and maintain pH above 7.0. Indeed, when tumors are heated in experimental animals followed by tumor excision and assay of cell survival in vitro (see Chap. 13, Sec. 13.3.5), the tumor cells heated in vivo are more sensitive than the same cells cultured and heated in vitro (Fig 19.7). Increased sensitivity is also observed in tumor cells that are heated in vitro immediately after removal from the tumor. However, when the cells from the tumors are cultured for a few hours before heating, they rapidly assume the sensitivity of long-term cultured cells (Rhee et al., 1990; Li et al., 1992). Furthermore, cells heated in vitro immediately after removal from a tumor are not sensitized to heating by acid pH, suggesting that they have already adapted to acidic conditions in vivo. These results are consistent with the hypothesis that the tumor microenvironment sensitizes tumor cells to heating, and this is most likely to occur in nutrient-deprived regions of tumors.

If experimental tumors are left in situ for 24 to 48 h after heating, there may be further cell death (Song et al., 1980; Hahn, 1982). This is probably due to nutrient deprivation as a result of vascular damage caused by the heating (see Sec. 19.1.6). Thus, the response of tumors to heat treatment may be dependent on heat-induced changes in tumor blood vessels, on the effect of poor nutrient conditions on the tumor cells, as well as on the heat sensitivity of the tumor cells themselves (Li et al., 1992). Such factors are less likely to influence normal tissue sensitivity, since the vasculature in normal tissues is adequate to maintain nutritive supply and is less sensitive to damage by heating (see Sec. 19.1.6).

ditions is the intracellular pH (pH_i) (Chu and Dewey, 1988; Song et al., 1993). During heating, pH_i drops, and there appears to be a linear relationship between survival fraction and pH_i level following a given heat treatment (Liu et al., 1996b; Li and Liu, 1997). The primary regulators of acidic pH_i for cells in a tumor microenvironment are two membrane pumps; the Na^+/H^+ antiport, and the Na^+-dependent HCO_3^-/Cl^- exchanger. Inhibition of the function of these exchangers is one strategy that enhances heat-induced cytotoxicity (Lyons and Song, 1992; Song et al., 1994).

8. Exposure of cells to heat in a nutrient-deprived environment (such as balanced salt solution or glucose-free medium) can also sensitize them to heat treatment. This effect appears to correlate with changes in the cellular ATP level (Gerweck, 1988). Initially it was thought that cells treated under hypoxic conditions were also more sensitive to heat. These early findings were probably

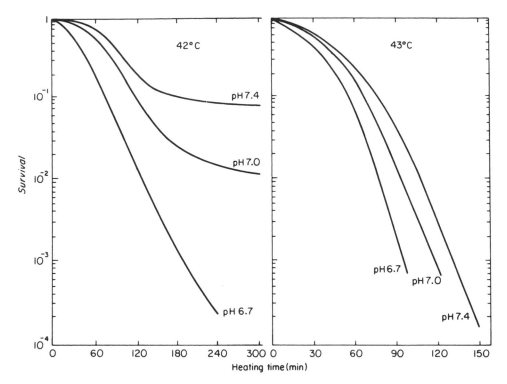

Figure 19.6. Survival of cells following heating for various times at different pH conditions. (Modified from Gerweck, 1977.)

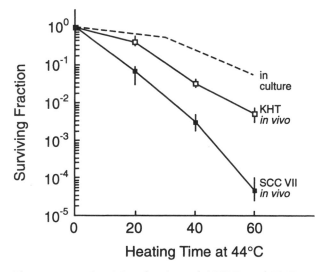

Figure 19.7. Surviving fraction of SCCVII and KHT tumors heated in vitro, compared with tumors heated in vivo first, excised, and then plated for growth. Dashed line shows approximate survival of SCCVII and KHT cells heated in culture at 44°C. (Modified from Li et al., 1992).

19.1.3 Fractionation of Heat Treatment, Thermotolerance, and Step-Down Heating

Cells have the capacity to develop transient resistance to heat treatment, a phenomenon known as *thermotolerance*. The resistant tail on the survival curves for lower temperatures shown in Figs. 19.1 and 19.4 is a manifestation of this effect. Thermotolerance can also be induced at higher temperatures, but its effect is not seen in Fig. 19.1 because it requires that cells be maintained for a few hours at 37°C after heating. In fact, cells heated at higher temperatures (>43°C) are more sensitive to heating at a lower temperature if the second heating occurs immediately after the initial treatment, before the development of thermotolerance (Henle, 1980). This effect, known as *step-down* heating, is probably related to the inhibition of protein synthesis by the initial treatment, which prevents the production of heat-shock proteins (see Sec. 19.1.4) during heating at the lower temperature.

Thermotolerance leads to a high level of resistance 12 to 48 h after heat exposure, but its effect starts to decay by about 72 h. Cells at lower pH (6.0 to 6.5) are less able to develop thermotolerance than cells at normal pH (see Fig. 19.6). Thermotolerance develops in vivo in both tumors and normal tissues, giving a large amount of protection against a second heat dose, but it appears to take longer to decay in vivo—e.g., up to 2 weeks in melanoma xenografts (Fig. 19.8), and both the time of the peak effect and the time for decay are dependent on the initial treatment (Law, 1988; Rofstad 1989). The only (indirect) information on thermotolerance in human tumors suggests that it may persist for up to 3 weeks after initial heat exposure (Liu et al., 1996a).

Because of thermotolerance, the efficacy of fractionated heat treatment is critically dependent on the interval between the fractions. Several prospectively randomized trials have compared from 2 to 10 heat treatments delivered throughout a course of radiation therapy over several weeks for the treatment of a variety of cancers (Valdagni 1988; Leopold et al., 1989; Kapp et al., 1990; Emami et al., 1992; Engin et al., 1993). With the exception of one trial (Leopold et al., 1989), they have demonstrated no advantage of more than two to four heat treatments scheduled with at least a 1-week interval during a course of radiation therapy. This result is consistent with the development and slow decay of thermotolerance and indicates that in contrast to radiation therapy, daily heat treatments are not useful.

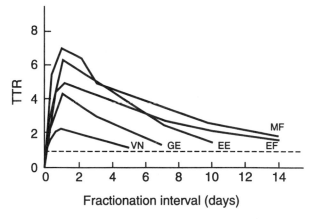

Figure 19.8. Thermotolerance ratio (TTR; i.e., the ratio of the slopes of the heat-survival curves for non-preheated versus preheated tumors) as a function of fractionation interval for five melanoma xenografts, grown in nude mice. Conditioning treatment was 43.5°C for 30 min; and then the tumors were re-treated at 43.5°C. (Modified from Rofstad, 1989.)

19.1.4 Mechanisms of Heat-Induced Cell Death

The nature of the critical lesion(s) that leads to death of cells following heat treatment remains unknown. There is evidence to implicate membrane damage, protein denaturation, chromosome damage, and the inhibition or stimulation of a variety of cellular biochemical pathways. The primacy of one particular type of lesion has not been established, although the weight of evidence favors membrane and cytoskeletal damage. One plausible hypothesis is that damage to membrane proteins affects the function of surface receptors, that heat-induced changes in signaling proteins disrupt the flow of information in the cell, and that these together disrupt regulation of the cytoskeleton, protein synthesis, and DNA replication (see Leeper, 1985; Henle and Roti-Roti, 1988; Yatvin and Cramp, 1993). Recently, the SAPK and p38^{HOG} stress-activated signal-transduction pathways (Chap. 6, Sec. 6.4) have been demonstrated to be important mediators of heat-induced cytotoxicity (Kyriakis et al., 1994; Raingeaud et al., 1995). Transfection experiments whereby the SAPK pathway was interrupted resulted in heat-resistance (Zanke et al., 1996), indicating that an intact SAPK cascade is important to mediate heat-induced cytotoxicity.

Another important cellular response to heat treatment is the induction of heat-shock proteins (HSP). These proteins are produced during heating at temperatures below about 43°C and/or within a few hours (at 37°C) after heating at higher temperatures, even though protein synthesis is reduced to a few percent of normal. Heat-shock proteins are synthesized by a wide range of organisms in response to heat (or exposure to a range of other stresses), and their appearance and disappearance is often correlated with the development and loss of thermotolerance (Li and Werb, 1982; Landry et al., 1982). Transfection of genes (Chap. 3, Sec. 3.3.10) encoding for two of these proteins (HSP-70, HSP-27) into recipient cells has demonstrated that the products of these genes can confer heat resistance, further implicating HSP production in the development of thermotolerance (Crete and Landry, 1990; Li et al., 1991). Following heat treatment, some of the proteins migrate to the nucleus while others remain in the cytoplasm. The function of HSPs is uncertain, but many of them are also constitutively expressed in cells and have been implicated in helping other cellular macromolecules to fold properly after synthesis, leading to the term *chaperone proteins* (Morimoto, 1993). Thus HSPs may function to stabilize the structure of proteins damaged or partially denatured during heating by binding to them, allowing damaged bonds to re-form or be repaired. As discussed in Chap. 12, Sec. 12.2.3, HSP-90 also appears to be involved in control of the expression of genes regulated by steroid hormones.

It is possible that HSPs and the SAPK/p38^{HOG} pathways are interlinked. For example, the heat-resistant cell line TR-4 (Hahn and van Kersen, 1988) is deficient in SAPK activation, and the cells have high basal levels of HSP and demonstrate a rapid induction of HSP production when exposed to heat (Park et al., 1989). In addition, recent experiments have demonstrated that overexpression of HSP70 not only resulted in thermotolerance but also suppressed activation of SAPK and p38^{HOG}, suggesting that HSP70 may somehow regulate the response of the signal-transduction cascades to stress stimuli such as heat shock (Gabai et al., 1997).

19.1.5 Influence of Time and Temperature

The biological effects of heat are dependent on both the temperature and duration of heating. If results such as those shown in Fig. 19.1 are presented as an isoeffect plot of times and temperatures that give the same level of cell killing, then a relationship of the form shown in Fig. 19.9A is obtained. Here, the heating time is plotted on a logarithmic scale and temperature on a linear scale. The rela-

tionship has two straight-line segments with a change in slope in the temperature range 42 to 43°C, which probably reflects the development of thermotolerance during the longer heating times required at lower temperatures. At temperatures above 42 to 43°C, the lines are all approximately parallel to one another and indicate that a change of 1°C is equivalent to a change of heating time by a factor of 2. Below this temperature there is more variability, but a change of 1°C is equivalent to changing the heating time by a factor of about 4 to 6 (Sapareto and Dewey, 1984). Although the isoeffect relationships shown in Fig. 19.9B are similar in shape, the absolute sensitivity of tissues to heat varies widely.

The similarity in the isoeffect relationships shown in Fig. 19.9B suggests that different heat doses (times and temperatures) can be expressed in terms of the equivalent amount of time at a reference temperature (e.g., 43°C) that would be expected to induce the same level of biological damage (Field and Morris, 1983; Sapareto and Dewey, 1984). This concept of equivalent heat dose allows estimation of an effective dose of heat for treatments during which the temperature varies. It could also allow the conversion of a measured temperature distribution into a distribution of equivalent heat doses (Oleson et al., 1993), analogous to isodose lines in radiotherapy. This type of analysis was successfully undertaken for the thermal dose data from the recent In-

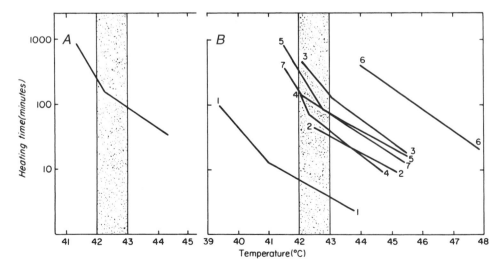

Figure 19.9. Relationship between temperature and heating time required to give a constant level of biological damage (A) for a given level of cell survival and (B) for different types of tumor or normal tissue: (1) mouse testis, (2) 9L rat tumor, (3) mouse foot skin, (4) mouse jejunum, (5) mouse mammary tumor, (6) pig and human skin, (7) mouse ear skin. (Modified from Field and Morris, 1983.)

ternational Collaborative Trial and demonstrated an association between equivalent heat dose and probability of complete response (Sherar et al., 1997).

19.1.6 Blood Flow

Blood flow is of major importance when tissue is heated, since it is the principal route by which heat is removed from tissues. Important findings related to the effect of heating on blood flow in animal tumors and normal tissues (Song, 1984; Vaupel and Kallinowski, 1987; Reinhold, 1988) may be summarized as follows (Fig. 19.10):

1. A large increase (five- to tenfold) in blood flow can occur in normal tissue (skin or muscle) during heating, but only a small if any increase occurs in large tumors.
2. Heating to high temperatures in rodent tumors can lead to a reduction in blood flow due to collapse of the microcirculation; but there is often restoration over the next few days, depending on the severity of the heat treatment. There is evidence that tumor blood vessels may be more sensitive to heat (particularly high temperatures) than are blood vessels in surrounding normal tissue, which in theory could lead to a temperature

differential between tumor and surrounding normal tissue.

3. Tumor vasculature is heterogeneous and may respond differently to heat in different regions of a tumor; it is often much easier to attain higher temperatures in the center of the tumor than at the periphery. In human tumors, the temperature differential between normal and tumor tissues is not as great as has been demonstrated in the rodent system (Vaupel et al., 1988; Levin et al., 1994). Studies of blood flow in human tumors demonstrated that between 41 and 44°C, blood flow increased by around 10 to 15 percent during the first 15 to 30 min of treatment and remained relatively constant thereafter (Waterman et al., 1991). Vascular collapse is generally not observed unless temperatures exceed 44°C.
4. There are recent data demonstrating that low-temperature heating (38 to 41.5°C for 1 h) can improve oxygenation (as measured by a polarographic probe) in rodent tumors (Horsman and Overgaard, 1997), which suggests an improvement in blood flow, although the mechanism remains uncertain. This effect has also been shown to occur in human sarcomas treated with combined radiation and hyperthermia (Brizel et al., 1996), implying that one of the potential mechanisms of interaction when heat is combined with radiation may be through radiosensitization by improved tumor oxygenation.

19.1.7 Hyperthermia and Radiation

The combination of hyperthermia and radiation results in greater cytotoxicity than either modality alone, with a reduction in both the shoulder and the slope of the radiation survival curve (Fig 19.11). The magnitude of sensitization depends on time-temperature exposure, but this thermosensitization is observed even at low temperatures (40°C) when no significant cytotoxicity is normally expected. Thermosensitization is observed when cells are heated and irradiated under acid pH conditions and also when cells have been rendered thermotolerant. The magnitude of the radiosensitization is expressed by the thermal enhancement ratio (TER), which is defined as the ratio of the radiation dose required to give the same level of cell killing at normal temperature to that at the elevated temperature. Most in vitro studies yield TER values of up to about 2 if the results are normalized to account for cytotoxicity from heat alone (Raaphorst, 1989).

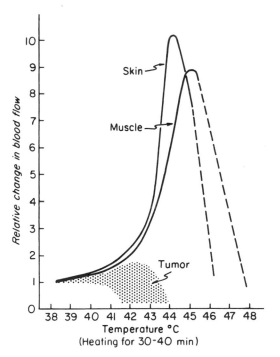

Figure 19.10. Relative changes in blood flow induced by heat treatment plotted as a function of the temperature of heating (for 30 to 40 min). A compilation of results largely from studies of mice or rats. (Modified from Song, 1984.)

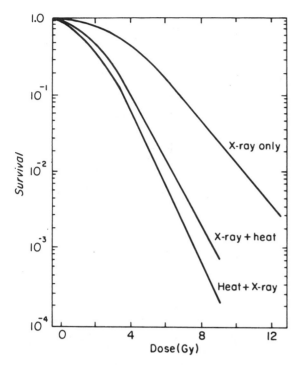

Figure 19.11. Survival of cells plotted as a function of radiation dose. Heat treatment (60 min at 43°C) was given immediately before or after the radiation treatment. (Modified from Li and Kal, 1977.)

The mechanisms by which heat and radiation interact to cause cell death are not clearly understood, but heat reduces repair of sublethal radiation damage, and this effect is dependent on heat dose and sequence, with a greater effect if the heat treatment is given immediately after the irradiation (Raaphorst, 1989). Repair of potentially lethal damage is also inhibited by heat treatment, and again, heat after irradiation is much more effective.

Maximal thermal enhancement of radiation cytotoxicity is observed when the two modalities are administered simultaneously. Laboratory data suggest that as the time interval between the two modalities is increased, regardless of the sequence of the modalities, the TER declines, both for cells in vitro and for tumors and normal tissues in vivo (Fig. 19.12). This decline is probably due to the repair of potentially lethal damage induced by one modality, which can be prevented by the other. Because of thermotolerance, there is no advantage of delivering daily external heat treatments with radiation therapy, and a 1-week interval between heat treatments appears to be the minimum time to allow decay of thermotolerance.

A compilation of data from clinical studies of combined hyperthermia and radiation therapy

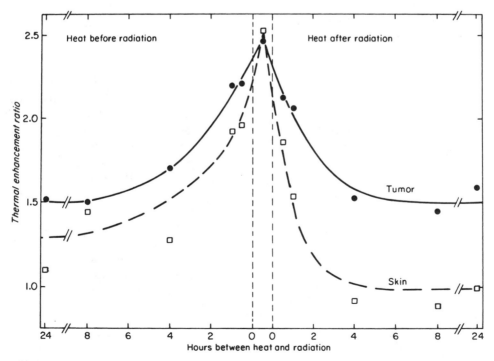

Figure 19.12. Thermal enhancement ratio for treatment of mouse mammary tumors or foot skin with radiation and heating (42.5°C for 1 h) given with various time intervals. (Adapted from Overgaard, 1980.)

(Overgaard, 1989) has indicated TER values in the range of 1.5 to 1.6 (Fig. 19.13). Acute normal-tissue responses are enhanced in patients when treatment is simultaneous or closely sequenced, but it appears that increased damage to late normal tissues is not a significant problem (International Collaborative Hyperthermia Group 1996; Overgaard et al., 1996).

Recent data in human cancer cell lines have indicated that long-duration, mild-temperature heating (around 41°C) can result in thermosensitization for irradiation at low dose rates (Fig 19.14; Armour et al.; 1991, Wang et al., 1992). This probably occurs because inhibition of repair eliminates the dose-rate effect for radiation treatment (see Chap. 14, Sec. 14.3.5). Low dose-rate radiation (0.3 to 1 Gy/h) is conventionally used in (brachytherapy) treatment of human tumors; therefore, this observation suggests a possible advantage from combining brachytherapy with mild hyperthermia to treat human tumors.

Four randomized trials have been conducted in recent years comparing hyperthermia plus radiation therapy with radiation therapy alone for treatment of various superficial cancers. Three of these trials demonstrated a significant benefit for control of local tumor with the combined-modality treatment and one showed no difference (Table 19.1). Hyperthermia added to radiation therapy increases the initial complete response rate. Since these complete responses are durable, this translates into an improved rate of local tumor control. All three positive

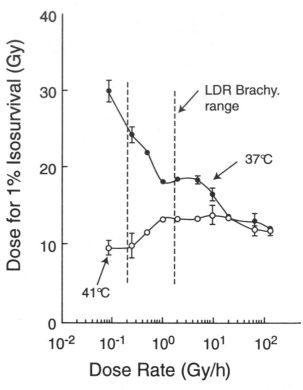

Figure 19.14. Plot of the 1 percent iso-survival dose $(D_{1\%})$ against the dose rate of ionizing radiation at temperatures of 37 or 41°C. The dose-rate effect observed at 37°C is eliminated with low-temperature heating at 41°C. (Modified from Wang et al., 1992.)

trials were conducted at large cancer centers on a single tumor type and site (Valdagni et al., 1988; Overgaard et al., 1995; International Collaborative Hyperthermia Group 1996). The single negative trial was conducted at multiple centers, with poor quality control of hyperthermia, and there was a mixture of different tumor types and sites of disease (Perez et al., 1991). Thus the evidence supports the use of hyperthermia plus radiation but suggests that appropriate technical support for delivering well-controlled hyperthermia treatments is important. Only two clinical trials have reported improved survival following combined treatment with radiation and hyperthermia (Valdagni and Amichetti 1993; van der Zee, 1997).

19.1.8 Hyperthermia and Drugs

Extensive studies of the interactions between heat and drugs in cells growing in vitro have been carried out by Hahn (1982), who classified drugs into

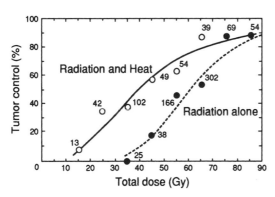

Figure 19.13. Combined results of treatments of neck nodes, from head and neck tumors, with hyperthermia plus radiation or with radiation alone. Numbers represent the number of nodes contributing to each point. Radiation doses were normalized to be equivalent to daily fractions of 2 Gy using the approach described in Chap. 16, Sec. 16.3.8. The displacement of the curve for radiation and heat to lower radiation doses is consistent with a TER of about 1.5. (Redrawn from Overgaard, 1989.)

Table 19.1. Summary of the Results of Phase III Trials of Radiation Alone (XRT) versus XRT plus Hyperthermia (XRT + HT) Performed in Human Patients

Tumor Site	Number of Patients	CR Rate		p Value	Reference
		XRT	XRT + HT		
Head/Neck (primary)	41	37%	82%	.015	Valdagni et al., 1988
Mixed (recurrent/mets)	245	30%	32%	NS	Perez et al., 1991
Melanoma (recurrent/mets)	70	28%	46%	.008	Overgaard et al., 1995
Breast (primary/recurrent)	306	41%	59%	.001	International Collaborative Group, 1996

four general categories. For alkylating agents, there is a continuous increase in drug sensitivity as the temperature is raised, demonstrated by an increasing slope of the cell-survival curve. Other drugs, such as the antibiotics doxorubicin and bleomycin, demonstrate a threshold effect, and their cytotoxicity is not enhanced unless the temperature is raised above 42 to 43°C. The cytotoxicity of antimetabolites, such as methotrexate, 5-fluorouracil, and the vinca alkaloids, seems to be affected little by increased temperature. Various agents, such as SH-containing compounds, ethanol, polyamines, and lidocaine, which have little toxicity at 37°C, act as heat sensitizers. More recent work has demonstrated sensitization with platinum complexes in both monolayer and spheroid models (Kubota et al., 1993); hyperthermia may be able to overcome resistance of cells to these drugs (Hettinga et al., 1997). Microenvironmental conditions such as pH and oxygen levels have been reported to alter the degree of thermochemosensitization (Dewhirst, 1993). Induction of thermotolerance may also increase the resistance of cells to certain drugs (Hahn, 1982), but the intervals of 1 to 3 weeks between courses of chemotherapy in the clinic should obviate this as a concern in therapeutic applications in humans.

The mechanisms by which heat acts to enhance drug toxicity are likely to be different for different drugs. Studies of the interaction of heat and alkylating agents have demonstrated an increase in the number of DNA breaks and cross-links and inhibition of repair of these lesions. Changes in drug delivery to and clearance from a heated tumor, as a result of changes in vasculature, may also be involved. For the antibiotics, mechanisms probably include inhibition of repair of potentially lethal damage and changes in the membrane permeability to the drug. The mechanisms by which heat may sensitize cells to cisplatin are unknown but may involve effects on intracellular drug accumulation, adduct formation, and processing (Hettinga et al., 1997; Raaphorst et al., 1996). Many other drugs may interact with heat to cause damage to the cell membrane.

Combined use of heat and cytotoxic drugs to treat tumors in experimental animals has generally confirmed the in vitro findings. Several phase I and phase II clinical studies that examined combinations of hyperthermia and drug treatment reported good disease response for treatment of limb melanoma (Engelhardt, 1987), pelvic tumors (Rietbroek et al., 1997), intra-peritoneal metastases (Alexander and Fraker, 1996), and other refractory tumors (Robins et al., 1997). No randomized studies have been reported.

Recently, extensive studies of trimodality therapy (combined heat, radiation, and chemotherapy) using murine tumors have indicated that the most effective drug was cisplatin, with the sequencing of drug followed by heat and then irradiation giving the greatest effect (Herman and Teicher, 1994). The experience with trimodality therapy in patients indicates substantial toxicity to the normal tissues; controlled clinical trials are needed (Herman and Teicher, 1994).

19.2 PHOTODYNAMIC THERAPY

19.2.1 Introduction

Photodynamic therapy (PDT) involves the use of light-activated drugs (photosensitizers), usually in the presence of oxygen, to cause cell or tissue destruction or modification. Although the principle of PDT was described early this century, current interest was sparked by the development, in the 1960s, of hematoporphyrin derivative (HpD), a particular photosensitizer that showed selective localization in a variety of solid tumors, as demonstrated by its red fluorescence when activated by short-wavelength visible light (Lipson et al., 1967). Subsequently, work by Dougherty et al. (1975) demonstrated that, upon activation by light, HpD could effect selective destruction and local control of transplanted rodent tumors. Since that time PDT has been used as an investigational clinical therapy for attempted cure, palliation, or prophylaxis of virtually all types of solid tumors, either as a stand-alone modality or adjunctively to radiation therapy and surgery, with treatment of several thousand patients reported (Buskard and Wilson 1994; Dougherty 1996).

The majority of clinical treatments have utilized HpD as the photosensitizer, now known commercially as Photofrin® (porfimer sodium). A typical HpD-mediated PDT treatment involves (1) administering the photosensitizer intravenously, (2) waiting for 24 to 72 h to allow selective localization in the tumor, and (3) irradiating the target volume with light at a wavelength selected both to activate the photosensitizer and to give adequate tissue penetration (usually red light around 630 nm). Treatment of deep-seated tumors has been made possible by endoscopic, intracavitary, or interstitial delivery of light via optical fibers from a laser source. A troublesome side-effect has been general skin photosensitivity, which may last for several weeks after HpD administration.

Porphyrin-mediated PDT has been approved in different countries for prophylaxis of recurrent papillary bladder carcinoma, as a palliative treatment for obstructing bronchial and esophageal tumors, and as a potentially curative modality for early-stage endobronchial, esophageal, gastric, and cervical cancers. However, relatively few prospectively randomized clinical trials have been reported. Examples of clinical findings for various sites are presented in Table 19.2. Attempts to improve the selectivity and/or efficacy of PDT, to extend its range of applications, and to reduce or eliminate the inconvenience of extended skin photosensitivity with HpD have resulted in the development of "second-generation" photosensitizers. Those being evaluated in clinical trials are listed in Table 19.3; they include porphyrins, chlorins, and purpurins in addition to aminolevulinic acid (ALA), a photosensitizer precursor.

No significant interactions have been noted, either synergistic or antagonistic, between PDT and surgery, radiotherapy, or chemotherapy. Indeed, PDT is used adjunctively either before, during, or after these modalities. It is presumed that the non-DNA targeting of PDT is an important factor in this regard (see Sec. 19.2.4). Hyperthermia and PDT may be interactive, depending on the time interval and sequencing (Chen et al., 1996). Treatment with PDT can be used multiple times to retreat the same lesion without apparent resistance. Fractionated light treatments within a single photosensitizer administration may be effective in increasing the tissue response, due variously to drug redistribution, resynthesis (with ALA), or reoxygenation. The healing of normal tissues in the target volume is very effective, resulting in excellent cosmesis and structural integrity. This is probably due to preservation of the collagen architecture (Barr et al.,1987).

Although historically PDT has been developed mainly for therapy of solid tumors, many other clinical applications are now under investigation, including the ablation of diseased tissue in psoriasis, vascular dermal lesions, dysplasia (e.g., cervix, lung, esophagus), age-related muscular degeneration of the retina (choroidal neovascularization), and endometriosis. Ex vivo photodynamic purging of autologous bone marrow transplants for treatment of leukemias and lymphomas has been reported (Mulroney et al., 1994), and there is potential for PDT to inactivate viruses, including HIV, in blood or blood products (North et al., 1993). A critical issue is to match the characteristics of the specific photosensitizer being used with the intended biological target. The majority of applications involve second-generation photosensitizers. Only the application of PDT for solid tumor destruction is considered here.

19.2.2 Photophysics and Photochemistry

As illustrated in Fig. 19.15, upon absorption of a light photon (energy ~2 eV) the ground-state (S_0) photosensitizer is raised to an electronic excited singlet state (S_1). Depending on its molecular structure and the local microenvironment (pH, temperature, substrate binding), the photosensitizer may then return to the ground-state nonradiatively or by fluorescence emission of a longer wavelength photon, or it may undergo an internal transition to an excited triplet (T_1) state. This is relatively long-lived ($> 10^{-4}$ s) and may transfer its excess energy to molecular oxygen to produce highly reactive singlet-state oxygen, $^1O_2$. While other cytotoxic pathways, either oxygen-dependent or independent, may also

Table 19.2. Results of Some Clinical Trials of Photodynamic Therapy Using HpD (Photofrin)

Tumor Site Stage	Number of Evaluable Patients/ Number of Lesions	Responses	Comments	Reference
Lung/early	49/59	CR = 85% mean duration = 14 months (range 2–32)		Futurse et al., 1993
Lung/early	30/39	CR = 72% mean survival = 10 months (range 2–95)	One or two PDT treatments	Sutedja et al., 1994
Esophagus/ advanced	218/[a]	CR + PR = 32% PDT 20% YAG	Palliative intent, comparison with YAG laser ablation	Lightdale et al., 1995
Esophagus/ dysplasia in Barrett's	45/[a]	CR = 78% assessed at 6 months	Normalization of epithelium in 75–80% of cases	Overholt and Panjehpour, 1996
Malignant glioma/ de novo	20/[a]	1-year survival = 30% low light dose 50% high light dose	Intraoperative PDT post–surgical resection	Muller and Wilson, 1996
Skin/ basal cell	37/151	CR = 88% RR = 8.7% for primary lesions		Wilson et al., 1992
Bladder/ carcinoma in situ	37/[a]	CR = 88% 25% recurrence over 12–60 months	Whole-Bladder irradiation	Nseyo, 1992
Bladder/ superficial papillary	34/[a]	RR = 81% control 39% PDT time to recurrence: 91 days control 394 days PDT	Post-transurethral resection	Dugan et al., 1991

Key: CR = complete response; PR = partial response; RR = recurrence rate.

[a] No. of lesions not reported.

contribute to tissue toxicity, $^1O_2$ production is believed to be dominant for HpD and most of the other photosensitizers being evaluated clinically.

Singlet oxygen can be detected in solution by its near-infrared luminescence emission at 1270 nm. However, in vitro and in vivo, this is not technically feasible at present, since its lifetime is greatly shortened due to its high biomolecular reactivity (Patterson et al., 1990). As a result, the distance over which $^1O_2$ diffuses is very small (< 0.1 μm; Moan, 1990), so that the microlocalization of the photosensitizer within cellular and subcellular compartments is a primary determinant of the initial targets for photodynamic damage (see Sec. 19.2.4). Since many photodynamic sensitizers appear to be membrane-

bound (Kessel, 1997), membrane peroxidation has been reported as an initial biochemical event in PDT damage of mammalian cells. This, in turn, leads to changes in membrane permeability and fluidity, cross-linking of proteins and lipids, and inactivation of membrane-associated enzymes and receptors (Girotti, 1990). In solid tumors, this initial damage may occur either in the tumor cells or in endothelial cells of the microvasculature.

As long as the excitation photon energy is high enough to produce the S_1 state, the subsequent photophysical and photochemical events are independent of the wavelength. However, the probability of photon absorption by the photosensitizer is strongly dependent on wavelength, as illustrated in

Table 19.3. Clinically Used Photosensitizers

Photosensitizers	Approximate Main Activation Wavelength, nm	Approximate Molar Extinction Coefficient at This Wavelength, ($\times 10^3$ cm^{-1}M^{-1})	General References
Hematoporphyrin derivative (porfimer sodium)	630	2–5[a]	Pass and Delaney, 1993
5-Aminolevulinic acid (protoporphyrin IX)	630	< 10 (PpIX)	Kennedy et al., 1996; Peng et al., 1997
Tin ethyletiopurpurin (SnET$_2$)	650	40	Wilson et al., 1995 Garbo et al., 1996
Mono-1-aspartyl- chlorin e$_6$ (NPe6)	660	60	Katsumi et al., 1996 McMahon et al., 1994
Meta-tetra (hydroxyphenyl) chlorin (mTHPc)	650	20	Ris et al., 1993
Benzoporphyrin derivative-monoacid ring A (BPD)	690	40	Richter et al., 1993
Lutetium texafrin	730	30	Young et al., 1996

[a]Depending on oligomeric state and porphyrin composition.

Figure 19.16*B*. Unfortunately, the maximum absorption for HpD is at shorter wavelengths, where—due to absorption by other tissue chromophores (particularly hemoglobin) and high optical scattering due to the tissue microstructure (Star et al., 1992)—the light penetration in tissue is poorest. This limits the tumor volume or thickness that can be treated effectively.

As seen in Fig. 19.16*A*, light penetration into tissue increases with wavelength, particularly between 600 and 800 nm: for example, the depth at which the light fluence is 10 percent of the incident value may be 1 cm or greater at the longer wavelengths. Hence, in the synthesis of new photosensitizers, both activation at wavelengths longer than 630 nm and, particularly, much higher light absorption

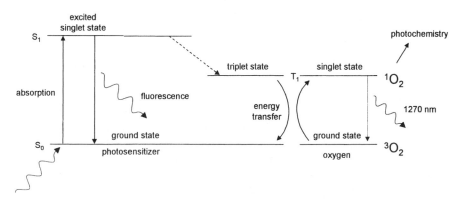

Figure 19.15. Energy level diagram for photosensitizer activation, showing the singlet ground-state (S$_0$), excited singlet state (S$_1$), and excited triplet state (T$_1$). Decay of S$_1$ to S$_0$ may result in emission of a fluorescent photon, as shown. Also shown is the energy exchange from the photosensitizer T$_1$ state to (triplet) ground-state oxygen (^{3}O$_2$), producing excited singlet-state oxygen (^{1}O$_2$).

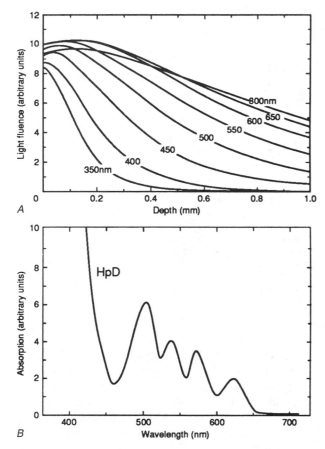

Figure 19.16. A. Curves demonstrating the penetration of light of different wavelengths into tissue. The light fluence is plotted as a function of depth into the tissue. (Modified from Russo et al., 1989.) B. The absorption spectrum of HpD over the wavelength range from 400 to 700 nm.

ceed the diffusion of molecular oxygen from the tumor capillary bed (Foster and Gao, 1992). This effect can be overcome by pulsing (chopping) the light, typically with a 1- to 30-s on-off cycle, to allow reperfusion to take place during the dark phases. Hence, the PDT effect on poorly perfused tumor tissue can be enhanced relative to well-perfused normal host tissue in which there is no photochemical oxygen depletion.

19.2.3 Properties of Photosensitizers

In general, the desirable characteristics of PDT photosensitizers can be grouped into physical, pharmacologic, and biological. For most solid tumor applications, the "ideal" photophysical properties include high absorption at long wavelength, high singlet-oxygen quantum yield, and moderate photobleaching. Therapeutic selectivity in PDT is the result of selective uptake of the drug in tumors and targeting of the light. The "dark toxicity" of the photosensitizers is minimal at the doses used. For HpD administered systemically, tumor-to-host tissue ratios of about 5–10 to 1 at the time of light irradiation are achievable in extracranial human tumors (Moore et al., 1997).

Numerous mechanisms have been invoked to explain the selective uptake or retention of photosensitizers in tumor tissue (Boyle and Dolphin, 1996; Ochsner, 1997). These include low tumor pH causing preferential disaggregation and cellular internalization of oligomeric drugs such as HpD, transport by serum low-density lipoproteins with subsequent preferential targeting to membrane receptors, and pinocytosis by macrophages. Lipophilicity appears to be an important feature of selective tumor concentration of many sensitizers, and this also affects the relative contributions of direct tumor cell and microvascular damage due to the drug microlocalization (see Sec. 19.2.4). For hydrophobic photosensitizers used systemically, liposomes or emulsions have successfully served as drug delivery vehicles (Reddi, 1997). In this case, the pharmacokinetics and microlocalization are determined primarily by the delivery vehicle rather than by the photosensitizer. Generally, intratumoral administration has not been successful, but antibody-photosensitizer conjugates have been explored experimentally for targeting disseminated intraperitoneal ovarian cancer (Goff et al., 1994)

An alternative approach (reviewed by Peng et al., 1997) has been to use the "pro-drug" 5-aminolevulinic acid (ALA). While not a photosensitizer itself, ALA supplied exogenously results in increased

(molar extinction) at these wavelengths compared to HpD have been sought. (For some applications — e.g., treatment of dysplasia or carcinoma in situ — short-wavelength treatment may be preferred in order to spare underlying normal structures.) If the tissue concentration or molar extinction coefficient of the photosensitizer at the treatment wavelength is too great, then the light penetration may also be limited by absorption due to the photosensitizer itself. This can be mitigated if the sensitizer is destroyed ("photobleached") during the treatment (Wilson et al., 1997) due either to direct photochemical action or to singlet oxygen. In fact, rapid photobleaching may give a practical advantage, since the treatment can then become self-limiting. A further factor in treatment optimization is that photochemical depletion of oxygen occurs at high drug absorption and light fluence rate, and this can exceed heme synthesis, the penultimate step of which produces the photosensitizer protoporphyrin IX (PpIX). Preferential PpIX concentration is observed in various tumors, possibly due to reduced ferrochelatase, which converts PpIX to heme in normal tissues. A specific characteristic of ALA is the highly selective PpIX production/accumulation in different components of normal tissues—e.g., mucosa relative to submucosa and muscularis in hollow organs. Aminolevulinic acid may be applied topically, orally, or intravenously, depending on the tumor site.

With all photosensitizers and/or delivery vehicles, the time course of tissue uptake and clearance is strongly drug- and tissue-dependent. For example, the optimum time interval between photosensitizer administration and light irradiation ranges from only a few minutes where neovasculature is targeted to several days with some photosensitizers used for destruction of solid tumors. High variability has been reported (Braichotte et al., 1995a,b) from patient to patient and site to site in the time for the photosensitizer to reach its peak concentration in tumor tissue and in the ratio of the peak concentration in tumor to that in normal tissues, even for the same photosensitizer dose. Thus, in situ drug measurement may be important to optimize treatments in individual patients (Wilson et al., 1997).

19.2.4. Mechanisms of Action

The in vivo response of any tissue to PDT depends on the photosensitizer and route of administration, on the time interval before light irradiation, on the wavelength and intensity of the light treatment, and on tissue oxygenation (Henderson and Dougherty, 1992; Moore et al., 1997). The detailed mechanisms of action are not well established, even for HpD, so only the general mechanistic features are discussed here.

Direct effects of PDT on cells can be studied in vitro. Figure 19.17 shows typical PDT cell survival curves, which are similar for fixed light and varying drug doses or vice versa. Although different cell lines show large photosensitizer-dependent differences in PDT sensitivity in vitro, no marked systematic difference between the responses of malignant and normal cells has been reported. A shoulder region is often but not always seen. Unlike ionizing radiation (Chap. 13, Sec. 13.4.1), however, this is more likely due to a "threshold" effect, ie., to there being a minimum $^1O_2$ concentration required for cytotoxicity, rather than to repair of sublethal damage. The cytotoxicity is strongly dependent on the

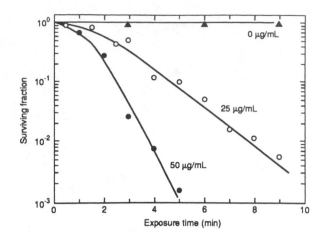

Figure 19.17. Survival curves for CHO cells incubated with two different concentrations (25 or 50 µg/mL) of HpD for 2 h before being exposed for various times to red light (4 mW/cm²). Without HpD, there is no toxicity. (Redrawn from Gomer and Smith, 1980.)

oxygen concentration (Chapman et al., 1991), falling off rapidly below about 1 to 2 percent O_2 (Fig. 19.18). In vivo, both direct photocytotoxicity to the tumor cells and indirect tumor cell death, primarily through vascular shutdown and subsequent tissue ischemia, can contribute to the immediate tissue response (Fingar, 1996). This is usually manifest as gross hemorrhagic necrosis and is usually complete within a few days of treatment. Figure 19.19 demonstrates that the in vitro clonogenicity of tumor cells after in vivo treatment may decrease with the time that the tumor is left in situ (Henderson et al., 1985), corresponding to a delayed ischemic response (or possibly other secondary biochemical or immune factors). Not all photosensitizers show a vascular effect; e.g., some phthalocyanines and cationic drugs appear to work in vivo by direct cell killing only (Henderson and Dougherty, 1992). The in vivo response, both in tumor and normal tissues, shows a threshold behavior with a minimum singlet oxygen concentration (and, hence, photosensitizer–light dose product) being required to produce damage. Thus, the boundary between viable and damaged tissue is often sharply demarcated, despite an exponential fall-off in light fluence with depth (Lilge et al.,1996)

With lipophilic anionic photosensitizers such as HpD, there is marked localization in membranes; in the plasma membrane at short incubation times and in mitochondrial membranes at the longer incubation times typical of treatment protocols (Kessel, 1997). Supporting evidence for mitochondria as pri-

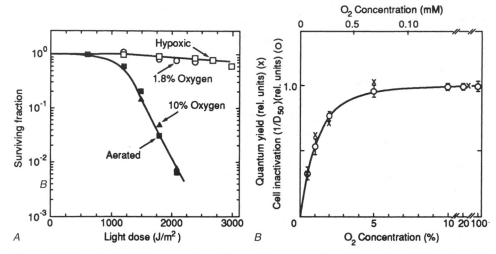

Figure 19.18. *A.* Survival curves for Chinese hamster ovary cells incubated for 2 h with DHE (purified version of HpD) (25 μg/mL) before exposure to red light under different oxygen levels as indicated. (Modified from Mitchell et al., 1985.) *B.* Relative quantum yield of singlet oxygen formation in 50 μM hematoporphyrin solution in PBS and relative HpD-sensitized phototoxicity for NHIK 3025 cells determined at different oxygen levels. Phototoxicity is plotted as the inverse of the time of exposure to 410 nm light (1.5 mW/cm²) required to inactivate 50 percent of the cells (D_{50}), after incubation in 25 μg/mL HpD for 18 h. (Redrawn from Moan and Sommer, 1985.)

mary targets of PDT damage comes from the demonstration of early changes in enzymes such as cytochrome-*C* oxidase and succinate dehydrogenase, following porphyrin-mediated PDT (Gibson et al., 1989), and from structural and functional changes in mitochondria of tumor cells in which

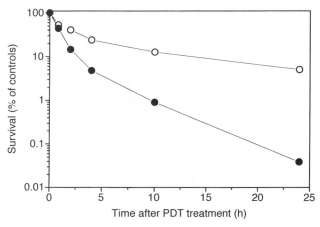

Figure 19.19. In vitro clonogenic survival of tumor cells at different time intervals following in vivo PDT treatment of EMT6 solid tumors in BALB/c mice (HpD 7.5 mg/kg IP, 200 J/cm² of 630 nm light at 24 h after HpD administration). ○, plating efficiency; ●, clonogenic cells per gram of tumor. (Adapted from Henderson et al., 1985.)

PDT resistance has been induced (or selected) by multiple cycles of treatment and regrowth of survivors in vitro (Sharkey et al., 1993). (Note, however, that induced PDT resistance has not been reported in vivo, either clinically or preclinically.) Although DNA damage (e.g., DNA single-strand breaks) can be induced, PDT is not significantly mutagenic relative to ionizing radiation at equitoxic doses, and DNA is not generally thought to be a major target for toxicity (Evans et al., 1989).

There have been limited studies of molecular events in PDT-treated cells. Some stress proteins (HSP-70, GRP-78) can be induced at the transcriptional level (Gomer et al., 1996), and cytokine release has been noted, depending on the photosensitizer and incubation conditions. In addition to necrotic cell death, apoptosis of tumor cells has been observed following PDT treatment with various photosensitizers in vitro (Noodt et al., 1996), likely involving specific signal transduction pathways triggered by the initial membrane lipid peroxidation. Tumor and normal cell apoptosis has also been noted in vivo (Zaidi et al., 1993), but the significance of this in the overall tissue response is not known.

The indirect, vascular-mediated response in vivo is most likely due to damage to capillary endothelial cells. In models where tumor vasculature can be observed directly, as in implanted window chambers (Star et al., 1986), a sequence of transient and then irreversible vascular stasis and occlusion has been reported; this may be due to platelet aggregation and thrombosis following initial endothelial cell damage and exposure of the basement membrane (Fingar, 1996). These vascular effects are likely mediated by release of factors such as prostaglandins, lymphokines, and thromboxanes by damaged endothelial cells. The effect of PDT-induced hypoxia in tissue due to this vascular response allows the hypoxic cell cytotoxin misonidazole to increase the PDT response in vivo (Gonzales et al.,1986).

19.2.5 Technologies

A typical PDT treatment requires about 100 J of total light energy per cm^2 of surface area, either at a single wavelength or at about a ±10 nm interval. (In terms of absorbed energy, this is several orders of magnitude higher than for ionizing radiation; see Chap. 13, Sec. 13.2.1.) Thus, for a superficial tumor of about 10 cm^2, a source delivering a power of at least 1 W is required for treatment in about 15 min; whereas several watts may be needed for thick tumors or endoscopic or intraoperative applications. Although nonlaser sources, including filtered arc lamps or light-emitting diode (LED) arrays, are available with such outputs, a laser is generally required for efficient light coupling into small-core optical fibers. For light of 630 nm (HpD, PpIX) and above, a tunable dye laser has traditionally been employed, but these are large and expensive and are now being replaced by compact diode lasers.

A variety of fiberoptic applicators are available with which the output light distribution can be tailored to give approximately uniform illumination of the target tissue volume. These include external surface applicators and interstitial point or line (cylindrical) diffusers. For larger solid tumors, the limited penetration can be mitigated by using multiple interstitial sources or light treatment applicators specially designed to match the target tissue shape and volume. These approaches are analogous, at least in terms of physical dosimetry, to brachytherapy, and many of the same issues pertain in optimal source arrangement and treatment planning.

Since PDT involves several interdependent elements, namely light, photosensitizer, and oxygen, dosimetry is complex and much less developed than in radiation therapy (Wilson et al., 1997). Fiberoptic microprobes may be used to measure local light fluences in or on target tissues (Lilge et al., 1992; Star,

1997), while optical fiber–based absorption or fluorescence spectroscopy are used increasingly for invasive or noninvasive photosensitizer measurements in situ and for monitoring photobleaching during treatment (Weersink et al., 1997).

19.2.6. Detection of Tumors with Fluorescence

As seen in Fig. 19.15, the fluorescence de-excitation pathway competes with the therapeutic pathway. Photosensitizer fluorescence is useful for de novo detection of early tumors, for localization and targetting prior to light irradiation, and for quantifying photosensitizer concentration and monitoring photobleaching in PDT dosimetry (Wilson et al., 1997). It may be used either as a surface or endoscopic imaging technique or with noninvasive or interstitial optical fiber point measurements. Usually two or more excitation or emission wavelengths are used in order to correct for the tissue autofluorescence background (Braichotte et al., 1995b). In vivo detection of micrometastases and of lymphatic spread of tumors has been demonstrated (Mang et al., 1993). Fluorescence may be particularly useful for defining tumor margins for surgical resection and for detection of premalignant dysplasia or carcinoma in situ for subsequent photodynamic therapy. However, at least for early bronchial lesions, detectability may be achieved using tissue autofluorescence alone, without administering an exogenous photosensitizer (Lam et al., 1993).

19.3 SUMMARY

Heating to temperatures above about 40°C results in cell killing by mechanisms that are not well understood but probably involve membrane damage and activity of cell signaling pathways, such as the SAPK pathway. Both temperature and duration of heating are important, and small changes in either can have large biological effects. Cells are more sensitive to heat under conditions of acid pH and nutritional deprivation. Cells can develop a state of thermotolerance (within 1 day) in which they become more resistant to the cytotoxic effects of subsequent heat treatments. Hyperthermia sensitizes cells and tissues to treatment with ionizing radiation, by interfering with DNA repair mechanisms. It also interacts with many cytotoxic drugs for reasons that probably depend both on the particular drug action and on heat effects such as membrane damage. The maximum interactive effect of heat with radiation or drugs occurs when the two treatments are given close together and is small or absent if more than a few hours elapse between the treatments. Blood flow, the major cooling mechanism for tissue, plays an important role during heat treatment, since a major difficulty in the introduction of hyperthermia as a cancer treatment modality is that it is not possible to produce uniform, well-controlled heating of tissue. Despite the inadequacies of heating methods and the variability in the heating distributions obtained, phase III trials have demonstrated improved treatment outcome for the addition of hyperthermia to radiation therapy, but these treatments must be delivered with appropriate technical expertise.

Photodynamic therapy using HpD has been shown to have some useful specific applications in the clinic and depends on the preferential uptake (and/or retention) of the photosensitizer in the tumor relative to normal tissue and targeting of the light irradiation. Direct cytotoxicity to tumor cells during PDT with HpD depends on the production of the highly reactive singlet oxygen by light activation of the photosensitizer and transfer of energy to the oxygen molecules in the tissue. Thus, cytotoxicity depends on photosensitizer concentration, light intensity and wavelength, and tissue oxygenation. Since HpD is taken up in cellular and mitochrondrial membranes, it is probable that cell killing is not caused by direct DNA damage, but the mechanisms of cytotoxicity are poorly understood. There is good evidence that the in vivo effects of PDT also arise in part as a result of vascular damage, which leads to stasis and hemorrhagic necrosis in the tumor. The next phase in PDT will exploit newer second-generation photosensitizers, which have better light absorption properties at long wavelengths (for which tissue penetration is better) and more user-friendly and cost-effective optical technologies. Improvements in tumor selectivity and photosensitizer–light dose optimization can be expected, but their exploitation will require a better understanding of the biological mechanisms that underlie PDT cytotoxicity.

REFERENCES

Alexander HR, Fraker DL: Treatment of peritoneal carcinomatosis by continuous hyperthermic peritoneal perfusion with cisplatin. *Cancer Treat Res* 1996; 81:41–50.

Armour EP, Wang Z, Corry P, Martinez A: Sensitization of rat 9L gliosarcoma cells to low dose irradiation by long duration 41°C hyperthermia. *Cancer Res* 1991; 51:3088–3095.

Armour EP, McEachern D, Wang Z, et al: Sensitivity of human cells to mild hyperthermia. *Cancer Res* 1993; 53:2740–2744.

Barr H, Tralau CJ, Boulos PB, et al: The contrasting mechanisms of colonic collagen damage between photody-

namic therapy and thermal injury. *Photochem Photobiol* 1987; 46:795–800.

Boyle RW, Dolphin D: Structure and biodistribution relationships of photodynamic sensitizers. *Photochem Photobiol* 1996; 64:469–485.

Braichotte DR, Wagnieres GA, Bays R, et al: Clinical pharmocokinetic studies of Photofrin by fluorescence spectroscopy in the oral cavity, the esophagus and the bronchi. *Cancer* 1995a; 75:2768–2778.

Braichotte DR, Savary J-F, Glanzmann T, et al: Clinical pharmacokinetic studies of tetra (meta-hydroxyphenyl) chlorin in squamous cell carcinoma by fluorescence spectroscopy at 2 wavelengths. *Int J Cancer* 1995b; 63:198–204.

Brizel DM, Scully SP, Harrelson JM, et al: Radiation therapy and hyperthermia improve the oxygenation of human soft tissue sarcomas. *Cancer Res* 1996; 56:5347–5350.

Buskard NA, Wilson BC, eds: The use of photodynamic therapy in cancer. *Semin Oncol* 1994; 21 (suppl 15): 1–27.

Chapman JD, Stobbe CC, Arnfield MR, et al: Oxygen dependency of tumor cell killing in vitro by light-activated Photofrin II. *Radiat Res* 1991; 126:73–79.

Chen Q, Chen H, Shapiro H, Hetzel FW: Sequencing of combined hyperthermia and photodynamic therapy. *Radiat Res* 1996; 146:293–297.

Chu GL, Dewey WC: The role of low intracellular or extracellular pH in sensitization to hyperthermia. *Radiat Res* 1988; 114:154–167.

Clegg ST, Das SK, Zhang Y, et al: Verification of a hyperthermia model method using MR thermometry. *Int J Hyperthermia* 1995; 11:409–424.

Crete P, Landry J: Induction of HSP 27 phosphorylation and thermoresistance in Chinese hamster cells by arsenite, cycloheximide, A23187, and EGTA. *Radiat Res* 1990; 121:320–327.

Dewey WC: Mechanism of thermal radiosensitization. In: Urano M, Double E, eds. *Hyperthermia and Oncology.* Utrecht, Netherlands: VSP; 1989(2):1–16.

Dewey WC, Hopwood LE, Sapareto SA, Gerweck LE: Cellular responses to combinations of hyperthermia and radiation. *Radiology* 1977; 123:463–474.

Dewhirst MW: Factors influencing hyperthermic enhancement of drug cytotoxicity. *Int J Radiat Oncol Biol Phys* 1993; 25:569–570.

Dougherty TJ, ed.: Photodynamic therapy. *J Clin Laser Med Surg* 1996; 14:219–348.

Dougherty TJ, Grindley GE, Fiel R, et al: Photoradiation therapy: II. Cure of animal tumors with hematoporphyrin and light. *J Natl Cancer Inst* 1975; 55:115–121.

Dugan M, Crawford E, Nseyo U, et al : A randomized trial of observation (OBS) vs photodynamic therapy (PDT) after transurethral resection (TUR) for superficial papillary bladder carcinoma (SPBC) (abstr). *Proc Amer Soc Clin Oncol* 1991; 10:554.

Emami B, Myerson RJ, Cardenes H, et al: Combined hyperthermia and irradiation in the treatment of superficial tumors: Results of a prospective randomized trial of hyperthermia fractionation (1/wk vs 2/wk). *Int J Radiat Oncol Biol Phys*,1992; 24:145–152.

Engelhardt R: Hyperthermia and drugs. *Rec Results Cancer Res* 1987; 104:136–203.

Engin K, Leeper DB, Cater JR, et al: Extracellular pH distribution in human tumours. *Int J Hyperthermia*, 1995; 11:211–216.

Engin K, Tupchong L, Moylan DJ, et al: Randomized trial of one versus two adjuvant hyperthermia treatments per week in patients with superficial tumours. *Int J Hyperthermia*, 1993; 9:327–340.

Evans HH, Rerko RM, Mencl J, et al: Cytotoxic and mutagenic effects of the photodynamic action of chloroaluminum phthalocyanine and visible light in L5178Y cells. *Photochem Photobiol* 1989; 49:43–47.

Fairbairn J, Khan M, Ward K, et al: Induction of apoptotic cell DNA fragmentation in human cells after treatment with hyperthermia. *Cancer Lett*, 1995; 89:183–188.

Field SB, Hand JW, eds: *An Introduction to the Practical Aspects of Clinical Hyperthermia.* London: Taylor and Francis; 1990.

Field SB, Morris CC: The relationship between heating time and temperature: Its relevance to clinical hyperthermia. *Radiother Oncol* 1983; 1:179–186.

Fingar VH. Vascular effects of photodynamic therapy. *J Clin Laser Med Surg* 1996; 14:323–326.

Foster TH, Gao L: Dosimetry in photodynamic therapy: Oxygen and the critical importance of capillary density. *Radiat Res* 1992; 130:379–383.

Futurse K, Fukuoka M, Kato H, et al: A prospective phase II study on photodynamic therapy with Photofrin II for centrally located early-stage lung cancer. *J Clin Oncol* 1993; 11:1852–1857.

Gabai V, Meriin A, Mosser D, et al: Hsp70 prevents activation of stress kinases. *J Biol Chem* 1997; 272:18033–18037.

Garbo GM: Purpurins and benzochlorins as sensitizers for photodynamic therapy. *J Photochem Photobiol* 1996; B34: 109–116.

Gerweck LE: Modification of cell lethality at elevated temperatures: The pH effect. *Radiat Res* 1977; 70:224–235.

Gerweck LE: Modifiers of thermal effects: Environmental factors. In: Urano M, Douple E, eds. *Hyperthermia and Oncology.* Utrecht, Netherlands: VSP; 1988; 1:83–98.

Gibson SL, Murant RS, Chazen MD, et al: In vitro photosensitization of tumour cell enzymes by Photofrin II administered in vivo. *Br J Cancer* 1989; 59:47–53.

Girotti AW: Photodynamic lipid peroxidation in biological systems. *Photochem Photobiol* 1990; 51:497–509.

Goff B, Hermanto U, Rumbaugh J, et al: Photoimmunotherapy and biodistribution with an OC125-chlorin immunoconjugate in an in vivo murine ovarian cancer model. *Br J Cancer* 1994; 70:474–480.

Gomer CJ, Smith DM: Photoinactivation of Chinese hamster cells by hematoporphyrin derivative and red light. *Photochem Photobiol* 1980; 32:341–348.

Gomer CJ, Luna M, Ferrario A, et al: Cellular targets and molecular responses associated with photodynamic therapy. *J Clin Laser Med Surg.* 1996; 14:315–322.

Gonzales S, Arnfield MR, Meeker BE, et al: Treatment of Dunning R 3327-AT rat prostate tumors with photodynamic therapy in combination with misonidazole. *Cancer Res* 1986; 46:2858–2862.

Hahn GM: *Hyperthermia and Cancer.* New York: Plenum Press; 1982.

Hahn GM, van Kersen I: Isolation and initial characterization of thermoresistant RIF tumor cell strains. *Cancer Res* 1988; 48:1803–1807.

Henderson BW, Dougherty TJ: How does photodynamic therapy work? *Photochem Photobiol* 1992; 55:145–157.

Henderson BW, Waldow SM, Mang TS, et al. Tumor destruction and kinetics or tumor cell death in two experimental mouse tumors following photodynamic therapy. *Cancer Res* 1985; 45:572–576.

Henle KJ: Sensitization to hyperthermia below 43°C induced in Chinese hamster ovary cells by step-down heating. *J Natl Cancer Inst* 1980; 64:1479–1483.

Henle KJ, Roti-Roti JL: Response of cultured mammalian cells to hyperthermia. In: Urano M, Douple E, eds. *Hyperthermia and Oncology.* Utrecht, Netherlands: VSP; 1988;1:57–82.

Herman TS, Teicher BA: Summary of studies adding systemic chemotherapy to local hyperthermia and radiation. *Int J Hyperthermia* 1994; 10:443–449.

Hettinga JV, Konings AW, Kampinga HH: Reduction of cellular cisplatin resistance by hyperthermia—A review. *Int J Hyperthermia* 1997; 13:439–457.

Hill CR, ter Haar GR: Review article: High intensity focused ultrasound—Potential for cancer treatment. *Br J Radiology* 1995; 68:1296–1303.

Hornback HB: Hyperthermia and cancer: *Human Clinical Trials Experience.* Boca Raton, FL: CRC Press; 1984. Vol. 1.

Horsman MR, Overgaard J: Can mild hyperthermia improve tumour oxygenation? *Int J Hyperthermia* 1997; 13:141–147.

International Collaborative Hyperthermia Group: Radiotherapy with or without hyperthermia in the treatment of superficial localized breast cancer—Results from five randomized controlled trials. *Int J Radiat Oncol Biol Phys* 1996; 35:731–744.

Kapp DS, Petersen IA, Cox RS, et al: Two or six hyperthermia treatments as an adjunct to radiation therapy yield similar tumor responses: Results of a randomized trial. *Int J Radiat Oncol Biol Phys*, 1990; 19:1481–1495.

Katsumi TA. Aizawa K. Kuroiwa Y, et al: Photodynamic therapy with a diode laser for implanted fibrosarcoma in mice employing mono-L-aspartyl chlorin E6. *Photochem Photobiol* 1996; 64:671–675.

Kennedy JC, Marcus SL, Pottier RH. Photodynamic therapy (PDT) and photodiagnosis (PD) using endogenous photosensitization induced by 5-aminolevulinic acid (ALA): Mechanisms and clinical results. *J Clin Laser Med Surg* 1996; 14:289–304.

Kessel D, ed: Symposium in print: Subcellular localization of photosensitizing agents. *Photochem Photobiol* 1997; 65:387–426.

Kubota N, Kakehi M, Inada T: Hyperthermic enhancement of cell killing by five platinum complexes in human malignant melanoma cells grown as monolayer cultures and mutlicellular spheroids. *Int J Radiat Oncol Biol Phys* 1993; 25:491–497.

Kyriakis JM, Banerjee P, Nikolakaki E, et al: The stress-activated protein kinase subfamily of c-jun kinases. *Nature* 1994; 369:156–160.

Landry J, Bernier D, Chretien P, et al: Synthesis and degradation of heat shock proteins during development and decay of thermotolerance. *Cancer Res* 1982; 42:2457–2461.

Law MP: The response of normal tissues to hyperthermia. In: Urano M, Douple E, eds. *Hyperthermia and Oncology*. Utrecht, Netherlands: VSP; 1988; 1:121–159.

Lam S, MacAulay C, Hung J, et al: Detection of dysplasia and carcinoma in situ with a lung imaging fluorescence endoscope. *J Thorac Cardiovasc Surg* 1993; 105:1035–1040.

Leeper D: Molecular and cellular mechanisms of hyperthermia alone or combined with other modalities. In: Overgaard J, ed. *Hyperthermia Oncology*, 1984. London: Taylor and Francis; 1985; 2:9–40.

Leopold KA, Harrelson J, Prosnitz L, et al: Preoperative hyperthermia and radiation for soft tissue sarcomas: Advantage of two vs one hyperthermia treatments per week. *Int J Radiat Oncol Biol Phys*, 1989; 16:107–115.

Levin W, Sherar MD, Cooper B, et al: The effect of vascular occlusion on tumour temperatures during superficial hyperthermia. *Int J Hyperthermia* 1994; 10:495–505.

Li GC, Kal HB: Effect of hyperthermia on the radiation response of two mammalian cell lines. *Eur J Cancer* 1977; 13:65–69.

Li GC, Li L, Lin Y-K, et al: Thermal response of rat fibroblasts stably transfected with the human 70 kDa heat shock protein-encoding gene. *Proc Natl Acad Sci USA* 1991; 88:1681–1685.

Li GC, Mak JY: Re-induction of hsp 70 synthesis: An assay for thermotolerance. *Int J Hyperthermia* 1989; 5:389–403.

Li G, Werb Z: Correlation between synthesis of heat shock proteins and development of thermotolerance in Chinese hamster fibroblasts. *Proc Natl Acad Sci USA* 1982; 79:3218–3222.

Li J-H, Liu F-F: Intracellular pH and heat sensitivity in two human cancer cell lines. *Radiat Oncol* 1997; 42:69–76.

Li XL, Brown SL, Hill RP: Factors influencing the thermosensitivity of two rodent tumors. *Radiat Res* 1992; 130:211–219.

Lightdale CJ, Heier SK, Marcon NE, et al: Photodynamic therapy with porfimer sodium versus thermal ablation therapy with Nd:Yag laser for palliation of esophageal cancer: A multicenter randomized trial. *Gastrointest Endosc* 1995; 42:507–512.

Lilge L, Haw T, Prahl S, et al: Miniature isotropic optical fiber probes for quantitative light dosimetry in tissue. *Phys Med Biol* 1992; 38:215–230.

Lilge L, Olivo M, Schatz S, et al: The sensitivity of normal brain and intracranially implanted VX2 tumour to interstitial photodynamic therapy. *Br J Cancer* 1996;73:332–343.

Lipson RL, Baldes EJ, Gray MJ: Hematoporphyrin derivative for detection and management of cancer. *Cancer* 1967; 20:2255–2257.

Liu F-F, Miller N, Levin W, et al: The potential role of hsp70 as an indicator of response to radiation and hyperthermia treatments for recurrent breast cancer. *Int J Hyperthermia* 1996a; 12:197–208.

Liu F-F, Sherar MD, Hill RP: The relationship between intracellular pH and heat sensitivity in a thermoresistant cell line. *Radiat Res* 1996b; 145:144–149.

Lyons JC, Kim GE, Song CW: Modification of intracellular pH and thermosensitivity. *Radiat Res* 1992; 129:79–87.

Lyons JC, Song CW: Enhancement of hyperthermia effect in vivo by amiloride and DIDS. *Int J Rad Oncol Biol Phys*, 1992; 25:95–103.

Mang TS, McGinnis C, Liebow C, et al: Fluorescence detection of tumors. Early diagnosis of microscopic lesions in preclinical studies. *Cancer* 1993; 71:269–276.

Mayer JL: The clinical efficacy of localized hyperthermia. *Cancer Res (Suppl)* 1984; 44:4745s–4751s.

McMahon KS, Wieman TJ, Moore PH, Fingar VH: Effects of photodynamic therapy using mono-L-aspartyl chlorin e6 on vessel constriction, vessel leakage and tumor response. *Cancer Res* 1994; 54:5374–5379.

Mitchell JB, McPherson S, De Graff W, et al: Oxygen dependence of hematoporphyrin derivative-induced photoinactivation of Chinese hamster cells. *Cancer Res* 1985; 45:2008–2011.

Moan J: On the diffusion length of singlet oxygen in cells and tissues. *J Photochem Photobiol* 1990: B6;343–347.

Moan J, Sommer S: Oxygen dependence of the photosensitizing effect of hematoporphyrin derivative in NHIK 3025 cells. *Cancer Res* 1985; 45:1608–1610.

Moore JV, West CML, Whitehurst C. The biology of photodynamic therapy. *Phys Med Biol* 1997; 42:913–935.

Morimoto, RI: Cells in stress: Transcriptional activation of heat shock genes. *Science* 1993; 259:1409–1410.

Morris CC, Myers R, Field SB: The response of the rat tail to hyperthermia. *Br J Radiol* 1977; 50:576–580.

Muller PM, Wilson BC: Photodynamic therapy for malignant newly diagnosed supratentorial gliomas. *J Clin Laser Med Surg* 1996; 14:263–270.

Mulroney CM, Gluck S, Ho AD: The use of photodynamic therapy in bone marrow purging. *Semin Oncol* 1994; 21 (suppl 15):24–27.

Noodt BB, Berk K, Stokke T, et al: Apoptosis and necrosis induced with light and 5-aminolevulinic acid–derived protoporphyrin IX. *Br J Cancer* 1996; 74:22–29.

North J, Neyndorff H, Levy JG: Photosensitizers as virucidal agents. *J Photochem Photobiol* 1993; B17:99–108.

Nseyo UO: Photodynamic therapy. *Urol Clin North Am* 1992; 19:591–599.

Ochsner M: Photophysical and photobiological processes in the photodynamic therapy of tumours. *J Photochem Photobiol* 1997; B39:1–18.

Oleson JR, Samulski TV, Leopold KA, et al: Sensitivity of

hyperthermia trial outcomes to temperature and time: Implications for thermal goals of treatment. *Int J Radiat Oncol Biol Phys* 1993; 25:289–297.

Overgaard J: Simultaneous and sequential hyperthermia and radiation treatment of an experimental tumor and its surrounding normal tissue in vivo. *Int J Radiat Oncol Biol Phys* 1980; 6:1507–1517.

Overgaard J: The current and potential role of hyperthermia in radiotherapy. *Int J Radiat Oncol Biol Phys* 1989; 16:535–543.

Overgaard J, Gonzalez-Gonzalez D, Hulshof MCCH, et al: Randomized trial of hyperthermia as adjuvant to radiotherapy for recurrent or metastatic malignant melanoma. *Lancet* 1995; 345:540–543.

Overgaard J, Gonzalez-Gonzalez D, Hulshof MCCH, et al: Hyperthermia as an adjuvant to radiation therapy of recurrent or metastatic malignant melanoma: A muticentre randomized trial by the European Society for Hyperthermic Oncology. *Int J Hyperthermia* 1996; 12:3–20.

Overholt BF, Panjehpour M: Photodynamic therapy in Barrett's esophagus. *J Clin Laser Med Surg* 1996; 14:245–249.

Park KYM, Mivechi NF, Auger EA, Hahn GM: Altered regulation of heat shock gene expression in heat resistant mouse cells. *Int J Radiat Oncol Biol Phys* 1989; 28:179–187.

Pass HI, Delaney TF: Photodynamic therapy. In: DeVita VT, Hellman S, Rosenberg SA, eds. *Cancer: Principles and Practice of Oncology*, 4th ed. Philadelphia: Lippincott; 1993:2678–2700.

Patterson MS, Madsen SJ, Wilson BC: Experimental tests of the feasibility of singlet oxygen luminescence monitoring in vivo during photodynamic therapy. *J Photochem Photobiol* 1990; B5:69–84.

Peng Q, Berg K, Moan J, et al: 5-Aminolevulinic acid-based photodynamic therapy: Principles and experimental research. *J Photochem Photobiol* 1997; 65:235–251.

Perez CA, Pajak T, Emami B, et al: Randomized phase III study comparing irradiation and hyperthermia with irradiation alone in superficial measurable tumors: Final report by the Radiation Therapy Oncology Group. *Am J Clin Oncol* 1991; 14:133–141.

Raaphorst GP, Romano SL, Mitchell JB, et al: Intrinsic differences in heat and/or x-ray sensitivity of seven mammalian cell lines cultured and treated under identical conditions. *Cancer Res* 1979; 39:396–401.

Raaphorst GP: Thermal radiosensitization in vitro. In: Urano M, Douple E, eds. *Hyperthermia and Oncology*. Utrecht, Netherlands: VSP; 1989; 2:17–51.

Raaphorst GP, Yang H, Wilkins DE, Ng CE: Cisplatin, hyperthermia and radiation treatment in human cisplatin-sensitive and resistant glioma cell lines. *Int J Hyperthermia* 1996; 12:801–812.

Raingeaud J, Gupta S, Rogers JS, et al: Pro-inflammatory cytokines and environmental stress cause p38 mitogen-activated protein kinase activation by dual phosphory-lation on tyrosine and threonine. *J Biol Chem* 1995; 270:7420–7426.

Reddi E: Role of delivery vehicles for photosensitizers in the photodynamic therapy of tumours. *J Photochem Photobiol* 1997; B37:189–195.

Reinhold HS: Physiological effects of hyperthermia. *Rec Results Cancer Res* 1988; 107:32–43.

Rhee JG, Eddy HA, Hamson GH, Salazar OM: Heat-sensitive state of mouse mammary carcinoma cells in tumors. *Radiat Res* 1990; 123:165–170.

Richter AM, Waterfield E, Jain AK, et al: Photosensitizing potency of structural analogues of benzoporphyrin derivative (BPD) in a mouse tumour model. *Br J Cancer* 1993; 63:87–93.

Rietbroek RC, Schilthuis MS, Bakker PJ, et al: Phase II trial of weekly locoregional hyperthermia and cisplatin in patients with a previously irradiated recurrent carcinoma of the uterine cervix. *Cancer* 1997; 79:935–943.

Ris NH, Altermatt HJ, Stewart JCM, et al: Photodynamic therapy with meta-tetrahydroxylphenylchlorin in vivo: Optimization of the therapeutic index. *Int J Cancer* 1993; 55:245–249.

Robins HI, Rushing D, Kutz M, et al: Phase I clinical trial of melphalan and 41.8 degrees C whole-body hyperthermia in cancer patients. *J Clin Oncol* 1997; 15:158–164.

Rofstad EK: Influence of cellular, microenvironmental, and growth parameters on thermotolerance kinetics in vivo in human melanoma xenografts. *Cancer Res* 1989; 49:5027–5032.

Russo A, Mitchell JB, Pass HI, Glatstein EJ: Photodynamic therapy. In: De Vita VT, Hellman S, Rosenberg SA, eds. *Cancer: Principles and Practice of Oncology*, 3d ed. Philadelphia: Lippincott; 1989:2449–2460.

Sapareto SA, Dewey WC: Thermal dose determination in cancer therapy. *Int J Radiat Oncol Biol Phys* 1984; 10:787–800.

Sharkey SM, Wilson BC, Moorehead R, Singh G: Mitochondrial alterations in photodynamic therapy resistant cells. *Cancer Res* 1993; 53:4994–4999.

Sherar M, Liu F-F, Pintilie M, et al: Relationship between thermal dose and outcome in thermoradiotherapy treatments for superficial recurrences of breast cancer: Data from a phase III trial. *Int J Radiat Oncol Biol Phys* 1997; 39:371–380.

Song CW: Effect of local hyperthermia on blood flow and microenvironment: A review. *Cancer Res (Suppl)* 1984; 44:4721s–4730s.

Song CW, Kang MS, Rhee JC, Levitt SH: Vascular damage and delayed cell death in tumors after hyperthermia. *Br J Cancer* 1980; 41:309–312.

Song CW, Lyons JC, Griffin RJ, et al: Increase in thermosensitivity of tumor cells by lowering intracellular pH. *Cancer Res* 1993 53:1599–1601.

Song CW, Kim GE, Lyons JC, et al: Thermosensitization by increasing intracellular acidity with amiloride and its analogs. *Int J Radiat Oncol Biol Phys* 1994; 30:1161–1169.

Star WM: Light dosimetry in vivo. *Phys Med Biol* 1997; 42: 763–788.

Star WM, Marijnissen HPA, ven den Berg-Blok AE, et al: Destruction of rat mammary tumor and normal tissue microcirculation by hematoporphyrin derivative photoradiation observed in vivo in sandwich observation chambers. *Cancer Res* 1986; 46:2532–2540.

Star WM, Wilson BC, Patterson MS: Light delivery and optical dosimetry in photodynamic therapy of solid tumors. In: Dougherty TJ, Henderson BW, eds. *Photodynamic Therapy*. New York: Marcel Dekker; 1992: 335–365.

Sutedja T, Lam S, LeRichie JC, Postmus PE: Response and pattern of failure after photodynamic therapy for intraluminal stage I lung cancer. *J Bronchol* 1994; 1:295–298.

Valdagni R: Two versus six hyperthermia treatments in combination with radical irradiation for fixed metastatic nodes: Progress report. *Rec Results Cancer Res* 1988; 107:123–128.

Valdagni R, Amichetti M: Report of long-term follow-up in a randomized trial comparing radiation therapy and radiation therapy plus hyperthermia to metastatic lymph nodes in stage IV head and neck patients. *Int J Radiat Oncol Biol Phys* 1993; 28:163–169.

Valdagni R, Amichetti M, Pani G: Radical radiation alone versus radical radiation plus microwave hyperthermia for N_3(TMN-UICC) neck nodes: A prospective randomized clinical trial. *Int J Radiat Oncol Biol Phys* 1988; 15:13–24.

van der Zee J: Radio-thermotherapy of deep pelvic tumours: Results of Dutch studies, Sixteenth Annual Meeting of the North American Hyperthermia Society, Providence, RI, p 9, May 3–7, 1997, p 9.

Vaupel P, Kallinowski F: Physiological effects of hyperthermia. *Rec Results Cancer Res* 1987; 104:71–109.

Vaupel P, Kallinowski F, Kluge M: Pathophysiology of tumors in hyperthermia. *Rec Results Cancer Res* 1988; 107:65–75.

Wang A, Armour EP, Corry PM, Martinez A: Elimination of dose-rate effects by mild hyperthermia. *Int J Radiat Oncol Biol Phys* 1992; 24:965–973.

Waterman FM, Tupchong L, Nerlinger RE, Mathews J: Blood flow in human tumors during local hyperthermia. *Int J Radiat Oncol Biol Phys* 1991; 20:1255–1262.

Weersink RA, Hayward JE, Diamond KR, Patterson MS: Accuracy of noninvasive in vivo measurements of photosensitizer uptake based on a diffusion model of reflectance spectroscopy. *Photochem Photobiol* 1997; 66: 326–335.

Wike–Hooley JL, Haveman J, Reinhold HS: The relevance of tumour pH to the treatment of malignant disease. *Radiother Oncol* 1984; 2:343–366.

Wilson BD, Patterson MS, Lilge L: Implicit and explicit dosimetry in photodynamic therapy: A new paradigm. *Lasers Med Sci* 1997; 12:182–199.

Wilson BD, Bernstein Z, Sommer C, et al: Photodynamic therapy for Kaposi's sarcoma using photofrin and tin ethyl etiopurpurin (SnET2). *Invest Dermatol* 1995; 104: 693–697.

Wilson BD, Mang TS, Stoll H, et al: Photodynamic therapy for the treatment of basal cell carcinoma. *Arch Dermatol* 1992; 128:1597–1601.

Yatvin MB, Cramp WA: Role of cellular membranes in hyperthermia: some observations and theories reviewed. *Int J Hyperthermia* 1993; 9:165–185.

Young SW, Woodburn KW, Wright M, et al: Lutetium texafrin (PCI-0123): A near-infrared, water-soluble photosensitizer. *J Photochem Photobiol* 1996; B63:892–897.

Zaidi SI, Oleinick NL, Zaim MT, Mukhtar H: Apoptosis during photodynamic therapy-induced ablation of RIF-1 tumors in C3H mice: Electron microscopic, histopathologic and biochemical evidence. *J Photochem Photobiol* 1993; B58:771–776.

Zanke BW, Boudreau K, Rubie E, et al: The stress-activated protein kinase pathway mediates cell death following injury induced by *cis*-platinum, UV irradiation or heat. *Curr Biol* 1996; 5:606–613.

20

Guide to Studies of Diagnostic Tests, Prognostic Factors, and Treatments

Martin R. Stockler, Norman F. Boyd, and Ian F. Tannock

20.1 INTRODUCTION
    20.1.1 Uncertainty, Random Error, and Bias

20.2 DIAGNOSIS
    20.2.1 Diagnostic Tests as Discriminators
    20.2.2 Sources of Bias in Evaluation of Tests
    20.2.3 Bayes' Theorem and Likelihood Ratios
    20.2.4 Diagnostic Tests for Screening of Disease

20.3 PROGNOSIS
    20.3.1 Sources of Bias in Prognostic Studies
    20.3.2 Evaluation of Prognostic Factors
    20.3.3 Uses and Limitations of Prognostic Information

20.4 TREATMENT
    20.4.1 Purpose of Clinical Trials

20.4.2 Sources of Bias in Clinical Trials
20.4.3 Allocation of Treatments: Randomization
20.4.4 Choice and Assessment of Outcomes
20.4.5 Survival Curves and Their Comparison
20.4.6 Statistical Issues
20.4.7 Meta-analysis
20.4.8 Assessment of Quality of Life
20.4.9 Clinical Decision Making
20.4.10 Economic Analyses

20.5 SUMMARY

REFERENCES

BIBLIOGRAPHY

20.1 INTRODUCTION

Clinical oncologists must be experts in the application of diagnostic tests, the estimation of prognosis, and the selection of therapy for people with cancer. They must therefore be able to select, evaluate, and interpret relevant clinical studies from the burgeoning literature of medical research. This chapter provides a critical overview of methods used in clinical research.

20.1.1 Uncertainty, Random Error, and Bias

The outcome of the treatment of individuals with cancer is inherently unpredictable. In a given individual, we cannot know beforehand whether a resected tumor is destined to relapse without adjuvant treatment or whether adjuvant treatment will prevent relapse. Individuals with similar types of cancer live for different lengths of time, develop different complications, react differently to them, and respond differently to the same treatments. Clinical studies are carried out with the intention of extrapolating results from a sample of individuals to the wider population of all individuals who appear to have disease of similar type. The results in the sample are used to *estimate* what will happen in a future population. As our knowledge of mechanisms of cancer growth and development has increased (see earlier chapters), so has our ability to define the relevant characteristics of our sample more precisely and hence to extrapolate more effectively to the wider population. However, substantial heterogeneity exists between individuals with ostensibly similar disease.

Random error is the imprecision that occurs when measurements of a parameter from a random sample of individuals are used to estimate the value of the parameter among all such individuals. Random error can be quantified and expressed with confidence intervals. The precision of an estimate depends on the degree of heterogeneity among the sample population (often unknown) and on the number of subjects on which it is based: the larger the number of subjects, the more precise the estimate. However, even substantial numbers of subjects produce estimates with wide ranges of plausible values. For example, an estimated response rate of 50 percent based on a sample of 100 patients will have a 95 percent confidence interval of 40 to 60 percent.

Bias is more sinister. A biased estimate is one that differs systematically from the truth. This occurs when the sample represents a systematically different population from the population of interest. Suppose we are interested in the response rate for a new anticancer drug in people with a particular type of cancer. Estimates of this response rate based on a sample of patients with good performance status and no comorbid disease are likely to overestimate the response rate among all patients with that cancer. The effect of bias is not reduced by increasing the number of subjects.

Good clinical studies are designed to provide reliable estimates by avoiding bias and accounting for random error.

20.2 DIAGNOSIS

Diagnostic tests are used to establish the existence or extent of cancer among people suspected of having cancer, screen for cancer among people who are symptom free, and follow changes in the extent and severity of the disease during therapy. The evaluation of diagnostic tests usually focuses on aspects of test performance—i.e., the ability of the test to detect or monitor disease. Although test performance is important, the usefulness of a test must be gauged by its impact on the lives of those being tested. The application of a test may influence both duration and quality of life. Unfortunately, these crucial outcomes are rarely evaluated.

20.2.1 Diagnostic Tests as Discriminators

Diagnostic tests are used to help distinguish between those people with a particular cancer (or sites of involvement by cancer) and those without it. Test results may be expressed quantitatively on a continuous scale or qualitatively on a categorical scale. The results of serum tumor marker tests, such as prostate-specific antigen (PSA), are usually expressed quantitatively as a concentration, whereas the results of imaging tests, such as a computed tomography (CT) scan, are usually expressed qualitatively as normal or abnormal.

If a quantitative test is to be used to distinguish subjects with or without cancer, then a cutoff point must be selected that distinguishes positive results from negative results. Quantitative test results are often reported with a normal or reference range. This is the range of values obtained from some arbitrary proportion, usually 95 percent, of apparently healthy individuals; the corollary is that 5 percent of apparently healthy people will have values outside this range. This statistical definition of normal is quite different from the clinical definition of normal: the absence of disease. Diagnostic test results are rarely conclusive about the presence or absence of disease such as cancer; more often they just raise or lower the likelihood that it is present.

The effects of choosing different cutoff points for a diagnostic test are shown in Fig. 20.1. A cutoff point at level *A* provides some separation of subjects with and without cancer, but because of overlap, there is always some misclassification. If the cutoff point is increased to level *C*, fewer subjects without cancer are misclassified but more people with cancer fall below the cutoff and will be incorrectly classified. A lower cutoff point at level *B* has the opposite effect: more subjects with cancer are correctly classified, but at the cost of misclassifying larger numbers of people without cancer. This tradeoff between the ability of a test to identify people with and

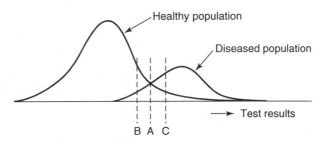

Figure 20.1. Interpretation of a diagnostic test (e.g., PSA for prostate cancer) requires the selection of a cutoff point that separates negative from positive results. The position of the cutoff point (which might be set at A, B, or C) influences the proportion of patients who are incorrectly classified as being healthy or having disease.

without disease correctly is a feature of all diagnostic tests.

The test for serum levels of prostate-specific antigen (PSA) provides a useful example. The reported normal range for serum PSA level is < 4 ng/mL, a definition based on the distribution of PSA levels in apparently healthy men. A level of PSA < 4 ng/mL lowers the likelihood of prostate cancer but does not rule it out, since some men with prostate cancer have low levels of PSA. A PSA level >8 ng/mL increases the likelihood of prostate cancer but does not make it certain, since some men without prostate cancer will have levels of this magnitude. Progressively higher levels of PSA are associated with progressively higher likelihood of prostate cancer.

To assess how well a diagnostic test discriminates between those with and without disease, it is necessary to have an independent means of classifying those with and without disease—a "gold standard." This might be the findings of surgery, the results of a biopsy, or the clinical outcome of patients after prolonged follow-up. If direct confirmation of the presence of disease is not possible, the results of another diagnostic test whose properties are known from previous studies may be the best standard available.

Simultaneously classifying the subjects into diseased (D +) and nondiseased (D −) according to the gold-standard test and positive (T +) or negative (T −) according to the diagnostic test being assessed defines four subpopulations (Fig. 20.2).

These are true positives (TP: people with the disease in whom the test is positive), true negatives (TN: people without the disease in whom the test is negative), false positives (FP: people without the disease in whom the test is positive), and false negatives (FN: people with the disease in whom the test is negative). The proportion of people with disease is referred to as *the prevalence of disease*. The prevalence of disease among those tested is usually higher than that in the general population, because diagnostic (or screening) tests are often applied to a population that is believed to have a higher risk of disease for some prior reason (e.g., suspicious symptoms, family history of cancer, or exposure to a specific risk factor).

Test performance can be described by indices calculated from the 2×2 table shown in Fig. 20.2. "Vertical" indices are calculated from the columns of the table and describe the frequency with which the test is positive or negative in people whose disease status is known. These indices include sensitivity (the proportion of people with disease who test positive) and specificity (the proportion of people without disease who test negative). These indices are characteristic of the particular test and do not depend on the prevalence of disease in the population being tested. The sensitivity and specificity of a test can be applied directly to populations with differing prevalence of disease.

"Horizontal" indices are calculated from the rows of the table and describe the frequency of disease in individuals whose test status is known. These indices

Disease Status

Test Result		Disease present (D+)	Disease absent (D−)
	Test positive (T+)	True positive (TP) T+D+	False positive (FP) T+D−
	Test negative (T+)	False negative (FN) T−D+	True negative (TN) T−D−

Figure 20.2. Selection of a cutoff point for a diagnostic test defines four subpopulations as shown. Predictive values (but not sensitivity and specificity) depend on the prevalence of disease in the population tested.

"Vertical properties" calculated from columns:

$$\text{Sensitivity} = \text{TP}/(\text{TP}+\text{FN})$$
$$\text{Specificity} = \text{TN}/(\text{TN}+\text{FP})$$
$$\text{False-negative rate} = \text{FN}/(\text{FN}+\text{TP})$$
$$\text{False-positive rate} = \text{FP}/(\text{FP}+\text{TN})$$

"Horizontal properties" calculated from rows:

$$\text{Prior probability (prevalence)} = (\text{TP}+\text{FN})/(\text{TP}+\text{FN}+\text{FP}+\text{TN})$$
$$\text{Posterior probability (positive predictive value)} = \text{TP}/(\text{TP}+\text{FP})$$
$$\text{Negative predictive value} = \text{TN}/(\text{TN}+\text{FN})$$

indicate the predictive value of a test—for example, the probability that a person testing positive has the disease (positive predictive value) or the probability that a person testing negative does not have the disease (negative predictive value). These indices depend on characteristics of both the test (sensitivity and specificity) and the population being tested (prevalence of disease). The predictive value of a test cannot be applied directly to populations with differing prevalence of disease.

Figure 20.3 illustrates the influence of disease prevalence on the performance of a hypothetical test assessed in populations with high, intermediate, and low prevalence of disease. Sensitivity and specificity are constant, since they are independent of prevalence. As the prevalence of disease declines— as it would, for example, if subjects in the general population were studied instead of patients in a hospital—the positive predictive value of the test declines. This occurs because, although the *proportions* of TP results among diseased subjects and FP results among non-diseased subjects remain the same, the *absolute numbers* of TP and FP results differ. In the high-prevalence population, the absolute number of false positives (10) is small in comparison with the absolute number of true positives (80): a positive result is eight times more likely to come from a subject with disease than a subject without disease, and the positive predictive value of the test is relatively high. In the low-prevalence population, the absolute number of false positives (1000) is large in comparison with the absolute number of true positives (80): a positive result is 12.5 times more likely to come from a subject without disease, and the positive predictive value is relatively low. For this reason, diagnostic tests that may be useful in patients where

there is already suspicion of disease (high-prevalence situation) may not be of value as screening tests in a less selected population (low-prevalence situation, see Sec. 20.2.4).

The 2×2 table and the indices derived from it (Fig. 20.2) provide a simple and convenient method for describing test performance at a single cutoff point; however, they give no indication of the effect of using different cutoff points. The effects on test performance of using different cutoff points can be assessed with several 2×2 tables, one for each cutoff point, but this is cumbersome. The receiver-operating-characteristic (ROC) curve is a powerful method for summarizing the effects of different cutoff points on sensitivity, specificity, and test performance.

Examples of ROC curves are shown in Fig. 20.4. The ROC curve plots the true-positive rate (TPR, which equals sensitivity) against the false-positive rate (FPR, which equals $1 -$ specificity) for different cutoff values. The "best" cutoff point is the one that offers the best compromise between TP and FP rates. This is represented by the point on the ROC curve closest to the upper-left-hand corner. The performance of a test across the range of cutoff points is summarized by the area under the ROC curve: the greater the area under the curve, the better the test. A worthless test, equivalent to tossing a coin, has an area under the curve of 0.5; a perfect test has an area under the curve of unity.

Altering the cutoff point for a test has opposite effects on its sensitivity and specificity. For example, lowering the cutoff point above which a serum PSA level is regarded as abnormal will increase its sensitivity for detecting prostate cancer (increases the number of true positives—men with prostate can-

High Prevalence (50%)

	D⁺	D⁻		
T⁺	80	10	Sensitivity	80%
			Specificity	90%
T⁻	20	90	Predictive Value (+)	89%

Intermediate Prevalence (~9%)

	D⁺	D⁻		
T⁺	80	100	Sensitivity	80%
			Specificity	90%
T⁻	20	900	Predictive Value (+)	44%

Low Prevalence (~1%)

	D⁺	D⁻		
T⁺	80	1000	Sensitivity	80%
			Specificity	90%
T⁻	20	9000	Predictive Value (+)	7.4%

Figure 20.3. Test properties and disease prevalence. Examples of application of a diagnostic test to populations in which disease has high, intermediate, or low prevalence. The predictive value of the test decreases when there is a low prevalence of disease.

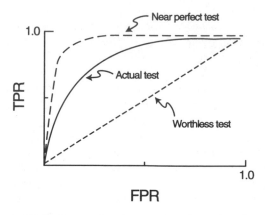

Figure 20.4. Curves showing receiver operating characteristics (ROCs) in which the true-positive rate (TPR) is plotted against the false-positive rate (FPR) of a diagnostic test as the cutoff point is varied. The performance of the test is indicated by the shape of the curve, as shown.

cer and with a PSA level above the cutoff) but will decrease its specificity (increases the number of false positives—men without prostate cancer but with a PSA level above the cutoff). This relationship is reflected by the the shape of the ROC curve.

20.2.2 Sources of Bias in Evaluation of Tests

The performance of a diagnostic test is usually evaluated in a research study to estimate its usefulness in clinical practice. Differences between the conditions under which a test is evaluated and the conditions under which it will be used may produce misleading results. Important factors relating both to the people being tested and the methods being used are summarized in Table 20.1 (see also Jaeschke et al., 1994). Important characteristics of the people being tested include the distribution among them of different disease states, the prevalence of comorbid conditions, and the range of pathologic subtypes. Important characteristics of the methods include how the diagnostic test was applied, how disease status was classified, and how test status and disease status were compared. Distortions in these factors often produce optimistic estimates of test performance (Ransohoff and Feinstein, 1978).

Diagnostic tests are used in clinical practice to help select those people who have a disease from a larger group of people who are suspected of having the disease. The suspicion of disease may be prompted by symptoms or signs suggesting the presence of disease, a history of exposure to a suspected risk-factor, or the presence of an associated condi-

tion. For example, the performance of a chest x-ray to diagnose lung cancer may be provoked by a history of hemoptysis, heavy smoking, or the presence of another tobacco-related disease. An adequate evaluation of test performance requires a sample of people who are representative of the people selected for testing in clinical practice.

If a test is to be used to identify patients with colon cancer, then the study sample should include people with both localized and advanced disease (a wide clinical spectrum). The sample should also include people with other clinical conditions that might be mistaken for colon cancer (e.g. diverticular disease) in order to evaluate the ability of the test to distinguish between these conditions. People with associated diseases that might complicate the detection and diagnosis of colon cancer (e.g., ulcerative colitis) should also be included (comorbid spectrum). If there are different histologic types of a cancer, then the test should be evaluated in a sample including these different histologic types (pathologic spectrum).

The evaluation of diagnostic test performance requires subjects to be classified by both disease status (diseased or nondiseased) and test status (positive or negative). For the evaluation to be valid, the two acts of classification must be independent. If either the classification of disease status is influenced by the test result or the interpretation of the test result is influenced by disease status, then there will be an inappropriate and optimistic estimate of test performance (see below and Table 20.1).

Table 20.1. Factors That May Distort the Estimated Performance of a Diagnostic Test

Spectrum of patients used for evaluation of the test
  Clinical spectrum: Should include patients with a wide range of features of the disease
  Comorbid spectrum: Should include patients with a wide range of other diseases
  Pathologic spectrum: Should include patients with a range of histological types of disease

Potential sources of bias in test evaluation
  Exclusion of equivocal cases
  Workup bias: Results of the test influence the choice of subsequent tests that confirm or refute diagnosis
  Test review bias: Results of the test influence the interpretation of subsequent tests to establish diagnosis
  Diagnostic review bias: Knowledge of the disease influences the interpretation of the test
  Incorporation bias: Test information is used as a criterion to establish diagnosis

Workup bias arises if the results of the diagnostic test under evaluation influence the choice of other tests used to determine the subject's disease status. For example, suppose that the performance of the serum tumor marker CA-125 is to be evaluated as an indicator of ovarian cancer by comparing it with the results of laparotomy. Workup bias will occur if only women with high CA-125 levels are selected for laparotomy, since ovarian cancer in women with normal CA-125 levels will remain undetected; this leads to an exaggerated estimate of the predictive value of CA-125 testing.

Test-review bias and *diagnostic-review bias* occur when the subjective interpretation of one test is influenced by knowledge of the result of another test. For example, a radiologist's interpretation of an abdominal CT scan might be influenced by knowledge of a surgeon's findings at laparotomy (test-review bias); alternatively, a surgeon's interpretation of the findings at laparotomy might be influenced by knowledge of the results of a preoperative CT scan. *Incorporation bias* is the most obvious violation of independence. It arises when the test being evaluated is itself incorporated into the classification of disease status.

20.2.3 Bayes' Theorem and Likelihood Ratios

The results of diagnostic tests are rarely conclusive about the presence or absence of disease; rather, they raise or lower the probability that disease is present (Jaeschke et al., 1994). Similar statements may be made about evidence relating to a prognostic factor (Sec. 20.3) or the results of a clinical trial (Sec. 20.4). Clinical trials rarely give definitive evidence that one treatment is better than another; they merely change the probability that this is so. These concepts are embodied in *Bayes' theorem*. This theorem allows an initial estimate of the probability that a disease is present (or, in a clinical trial, that one treatment is better) to be adjusted to take account of new information from a diagnostic test (or a clinical trial) to produce a revised estimate of the probability that the disease is present (or one treatment is better). The initial estimate is referred to as the *prior* or *pretest probability*; the revised estimate is the *posterior* or *posttest probability*.

For example, the pretest probability of breast cancer in a 45-year-old American woman presenting for screening mammography is about 3 in 1000 (pretest probability or prevalence of disease in women of this age). If her mammogram is reported as "suspicious for malignancy," then her posttest probability of having breast cancer rises to about 300 in 1000;

whereas if the mammogram is reported as "normal," then her posttest probability of having breast cancer falls to about 0.4 in 1000 (Kerlikowske et al., 1996).

Bayes' theorem describes the mathematical relationship between the new posttest probability, the former prior probability (i.e., the prevalence of disease in the tested population), and the additional information provided by the diagnostic test (or clinical trial). This relationship can be expressed with two formulas that look different but are logically equivalent. For a diagnostic test with the characteristics defined in Fig. 20.2, *the probability form of Bayes' theorem* can be expressed as

Posttest probability =

$$\frac{\text{sensitivity} \times \text{prevalence}}{(\text{sensitivity} \times \text{prevalence}) + (1 - \text{specificity})(1 - \text{prevalence})}$$

The alternative form of Bayes' theorem is expressed in terms of a likelihood ratio and is much easier to use. The *likelihood ratio* is a useful concept that for any test result represents the ratio of the probability that disease is present to the probability that it is absent. For a positive diagnostic test, the likelihood ratio is the likelihood that the positive test represents a true positive rather than a false positive:

Likelihood ratio of a positive test result
= true-positive rate/false-positive rate
= sensitivity/(1−specificity)

For a negative diagnostic test, the likelihood ratio is the likelihood that the negative result represents a false negative rather than a true negative (i.e., false-negative rate/true-negative rate).

Thus a good diagnostic test has a high likelihood ratio for a positive test (ideally greater than 10) and a low likelihood ratio for a negative test (ideally less than 0.1).

The alternative expression for Bayes' theorem also uses odds instead of probabilities. Odds and probabilities are closely related: the odds of an event is the probability of it happening divided by the probability of it not happening

Odds = probability/(1−probability)
Probability = odds/(odds+1)

For probabilities less than about 0.1, the odds and the probability are almost equal.

The *odds form of Bayes' theorem* relates the odds of disease in those who test positive (posterior or posttest odds) to the odds of disease before testing (prior or pretest odds) and the likelihood ratio of a positive test result:

Posterior odds = prior odds × likelihood ratio of a positive result

Similarly, for a negative test result:

Posterior odds = prior odds × likelihood ratio of a negative result

Usually we wish to know the probability that disease is present (rather than the odds), and interconversion between odds and probability is facilitated by using the nomogram shown in Fig. 20.5 (Fagan, 1975; Jaeschke et al., 1994). Returning to the example of mammography applied to a 45-year-old woman, the likelihood ratio of a mammogram reported as "suspicious for malignancy" is about 144, so that a mammogram reported in this way increases her probability of having breast cancer from about 3 in 1000 to about 300 in 1000 (30 percent). For a negative mammogram, the likelihood ratio is about 0.14, so that her probability of having breast cancer is reduced to about 0.4 in 1000. Unfortunately, most abnormal screening mammograms are reported as "additional evaluation needed"; a category that is associated with a likelihood ratio of about 7 and which raises the probability of breast cancer being present from about 0.3 percent to 2 percent (Kerilowski et al., 1966).

20.2.4 Diagnostic Tests for Screening of Disease

Death and recurrence of disease are the commonest outcomes measured in studies evaluating the impact of diagnostic tests in cancer. Diagnostic tests can also influence quality of life, but this is rarely assessed. For example, tests used for early diagnosis might lead to a reduction in the number of people suffering disease-related morbidity and might provide reassurance (perhaps false) for people with negative test results; however, these tests might also lead to an increase in the number of people suffering from treatment-related morbidity and might prolong the anxiety associated with the knowledge of having cancer.

Several types of bias may affect studies that evaluate the impact of diagnostic testing on survival. For example, the survival from diagnosis of women with breast cancer detected by screening mammography is superior to that of women with breast cancer detected in other ways; however, this does not necessar-

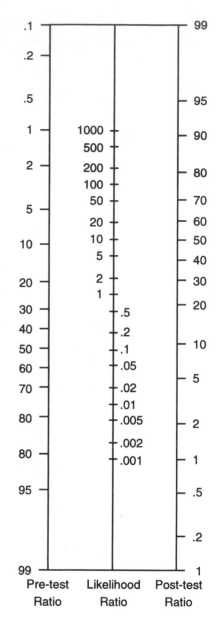

Figure 20.5. Nomogram for interpreting results of diagnostic tests, using the likelihood ratio (From Jaeschke et al., 1994, with permission.)

ily mean that mammography has prolonged their lives. Survival will appear to be better in the women diagnosed by mammography even if mammography and subsequent treatment have no effect on the clinical course of the disease. This paradox results from two types of bias: length-time bias and lead-time bias.

Length-time bias is illustrated in Fig. 20.6. The horizontal lines in the figure represent the length of time from the inception of disease to the death of the patient. Long lines indicate slowly progressing disease and short lines rapidly progressing disease.

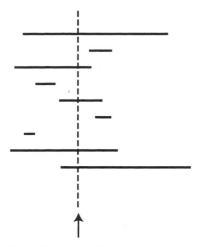

Point of application of screening test

Horizontal lines represent the length of time that disease is present prior to the death of the patient.

Figure 20.6. Illustration of length-time bias in a screening test. The test is more likely to detect disease that is present for a long time (i.e., slowly growing disease). Horizontal lines represent the length of time that disease is present prior to the death of the patient.

A single examination, such as screening for breast cancer with mammography (represented in the figure by the dashed vertical line), will intersect (detect) a larger number of long lines (people with indolent disease) than short lines (people with aggressive disease). Thus, a screening examination will selectively identify those people with slowly progressing disease.

Lead-time bias is illustrated in Fig. 20.7. The purpose of many diagnostic tests, and of all tests that are used to screen healthy people, is to allow clinicians to identify disease at an earlier point in its clinical course than would be possible without the test. Four critical time points in the clinical course of the disease are indicated in Fig. 20.7: the time of disease inception (0), the time at which the disease becomes incurable (1), the time of diagnosis under ordinary circumstances (2), and the time of death (3).

Many patients with common cancers are incurable by the time that their disease is diagnosed. The aim of screening tests is to advance the time of diagnosis to a point where the disease is curable. Even if the cancer is incurable despite the earlier time of diagnosis, survival will appear to be prolonged by early detection because of the additional time (the lead-time) that the disease is known to be present (Fig. 20.7). In screening for breast cancer with

mammography, the lead time is estimated to be about 2 years. Advancing the date of diagnosis may be beneficial if it increases the chance of cure. However, if it does not increase the chance of cure, then advancing the date of diagnosis may be detrimental, because patients spend a longer time with the knowledge that they have incurable disease.

Disease-specific mortality is the proportion of people in a population who die of a given disease in 1 year. For disease-specific mortality, the denominator is the whole population; it is therefore independent of factors that influence the time of diagnosis of disease. In contrast, the case fatality rate is the proportion of patients with the disease who die in 1 year; the denominator is the number of cases, which depends strongly on factors such as length and lead-time bias.

The strongest study design for evaluating the impact of a diagnostic or screening test involves the randomization of people to either have or not have the test. The end points assessed in such a trial should reflect the outcomes considered most important in that situation: overall survival, disease-specific survival, and quality of life. Randomized trials have demonstrated reductions in mortality rates associated with mammographic screening for breast

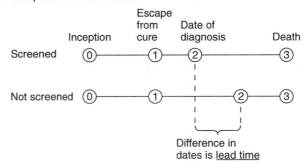

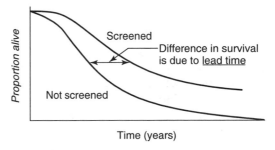

Figure 20.7. Illustration of lead-time bias. *A.* Application of a test may lead to earlier diagnosis without changing the course of disease. *B.* There is an improvement in survival when measured from time of diagnosis.

cancer in post-menopausal women (Nystrom et al., 1991; Kerlikowske et al., 1995) and with fecal occult blood testing for colorectal carcinoma (Hardcastle et al., 1996; Kronberg et al., 1996). Randomized trials have failed to demonstrate any benefit associated with screening for lung cancer (Eddy, 1989). Randomized trials to assess the usefulness of screening tests for prostate cancer are a major public health priority (Krahn et al., 1994).

Randomized trials can also be used to compare the utility of alternative approaches to follow-up. Here the goal is detection of recurrence or metastases following initial treatment of the primary cancer. Two recent studies compared the effects of two policies of follow-up testing on overall survival and quality of life following treatment for early breast cancer: intensive follow-up testing with routine x-rays, bone scans, and serum biochemistry versus less intensive follow-up with testing only when clinically indicated. Neither study demonstrated an advantage for more intensive follow-up testing (GIVIO Investigators, 1994; Rosseli Del Turco et al., 1994).

20.3 PROGNOSIS

A prognosis is a forecast of expected course and outcome. It may apply to the unique circumstances of an individual or to the general circumstances of a group. Individuals with apparently similar types of cancer live for different lengths of time, have different patterns of progression, and respond differently to the same treatments. Variables associated with the outcome of a disease that can account for some of this heterogeneity are known as *prognostic factors*.

Several variables related to the tumor, such as tumor size and extent, or to the host, such as physical performance status, are associated with the outcome of most types of cancer. An increasing number of biological factors, such as degree of tumor hypoxia or p53 status, have also been found to convey prognostic information. Differences in prognostic characteristics often account for bigger differences in outcome than do differences in treatment. For example, in women with primary breast cancer, differences in survival according to lymph node status are much greater than differences in survival according to treatment (Fig. 20.8). Imbalances in the distribution of such important prognostic factors in clinical trials which compare different treatments may produce biased results by either obscuring true differences or creating spurious ones. Furthermore, the effects of treatment may be different in patients with differing prognostic characteristics.

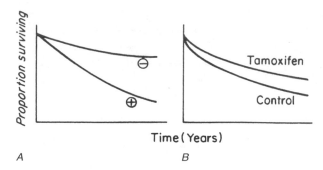

Figure 20.8. Factors that influence survival of postmenopausal patients with primary breast cancer. *A.* Involvement of axillary lymph nodes by disease. *B.* Treatment with tamoxifen. Note that the prognostic influence of nodal involvement is much greater than the effect of treatment.

20.3.1 Sources of Bias in Prognostic Studies

The prognosis of patients seen in clinical practice is usually based on studies of patients who are referred to academic centers and/or who participate in clinical studies. Differences between general clinical practice and clinical research may then lead to misleading conclusions. Patients who are referred to academic centers may differ systematically from others with the same type of malignancy, leading to *referral bias;* also, those who participate in clinical trials appear to have different (generally better) outcomes than those who do not participate in clinical trials, regardless of their allocated treatment (Antman et al., 1985; Davis et al., 1985; Karjalainen and Palva, 1989). Thus population-based data—for example, data from cancer registries—may provide more pertinent information regarding prognosis than data from highly selected patients referred to academic centers or enrolled in clinical trials.

The relative influence of a prognostic factor in a disease is less likely to be affected by referral bias than the absolute estimate of prognosis for that disease. For example, if hormone-receptor status influences survival, it is likely to do so within each center, even if the absolute survival of patients differs between centers. Ideally, a prognostic study should include all identified cases within a large, geographically defined area.

Study of the clinical course of a particular group of patients requires selection of a specific time in their disease history (called *zero time*) at which the patients will be characterized and from which their subsequent survival will be measured. Thus, in a study of the influence of estrogen receptors on the survival of patients with breast cancer, the zero time might be specified as the time of diagnosis of breast cancer; receptor status would be characterized at that time, and survival time would be recorded for patients with different receptor values. A group of such patients is referred to as an *inception cohort* (Feinstein, 1985). The zero-time point is often the time of diagnosis, but it could be some other suitable point in time. For example, for the study of prognosis of patients with metastatic breast cancer, zero time might be the date at which metastases were first identified.

Objective criteria, independent of knowledge of the patients' initial prognostic characteristics, must be used to assess the relevant outcomes such as disease recurrence or cause of death. Workup bias, test-review bias, and diagnostic review bias, discussed in Sec. 20.2.2, have their counterparts in studies of prognosis. For example, a follow-up bone scan in patients with breast cancer that is equivocal may be more likely to be read as positive (i.e., indicating recurrence of disease) if it is known that the patient initially had extensive lymph node involvement or that she subsequently developed proven bone metastases. To avoid these biases, all patients should be assessed with the same frequency, using the same tests, interpreted with the same explicit criteria and without knowledge of the patient's initial characteristics or subsequent course.

Complete follow-up is also important. Patients may be lost to follow-up for many reasons, some of which may be related to the outcome of their disease. For example, patients lost to follow-up may have died or sought treatment elsewhere. Both incomplete follow-up and incomplete information may introduce bias (see also Laupacis et al., 1994).

20.3.2 Evaluation of Prognostic Factors

Two broad approaches to the analysis of prognostic factors can be identified: exploratory and confirmatory (Tukey, 1977). In an exploratory analysis, the data are used to identify apparent patterns and relationships; the emphasis is on description and the generation of hypotheses. In confirmatory analyses, data are used to quantify the level of support for prespecified hypotheses; the emphasis is on criticism and the testing of hypotheses.

Most studies evaluate a number of "candidate" prognostic factors with varying levels of prior support. These candidate prognostic factors can be evaluated either one at a time in univariable analyses or simultaneously in multivariable analysis. (Strictly speaking, the terms *univariate* and *multivariate* are incorrect in this context, since they refer to the number of outcome variables, not the number of prognostic variables; the terms *univariable* and *multivariable* are preferable.)

In univariable analysis, the strength of association between each candidate prognostic factor and the outcome is assessed and expressed separately. Univariable analyses are simple to perform and interpret, but they fail to account for relationships between prognostic factors and do not indicate whether different prognostic factors are providing the same or different information. For example, in women with breast cancer, lymph node status and hormone receptor status are both found to be associated with survival duration in univariable analysis; however, they are also found to be associated with one another. Univariable analysis will not clarify whether measuring both factors provides more prognostic information than measuring either one alone.

Multivariable analyses account and adjust for the simultaneous effects of several variables on the outcome of interest. Variables that are significant when included together in a multivariable model provide independent prognostic information. The disadvantage of multivariable models is that they are more difficult to perform and interpret (Concato et al., 1993). Typically, a large number of candidate prognostic factors are assessed in univariable analyses, and those factors exhibiting some arbitrary minimum degree of association, often defined in terms of a p value $<.05$, are included in a starting set of variables for the multivariable analysis. The final multivariable model reported usually contains only the subset of these variables that remain significant when simultaneously included in the same model. Different methods have been used to select those variables that appear to give independent prognostic information; these methods may lead to the selection of different variables, particularly if the number of variables examined is large in relation to the number of outcome events. A rough but widely accepted guideline is a minimum of 10 outcome events for each prognostic factor assessed. Thus in a study assessing prognostic factors for survival in 200 patients of whom 100 have died, no more than 10 candidate prognostic factors should be assessed.

The results of a prognostic study are often reported in terms of the p values for the selected prognostic variables. The conventional interpretation of a p value as the probability of detecting an association if none existed is inappropriate in this setting. Prognostic studies typically involve large numbers of comparisons that greatly exaggerate the apparent significance of reported p values. The probability of detecting spurious associations due to chance increases dramatically with the number of comparisons. A single test at the .05 level has, by definition, a 5 percent probability of indicating an association when none exists. The probability of showing at least one spurious association at the .05 level rises to 10 percent with two tests, 23 percent with 5 tests, 40 percent with 10 tests, and 64 percent with 20 tests if the tests are assumed to be independent. A selection from a pool of 10 prognostic variables may involve the comparison of over a thousand different models. The number of comparisons is increased further if different cutoff points are examined for each variable, as with recursive partitioning and amalgamation—a recent addition to available strategies for multivariable prognostic factor analysis. Thus "significant" results should be regarded as hypothesis-generating rather than definitive, especially if p values are borderline.

20.3.3 Uses and Limitations of Prognostic Information

Methods of classifying cancer are based on factors known to influence prognosis, such as anatomic extent and histology of the tumor. The widely used TNM system for classifying or staging cancers is based on the extent of the primary tumor (T), the presence or absence of regional lymph node involvement (N), and the presence or absence of distant metastases (M). Other attributes of the tumor that have an influence on outcome, such as the estrogen-receptor concentration in breast cancer, are also included as prognostic factors in the analysis and reporting of therapeutic trials in these diseases. The identification of novel prognostic factors using the methods of molecular biology is an area of active investigation. Guidelines for selecting useful

prognostic factors have been suggested by Levine et al. (1991).

Prognostic classifications based solely on attributes of the tumor ignore patient-based factors known to affect prognosis such as performance status, quality of life, and the presence of other illnesses (comorbidity). Performance status, a measure of an individual's physical functional capacity, is one of the most powerful and consistent predictors of prognosis across the spectrum of malignant disease (Weeks, 1992). Studies in breast cancer (Coates et al., 1992), melanoma (Coates et al., 1993), lung cancer (Ganz et al., 1991) and prostate cancer (Tannock et al., 1996) have consistently demonstrated strong, independent associations between simple patient-based measures of quality of life and survival. Incorporation of these measures in clinical studies will reduce the heterogeneity that remains after accounting for attributes of the tumor.

The utility of a prognostic factor also depends on the accuracy with which it can be measured. For example, the size and extent of the primary tumor are important prognostic factors in men with early prostate cancer; however, studies have demonstrated substantial variability between observers in assessing these attributes (Smith and Catalona, 1995). This variation between observers contributes to the variability of prognosis in patients assigned to the same prognostic category by different observers. Random variation merely adds to imprecision, but systematic variation creates bias. Stage migration is an example of such systematic variation (see Fig. 20.9).

Stage migration occurs when patients are assigned to different clinical stages because of differences in the precision of staging rather than differences in the extent of disease. This can occur if patients staged very thoroughly as part of a research proto-

Figure 20.9. Stage migration. The diagram illustrates that a change in staging investigations may lead to the apparent improvement of results within each stage without changing the overall results. In the hypothetical example, patients are divided into six equal groups, each with the indicated survival. Introduction of more sensitive staging investigations moves patients into higher-stage groups, as shown, but the overall survival of 50 percent remains unchanged. (From Tannock, 1989, with permission; adapted from Bush and Hill, 1979.)

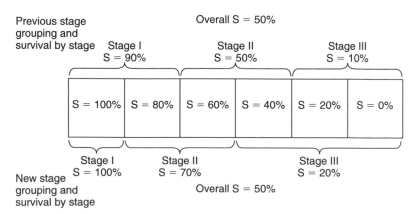

col are compared with patients staged less thoroughly in the course of routine clinical practice, or if patients staged with newer more accurate tests are compared with historical controls staged with older, less accurate tests. Stage migration is important because the introduction of new and more sensitive diagnostic tests produces apparent improvements in outcome for each anatomically defined category of disease in the absence of any real improvement in outcome for the disease overall (Bush, 1979; Feinstein et al., 1985). This paradox arises because, in general, the patients with the worst prognosis in each category are reclassified as having more advanced disease. As illustrated in Fig. 20.9, a proportion of those patients initially classified as having localized disease (stage I) will be found to have regional spread, and a proportion of those initially classified as having only regional spread (stage II) will be found to have systemic spread. The patients moving from the localized to the regional category will have a worse prognosis than the group they are leaving and a better prognosis than the group they are joining. The same applies for patients moving from the regional to the systemic category (stage III). As a consequence, the prognosis of each category of disease improves in the absence of any real improvement in the prognosis of the disease overall.

20.4 TREATMENT

20.4.1 Purpose of Clinical Trials

Clinical trials are research studies designed to assess the effects of interventions on the health of human beings. Possible interventions include treatment with drugs, radiation, or surgery; modification of diet, behavior, or environment; and surveillance with physical examination, blood tests, or imaging tests. This chapter focuses on trials of treatment.

The purpose of a clinical trial is to answer specific questions about the effects of a treatment. Different types of question require different types of trial. Schwartz et al. (1980) emphasized the distinction between *explanatory* trials, designed to evaluate the biological effects of treatment, and *pragmatic* trials, designed to evaluate the practical effects of treatment. This distinction is crucial, because treatments that have desirable biological effects (e.g., the ability to kill cancer cells and cause tumor shrinkage) may not have desirable effects in practice (i.e., may not lead to improvement in duration or quality of life). For example, some drugs with strong antitumor effects are so toxic that patients are unable to tolerate and derive benefit from them. The major differences between explanatory and pragmatic trials are listed in Table 20.2.

Table 20.2. Classification of Clinical Trials

Characteristic	Explanatory	Pragmatic
Purpose	The results will be used to guide further research and not to formulate treatment policy; the purpose of the work is to contribute new knowledge	The results will be used to select future treatment policy
Treatment	Choose treatment most likely to demonstrate the phenomenon under study	Choose treatment with tolerance of the target population in mind
Assessment criteria	Choose criteria that give biological information such as tumor response	Choose information of practical importance such as functional capacity or survival
	Use single or a small number of criteria	Take account of all practically important criteria, but require a *single* decision at the stage of analysis
Choice of patients	Choose patients most likely to demonstrate an effect	Choose patients who are representative of the population to whom the results of the research will be applied
	Patients are used as a "means to an end" in the research	The effect of treatment on patients is the end product of the research
	Idealized conditions	"Real-life" conditions

The evaluation of new cancer treatments usually involves progression through a series of clinical trials. Phase I trials are designed to evaluate the relationship between dose and toxicity and aim to establish a tolerable schedule of administration. Phase II trials are designed to screen treatments for their antitumor effects in order to identify those worthy of further evaluation. Phase III trials are designed to determine the usefulness of treatments in the management of patients. The designation "phase IV" is used for trials designed to monitor the effects of treatments that have been incorporated into clinical practice.

Phase I and II trials are explanatory—they assess the biological effects of treatment on host and tumor in small numbers of subjects to guide decisions about further research.

Phase I trials are designed to identify the maximum tolerable dose of a new drug. The focus is on the relationship between dosage and toxicity and on pharmacokinetics (Chap. 16, Sec. 16.2). Small numbers of patients are treated at successively higher doses until the maximum acceptable degree of toxicity is reached. Many variations have been used; a typical design is to us a low initial dose, unlikely to cause severe side effects, based on animal toxicology data by dividing the LD_{10} (the dose in milligrams per meter squared of body surface area causing death in 10 percent of the most sensitive animals tested) by a factor of 10. A modified Fibonacci sequence is then used to determine dose escalations: the second dose level is 100 percent higher than the first, the third is 67 percent higher than the second, the fourth is 50 percent higher than the third, the fifth is 40 percent higher than the fourth, and all subsequent levels are 33 percent higher than the preceding levels. Three patients are treated at each level in the absence of dose-limiting toxicity. Six patients are treated at any dose where dose-limiting toxicity is encountered. The maximum tolerable dose is defined as the maximum dose at which dose limiting toxicity occurs in less than one- third of the patients tested. This design is based on experience rather than data and is predicated on the assumption that the maximum tolerable dose is also the most effective anticancer dose.

Phase II trials are designed to determine whether a new treatment has sufficient activity to justify further evaluation. They usually include highly selected patients with a given type of cancer, exclude those with "nonevaluable" disease, and use tumor response rate as the primary measure of outcome. Their sample size is calculated to distinguish active from inactive therapies according to whether the re-

sponse rate is greater or less than some arbitrary level, often 20 percent. The resulting sample size is inadequate to provide a precise estimate of activity. For example, a phase II trial with 24 patients and an observed response rate of 33 percent has a 95 percent confidence interval of 16 percent to 55 percent. While tumor response rate is a reasonable end point for assessing the anticancer activity of a drug, it is not an adequate surrogate for patient benefit. Phase II trials are suitable for guiding decisions about further research but are not suitable for making decisions about patient management. The literature is confusing, however, because phase II trials are often reported and interpreted as if they did provide answers to questions about patient management (Tannock and Warr, 1988).

Phase III trials are pragmatic, since they are designed to answer questions about the usefulness of treatments in patient management. Their end points should reflect patient benefit, such as duration and quality of survival. Questions about patient management tend to be comparative, since they involve choices between alternatives—i.e., an experimental versus the current standard of management. The current standard may include other anticancer treatments or may be "best supportive care" without specific anticancer therapy. The aim of a phase III trial is to estimate the difference in outcomes associated with a difference in treatments, sometimes referred to as the *treatment effect*. Ideally, alternative treatments are compared by administering them to groups of patients that are equivalent in all other respects. Randomized controlled phase III trials are the best and often only reliable means of determining the usefulness of treatments in patient management. The following discussion focuses on randomized controlled phase III trials.

20.4.2 Sources of Bias in Clinical Trials

The characteristics of the patients enrolled in a clinical trial define the population to whom the results apply. Important characteristics include demographic data (e.g., age and gender), clinical characteristics (the stage and pathologic type of disease), the performance status of the patients, and other prognostic factors. The selection of subjects, inclusion criteria, and exclusion criteria must be described in sufficient detail for clinicians to judge the degree of similarity between the patients in a trial and the patients in their practice.

The distribution of prognostic factors is important because the outcomes of people with cancer often depend more on their initial prognostic characteristics than on their subsequent treatment (see Sec. 20.3 and Fig. 20.8). Imbalances in prognostic factors can have profound effects on the results of a trial. The reports of most randomized clinical trials include a table of baseline prognostic characteristics. The *p* values often reported in these tables are misleading, since any differences between the groups, other than the treatment assigned, *are known* to have arisen by chance. The important question is whether any such imbalances influence the estimate of the treatment effect. This question is best answered by an analysis that gives an estimate of the treatment effect adjusted for any imbalances in prognostic factors (see Sec. 20.4.5).

There is evidence that patients enrolled in clinical trials have better outcomes (even if receiving standard treatment) than patients who are seen in routine practice (Antman et al., 1985; Davis et al., 1985; Karjalainen and Palva, 1989). While patients in randomized trials may differ from those in clinical practice (because of differing prognostic characteristics, better compliance with treatment, better supportive care, or other unknown factors), this difference does not usually detract from the primary conclusion of a randomized trial. Randomized trials are designed to estimate differences between treatments rather than the absolute effect of individual treatments. This distinction is subtle but important.

Treatments must be described in sufficient detail to be replicated. This applies equally to treatment with drugs, radiation, or surgery. Reports of drug trials should include the starting doses; the frequency, mode, and route of administration; and adjustments for toxicity or impaired organ function. Differences between the treatment specified in the protocol and the treatment received by the patients should be reported clearly.

Compliance refers to the extent to which a treatment is delivered as intended. It depends on the willingness of physicians to prescribe treatment as specified in the protocol and the willingness of patients to take treatment as prescribed by the physician. Patient compliance with oral medication is variable (Lee et al., 1992) and may be a major barrier to the delivery of efficacious treatments.

Contamination occurs when people in one arm of a trial receive the treatment intended for those in another arm of the trial. This may occur if people allocated to placebo obtain active drug from elsewhere, as has occurred in trials of treatments for human immunodeficiency virus (HIV) infection. This type of contamination is rare in trials of anticancer drugs but common in trials of dietary treatments, vitamin supplements, or other widely available agents.

The effect of contamination is to blur distinctions between treatment arms.

Crossover is a related problem that influences the interpretation of trials assessing survival duration. It occurs when people allocated to one treatment subsequently receive the alternative treatment when their disease progresses. While defensible from pragmatic and ethical viewpoints, crossover changes the nature of the question being asked about survival duration. In a two-arm trial without crossover, the comparison is of treatment A versus treatment B; whereas with crossover, the comparison is of treatment A followed by treatment B versus treatment B followed by treatment A.

For example, a recent randomized trial compared chemotherapy with mitoxantrone plus prednisone to prednisone alone for men with advanced prostate cancer (Tannock et al., 1996). About 60 percent of men allocated to the prednisone-alone arm subsequently received mitoxantrone when their disease progressed, as recommended in the protocol. The trial's primary outcome was the proportion of patients achieving substantial pain relief during their initially allocated treatment, an end point unaffected by treatment following disease progression. The trial assessed survival duration as a secondary outcome. Survival duration may be affected by treatment given following disease progression. In terms of pain relief, the comparison is of mitoxantrone plus prednisone versus prednisone alone; in terms of survival duration, the comparison is of initial mitoxantrone plus prednisone versus initial prednisone with optional mitoxantrone on progression.

Cointervention occurs when treatments are administered that may influence outcome but are not specified in the trial protocol. Examples are blood products and antibiotics in drug trials for acute leukemia or radiation therapy in trials of systemic adjuvant therapy for breast cancer. Because cointerventions are not allocated randomly, they may be distributed unequally between the groups being compared and can contribute to observed differences in outcome.

20.4.3 Allocation of Treatments: Randomization

The ideal comparison of treatments comes from observing their effects in groups that are otherwise equivalent. Allocation to different treatments by clinical judgment is almost certain to generate groups that differ systematically in their baseline prognostic characteristics. Important factors that are measurable can be accounted for in the analysis; however, important factors that are poorly specified—such as comorbidity, a history of complications with other treatments, the ability to comply with treatment, or family history—cannot.

Comparisons based on historical controls are prone to bias due to changes over time in factors other than treatment. Changes in the spectrum of patients due to stage migration (see Fig. 20.9), better patient selection, or altered referral patterns can lead to spurious improvements in outcome that may be wrongly attributed to a new treatment. Improved outcomes due to better supportive care may also be wrongly attributed to a new treatment. These changes over time are difficult to assess and therefore difficult to adjust for in analysis. Such differences also tend to favor the most recently treated group and therefore to exaggerate the apparent benefits of new treatments (Sacks et al., 1983).

Randomization provides the best method for obtaining equivalence between the groups of patients to be compared. It is only ethical to allocate patients to treatments randomly when there is uncertainty about which treatment is best. The difficulty for individual clinicians is that this ambivalence usually resides among physicians collectively rather than within them individually (Freedman, 1987). Although the allocation of patients to physicians in clinical practice appears random, clinical judgment affects both the physicians to whom patients are referred and the treatments those physicians offer (Moore et al., 1988). For example, men with localized prostate cancer are more likely to be referred to surgeons and to be offered radical surgery if they are fit and to radiation oncologists if they have coexisting medical problems; nonrandomized comparisons of these treatments are likely to favor surgery.

Random allocation of treatment does not ensure that treatment groups are equivalent, but it does ensure that any differences in baseline characteristics are due to chance. Differences in outcome, therefore, must be due to either chance or treatment. Standard statistical tests estimate the probability (p value) that differences in outcome, as observed, might be due to chance alone. The lower the p value, the less plausible the *null hypothesis* that the observed difference is due to chance, and the more plausible the *alternate hypothesis* that the difference is due to treatment.

Randomization can be stratified and blocked to reduce imbalances in important prognostic factors. *Stratification* refers to the grouping of patients with similar prognostic characteristics into strata. For example, in a trial of adjuvant hormone therapy for breast cancer, patients might be stratified according to the presence or absence of lymph node involve-

ment, hormone receptor levels, and menopausal status. *Blocking* ensures that treatment allocation is balanced for every few patients within each stratum. This is practical only for a small number of strata. Randomization in multicenter trials is often blocked and stratified by treatment center to account for differences between centers; however, this carries the risk that when there is almost complete accrual within a block the physicians may know the arm to which the next patient(s) will be assigned. If feasible, it is preferable that both physicians and patients be unaware of which treatment is being administered. This optimal double-blind design prevents bias. Evidence for bias in nonblinded randomized trials comes from the observation that unblinded trials lead more often to apparent improvements in outcome from experimental treatment and that assignment sequences in randomized trials have sometimes been deciphered (Chalmers et al., 1983; Shulz, 1995).

Multivariable statistical methods can be used to adjust for imbalances in prognostic factors. For large trials in which the likelihood of major imbalance in baseline characteristics is small, stratified randomization and adjusted analysis are unlikely to affect the conclusions. Substantive differences between adjusted and unadjusted analyses suggest that the sample size was inadequate for reliable conclusions. The main purpose of these maneuvers is to provide reassurance that the results of the trial are not affected by differences in important prognostic variables.

20.4.4 Choice and Assessment of Outcomes

The measures used to assess a treatment should reflect the goals of that treatment. Much treatment for advanced cancer is given with palliative intent—to reduce symptoms or prolong survival without realistic expectation of cure. Survival duration is an unequivocal end point that should be measured in all clinical trials; if the aim of treatment is to improve quality of life, then quality of life should be measured. Anticancer treatments may prolong survival through toxic effects on the cancer or may shorten survival through toxic effects on the host. Similarly, anticancer treatments may improve quality of life by reducing cancer-related symptoms but may worsen quality of life by adding toxicity due to treatment. Patient benefit depends on the trade-off between these positive and negative effects, which can be assessed only by measuring duration of survival and quality of life directly.

Surrogate or indirect measures of patient benefit, such as tumor shrinkage or disease-free survival, can sometimes provide an early indication of efficacy, but they are not substitutes for more direct measures. For example, the use of disease-free survival rather than overall survival in adjuvant studies requires fewer subjects and shorter follow-up but ignores what happens following the recurrence of disease. Higher tumor response rates or advantages in disease-free survival do not always translate into longer overall survival or better quality of life. In trials of adjuvant chemotherapy for women with early-stage breast cancer, differences in disease-free survival have, in general, translated into smaller but nonetheless important differences in overall survival; this has not generally been the case for trials of adjuvant radiation therapy for breast cancer (Cuzick et al., 1994).

Changes in the concentrations of tumor markers in serum, such as PSA for prostate cancer and CA-125 for ovarian cancer, have been recommended as outcome measures in several types of cancer. Levels of these markers may reflect tumor burden in general, but the relationship is quite variable; there are individuals with extensive disease who have low levels of a tumor marker in serum. The relationship between serum levels of a tumor marker and outcome is also variable. In men who have received local treatment for early-stage prostate cancer, the reappearance of PSA in the serum indicates disease recurrence. In men with advanced prostate cancer, however, baseline levels of serum PSA are not associated with duration of survival, and changes in PSA following treatment are not related consistently to changes in symptoms (Tannock et al., 1996).

It is essential to assess outcomes for all patients who enter a clinical trial. It is common in cancer trials to exclude patients from the analysis on the grounds that they are "not evaluable." Reasons for nonevaluability vary, but may include death soon after treatment was started or failure to receive the full course of treatment. It may be permissible to exclude patients from analysis in explanatory phase II trials that are seeking to describe the biological effects of treatment; these trials indicate the effect of treatment in those who were able to complete it. It is seldom appropriate to exclude patients in pragmatic trials, which should reflect the conditions under which the treatment will be applied in practice. Such trials test a policy of treatment, and the appropriate analysis for a pragmatic trial is by intention to treat: patients should be included in the arm to which they were allocated regardless of their subsequent course.

For some events (e.g., death) there may be no doubt as to whether the event has occurred, but assignment of a particular cause of death (e.g., whether it was cancer-related) is a subjective matter, as is the assessment of tumor response, recognition of tumor recurrence, and therefore determination of disease-free survival.

The compared groups should be followed with similar types of evaluation so that they are equally susceptible to the detection of outcome events such as disease recurrence. Whenever the assessment of an outcome is subjective (i.e., cannot be assumed to be independent of the observer making the assessment), variation between observers should be examined. Variable criteria of tumor response and imprecise tumor measurement have been documented as causes of variability when this end point is used in clinical trials (Warr et al., 1984; Tonkin et al., 1985).

As described above, "blinding" of observers is always preferred to avoid bias but this may be difficult or impossible if different types of treatment with different side effects are compared.

20.4.5 Survival Curves and Their Comparison

Clinical trials usually accrue subjects over a prolonged period, often several years, and then follow them for an additional period. Subjects enrolled early in a trial are observed for a longer time than subjects enrolled later and are more likely to have died by the time the trial is analyzed. For this reason, the distribution of survival times is the preferred outcome measure for assessing the influence of treatment on survival. Survival duration is defined as the interval from some convenient "zero time," usually the date of enrolment in a study, to the time of death. Subjects who have died provide actual observations of survival duration. Subjects who were alive at last follow-up provide *censored* (incomplete) observations of survival duration: their eventual survival duration will be at least as long as the time to their last follow-up. Most cancer trials are analyzed before all subjects have died, so a method of analysis which accounts for censored observations is required.

Actuarial survival curves provide an estimate of the eventual distribution of survival duration (when everyone has died) based on the observed survival duration of those who have died and the censored observations of those still living. Actuarial survival curves are preferred to simple cross-sectional measures of survival because they incorporate and describe all of the available information.

The life-table method for construction of an actuarial survival curve is illustrated in Table 20.3. The period of follow-up after treatment is divided into

Table 20.3. Calculation of Actuarial Survival

Follow-up Interval (A)	Number at Risk (B)	Number Dying (C)	Number Withdrawn Alive (D)	Probability of Dying during Interval (E)	Probability of Surviving during Interval (F)	Overall Probability of Survival (G)
0	100	—	—	—	—	1
1	100	8	2	0.080	0.920	0.920
2	90	3	2	0.033	0.967	0.890
3	85	1	0	0.012	0.988	0.879
4	84	3	1	0.036	0.964	0.847
5	80	7	3	0.088	0.912	0.773
6	70	6	4	0.086	0.914	0.706
7	60	5	5	0.083	0.917	0.648
8	50	1	4	0.020	0.980	0.635
9	45	1	2	0.022	0.978	0.621
10	42	1	1	0.024	0.976	0.606

Note: A, Follow-up interval may be of any convenient size; usually days, weeks, or months. B, Number at risk means number of patients alive at the start of the interval. C, Number dying is number of patients dying during each interval. D, Number withdrawn alive refers to patients alive who have not been followed longer than the interval after randomization. E, Probability of dying during each interval is number of patients dying (C) divided by the number at risk (B). F, Probability of survival during each interval is the complement $(1-E)$ of the probability of dying. G, Overall probability of survival is the cumulative products of the probabilities in (F). The numbers in this column may be plotted against time as a survival curve.

convenient short intervals—for example, weeks or months. The probability of dying in a particular interval is estimated by dividing the number of people who died during that interval by the number of people who were known to be alive at its beginning $(E = C/B)$. The probability of surviving a particular interval, having survived to its beginning, is the complement of the probability of dying in it $(F = 1 - E)$. The actuarial estimate of the probability of surviving for a given time is calculated by cumulative multiplications of the probabilities of surviving each interval until that time.

The Kaplan-Meier method, also known as the product limit method, is identical except that the calculations are performed at each death rather than at fixed intervals. The Kaplan-Meier survival curve is depicted graphically by a step function with the probability of surviving on the y axis and time on the x axis: vertical drops occur at each death (Fig. 20.10). The latter part of a survival curve is often the focus of most interest, since it estimates the probability of long-term survival; however, it is also the least reliable part of the curve, since it is based on the fewest observations.

The validity of all actuarial methods depends on the time of censoring being independent of the time of death. The subsequent survival of subjects with censored observations can then be estimated from the observations of subjects who have been fol-

lowed longer. The most obvious violation of this assumption occurs if subjects are lost to follow-up because they have died or are too sick to attend clinics.

Overall survival curves do not take into account the cause of death. Cause-specific survival curves are constructed by considering only death from specified causes; patients dying from other causes are treated as censored observations at the time of their death. The advantage of cause-specific survival curves is that they focus on deaths due to the cause of interest. However, they may be influenced by uncertainty about the influence of cancer or its treatment on death due to apparently unrelated causes. Deaths due to cardiovascular causes, accidents, or suicides, for example, may all occur as an indirect consequence of cancer or its treatment.

The first step in comparing survival distributions is visual inspection of the survival curves. Ideally, there will be indications of both the number of censored observations, often indicated by ticks on the curve, and the numbers of people at risk at representative time points, often indicated beneath the curve (Fig. 20.10). Curves that cross are difficult to interpret, since this means that shorter-term survival is better in one arm, while longer-term survival is better in the other. Two questions must be asked of any observed difference: (1) whether it is clinically important and (2) whether it is likely to have arisen

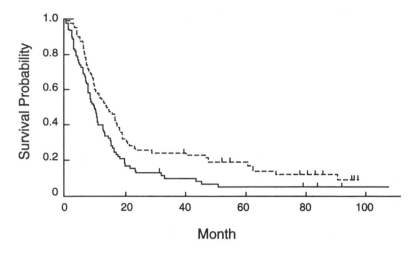

Figure 20.10. Illustration of Kaplan-Meier survival curves. The curves summarize the survival experience of patients with stage III non-small cell lung cancer treated with radiation (RT, solid line) alone or with chemotherapy prior to radiation (CT-RT, dashed line). (From Dillman et al., 1996, with permission.)

Number of patients at risk:

RT Only	38	13	7	4	3	1
CT-RT	48	25	18	12	7	3

by chance. The first is a value judgment that will be based on factors such as toxicity, baseline risk, and cost (See Sec. 20.4.10). The second is a question of statistical significance that depends on the the size of the difference and the sample size of the trial.

The size of any estimated difference in survival or other end point should always be described, preferably with an indication of its precision. The precision of an estimate is conveniently described by its *95 percent confidence interval.* Confidence intervals are closely related to *p* values: a 95 percent confidence interval that excludes a treatment effect of zero indicates a *p* value of less than .05. The usual interpretation of a 95 percent confidence interval is that we can be 95 percent confident that the true value lies within that range.

The *statistical significance* of a difference in survival distributions is expressed by a *p* value, which is the probability that a difference as large as or larger than that observed would have arisen by chance alone. Several statistical tests are available for calculating the *p* value for differences in survival distributions. The log-rank test and its variants are used most commonly under a variety of names (Mantel-Haenszel test, generalized Savage or Wilcoxon test). The log-rank test gives equal weight to each death; this results in *relatively* greater emphasis being given to deaths that occur late, when there are few individuals at risk (the least stable part of the curve). Peto's modification of the log-rank test gives more weight to deaths occurring early, where the survival curve is defined with greater certainty (Peto et al., 1976, 1977).

Survival analyses can be adjusted, in principle, for any number of prognostic variables. For example, a trial comparing the effects of two regimens of adjuvant chemotherapy on the survival of women with early-stage breast cancer might include women with or without spread to axillary lymph nodes and with or without hormone-receptor expression. An unadjusted analysis would compare the survivals of the two treatment groups directly. The estimate of the treatment effect can be adjusted for any imbalances in these prognostic factors by including them in the analysis. The log-rank test allows adjustment for prognostic variables that are categorical (e.g., presence or absence of involved lymph nodes). Cox's proportional hazards model is more versatile and more complex, allowing adjustment for continuous and time-dependent variables as well (Tibshirani, 1982). In large randomized trials, such adjustments rarely affect the conclusions, since the likelihood of major imbalances is small.

Differences in the distribution of survival times for two treatments compared in a randomized trial may be summarized in several ways: (1) the absolute difference in the proportion of patients that are expected to be alive at a specified time after treatment (e.g., at 5 or 10 years). (2) The hazard ratio, or the ratio of mean hazard functions for the two arms; the hazard function or time-specific mortality rate is the mortality rate at any given time among individuals who have survived until that time. (3) The odds ratio, or reduction in the odds of death, which is defined for each arm as the probability of dying in a given period divided by the probability of surviving in that period. In practice, the odds ratio (applied to short time intervals) will be almost identical to the hazard ratio. (4) The number of patients who would need to be treated for a given period of time to save one life.

Oncologists are often confused by these different ways of summarizing data. A substantial reduction in hazard or odds ratio may lead to a variable and quite small improvement in absolute survival and to a variable number of patients who would need to be treated to save one life; these values depend on the expected level of survival in the control group. For example, a 25 percent reduction in the annual odds of death has been found for use of adjuvant combination chemotherapy in younger women with breast cancer (Early Breast Cancer Trialists Collaborative Group, 1992). If this treatment effect is applied to node-positive women with a control survival at 10 years of less than 50 percent, it will lead to an absolute increase in survival of about 10 percent (Gelber et al., 1993); between five and eight women would need to be treated to save one life over that 10-year period (Chatellier et al., 1996). The same 25 percent reduction in hazard ratio would lead to about a 7 percent increase in absolute survival at 10 years for poor-risk node-negative women (e.g., about 65 to 72 percent), and about a 3 percent gain for good-risk node-negative women (e.g., about 87 to 90 percent; Gelber et al., 1993). Corresponding numbers of women that need to be treated to save one life over 10 years are about 14 and 30 (Chatellier et al., 1996). When presented with different summaries of trials, physicians may select the experimental treatment on the basis of what appears to be a substantial reduction in hazard or odds ratio but reject treatment on the basis of a smaller increase in absolute survival or a large number of patients that need to be treated to save one life, even though these represent different expressions of the same effect (Naylor et al., 1992). Note also that the reduction in hazard or odds ratio or death cannot be applied directly to the cumulative risk of dying over a long time interval (5 or 10 years), since the number of patients at risk changes with time; the absolute gain in survival is less than would be estimated by this calculation.

20.4.6 Statistical Issues

The number of subjects required for a randomized clinical trial where the primary end point is duration of survival depends on several factors:

1. The minimum difference in survival rates that is considered clinically important: the smaller the difference, the larger the number of subjects required.
2. The number of deaths expected with the standard treatment used in the control arm of the study: the larger the number of deaths, the smaller the number of subjects required. Since more patients will have died during longer follow-up, fewer subjects are required for trials with longer follow-up.
3. The probability of (willingness to accept) a false-positive result (alpha, or type I error): the lower the probability, the larger the number of subjects required.
4. The probability of (willingness to accept) a false-negative result (beta, or type II error): the lower the probability, the larger the number of subjects required.

The minimum difference that is clinically important is the smallest difference that would lead to the adoption of a new treatment. This judgment will depend on the severity of the condition being treated and the feasibility, toxicity, and cost of the treatment(s). Methods are available to help quantify such judgments. For example, the practitioners who will be expected to make decisions about treatment based on the results of the trial can be asked what magnitude of improvement would be sufficient for them to change their practice by adopting the new treatment. Based on such information, the number of patients required to be entered into a trial can be estimated from tables similar to Table 20.4.

In a trial assessing survival duration, it is the number of deaths, not the number of subjects, that determines the reliability of its conclusions. For example, a trial with 1000 subjects and 200 deaths will be more reliable than a trial with 2000 subjects and 150 deaths. From a statistical point of view, this means that it is more efficient to perform trials in subjects at a higher risk of death than at a lower risk of death. It also explains the value of prolonged follow-up—longer follow-up means more deaths, which produce more reliable conclusions.

The acceptable values for the error probabilities are matters of judgement. Values of 0.05 for alpha (false positive error) and 0.1 or 0.2 for beta (false negative error) are well-entrenched. There are good arguments for using lower (more stringent) values (Peto et al, 1976, 1977).

Power refers to the ability of a trial to detect a difference between treatments when in fact they do

Table 20.4. Number of Patients Required to Detect or Exclude an Improvement in Survival[a]

		Expected Survival in Experimental Group										
		0	0.1	0.2	0.3	0.4	0.5	0.6	0.7	0.8	0.9	1.0
	0		150	75	50	35	30	25	20	15	15	10
	0.1			430	140	75	50	35	25	20	15	15
	0.2				625	185	90	55	40	30	20	15
Expected	0.3					755	210	100	60	40	25	20
survival in	0.4						815	215	100	55	35	25
control	0.5							815	210	90	50	30
group	0.6								755	185	75	35
	0.7									625	140	50
	0.8										430	75
	0.9											150
	1.0											

[a] $\alpha = 0.05$; power, $1 - \beta = 0.90$.

Source: Adapted from Walter, 1979.

differ. The power of a trial is the complement of beta, the type II error (power = 1 − beta). The relationship between expected difference between treatments and the number of patients required is shown in Table 20.4. A randomized clinical trial that seeks to detect an absolute improvement in survival of 20 percent, compared with a control group receiving standard treatment whose expected survival is 40 percent, will require about 108 patients in each arm at $\alpha = 0.05$ and a power of 0.9. This means that a clinical trial of this size has a 90 percent chance of detecting an improvement in survival of this magnitude. Detection of a smaller difference between treatments — for example, a 10 percent absolute increase in survival — would require about 410 patients in each arm. A substantial proportion of published clinical trials are too small to detect clinically important differences reliably (Freiman et al., 1978). The selection of β is subjective and is influenced by the number of patients that are available to enter a trial. If there are insufficient patients to have an 80 to 90 percent chance of detecting a worthwhile difference in survival, then a trial should probably not be undertaken.

Clinical trials are analogous to diagnostic tests (Sec.20.2.1): they generate both false positives (positive trial despite no true advance) and false negatives (negative trial despite a true advance) as well as true positives and true negatives. The positive predictive value of a clinical trial—i.e., the probability of a true advance given a positive trial—will depend not only on the nature of the trial (sensitivity and specificity) but also on the background prevalence of true advances. If the prevalence of true gains in survival is as low as has been found generally for new treatments of cancer such as breast cancer (Chlebowski and Lillington, 1994), then apparently positive trials will often be false positives.

The probability of a false-positive result increases with the number of different end points (outcomes) assessed. The usual interpretation of a p value is predicated on the performance of a single statistical test per study. The probability of detecting a difference at the .05 level in the absence of a true difference is 5 percent for a single test, 10 percent for two tests, 23 percent for five tests, and 40 percent for ten tests, assuming that the tests are independent. A single trial might assess overall survival, disease-specific survival, progression-free survival, tumor response rate, various measures of treatment toxicity, and multiple dimensions of quality of life. The number of tests increases further if interim analyses are performed during the course of a trial, which might be used for early stopping and analysis. The number of statistical comparisons reported in a typical cancer clinical trial is large and many more tests are performed than are reported (Tannock, 1996). Ideally, a single primary end point and time of analysis should be specified in a trial protocol and identified in the final report. Other comparisons (e.g., analysis of subgroups) may be important in generating new hypotheses but should not be regarded as giving definitive information.

P values should not be interpreted as dichotomous criteria for acceptance ($p > .05$) or rejection ($p < .05$) of a null hypothesis, nor should they be interpreted as indicating the chance that a null hypothesis is true; p values are best interpreted as indicators of support for competing hypotheses. The lower the p value, the less the support for the null hypothesis and the greater the support for the alternative hypothesis that an observed difference between treatments is real.

20.4.7 Meta-analysis

Meta-analysis is a method by which data from individual randomized clinical trials that test similar treatments (e.g., adjuvant chemotherapy for breast cancer versus no chemotherapy) are combined to give an overall estimate of treatment effect. Meta-analysis can be useful because (1) the results of individual trials are subject to random error and may give misleading results and (2) a small effect of a treatment (e.g., about 5 percent absolute improvement in survival for node-negative breast cancer from use of adjuvant chemotherapy) may be difficult to detect in individual trials because of a requirement for several thousand patients to be randomized, yet it may be of sufficient importance to recommend adoption of the new treatment as standard.

The principles of meta-analysis involve the identification and selection of trials addressing the question of interest. Data from these trials are extracted and combined. The preferred method involves collection of data on individual patients (date of randomization, date of death, or date last seen if alive) that were entered in individual trials. The trials will, in general, compare related strategies of treatment to standard management (e.g., radiotherapy with or without chemotherapy for stage III non-small-cell lung cancer) but will not be identical (e.g., different types of chemotherapy might be used). Composite actuarial survival curves for experimental and control groups are derived and treatment effect is estimated usually by the odds ratio and its 95 percent confidence interval (see Sec. 20.4.5). Data are presented typically as in Fig. 20.11, which illustrates the comparison of a strategy (in this example ovarian ablation as adjuvant therapy for breast cancer) used alone versus no such treatment (upper part of fig-

ure) and a related comparison where patients in both arms also receive chemotherapy (lower part of figure). Here, each trial included in the meta-analysis is represented by a symbol, proportional in area to the number of patients on the trial, and by a horizontal line representing its confidence interval. A vertical line represents the null effect, and a diamond beneath the individual trials represents the overall treatment effect and confidence interval. If this diamond symbol does not intersect the vertical line representing the null effect, a significant result is declared.

Meta-analysis is an expensive and time-consuming procedure. Important considerations are as follows:

1. The question addressed must be important and influence fundamental decisions about treatment.
2. The included trials must be of high quality. Bias in individual trials will influence the results of a meta-analysis, although the relative influence of such trials may be smaller.
3. Attempts should be made to include the latest results of all trials; unpublished trials should be included to avoid publication bias.
4. Because of publication bias and other reasons, meta-analyses obtained from reviews of the literature tend to overestimate the effect of experimental treatment as compared with a meta-analysis based on data for individual patients obtained from the investigators (Stewart and Parmar, 1993).
5. Since meta-analysis may combine trials with related but different treatments (e.g. less effective and more effective chemotherapy) the results may underestimate the effects of treatment that could be obtained under optimal conditions.

There is extensive debate in the literature about the merits and problems of meta-analyses and their advantages and disadvantages as compared with a single large well-designed trial (Eysenck, 1994; Cappelleri et al., 1996; Parmar et al., 1996). However, a well-performed meta-analysis uses all the available data, recognizes that false-negative and false-positive trials are likely to be common, and may limit the inappropriate influence of individual trials on practice.

20.4.8 Assessment of Quality of Life

Quality of life is an abstract, multidimensional concept reflecting physical, psychological and social aspects, that includes but is not limited to the concept

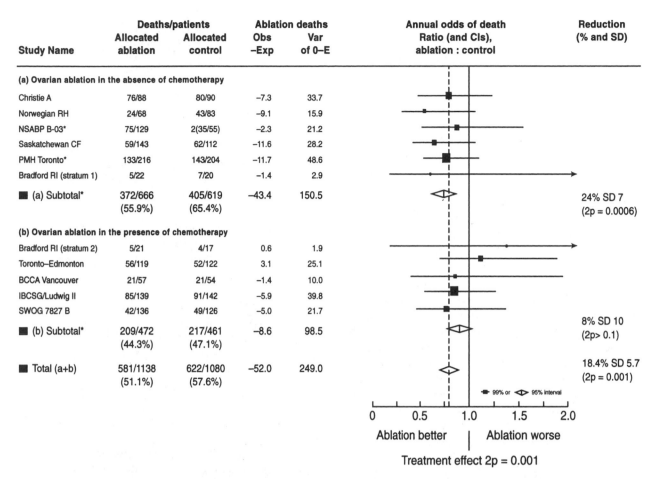

Figure 20.11. Typical presentation of results of a meta-analysis. Each trial is represented by a square symbol, whose area is proportional to the number of patients entered, and by a horizontal line. These represent the mean and 99 percent confidence interval for the ratio of annual odds of death in the experimental and standard arms. A vertical line drawn through the odds ratio 1.0 represents no effect. The trials are separated into those asking a simple question (in this example: ovarian ablation versus no adjuvant treatment for early breast cancer) and a related but more complex question (ovarian ablation plus chemotherapy versus chemotherapy alone). Diamonds represent overall mean odds ratios and their 95 percent confidence intervals for the two subsets of trials and for overall effect. The vertical dashed line represents mean reduction in annual odds of death for all trials. (Adapted from Early Breast Cancer Trialists Collaborative Group, 1996.)

of health. It reflects an individual's perception of and response to his or her unique circumstances. This definition gives primacy to the individual's views and identifies self-assessment as essential. *Instruments* (questionnaires) addressing differing aspects of quality of life from a variety of perspectives are now available. These range from generic instruments designed for heterogenous populations typical of health services research to instruments designed for patients with a specific type and stage of cancer.

Examples from the most generic through increasing degrees of specificity include the Medical Outcomes Study Short Form 36 (MOS SF-36, Ware et al., 1993), the Functional Living Index–Cancer (FLIC), developed for people with cancer (Schipper et al., 1984); the European Organisation for Research and Treatment of Cancer Core Quality of Life Questionnaire (EORTC QLQ-C30), developed for people with cancer participating in international clinical trials (Aaronson et al., 1993); the Functional Assessment of Cancer Therapy–General (FACT-G), developed for people receiving cancer treatments (Cella et al., 1993); and the Prostate Cancer–Specific Quality-of-Life Instrument (PROSQOLI), developed for men receiving treatment for advanced prostate cancer

(Tannock et al., 1996). Several of these instruments combine a core questionnaire relevant to most patients with cancer, as well as additional disease or trial-specific items.

The *validity* of an instrument refers to the extent to which it measures what it is supposed to measure. The validity of a quality-of-life instrument is always open to question, since there is no objective, external gold standard for comparison. Instead, a variety of indirect methods are used to gauge the validity of quality-of-life instruments (Aaronson et al., 1993). Examples include *convergent validity*, the degree of correlation between instruments or scales purporting to measure similar attributes; and *discriminant validity* or the degree to which an instrument can detect differences between different aspects of quality of life. *Face validity* and *content validity* refer to the extent to which an instrument addresses the issues that are important. *Responsiveness* refers to the detection of changes in quality of life with time, such as those due to effective treatment, while *predictive validity* refers to the prognostic information of a quality-of-life scale in predicting an outcome such as duration of survival. Validated quality-of-life scales are often strong predictors of survival (see Sec. 20.3.3).

Validity is *conditional*—it cannot be judged without specifying for what and for whom it is to be used. The context may be very narrow, as is the case of the Prostate Cancer Specific Quality-of-Life Instrument, or very broad, as is the case of the Medical Outcomes Study Short Form 36. Good validity in symptomatic men with advanced hormone-resistant prostate cancer does not guarantee good validity in men with earlier-stage prostate cancer, for whom pain might be less important and sexual function more important. Good validity in either or both of these populations will not guarantee good validity across the spectrum of all prostate cancer or for patients with other types of cancer. Even within the same population of subjects, differences between interventions, such as toxicity profiles, might influence validity. For example, nausea and vomiting might be important in a trial of doxorubicin or cisplatin, whereas sexual function might be more important in a trial of hormonal therapy. The context in which an instrument is to be used and the context(s) in which its validity was assessed must be re-examined for each application. Quality of life also changes over time, often dramatically in people with cancer. The pace and magnitude of these changes are highly variable and there may be changes in a patient's frame of reference as to what is considered "normal" quality of life (Sprangers, 1996).

20.4.9 Clinical Decision Making

Decision making is the process of choosing among alternatives. Ideally, clinical decisions should reflect the logical application of accurate information about the cancer and its treatment to the salient details of individual cases. Good clinical decisions require an understanding of the generic data regarding disease and treatment, the specifics of the individual problem, the nature of trade-offs, the individual patient's preferences, and uncertainty. Clinical decisions can be considered either diagnostic or therapeutic.

Formal models of decision making have been applied to a variety of medical problems. The aim of such models is to describe available alternatives and their outcomes in terms of their probabilities and utilities. A *utility* is a measure of preference for a particular health state rated on a scale from 0 to 1, where 0 represents immediate death and 1 represents perfect health. For decision making, a decision tree is constructed: at each branch of the tree, alternative options for diagnosis or treatment are listed, and further branches indicate possible outcomes: the *expected value* of each alternative is calculated by adding the products of the probability and utility of each of its possible outcomes. The alternative with the highest expected value is the preferred option. A simple example of a decision tree relating to options for early-stage Hodgkin's disease is shown in Fig. 20.12 (de Haes and Zittoun, 1995). In this hypothetical example, the expected value for the strategy of immediate treatment with chemotherapy and radiation (.86) is lower than that for first undertaking a staging laparotomy (.875); however, small changes in outcome or in estimates of utility could change the decision and suggest immediate chemotherapy and radiation as preferred treatment.

Three methods have been used for calculating utilities (Torrance, 1987):

1. *The standard gamble,* in which a subject in a given health state is asked to make a hypothetical "gamble" between remaining in this health state, or of accepting a probability (p) of perfect health and a probability ($1-p$) of sudden death. The probability p at the point of indecision represents the utility of that health state.

2. *The time trade-off method,* in which a subject in a given health state is asked to "select" between the hypothetical option of a given period of survival (T) in that health state or a shorter period of survival (t) in perfect health. At the point of indecision, the utility is given by the ratio t/T.

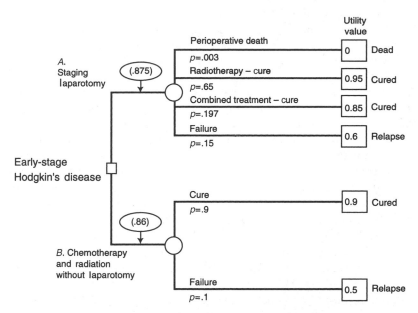

Figure 20.12. Example of a decision tree. For early-stage Hodgkin's diseases one might choose to base treatment decisions on the basis of a staging laparotomy (option *A*), which might avoid use of chemotherapy or to treat immediately with chemotherapy and radiation, which avoids a laparotomy (option *B*). The outcomes and estimates of their utility are shown at right. (Relapse has a higher utility for arm *A*, because of higher chance of salvage with chemotherapy). In this example the expected value (*ringed*) for strategy *A*, calculated by summing the products of various outcomes and their utilities is 0.875 ($0.65 \times 0.95 + 0.197 \times 0.85 + 0.15 \times 0.6$). For option *B*, the expected value is 0.86 ($0.9 \times 0.9 + 0.1 \times 0.5$). Option *A* would be preferred in this hypothetical example. (Modified from deHaes and Zittoun, 1995.)

3. *Conversion of a scale for overall quality of life* (e.g., by a scaling factor) to represent utility.

The methods outlined above do not often lead to similar values of utility. The first two methods can be criticized because they represent unreal situations, but they do reflect the element of choice that is essential to clinical decision making. Conversion of a quality-of-life scale usually leads to an underestimate of utility as calculated by the other methods; quality of life is important when the goal of treatment is palliation, but even very sick patients are unwilling to "trade" much survival time for improved quality of life (e.g., Slevin et al., 1990).

Formal clinical decision models are useful for revealing key factors that may influence choices between different treatments. However, the strength of their conclusions is often limited by the lack of high-quality data relating to the efficacy and toxicity of alternative strategies. Such decision models can stimulate the design of clinical trials to provide this missing information.

20.4.10 Economic Analyses

Rising costs have focused attention on the economics of health care and on the need to make choices between treatments based on cost as well as on outcome. Two types of analysis predominate.

Cost-outcome studies are descriptive and indicate the costs associated with a particular disease or treatment strategy. The usefulness of such studies is often limited by the lack of information about efficacy and the lack of a suitable comparison. For example, the median cost of treating women with advanced ovarian cancer with second-line and subsequent chemotherapy in Canada was estimated to be about $37,000; however, costs and outcomes in the absence such treatment were not available (Doyle et al., 1997).

Cost-effectiveness studies compare the incremental cost of one treatment over another with the incremental benefit (Detsky and Naglie, 1990). For treatments that influence survival, the cost can be expressed in terms of life-years gained. Since the gain in survival may occur when the patient is in a state of imperfect health because of the effects of the cancer or its treatment, the life-years gained may be multiplied by the utility of the health state (see Sec. 20.4.9) to give quality-adjusted life years (QALYs). The concept of a QALY may also be applied to palliative treatments that improve quality of life but do not influence overall survival. If benefit is measured in QALYs gained, then the cost-effectiveness is expressed in additional dollars spent per QALY gained. For example, in the United States, the incremental cost of adjuvant chemotherapy for node-negative breast cancer in premenopausal women has been estimated to be about $10,000 per QALY gained (Hillner and Smith, 1991).

Guidelines are available for the interpretation and appraisal of economic evaluations (Mason et al., 1993). The concept of cost per QALY allows, in theory, health providers to choose between funding different treatment strategies in quite different areas of medicine. For example, should one use limited resources to fund wider use of dialysis in kidney failure or bone marrow transplantation for leukemia? In general, wealthier countries can regard treatments that cost less than U.S.$20,000 per QALY gained as highly cost-effective and those that cost more than U.S.$100,000 per QALY gained as cost-ineffective, with a gray zone between. While economic analyses are critical for decision making at the community level, their role in decision making at the individual level is controversial.

20.5 SUMMARY

Diagnostic tests are used to distinguish patients with and without disease or to evaluate the extent or progress of disease. Their performance may be described by their sensitivity and specificity, which are independent of the prevalence of disease, or by the more clinically relevant properties of predictive values for positive and negative tests, which depend on prevalence. Likelihood ratios and ROC curves provide more comprehensive methods for assessing the performance of diagnostic tests. It is important to assess the impact of screening tests on health outcomes, such as survival and quality of life, preferably by means of randomized controlled trials.

Knowledge of prognostic factors is important for planning and analyzing clinical trials. Prognostic factors are often interdependent and may exert larger effects on survival than treatment. Estimates of prognosis from referral centers may be biased if the patients studied are not representative of those with the disease.

Clinical trials of treatment may be grouped into those that seek to detect the biological effects of treatment (explanatory trials, including phase I and II trials of new agents) and those that seek to determine whether patients benefit from receiving treatment (pragmatic trials, including most phase III trials). Pragmatic trials of cancer treatment require randomization to prevent bias in the allocation of treatment, and use direct assessment of patient-benefit by measuring survival duration and quality of life. The number of patients required in trials is determined by the size of the minimum clinically important difference, the variability of the outcome, and the probability of false-positive and false-negative results that are accepted by the investigators.

Good clinical decisions are based on an understanding of the generic data regarding disease and treatment, the specifics of the individual problem, the individual patient's preferences, the nature of trade-offs, and uncertainty. Quantity and quality of life are crucial outcomes that should always be considered. Economic considerations are important in decisions about the allocation of scarce resources, but their role in decisions about individual patients is controversial.

REFERENCES

Aaronson NK, Ahmedzai S, Bergman B, et al: The European Organisation for Research and Treatment of Cancer QLQ-C30: A quality of life instrument for use in international clinical trials in oncology. *J Natl Cancer Inst* 1993; 85:365–376.

Antman K, Amato D, Wood W, et al: Selection bias in clinical trials. *J Clin Oncol* 1985; 3:1142–1147.

Bush RS: Cancer of the ovary: natural history. In: Peckham MJ, Carter RL, eds. *Malignancies of the Ovary, Uterus and Cervix: The Management of Maligant Disease, Series #2*, London, England: Edward Arnold; 1979: 26–37.

Cappelleri JC, Ioannidis JPA, Schmid CH, et al: Large trials vs meta-analysis of smaller trials: How do their results compare? *JAMA* 1996; 276:1332–1338.

Cella DF, Tulsky DS, Gray G, et al: The Functional Assessment of Cancer Therapy scale: development and validation of the general measure. *J Clin Oncol* 1993; 11:570–579.

Chalmers TC, Celano P, Sacks HS, Smith H Jr: Bias in treatment assignment in controlled clinical trials. *N Engl J Med* 1983; 309:1358–1361.

Chatellier G, Zapletal E, Lemaitre D, et al: The number needed to treat: A clinically useful nomogram in its proper context. *Br Med J* 1996; 312:426–429.

Chlebowski RT, Lillington LM: A decade of breast cancer clinical investigation: Results as reported in the Program/Proceedings of the American Society of Clinical Oncology. *J Clin Oncol* 1994; 12:1789–1795.

Coates A, Gebski V, Murray P, et al: Prognostic value of quality of life scores during chemotherapy for advanced breast cancer. *J Clin Oncol* 1992; 10:1833–1838.

Coates A, Thompson D, McLeod GRM, et al: Prognostic value of quality of life scores in a trial of chemotherapy with or without interferon in patients with metastatic malignant melanoma. *Eur J Cancer* 1993; 29A: 1731–1734.

Concato J, Feinstein AR, Holford TR: The risk of determining risk with multivariable models. *Ann Intern Med* 1993; 118:201–210.

Cuzick J, Stewart H, Rutqvist L, et al: Cause-specific mortality in long-term survivors of breast cancer who participated in trials of radiotherapy. *J Clin Oncol* 1994; 12:447–453.

Davis S, Wright PW, Schulman SF et al: Participants in prospective randomized trials for resected non-small cell lung cancer have improved survival compared with nonparticipants in such trials. *Cancer* 1985; 56: 1710–1718.

De Haes JCJM, Zittoun RA: Quality of Life. In: Peckham M, Pinedo HM, Veronesi V, eds. *Oxford Textbook of Oncology,* Oxford England: Oxford University Press; 1995:2400–2408.

Detsky AS, Naglie IG: A clinicians guide to cost-effectiveness analysis. *Ann Intern Med* 1990; 113:147–154.

Dillman RO, Herndon J, Seagreen SL, et al: Improved survival in stage III non-small cell lung cancer: Seven-year follow-up of Cancer and Leukemia Group B (CALGB) 8433 trial. *J Natl Cancer Inst* 1996; 88:1210–1215.

Doyle C, Stockler M, Pintilie M, et al: Resource implications of palliative chemotherapy for ovarian cancer. *J Clin Oncol* 1997; 15:1000–1007.

Early Breast Cancer Trialists' Collaborative Group: Systemic treatment of early breast cancer by hormonal, cytotoxic or immune therapy: 133 randomized trials involving 31000 recurrences and 24000 deaths among 75000 women. *Lancet* 1992; 339:1–5, 71–85.

Early Breast Cancer Trialists' Collaborative Group: Ovarian ablation in early breast cancer: Overview of the randomised trials. *Lancet* 1996; 348:1189–1196.

Eddy DM: Screening for lung cancer. *Ann Intern Med* 1989; 111:232–237.

Eysenck HJ: Meta-analysis and its problems. *Br Med J* 1994; 309:789–792.

Fagan TJ: Nomogram for Bayes theorem. *N Engl J Med* 1975; 293:257.

Feinstein AR: *Clinical Epidemiology: The Architecture of Clinical Research.* Philadelphia: Saunders; 1985.

Feinstein AR, Sosin DM, Wells CK: The Will Rogers phenomenon: Stage migration and new diagnostic techniques as a source of misleading statistics for survival in cancer. *N Engl J Med* 1985; 312:1604–1608.

Freedman B: Equipoise and the ethics of clinical research. *N Engl J Med* 1987; 317:141–145.

Freedman LS: Tables of the number of patients required in clinical trials using the log rank test. *Stat Med* 1982; 1:121–129.

Freiman JA, Chalmers TC, Smith H Jr, et al: The importance of beta, the type II error and sample size in the design and interpretation of the randomized control trial: Survey of 71 "negative" trials. *N Engl J Med* 1978; 299:690–694.

Ganz PA, Lee JJ, Siau J: Quality of life assessment: An independent prognostic variable for survival in lung cancer. *Cancer* 1991; 67: 3131–3135.

Gelber RD, Goldhirsch A, Coates AS, for the International Breast Cancer Study Group: Adjuvant therapy for breast cancer: Understanding the overview. *J Clin Oncol* 1993; 11:580–585.

GIVIO Investigators: Impact of follow-up testing on survival and health-related quality of life in breast cancer patients: A multicenter randomized controlled trial. *JAMA* 1994; 271:1587–1592.

Hardcastle JD, Chamberlain JO, Robinson MHE, et al: Randomized controlled trial of faecal-occult-blood screening for colorectal cancer. *Lancet* 1996; 348:1472–1477.

Hillner BE, Smith TJ: Efficacy and cost-effectiveness of adjuvant chemotherapy in women with node-negative breast cancer: A decision analysis model. *N Engl J Med* 1991; 324:160–168.

Jaeschke R, Guyatt GH, Sackett DL, for the Evidence-Based Medicine Working Group: Users' guides to the medical literature: III. How to use an article about a diagnostic test. *JAMA* 1994; 271:389–391, 703–707.

Karjalainen S, Palva I: Do treatment protocols improve end results? A study of survival of patients with multiple myeloma in Finland. *Br Med J* 1989; 299: 1069–1072.

Kerlikowske K, Grady D, Barclay J, et al: Likelihood ratios for modern screening mammography: Risk of breast cancer based on age and mammographic interpretation. *JAMA* 1996; 276:39–43.

Kerlikowske K, Grady D, Rubin SM, et al: Efficacy of screening mammography: A meta-analysis. *JAMA* 1995; 273:149–154.

Krahn MD, Mahoney JE, Eckman MH, et al: Screening for prostate cancer: A decision analytic view. *JAMA* 1994; 272:773–780.

Kronberg O, Fenger C, Olsen J, et al: Randomized study of screening for colorectal cancer with faecal-occult-blood test. *Lancet* 1996; 348:1467–1471.

Laupacis A, Wells G, Richardson S, et al, for the Evidence-Based Medicine Working Group: Users' guides to the medical literature: V. How to use an article about prognosis. *JAMA* 1994; 272:234–237.

Lee CR, Nicholson PW, Souhami RL, Deshmukh AA: Patient compliance with oral chemotherapy as assessed by a novel electronic technique. *J Clin Oncol* 1992; 10:1007–1013.

Levine MN, Browman GP, Gent M, et al: When is a prognostic factor useful? A guide for the perplexed. *J Clin Oncol* 1991; 9:348–356.

Mason J, Drummond M, Torrance G: Some guidelines on the use of cost-effectiveness league tables. *Br Med J* 1993; 306:570–572.

Moore MJ, O'Sullivan B, Tannock IF: How expert physicians would wish to be treated if they had genitourinary cancer. *J Clin Oncol* 1988; 6:1736–1745.

Naylor CD, Chen E, Strauss B: Measured enthusiasm: does the method of reporting trial results alter perceptions of therapeutic effectiveness? *Ann Intern Med* 1992; 117:916–921.

Nystrom L, Rutqvist LE, Wall S, et al: Breast Cancer Screening with mammography: Overview of Swedish randomized trials. *Lancet* 1991; 341:973–978.

Parmar MKB, Stewart LA, Altman DG: Meta-analyses of randomised trials: When the whole is more than just the sum of the parts. *Br J Cancer* 1996; 74:496–501.

Peto R, Pike MC, Armitage P, et al: Design and analysis of randomized clinical trials requiring prolonged observation of each patient: I. Introduction and design. *Br J Cancer* 1976; 34:585–612.

Peto R, Pike MC, Armitage P, et al: Design and analysis of randomized clinical trials requiring prolonged observation of each patient: II. Analysis and examples. *Br J Cancer* 1977; 35:1–39.

Ransohoff DF, Feinstein AR: Problems of spectrum and bias in evaluating the efficacy of diagnostic tests. *N Engl J Med* 1978; 299:926–930.

Rosseli Del Turco M, Palli D, Cariddi A, et al: Intensive diagnostic follow-up after treatment of primary breast cancer: A randomized trial. *JAMA* 1994; 271:1593–1597.

Sacks HS, Chalmers TC, Smith H: Sensitivity and specificity of clinical trials: Randomized v historical controls. *Arch Intern Med* 1983; 143:753–755.

Schipper H, Clinch J, McMurray A, Levitt M: Measuring the quality of life of cancer patients: The Functional Living Index—Cancer: development and validation. *J Clin Oncol* 1984; 2:472–483.

Schwartz D, Flamant R, Lellouch J: *Clinical Trials.* London: Academic Press; 1980.

Shulz KF: Subverting randomization in controlled trials: *JAMA* 1995; 274:1456–1458.

Slevin ML, Stubbs L, Plant HJ, et al: Attitudes to chemotherapy: Comparing views of patients with cancer and those of doctors, nurses, and general public. *Br Med J* 1990; 300:1458–1460.

Smith DS, Catalona WJ: Interexaminer variability of digital rectal examination in detecting prostate cancer. *Urology* 1995; 45:70–74.

Sprangers MAG: Response-shift bias: A challenge to the assessment of patients' quality of life in cancer clinical trials. *Cancer Treat Rev* 1996; 22(supplA):55–62.

Stewart LA, Parmar MKB: Meta-analysis of the literature or of individual patient data: Is there a difference? *Lancet* 1993; 341:418–422.

Tannock IF: Combined modality treatment with radiotherapy and chemotherapy. *Radiother Oncol* 1989; 16:83–101.

Tannock IF: False positive results in clinical trials: Multiple significance tests and the problem of unreported comparisons. *J Natl Cancer Inst* 1996; 88:206–207.

Tannock IF, Osoba D, Stockler MR, et al: Chemotherapy with mitoxantrone plus prednisone or prednisone alone for symptomatic hormone-resistant prostate cancer: A Canadian randomized trial with palliative endpoints. *J Clin Oncol* 1996; 14:1756–1764.

Tannock I, Warr D: Non-randomized trials of cancer chemotherapy: Phase II or III? *J Natl Cancer Inst* 1988; 80:800–801.

Tibshirani R: A plain man's guide to the proportional hazards model. *Clin Invest Med* 1982; 5:63–68.

Tonkin K, Tritchler D, Tannock I: Criteria of tumor response used in clinical trials of chemotherapy. *J Clin Oncol* 1985; 3:870–875.

Torrance GW: Utility approach to measuring health-related quality of life. *J Chronic Dis* 1987; 40:593–600.

Tukey JW: *Exploratory Data Analysis.* Reading, MA: Addison-Wesley; 1977.

Walter S: In defense of the arcsine approximation. *Statistician* 1979; 28:219–222.

Ware JE Jr, Snow KK, Kosinski M, Gandek B: *SF-36 Health Survey: Manual and Interpretation Guide.* Boston: The Health Institute, New England Medical Center; 1993.

Warr D, McKinney S, Tannock I: Influence of measurement error on assessment of response to anticancer chemotherapy: Proposal for new criteria of tumor response. *J Clin Oncol* 1984; 2:1040–1046.

Weeks J: Performance status upstaged? *J Clin Oncol* 1992; 10:1827–1829.

BIBLIOGRAPHY

Armitage P, Berry G: *Statistical Methods in Medical Research.* Oxford, England: Blackwell; 1987.

Drummond MF, Stoddart GL, Torrance GW: *Methods for the Economic Evaluation of Health Care Programmes.* New York: Oxford University Press; 1987.

Hennekens CM, Buring JE: *Epidemiology in Medicine.* Boston: Little, Brown; 1987.

Morrison AS: *Screening in Chronic Disease.* New York: Oxford University Press; 1986.

Sackett DL, Haynes RB, Guyatt GH, Tugwell P: *Clinical Epidemiology: A Basic Science for Clinical Medicine.* Boston: Little, Brown; 1991.

Sackett DL, Richardson WS, Rosenberg W, Haynes RB: *Evidence Based Medicine: How to Practice and Teach EBM.* London: Churchill Livingstone; 1997.

Symposium on Methodology and Quality Assurance in Cancer Clinical Trials. *Cancer Treat Rep* 1985; 69:1039–1129.

Glossary

Terms set in boldface are defined in the Glossary.

Accelerated fractionation: A schedule used in radiation therapy whereby the total treatment time is reduced to less than the conventional time (5 to 6 weeks), usually by giving more than one radiation fraction per day. (See Chap. 14, Sec. 14.4.1.)

Acute transforming virus: A virus that contains an **oncogene** and, following integration into the host-cell DNA, can cause malignant **transformation** of normal cells quite rapidly. (See Chap. 5, Sec. 5.3.2.)

Active immunotherapy: A treatment strategy that attempts to generate or stimulate an antitumor response by the host's own immune system. (See Chap. 18, Sec. 18.4.)

Active transport: The transport of molecules into a cell by an energy-dependent process. This process can transport molecules against a concentration gradient.

Adaptor protein: A small molecule that may act in **signal transduction** in cells by facilitating the association between other molecular components of signaling pathways. (See Chap. 6, Sec. 6.3.3.)

Additivity: The range of effects that might be expected when two or more cytotoxic agents are used in combination for treatment of cells or tumors when there is no specific interaction between them. This range of additivity can be defined from dose-response curves for the individual agents. (See Chap. 17, Sec. 17.3.2.)

Adjuvant: A substance that will enhance an immunologic response. An example is bacille Calmette-Guérin (BCG). A probable mechanism is stimulation of the secretion of **cytokines** that aid in the activation of an acquired immune response. (See Chap. 11, Sec. 11.2.1.)

Adjuvant chemotherapy: Drug treatment given to patients following surgical removal of their primary tumor and/or radiotherapy to it, when there is known to be a high risk of occult micrometastases but no clinical or radiological evidence of metastatic disease. If chemotherapy is given prior to treatment of the primary tumor, this therapy is referred to as "neoadjuvant chemotherapy." (See Chap. 17, Sec. 17.1.3.)

Adoptive immune therapy: A treatment strategy in which active immune cells are transferred to a tumor-bearing host; these cells have the capacity for stimulating tumor rejection. (See Chap. 18, Sec. 18.3.2.)

Alkylating agent: A compound that has positively charged (i.e., electron-deficient) groups or that may be metabolized to form such groups. These reactive ("**electrophilic**") groups can form covalent linkages with negatively charged chemical groups on biologic molecules such as those on the bases of DNA. A monofunctional alkylating agent can form a single adduct, whereas bifunctional alkylating agents can form two adducts, leading to inter- or intrastrand DNA–DNA **cross-links** or to DNA-protein cross-links. Alkylating agents include commonly used anticancer drugs such as cyclophosphamide. They may also have **mutagenic** and **carcinogenic** properties. (See Chap. 8, Sec. 8.2, and Chap. 16, Sec. 16.3.)

Alleles: Different forms of a **gene** that represent the same genetic locus on homologous **chromosomes.**

Allograft: Tissue that is transplanted between genetically different individuals of the same species.

Alpha error: Another term for **type I error.**

Ames assay: A widely used short-term assay for detecting mutagenic substances that uses a mutant bacterial strain *Salmonella typhimurium,* which is unable to synthesize the essential amino acid histidine. The assay detects revertant colonies that can grow because of **mutations** rendering them independent of histidine. (See Chap. 8, Sec. 8.3.1.)

Anaplasia: Histopathologic appearance of a tumor that lacks features allowing easy identification with the tissue of origin. Anaplastic tumors are usually rapidly growing and have a large number of cells in mitosis. (A synonym is "undifferentiated").

Anchorage-independence: A property of most cells that have undergone malignant transformation and of normal hemopoietic cells. These cells can proliferate in semisolid media such as agarose or methylcellulose without adherence to glass or specially coated tissue-culture plates.

Angiogenesis: Formation of new blood vessels. This process is essential for tumor growth and appears to be stimulated by endothelial cell **growth factor(s).** (See Chap. 9, Sec. 9.3.)

Antibody: A soluble protein molecule produced by plasma cells in response to an **antigen** and capable of specifically binding to that antigen. (See Chap. 11, Sec. 11.2.6.)

Antigen: An agent that is foreign (i.e., "nonself") to an animal and that is recognized by the immune system.

Antigen-presenting cell (APC): A cell that can present peptide antigens on its cell surface in association with molecules of the **major histocompatibility complex.** "Professional APCs" include **dendritic cells,** Langerhans cells in the skin, macrophages, and activated **B lymphocytes;** these cells are capable of fully activating lymphocytes and inducing an immune response. (See Chap. 11, Secs. 11.2 and 11.3; and Chap. 18, Sec. 18.4.5.)

Antimetabolite: A type of anticancer drug that is an analogue of a normal metabolite. Antimetabolites may inhibit metabolic pathways or may be mistaken for normal metabolites during the synthesis of macromolecules such as DNA or RNA. Examples are methotrexate and 5-fluorouracil, which are analogues of folic acid and thymine (or uracil), respectively. (See Chap. 16, Sec. 16.4.)

Antisense RNA: An RNA molecule with a sequence that is **homologous** to that contained within a target **gene.** These molecules can hybridize specifically with the complementary sequences in the mRNA which is transcribed from this gene, and prevent the production of the corresponding protein. (See Chap. 3, Sec. 3.3.11.)

Apoptosis: A process resulting in cell death due to the activation of a genetic program that causes cells to lose viability before they lose membrane integrity. The process involves **endonuclease**-mediated cleavage of the DNA into fragments of specific lengths, leading to a **"DNA ladder"** when it is subjected to gel **electrophoresis.** Apoptosis is also called **programmed cell death** and is important in maintaining tissue **homeostasis;** it may be important in the response to therapeutic agents. (See Chap. 7, Sec. 7.3.)

Area under the curve (AUC): A measure of the total exposure of blood or tissue to a chemical agent such as a toxin or anticancer agent. The AUC is obtained by plotting the concentration of the agent as a function of time and obtaining the AUC by integration. (See Chap. 16, Sec. 16.2.1.)

Ataxia telangiectasia (AT): A clinical syndrome in which patients have a variety of symptoms including ataxia (unstable gait) and telangiectasia (prominent and tortuous blood vessels). Cells from such individuals are sensitive to ionizing radiation and defective in **repair of DNA** damage. The AT patients have a high incidence of lymphoma. (See Chap. 4, Sec. 4.4.1.)

Autocrine: Refers to the production of substances (i.e., **growth factors** or hormones) that can influence the metabolism of the cell producing them.

Autoradiography: A technique to identify where a radioactive isotope is localized in cells or subcellular components. The process involves covering biological material with photographic film or emulsion. The radioactivity produced by the isotope then causes local exposure of the overlying film or emulsion, which, upon development, can be detected as dark grains close to the location of the isotope. (See Chap. 7, Sec. 7.4.1.)

Autosome: Any **chromosome** other than the sex chromosomes.

B cell (or B lymphocyte): A lymphocyte that is a precursor of antibody-producing plasma cells and expresses an **antibody** molecule (**immunoglobulin**) on its cell surface. (See Chap. 11, Sec. 11.2.6.)

Bacteriophage: A virus that infects bacteria. Bacteriophages are commonly used as carriers of **cloned genes.**

Base excision: A mechanism of **DNA repair** whereby a single damaged base is removed from the DNA. (See Chap. 4, Sec. 4.4.5.)

Basement membrane: A membranous tissue that surrounds nests of epithelial or endothelial cells and provides a structural framework for their organization. A basement membrane may also surround certain types of mesenchymal cells.

Bayes' theorem: Bayes' theorem is used in the interpretation of diagnostic tests to estimate the probability that disease may be present, based on previous knowledge of the probability that such disease is present and the new information gained in the diagnostic test. (See Chap. 20, Sec. 20.2.3.)

Bcl-2/Bax: **Genes** involved in the control of **apoptosis.** Their products form **dimers,** and increased *bcl-2* expression is associated with inhibition of apoptosis, whereas increased expression of *bax* is associated with stimulation of apoptosis. *bcl-2* may be an **oncogene.** (See Chap. 7, Sec. 7.3.3.)

Bcr/Abl: A fusion **gene** formed by the **translocation** of the *bcr* (break-point cluster region) gene on chromosome 22 next to the *c-abl* sequences on chromosome 9. This **reciprocal translocation,** which gives rise to the characteristic **Philadelphia chromosome,** occurs in chronic myelogenous leukemia. (See Chap. 4, Sec. 4.3.2; and Chap. 5, Sec. 5.4.4.)

Beta error: Another term for **type II error.**

Bias: Systematic departure from the true state (as compared to error, which is random departure from the true state). Faulty design may lead to the presence of many types of bias in trials of cancer causation and cancer treatment.

Bioassay: Quantitation of an agent by measuring the extent of its interaction with living organisms whose dose response has been predetermined. Examples are the assessment of the quantity of active metabolites of a drug in human serum by the toxicity of that serum for cells of known sensitivity, or the assessment of the level of a **growth factor** by measuring the stimulation of growth of sensitive cells.

Bioavailability: The proportion of an administered drug that is delivered to its site of action. For most agents, this is the proportion of drug entering the circulation. Bioavailability may be low if a drug is given orally. (See Chap. 16, Sec. 16.2.1.)

Biological response modifier: A biological agent that either (1) influences the host's own defense mechanisms to act against cancer cells or (2) modifies the response to another therapeutic agent. Examples of such agents are **interferons, interleukins,** and hemopoietic **growth factors.**

Bioreduction: The reductive metabolism of (usually) inactive precursor drugs to form metabolites that may be active in vivo. Bioreduction may take place in hypoxic regions of tumors. (See Chap. 15, Sec. 15.3.4.)

Cadherins: Membrane proteins that can interact to allow cell-cell adhesion. (See Chap. 9, Sec. 9.2.4.)

Carcinoembryonic antigen (CEA): A **glycoprotein** produced in the embryo and in lower concentrations in the adult colon. It may also be produced in higher concentrations by certain types of tumor cells, such as those originating in the colon or rectum. CEA is one example of substances that are known generally as **oncofetal antigens** and are used as tumor **markers.**

Carcinogen: A substance that causes cancer. Some chemical carcinogens can act directly, but others require metabolism in vivo before becoming effective. Most carcinogens are **mutagens.** (See Chap. 8.)

Carcinoma: Type of cancer arising in epithelial tissue (i.e., tissue lining internal or external organs, or glandular tissue). Most human cancers are carcinomas.

Carcinoma in situ: A pathologic description of tissue that has undergone changes in cellular features characteristic of malignant **transformation** but without invasion through the epithelial **basement membrane.**

Case-control study: An epidemiologic study in which individuals with disease (cases) are matched with those who are not diseased (controls), followed by assessment of these individuals for their previous exposure to putative causative agents such as **carcinogens.** (See Chap. 2, Sec. 2.2.4.)

Caspases: A family of molecules that effect **programmed cell death** or apoptosis. Also known as **ICE proteases.**

cDNA: A DNA copy complementary to mRNA sequences transcribed from a given **gene** or genes. cDNA therefore will **hybridize** with the DNA of the nontranscribed strand of these genes and, if radiolabeled, will allow their detection in **chromosomes ("in situ hybridization")** or in DNA or mRNA extracted from cells and separated by **electrophoresis** (in **Southern** or **Northern blots,** respectively). (See Chap. 3, Sec. 3.3.)

Cell adhesion molecules (CAMs): Molecules that are expressed on the surface of cells and that mediate the attachment of cells to the extracellular matrix and/or to other cells. Such molecules may be attached to the **cytoskeleton** and may also be involved in **signal transduction** pathways. (See Chap. 9, Sec. 9.2.)

Cell differentiation (CD) antigens: A classification for **antigens** expressed on the surface of different types of cells. The identification of CD antigens (usually with **monoclonal antibodies**) provides information about the nature and function of a particular cell. This classification has been particularly useful in differentiating the function of various hematologic precursor cells and of cells involved in the immune response.

Cell-mediated immunity: Immunologic defense against foreign agents that is mediated by cells (e.g., various types of lymphocytes) rather than by **antibodies.** (See Chap. 11, Sec. 11.3.)

Cell survival: A major determinant of the efficacy of anticancer drugs or radiation. Cell survival is determined by the ability of treated cells to proliferate to form a colony or **clone.** A **cell-survival curve** relates cell survival (usually plotted on a logarithmic scale) to dose of radiation or anticancer drug. (See Chap. 13, Secs. 13.3 and 13.4; and Chap. 15, Sec. 15.2.3.)

Centromere: The region of the **chromosome** at which the two identical components after DNA replication (known as **chromatids**) are held together, prior to their separation at mitosis. (See Chap. 3, Sec. 3.2.)

Chromatin: The DNA and associated proteins seen in the nucleus of cells in **interphase.**

Chromosome: The structural unit containing the genetic material (DNA) and associated proteins within a cell. Human cells usually have 46 chromosomes consisting of 22 pairs of **autosomes** plus the sex chromosomes (XX in females, XY in males). Different chromosomes may be recognized in metaphase cells by their shape and by the application of various stains that lead to the production of characteristic **bands.** After DNA replication, each chromosome contains a pair of **chromatids** joined at the **centromere.** Alterations in the structure of chromosomes are known as **aberrations.** They are common in cancer cells. (See Chap. 3, Sec. 3.2.)

Chromosome banding/G-banding: A method of staining **chromosomes** from metaphase cells to facilitate their recognition. G-banding is obtained by application of the

Giemsa stain to metaphase chromosomes that have been treated briefly with the proteolytic enzyme trypsin. (See Chap. 3, Sec. 3.2.)

Chronic Tumor Virus: A virus that can cause malignant **transformation** in target cells through integration into the host-cell DNA and the aberrant activation of adjacent cellular **genes.** In contrast to an **acute transforming virus,** a chronic tumor virus does not contain an **oncogene** and transformation takes place more slowly. (See Chap. 5, Sec. 5.3.3.)

Clonal evolution/Clonal selection: There is evidence that most tumors originate from a single cell (i.e., are clonal), but ongoing genetic changes during tumor growth lead to the generation of different subclones. "Clonal evolution/selection" refers to the growth advantage of certain **clones** within the tumor, generally those expressing more malignant properties. (See Chap. 10, Sec. 10.1.)

Clone: A family of cells all derived from one parent cell. A clonal marker (e.g., an abnormal **chromosome** or protein product) may identify all of the cells within a given clone. Most human tumors appear to arise from a single cell and hence are clonal.

Cloned gene: A **gene** that has been isolated and inserted into a **"vector,"** such as a **plasmid** or **bacteriophage** virus. The vector containing the gene can be produced in large amounts, thereby providing many copies of the gene suitable for assays and studies of its function. Cloned genes can be used to produce large quantities of pure protein products of cells (e.g., insulin, **interferons**). (See Chap. 3, Sec. 3.3.3.)

Clonogenic assay: An experimental method that assesses the probability of survival of colony-forming (i.e., **clonogenic**) cells after some form of treatment, as with radiation or anticancer drugs. (See Chap. 13, Sec. 13.3; and Chap. 15, Sec. 15.2.3.)

Clonogenic cell: A cell that has the ability to generate progeny which form a colony of predetermined minimum size when plated in appropriate growth conditions. Such a cell is also referred to as a colony-forming unit (CFU). Clonogenic cells may be identified in assays of **cell survival.** The term "CFU" is most often applied to progenitor cells in the bone marrow that may produce **clones** of cells in one or more pathways of **differentiation.**

Coding region: The coding region is that part of a gene which codes for a protein. The part of the DNA molecule that is initially transcribed into messenger RNA (mRNA) contains both **introns** and **exons.** The **introns** are regions of mRNA that are **spliced** out during posttranscriptional processing. The **exon** regions in the mRNA comprise the processed message; they contain the coding regions and therefore are the "expressed" portion of the **gene.** The processed mRNA usually contains untranslated regions both 5' and 3' to the region that codes the protein being made; some of these untranslated regions contain important regulatory signals.

Codon: A group of three DNA or mRNA bases that code for a given amino acid. Codons thus form the "words" of the genetic code.

Cohort study: An epidemiologic study whereby subsets of a given population are defined on the basis of exposure or nonexposure to a factor suspected of increasing the risk of disease (such as cancer) and then followed forward in time to observe the development of the disease. (See Chap. 2, Sec. 2.2.3.)

Colony-forming assay: Another term for **clonogenic assay.**

Colony-stimulating factor: A **growth factor** that stimulates the formation of colonies of progeny from certain types of cell. The term is used most commonly to describe growth factors that act on precursors of hemopoiesis. (See Chap. 7, Sec. 7.5.1.)

Complementation: A technique that can assist in localizing a defective **gene.** Two types of cell containing different genetic defects are **hybridized** and complementation is said to occur if the hybrid cell lacks these genetic defects. This result indicates that the genes are on different parts of **chromosomes,** so that the normal chromosomal component provided by the other cell complements the defect. (See Chap. 3, Sec. 3.4.2; and Chap. 4, Sec. 4.4.2.)

Comparative genomic hybridization (CGH): A method that allows detection of amplified or deleted segments of DNA. In this technique, DNA from two different types of cells is labeled with two different fluorochromes and then **hybridized** simultaneously to normal chromosomal metaphase spreads. Regions of gain or loss of DNA sequences in one cell as compared with the other are seen as changes in the ratio of the intensities of the two fluorochromes along the target chromosome. (See Chap. 3, Sec. 3.4.5.)

Cosmid: A circular piece of DNA that has properties similar to those of a **plasmid.** It is larger than a plasmid and may contain different regulatory elements.

Costimulatory molecule: A molecule expressed on the surface of **antigen-presenting cells** that provides a second signal (augmenting the primary signal initiated by the **antigenic** peptide presented by a **major histocompatibility molecule**) for stimulation of an immune response. (See Chap. 11, Sec. 11.3.5.)

Cross-links: Abnormal bonding between (interstrand) or within (intrastrand) DNA strands or between DNA strands and proteins (DNA-protein) that can be induced by radiation or anticancer drugs.

Cyclin/cyclin-dependent kinase: Cyclins are proteins whose activity varies around the cell cycle. Cyclins bind to cyclin-dependent kinases (CDKs), which are small serine/threonine kinases expressed at relatively constant levels through the cell cycle. Activation of cyclins in these complexes is associated with progression of cells from one cell cycle phase to the next. Different cyclins and CDKs are involved in different phases of the cell cycle. (See Chap. 7, Sec. 7.2.2.)

Cyclin-dependent kinase (CDK) inhibitor: A protein that inhibits the function of **cyclin–dependent kinases** and thereby inhibits cell cycle progression. CDK inhibitors are members of two families known as the KIP (*Kinase Inhibitor Protein*) family and the INK-4 (*Inhibitor of CDK-4*) family. (See Chap. 7, Sec. 7.2.3.)

Cytochrome P-450: A large family of drug metabolizing enzymes that are particularly important in the activation of **carcinogens.** (See Chap. 8, Sec. 8.2.2.)

Cytokine: A protein molecule that is secreted by cells and acts to modify the proliferation, **differentiation,** or function of other cells that express specific **receptors.** Cytokines are particularly important in the generation and control of immune responses.

Cytoskeleton: The group of molecules that provides physical structure and defines the form and shape of cells.

Cytotoxic T lymphocytes: Activated T lymphocytes responsible for the killing of target cells during a cell-mediated immune response. (See Chap. 11, Sec. 11.3.3.)

Deletion: Loss of DNA. Deletions can be small, affecting only a small part of a single **gene,** or large—for example, a **chromosomal** deletion involving many genes.

Dendritic cell: A cell derived from the bone marrow that expresses high cell surface levels of critical **major histocompatibility antigens** as well as **costimulatory** and adhesive molecules that render it an efficient **antigen-presenting cell.** Purified dendritic cells are being used in approaches to immunotherapy. (See Chap. 18, Sec. 18.4.5.)

DNA adduct: A chemical group bound to DNA that will usually interfere with DNA replication and/or transcription.

DNA arrays: A matrix of a large number of known DNA molecules (or parts of molecules) attached to an inert substrate. Such matrices can be **hybridized** with unknown mixtures of mRNAs or DNAs to identify which **genes** are being expressed or are the subject of genomic imbalance in the cells from which the mixtures were derived.

DNA ladder: A pattern seen in **electrophoresis** of DNA from apoptotic cells. **Endonucleases** induced during **apoptosis** cut DNA into fragments that are multiples of about 180 base pairs. When the DNA of such cells is subjected to gel **electrophoresis,** a characteristic ladder-like pattern of DNA fragments is produced. (See Chap. 7, Sec. 7.3.1.)

DNA methylation: Bases in DNA, particularly cytosine, may become methylated. This can modify or inhibit the transcription of a gene. Such methylations are potentially reversible and are often referred to as "**epigenetic** changes" to distinguish them from **mutations** involving changes in DNA bases.

DNA repair: The process whereby damaged DNA acts as a substrate for enzymes that attempt to restore its normal structure and the original base sequence. It is a complex process involving many enzymes and may lead to repair of damage in one or both strands. Repair may lead to complete restoration of the DNA (error-free repair) or may result in alteration or deletion of bases (error-prone repair). (See Chap. 4, Sec. 4.4.)

Dicentric chromosome: An abnormal chromosome that contains two **centromeres.**

Differential display analysis: A technique for detecting differences in the expression levels of mRNAs in different cells. This electrophoresis-based technique allows the identification of differences in expression of unknown mRNAs, which can then be isolated and sequenced. (See Chap. 3, Sec. 3.3.9.)

Differentiation: The development by cells of specific characteristics that allow the normal function of tissues. Tumors may show varying degrees of differentiation, depending on their similarity to the structure of the organ from which the tumor was derived. **Terminal differentiation** is said to occur when cells form progeny that are no longer capable of division.

Dimer: A molecule formed by the joining of two substituent molecules. In a homodimer, the constituent molecules are identical; in a heterodimer, they are different.

Diurnal rhythm: Variation in the biological properties of an organism throughout the day. Many properties—such as the concentration of hormones or the activity of certain enzymes—may show diurnal variation.

Double minute: A small amount of genetic material seen in some cells as a paired body resembling a very small **chromosome** without a **centromere.** Because they lack a centromere, double minutes distribute themselves randomly at mitosis and are easily lost during cell growth. Double minutes have been shown to contain amplified **genes.** (See Chap. 4, Sec. 4.3.1.)

Double-strand break (DSB): A lesion causing interruption of both strands (sugar-phosphate "backbone") of a DNA molecule. Such DSBs are believed responsible for the cytotoxic effects of ionizing radiation. (See Chap. 4, Sec. 4.4.6; and Chap. 13, Sec. 13.2.3.)

Doubling time: The time taken for an exponentially growing tumor (or cell population) to double its volume (or number of cells). (See Chap. 7, Sec. 7.6.1.)

Dysplasia: Abnormal morphologic changes in the cells of a tissue involving their nuclei, organization, and maturation.

Ectopic hormone: A hormone produced by cells that do not usually produce it. The cells of several types of tumor may produce ectopic hormones.

Electrophile: A molecule or chemical group that is positively charged and attracts electrons. Electrophiles, therefore, interact with negatively charged electron-rich groups on biological molecules such as DNA. The active forms of many **carcinogens** are electrophiles and therefore can bind to DNA. (See Chap. 8, Sec. 8.2.)

Electrophoresis: The separation of molecular components (peptides, proteins, or pieces of DNA or RNA) by their different rates of migration in an electric field. **Gel electrophoresis** refers to electrophoresis through an agarose or polyacrylamide gel and is used commonly in molecular technology. Molecules of lower molecular weight usually migrate more rapidly under electrophoresis.

Electroporation: A process whereby cells are exposed to an electric field that causes the formation of temporary pores in the cell membrane, allowing large molecules such as DNA or antibodies, which would normally be excluded, to enter the cell.

Endocrine: A gland at one site in the body that releases a hormone into the bloodstream to act on tissues distant to that site is known as an endocrine gland. An example of an endocrine gland is the thyroid gland. (See Chap. 12.)

Endonuclease: An enzyme that can cut an intact strand of DNA or RNA at some point in the strand other than at an end. Endonucleases are important in **DNA repair** (see Chap. 4, Sec. 4.4) and are responsible for cutting of DNA during **apoptosis.** (See Chap. 7, Sec. 7.3.)

Enhancer: A DNA sequence that increases the activity of **promotor** sequences or initiators of mRNA transcription. Enhancers can be located anywhere in the noncoding regions of a gene.

Enzyme-linked immunoadsorbent assay (ELISA): A sensitive method for measuring the amount of a substance. The method requires the availability of an **antibody** to the substance and depends on measuring the activity of an enzyme (e.g., alkaline phosphatase) bound to the antibody.

Epidermal growth factor (EGF): A **growth factor** that binds to a specific **receptor** (EGFR) that can initiate **signal transduction** in target cells of the epidermis and other normal or malignant epithelial tissues. (See Chap. 6, Sec. 6.2.)

Epigenetic: Epigenetic changes alter the expression of **genes** without causing permanent base damage. **DNA methylation** represents one form of epigenetic change in DNA.

Episome: A circular form of DNA that replicates in cells independent of the **chromosomes.** Viral DNA may form episomes in cells. **Plasmids** used for gene cloning grow as episomes in bacteria.

Epitope: A small part of a molecule that can be recognized by **antigen receptors** on lymphocytes and which elicits an immune response against that molecule. (See Chap. 11, Sec. 11.2.3.)

Epstein-Barr virus: A DNA virus associated with Burkitt's lymphoma, nasopharyngeal cancer, and Hodgkin's disease. (See Chap. 5, Sec. 5.2.4.)

Erythropoietin: A hormone produced by the kidney that stimulates the proliferation of red cell precursors in the bone marrow. It is now being used to treat anemia.

Exocrine: A gland that releases substances to act locally through a duct is known as an exocrine gland. An example of such a gland is the **sweat gland.**

Exons: The regions of a **gene** that contain the DNA sequences necessary to direct translation of the polypeptide gene product. These sequences, which include the **coding region,** are preserved in the processed mRNA.

Exonuclease: An enzyme that catalyzes the base-by-base destruction of DNA or RNA starting at one end of a strand.

Experimental metastasis assay: A technique for studying the ability of cells to form **metastases** in experimental animals after intravenous injection. (See Chap. 10, Sec. 10.3.1.)

Extracellular matrix: The complex group of molecules that exist in tissue outside the cells. (See Chap. 9, Sec. 9.1.1.)

Facilitated diffusion: A process in which the diffusion of certain substances into cells is enhanced. Specific molecules in the cell membrane (permeases) bind to the substance and assist its diffusion through the membrane down a concentration gradient from outside to inside the cell.

First pass: "First pass" refers to the absorption of orally applied drugs into the intestinal circulation and their subsequent passage (first pass) through the liver, where metabolism can occur, before they reach the general circulation. This first-pass metabolism can account for differences in **bioavailability** between orally and intravenously administered drugs. (See Chap. 16, Sec. 16.2.1.)

Fluorescence-in-situ hybridization (FISH): A technique in which a fluorescent-labeled DNA probe binds to the **complementary gene** segment in **chromosomes** of metaphase spreads. FISH, therefore, allows the localization of genes to specific chromosomes. The technique can also be used in interphase cells to determine the number of copies of the gene that the cells contain. Using chromosome-specific probes the technique can identify chromosome aberrations, particularly **translocations.** (See Chap. 3, Sec. 3.4.4.)

Flow cytometry: A technique in which cells are tagged with a fluorescent dye and then directed in single file through a laser beam. The intensity of fluorescence induced by the laser light is detected and the number of cells exhibiting different levels of fluorescence is recorded. The method is used frequently to study cell-cycle properties, since several dyes are available whose binding in cells—and hence fluorescence intensity—is proportional to DNA content. Cells may also be separated according to the intensity of their fluorescence in a process known as fluorescence-activated cell sorting (FACS). (See Chap. 7, Sec. 7.4.)

Frameshift mutation: A DNA mutation that leads to a change in the initiation point of translation of the mRNA transcript, such that the normal reading frame for the **codons,** which define the amino acid sequence of the protein product, is shifted by one or two bases, resulting in a different amino acid sequence.

Free radical: An unstable chemical species that is highly reactive due to the presence of an unpaired electron. It may be formed when drugs or radiation interact with tissue. Free radicals may be responsible for much of the biological damage that occurs after such interactions.

Fusion protein: A protein formed by transcription from fused genetic segments of two or more **genes.** Fusion proteins may occur naturally (for example, the *bcr/abl* protein formed by **translocation** in chronic myelogenous leukemia) or may be genetically engineered to produce a protein of desired characteristics (for example, a protein that is fused from components that are (1) toxic and (2) bind to a **receptor** on a tumor cell). (See Chap. 17, Sec. 17.1.4; and Chap. 18, Sec. 18.3.4.)

G proteins: A family of proteins that bind to guanosine triphosphate (GTP) and include the products of the *ras* **oncogenes.** (See Chap. 6, Sec. 6.3.4.)

G418: An analogue of the cytotoxic antibiotic neomycin that is used commonly to select for cells that have been **transfected** with genetic constructs containing the *neo*^{R} (neomycin resistance) **gene.**

Gene: A sequence of DNA that codes for a single polypeptide or protein. This sequence includes **coding** and noncoding regions as well as regulatory regions. Genes may sometimes be overlapping, so that the same sequence contributes to two different proteins. **Gene amplification** may occur through multiplication of the DNA sequences of the gene; a large amount of amplification can often be recognized by the presence of either **homogeneously staining regions** (HSRs) on **chromosomes** or by the presence of **double minutes.**

Genetic epidemiology: Study of the distribution among populations of various genetic defects such as those predisposing to various types of cancer (e.g., *BRCA-1* or retinoblastoma gene mutations).

Glutathione: A small molecule composed of three amino acids (glycine, cysteine, glutamate) that is prevalent within cells and can bind to reactive compounds and aid in their excretion. (See Chap. 17, Sec. 17.2.6.)

Glycoprotein: A protein to which various types of sugar molecule have been attached. Glycoproteins are important components of the cell surface.

Grade: The histopathologic appearance of a tumor in terms of its degree of **differentiation.** A low-grade tumor is well differentiated and a high-grade tumor tends to be **anaplastic.**

Growth factor: A polypeptide produced by cells that acts to stimulate or inhibit proliferation by either the same cell or other cells. Several types of growth factor have been isolated and some of these may be associated with abnormal regulation of growth in **transformed** cells. Growth factors interact with cells through specific **receptors** in the cell membrane.

Growth fraction: The proportion of cells within a tumor that are actively proliferating (i.e., progressing through the cell cycle). (See Chap. 7, Sec. 7.4.1.)

Half-life (plasma): The plasma clearance curve that describes the concentration of a drug in plasma as a function of time after administration frequently has components that are approximately exponential. Plasma half-lives characterize the exponentially decreasing components of these clearance curves and represent the time for drug concentration to decrease by 50 percent. (See Chap. 16, Sec. 16.2.1.)

Half-life (radioactivity): Radioactive isotopes decay randomly, so that on average there is a constant time for the activity to decay to half of its starting value. This time is the half-life.

Heat-shock proteins: A family of stress proteins whose synthesis is stimulated by the exposure of cells to heat or various other stimuli, including hypoxia and hypoglycemia. Heat-shock proteins have diverse functions; for example, the 90-kDa heat-shock protein binds to the steroid hormone receptor and plays a part in regulating its function, while other HSPs may act as "chaperone" proteins that bind to and assist other proteins to fold correctly. (See Chap. 12, Sec. 12.2.3; and Chap. 19, Sec. 19.1.4.)

Heterogeneity: Variability in the properties of cells within an individual tumor. Wide heterogeneity of many properties is found among cancer cells. (See Chap. 10, Sec. 10.1.)

Histocompatibility antigen: Rejection of foreign tissue is determined by differences in histocompatibility antigens on cells of the donor and host tissues. One locus (which includes several **genes**) is associated with strong rejection and is known as the **major histocompatibility complex (MHC).** MHC molecules present peptide fragments from degraded molecules as antigens on the surface of **antigen-presenting cells.** Class I MHC molecules present peptide fragments from degraded intracellular molecules, whereas class II MHC molecules present fragments of extracellular peptides that have been endocytosed into the cell. (See Chap. 11, Sec. 11.3.2.)

Homeostasis: The maintenance of a normal physiologic state. Homeostasis is often maintained through feedback systems employing signals (e.g., hormones or **growth factors**) that have opposite effects.

Homogeneously staining region (HSR): A region appearing uniform on **chromosomes** that have been stained to examine their banding pattern. It often represents amplification of **genes.** HSRs tend to be stably inherited by daughter cells. (See Chap. 4, Sec. 4.3.1.)

Homologous recombination: The crossing over and rejoining of corresponding (homologous) regions of DNA on opposite **chromosomes** that occur normally during meiosis. A similar process can occur between a segment of DNA introduced into a cell and the homologous region on one of the chromosomes, or during **repair of DNA** damage.

Homology: Correspondence of the sequence of bases on different strands of DNA or RNA such that either strand will **hybridize to** complementary sequences.

Homozygosity (homozygous): When the two **alleles** of a **gene** on the two copies of the same **chromosome** in a cell are identical. (**Heterozygosity** refers to the presence of different alleles of a gene on the two copies of the same chromosome).

Human antimouse antibody (HAMA) response: The rejection response that can occur when **monoclonal antibodies** derived from murine cells are injected into humans for immunotherapy or immunodiagnosis. (See Chap. 18, Sec. 18.3.4.)

Humoral immunity: Immunologic defenses mediated by **antibodies.** (See Chap. 11, Sec. 11.2.6.)

Hybridization: (1) The fusion of two somatic cells to form a single cell. (2) The binding of complementary sequences of DNA or RNA. Such complementary binding may take place under different conditions (degrees of stringency) that dictate the extent of complementarity required for binding to occur. Radiolabeled pieces of DNA or RNA can be used as **probes** to identify the presence of specific DNA sequences by hybridization. The technique may also localize **genes** to specific **chromosomes** in a process known as "in situ hybridization."

Hybridoma: The term is used most commonly to describe a population of hybrid cells that produces **monoclonal antibodies.** Such a cell is produced by fusing an antibody-producing normal cell and a non-antibody-secreting myeloma cell. (See Chap. 18, Sec. 18.3.3.)

Hydrophilic: A molecule or chemical group that has high solubility in water primarily because of its polarity.

Hydrophobic: A molecule or chemical group that has low solubility in water, usually because it is nonpolar. Such molecules usually have higher solubility in lipids.

Hyperfractionation: A schedule used in radiation therapy where multiple (two or three) small dose fractions are given each day. (See Chap. 14, Sec. 14.4.1.)

Hyperplasia: An increase in the number of normal cells in a tissue. Hyperplasia can be either a normal (physiologic) or an abnormal (pathologic) process.

Hyperthermia: The use of elevated temperature as an anticancer treatment. (See Chap. 19, Sec. 19.1.)

Hypoxic cell: A cell, often within a tumor, that lacks oxygen. Such cells are important because they are resistant to the effects of radiation therapy and are usually in regions with poor vascular supply.

Idiotype: The variable (V) region of an **antibody** or **T cell receptor.** The idiotype is, itself, **antigenic,** and anti-idiotype responses have been used in the treatment of lymphomas. (See Chap. 11, Sec. 11.2.6; and Chap. 18, Sec. 18.4.1.)

Immortalization: The process that allows cells to form a cell line (i.e., to be able to proliferate indefinitely) in culture. Normal cells will proliferate for only a limited number of passages in culture before they undergo **senescence** and die. Immortalization appears to be a necessary but not sufficient step for **transformation** to a **malignant** state.

Immune surveillance: A proposed mechanism whereby the immune response recognizes the development of **malignant** cells at an early stage and inactivates them before they can develop into tumors. (See Chap. 11, Sec. 11.4.2.)

Immunogen: Any molecule that can elicit an immune response.

Immunoglobulin: An **antibody** molecule. In general, immunoglobulins consist of two heavy chains and two light chains linked by disulfide bonds (IgM-class immunoglobulins have 10 heavy and 10 light chains). The **immunoglobulin superfamily** consists of molecules with related structure and sequence that are found as components of a number of protein molecules, including those involved in cellular interactions with the **extracellular matrix.** (See Chap. 11, Sec. 11.2.6.)

Immunohistochemistry: A histologic process whereby a colored stain is linked to an **antibody** (usually a **monoclonal antibody**) that recognizes specific **receptors** on cells in tissue.

Immunosuppression: A state in which immune responses are impaired. This may occur in patients with some types of cancer, following treatment with drugs and radiation, or following treatment given as part of the preparation for organ transplantation. Certain inbred strains of mice may be immunosuppressed (or immune-deprived) by virtue of

mutations that they carry in their genome [e.g., **nude** mice or mice with severe combined immunodeficiency (**SCID**)].

Immunotoxin: A molecule that recognizes and binds to target cells by immune-mediated mechanisms and which has a toxic component that can inactivate target cells. The term is used most commonly to describe a hybrid molecule consisting of a **monoclonal antibody** that is conjugated or fused to a toxin. (See Chap. 18, Sec. 18.3.4.)

Imprinting: A process whereby a specific **gene** or **allele** is silenced (prevented from producing a product), usually by **methylation** of cytosine bases. This usually occurs in the embryo and is often tissue-specific. (See Chap. 4, Sec. 4.2.1.)

Innate immunity: A component of the immune system that is nonspecific and present at all times in normal individuals. It depends on a group of cells and released factors that provide natural resistance as the first-line of defense against invading pathogens. (See Chap. 11, Sec. 11.2.1.)

Incidence: A term used in epidemiology to describe the number of new cases (e.g., of cancer) observed in a population in a given unit of time, usually 1 year. (See Chap. 2, Sec. 2.2.1.)

Initiation: The first stage in the process of carcinogenesis. It involves interaction of the **carcinogen** with the DNA of the target cells to produce, after DNA replication, a permanent lesion. Subsequent steps include **promotion** and **progression.** (See Chap. 8, Sec. 8.2.1.)

Insertional mutagenesis: The process in which there is a change (or loss) of function of a **gene** as a result of the incorporation of a piece of exogenous DNA (often from a virus or **plasmid** introduced into the cell) into the DNA of that gene, thereby disrupting its normal transcription and translation or the control of these processes.

Integration: The process by which viral or **plasmid** DNA, or DNA copies of the RNA of a **retrovirus,** are incorporated into the chromosomal DNA of a cell.

Integrins: A family of membrane **glycoproteins** that can bind to a range of molecules present in the **extracellular matrix** (or on the surface of other cells) and that can mediate adhesion between a cell and the extracellular matrix or between cells. Integrins can also initiate **signal transduction.** (See Chap. 9, Sec. 9.2.1.)

Interferon: A protein produced by cells in response to viral infection. Several types of interferon have been identified and they have multiple effects on the host immune response as well as more general effects on cell growth and **differentiation.** Interferons are examples of **biological response modifiers.**

Interleukins: A family of molecules that are secreted, most often by lymphocytes, and which regulate the proliferation, **differentiation,** or function of hemopoietic cells or cells of the immune system.

ICE proteases: A family of molecules that effect **programmed cell death** or **apoptosis.** (ICE = *I*nterleukin 1B–Converting *E*nzyme). The enzymes are now also known as caspases. (See Chap. 7, Sec. 7.3.3.)

Interphase: The phases of the cell cycle other than mitosis. Thus, G1, S, and G2 phase are all components of interphase.

Intron: A noncoding region in the internal portion of a **gene.** Sequences transcribed from these regions are **spliced** out during processing of the initial mRNA transcript.

Invasion: Infiltration by cancer cells into neighboring normal tissues. It is one of the distinguishing features of malignancy.

Ionizing radiation: Radiation (e.g., x- or γ-rays) that is sufficiently energetic for its interactions with matter (tissue) to cause the formation of ions. (See Chap. 13, Sec. 13.2.1.)

Isobologram: A diagram in the format of a graph whose axes represent doses of two cytotoxic agents A and B. The isobologram joins points at which the combination of different doses of A and B produce an equal level of biological damage. The diagram is useful in determining whether the effects of two agents may be **additive,** subadditive (or antagonistic), or supraadditive (or **synergistic**). (See Chap. 17, Sec. 17.3.2.)

Isoeffect curve: An isoeffect curve indicates graphically the relationship between different dose schedules of a treatment that produce the same biological effect. The curve is used mainly to represent the effects of radiation treatments given as different numbers of fractions or in different overall times. The total radiation dose is plotted as a function of the fraction number, fraction size, or treatment time. (See Chap. 14, Sec. 14.3.7.)

Isomer: One structural form of a chemical compound that can occur naturally in a number of different structural forms. An example is diammine dichloroplatinum II, in which a different arrangement of the attachment of the amine and chloride groups to the platinum atom gives rise to the *cis*- and *trans*-isomers, which have very different biological activities.

Isozyme (isoenzyme): One of several chemical forms of an enzyme that have the same biological function. Tumor cells often produce one particular isozyme, frequently that associated with fetal tissue.

Karyotype: The **chromosome** content of a particular cell. The karyotype is usually displayed by imaging the chromosomes in a metaphase cell and ordering them according to a standard notation. (See Chap. 3, Sec. 3.2.)

Knockout mouse: A mouse derived from an embryonic stem (ES) cell that has been manipulated to cause a dysfunctional (knockout) mutation in a specific **gene.** (See Chap. 3, Sec. 3.3.12.)

Knudson's hypothesis: The hypothesis that at least two genetic events are required in order to transform a normal cell into a **malignant** cell. It was postulated originally by Knudson to explain the inheritance pattern of retinoblastoma, a rare childhood malignancy. (See Chap. 4, Secs. 4.2.2 and 4.5.1.)

Labeling index: The proportion of cells in any tissue that are synthesizing DNA and that, therefore, can be recognized as labeled by uptake of DNA precursors such as ^{3}H-thymidine or bromodeoxyuridine (BrdUrd). (See Chap. 7, Sec. 7.4.1.)

Late effects: Toxicity to normal tissues that becomes apparent at a time long after (months to years) the application of radiation therapy. Late effects usually limit the dose of radiation that can be given. (See Chap. 14, Sec. 14.2.2.)

Lead-time bias: A type of **bias** that can confound the interpretation of screening studies. Screening will usually detect disease at an earlier stage, and survival from the time of diagnosis will therefore be increased by the lead time that is gained by the screening assay. This is independent of any change in survival due to earlier initiation of therapy. (See Chap. 20, Sec. 20.2.4.)

Lectins: Naturally occurring proteins that can bind to specific oligosaccharide structures on cell-surface **glycoproteins** and glycolipids. They may have two or more binding sites and hence can cause cell agglutination.

Leucine-zipper domain: The part of a protein in which every seventh amino acid is leucine. These leucine residues protrude from the same side of the α-helical secondary structure of the protein and interact **hydrophobically** with similar domains on another protein to form molecules that are **homo-** or **heterodimers.** Such domains are usually found in proteins that are **transcription factors.** (See Chap. 6, Sec. 6.3.6.)

Length-time bias: A type of **bias** in screening studies that arises because a test performed at fixed intervals is more likely to detect slower-growing disease (that which is present for a longer time) than rapidly progressive disease. Thus, patients whose disease is detected by such a screening test may have a better prognosis. (See Chap. 20, Sec. 20.2.4.)

Lethal dose 50 percent (LD$_{50}$): The dose of radiation or of a drug that will, on average, cause 50 percent of animals receiving it to die.

Ligand: A molecule that binds to a **receptor.**

Likelihood ratio: The ratio of the probability that disease is present and the probability that it is absent following application of a diagnostic test. (See Chap. 20, Sec. 20.2.3.)

Linear energy transfer (LET): A measure of the density of energy deposition along the track of a given type of **ionizing radiation** in matter. The deposition of energy in matter by ionizing radiation occurs randomly along the parti-

cle track and in different amounts, hence LET is a quantity usually averaged over segments of the track length (track-averaged LET). (See Chap. 13, Sec. 13.2.2.)

Linear quadratic equation: An equation describing biological effect as a function of dose of a cytotoxic agent, such as radiation, which contains both linear and quadratic (squared) terms of dose with constants α and β respectively. It provides a useful model for describing the shape of radiation **survival curves** and for comparing **isoeffective** radiation treatments. (See Chap. 13, Sec. 13.4.3; and Chap. 14, Sec. 14.3.8.)

Linkage: A measure of the proximity of two **genes** on a **chromosome.** The more closely linked the two genes the less likely they are to be separated by crossing over of chromosomes during meiosis and hence the more likely they are to be inherited together.

Lipophilic: A substance that is lipid-soluble. Lipophilic substances penetrate readily into cells, since they are soluble in the cell membrane.

Liposome: A small vesicle containing fluid surrounded by a lipid membrane. Liposomes may be constructed to have varying lipid content in their membranes and to contain various types of drugs or other molecules. (See Chap. 17, Sec. 17.1.4.)

Loss of heterozygosity (LOH): An individual with two different **alleles** of a **gene** is said to be **heterozygous** for that gene. Loss of heterozygosity signifies loss of one of the alleles. This may occur by simple loss of an allele or by replacement of one allele with a duplicated copy of the other allele. In a tumor cell, LOH may indicate that the tumor suppressor gene of a normal allele has been replaced by a mutant allele. (See Chap. 4, Sec. 4.5.3; and Chap. 5, Sec. 5.5.1.)

Lymphokine: A substance usually produced by lymphocytes (or monocytes) that has an effect on other lymphocytes. An example is **interleukin**-2 (IL-2), also known as T-cell **growth factor,** which is required for the growth of **T lymphocytes.**

Lymphokine-activated killer (LAK) cells: Lymphocytes that have been incubated in vitro with high levels of **interleukin-2** proliferate and **differentiate** into aggressive killer cells with antitumor activity. These cells have been used in approaches to immunotherapy of human tumors. (See Chap. 11, Sec. 11.3.7; and Chap. 18, Sec. 18.3.2.)

Major histocompatibility complex (MHC): The complex locus of genes transcribed into proteins (**histocompatibility antigens**) that are expressed on cells and are responsible for the rejection of foreign tissue. (See Chap. 11, Sec. 11.3.2.)

Malignancy: The essential property of cancer cells that is demonstrated by their ability to proliferate indefinitely, to invade surrounding tissue, and to **metastasize** to other organs.

Marker: A substance produced by tumor cells and released into the blood such that the concentration in blood may be related to the bulk of tumor present in the individual.

Meta-analysis: A statistical technique for combining the results of clinical trials evaluating similar strategies. The technique facilitates the detection of small but clinically important differences between experimental and standard therapies. (See Chap. 20, Sec. 20.4.7.)

Metalloproteinases: Proteolytic enzymes secreted by cells that may cause degradation of components of **the extracellular matrix.** These enzymes may be involved in the process of **metastasis.** (See Chap. 10, Sec. 10.5.2.)

Metastasis: The spread of cells from a primary tumor to a noncontiguous site, usually via the bloodstream or lymphatics, and the establishment of a secondary growth.

Microenvironment: The environment surrounding cells in solid tissue. The microenvironment may change quite markedly over short distances with respect to metabolic factors such as level of oxygen and pH as well as in the consistency of the **extracellular matrix.**

Mismatch repair: A mechanism for **repair of DNA** that contains single-base mispairs or small insertions or **deletions.** Defects in mismatch repair **genes** may predispose to cancer and to progressive genetic changes in malignant cells. (See Chap. 4, Sec. 4.4.4, and Chap. 10, Sec. 10.1.)

Mitogen: A substance that stimulates the proliferation of cells.

Mitogen-activated protein kinase (MAPK) pathway: A signaling pathway that transmits signals imparted by **growth factors** or other **mitogens** at the cell surface to influence proliferation-related **genes** in the cell nucleus. (See Chap. 6, Sec. 6.3.5.)

Mitotic death: The degradation and lysis of cells in mitosis. This is observed frequently following radiation. (See Chap. 13, Sec. 13.3.3.)

Mitotic delay: Delay in the passage of a cell through its growth cycle (particularly mitosis) that is induced by radiation or some anticancer drugs. (See Chap. 13, Sec. 13.3.2.)

Mitotic index: The proportion of cells in a tissue that are in mitosis at any given time.

Monoclonal antibody: An **antibody** of a single defined specificity, most commonly obtained from a single clone of antibody-producing cells or **hybridoma.** A monoclonal antibody binds to a specific **epitope** of the foreign protein it recognizes. (See Chap. 18, Sec. 18.3.3.)

Mucositis: Inflammation of the mucous membranes, especially in the mouth, which may occur after treatment with radiation or anticancer drugs.

Multiple drug resistance: Resistance to a group of chemically unrelated drugs that develops in cells and may be induced or selected for by exposure of the cells to any one of the drugs. One form of multiple drug resistance is caused by expression of **P-glycoprotein** in the cell surface, which is encoded by *mdr* **genes.** (See Chap. 17, Sec. 17.2.4.)

Multiple drug resistance–associated protein (MRP): A protein expressed on the surface of some drug-resistant cells that facilitates the excretion of certain anticancer drugs, either alone or in association with glutathione, thereby increasing the dose of the drug required for toxicity. Expression of MRP is one cause of **multiple drug resistance.** (See Chap. 17, Sec. 17.2.4.)

Multivariate (multivariable) analysis: A statistical method that allows analysis of the influence of several factors on prognosis or outcome after treatment to determine which factors may be independently predictive of that outcome. (See Chap. 20, Sec. 20.3.2.)

Mutation: A change in one or more of the DNA bases in a **gene.** Changes can include insertion of extra bases or **deletion** of a base or bases. Mutations in coding **exons** may lead to altered protein products; mutations in noncoding regions can lead to altered amounts of protein. **Missense mutation:** A mutation that leads to a nonfunctioning protein or to nonproduction of protein. **Germline mutation:** A mutation in the germline cells that is, therefore, inherited.

Mutation hot spot: A region of a **gene** where mutations are found more frequently than in the rest of the gene.

Myelosuppression: A reduction in mature blood cells in the peripheral circulation, particularly granulocytes, that may occur after treatment with anticancer drugs. (See Chap. 15, Sec. 15.4.1.)

Natural killer cell: A lymphocyte that can kill certain types of malignant cells without prior specific sensitization. (See Chap. 11, Sec. 11.3.7.)

Necrosis: Death of cells. It often occurs in solid tumors, leading to areas containing degenerating or pyknotic cells.

Neoplasm: Literally, a new growth or tumor. Often used to describe a **malignant** tumor or cancer.

Northern blot analysis: A technique for determining the presence of specific mRNA sequences in cells. Messenger RNA molecules are separated by **electrophoresis** and then blotted onto nitrocellulose paper. A labeled **probe,** containing DNA sequences (**cDNA**) complementary to the mRNA that is to be detected, is applied to the blot and allowed to **hybridize.** The labeled cDNA is then detected by a technique such as **autoradiography,** phosphoimaging, or chemiluminescence. (See Chap. 3, Sec. 3.3.4.)

Nucleophile: A substance which can interact with negatively charged molecules such as DNA. (See also **Electrophile.**)

Nucleotide excision: A **DNA repair** process that involves excision of a group of nucleotides containing a damaged or altered base in one strand of a DNA molecule and its replacement by synthesis of new DNA using the opposite strand as a template. (See Chap. 4, Sec. 4.4.5.)

Nude mouse: A mouse that congenitally lacks a thymus and hence has no mature **T cells. Xenografts** of human tumors will often grow in such immune-deficient animals. These mice are also hairless, hence the term "nude."

Null hypothesis: A statistical term used in testing the significance of a difference between two samples. The null hypothesis assumes that the two samples are drawn at random from the same population. The null hypothesis is rejected if the probability that a difference of the magnitude observed could arise by chance is very low, usually less than 5 percent (1 in 20).

Oligonucleotide: A short piece of DNA or RNA usually containing a defined sequence of bases.

Oligomer: A molecular complex made up of a number of copies of the same molecule (e.g., the form of **p53** that binds to DNA is a tetramer of four p53 protein molecules).

Oncofetal antigen: A protein produced by fetal tissue that is usually present at very low levels in the adult. Many tumors produce oncofetal antigens (e.g., **carcinoembryonic antigen**), which have been used as **markers** of tumor bulk.

Oncogene: A **gene** whose protein product may be involved in processes leading to **transformation** of a normal cell to a **malignant** state. The gene may be known as a **viral oncogene,** if it was detected in a transforming virus.

Orthotopic: Literally, of the same type. Tumor cells are said to be transplanted orthotopically if they are inoculated into an organ of the same tissue type (e.g., breast carcinoma cells transplanted into a mammary gland).

Oxygen enhancement ratio: The ratio of the radiation dose given in the absence of oxygen required to produce a given level of cell killing or tissue damage divided by the dose required to give the same level of killing or damage in the presence of oxygen. (See Chap. 13, Sec. 13.5.2.)

Oxygen radical: An oxygen molecule that is highly reactive with other biological molecules because it has an unpaired electron.

p53 **gene:** A **tumor suppressor gene,** so named because of the molecular weight of the corresponding protein (~53 kDa). The p53 protein is involved in control of progression of cells through the cell cycle, particularly, the transition from G1 phase to S phase. It appears to be active in preventing cells with DNA damage from progressing into S phase. (See Chap. 5, Sec. 5.5.2.)

Palliation: Treatment for the relief of symptoms of disease as opposed to treatment for cure of the disease (radical treatment).

Papillomavirus: A family of DNA-containing viruses, some of which are capable of inducing **malignant transformation** of cells. Some papillomaviruses are implicated in causing human cervical and anal cancers. (See Chap. 5, Sec. 5.2.3.)

Paracrine: Refers to the production of substances (usually hormones or **growth factors**) produced by one cell and secreted to act on a neighboring cell.

Paraneoplastic syndrome: Signs or symptoms occuring in a patient with cancer that are not due directly to the local effects of the tumor cells. Examples include the effects of **ectopic** production of hormones by cancer cells.

Parenchyma: The cells of a tissue that are responsible for its various functions, as distinct from **stroma,** which refers to blood vessels and connective tissue.

Passive diffusion: A process by which substances enter or leave cells as a result of a concentration gradient into or out of the cells.

Passive immunotherapy: Nonspecific stimulation of the host immune system to induce an immune reaction against a tumor, or transfer into the body of **antibodies** or immune cells, reactive against the tumor, that were created outside the body. (See Chap. 18, Sec. 18.3.)

P-glycoprotein: A membrane protein of molecular weight 180 kDa that has been implicated in the development of **multiple drug resistance** of tumor cells. High levels of P-glycoprotein are effective in pumping cytotoxic drugs and other foreign substances out of the cells. (See Chap. 17, Sec. 17.2.4.)

Pharmacodynamics: The effects of a drug within the body. (See Chap. 16, Sec. 16.2.)

Pharmacokinetics: The time course of drug absorption, distribution, metabolism, and excretion within the body. (See Chap. 16, Sec. 16.2.)

Phase I, phase II, and phase III trials: Designation of different types of clinical trials according to their purpose. (See Chap. 20, Sec. 20.4.1.) **Phase I trials** seek to determine the maximum tolerated dose and an appropriate schedule for administration of a new drug. **Phase II trials** seek evidence of biological effect. **Phase III trials** evaluate benefit to patients, usually by comparing experimental and standard therapy in a randomized trial.

Phenotype: Characteristics of a cell or tissue resulting from the expression of specific **genes.**

Philadelphia chromosome: A characteristically altered copy of chromosome 22 that is found in chronic myelogenous leukemia cells and is the result of a specific **chromo-**

some translocation involving chromosomes 9 and 22. The translocation provides a **fusion** between the *bcr* and *abl* genes. (See Chap. 4, Sec. 4.3.2; and Chap. 5, Sec. 5.4.4.)

Phosphoimaging: A technique for detecting and quantitating low levels of radioactivity found in **Southern, Northern,** or **Western blots.**

Photobleaching: Decreased fluorescence from a fluorescent molecule as a result of exposure to high levels of absorbed light; this reduces, permanently or temporarily, the fluorescent properties of the molecule. (See Chap. 19, Sec. 19.2.2.)

Photosensitizer: A drug or chemical that sensitizes cells or tissues to light. (See Chap. 19, Sec. 19.2.)

Plasmid: A circular piece of DNA that may reproduce separately from chromosomal DNA within cells, bacteria, or other organisms.

Plating efficiency: The fraction of **clonogenic** cells in a population.

Ploidy: A description of the **chromosome** content of the cell. Normal mammalian cells contain two copies of each chromosome (except for the sex chromosomes in males) and are diploid. Germ cells contain only one copy of each chromosome and are haploid. Cells in tumors often have missing or additional chromosomes (aneuploidy) and/or may have one or more **chromosome aberrations.** (See Chap. 3, Sec. 3.2.)

Polymerase chain reaction (PCR): A method by which a given segment of DNA is amplified multiple times by the synthesis of complementary strands. **RT-PCR** is a method for amplifying mRNA, that involves an initial **reverse transcription** of the mRNA to **cDNA** before amplification by PCR.

Polymorphism: An altered DNA base sequence in a gene, either between the two alleles in one individual or between different individuals, that occurs naturally in the population and usually does not lead to changes in the function of the coded protein.

Potential doubling time (T_{pot}): The predicted doubling time of a population of cells (usually a tumor) calculated from measured parameters such as the labeling index (LI) and the length of S phase (T_S) and based on the assumption that no cells are lost from the growing population. (See Chap. 7, Secs. 7.4.3 and 7.6.3.)

Potentially lethal damage: Damage to a cell that may be caused by radiation or drugs and that may or may not be repaired depending on the environment of the cell following treatment.

Power: The probability that a clinical trial will be able to detect a real difference between two treatments. The power of a study depends strongly on its sample size. (See Chap. 20, Sec. 20.4.6.)

Predictive assay: An assay which measures a specific biological parameter, the value of which is expected to be predictive for the outcome of treatment. (See Chap. 14, Sec. 14.5; and Chap. 15, Sec. 15.3.3.)

Premature chromosome condensation: A technique for inducing condensation of the chromosomal DNA of a cell that is not in mitosis; it involves fusing the cell of interest with a cell in mitosis.

Prevalence: The frequency of disease in a population at a given time. (See Chap. 2, Sec. 2.2.1.)

Probe: A **cloned gene** or fragment of a cloned gene that can be labeled and used to detect **homologous** DNA (**Southern blot** or in situ hybridization) or RNA (**Northern blot**). (See Chap. 3, Sec. 3.3.1.)

Procarcinogen: A chemical that can be metabolized in the body to form a **carcinogenic** compound. (See Chap. 8, Sec. 8.2.2.)

Prognosis: The expected outcome (e.g., chance of survival) for a patient with a particular type and stage of disease.

Prognostic factor: A detectable feature of a cancer or patient that can be used to predict the likely outcome of treatment of the cancer. (See Chap. 20, Sec. 20.3.)

Programmed cell death: An orderly process by which cells die. Also known as **apoptosis.** (See Chap. 7, Sec. 7.3.)

Progression: The tendency of tumors to become more **malignant** as they grow.

Progression delay: The delay in passage through phases of the cell cycle that may occur after (nonlethal) treatment with drugs or radiation. Also known as **Division delay.** (See Chap. 13, Sec. 13.3.2; and Chap. 15, Sec. 15.2.4.)

Proliferation-dependent antigen: A molecule that is expressed selectively in actively cycling cells. (See Chap. 7, Sec. 7.4.1.)

Promoter (or promotor): (1) A DNA sequence involved in the initiation of transcription. Promoters, in contrast to **enhancers,** have direction and are always located near the beginning of the first **exon.** (2) A compound that may not itself be **carcinogenic** but that stimulates the proliferation of **initiated** cells to form a cancer. Promotion is reversible and is normally a slow process. (See Chap. 8, Sec. 8.2.1.)

Protein denaturation: Destruction, usually by heating, of the three-dimensional structure of a protein required for its function.

Protein kinase: An enzyme that catalyzes the phosphorylation of proteins. Phosphorylation and dephosphorylation of proteins appear to be major mechanisms controlling their function. Many **oncogenes** code for protein kinases.

Protein truncation assay: A technique used to detect **mutations** in a **gene** that lead to the production of a truncated or smaller-than-normal protein. (See Chap. 3, Sec. 3.3.8.)

Proteolytic enzyme: An enzyme that can catalyze the breakdown of other proteins.

Proto-oncogene: A **gene,** in a normal cell, **homologous** to a viral transforming gene. Some proto-oncogenes encode proteins that influence the control of cellular proliferation and **differentiation. Mutations, amplifications, rearrangements,** etc., of proto-oncogenes may allow them to function as **oncogenes,** i.e., genes whose products are involved in cell **transformation.** (See Chap. 5, Sec. 5.4.)

Provirus: A DNA copy of the RNA of a **retrovirus,** which is integrated into the chromosomal DNA of a cell. (See Chap. 5, Sec. 5.3.1.)

Pyrimidine dimer: The formation of chemical bonds between two adjacent pyrimidine bases (thymine or cytosine) in DNA results in a pyrimidine dimer. This can be caused by exposure to ultraviolet light. (See Chap. 4, Sec. 4.4.3.)

Quality of life: A measure of the overall health of a patient during and after treatment that addresses symptoms and function rather than the state of the disease being treated. (See Chap. 20, Sec. 20.4.8.)

Radioimmunoassay (RIA): A sensitive method that may be used for the quantitation of any substance recognizable by an **antibody.** It depends on the binding of radiolabeled antibodies to the substance.

Radiosensitizer: A compound that increases the sensitivity of cells to ionizing radiation. (See Chap. 14, Sec. 14.4.3.)

Randomization: A process by which patients (or other experimental subjects) are assigned to treatment groups on the basis of random selection, so that the selection is not subject to **bias** by any unknown variables. This process is part of **phase III clinical trials.** (See Chap. 20, Sec. 20.4.3.)

Ras **gene:** A gene involved in signal transduction pathways that can induce cell proliferation. It is an oncogene that is commonly mutated in human cancers. (See Chap. 5, Sec. 5.4.1; and Chap. 6, Sec. 6.3.4.)

Rearrangement: Changes in the sequence of **genes** or of DNA sequences within genes that lead to alteration in their protein products. Rearrangement of genes is important in such processes as the generation of diversity of **antibody** molecules. Abnormal rearrangements between different genes appear to be important in **malignant transformation**—e.g., the **Philadelphia chromosome** in chronic myelogenous leukemia.

Receiver-operating-characteristics (ROC) curve: A technique for assessing the efficacy of a diagnostic test based on knowledge of the true-positive and false-positive rates for the test in question. (See Chap. 20, Sec. 20.2.1.)

Receptor: A molecule inside or on the surface of cells that recognizes a specific hormone, **growth factor,** or other biologically active molecule. The receptor also mediates transfer of signals within the cell.

Reciprocal translocation: A **chromosomal** aberration that involves the reciprocal exchange of parts of two chromosomes without loss of genetic material.

Recombination (DNA): A process that results in exchange of segments between two DNA molecules. **Homologous recombination** occurs when the segments have matching (homologous) sequences over at least part of the segment (usually at both ends). **Nonhomologous recombination** is said to occur when there is little or no homology between the exchanged segments. This latter process is believed to occur when a **provirus** is integrated into the cellular DNA.

Redistribution: When treatment (with radiation or drugs) is differentially toxic to cells in different parts of the cell cycle, the treatment will cause partial synchrony of the cells surviving the treatment. Between treatments, these surviving cells will redistribute around the cell cycle. (See Chap. 14, Sec. 14.3.3.)

Regional chemotherapy: Treatment with chemotherapy in which the drug is introduced directly into the tumor-bearing region of the body by, for example, intra-arterial infusion or intra-thecal injection. (See Chap. 16, Sec. 16.2.2.)

Relative biological effectiveness (RBE): A measure of the relative effectiveness of a given type of radiation. RBE is defined as the ratio of the dose of a commonly used type of radiation (e.g., γ-rays) to the dose of the test radiation that gives the same biological effect. (See Chap. 13, Sec. 13.5.1.)

Relative risk: The ratio of disease frequency in exposed and unexposed members of a population. (Exposure implies any attribute, personal, environmental, or genetic, that may cause or protect against disease). (See Chap. 2, Sec. 2.2.1.)

Remission: Decrease in tumor volume (or cell number) following treatment. Complete remission indicates that disease cannot be detected by physical examination or clinical tests but does not necessarily imply that the disease has been cured. Partial remission is usually defined as shrinkage by at least 50 percent of the cross-sectional area of measurable tumors.

Reoxygenation: A process by which cells in a tumor that are at low oxygen levels because of poor blood supply, and hence are resistant to radiation, gain access to oxygen following a treatment so that they become more sensitive to a subsequent radiation treatment. (See Chap. 14, Sec. 14.3.4.)

Repopulation: Proliferation of surviving cells in a tumor (or normal tissue) during or following cytotoxic treatment. Repopulation during a course of fractionated radiation therapy may lead to a requirement for an increased total dose of radiation to eradicate the tumor. (See Chap. 14, Sec. 14.3.2.)

Restriction enzymes: Enzymes obtained from bacteria that make cuts at specific sequences of four to eight bases in double-stranded DNA. (See Chap. 3, Sec. 3.3.2.)

Restriction-fragment-length polymorphism (RFLP) analysis: A method, based on **Southern blot analysis,** that may be used to identify unique DNA sequences within a cell. (See Chap. 3, Sec. 3.3.5.)

Retinoblastoma gene: A **tumor suppressor gene** that was identified initially because it was **mutated** in inherited cases of retinoblastoma (a childhood eye tumor). The gene is now known to be involved in controlling the movement of cells through the cell cycle, in particular the transition from the G1 phase to S phase. (See Chap. 4, Sec. 4.5.2.)

Retrovirus: A virus in which the genome comprises RNA. (See Chap. 5, Sec. 5.3.)

Reverse transcriptase: An enzyme, found mostly in **retroviruses,** that catalyzes the production of a complementary DNA (**cDNA**) strand from an RNA strand.

RGD sequence: A sequence of three consecutive amino acids (R = arginine, G = glycine, D = aspartic acid) that acts as a binding site for **cell adhesion molecules,** such as **integrins,** to molecules of the **extracellular matrix,** such as fibronectin or vitronectin. (See Chap. 9, Sec. 9.1.1.)

RNAse protection: A technique for detecting **mutations** in any **gene** that has been **cloned** and **sequenced.** The technique depends on a mismatch between the complementary RNA (to the gene of known sequence) and the DNA of the mutant gene and on the ability of RNAse to cut single-strand RNA at the site of the mismatch. The technique is also used for quantitation of specific RNAs by using a labeled probe that can hybridize to the RNA of interest and protect it from degradation by RNAse. (See Chap. 3, Sec. 3.3.8.)

Sarcoma: A **malignant** tumor derived from mesenchymal cells (e.g., connective tissue, vascular tissue, bone).

SCID mouse: A mouse that has *s*evere *c*ombined *i*mmuno*d*eficiency by virtue of having no functioning **T** or **B** lymphocytes because of a **mutation** that prevents effective **rearrangement** of the **immunoglobulin and T-cell receptor genes.** Such mice will allow the growth of human tumor **xenografts** because of their immunodeficiency.

Screening: (1) The application of a test (e.g., mammography) that may detect disease in a population of individuals having no symptoms of the disease. (2) The use of assays for detecting antitumor activity of compounds.

Second messenger: A substance involved in transmission of information (i.e., **signal transduction**) between the surface of the cell and its interior, often leading to changes in the expression of specific **genes.** Nonsteroidal hormones stimulate second messengers such as cyclic AMP or phosphoinositides to influence the behavior of cells.

Self-renewal: Proliferation of a cell to produce two daughter cells, at least one of which retains the properties of the original cell. Usually applied to **stem cells.**

Senescence: The slow loss of proliferative potential and eventual death that occurs when normal cells are grown over periods of time in culture. Immortalized cells have overcome this effect and can grow indefinitely in culture. Senescence is believed to be associated with the shortening of **telomeres** during multiple rounds of proliferation; immortalized cells have upregulated **telomerase** activity, which can prevent this from occurring. (See Chap. 7, Sec. 7.3.5.)

Sensitivity: The probability that a diagnostic test will identify those patients who have a given disease or attribute. (See Chap. 20, Sec. 20.2.1.)

SH2 and SH3 domains: The *Src-H*omology domains are homologous to regions in src family protein kinases. They are present in many proteins involved in signal transduction and give the proteins the ability to bind to other proteins in a manner facilitating **signal transduction.** (See Chap. 6, Sec. 6.3.2.)

Signal transduction: A process by which information is transmitted from the surface of the cell to the nucleus. It involves a series of molecular components (proteins), that activate subsequent members of the cascade (usually by phosphorylation), resulting in activation of **transcription factors.** (See Chap. 6.)

Single-strand break: A break in one of the sugar-phosphate backbones of a double-stranded DNA molecule.

Single-strand conformation polymorphism (SSCP): A technique for detecting **mutations** in **genes** by virtue of changes in the migration of the DNA under **gel electrophoresis.** (See Chap. 3, Sec. 3.3.8.)

Site-directed mutagenesis: A technique for introducing a change in DNA sequence at a given site in DNA. (See Chap. 3, Sec. 3.3.11.)

Somatic cell hybrid: The fusion of two somatic (nongerm) cells to produce a **hybrid** cell that retains all (or some selected fraction) of the DNA of both of the parent cells. Such cells can be used in genetic studies, particularly those involving **complementation** analysis. (See Chap. 3, Sec. 3.4.2.)

Southern blot analysis: A technique used for detecting specific DNA sequences in cells. DNA is extracted from cells and cut with one or more **restriction enzymes.** The DNA fragments are separated by gel **electrophoresis** and blotted onto nitrocellulose paper. The DNA is then **hybridized** using a labeled DNA **probe** with a sequence complementary to the specific sequence to be detected. The

DNA fragments that hybridize with the probe can be detected by techniques such as **autoradiography, phosphoimaging,** or chemiluminescence. (See Chap. 3, Sec. 3.3.4.)

Specificity: The probability that a negative diagnostic test will correctly identify those patients who do not have a given disease or attribute. (See Chap. 20, Sec. 20.2.1.)

Spheroid: A spherical aggregation of cells that can be grown in tissue culture and provides a useful model for studying the properties of solid tumors. (See Chap. 7, Sec. 7.6.3.)

Splicing (RNA): The process in which the initial RNA copy made from DNA during transcription is modified to remove certain sections (such as **introns**) prior to use as a template for translation. Many **genes** can undergo **alternative splicing,** which can remove some **exons** (as well as the **introns**), resulting in mRNAs of different length that may be translated to produce proteins of different sizes.

Stem cell: A cell that has the capacity to repopulate functional units within a tissue. The term is most aptly applied to renewal tissue such as the bone marrow, where it is possible to demonstrate the presence of a cell that can regenerate all the various **differentiated** cells in blood. The term is also used to describe a cell in a tumor that can produce a very large number of progeny and which, if it survives, can regenerate the tumor after treatment.

Stem-cell transplantation: Injection of (bone marrow) stem cells into the circulation of an animal or human in order to replace **stem cells** killed by cytotoxic treatment. (See Chap. 15, Sec. 15.4.2.)

Stress-activated protein kinase (SAPK): A protein kinase that is part of the signal transduction pathway of the same name. This pathway is activated by exposure of the cell to stress, such as that caused by cytotoxic agents, heat, or hypoxia. (See Chap. 6, Sec. 6.4.)

Stroma: The part of tissue that provides the supporting structure for the **parenchymal** (functional) cells of that tissue. Stroma includes blood vessels, connective tissue such as fibroblasts, and the **extracellular matrix** (ECM).

Sublethal damage: Damage to a cell that may be caused by radiation or drugs and that can be repaired within a few hours after the treatment. Classically, repair of sublethal damage is revealed by giving two treatments separated by a variable time interval. (See Chap. 14, Sec. 14.3.1.)

Survival curve: (1) See **cell survival curve.** (2) A graph indicating the proportion of patients who are alive at different times after treatment (or diagnosis).

Surviving fraction: The fraction of cells that retain long-term proliferative potential (i.e., usually **clonogenic** cells) following treatment with a cytotoxic agent.

Synchronized cells: A population of cells most of which are at a given stage of the growth cycle at any one time and that move through the cell cycle as a cohort. Drugs that kill cells at a given phase of the cell cycle cause partial synchrony among the survivors.

Synergy: An interaction between two agents that is greater than would be predicted from the activity of either alone. This word is commonly misused in describing the interaction between drugs or between drugs and radiation, since there is a range of effects that would be predicted as being **additive.** (See Chap. 17, Sec. 17.3.2.)

T cell (or T lymphocyte): A lymphocyte that has been processed by the thymus which may have cytotoxic or regulatory functions in the immune response. T cells express the **T-cell receptor** on their surface. (See Chap. 11, Sec. 11.3.3.)

T-cell receptor: A receptor on the surface of **T lymphocytes** that is required for them to recognize **antigens** presented on the surface of **antigen-presenting cells** and to interact with other cells of the immune system. (See Chap. 11, Sec. 11.3.4.)

T-helper cells: A subset of T lymphocytes that can be activated to secrete **cytokines,** which stimulate other cells of the immune system to mount an immune response. (See Chap. 11, Sec. 11.3.3.)

Taq polymerase: A DNA polymerase, isolated from a thermoresistant bacterium (*Thermus aquaticus*), which is thermostable at temperatures used in PCR to denature the double strands of DNA. (See Chap. 3, Sec. 3.3.7.)

Telomere: The ends of **chromosomes** which contain multiple repeats of specific DNA sequences and associated proteins. The DNA replication machinery in most normal cells has difficulty replicating these ends completely. Shortening of the telomeres may lead eventually to **senescence** and cell death. (See Chap. 7, Sec. 7.3.5.)

Telomerase: An enzyme that can act to replicate the **telomeres** of **chromosomes.** The enzyme may be upregulated in tumors and prevent the **senescence** observed in normal cells. (See Chap. 7, Sec. 7.3.5.)

Therapeutic index (therapeutic ratio): The dose of a therapeutic agent required to produce a given level of damage to a critical normal tissue divided by the dose of the agent required to produce a defined level of antitumor effect. Therapeutic index is therefore a measure of the relative efficacy of therapy against tumors as compared with the normal tissue damage caused. (See Chap. 14, Sec. 14.2.3; and Chap. 17, Sec. 17.1.1.)

Thermotolerance: The development of resistance to the effects of further heating induced by initial heating of cells or tissues. (See Chap. 19, Sec. 19.1.3.)

Tissue inhibitors of metalloproteinases (TIMPS): Proteins that can bind to and inhibit the proteolytic action of **metalloproteinases.** (See Chap. 10, Sec. 10.5.2.)

Tolerance: A term used in immunology to indicate the process whereby specific **antigens** fail to elicit an immunologic response. Tolerance is required to prevent a response against "self-antigens"; it can also be induced against foreign antigens. (See Chap. 11, Sec. 11.2.5.)

Topoisomerases: Enzymes that allow breakage of one or both DNA strands, unwinding of DNA, and resealing of the strands. The enzymes are required for DNA and RNA synthesis and are important for the action of some anticancer drugs. Decreased activity of topoisomerases is a cause of **multiple drug resistance.** (See Chap. 17, Sec. 17.2.5.)

Transactivation: The process by which the transcription of a gene is increased by proteins that interact with the **promoter** DNA of the transcribed gene.

Transcription factors: Proteins that can bind to DNA (often after their association to form **dimers**) and that control the **transcription** of genes. (See Chap. 6, Sec. 6.3.6.)

Transduction: The process by which the behavior of a cell is modified by introduction of foreign DNA.

Transfection: The direct transfer of DNA molecules into a cell. Transfection of specific **genes** is a powerful tool for determining their function.

Transformation: Commonly used to describe the conversion of normal cells to those with abnormalities in cellular appearance and growth regulation in tissue culture (morphologic transformation). **Malignant transformation** indicates that the cells can produce a tumor in an appropriate animal.

Transforming growth factors α and β (TGF-α, and TGF-β): Growth factors that were originally isolated from tumor cells and believed to be responsible for their growth, hence their name as **transforming** growth factors. TGF-α is now known to be related to **epidermal growth factor** (EGF) and to bind to and stimulate its **receptor** (EGFR) on cells. TGF-β is a multifunctional growth factor that can both inhibit and stimulate the growth of different cell types and can induce **differentiated** functions in cells, such as the production of collagen by fibroblasts.

Transgenic mouse: A mouse produced from a germline cell into which a specific **gene** has been introduced. All cells of such mice carry this gene, including the germline. (See Chap. 3, Sec. 3.3.12.)

Translocation: The displacement of one part of a **chromosome** to a different chromosome or to a different part of the same chromosome. An example is the translocation between chromosomes 9 and 22, which leads to the appearance of the **Philadelphia chromosome** in chronic myelogenous leukemia.

Tritiated thymidine (^{3}H-TdR): Thymidine is one of the bases of DNA. Tritiated thymidine contains radioactive tritium (an isotope of hydrogen) and has been used widely in studies of cell proliferation, since it is taken up into cells and incorporated into newly synthesized DNA. High specific activity (highly labeled) tritiated thymidine can be used to kill S-phase cells, since cells engaged in DNA synthesis incorporate sufficient radioactivity to kill themselves. (See Chap. 7, Sec. 7.4.1.)

Tumor antigen: An antigenic determinant on the surface of a tumor cells that is not usually expressed by normal cells of the same histopathologic type. Such antigens may or may not be **immunogenic.** (See Chap. 11, Sec. 11.4.1; and Chap. 18, Sec. 18.1.1.)

Tumor infiltrating lymphocytes (TIL cells): T lymphocytes found in tumors. These cells may be reacting against **tumor antigens** and, after extraction from the tumor and expansion in vitro, have been used for active immunotherapy. (See Chap. 18, Sec. 18.3.2.)

Tumor suppressor gene: A gene whose mutation or loss may lead to cellular **transformation** and to the development of cancer. (See Chap. 4, Sec. 4.5; and Chap. 5, Sec. 5.5.)

TUNEL assay: A technique (*T*erminal deoxynucleotidyl transferase d*U*DP *N*ick *E*nd *L*abeling) widely used to detect cells that are undergoing **apoptosis.** (See Chap. 7, Sec. 7.3.1.)

Type I and type II error: Types of error associated with assessing the statistical significance of a clinical trial (or a set of experimental observations). Type I error (also known as the **alpha error**) relates to the probability that different outcomes between two different treatment arms in a clinical trial (or in an experimental study) could arise by chance. If this probability (p value) is less than 5 percent (i.e., less than 1 in 20 that the result could have occurred by chance), the result is usually regarded as statistically significant, although the cutoff value for statistical significance may have to be reduced if multiple comparisons are being made. Type II error (also known as the **beta error**) relates to the probability that, by chance, the trial will fail to demonstrate a statistically significant difference even though a real difference between the two treatment arms actually exists. (See Chap. 20, Sec. 20.4.6.)

Tyrosine kinase: An enzyme that has the ability to phosphorylate proteins on the amino acid tyrosine. The phosphorylation is often highly specific for individual tyrosine residues, depending on the amino acids surrounding the tyrosine in the protein. (See Chap. 6, Sec. 6.3.)

Vascular endothelial growth factor (VEGF): A **growth factor** that acts on endothelial cells to promote their proliferation as part of new vessel formation (**angiogenesis**). This factor induces increased vascular permeability and is also known as "vascular permeability factor" (VPF). (See Chap. 9, Sec. 9.3.2.)

Vector: A short piece of DNA or RNA, such as a DNA **plasmid** or RNA virus, into which genetic material of interest is incorporated and which is used to transfer this genetic material into a cell for either transient or long-term expression.

Western blot analysis: A procedure analogous to **Southern** and **Northern blot** analyses that allows the detection of specific proteins. Proteins are separated by **electrophoresis** and transferred onto a membrane. They are usually detected following binding with labeled antibodies. (See Chap. 3, Sec. 3.3.4.)

Wild type: The usual or normal configuration of a **gene** or protein (as compared with a mutant form).

Xenobiotic: A substance (usually a chemical) that is foreign to the body.

Xenograft: Tissue that is transplanted from one species of animal into another. Most commonly this refers to the transplantation of a human tumor into an immune-deficient mouse (e.g., a **nude mouse** or **SCID mouse**). (See Chap. 15, Sec. 15.3.2.)

Xeroderma pigmentosum: A human genetic disease characterized by extreme sensitivity to sunlight and the early onset of skin cancers. The genetic defect lies in the ability of the individual's cells to **repair DNA** damage caused by ultraviolet light. (See Chap. 4, Sec. 4.4.1.)

X-ray crystallography: A technique for imaging the three-dimensional structure of molecules. The substance is allowed to form a crystal in which the molecules have a repeating alignment. The crystal is then exposed to x-rays and the diffraction pattern of the crystal is used to deduce the structure.

Zinc-finger domain: The region of a protein that is formed into a finger-like projection by binding of some of the amino acids (cysteines or histidines) to a zinc atom. This configuration usually provides a DNA-binding region and is often found in **transcription factors.** (See Chap. 6, Sec. 6.3.7.)

Index

Note: Numbers followed by an "f" refer to figures; numbers followed by a "t" refer to tables.

Absorption of drugs, 370–371
Accelerated fractionation, 493
2-Acetylaminofluorene, 167f
Acetylaminofluoreneguanine, 174
Acoustic neuroma, genetics of, 73
Acquired drug resistance. *See* Drug resistance
Acquired immunodeficiency syndrome (AIDS), 245, 252
  apoptosis and, 145
Acridine orange, 147, 148f
Acrolein, 375, 375f
ACTH (adrenocorticotropic hormone), 265
Active immunotherapy. *See* Immunotherapy, active
Active transport, 493
Acute leukemia(s)
  lymphoblastic, 96–98, 98f
  myeloblastic, 96–98, 157
  myelocytic, 96
  myelogenous, 432
  prognosis for, 160t
Acute (rapidly) transforming viruses, 88, 88f, 493, 496
Adaptive response to radiation, 316
Adaptor protein, 493
ADCC (antibody-directed cellular cytotoxicity), 246, 246f, 430, 430f
Additivity, drug, 410–412, 411f, 493
Addressins, 256
Adenine, chemical carcinogenesis and, 173f
Adeno-associated viruses, for gene transfer, 424–425
Adenoma polyposis coli (APC), 74, 74f, 206
Adenomas, genetics of, 57t, 58
Adenosine, structure of, 382f
Adenosine arabinoside (ara-A), 381–382

Adenosine deaminase (ADA), 382
Adenoviruses, 37, 83
  for gene transfer, 424, 425t
ADEPT (antibody-dependent enzyme-activated prodrug therapy), 396
Adhesion molecules. *See* Cell adhesion molecules
  and metastases, 232
Adjuvant chemotherapy, 393–395, 493
Adoptive immune therapy, 493
Adrenal hormones, 263–264. *See also* Hormones
Adrenocorticotropic hormone (ACTH), 265
Adult T-cell leukemia (ATL), 89–90, 90t, 91f, 102
AEV (avian erythroblastosis virus) transforming protein (v-erb-B), 125
AF2a transcriptional activator, 287
Aflatoxin B1, 166, 167f, 170–171, 171f, 174, 179t
  metabolic activation for, 171f
AF-1 transcriptional activator, 287
Age
  and breast cancer, 275t, 276
  and incidence of cancer, 49f, 49–50
  at menarche, and breast cancer, 275, 276t
  of parity, and breast cancer, 275, 275t
  and prostate cancer, 279, 279t
Age distribution, in epidemiology, 16, 17f
Age-standardized incidence rates, 7–8, 8f, 49, 49f
AGM1470 (TNP-470), 214t
AIDS (acquired immunodeficiency syndrome), 245, 252
  apoptosis and, 145

Alcohol, as risk factor for cancer, 17t, 18, 18f
Aldophosphamide, 375, 375f
Aldosterone, 266
  structure of, 266f
Alkylating agents, 62–63, 170–171, 171f, 173, 173f, 350–351, 351f, 354, 354f, 493. *See also individual drugs*
  carcinogenic properties of, 364
  hyperthermia and, 453
  pharmacology of, 373–377
  resistance to, 397, 397t, 407–408, 409
O^6-Alkylguanine DNA alkyltransferase (AGAT), 408
Alkyl transferase repair, 63, 64f
Alleles, 249, 493
Allelic polymorphism, 249
Allogeneic transplantation, 248
Allograft, 493
All-trans retinoic acid, 366
Alpha error, 484, 493
Alternative splicing, 508
ALV (avian leukemia virus), 89
Ames assay, 176, 178f, 493
Amifostine, 412
9-Aminocamptothecin, 388
  structure of, 387f
Aminoglutethimide, 285, 288–289
5-δ-Aminolevulinic acid (ALA), 456t, 457–458
2-Amino-3-methylimidazo[4,5-*f*] quinoline (IQ), 166–167, 167f
Amphiregulin, 273, 274t
Amplicons, 54
Anal tumors, 91
Analytic epidemiology, 7, 8
Anaplasia, 493
Anaplastic large-cell kinase (ALK), 126
Anastrozole, 285

Anchorage-independence, 93, 93f, 176t, 493
Androgen ablation, for prostate cancer, 287–288
Androgen receptor, 289
Androgen resistance, and prostate cancer, 289–290
Androgens, 267, 267f
    anti-, 288
    inhibition of synthesis of, 288–289
Androstenedione
    and prostate cancer, 280
    structure of, 266f
Aneuploid tumors, 149–150, 159
    prognosis for, 159–160, 160t
Angiogenesis, tumor, 4–5, 159, 200f, 208–215, 357, 494
    chemotherapy against, 208, 366
    dependence of tumors on blood supply, 208, 357
    growth factors and growth-factor receptors, 208–211, 209f, 210t, 212t
    inhibitors of, 211–215, 214t, 215f
        endogenous and exogenous, 214t
    integrins and, 205
    and metastases, 200, 200f, 205, 232
    as prognostic indicator, 215
    vascular endothelial growth factor and, 125, 211
Angiogenin, 210t
Angiopoietin-1, 211, 212t
Angiopoietin-2, 211, 212t
Angiostatin, 213, 214t
Animal models
    of breast cancer, 277, 278–279
    of chemical carcinogenesis, 177, 177t, 177–180
    of radiation carcinogenesis, 187–189, 188t, 189f
    transgenic and knockout mice, 3, 39–41, 40f, 81, 509
Anoikis, 213
Anthracenediones, pharmacology of, 383–385
Anthracyclines, 351, 351f. See also individual drugs
    pharmacology of, 383–385
    resistance to, 397t, 402t
    toxicity of, 364, 384–385
Antiandrogens, for prostate cancer, 288
Antibodies, 241, 245f, 245–248, 494
    chimeric, 429, 429f, 431–432
    classes of, 246t
    complement-mediated lysis, 246, 246f

constant (C) region, 246
    heavy (H) chain, 245f, 245–246
    light (L) chain, 245f, 246
    monoclonal, 495, 500, 503
        bispecific, 433
        chimeric, 429, 429f, 431–432
        cytokine enhancement of, 433
        fluorescent-labeled, 150
        immunotherapy with, 428f–430f, 428–433, 431t
        immunotoxins and, 432–433
        production of, 428f, 428–430
        radiolabeled, 432
    opsonization by, 246, 246f
    polyclonal, 503
    variable (V) region, 246
Antibody-dependent enzyme-activated prodrug therapy (ADEPT), 396
Antibody-directed cellular cytotoxicity (ADCC), 246, 246f, 430, 430f
Anticancer drugs. See Chemotherapy and individual drugs
Anticoagulants, and inhibition of metastases, 229, 235
Antiestrogens, 283f, 283–284, 284f
Antigenic agents, 240
Antigenic cross-reactivity, 430–431, 431t
Antigenic modulation, 431, 431t
Antigen-presenting cells (APCs), 241, 242–243, 244f, 249, 254, 255f, 256, 422f, 494, 497, 499
Antigen-pulsed dendritic cells, 438–440, 439f
Antigen receptors, 498
    lymphocyte, 122–123
    signaling through, 122–123
Antigen recognition activation motif (ARAM), 122–123, 127
Antigens, 494
    cell differentiation, 495
    histocompatibility (H), 248, 499–500
    human leukocyte (HLA), 249
    oncofetal, 495, 503
    tumor, 257–258, 509
    tumor-rejection (TRAs), 420–421, 421t, 422, 422f, 433–434, 434f, 436
Antimetabolites, 350, 351, 351f, 353, 494. See also individual drugs
    pharmacology of, 377–383
    resistance to, 397t, 398–400
Antimetastatic drugs, 235–236. See also Chemotherapy
Antioxidants, 183

Antiprogestins, 284
Antisense RNA, 39, 494
APC (adenoma popyposis coli) gene, 53t, 74, 74f, 206
APCs (antigen-presenting cells), 241, 242–243, 244f, 249, 254, 255f, 256, 422f, 494, 497, 499
Aphidicolin, 408
Apoptosis, 3, 134, 140–145, 158, 161, 242, 263, 270, 494, 495, 497
    assays of, 3–4
    and cancer, 144–145
    cellular injury and, 142
    from chemotherapy, 351–352
    death domains, 142
    degradation phase of, 142, 143f, 144
    direct death signals, 142
    drug resistance and, 408–409
    effector phase of, 142, 143f, 144
    induction phase of, 142–143
    radiation-induced, 303, 327, 344. See also Radiation; Radiotherapy
    regulation of, 143–144
Apoptotic cells, ultrastructure of, 141, 141f
Apparent volume of distribution of drugs, 371t
Ara-C. See Cytosine arabinoside
Aralkylating agents, 170, 171f, 172, 172f, 174. See also specific agents
ARAM (antigen recognition activation motif), 122–123, 127
Area under the curve (AUC), 371t, 372, 372f, 494
Arginine-glycine-aspartic acid (RGD) sequence, 198
Aromatase, 267
Aromatase inhibitors, 285
Aromatic amides, 171–172, 172f
Aromatic amines, 171–172, 172f
    metabolic activation for, 172f
Aromatic hydrocarbons, cancer and, 17t
Arylaminating agents, 170, 171f, 171–172, 172f, 173. See also specific agents
Asbestos, cancer and, 19
Ascites, malignant, 222–223
L-Asparaginase, 389
Aspirin, 235
Assay(s)
    Ames, 176, 178f, 493
    anchorage-independent growth, 93, 93f
    of antitumor effects of chemotherapy, predictive, 356–357, 357t

of apoptosis, 3–4
avidin-biotin-peroxidase immunohistochemical, 272f, 273
bio-, 495
cell adhesive matrix (CAM)
  of chemotherapy, 357
  for radiation-exposed cells, 304–305, 342–343, 343f
of cell proliferation, after radiation
  in vitro, 303–305, 304f
  in vivo, 305f, 305–306, 306f
of cell transformation
  in chemical carcinogenesis, 175–176
  in radiation carcinogenesis, 185f, 185–186
of cellular effects of chemotherapy
  colony-forming, 352t, 352–353, 353f
  nonclonogenic, 351–352, 352t
of chemical carcinogenesis, in vitro, 175–177
clonogenic, 3–4, 496
  of chemotherapy effects, 351, 355, 356f
  for radiation-exposed cells, 304, 304f, 325, 325f, 342–343
colony-forming of chemotherapy, 352t, 352–353, 353f, 496
comet, 300t
crypt stem cell survival, 305, 306f
of DNA radiation damage, 300t
of DNA strand breaks, 312t
end-point dilution, 305, 305f
enzyme-linked immunosorbent (ELISA), 498
filter elution, 300t
focus formation, 93, 93f
heteroduplex mobility shift, 35
histomorphometric, 312t
of intratumoral hypoxia, 312t
lung-colony, 305
of metastasis, 223–228
  experimental, 224f, 224–225
  spontaneous, 223–224, 224f, 225
  in vitro, 226, 226f
  in vivo, 223–225, 224f
MTT, 352, 365
  for radiation-exposed cells, 304
nucleoid sedimentation, 300t
polarographic oxygen electrode, 312t
predictive, 505
  for chemotherapy, 356–357, 357t
  for radiotherapy, 342–344

protein truncation, 36, 506
Salmonella mutagenicity, 177t, 178f
spleen-colony, 305
  of chemotherapy, 353
SRB (sulforhodamine B), 352, 365
sucrose velocity sedimentation, 300t
TDT-mediated dUTP nick-end labeling (TUNEL), 141–142, 142f, 509
of transfection, 95
tumor formation, 93, 93f
Ataxia telangiectasia (AT), 494
  clinical and cellular characteristics of, 58–60, 59t, 69, 70
Atomic bomb exposure, 20, 188, 189–190, 191, 191f
ATP-binding cassette, 401f, 401–402
ATP-dependent transporters, 250, 251f, 256
AUC (area under the curve), 371t, 372, 372f, 494
Autocrine, 494
Autoimmune diseases, 240–241, 245, 252
Autoradiography of cells, 145–146, 148, 494, 503, 508
Autosomal dominant traits, 52
Autosome, 494, 495
Avian erythroblastosis virus (AEV) transforming protein (v-erbB), 125
Avian leukemia virus (ALV), 89
Avidin-biotin-peroxidase immunohistochemical assay, 272f, 273
awd gene, 234
Azathioprine, 381–382

B16 murine melanoma
  cells in, 226, 226f, 227, 229f
  integrins and, 204
Bacille Calmette-Guérin (BCG), 241, 433, 493
Bacteriophage, 494, 496
B7-1 and B7-2 costimulatory molecules, 438, 439
Basal cell carcinoma, cadherins and, 205
Base excision, 65–67, 66f, 494
Basement membrane, 494
  and metastases, 230–231
Basophils, 241
Batimastat (BB-94), 214t
Bax gene, 494
Bayes' theorem, 471–472, 494
BB2516 (matimastat), 214t

B cell(s), 123, 241, 494
  activation of, 241, 245–248
  clonal selection hypothesis of, 242
B-cell lymphomas, 433
  ALV-induced, 89
  clonal markers of, 156
  flow cytometry of, 150
B-cell receptor (BCR), 247
BCG (bacille Calmette-Guérin), 241, 433, 493
bcl-2 gene, 93t, 99, 144, 289, 409, 494
bcl-6 gene, 128
Bcl-2 protein, 145
bcl-x_L and *bcl*-x_S genes, 144, 145
BCNU. *See* Carmustine (BCNU)
bcr-abl gene, 43, 44f, 45, 54, 93t, 96, 97, 98f, 124t, 126–127, 257, 421, 421t, 426, 494, 499
BDNF, 108t
Benign tumors, classification of, 2
Benzidine, structure of, 167f
Benzo[a]pyrene (BP), 166, 168, 171f, 178f, 180, 183
  metabolic activation of, 172f
  structure of, 167f
Benzo[a]pyrene-guanine, 174
Benzoporphyrin derivative-monoacid ring A, 456t
Berkson's bias, 12
Beta carotene, 19, 184
Beta error, 484, 494
β2 microglobulin, 256
BHA (butylated hydroxyanisole), 183
BHT (butylated hydroxytoluene), 183
Bias, 494
  Berkson's, 12
  in clinical trials, 478–479
  detection, 13
  in diagnostic tests, 470t, 470–471
  in epidemiology, 12–13
  information, 13
  lead-time, 473, 473f, 502
  length-time, 472–473, 473f, 502
  prevalence-incidence (length), 12
  in prognostic studies, 474–475
  recall, 13
  selection, 12
  in studies and tests, 466–467
Bicalutamide, 288
Bioassay, 495
Bioavailability of drugs, 370, 495, 498
Biological response modifier, 495, 501

Biological therapy, 420–442
  active immunotherapy, 433–440, 493
    antigen-pulsed dendritic cells, 438–440, 439f
    DNA immunogens, 435f, 435–436
    protein immunogens, 433–434, 434f
    with tumor cells, 436
      genetically modified, 436–438, 437f
  gene therapy, 422–426
    approaches to, 323f, 422–423
    clinical studies of, 426
    physical methods for gene transfer, 425–426
    viral methods for gene transfer, 423–425, 425t
  molecular and cellular requirements for immune activation, 422, 422f
  passive immunotherapy, 426–433, 504
    adoptive cellular therapy, 427–428
    cytokines, 426–427
    monoclonal antibodies, 428f–430f, 428–433, 431t
Bioreduction of drugs, 340, 359, 495
Biotin, 43
Biotransformation of chemical carcinogens, 169–170
Bis-chloroethylnitrosurea (BCNU, carmustine), 354, 361, 371
Bladder, radiation damage to, 326t
Bladder cancer
  cadherins and, 205
  chemicals and, 179f
  genetics of, 73, 173
  photodynamic therapy for, 454, 455t
  prognosis for, 160t
  smoking and, 17
Blast transformation, 243
Bleomycin, 354, 354f, 385
  hyperthermia and, 453
  pharmacology of, 385
  toxicity of, 363, 385, 410, 415t
Blocking (in treatment allocation), 480
Blood supply
  dependence of tumors on, 5, 221. See also Angiogenesis, tumor; Vasculature of tumors
  in hyperthermia, 450, 450f
  and metastasis of tumors, 221, 228, 230, 230f

Bloom's syndrome (BS), clinical and cellular characteristics of, 58–60, 59t, 69
B lymphocyte(s). See B cell(s)
Bone, metastases to, 221, 222t
Bone marrow
  chemotherapy toxicity to, 360f, 360–361, 362f, 410
  radiation damage to, 326f, 326t
  transplantation of, 361–363
Boron neutron capture therapy (BNCT), 342
Bovine leukemia virus (BLV), 127
BP. See Benzo[a]pyrene
Brachytherapy, and hyperthermia, 452
Bragg peak, 297f, 298, 341
Brain, metastases to, 221, 222t
Brain cancer, estimates of T_S, T_C, and T_{POT} for, 158t
BRCA1/BRCA2 genes, 2, 3, 22, 53t, 75
BrdUrd (5-bromodeoxyuridine), 148, 149f, 157
Breast cancer
  adjuvant chemotherapy for, 394, 395f
  alcohol and, 18
  breast tissue xenograpt studies, 278
  cadherins and, 205
  chemically induced models of, 277
  cyclin overexpression in, 140
  diet and, 18, 276
  doubling time of, 155t
  epidemiology of, 15, 17f, 22, 22t
  epidermal growth factor receptor and, 273
  estimates of T_S, T_C, and T_{POT} for, 158t
  estrogens and, 267
  experimental models of, 277–279
  genetics of, 2, 3, 22, 48, 51t, 75. See also BCRA1/BRCA2 genes
  growth factors and, 273
  hormonal replacement therapy and, 277
  hormonal risk factors for, 19–20, 127–128, 273, 274t, 274–277, 275t
  integrins and, 204
  metastasis-associated genes and, 234, 235t
  metastatic, 222t
  obesity and, 267, 275t, 275–276
  oral contraceptives and, 20
  prognosis for, 160t
  radiotherapy for, 325t
    with hyperthermia, 453t
  risk factors for, 22, 22t, 274–277
  spread of, 221

therapy for, 268, 380
  endocrine, 282t, 282–285
    resistance to, 285–287, 286f
  radiotherapy, 325t, 453t
  transgenic mice models of, 278–279
  virally-induced rodent models of, 277
5-Bromodeoxyuridine (BrdUrd), 148, 149f, 157
BSO (buthionine sulfoximine), 408
Burkitt's lymphoma, 20f, 21, 55t, 84–85, 127
  chromosomal abnormality in, 55t, 56
Buserelin acetate, 283, 287
Busulfan, 376–377
  resistance to, 401
  structure of, 377f
  toxicity of, 361, 377
Buthionine sulfoximine (BSO), 408
Butylated hydroxyanisole (BHA), 183
Butylated hydroxytoluene (BHT), 183

Cadherins, 201f, 205–206, 495
  and metastases, 232
Calcinurin, 123
Calcium channel blockers
  antimetastatic activity of, 235
  and P-glycoprotein, 403
Calcium phosphate precipitation, 37
Calmodulin, 144
  and p-glycoprotein, 403
Calreticulin, 201f, 203f
CAM(s). See Cell adhesion molecules
Camptothecin, 351, 406
  derivatives of, 387–388
  structure of, 387f
Capillary electrophoresis, 34
Capillary-leak syndrome, 427
Carboplatin, 351, 389
  pharmacology of, 371, 372, 388–389
  structure of, 388f
Carboxyphosphamide, 375, 375f
Carcinoembryonic antigen (CEA), 201f, 207, 428, 495
Carcinogenic drugs, 364, 493, 495. See also Drug toxicity
Carcinomas, 495
  genetics of, 57t, 58
Cardiotoxicity of drugs, 380, 384–385, 412
Carmustine (BCNU), 354, 371, 376, 376f
  resistance to, 401
  toxicity of, 361

Cartilage-derived inhibitor (CDI), 212
Case-control studies, 10–12, 11f, 495
Caspases, 144, 495
Castleman's disease, 92
Castration, 279, 279t
  for prostate cancer, 287–288
Catecholamine hormones, 265
Catenins, 201f, 206
CBP protein, 82
CCNU (lomustine), 376, 376f, 401
cdc25 phosphatase, 136f, 137
CD44 hyaluronate-binding proteins, 201f, 207–208
CDKN2 gene, 53t, 102
cdks. *See* Cyclin-dependent kinases
CD2 molecule, 255–256
CD3 molecule, 122, 122f, 253–254, 259, 427
CD4 molecule, 122f, 122–123, 247, 251–252, 254, 255f, 256, 435
CD5 molecule, 255
CD7 molecule, 255
CD8 molecule, 122f, 122–123, 247, 251–252, 254, 255f, 256, 420, 423
CD19 molecule, 123
CD21 molecule, 123
CD28 molecule, 242–243, 247, 254, 255, 255f, 256
CD40 molecule, 242–243, 251, 439
CD45 molecule, 122f, 123, 247, 254
CD45R0, 254
CD45RA, 254
cDNA (complementary DNA), 30, 31f, 61, 495, 503
CDR engraftment, 429
ced-3; ced-4; ced-9 genes, 144
Cell adhesion molecules (CAMs), 199–208, 201f, 247, 495, 507
  cadherins, 201f, 205–206, 232, 495
  carcinoembryonic antigen (CEA), 201f, 207, 428, 495
  CD44 hyaluronate-binding proteins, 201, 207–208
  of immunoglobulin superfamily, 206–207
  integrins, 200, 201f, 202
    signal transduction by, 202–204, 203f
    in tumor progression and metastasis, 204–205
  and metastases, 232, 294–205
Cell adhesive matrix (CAM) assay
  of chemotherapy, 357
  for radiation-exposed cells, 304–305, 342–343, 343f

Cell cycle, 134–135, 135f
  and cancer, 139–140
  chemotherapy effects on, 353–355, 354f
  cyclin-dependent kinases and, 135–137, 136f, 497
  cyclins and, 135–137, 136f
  flow cytometry and, 148–149, 149f
  G0, G1, G2 phases, 135, 135f, 136, 136f
  inhibitors of progression of, 137f, 137–139, 139t
  mean time of, 152
  M phase, 135, 135f, 136, 136f
  radiation and, 301f, 301–303, 343
    position in, and survival after, 313–314, 314f
  regulation of, 134–140
  S phase, 135, 135f, 136, 136f, 148, 152, 158t, 159
    and prognosis, 160t
Cell-cycle time of tumors, 157–158, 158t
Cell death, 3, 4–5, 134–165. *See also* Cell survival
  programmed. *See* Apoptosis
  radiation-induced, 303, 343–344. *See also* Radiation; Radiotherapy
Cell differentiation, 497
  chemotherapy and, 366–367
  extracellular matrix and, 199
  growth factors and, 116–117
Cell differentiation (CD) antigens, 495
Cell kinetics. *See also* Cell proliferation
  assessment of, 145–150
    by flow cytometry, 148–149, 149f
  tumor growth and, 153–161
  radiotherapy and, 343–344
Cell loss rate, from tumors, 146
Cell-mediated immunity, 241, 248–257, 495
  inter- and intracellular signaling, 254–256, 255f
  major histocompatibility complex, 249f, 249–251, 251f
  natural killer cells, 256–257
  T-cell receptors, 252–254, 253f
  T cells, 251–252. *See also* T cell(s)
    activation of, 254–256, 255f
    geography of, 256
  transplantation, 248–249
Cell necrosis, 140, 158, 159f, 503
Cell proliferation, 134–165, 135f. *See also* Cell cycle; Cell death; Cell kinetics

after radiation, 330–331, 344
  in vitro assays for, 303–305, 304f
  in vivo assays for, 305f, 305–306, 306f
  chemotherapy effects on, 351, 353–355, 366
  growth factor signaling pathways and, 115–116
  hypoxia and, 159
  in intestine, 152–153, 153f
  in normal tissues, 150–153
  prognosis and, 159–161, 160t
  therapy and, 159–161, 160t
  in tumors, 157–159, 158t, 159f
Cell redistribution, after radiation, 331–332, 332f, 334
Cell repopulation, 506–507
  after radiation, 330f, 330–331, 331f
Cell survival
  crypt stem cell assay, 305, 306f
  hyperthermia and, 443–446, 444f–447f
  radiation and
    growth factors and, 316–317
    linear-quadratic model, 308, 308f, 336–337
    mean inactivation dose and, 308
    models of, 306–308
    molecular and cellular repair, 314–316, 315f, 316f
    multitarget, single-hit model, 307
    oxygen, 309–313, 310f, 344
    position in cell cycle, 313–314, 314f
    quality of radiation, 309, 309f
    relative biological effectiveness (RBE), 309, 309f
    single-hit, single-target, 307, 307f
    target theory, 306–308
    tumor suppressor genes and, 316–317
Cell-survival curves, 495, 496
  chemotherapy and, 352t, 352–353, 353f
  radiation and, 304–308
Cell transformation assays
  in chemical carcinogenesis, 175–176
  in radiation carcinogenesis, 185f, 185–186
Cellular oncogenes (proto-oncogenes), 92–100, 93t. *See also* Oncogenes
Cellular requirements, for immune activation, 422, 422f
Cellular responses to radiation, 300–306

Cellular senescence, 138, 140, 145, 500, 507
Central nervous system, radiation damage to, 326t
Centrifugal elutriation, 149
Centromere, 495, 497
c-*erb*-B gene, 89, 96, 273
Cervical cancer, 83
  photodynamic therapy for, 454
  radiotherapy and oxygenation of, 339t
  smoking and, 17
Cervical intraepithelial neoplasia, 83, 91
c-*fms* gene, 89
cftr gene, 401f
CGH (comparative genomic hybridization), 43, 45f, 58, 496
Chaperone proteins, 448–449
CHART (combined hyperfractionated accelerated radiation therapy), 338
Chemical carcinogenesis, 2, 166–185. *See also individual agents*
  alkylating agents, 170–171, 171f
  aralkylating agents, 171f, 172, 172f
  arylaminating agents, 171f, 171–172, 172f
  biological processes in, 167–175
  biotransformation in, 169–170
  chemoprevention of, 183–185
  genetic polymorphisms of enzymes, 173
  identification of agents, 175–183, 176t
    challenges in, 180, 181f
  initiation of, 167–168
  metabolism of carcinogens, 169f, 169–172, 170t, 171f
  molecular epidemiology, 180–181, 181f
  multistep model of, 167–169
  range of potencies of various chemicals, 179, 179f
  risk assessment and management, 182–183
  targets of, 175
  tumor progression in, 169
  tumor promoters and, 168, 168f
  in vitro assays for, 175–177
Chemokines, 241
Chemoprevention of cancer, 183–185
  human trials, 184–185
Chemotherapy, 2, 3, 4, 350–410. *See also under* Drug *and individual drugs*
  adjuvant, 393–395, 493
  angiogenesis and, 208

antimetastatic, 235–236
antitumor effects of, 355–360
  predictive assays, 356–357, 357t
  in situ assessment, 355, 356f
  tumor microenvironment and, 357–360, 358f, 359f
  xenografts, 355–356
cellular effects of, 351–355
  cell-cycle effects, 353–355, 354f
  colony-forming assays and cell survival curves, 352t, 352–353, 353f
  nonclonogenic assays, 351–352, 352t
  types of cell damage, 351
classification of major drugs, 352f
directed drug delivery, 395–396
discovery and design of new drugs, 364–367
  new targets, 365–367
  screening for activity, 364–365
experimental, 4, 396–410
high-dose, 361–363
hyperthermia and, 452–453
multiagent, 410–415
neoadjuvant, 395, 414, 493
new targets for, 365–367
  angiogenesis, 366
  cellular differentiation, 366–367
  ras gene, 365–366
pharmacology of agents, 370–391. *See* Pharmacology of anticancer drugs
principles of, 392–396
and prognosis, 160
regional, 372–373, 506
resistance to, 4, 5, 396–410
therapeutic index, 392–393, 393f, 508
toxicity of, 360–364
  to bone marrow, 360f, 360–361, 362f
  carcinogenesis, 364
  determinants of, 363–364
  high-dose with stem-cell transplantation, 361–363
  nausea and vomiting, 364
  to other proliferative tissues, 363
  tumor remission vs. cure, 393, 394f
Chernobyl nuclear accident, 98, 190
Chimeric antibodies, 429, 429f
Chimney sweeps, cancer in, 1, 8, 166
Chlorambucil
  pharmacology of, 374
  resistance to, 401
  structure of, 374f
2-Chlorodeoxyadenosine (2CdA), 377, 382
  structure of, 382f

Chloroquine, 403
Cholesterol, structure of, 266f
c-H-*ras* gene, 89. *See also* H-*ras* gene
Chromatids, 495
Chromosomal abnormalities
  in lymphoid and myeloid malignancies, 55t, 55–57
  molecular genetic consequences of, 53–55
  in tumors, 53–58, 55t, 57t
Chromosomal addition, 28t
Chromosomal analysis, 26–27, 28f, 28t. *See also* Genetic analysis
  nomenclature in, 28t
Chromosomal deletions, 28t, 43
Chromosomal gain, 28t
Chromosomal inversion, 28t
Chromosomal location of tumor suppressor genes, 53t
Chromosomal loss, 28t
Chromosomal translocation(s), 28t, 96–99, 97f, 98f, 257
  1;9, 98
  1;19, 127
  2;5, 126
  2;14, 99
  8;14, 99, 127
  9;22, 2, 28f, 96, 97f, 505
  14;18, 99
  15;17, 96, 128
  22;14, 99
  in lymphoid and myeloid malignancies, 55t, 56–57
  reciprocal, 494
  in solid tumors, 57t, 57–58
Chromosome, 495
Chromosome banding, 495–496
Chronic myeloid leukemia, 55t, 56
Chronic tumor viruses, 88–89, 496
Cicaprost, antimetastatic activity of, 235
Ciliary neurotrophic factor (CNTF), 120, 120f
Cisplatin, 351, 354, 354f, 355, 388–389
  metabolism of, 371
  pharmacology of, 388–389
  resistance to, 397, 397t, 401, 408
  structure of, 388f
  toxicity of, 408, 410, 415t
c-*jun* gene, 117, 118f
c-kit receptor, 151
c-K-*ras* gene, 89. *See also* K-*ras* gene
CLA (cutaneous leukocyte antigens), 256
Clearance of drugs, 371t
Clinical decision making, 488–489, 489f

Clinical trials, 485
    classification of, 477, 477t
    cointervention in, 479
    compliance in, 479
    contamination in, 479
    crossover in, 479
    explanatory, 477, 477t
    phase I, 478, 504
    phase II, 478, 504
    phase III, 478, 504
    pragmatic, 477, 477t
    purpose of, 477–478
    source of bias in, 478–479
    treatment effect in, 478
Clonal evolution of tumors,
        155–157, 219–220, 220f
    and metastases, 227f, 227–228
Clonal markers, 156
Clonal selection hypothesis, 242, 242f
Cloned gene, 496, 505
Cloned probes, 494, 505
    generation of, 30, 31f
Clonogenic assays, 3–4, 496
    for chemotherapy effects, 351, 355,
        356f
    for radiation-exposed cells, 304,
        304f, 325, 325f, 342–343
Clonogenic cells, 149, 304–305, 496.
        See also Stem cells
CM101, 214t
c-mos gene, 89
c-myb gene, 89, 426
c-myc gene. See myc gene
Cockayne's syndrome, clinical and
        cellular characteristics of, 59t,
        60, 69
Coding region, 496
Codon, 496, 498
Cohort studies, 9f, 9–10, 10t, 496
Cointervention in clinical trials, 479
Colon carcinoma. See Colorectal
        cancer
Colony-forming assays
    for chemotherapy, 352t, 352–353,
        353f, 496
    for radiation, 303–306
Colony forming units, 151, 151f
Colony-stimulating factors (CSF),
        119, 151f, 151–152, 412, 496
    granulocyte, 119, 121, 126, 151f,
        151–152, 152t, 210t, 412, 439
    granulocyte-macrophage, 120,
        120f, 126, 151f, 151–152,
        152t, 252, 258, 412, 433, 439
    macrophage, 126
Colorectal cancer
    cadherins and, 205
    carcinoembryonic antigen and,
        207

clonality and, 157
cyclin overexpression in, 140
doubling time of, 155t
epidemiology of, 15
estimates of T_S, T_C, and T_{POT} for,
        158t
genetics of, 48, 74f, 74–75, 169
integrins and, 204
oncogenes and, 99
prognosis for, 160t
response to radiotherapy, 325t
Combined hyperfractionated
        accelerated radiation therapy
        (CHART), 338
Comet assay, 300t
Comparative genomic hybridization
        (CGH), 43, 45f, 58, 496
Complementation, 496
Complement-mediated lysis, 246,
        246f
Compliance in clinical trials, 479
Compton effect, 296
c-onc genes. See Proto-oncogenes
Conditional validity (in studies), 488
Confounding in epidemiology, 13
Contactin, 206
Contamination in clinical trials, 479
Content validity (in studies), 488
Corticotropin releasing factor (CRF),
        265
Cortisol, 265
    structure of, 266f
Cosmid, 496
Cost-effectiveness studies, 490
Costimulatory molecule, 496
Cost-outcome studies, 489–490
Coumarin, antimetastatic activity of,
        235
Covergent validity (in studies), 488
Cox's proportional hazards model,
        483
CPP35 (prICE), 144
CPT-11, 387, 388, 406
    structure of, 387f
CREB (cAMP response
        element–binding) protein, 82
Cross-links, 298, 373, 493, 496
Crossover in clinical trials, 479
Crypt stem cell survival assay, 305,
        306f
CS-1, 198
CSF (cerebrospinal fluid), regional
        chemotherapy via, 372–373
CSF (colony-stimulating factors). See
        Colony stimulating factors
csk (cytoplasmic kinases), 93t, 112
CTLs. See Cytotoxic T lymphocytes
Cure, remission of tumor vs., 393,
        394f

Cutaneous leukocyte antigens
        (CLA), 256
Cyclin(s), 496
    and cell cycle, 135–137, 136f
    chemotherapy and, 366
    overexpression of, 139–140
    subfamilies of, 136
Cyclin A, overexpression of, 140
Cyclin B, radiation and, 302
Cyclin D, 138
    overexpression of, 140, 366
Cyclin-dependent kinases (cdks), 3,
        102, 366, 496–497
    activation of, 135
    cdk1, 136f, 137
    cdk2, 136, 136f, 137, 137f
    cdk4, 138, 139t
    cdk6, 139t
    and cell cycle, 135–137, 136f
    inhibitors of, 3, 137f, 137–139, 497
Cyclin E, overexpression of, 140
Cyclophosphamide, 350, 354, 427
    in combination therapy, 410
    metabolism of, 371, 375f
    pharmacology of, 375
    resistance to, 213, 401
    structure of, 374f
    toxicity of, 360–361, 375–376, 415t
Cyclosporin A, 123
CYP19, 277
CYP1A1, 21, 170t, 180, 181f
CYP1A2, 21, 170t, 176, 183, 184
CYP3A4, 170t
CYP1B1, 170t
CYP2B1, 183
CYP2C19, 173
CYP1D6, 21
CYP2D6, 173
CYP2E1, 170t, 183
Cyproterone acetate, 288, 288f
Cytidine analogues, 380–381
    toxicity of, 381
Cytochrome P450 enzymes, 170,
        170t, 171, 173, 497. See also
        under CYP
Cytokine(s), 106, 241, 244f, 251, 495,
        497. See also Growth factors
        and specific cytokines
    and cell proliferation, 366
    chemotherapy and, 366
    enhancement of monoclonal
        antibodies, 433
    growth inhibitory, 138
    immunotherapy with, 426–427,
        436, 493
Cytokine receptors, signaling
        through, 119–122, 121f
Cytokine-receptor superfamily, 119,
        497

Cytokine suppressive anti-inflammatory drugs (CSAIDS), 119
Cytometry, flow. *See* Flow cytometry
Cytoplasmic kinases (csk), 93t, 112
Cytoplasmic proteins, 93t, 100
Cytoplasmic signaling, 123
Cytoplasmic signaling transducers, abnormalities of, 126–127
Cytosine, chemical carcinogenesis and, 173f
Cytosine arabinoside (Ara-C), 353, 354f, 377, 380–381, 408
   metabolism of, 380–381, 381f
   resistance to, 399
   structure of, 381f
   toxicity of, 363
Cytoskeleton, 495, 497
Cytotoxic drugs. *See* Chemotherapy *and specific drugs*
Cytotoxic T lymphocytes (CTLs), 241, 251, 254, 255f, 258, 259f, 426, 497
   tumor rejection antigens and, 420–421

Dacarbazine (DTIC), 377
Daunorubicin, structure of, 384f
DDT, cancer and, 19
DEAE-dextran transfections, 37
Death domains, 142
Dehydroepiandrosterone (DHEA)
   anticancer effects, 184, 288
   structure of, 266f
Deleted in colon carcinoma, 206–207
Deleted in colon carcinoma (DCC) gene, 74, 206–207
Deletion, 497. *See also* Chromosomal deletions
Dendritic cells, 241, 494, 497
   antigen-pulsed, 438–440, 439f
Deoxycoformycin, 382
   structure of, 382f
Deoxycytidine, structure of, 381f
Deoxynucleotide triphosphates, 33
Deoxyribonucleic acid. *See* DNA
Deoxyuridine monophosphate (dUMP), 377, 399
DER (dose-effect ratio) of chemotherapy and radiotherapy, 414–415
Descriptive epidemiology, 14–16
   age distribution, 16, 17f
   data sources and trends, 14–15, 15f
   geographic distribution, 15–16, 16f, 17f

Detection bias, 13
Dexamethasone, 265, 358
Dexrazoxane, 385, 412
DHFR (dihydrofolate reductase), 377, 400, 400f
DHT. *See* Dihydrotestosterone
Diacylglycerol (DAG), 111, 123
Diagnostic tests, 467–474, 485
   Bayes' theorem, 471–472
   as discriminators, 467f–470f, 467–470
   disease-specific mortality and, 473
   guide to, 467–474
   lead-time bias in, 473, 473f
   length-time bias in, 472–473, 473f
   likelihood ratios in, 471–472, 472f
   for screening, 472–474, 473f
   sources of bias in evaluation of, 470t, 470–471
Dialkylnitrosamines, 170–171, 171f
Diallyl sulfide, 183
Dicentric chromosome, 497
Dideoxy-chain termination, 33, 33f
Dideoxy CTP (ddCTP), 33
Diet
   and breast cancer, 18, 276
   and prostate cancer, 279t, 280
   as risk factor for cancer, 15, 18–19, 19f, 22
Dietary risk factors, for breast cancer, 276
Diethylstilbestrol, 8, 14. *See also* Stilbestrol
Differential display analysis, 497
Differential display mRNA, 36, 37f
Differentiation, cell. *See* Cell differentiation
Differentiation factors (DFs), 243, 244f
7,8-Dihydrodiol, 172, 172f
Dihydrofolate reductase (DHFR), 377, 400, 400f
Dihydropyrimidine dehydrogenase (DPD), 363
Dihydrotestosterone (DHT), 267
   and prostate cancer, 280
   structure of, 266f
   sulfate (DHEA-S), 267
Dimer, 497
Dimethylbenzanthracene (DMBA), 95, 277
Dimethylcarbamyl chloride, structure of, 167f
Dimethylnitrosamine, 174
   metabolic activation for, 171f
   structure of, 167f, 171f
Diphtheria exotoxin, 432, 433
Diploid tumors, 149–150, 159

Dipyridamole, antimetastatic activity of, 235
Direct death signals, 142
Directed drug delivery, 395–396
Division delay, 505
DMBA (dimethylbenzanthracene), 95, 277
DNA (deoxyribonucleic acid)
   amplified, 54
   of apoptotic cells, 141, 141f
   complementary (cDNA), 30, 31f, 61, 495, 503
   cross-links, 298, 373, 493, 496
   damage reversal, 62–63, 64f
   double-stranded, 39, 67f, 67–69, 497
   heteroduplex, 35
   messenger (mDNA), 30
   repair of, 58–70, 497, 498
      after radiation, 314–316, 315f, 316f, 329–330
      base excision, 65–67, 66f, 494
      chemical carcinogenesis and, 173f, 173–175
      chemotherapy and, 363–364
      daughter strand gap, 68, 68f
      deficiency diseases, 58–60, 59t, 363–364
         mutations leading to, 59t, 60–62, 61f, 62t, 63t
      drug resistance and, 408
      mismatch, 63–65, 65f
      nucleotide excision repair (NER), 65–67, 66f, 174
   sequencing of, 33f, 33–34
   single-stranded, 67–69, 507
   Southern blot, 29, 30–32, 31f, 42, 94, 97f, 127, 495, 505, 507, 510
   strand breaks of, 67f, 67–69
      in apoptotic cells, 141f, 141–142, 142f
      assays of, 312t
      double (DSB), 67f, 67–69, 497
      ionizing radiation and, 67–69
      single (SSB), 67–69, 507
   transfection of, 95, 99
   tumor viruses. *See* DNA tumor viruses
DNA adducts, 497
   chemical carcinogenesis and, 173f, 173–175, 174f
DNA arrays, 45–46, 497
DNA damage
   cdk inhibitors and, 139
   cell apoptosis and, 141
   by radiation, 2, 187, 298–299, 299t
   assays, 300t

DNA-dependent protein kinase
(DNA-PK), 69, 70
DNA-DNA cross-links, 493, 496
DNA immunogens, 435f, 435–436
DNA ladder, 497
DNA methylation, 50, 497, 498
DNA mutations in tumors, 35–36
DNA probes, 29, 31, 31f, 500
generation of, 30
DNA strand breaks. See DNA, strand
breaks of
DNA triple helix formation, 39
DNA tumor viruses, 79, 80–86. See
also individual viruses
Epstein-Barr virus, 84–85
hepatitis B virus, 85–86
human adenoviruses, 83
human papillomaviruses, 83–84,
84f
polyomavirus, 80–83
Simian virus 40, 80–83, 81f, 82f
Docetaxel, 351, 354, 354f, 386f,
386–387
pharmacology of, 386–387
structure of, 386f
toxicity of, 386–387
Dominantly acting oncogenes, 2,
92–100
Dopamine, 265
Dormancy, tumor, 209
Dose-effect ratio (DER) of
chemotherapy and
radiotherapy, 414–415
Dose-response curve
chemotherapy, 355, 356f
radiation carcinogenesis, 188–189,
189f
Double minutes (DMs), 44f, 54, 58,
96, 400, 497, 499
Double (DSB) strand breaks, 67f,
67–69, 497
Doubling time of tumor, 3, 497
potential (T$_{pot}$), 146, 148, 158,
158t, 344, 505
radiotherapy and, 343–344
volume, 154, 155t, 161
radiotherapy and, 343–344
Doxorubicin, 351, 354, 354f, 356f,
358, 359f, 384–385, 404
in combination therapy, 410
hyperthermia and, 453
metabolism of, 371
resistance to, 397, 397t, 398t,
407–408
structure of, 384f
toxicity of, 360–361, 364,
384–385, 415t
DPC4 gene, 102

Droloxifene, 283
Drug absorption, 370–371
Drug additivity, 410–412, 411f, 493
Drug clearance, 371t
Drug concentration, 371t
Drug distribution, 370
Drug influx, impaired, resistance due
to, 400–401
Drug metabolism, 370–371. See also
individual drugs
Drug penetration, studies of,
357–360
Drug pharmacology. See
Pharmacology
Drug resistance, 396–410
to antimetabolites, 397t, 398–400,
400f
apoptosis and, 408–409
combination therapy and, 410
DNA repair and, 408
gene transfer and, 426
glutathione and, 407f, 407–408
from impaired drug influx,
400–401
lung-resistance protein (LRP) and,
402, 402t, 404f, 404–405
mechanisms of, 397t, 397–398,
398t
multidrug-resistance protein
(MRP) and, 401f, 401–402,
402t, 404, 405, 426, 503
multiple, 401–405
P-glycoprotein and, 401, 402t,
402–403, 403f, 404
topoisomerases and, 387, 405f,
405–406, 406f
in vivo, 409–410
Drug synergy, 410–412, 411f, 508
Drug therapy. See Chemotherapy and
individual drugs
Drug toxicity, 360–364
of alkylating agents, 375–376, 377
of anthracyclines, 364, 384–385
of bleomycin, 363, 385
to bone marrow, 360f, 360–361,
362f
carcinogenesis, 364
of cytidine analogues, 381
determinants of, 363–364
of doxorubicin, 360–361, 364,
384–385
of epipodophyllotoxins, 387
of 5-flourouracil, 363, 379, 380
high-dose with stem-cell
transplantation, 361–363
of methotrexate, 363, 379, 380
of mitomycin C, 388
multidrug therapy and, 410

nausea and vomiting, 364
to other proliferative tissues, 363
of purine antimetabolites, 382
radiotherapy and, 414–415, 415t
of taxanes, 386–387
of thymidylate synthase inhibitors,
383
of vinca alkaloids, 386
Drug transport, 371
resistance due to impaired,
400–401
DTIC (dacarbazine), 377
dTMP (thymidine monophosphate),
377
Dunning (R3327) rat tumor, 280,
281f
Dysplasia, 497
Dysplastic nevi, 23

E1A protein, 81, 82f, 83
E1B protein, 82f, 83
Early region gene(s)
E1A, 82f, 83, 233
E2A, 98
E1B, 82f, 83
EBNA-1; EBNA-2 gene, 85
E-cadherin, 205
Economic analyses, 489–490
Ectopic hormone, 498
Effective dose-50 (ED-50), 393
Effect modification, in epidemiology,
13
EGF. See Epidermal growth factor
EJ bladder cancer, 94
Electrons, 296, 297t
Electrophiles, 169–172, 493, 498
Electrophoresis, 31, 31f, 32, 494, 495,
497, 498, 503
Electrophoretic mapping methods,
42
Electroporation, 37, 498
ELF-1, 108t
Elimination half-life of drug, 371t,
372, 499
ELK-L3, 108t
Embryonic stem (ES) cells, 39–41,
40f
Endocrine signaling, 264, 264f
Endocrine system, 263–264, 264f,
498. See also Hormones
classical, 263
diffuse, 263
Endocrine therapy, for breast cancer,
282t, 282–285
resistance to, 285–287, 286f
acquired, 285
intrinsic, 285

Endometrial cancer, hormones and, 19–20
Endonucleases, 63, 65, 66f, 141, 143f, 144, 497, 498. *See also* Restriction enzymes
Endostatin, 213, 214t
End-point dilution assay, 305, 305f
Energy
    absorption of, 296–298
    linear transfer of, 296–298, 297t
Enhanced chemiluminescence (ECL), 32
Enhancer, 498
Enhancer insertion, 89, 89f
env gene, 88, 90
Environmental epidemiology, 7
Environmental risk factors for cancer, 7, 15, 17t. *See also specific factors*
    alcohol, 17t, 18, 18f
    diet, 18–19, 19f
    occupational exposures, 19, 20t
    tobacco, 8, 12, 13, 14, 17t, 17–18, 18f, 21, 182, 182f
Enzyme-linked immunosorbent assay (ELISA), 498
EORTC QLQ-C30, 487
Eosinophils, 241
Epidemiology, 1–2, 6–25
    analytic, 7, 8
    bias in, 12–13
    of breast cancer, 22, 22t
    case-control studies, 10–12, 11f
    causal associations in, criteria for determining, 13–14
    cohort studies, 9f, 9–10, 10t
    confounding and effect modification in, 13
    definition of, 6
    descriptive, 14–16
        age distribution, 16, 17f
        data sources and trends, 14–15, 15f
        geographic distribution, 15–16, 16f, 17f
    environmental, 7, 15, 17t
    generation and testing of hypotheses about cancer causation, 8–9
    genetic, 7
    of lung cancer, 21
    measures for, 7–8, 8f
    of melanoma, 22–23
    methods of, 7–14
    molecular, 7
    nutritional, 7
    observation in, 7
    principles of, 7

random error in, 12
risk factors for cancer, 16–21, 17t
    alcohol, 17t, 18, 18f
    diet, 18–19, 19f
    environmental, 15, 17t
    hormonal and reproductive, 19–20, 20t
    occupational exposures, 19, 20t
    tobacco, 8, 12, 13, 14, 17t, 17–18, 18f, 21, 182, 182f
    scope of, 6–7
Epidermal growth factor (EGF), 107, 108t, 117, 210t, 213, 265, 498
    and breast cancer, 273, 274t
    and radiation, 301, 317
Epidermal growth-factor receptor (EGFR), 115, 273
    abnormalities of, 125
Epidermal growth-factor receptor (EGFR) gene, 89
Epigenetic, 498
Epinephrine, 265
Epipodophyllotoxins, pharmacology of, 387
Epirubicin, 364, 383
    structure of, 384f
Episome, 498
Epitopes, 242, 498, 503
Episteride, 289
Epstein-Barr virus (EBV), 17t, 21, 84–85, 127, 498
erb-A gene, 93t, 128
erb-B1 gene, 58, 93t, 125
erb-B2/*neu* gene, 58, 109f, 125, 273, 396
Erbstatin, 366
ERK kinase (SEK), 117f, 118
Error
    alpha, 493, 509
    beta, 494, 509
    random, 12
        in epidemiology, 12
        in tests and studies, 467
    type I, 493, 509
    type II, 494, 509
Erythropoietin, 151, 152t, 498
    radiation and, 317
E-selectin, 256
Esophageal cancer
    photodynamic therapy for, 454, 455t
    smoking and, 17
Esterase D (ESD) enzyme, 41, 41f
17β-Estradiol, 183, 184, 267, 268, 270–271, 283
    action in cells, 283, 284f
    structure of, 266f, 283f
Estrogen receptor, 268, 268f, 269f, 270, 271, 273

aberrant post-translational modification of, 286–287
and breast cancer, 273, 282, 282t, 285
ERδE3, 285
ERδE5, 285
loss or mutation of, 286
quantitation of, 271
Estrogen response element (ERE) modification, 287
Estrogens, 17t, 20, 267, 267f
    for prostate cancer, 287–288
    and tumor growth, 17t, 20, 273
Estrone, structure of, 266f
Etanidazole (SR2508), 340
    structure of, 340f
Ethacrynic acid, 408
Ethidium bromide, 147
Ethnicity
    and breast cancer, 275t, 276
    and prostate cancer, 279t, 279–280
Ethylene vinyl acetate (EVA), 45
Etoposide (VP-16), 364
    resistance to, 397t, 402t
ets gene, 93t
Ewing sarcoma, genetics of, 57t
Excitation, 296
Exocrine, 264, 264f, 498
Exons, 30, 496, 498, 503
Exonuclease, 498
Experimental metastasis assay, 224f, 224–225, 498
Extracellular environment, 4–5, 197–218
    interaction with cells, 197–199
Extracellular growth factors. *See* Growth factors
Extracellular matrix (ECM), 197–199, 498, 500
    and metastases, 231
Extracellular regulated kinases (ERKs), 114, 114f, 117, 121f
    signaling pathways, 117, 119

Face validity (in studies), 488
Facilitated diffusion, 498
FACT-G (functional Assessment of Cancer Therapy–General), 487–488
Factor VII, antimetastatic activity of, 235
FAK (focal adhesion kinase), 201f, 202, 203, 203f
Familial medullary thyroid carcinoma (FMTC), 98
Family studies, 2
    of breast cancer, 22

Fanconi's anemia (FA), clinical and cellular characteristics of, 58–60, 59t

FAPs (focal adhesion plaques), 202, 203, 203f

Farnesyl protein transferase inhibitors, 365

Fas-Fas ligand interactions, 258

Fat, dietary
  and breast cancer, 276
  and cancer, 18–19, 19f

F$_c$ receptors (FcRs), 246, 246f, 430

fes/fps gene, 93t

FGF. *See* Fibroblast growth factor

fgr gene, 93t

FHIT gene, 53t

Fiber, dietary, and breast cancer, 276

Fibroblast(s)
  primary, 99
  properties of normal and transformed, 176, 176t

Fibroblast growth factor (FGF), 107, 108t
  3 (FGF-3/*int*-2), 210t
  4 (FGF-4/*hst*K-FGF), 210t
  abnormalities of, 124t, 125
  acidic (aFGF), characteristics of, 210t
  basic (bFGF)
    characteristics of, 209, 210t, 211, 212–213
    extracellular matrix and, 199
    and metastases, 232
    radiation and, 301, 327

Fibronectin, 206, 213
  and signal transduction, 199, 199f
  structure of, 198, 198f

Filter elution assay, 300t

Finasteride, 289

First pass, 370, 498

FISH. *See* Fluorescence in situ hybridization

FITC (fluorescein isothiocyanate), 42

FK506, 123

FKHR gene, 57t, 58

Flavonoids, 366

Flaxseed, 276

FLIC (Functional Living Index–Cancer), 487

Flk-1 receptor, 209, 210t, 211
  function of, 213t

Flk-2/Flk-3 receptor, 151

Flow cytometry, 146, 498–499
  analysis of cell kinetics by, 148–149, 149f
  chemotherapy and, 354
  other applications of, 149–150
  principles of, 146–148, 147f, 148f

flt-1 receptor, 209, 210t, 211
  function of, 212t

FLT-3 (fms-like tyrosine kinase), 124t, 126

flt-3 ligand, 124t, 126, 439

Fludarabine, 382
  structure of, 382f

Fluorescein dyes, 43

Fluorescein isothiocyanate (FITC), 42

Fluorescence, photosensitizer, 460

Fluorescence in situ hybridization (FISH), 27, 42–43, 44f, 58, 300t, 498
  flow cytometry and, 150

Fluorescent dyes
  and chemotherapy, 358–359, 359f
  for cytometry, 147–148, 148f

9α-Fluorocortisol (fludrocortisone), 266

5-Fluorodeoxyuridine (5-FUdR), 373

5-Fluorouracil (5-FU), 351, 354, 363, 365, 377, 379–380
  pharmacology of, 379f, 379–380
  resistance to, 399
  structure of, 379f
  toxicity of, 363, 379, 380, 415t

Flutamide, 288, 288f

FLV (Friend leukemia virus), 52–53

fms gene, 93t, 95, 126

Fms-like tyrosine kinase (FLT-3), 124t, 126

Focal adhesion kinase (FAK), 201f, 202, 203, 203f

Focal adhesion plaques (FAPs), 202, 203, 203f

Focus formation assay, 93, 93f

Folic acid, structure of, 378f

Folinic acid, 378

Follicle-stimulating hormone (FSH), 267

Folylpolyglutamate hydrolase, 399

Folylpolyglutamate synthase, 399

Food preservatives, cancer and, 19

Formestane, 285

5-Formyltetrahydrofolate, 378

Forskolin, antimetastatic activity of, 235

fos gene, 2, 93t, 117f, 128, 284, 300, 426

Fractionation
  accelerated, 338, 493
  of heat treatment, 447–448
  of radiotherapy, 329–337
    accelerated, 338, 493
    altered schedules for, 337–338
    combined hyperfractionated accelerated radiation therapy, 338

conventional, 338
hyper, 337–338
isoeffect curves, 335f, 335–336, 336f
low-dose-rate irradiation, 333–334, 334f
redistribution, 331–332, 332f
reoxygenation, 332–333, 333f, 338–339
repair, 329f, 329–220
repopulation, 330f, 330–331, 331f, 506–507
time and dose relationships, 334–335, 335t

Frameshift mutation, 499

Free radical, 499

Frequency, definition of, 7

Friend leukemia virus (FLV), 52–53

FSH (follicle-stimulating hormone), 267

5-FU. *See* 5-Fluorouracil

5-FUdR (5-Fluorodeoxyuridine), 373

Functional Assessment of Cancer Therapy–General (FACT-G), 487–488

Functional Living Index–Cancer (FLIC), 487

Fusion protein, 499

G418, 499

GADD45 gene (and protein), 69, 101–102

GADD (*growth arrest after DNA damage*) genes, 301

gag gene, 88, 90

Gamma rays. *See* Ionizing radiation; Radiation; Radiotherapy

GAPs (GTPase-activating proteins), 113–114, 126

GAS6, 108t

Gastrointestinal cancer
  age and, 49
  5-FU for, 380
  metastatic, 222t

Gastrointestinal tract, radiation damage to, 326t

G-banding, 27, 28f, 495–496

G-CSF (granulocyte colony-stimulating factor), 119, 121, 126, 151f, 151–152, 152t, 210t, 412, 439

GD-AIF (glioma-derived angiogenesis inhibitory factor), 213

GDP (guanosine diphosphate), 113, 113f

Gel electrophoresis, 498. *See also* Electrophoresis

Gemcitabine, 381
    structure of, 381f
Gene(s), 499. *See also individual genes*
    cloned, 496, 505
    oncogenes, 27, 79, 92–100, 257,
        493, 504. *See also* Oncogenes
    proto-oncogenes, 52, 99–100,
        123–124, 506. *See also* Proto-
        oncogenes
    tumor suppressor, 3, 52, 53t,
        54–55, 73–74, 79, 80,
        100–102, 257, 509. *See also*
        Tumor suppressor genes
Genealogical index, 52, 52t
Gene amplification, 43, 54, 54f, 96,
    499
Gene chip hybridization, 45–46
Gene families, 34
Gene mapping, 41–46. *See also*
    Genetic analysis, gene
    mapping
Gene therapy, 422–426
    approaches to, 323f, 422–423
    clinical studies of, 426
    physical methods for gene transfer,
        425–426
    viral methods for gene transfer,
        423–425, 425t
Genetic analysis, 26–47. *See also*
    Genetics of cancer
    chromosomal, 26–27, 28f, 28t
    nomenclature in, 28t
    gene mapping and tumor analysis,
        41–46
        comparative genomic
            hybridization, 43, 45f
        electrophoretic mapping
            methods, 42
        fluorescence in situ
            hybridization (FISH), 42–43,
            44f
        linkage analysis, 41f, 41t, 41–42
        somatic cell hybrids, 42
        tissue sections and single cells,
            43–46
    molecular, 27–41
        DNA sequencing, 33f, 33–34
        hybridization of nucleic acid
            probes, 28–29, 29f
        identification of mutations in
            tumors, 35–36, 36f
        manipulation of genes and
            generation of cloned probe,
            30, 31f
        polymerase chain reaction,
            34–35, 35f
        specialized application of,
            36–37, 37f

putting new genes into cells,
    37–38
restriction enzymes, 29f, 29–30,
    30f
restriction fragment length
    polymorphism, 32, 32f
site-directed mutagenesis, 38f,
    38–39
Southern blot, 30–32, 31f
transgenic and knockout mice,
    39–41, 40f
Genetic epidemiology, 7, 11–12, 499
Genetic linkage analysis, 41f, 41t,
    41–42
Genetic markers, 2
Genetic mutations, 2
    and risk for cancer, 51–53
Genetics of cancer, 1, 2–3, 15,
    48–77, 49t, 413, 413t. *See also*
    Genetic analysis; Oncogenes;
    Tumor suppressor genes
    age and incidence of cancer, 49f,
        49–50
    basic concepts in, 49–53
    bladder, 73, 173
    breast, 2, 3, 22, 48, 51t, 75–76
    carcinomas, 57t, 58
    chromosomal abnormalities,
        53–58, 55t
    colon/colorectal, 48, 74–75, 169
    DNA repair, 58–70
    hematologic malignancies,
        55–57
    heritability, 70–75
    lung, 21, 57t, 173, 181f
    metastases, 234t, 234–235
    model of, 50f, 50–51
    mutations and, 51–52
    neuroblastoma, 57t, 58, 73, 127
    progenitor cells, 50
    renal cell carcinoma, 57t, 73
    retinoblastoma, 70–73
    rhabdomyosarcoma, 57t, 57–58
    risk factors and, 51, 51t
    sarcomas, 57t, 57–58
    solid tumors, 57t, 57–58
Genetics of drug resistance,
    397–398, 399f
Gene transduction, 423
Gene transfer
    physical methods for, 425–426
    viruses for, 423–425, 425t
Genistein, 366
Genomic hybridization, comparative,
    43, 45f
Geographic distribution of cancer, 8,
    15–16, 16f, 17f
Germ cell tumor, genetics of, 57t

Germinal centers, 248
Germline mutation, 503
Giemsa stain, 27
gli gene, 58
Glioblastoma, response to
    radiotherapy, 325t
Glioblastoma multiforme, genetics
    of, 57t
Glioma-derived angiogenesis
    inhibitory factor (GD-AIF),
    213
Glucocorticoid receptor, 269f
Glucocorticoids, 265
    structure of, 266f
Glucose-6-phosphate dehydrogenase
    (G6PD), 2, 156, 156f
Glutathione (GSH), 499
    and drug resistance, 407f,
        407–408
    metabolism of, 407, 407f
Glutathione S transferases (GSTs),
    183, 407
GM-CSF (granulocyte-macrophage
    colony-stimulating factors),
    120, 120f, 126, 151f,
    151–152, 152t, 252, 258, 412,
    433, 439
Goldie-Coldman model, 398
Goserelin acetate, 283
    for prostate cancer, 287
gp100, 421t
gp130 (IL-6Rβc), 119–120, 120f,
    121f
gp160, 435
G6PD (glucose-6-phosphate
    dehydrogenase), 2, 156, 156f
G0, G1, G2 phases of cell cycle, 135,
    135f, 136, 136f
G proteins, 113, 113f, 499
Grade, 499
Graft-versus-host disease, 361–362
Granisetron, 364
Granulocyte(s)
    differentiation of, 150
    drug toxicity to, 360–361
Granulocyte colony-stimulating
    factor (G-CSF), 119, 121, 126,
    151f, 151–152, 152t, 210t,
    412, 439
Granulocyte-macrophage colony-
    stimulating factor (GM-CSF),
    120, 120f, 126, 151f, 151–152,
    152t, 252, 258, 412, 433, 439
Grays, 296
GRB2 (growth-factor receptor
    binding protein 2), 112, 113
Growth arrest after DNA damage
    (GADD), 301

Growth factor(s), 4, 93t, 100, 106–133, 499. *See also* Cytokine(s) *and individual factors*
  angiogenic, 208–211, 209f, 210t, 212t
  and breast cancer, 273
  and cell differentiation, 116–117
  and cell proliferation, 150–152, 151f, 152t
  and cell survival after radiation, 316–317
  chemotherapy and, 361
  epidermal (EGF), 107, 108t, 117, 210t, 213, 265, 498
    and breast cancer, 273, 274t
    and radiation, 301, 317
  extracellular matrix and, 199
  fibroblast (FGF), 107, 108t, 124t, 125, 210t
    basic
      characteristics of, 209, 210t, 211, 212–213
        extracellular matrix and, 199
        and metastases, 232
        radiation and, 301, 327
  hepatocyte/scatter factor (HGF/SF), 210t
  insulin-like, 108t, 274t, 317
  malignant transformation and, 116
  placental (PIGF), 210t
  placental (PlGF), 210t
  platelet-derived (PDGF), 107, 108t, 110f, 122, 124t, 124–125, 210t, 212t, 301
  point mutations and, 116
  properties of, 108t
  radiation and, 301, 327
    cell survival, 316–317
  receptor-substrate complexes, 111f, 111–113
  signaling pathways triggered by, 107–117, 109f, 109t, 110f
  signal propagation, 111f, 111–113
  steroid hormones and, 273–274
  transforming α, 108t, 210t, 211, 252, 273, 274t, 301, 509
  transforming β, 107, 108t, 138–139, 139t, 153, 199, 210t, 211, 212t, 242, 259, 273, 274t, 509
  vascular endothelial (VEGF), 5, 124, 124t, 125, 209–211, 210t, 212t, 213, 232, 234, 509
Growth-factor receptor binding protein 2 (GRB2), 112, 113

Growth-factor receptors, 93t, 100, 107, 109f, 109t, 110f, 208–211, 209f, 210t, 212t, 243, 244f, 499. *See also* individual growth-factor receptors
  abnormalities of, 125–126
  angiogenic, 208–211, 209f, 210t, 212t
  binding to cytoplasmic proteins, 107, 109–111
  and cell proliferation, 138
  epidermal (EGFR), 115, 273
  neuronal, 115, 119
Growth factor stimulated signaling pathways, 107–117, 109f, 109t, 110f
  function of, 115–117
  stress activated, 117–119
Growth fraction, 146, 499
  flow cytometry and, 148
Growth inhibitory cytokine, 138
GRP-78, 459
GSH. *See* Glutathione
GSTs (glutathione S transferases), 183, 407
GTBP/P160 gene, 64
GTP (guanosine triphosphate), 113, 113f
GTPase-activating proteins (GAPs), 113–114, 126
Guanine
  chemical carcinogenesis and, 173f
  structure of, 382f
Guanosine diphosphate (GDP), 113, 113f
Guanosine triphosphate (GTP), 113, 113f

Hair loss from chemotherapy, 363
Half-life of drug, 371t, 372, 499
HAMA (human antimouse antibodies), 428, 431t, 432, 500
HAMA response, 428, 431t, 432, 500
H (histocompatibility) antigens, 248, 499–500
Harvey sarcoma virus, 94
HAT (hypoxanthine, aminopterin, and thymidine) medium, 428
Hazard ratio, 483
HBV (hepatitis B virus), 17t, 85–86
HBx gene, 86
HCC (human hepatocellular cancer), hepatitis B and, 20–21, 86
hck gene, 93t

Head and neck cancer
  estimates of T_S, T_C, and T_{POT} for, 158t
  radiotherapy for
    with hyperthermia, 453t
    and oxygenation, 339t
Heat, cell sensitivity to, 443–446, 444f–447f
Heat-induced cytotoxicity, mechanisms of, 448–449
Heating, step-down, 447–448
Heating time, influence of, in hyperthermia therapy, 449f, 449–450
Heat-shock proteins (HSPs), 114f, 117f, 268f, 269, 270f, 434, 448–449, 459, 499
Heat therapy. *See* Hyperthermia
Helix-loop-helix (HLH) transcription factors, 115, 116f
  abnormalities of, 127
Helix-turn-helix (HTH) transcription factors, 115, 116f
  abnormalities of, 127
Hematologic malignancies, cytogenetics of, 55t, 55–57
Hematoporphyrin derivative (HpD), 454, 456t
Hemopoietic cells, differentiation of, 150–152, 151f
Hepatitis, chronic, 86
Hepatitis B virus (HBV), 17t, 85–86
Hepatocellular cancer, hepatitis B and, 20–21, 86
Hepatocyte growth factor/scatter factor (HGF/SF), 210t
Hereditary nonpolyposis colon cancer (HNPCC), clinical and cellular characteristics of, 59t, 60, 64–65
Heritable cancer, 70–76
HER-2/neu gene, 95–96, 107, 125, 258, 273, 281–282, 396
Herpes simplex virus thymidine kinase (HSV-TK), 426
Herpes simplex virus (HSV) type 2, 84
Heteroduplex mobility shift assay, 35
Heterogeneity of tumors, 220, 430, 431t, 499
  and metastasis, 227–228
Heterozygosity, 500
  loss of (LOH), 73, 100, 102, 502
Hexamethylmelamine, 377
  resistance to, 401
HGF/SF (hepatocyte growth factor/scatter factor), 108t, 210t

HHV-8 (human herpesviruses-8), 92
High osmolarity glycerol (HOG), 118
Hirschsprung disease, 98
Histocompatibility (H) antigens, 248, 499–500
Histomorphometric assays, 312t
HLA (human leukocyte antigens), 249
HLA-B7, 436
HLH (helix-loop-helix) transcription factors, 115, 116f
    abnormalities of, 127
hMLH1 gene, 53t, 64, 65
hMSH2 gene, 53t, 64, 65, 65f
HNPCC (hereditary nonpolyposis colon cancer), clinical and cellular characteristics of, 59t, 60, 64–65
Hodgkin's disease
    chemotherapy for, 361, 374
    Epstein-Barr virus and, 85
Hoechst 33342, 147, 358, 359f
Homeostasis, 220, 494, 500
Homogeneously staining regions (HSRs), 44f, 54, 96, 499, 500
Homologous recombination, 39–40, 500, 506
Homology, 500
Homozygosity, 500
Hormonal risk factors for cancer, 19–20, 20t
    of breast, 273, 274t, 274–277, 275t
    of prostate, 279t, 279–280
Hormonal therapy, 3
    for breast cancer, 277
    for prostate cancer, 287–289
Hormone response element (HRE), 268
Hormones, 263–294
    adrenal, 263–264
    adrenocorticotropic (ACTH), 265
    and carcinogenesis, 274–282
    catecholamine, 265
    ectopic, 498
    endometrial cancer and, 19–20
    follicle-stimulating (FSH), 267
    inter- and intracellular signaling, 264f, 264–265
    luteinizing (LH), 267
    luteinizing hormone releasing (LHRH), for prostate cancer, 287
    manipulation of, against chemical carcinogenesis, 184
    nonsteroid, 263–264
    oncogenes and, 281–282
    pharmacologic applications in cancer, 282–290

and prostate cancer, 19–20
    steroid, 263–264, 265–274
        anticancer effects, 184
        growth factors and, 273–274
        interaction with growth factors, 273–274
        receptors, 268f, 268–271, 269f
            DNA-binding domain of, 268
            N-terminal region of, 268–269
            quantitation of, 271–273, 272f
                dextran-coated charcoal method, 271, 272f
                immunocytochemical method, 272f, 273
                immunohistochemical method, 272f, 273
            structure and classification of, 265–267, 266f, 267f
            transport of, 267–268
        thyroid, receptors, 269f
        types of, 263–264
Horseradish peroxidase (HRP), 32
HpD (hematoporphyrin derivative), 454, 456t
HPV (human papillomaviruses), 83–84, 84f, 504
    cancer and, 17t, 20, 53
H-*ras* gene, 89, 93t, 94, 95, 126
    and metastases, 233, 234
H-ras protein, 94, 96, 113–114, 123
HRE (hormone response element), 268
HSPs (heat-shock proteins), 114f, 117f, 269, 270f, 434, 448–449, 459, 499, 628f
    HSP27, 448
    HSP70, 434, 448, 459
    HSPgp96, 434
HSRs (homogeneously staining regions), 44f, 54, 96, 499, 500
HST1 gene, 58
HSV-TK (herpes simplex virus thymidine kinase), 426
HSV (herpes simplex virus) type 2, 84
HTH (helix-turn-helix) transcription factors, 115, 116f
    abnormalities of, 127
HTLV-1 (human T-cell leukemia virus 1), 89–90, 90t, 91f, 102
HTLV-2 (human T-cell leukemia virus 2), 90–91
Human antimouse antibodies (HAMA), 428, 431t, 432, 500
Human genome project, 34, 41, 41t
Human hepatocellular cancer (HCC), hepatitis B and, 20–21, 86

Human herpesviruses-8 (HHV-8), 92
Human immunodeficiency virus (HIV), 86, 245, 252
Human leukocyte antigens (HLA), 249
Human papillomaviruses (HPV), 83–84, 84f, 504
    cancer and, 17t, 20, 53
Human T-cell leukemia virus 1 (HTLV-1), 89–90, 90t, 91f, 102
Human T-cell leukemia virus 2 (HTLV-2), 90–91
Humoral immunity, 241, 500
Hyaluronidase, 410
Hybridization, 28–29, 500
    comparative genomic, 43, 45f, 58, 496
    FISH. *See* Fluorescence in situ hybridization
    gene chip, 45–46
    of nucleic acid probes, 28–29, 29f
    in situ, 43–46, 495
    subtraction, 36–37, 37f
Hybridoma, 428–430, 429f, 500, 503
Hydralazine, 359
Hydrocortisone, 265
Hydrophilic, 500
Hydrophobic, 500
4-Hydroxycyclophosphamide, 375, 375f
8-Hydroxyguanine, 174
O^2-Hydroxymethylcytosine, 174
Hydroxyurea, 146, 354f, 389, 408
Hyperbaric oxygen to tumor cells, 338–339
Hyperfractionation, 500. *See also* Radiotherapy
Hyperimmunoglobulin M, X-linked, 251
Hypernephroma, response to radiotherapy, 325t
Hyperplasia, 500
Hyperthermia, 443–453
    blood flow and, 450, 450f
    cell sensitivity to heat, 443–446, 444f–447f
    cell survival and, 443–446, 444f–447f
    chemotherapy and, 452–453
    influence of heating time and temperature in, 449f, 449–450
    mechanisms of cytotoxicity, 448–449
    radiotherapy and, 450–452, 451f
Hypoxanthine, aminopterin, and thymidine (HAT) medium, 428

Hypoxia
assays for intratumoral, 312t
and tumor growth, 159, 208
Hypoxic cell(s), 500
chemotherapy against, 358–360
chronically, 311–312
combination therapy against, 413, 413t, 414
radiation resistance of, 208, 309–313, 310f, 311f, 312t, 313f, 332–333, 333f, 338–339, 344, 357
reoxygenation after radiotherapy, 332–333, 333f, 338–339, 344
trials of oxygen sensitization of, 339t
Hypoxic cell markers, 312t
Hypoxic cell radiosensitizers, 339t, 339–340, 340f

ICAMs (intracellular adhesion molecules), 206, 439
ICE (interleukin 1β converting enzyme), 144
ICE proteases, 144, 495, 501
Idarubicin, 383, 384
Idiotype, 248, 500
IFN. See Interferon(s)
Ifosfamide
pharmacology of, 376
structure of, 374f
toxicity of, 376
IGF (insulin-like growth factor), 108t, 274t, 317
IL. See Interleukin(s)
Immortalization, 145, 176, 185–186, 500
Immune activation, molecular and cellular requirements for, 422, 422f
Immune response
biology of, 241–248
cell-mediated, 241, 248–257
defects in, and monoclonal antibody therapy, 431, 431t
failure of, 258–260
self-nonself discrimination, 243–245
specificity and clonal selection of, 242, 242f
time course of, 242–243, 243f, 244f
Immune surveillance, 3, 241, 258, 260, 500
Immunity
acquired, 241
innate, 241

Immunity of tumors, 257–260
Immunogen, 500
Immunogenic agents, 240
Immunoglobulin, 494, 500. See also Antibodies
surface (sIg), 247
Immunoglobulin domain, 247
Immunoglobulin receptors, 245–248
Immunoglobulin superfamily, 34, 248. See also Antibodies
adhesion molecules of, 206–207
Immunohistochemistry, 272f, 500
Immunology, 240–262
Immunoregulation, 243–245
Immunosuppression, 259, 500–501
Immunotherapy
active, 433–440, 493
antigen-pulsed dendritic cells, 438–440, 439f
DNA immunogens, 435f, 435–436
protein immunogens, 433–434, 434f
with tumor cells, 436
genetically modified, 436–438, 437f
passive, 426–433, 504
adoptive cellular therapy, 427–428
cytokines, 426–427
monoclonal antibodies, 428f–430f, 428–433, 431t
Immunotoxins, 432–433, 501
Imprinting, 50, 501
Inception cohort, 475
Incidence, 501. See also Epidemiology
age and, 49f, 49–50
definition of, 7
Incidence rate
age-standardized, 7–8, 8f, 49, 49f
definition of, 7
Indole-3-carbinole (I3C), anticancer effects, 184
Indomethacin, 184, 408
Infertility from chemotherapy, 363
Information bias, 13
Inhibitor of cdk4 (INK4), 138, 140
Initiation, 501
Innate immunity, 501
Inositol 1,4,5 triphosphate (ITP), 111, 123
Insertional mutagenesis, 88–89, 501
In situ hybridization, 495
In situ nick translation, 141–142, 142f
Insulin-like growth factor (IGF), 108t
and breast cancer, 274t
radiation and, 317

Insulin-receptor substrate, 113
Integration, 501
Integrin linked kinase (ILK), 201f
Integrins, 200, 201f, 202–204, 213, 501
and metastases, 232
signal transduction by, 202–204, 203f
in tumor progression and metastasis, 204–205
Interaction (effect modification), 13
Intercellular signaling, immunity and, 254–256, 255f
Interferon(s), 119, 241, 495, 496, 501
antitumor activity of, 426–427
Interferon alpha (IFN-α), 214t
antitumor activity of, 426–427
Interferon gamma (IFN γ), 214t, 243, 250, 254, 433, 437
Interleukin(s), 119, 241, 495, 501
Interleukin-1, 117, 151, 152t
radiation and, 327
Interleukin-2, 89, 91f, 120, 256, 422, 433, 502
antitumor activity of, 427, 436–437
Interleukin-2 receptor, 120
Interleukin-3, 89, 120, 126, 151, 152t, 252
radiation and, 317
Interleukin-4, 252, 256
antitumor activity of, 427, 437
Interleukin-4 receptor, 120
Interleukin-5, 120, 252
Interleukin-6, 119–120, 151, 152t, 438
Interleukin-7, 438
Interleukin-7 receptor, 120
Interleukin-9 receptor, 120
Interleukin-10, 252, 256
Interleukin-11, 120
Interleukin-12, 214t, 439
antitumor activity of, 427, 438
Interleukin-13, 252
Interleukin-15 receptor, 120
Interleukin 1β converting enzyme (ICE), 144
Interphase, 501
Interstitial pressure in tumors, 358
Intestine, cell proliferation in, 152–153, 153f
int gene, 93t
int-2 gene, 58, 124t, 125, 282
int-5/aromatase, 277
Intracellular adhesion molecules (ICAMs), 106–128, 206, 439. See also Adhesion molecules
Intracellular signaling
chemotherapy and, 366
immunity and, 254–256, 255f

Intracrine signals, 264, 264f
Intrahepatic drug infusions, 373
Intravital videomicroscopy (IVVM),
        of metastases, 225f, 225–226,
        229–230, 231
Introns, 30, 496, 501
Invasion, 200f, 228–233, 501
Iodine 131 radioisotope, 432
Iododeoxyuridine (IUdR), 414
Ionizing radiation, 296, 501. *See also*
        Radiation; Radiotherapy
    DNA damage, 67–69, 298–299,
        299t
        assays for, 300t
        molecular and cellular responses
            to, 300–306
Ionizing radiation carcinogenesis,
        167, 185–186, 187–189
    in animals, 187–189, 188t, 189f
    dose-response curve, 188–189,
        189f
    in humans, 189–192
IRS (insulin-receptor substrate), 113
Isobologram analysis, 411–412, 412f,
        501
Isochromosome, 28t
Isoeffect curves, 501
    of radiotherapy, 335f, 335–336,
        336f
Isomer, 501
Isothiocyanates, 183
Isozyme, 501
ITP (inositol 1,4,5 triphosphate),
        111, 123
IUdR (iodo-deoxyuridine), 414
IVVM (intravital videomicroscopy),
        225f, 225–226, 229–230, 231

Janus family tyrosine kinases (JAKs),
        120, 121f, 122
    activation of, 121–122
Joules, 296
jun gene, 93t, 128
Juxtacrine factors, 264

KAI-1 gene, 234t
Kaplan-Meier method, 482, 483f
Kaposi's sarcoma (KS), 91, 92, 102
Kaposi's sarcoma–associated
        herpesvirus (KSHV), 92
Karyotype, 501
K1735 cell line, 438
KDR receptor, 209, 210t, 211
Ketoconazole, 288–289
4-Ketocyclophosphamide, 375, 375f
Ki-67 antigen, 148, 160

Kidney, radiation damage to, 326t
Kidney cancer. *See also* Renal cell
        carcinoma
    smoking and, 17
Kinase inhibitory protein (KIP),
        137f, 137–138, 139t
Kirsten *ras (K-ras)* proto-oncogene,
        74, 93t, 94, 95, 188
Kirsten sarcoma virus, 94
KiSS-1 gene, 234t
kit gene, 93t, 126
Kit ligand (stem-cell factor), 126,
        151, 152t
Klenow fragment, 29, 29f
Knockout mice, 3, 39–41, 40f, 501
Knudson's hypothesis, 70–71, 502
K-*ras* gene, 74, 93t, 94, 96, 188
K-ras protein, activation of, 113–114
k-rev gene, 233
KXGFFKR motif, 202

Labeling index (LI), 145, 157–158,
        502
Lactation, 265
LAK (lymphokine-activated killer)
        cells, 257, 427, 502
Laminin, 198, 204
Langerhans cells, 241
Large granular lymphocytes, 241
Laser capture microdissection, 45
Late effects, 326–328, 335–336, 414,
        502
Latency of tumor, 3
Latent membrane protein 2 (LMP2),
        85, 127
L-CAM, 205
lck (leukocyte kinase), 112, 123, 256
lck gene, 93t, 256
Lead-time bias, 473, 473f, 502
Lectins, 502
Leishmania, 252
Length-time bias, 472–473, 473f, 502
LET. *See* Linear energy transfer
Lethal dose 50 percent (LD$_{50}$), 326,
        326f, 502
Letrozole, 285
Leucine-zipper domain, 502
Leucine-zipper transcription factors,
        115, 116f
    abnormalities of, 128
Leucovorin, 378
Leukemia(s)
    acute, prognosis for, 160t
    acute lymphoblastic, 97–98, 98f
    acute myeloblastic, 96–98, 157
    acute myelocytic, 96
    acute myelogenous, 432

adult T-cell, 89–90, 90t, 91f
cell proliferation in, 157
chemotherapy for, 361–362
chemotherapy-induced, 364
chromosomal analysis in, 27, 44f
chronic myelogenous, 96, 98f, 157,
        432
estimates of T$_S$, T$_C$, and T$_{POT}$ for,
        158t
flow cytometry of, 150
ionizing radiation and, 190
lymphocytic, chromosomal
        abnormalities in, 55t, 55–57
myeloid, 43, 188
    chromosomal abnormalities in,
        55t, 55–57
oncogenes and, 54, 96–99
promyelocytic, 96
    chemotherapy for, 366
stem-cell transplantation for, 361
Leukemia inhibitory factor (LIF),
        120, 120f
Leukocyte functional antigen-3 (LFA-
        3), 256
Leukocyte kinase (lck), 112, 123, 256
Leupeptide, antimetastatic activity of,
        235
Leuprolide, 283
    for prostate cancer, 287
Lewis lung tumors, 223, 359f
LFA-3 (leukocyte functional antigen-
        3), 256
LH (luteinizing hormone), 267
LHRH analogues, 283
LHRH (luteinizing hormone
        releasing hormone) for
        prostate cancer, 287
Liarozole, 285, 289
LIF (leukemia inhibitory factor),
        120, 120f
Li-Fraumeni syndrome, 2, 74, 101
Ligand, 502. *See also individual*
        ligands
Likelihood ratios, 502
    in diagnostic tests, 471–472, 472f
Linear energy transfer (LET),
        296–298, 297t, 502
    high-LET radiation, 340–342,
        341f, 342f
Linear-quadratic (LQ) model of cell
        killing by radiation, 308, 308f,
        336–337, 502
Linkage, 502
Lipofection, 37
Lipoma, genetics of, 57t
Lipophilic, 502
Lipopolysaccharide (LPS), 119
Liposarcomas, genetics of, 57t

Liposomes, 502
  drug entrapment in, 395–396
  and gene transfer, 425t, 425–426
Liver
  metastases to, 221, 222, 222f, 222t
  radiation damage to, 326
Liver cancer, chemical carcinogens
    and, 175, 179f
LMP(latent membrane protein), 85,
    127
L-myc gene, 93t, 96
LNCaP cells, 281, 289
Log-rank test, 483
Lomustine (CCNU), 376, 376f
  resistance to, 401
Long terminal repeats (LTRs),
    87–88
Loss of heterozygosity (LOH), 73,
    100, 102, 502
LPS (lipopolysaccharide), 119
LQ model. See Linear-quadratic (LQ)
    model of cell killing by
    radiation
LRP (lung-resistance protein), 402,
    402t, 404f, 404–405
L-selectin, 256
Lung
  metastases to, 221, 222, 222f, 222t
  radiation damage to, 326t, 327
Lung cancer
  chemotherapy for, 359
  doubling time of, 155t
  epidemiology of, 21
  estimates of T_S, T_C, and T_{POT} for,
    158t
  genetics of, 57t, 173, 181f
  metastatic, 222t, 223
    doubling time of, 155t
  photodynamic therapy for, 455t
  radiotherapy for, 325t
  smoking and, 8, 12, 17t, 17–18,
    18f, 21, 182, 182f
Lung-colony assay, 305
Lung-resistance protein (LRP), 402,
    402t, 404f, 404–405
Luteinizing hormone (LH), 267
Luteinizing hormone releasing
    hormone (LHRH) for
    prostate cancer, 287
Lutetium texafrin, 456t
LY231514, 382–383
  structure of, 383f
lyl-1 transcription factor, 127
Lymph nodes
  germinal centers of, 248
  metastases to, 221, 222t
  spread of tumor via, 221, 221f, 223,
    223f, 228

Lymphoblastic leukemia, acute
    (ALL), 97, 98, 98f
Lymphocyte antigen receptors,
    122–123
Lymphocytes, 241. See also B cell(s);
    T cell(s)
  activation of, 242–243, 243f,
    244f
  adoptive transfer of, 427
  blast transformation of, 243
Lymphocytic leukemia,
    chromosomal abnormalities
    in, 55t, 55–57
Lymphokine, 502
Lymphokine-activated killer (LAK)
    cells, 257, 427, 502
Lymphoma(s)
  chromosomal analysis in, 27
  doubling time of, 155t
  estimates of T_S, T_C, and T_{POT} for,
    158t
  flow cytometry of, 150
  ionizing radiation and, 190
  lymphocyte activation and, 248
  non-Hodgkin's, 91
    prognosis for, 160t
  oncogenes and, 54
  pleural effusion, 92
  response to radiotherapy, 325t
  T-lymphocyte anaplastic large-cell,
    126

Macrophage colony-stimulating
    factor (M-CSF), 126
Macrophages, 241
MAG (myelin-associated
    glycoprotein), 206
MAGE antigens, 257, 421, 421t, 434
Major histocompatibility complex
    (MHC), 123, 248, 249f,
    249–251, 251f, 421, 439, 439f,
    494, 497, 499, 502
  class I, 249, 250, 257, 259, 439
  class II, 249–250, 439
  class III, 249
Malignancy, 502
Malignant glioma, photodynamic
    therapy for, 455t
Malignant transformation, 93, 93f,
    175–177, 185–187, 509
  growth factors and, 116
Malignant tumors, classification of,
    2
Mammogram density, and breast
    cancer, 275t, 276
Mammographic screening, 22
Mantel-Haenszel test, 483

MAPK (mitogen-activated protein
    kinase), 114f, 114–115, 117f,
    117–118, 202, 203f, 255, 503
Map kinase kinase 1 (MKK1), 118
Map kinase kinase 3 (MKK3), 118,
    119
Map kinase kinase 4 (MKK4), 118
Map kinase kinase 6 (MKK6), 118
Map kinase phosphatase-1 (MKP-1),
    119
MAP-kinases, 300–301
MAPKK kinase (MAPKKK), 114,
    114f, 117f, 117–118
Marker, 2, 503
MART 1 antigen, 421t
Matimastat (BB2516), 214t
MBP (myelin basic protein),
    244–245
3-MC (3-methylcholanthrene), 178,
    178f
mcl-2 gene, 144
M-CSF (macrophage colony-
    stimulating factor), 126
MDM2 gene, 58
mdr1 gene, 401f, 402
mdr2 gene, 402
mdr3 gene, 401f
Mechlorethamine. See Nitrogen
    mustard
Medical Outcomes Study Short Form
    36, 487
Medroxyprogesterone, 284
Medullary thyroid carcinoma,
    familial, 125
Megakaryocytes, differentiation of,
    150m151f
Megestrol acetate, 284
MEK-1 cells, 116
MEKK (MEK kinase), 114f, 115, 118
Melanoma, 22–23
  CD44v and, 208
  cyclins and, 140
  epidemiology of, 8, 22–23
  estimates of T_S, T_C, and T_{POT} for,
    158t
  integrins and, 204–205
  metastatic, 222t
  progression of, 232
  radiotherapy for, 324, 324f, 325t
    with hyperthermia, 453t
  UV exposure and, 192–193
  vaccines for, 433, 436
Melatonin, 108t
Melphalan, 354
  pharmacology of, 374–375
  resistance to, 401, 407–408
  structure of, 374f
  toxicity of, 361

Membrane-associated guanine nucleotide–binding proteins, 93t, 100
Memory cells, 242, 243
Menarche, age at, and breast cancer, 275, 275t
MEN1 gene, 53t
Meningioma, genetics of, 57t
Menstruation, chemotherapy effects on, 363
MEN (multiple endocrine neoplasia) type 2, 98, 125–126
6-Mercaptopurine (6-MP), 353, 381–382
  resistance to, 399
  structure of, 382f
Mesenchymal cells, 198
Meta-analysis, 340, 486, 487f
Metabolism of chemical carcinogens, 169f, 169–172, 170t, 171f
Metal ion-dependent adhesion site (MIDAS), 200
Metalloproteinases, 503
  and metastases, 232–233
  tissue inhibitors of (TIMPs), 4, 212, 214t, 508
    and metastases, 233
Metallothionein gene, 408
Metanalysis, 503
Metaphase chromosomal analysis, 27
Metastasis, 220–236, 502, 503. *See also* Progression of tumors
  arrest and extravasation in, 228–231, 230f, 231f
  CD44v and, 208
  cell adhesion molecules and, 232
  classification of, 2
  clonal populations and heterogeneity, 227f, 227–228, 229f
  detachment from primary tumor and, 228
  establishment of new growth, 231–232
  experimental approaches in study of, 223–228
  extracellular matrix and, 199
  genes associated with, 234t, 234–235, 235t
  host defense mechanisms to, 228
  of human tumors, 221–222, 222f, 222t
  inefficiency of, 222–223, 223f
  integrins in, 204–205
  intravital videomicroscopy of, 225f, 225–226
  lung cancer, doubling time of, 155t
  model of major steps in, 199, 200f

molecular mechanisms of, 232–235
  oncogenes and, 233t, 233–234
  organ specificity of, 227
  proteolytic enzymes and, 232–233
  routes of, 221, 221f
  selection of cell populations with specific properties, 226f, 226–227
  to specific organs, 222t
  steps in process of, 228–232
  therapeutic strategies for, 235–236
  treatment of, 4
  in vitro assays of, 226, 226f
  in vivo assays of, 223–225, 224f
Metastasis assays, 223–228
  experimental, 224f, 224–225
  spontaneous, 223–224, 224f, 225
  in vitro, 226, 226f
  in vivo, 223–225
Metastasis-associated genes, 234t, 234–235
Meta-tetra (hydroxyphenyl) chlorin (mTHPc), 456t
met gene, 93t
Methotrexate, 146, 351, 353, 354f, 358, 377–379
  5-FU interaction with, 380
  metabolism of, 371, 378, 378f
  pharmacology of, 377–379
  resistance to, 398–400
  structure of, 378f
  toxicity of, 363, 379, 380, 415t
2-Methoxyestradiol, 214t
3-Methyladenine, 174
3-Methyladenine DNA glycosylase (GLY), 408
7-Methyladenine, 174
Methyl-CCNU, 354, 364, 376
3-Methylcholanthrene (3-MC), 178, 178f
Methylguanine-DNA methyltransferase (MGMT), 174
Metronidazole
  as radiosensitizer, 340
  structure of, 340f
MGMT (methylguanine-DNA methyltransferase), 174, 408
MHC. *See* Major histocompatibility complex
Microenvironment of tumors, 503
  chemotherapy effects on, 357–360, 358f, 359f
MIDAS (metal ion-dependent adhesion site), 200
Mifepristone, 284
Mineralocorticoid receptor, 269f

Mineralocorticoids, 266f
Minocycline, 214t
Mismatch repair (MMR), 63–65, 65f, 503
Misonidazole, 339t
  as radiosensitizer, 340, 340f
  structure of, 340f
Missense mutation, 503
Mithramycin, 147
Mitogen, 503
Mitogen-activated protein kinase (MAPK), 114f, 114–115, 117f, 117–118, 202, 203f, 255, 503
Mitomycin C, 340, 359, 388
  pharmacology of, 388
  structure of, 341f
  toxicity of, 388, 415t
Mitotic death, 503
Mitotic delay, 503
Mitotic index, 27, 503
Mitoxantrone, 385, 402t
MKK. *See* Map kinase kinase
MKP-1 (map kinase phosphatase-1), 119
MLH1 gene, 102
MMR (mismatch repair), 63–65, 65f, 503
MMTV (murine mammary tumor virus), 277–278
MMTV-LTR (mouse mammary tumor virus long-terminal repeat), 278
MNNG (*N*-methyl*N'*-*nitro-N*-nitrosoguanidine), 174
Molecular biology, 2
Molecular epidemiology, 7
  of chemical carcinogens, 180–181, 181f
Molecular genetic analysis, 27–41
  DNA sequencing, 33f, 33–34
  hybridization of nucleic acid probes, 28–29, 29f
  identification of mutations in tumors, 35–36, 36f
  manipulation of genes and generation of cloned probe, 30, 31f
  polymerase chain reaction, 34–35, 35f
    specialized application of, 36–37, 37f
  putting new genes into cells, 37–38
  restriction enzymes, 29f, 29–30, 30f
  restriction fragment length polymorphism, 32, 32f
  site-directed mutagenesis, 38f, 38–39

Southern blot, 30–32, 31f
transgenic and knockout mice, 39–41, 40f
of tumor progression, 220
Molecular requirements for immune activation, 422, 422f
Molecular responses to radiation, 300–306
Mono-1-aspartyl-chlorine₆, 456t
Monoclonal antibodies, 495, 500, 503
  bispecific, 433
  chimeric, 429, 429f, 431–432
  cytokine enhancement of, 433
  fluorescent-labeled, 150
  immunotherapy with, 428f–430f, 428–433, 431t
  immunotoxins and, 432–433
  production of, 428f, 428–430
  radiolabeled, 432
Monosomy, 43
MOPP regime, 361, 374
Mormons, risk for cancer among, 51–52, 52t
mos gene, 93t
  and metastases, 233
Mouse mammary tumor virus long-terminal repeat (MMTV-LTR), 278
6-MP. *See* 6-Mercaptopurine
M phase of cell cycle, 135, 135f, 136, 136f
MRP (multidrug-resistance protein), 401f, 401–402, 402t, 404, 405, 407, 426, 503
mrp gene, 401f
MSH2 gene, 102, 175
M13 virus, 33, 39
mTHPc (meta-tetra (hydroxyphenyl) chlorin), 456t
mts-1 gene, 234t
MTT assay, 352, 365
  for radiation-exposed cells, 304
MUC 1 antigen, 421t
Mucosal ulceration from chemotherapy, 363, 379
Mucositis, 363, 503
Multicellular membrane studies, 357–358, 358f
Multidrug chemotherapy, 410–415
  isobologram analysis, 411–412, 412f
  modifiers, 412
  radiation and, 412–415, 413f, 413t, 415t
  synergy and additivity, 410–412, 411f, 412f, 508
  and therapeutic index, 410
Multidrug resistance, 401–409, 503

Multidrug-resistance protein (MRP), 401f, 401–402, 402t, 404, 405, 407, 426, 503
"Multihit" concept of carcinogenesis, 55, 74–75
Multiple endocrine neoplasia (MEN) type 2, 98, 125–126
Multiple myeloma, 156, 247
  chemotherapy for, 374
  ionizing radiation and, 190
  prognosis for, 160t
Multivariable analysis, 475, 480, 503
Murine mammary tumor virus (MMTV), 277–278
Muscle cell differentiation, 138
Mutagenesis, site-directed, 38f, 38–39
Mutagenic drugs, 493. *See also* Drug toxicity
Mutation, 503
  DNA repair deficiency states and, 59t, 60–62, 61f, 62t, 63t
  of estrogen receptor, 286
  frameshift, 499
  germline, 503
  missense, 503
  oncogene activation by, 95
  point, 116
  and risk for cancer, 51–53
  somatic hyper, 248
  in tumors, 35–36
    identification of, 35–36, 36f, 493
Mutation hot spot, 175, 220, 503
myc gene, 2, 29, 30f, 32, 43, 44f, 56, 58, 85, 88, 88f, 89, 89f, 93t, 96, 99, 101, 117f, 124t, 127, 284, 300, 316
  and metastases, 233, 234
Myelin-associated glycoprotein (MAG), 206
Myelin basic protein (MBP), 244–245
Myeloblastic leukemia, acute, 96–98, 157
Myeloblasts, differentiation of, 150, 151f
Myelocytic leukemia, acute, 96
Myelodysplastic syndromes, 96
Myelogenous leukemia, chronic, 96, 98f, 157, 432
Myeloid leukemia(s), 43, 188
  chromosomal abnormalities in, 55t, 55–57
Myeloma. *See* Multiple myeloma
Myeloma cell lines, for production of monoclonal antibodies, 428f, 428–429
Myeloma protein, 247

Myelosuppression, 503
  of chemotherapy, 360f, 360–361, 362f, 375, 379
MyoD, 138

N-acetylcysteine (NAC), 184
N-acetyltransferase 2 (NAT2) gene, 173
Nafazatrom, antimetastatic activity of, 235
β-Naphthylamine, 171f
  structure of, 167f
Nasopharyngeal cancer (NPC), 21, 84, 85
Natural killer (NK) cells, 234f, 241, 246, 256–257, 258, 259, 426, 430, 439, 503
  and inhibition of metastases, 228
Natural products, cytotoxic, 383–388. *See also individual drugs*
  anthracenediones, 383–385, 384f
  anthracyclines, 383–385, 384f
  bleomycin, 385
  camptothecin derivatives, 387f, 387–388
  epipodophyllotoxins, 387
  mitomycin C, 388
  taxanes, 386f, 386–387
  vinca alkaloids, 385f, 385–386
Nausea and vomiting from chemotherapy, 364
N-CAM (neural cell adhesion molecule), 206
NDF (neu differentiation factor), 125
Necrosis, cell, 140, 158, 159f, 503
Neoadjuvant chemotherapy, 395, 414, 493
neo gene, 427–428, 499
Neomycin, resistance to, 427–428
Neoplasm, definition of, 503
Nephrotoxicity of methotrexate, 378, 379
NER (nucleotide excision repair), 65–67, 66f, 504
Neu differentiation factor (NDF), 125
*neu/erb*B-2 gene, 93t, 95–96, 124t, 125
neu gene, 96, 125
Neural cell adhesion molecule (N-CAM), 206
Neuroblastoma
  genetics of, 57t, 58, 73, 127
  metastatic, 222t
  response to radiotherapy, 325t

Neurocrine signaling, 264, 264f
Neurodegenerative diseases,
      apoptosis and, 144–145
Neuronal growth factor receptor,
      115, 119
Neurotransmitters, 264f
Neutrons, 296, 297t
Neutrophils, 241
Neutrophins, 108t
NF-kappaB transcription factor, 409
NF-1/NF-2 gene, 53t
NGF, 108t
N1H/3T3 cells, 99, 115–116
   and metastases, 233
Nilutamide, 288
Nimorazole
   as radiosensitizer, 340
   structure of, 340f
Nitrites, cancer and, 19
Nitrogen mustard, 350, 351f
   pharmacology of, 373–376
   resistance to, 397t, 401, 407
   structure of, 167f, 374f
   toxicity of, 408
Nitrosomethylurea (NMU), 95, 96,
      174, 175, 207, 277
Nitrosureas, 354, 354f
   pharmacology of, 376
   structure of, 376
NK cells. See Natural killer cells
N-methylN'-nitro-N-nitrosoguanidine
      (MNNG), 174
N-methylN-nitrosurea (NMU), 95,
      174, 175, 207, 277
nm23 gene, and metastases, 233, 234,
      234t, 235t
NMU (nitrosomethylurea), 95, 174,
      175, 207, 277
N-myc gene, 93t, 96
NNK, 170, 183
   structure of, 167f
Nomenclature of chromosomes, 28t
Nonclonogenic assay of cellular
      effects of chemotherapy,
      351–352, 352t
Non-Hodgkin's lymphoma, 91
   prognosis for, 160t
Nonhomologous recombination, 506
"Non-self" proteins, 3
Nonsteroidal anti-inflammatory
      drugs (NSAIDs), anticancer
      effects, 184
Nonsteroid hormones, 263–264
Norepinephrine, 265
Normal cells
   radiation damage to, 325f–327f,
      325–328, 326t
   repair of, 329–330

radiation sensitivity of, 342–343
Northern blot, 32, 97f, 402–403, 495,
      503, 505, 510
Nowell's model, 220, 226
NPC (nasopharyngeal cancer), 21,
      84, 85
NPYX motif, 200–201
N-ras gene, 93t, 94–95, 99, 126
N-ras protein, activation of, 113–114
Nuclear factor kappa B protein, 265,
      300
Nuclear transcription factors,
      abnormalities of, 127–128
Nucleic acid probes, hybridization of,
      28–29, 29f
Nucleoid sedimentation assay, 300t
Nucleotide, 503
Nucleotide excision repair (NER),
      65–67, 66f, 174, 504
Nude mouse, 355, 504
Null hypothesis, 480, 504
Nutrient deprivation, hyperthermia
      therapy and, 446–447, 447f
Nutritional environment of tumors
   chemotherapy and, 357–358, 358f
   hyperthermia therapy and,
      446–447, 447f
Nutritional epidemiology, 7

Obesity
   and breast cancer, 267, 275t,
      275–276
   and prostate cancer, 279t, 280
Observational cohort studies, 9f,
      9–10, 10t
Occupational exposures as risk factor
      for cancer, 19, 20t
Odds ratio, 11, 11f, 483–484
OER (oxygen enhancement ratio),
      310, 310f, 328, 504
Oligomer, 504
Oligonucleotide, 504
Oltipraz, 184–185
Oncofetal antigens, 495, 503
Oncogenes, 27, 79, 92–100, 257, 493,
      504. See also individual genes
   activation by mutation, 95
   amplification of, 96
   and cell survival after radiation,
      316–317
   chromosomal translocation,
      96–99, 97f, 98f
   dominantly acting, 2, 53–54, 54f
   and hormones, 281–282
   identification by transfer of DNA,
      92–95
   and metastases, 232, 233t, 233–234

multiple, 99
   protein products of, 99–100
   recessive. See Tumor suppressor
      genes
   transduction, 80
Oncostatin M (OM), 120, 120f
Ondansetron, 364
Oophorectomy, 284
Opsonization, 246, 246f
Oral contraceptives
   and breast cancer, 20
   cancer and, 20
Orchiectomy for prostate cancer,
      287–288
"Organ preference" hypothesis of
      metastasis, 221, 231
Oropharyngeal cancer, smoking and,
      13
Orthotopic, 504
Osteosarcoma, response to
      radiotherapy, 325t
12-O-tetradecanoyl-phorbol-13-
      acetate (TPA), 193
Outcomes, choice and assessment of,
      480–481
Ovarian function, ablation of,
      282–283
Oxaliplatin, 389
   structure of, 388f
Oxygen. See also Hypoxia
   increased delivery to tumor cells,
      338–339
   and radiation survival of cells,
      309–313, 310f, 344
   reoxygenation after radiotherapy,
      332–333, 333f, 338–339
Oxygen enhancement ratio (OER),
      310, 310f, 328, 504
Oxygen probes, 344

Paclitaxel, 351, 354, 354f, 358,
      386–387
   pharmacology of, 386–387
   structure of, 386f
   toxicity of, 386–387
PAHs (polycyclic aromatic
      hydrocarbons), 167, 172, 172f
Palliation, 504
Pancreatic carcinoma, response to
      radiotherapy, 325t
Papillomaviruses. See Human
      papillomaviruses
Papovaviruses, 80–83
P91A protein, 421
Paracrine, 504
Paracrine signals, 264, 264f
Paraformaldehyde, 44–45

Paraneoplastic syndrome, 504
Parenchyma, 504
Parity, age of, and breast cancer, 275, 275t
Passive diffusion, 504
Passive immunotherapy. *See* Immunotherapy, passive
pbx-1/E2A gene, 124t
PCC (premature chromosome condensation), 298, 300t, 505
PC-3 cells, 281
PC-12 cells, 117
PCNA (proliferating cell nuclear antigen), 66, 101–102, 139, 148, 160, 505
PCR. *See* Polymerase chain reaction
PDT. *See* Photodynamic therapy
Pentosan polysulfate, 214t
PE (plating efficiency) of cells, 304, 505
Percent-labeled mitosis (PLM), 146, 157
Perforin, 258
Peritoneal cavity, regional chemotherapy via, 373
Peto's modification of log-rank test, 483
PF4 (platelet factor 4), 213, 214t
PFGE (pulsed-field gel electrophoresis), 42, 298, 300t
p15 gene (and protein), 138, 139, 139t, 140
p16 gene (and protein), 138, 140
p18 gene (and protein), 138
p19 gene (and protein), 138
p21 gene (and protein), 69, 137, 138, 140, 233
*p21*ʳᵃˢ, 94, 96, 113, 123, 233
*p21*ᵂᴬᶠ¹/ᶜ¹ᴾ¹ gene (and protein), 69, 137, 138, 140, 302
p27 gene (and protein), 137, 139, 139t, 140, 410
p34 gene (and protein), 301
*p38*ᴴᴼᴳ gene (and protein), 118–119
p53 gene (and protein), 2, 3, 52, 53t, 67, 69, 70, 73–74, 75, 80, 81, 82f, 101–102, 139, 145, 175, 188, 193, 213, 233, 289, 300, 302, 302f, 316–317, 409, 421, 421t, 422, 426, 504
p57 gene (and protein), 137
*p59*ᴴᴸᴷ gene (and protein), 203, 204
p70 zeta-associated protein kinase (ZAP-70), 123
*p120*ᴳᴬᴾ gene (and protein), 113
*p125*ᶠᴬᴷ gene (and protein), 201f, 202, 203f

P-glycoprotein, 150, 504
  and drug resistance, 401, 402t, 402–403, 403f, 404
pGm21 gene, 234t
Phage display, 429–430
Phagocytes, 241
Pharmacodynamics, 370–373, 504. *See also individual drugs*
Pharmacokinetics, 370–373, 504. *See also individual drugs*
  terminology of, 371t
Pharmacology
  absorption, 370–371
  area under the curve, 371t, 372, 372f, 494
  bioavailability, 370, 495, 498
  clearance, 371t
  metabolism, 370–371
Pharmacology of anticancer drugs, 370–391. *See also individual drugs*
  alkylating agents, 373–377
  anthracenediones, 383–385
  anthracyclines, 383–385
  antimetabolites, 377–383
  bleomycin, 385
  camptothecin derivatives, 387–388
  carboplatin, 388–389
  cisplatin, 388–389
  epipodophyllotoxins, 387
  mitomycin C, 388
  taxanes, 386–387
  vinca alkaloids, 385–386
Phase I, II, and III clinical trials, 478
Phase I and II enzymes, 170
Phenethyl isothiocyanate, 183
Phenobarbital, 168, 168f
Phenotype, 2, 504
Philadelphia (Ph) chromosome, 2, 28f, 41, 44f, 54, 56, 97f, 97–98, 98f, 126–127, 156, 494, 504–505, 506
  and acute lymphoblastic leukemia, 97–98, 98f
  and chronic myelogenous leukemia, 96, 98f
Phosphatidylinositol 4,5-diphosphate (PIP₂), 111
Phosphatidylinositol 3 kinase, 69, 111–112
Phosphoimaging, 505
Phospholipase A2 (PLA2), 111
Phospholipase C (PLC), 111
Phospholipase C gamma, 111, 111f, 114, 123, 254–255
Phospholipase D (PLD), 111
Phospholipases, 111
Phosphoramide mustard, 375f

Photobleaching, 456, 505
Photochemistry, 454–457, 456f, 457f
Photodynamic therapy (PDT), 453–461
  mechanisms of action, 458f, 458–461, 459f
  technologies for, 460
Photoelectric effect, 296
Photofrin, 454
Photons, 297t
Photophysics, 454–457, 456f, 457f
Photoreactivation, 62
Photosensitizer fluorescence, 460
Photosensitizers, 453–454, 455t, 505
  detection of tumors, 460
  mechanisms of action, 458f, 458–461, 459f
  properties of, 457–458
pim gene, 93t
PIP₂ (phosphatidylinositol 4,5-diphosphate), 111
PKC (protein kinase C), 111, 111f, 114, 202, 270, 273
PLA2 (phospholipase A2), 111
Placental growth factor (PIGF), 210t
Plakoglobin, 206
Plasma cells, 247, 248
Plasma membrane (PM), 201f
Plasmid, 496, 498, 505
Plasminogen, 213
Plasminogen activator
  and metastases, 233, 236
  and radiation, 301
Plasminogen activator inhibitor (PAI), 233
Platelet(s), differentiation of, 150, 151f
Platelet-derived growth factor (PDGF), 107, 108t, 110f, 122, 210t, 212t
  abnormalities of, 124t, 124–125
  radiation and, 301
Platelet factor 4 (PF4), 213, 214t
Plating efficiency (PE) of cells, 304, 505
PLC (phospholipase C), 111
PLC gamma, 111, 111f, 114, 123, 254–255
PLDR (potentially lethal damage repair), 315, 505
Pleiotrophin, 210t
Pleural effusion lymphoma, 92
PLM (percent-labeled mitosis), 146, 157
pLm59 gene, 234t
Ploidy, 505
  of tumor, 149–150
pMeta-1 gene, 234t

pml gene, 55t, 56, 98, 128
PMS2 gene, 102
Podophyllotoxins, 364
PODs (PML oncogenic domains), 98
Point mutations, growth factors and, 116
Polarographic oxygen electrode, 312t
pol gene, 88, 90
Polyclonal antibodies, 503
Polycyclic aromatic hydrocarbons (PAHs), 167, 172
  metabolic activation of, 172f
Polymerase chain reaction (PCR), 34–35, 35f, 42, 127, 505
  random, 45
  reverse transcriptase (RT-PCR), 34–35, 505
    in-cell, 45
  specialized application of, 36–37, 37f
Polymorphism, 505
Polyomavirus, 80–83
Polyposis coli, genetics of, 51t
Porfimer sodium, 454
Porfiromycin, 340
  structure of, 341f
Potential doubling time of tumor (T_{pot}), 146, 148, 158, 158t, 344, 505
Potentially lethal damage repair (PLDR), 315, 505
Pott, Sir Percival, 1, 8, 166
Power, 505
PRAD-1 gene, 282
pRB (retinoblastoma protein), 71–73, 81, 82, 82f
  phosphorylation of, 136f, 136–137, 139
  radiation and, 302, 302f
Predictive assays, 505
  for chemotherapy, 356–357, 357t
  for radiotherapy, 342–344
Predictive validity (in studies), 488
Prednisone, 265
Pregnancy, ionizing radiation in, 189–190
Pregnenolone, structure of, 266f
Premature chromosome condensation (PCC), 298, 300t, 505
preS2/S gene, 86
Prevalence, 7, 8, 505. *See also* Epidemiology
  definition of, 7
Prevalence-incidence (length) bias, 12
prICE (CPP35), 144
Probe, 505. *See also* DNA probes

Procarbazine, 377
  resistance to, 401
Procarcinogen, 505
Product limit method, 482, 483f
Progesterone, 266
  structure of, 266f
Progesterone receptor (PR), 267, 269f, 271, 273
  and breast cancer, 282, 282t, 284
  quantitation of, 271
Progestins, 266, 271, 284
Prognosis, 505
  angiogenesis and, 215
  cell proliferation and, 159–161, 160t
Prognostic factors, 474, 505
  evaluation of, 475–476
Prognostic studies
  guide to, 474f, 474–477
  inception cohort in, 475
  multivariable analysis in, 475
  referral bias in, 474
  source of bias in, 474–475
  stage migration in, 476f, 476–477
  univariable analysis in, 475
  uses and limitations of, 476f, 476–477
  zero time in, 474
Progression delay, 505
Progression of tumors, 219–220, 505. *See also* Metastasis
  angiogenesis and, 208–211
  clinical, 219
  clonal evolution, 219–220, 220f
  integrins and, 204–205
  molecular genetics of, 220
Prolactin, 213, 214t
Proliferating cell nuclear antigen (PCNA), 66, 101–102, 139, 148, 160, 505
Proliferative senescence, 145
Proliferin, 210t
Proliferin-related protein (PRP), 214t
Promoter, 498, 505
Promoter insertion, 89, 89f
Promyelocytic leukemia, 96, 128
Propidium iodide, 147, 148
β-Propiolactone, structure of, 167f
PROSQOLI, 488
Prostacyclin, antimetastatic activity of, 235
Prostate cancer
  androgen resistance in, 289–290
  epidemiology of, 15
  experimental models of, 280–281
    human cell lines, 281
    rodent, 280–281, 281f

hormones and, 19–20
  prognosis for, 160t
  risk factors for, 279t, 279–280
  treatment of, 287f, 287–289
Prostate Cancer–Specific Quality-of-Life Instrument, 488
Prostate-specific antigen (PSA), 281
Protein(s)
  adaptor, 112–113, 493
  fusion, 499
  G, 499
  produced by oncogenes, 93t, 99–100
Proteinases, and metastases, 232–233
Protein denaturation, 505
Protein immunogens, 433–434, 434f
Protein kinase C (PKC), 111, 111f, 114, 202, 270, 273
  and breast cancer, 273
Protein kinase signaling pathways, mitogen-activated, 114f, 114–115
Protein truncation assay, 36, 506
Protein tyrosine kinases, 107, 111, 111f, 113
  chemotherapy research and, 366
Protein tyrosine phosphatases (PTP), 111, 111f, 112
Proteolytic enzymes, 506
  and metastases, 232–233
Proteosome, 250
Protocadherins, 205
Protons, 296
Proto-oncogenes, 52, 99–100, 123–124, 506. *See also* Oncogenes
  activation of, 80
  amplification of, 96
  and hormones, 281–282
  protein products of, 93t, 99–100
  viral oncogenes vs., 88
Protoporphyrin IX, 458
Provirus, 87, 506
PRP (proliferin-related protein), 214t
PSA (prostate-specific antigen), 281
Pseudomonas exotoxin, 432
PTEN/MMAC1 gene, 53t
PTP (protein tyrosine phosphatases), 111, 111f, 112
Pulsed-field gel electrophoresis (PFGE), 42, 298, 300t
Purine antimetabolites, 381–382
  structure of, 382f
  toxicity of, 382
P values, 484–486
Pyrimidine, 299, 506
Pyrimidine-pyrimidine cyclobutane dimers, 62

QALYs (quality-adjusted life years), 490

Quality-adjusted life years (QALYs), 490

Quality of life, 506
  assessment of, 487–488
  conversion of a scale for overall, 489

Quercetin, 366

Quiescent tumor cells, 3, 146

Quinidine, 403

Race
  and breast cancer, 275t, 276
  and prostate cancer, 279t, 279–280

RAD genes, 67–68

Radiation. *See also* Radiotherapy; Ultraviolet light
  adaptive response to, 316
  cell adhesive matrix assays, 304–305, 342–343, 343f
  cell death induced by, 303
  cell proliferation after
    in vitro assays for, 303–305, 304f
    in vivo assays for, 305f, 305–306, 306f
  cell survival after
    cell-cycle position and, 313–314, 314f
    curves of, 306, 306f
    factors influencing, 309–317
    fraction following 2Gy (SF2), 308
    linear-quadratic model, 308, 308f, 336–337
    mean inactivation dose (MID), 308
    models of, 306–308
    molecular and cellular repair, 314–316, 315f, 316f
    multitarget, single-hit, 307
    oncogenes, tumor suppressor genes, and growth factors, 316–317
    oxygen effect and hypoxia in, 309–313, 310f, 311f, 312t, 313f
    quality of radiation and, 309, 309f
    relative biological effectiveness (RBE) and, 309, 309f
    single-hit, single-target, 307, 307f
    target theory, 306–308
  clonogenic assays, 304, 304f, 325, 325f, 342–343
  damage to normal cells, 325f–327f, 325–328, 326t
    repair of, 329f, 329–330

electromagnetic (EM), 295–296, 296f
interaction with matter, 295–299
ionizing, 296, 501
  carcinogenesis, 167, 185–186, 187–189
    in animals, 187–189, 188t, 189f
    dose-response curve, 188–189, 189f
    in humans, 189–192
  DNA damage, 67–69, 298–299, 299t
    assays for, 300t
  molecular and cellular responses to, 300–306
measurement of, 296
relative biological effectiveness (RBE) of, 309, 309f, 328, 340–341
therapeutic ratio, 328f, 328–329
types of, 295–296

Radiation carcinogenesis, 17t, 20, 167, 185–193
  cell transformation, 185f, 185–186
    mechanisms of, 186–187
  dose-response curve, 188–189, 189f
  ionizing, 167, 185–186, 187–189, 188t, 189f
    in animals, 187–189, 188t, 189f
    in humans, 189–192
  ultraviolet light, 17t, 20, 167, 186, 192–193

Radiation DNA damage, 2, 187, 298–299, 299t
  assays for, 300t

Radiation-response genes, activation of, 300–301

Radical
  hydroxyl, 298
  oxygen, 454–455, 504

Radioimmunoassay (RIA), 506

Radiolabeled monoclonal antibodies, 432

Radioresponsive tumors, 325

Radiosensitizers, 412, 413f, 506
  hypoxic-cell, 339t, 339–340, 340f

Radiotherapy, 3, 295–349. *See also* Ionizing radiation; Radiation
  angiogenesis and, 208
  cell redistribution after, 331–332, 332f
  cell repair after, 329f, 329–330
  cell repopulation after, 330f, 330–331, 331f
  chemotherapy and
    adjuvant, 393–395

multidrug, 412–415, 413f, 413t, 415t
dose response to, 322–325, 324f, 328f
  chemotherapy and, 414–415
  growth delay, 323, 323f
experimental, 322–349
fractionation, 329–337
  accelerated, 338
  altered schedules for, 337–338
  combined hyperfractionated accelerated radiation therapy (CHART), 338
  conventional, 338
  hyper, 337–338
  isoeffect curves, 335f, 335–336, 336f
  redistribution, 331–332, 332f
  reoxygenation, 332–333, 333f, 338–339
  repair, 329f, 329–220
  repopulation, 330f, 330–331, 331f
  time and dose relationships, 334–335, 335t
high-LET, 340–342, 341f, 342f
and hyperthermia, 450–452, 451f
intrinsic sensitivity to, 342–343
isoeffect curves for, 335f, 335–336, 336f
models for, 336–337
low-dose-rate, 333–334, 334f
molecular and cellular basis of, 295–321. *See also* Radiation
nominal standard dose (NSD), 336
normal tissue response to, 325f–327f, 325–328, 326t
predictive assays, 342–344
and prognosis, 161
reoxygenation after, 332–333, 333f, 338–339
therapeutic ratio, 328f, 328–329
  altered fractionation schedules, 337–338
  approaches to improving, 337–342
  high-LET radiation, 340–342, 341f, 342f
  oxygen delivery and, 338–339, 339t
  sensitizers and, 339–340, 340f
  time-dose relationships, 334–335, 335t

Radon gas, 190–191

raf/mil gene, 93t

Raf-1 protein, 114, 115

Random error
  in epidemiology, 12
  in tests and studies, 467

Randomization, 506
  in treatment, 479–480
Randomized trials, 9
Random PCR, 45
Rapidly transforming viruses, 88, 88f
RARA-PML gene, 55t, 56, 98
RasGAP molecule, 113, 113f, 212t
ras gene, 2, 113, 113f, 124t, 126, 316,
    421t, 499, 506
  and metastases, 233, 233t
ras protein
    activation of, 113–114
    chemotherapy against, 365–366
RBE (relative biological
    effectiveness) of radiation,
    309, 309f, 317, 328, 340–341,
    506
RB gene, 2, 3, 30f, 41, 41f, 48, 53t,
    71–73, 80, 100, 507
Rearrangement, 247, 247f, 506. *See
    also* Chromosomal
    translocation
Recall bias, 13
Receiver-operating-characteristics
    (ROC) curve, 469–470, 470f,
    506
Receptor, 506
    androgen, 289
    antigen, 122–123, 498
    B-cell, 247
    c-kit, 151
    cytokine, 119–122, 121f
    epidermal growth-factor, 115, 125,
        273
    estrogen, 268, 268f, 269f, 270, 271,
        273. *See also* Estrogen receptor
    Fc, 246, 246f, 430
    flk, 151, 209, 210t, 211
    flt, 209, 210t, 211, 212t
    glucocorticoid, 269f
    growth-factor, 93t, 100, 107, 109f,
        109t, 110f, 208–211, 209f,
        210t, 212t, 243, 244f, 499. *See
        also* Growth-factor receptors
    immunoglobulin, 245–248
    interleukin, 120
    KDR, 209, 210t, 211
    lymphocyte antigen, 122–123
    mineralocorticoid, 269f
    neuronal growth factor, 115, 119
    progesterone, 267, 269f, 271, 273.
        See also Progesterone receptor
    retinoic acid, 269f
    steroid hormone, 268f, 268–271,
        269f. *See also* Steroid hormone
        receptors
    T-cell, 122f, 247, 252–254, 253f,
        255f, 256, 508

    thyroid hormone, 269f
    tie-1, 211, 212t
    tyrosine kinase, 107, 109f, 151
    vascular endothelial growth factor,
        210t, 211
    vitamin D, 269f
Receptor protein tyrosine kinases
    (RPTKs), 107, 111, 111f, 113
Recessive oncogenes. *See* Tumor
    suppressor genes
Reciprocal translocation, 506. *See also*
    Chromosomal translocation
Recombination, 67–69, 68f, 506
Red blood cells, differentiation of,
    150
Redistribution, 506. *See also under*
    Radiotherapy
5α-reductase inhibitors, 289
Regional chemotherapy, 372–373,
    506
Relative biological effectiveness
    (RBE) of radiation, 309, 309f,
    317, 328, 506
Relative risk, 8, 506
rel gene, 93t
Remission of tumor, 506
    vs. cure, 393, 394f
Renal cell carcinoma
    genetics of, 57t, 73
    metastatic, 222, 222t
Renal toxicity of methotrexate, 378,
    379
Reoxygenation, 506
    after radiotherapy, 332–333, 333f,
        338–339
Replication error repair (RER),
    63–65, 65f
Replication factor C (RFC), 66, 66f
Repopulation, 506–507
    after radiation, 330f, 330–331,
        331f
Reproductive risk factors for cancer,
    19–20, 20t
Resistance to therapy, 4
Responsiveness (in studies), 488
Restriction enzymes, 29f, 29–30, 30f,
    507
Restriction fragment length
    polymorphism (RFLPs), 32,
    32f, 58, 71, 71f, 507
ret gene, 53t, 93t, 98, 188
    abnormalities of, 125–126
Retinoblastoma, 48, 51t, 70–71, 71f,
    72f, 100
Retinoblastoma *(RB)* gene, 2, 3, 30f,
    41, 41f, 48, 53t, 71–73, 80,
    100, 507
Retinoblastoma protein. *See* pRB

Retinoic acid receptor, 269f
Retinoic acid receptor α *(RARα)*
    gene, 98, 124t, 128
Retinoids, 184, 366
Retroviruses, 37, 79, 86–92, 507
    acute transforming, 88, 88f
    chronic, 88–89, 89f
    for gene transfer, 423–424, 425t
    HIV, 90–92, 92f
    human T-cell leukemia virus,
        89–90, 90t, 91f, 92f
    life cycle of, 86–88, 87f
Reverse transcriptase, 86–87, 87f,
    507
Reverse transcriptase polymerase
    chain reaction (RT-PCR),
    34–35
    in-cell, 45
Reverse transcription, 86–87
Rex protein, 90
Rex RNA response element, 90
RFLPs (restriction fragment length
    polymorphisms), 32, 32f, 58,
    71, 71f, 507
RGD (arginine-glycine-aspartic acid)
    sequence, 198, 507
Rhabdomyosarcoma
    genetics of, 57t, 57–58
    integrins and, 204
Rhenium 186 radioisotope, 432
Rhodamine, 43
rho gene, 118
Rho protein, 204
Ribonucleic acid. *See* RNA
Ricin exotoxin, 432–433
RIF-1 cells, 409
Risk, relative, 8
Risk assessment, for chemical
    carcinogens, 182–183
Risk factors for cancer, 16–21, 17t
    alcohol, 17t, 18, 18f
    of breast, 22, 22t, 274–277
    diet, 18–19, 19f
    environmental, 17t
    genetic, 51, 51t
    hormonal and reproductive,
        19–20, 20t
    occupational exposures, 19, 20t
    of prostate, 279t, 279–280
    tobacco, 8, 12, 13, 14, 17t, 17–18,
        18f, 21, 182, 182f
RNA
    antisense, 39, 494
    splicing of, 508
RNA-containing tumor viruses. *See*
    Retroviruses
RNA probes, 35–36
    single-stranded, 45

RNase protection, 35–36, 36f, 507
ROC (receiver-operating-characteristics) curve, 469–470, 470f, 506
ros gene, 93t
RPTKs (receptor protein tyrosine kinases), 107, 111, 111f, 113
RT-PCR (reverse transcriptase polymerase chain reaction), 34–35, 45
R3327 tumor, 280, 281f
RU486 (mifepristone), 284

Saccharin, 179, 179f
Salmonella mutagenicity assay, 177t, 178f
SAPK (stress-activated protein kinase), 114f, 117f, 117–118, 300–301, 409, 508
  signaling by, 118–119
Sarcoma(s), 507. *See also individual sarcomas*
  genetics of, 57t, 57–58
  oncogenes and, 54
Savage test, 483
SCF (stem-cell factor), 126, 151, 152t, 317
SCID mouse, 507
Screening, 507
  diagnostic tests for, 472–474, 473f
Scrotal cancer, 1, 8, 166
Second messengers, 264, 507
Selectins, 256
Selection bias, 12
Self-nonself discrimination, 243–245
Self-renewal, 155f, 507
Self-tolerance, 240–241, 243–244
Senescence
  cellular, 138, 140, 145, 500, 507
  proliferative, 145
Sensitivity, 468f, 469, 469f, 471, 507
Sensitizer enhancement ratio (SER) in radiotherapy, 339
Sensitizers, hypoxic cell, 339t, 339–340, 340f
Serotonin antagonists, 364
Severe combined immunodeficiency, 316, 355–356
Sex hormone binding globulin (SHBG), 268
Sexual behavior, prostate cancer and, 279, 279t
SH2 (Src homology-2) domain, 109–110, 110f, 112–113, 120, 121, 507
SH3 (Src homology-3) domain, 109, 110–111, 112, 507

Shionogi mouse mammary tumor, 281
SH-PTP1 (Src homology 2-protein tyrosine phosphatase 1), 112
SH-PTP2 (Src homology 2-protein tyrosine phosphatase 2), 112, 113, 115
Signaling pathways
  antigen receptors and, 122–123
  inter-pathway control of, 119
  triggered by growth factors, 107–117, 109f, 109t, 110f
Signaling through cytokine receptors, 119–122
Signaling transducers, cytoplasmic, abnormalities of, 126–127
Signal transducers and activators of transcription (STAT), 121, 121f
  activation of, 121, 121f
Signal transduction, 2, 123–128, 263, 493, 495, 498, 507
  by integrins, 202–204, 203f
  and metastases, 236
Simian sarcoma virus (SSV), 124
Simian virus 40, 80–83, 81f, 82f
  large-T antigen gene, 81–82, 82f
Single cell analysis, 43–46
Single-strand break, 67–69, 507
Single-strand conformational polymorphism (SSCP), 35, 507
sis gene, 93t
Site-directed mutagenesis, 38f, 38–39, 507
ski gene, 93t
Skin, radiation damage to, 326t, 327f
Skin cancer, 167
  melanoma, 22–23. *See also* Melanoma
  photodynamic therapy for, 455t
  UV light and, 192–193
"SKY" technique, 43
SLDR (sublethal damage repair), 314–315, 508
Slowly transforming viruses, 88–89
Smad4/DPC4 gene, 53t
Small bowel, radiation damage to, 326, 326t
Small-cell carcinoma, genetics of, 73
Smoking
  passive, 18
  and prostate cancer, 280
  as risk factor for cancer, 8, 12, 13, 14, 17t, 17–18, 18f, 21, 182, 182f
"Soil and seed" hypothesis of metastasis, 221, 231

Solid tumors. *See also individual tumors*
  cytogenetics of, 57t, 57–58
  microenvironment of, 4, 158–159, 197–199, 357–360, 358f
Somatic cell hybrids, 42, 507
Somatic hypermutation, 248
Son of sevenless (SOS), 113, 113f, 115
Southern blot, 29, 30–32, 31f, 42, 94, 97f, 127, 495, 505, 507, 510
Specificity, 508
Spermatogenesis, chemotherapy effects on, 363
S phase of cell cycle, 135, 135f, 136, 136f, 148, 152, 158t, 159
Spheroids, 357–358, 508
Spheroplast fusion, 37
Spinal cord, radiation damage to, 326t, 327f
Spleen-colony assay, 305
  of chemotherapy, 353
Splicing, 508
Squamous cell carcinoma
  cadherins and, 205
  response to radiotherapy, 325t
SR2508 (etanidazole), 340, 340f
SRB (sulforhodamine B) assay, 352, 365
src gene, 2, 93t, 112
  and metastases, 233
Src homology-2 (SH2) domain, 109–110, 110f, 112–113, 120, 121, 507
Src homology-3 (SH3) domain, 109, 110–111, 112, 507
Src kinases, 111, 112, 123
SSCP (single-strand conformational polymorphism), 35, 507
Stage migration, 476f, 476–477
Standard gamble (in utilities), 488
STAT (signal transducers and activators of transcription), 121, 121f
Statistical association, 9
Statistical significance, 483
Stefin A, 233
Stem-cell factor (SCF), 126, 151, 152t
  radiation and, 317
Stem cells, 508
  chemotherapy effects on, 352t, 352–353, 361–363, 362f
    toxicity, 361
  estimation of proliferation of, 146
  self-renewal of, 155f, 507
  transplantation of, 508
    chemotherapy and, 361–363
  and tumor growth, 155–157
  response to radiation, 323–325

Step-down heating, 447–448

Steroid hormone receptors, 268f, 268–271, 269f

DNA-binding domain of, 268

N-terminal region of, 268–269

quantitation of, 271–273, 272f

dextran-coated charcoal method, 271, 272f

immunocytochemical method, 272f, 273

immunohistochemical method, 272f, 273

Steroid hormones, 263–264, 265–274

anticancer effects, 184

interaction with growth factors, 273–274

structure and classification of, 265–267, 266f, 267f

transport of, 267–268

Steroid nucleus, 265

st-3 (stromelysin-3) gene, 234t, 235

"Sticky ends," 30

Stilbestrol, 13. See also Diethylstilbestrol

Stomach cancer. See also Gastrointestinal cancer

estimates of T_S, T_C, and T_{POT} for, 158t

Stratification (in treatment allocation), 480

Streptozotocin, 376

Stress-activated protein kinase (SAPK), 114f, 117f, 117–118, 409, 508

signaling by, 118–119

Stroma, 508

Stromelysin (st-3), 234t

and metastases, 233

Stromelysin-3 gene, 234t, 235

Subclones, 220, 220f

Sublethal damage repair (SLDR), 314–315, 508

Subtraction hybridization, 36–37, 37f

Sucrose velocity sedimentation assay, 300t

Sulforhodamine B (SRB) assay, 352, 365

Suramin, 214t

Surface immunoglobulin (sIg), 247

Surgery, adjuvant chemotherapy and, 393–395

Surveillance, Epidemiology and End Results (SEER) program, 14–15

Survival curves, 481–484, 482t, 508. See also Cell survival curves

actuarial, 481–482, 482t

cause-specific, 482–483

90 percent confidence interval, 483

statistical significance, 483

treatment studies, 481–484, 482t

Surviving fraction, 508. See also Cell survival

Sweat gland, 498

Synchronized cells, 313–314, 353–355, 508

Synergy, 410–412, 411f, 508

Syngeneic transplantation, 248

Systemic lupus erythematosus (SLE), 252

TAF (tumor angiogenesis factor), 208–209, 209f

tal-1 gene, 93t, 99

tal-1/scl transcription factor, 127

tal-2 transcription factor, 127

Tamoxifen, 184, 268, 283

action in cells, 283, 284f

metabolism of, 285–286

resistance to, 285–287, 286f

structure of, 283f

TAPs (ATP-dependent transporters), 250, 251f, 256

Taq polymerase enzyme, 34, 508

TAR (transactivation response element), 91–92

Target theory of cell killing by radiation, 306–308

tat gene, 91

Taxanes, 351, 351f

pharmacology of, 386–387

resistance to, 397t, 402t

tax gene, 90, 91f, 92f

Tax protein, 90, 92f

TCDD (2,3,7,8-tetrachlorodibenzo-p-dioxin), 168, 168f

T cell(s), 123, 241, 251–252, 508

activation of, 254–256, 255f

geography of, 256

clonal selection hypothesis of, 242, 243f

cytotoxic, 241, 251, 254–255, 258, 259f

development of, 247

helper, 241, 243, 244f, 251–252, 254, 258, 259, 259f, 260, 417, 508

and inhibition of metastases, 228

memory, 242, 243, 256

positive selection, 244

suppressor, 242, 252

and tumor rejection antigens, 420–421, 421t, 422

T-cell leukemia, 127

T-cell lymphomas, clonal markers of, 156

T-cell receptor genes, 54

T-cell receptors (TCRs), 122f, 243, 244, 247, 252–254, 253f, 255f, 256, 508

αβ, 252–253, 253f, 256

τδ, 257, 258

MHC-restricted, 244, 251

TCRs. See T-cell receptors

TDT-mediated dUTP nick-end labeling (TUNEL) assay, 141–142, 142f, 509

Tecogalan, 214t

tek/tie-2, 212, 213t

Telomerase, 4, 145, 366, 507

Telomere, 507, 508

Temozolomide, 377

Temperature level, influence of, in hyperthermia therapy, 449f, 449–450

Teniposide, 387

TER (thermal enhancement ratio), 450–452, 451f, 452f

Terminal differentiation, 497

Testosterone, 265, 267

structure of, 266f, 288f

suppression, for prostate cancer, 287–288

2,3,7,8-Tetrachlorodibenzo-p-dioxin (TCDD), 168, 168f

Tetradecanoyl phorbol acetate (TPA), 168, 168f, 193

TEY motif, 114–115

TF11H transcription factor, 66, 69

6-TG (6-thioguanine), 353, 377, 381–382, 382f

TGF. See Transforming growth factor

TGY, 118

Thalidomide, 214t

Therapeutic index (ratio) for drugs, 392–393, 393f, 508

Therapy. See also Treatment studies

biological. See Biological therapy

cell proliferation and, 159–161, 160t

drug. See Chemotherapy

heat. See Hyperthermia

photodynamic. See Photodynamic therapy

radiation. See Radiotherapy

Thermal enhancement ratio (TER), 450–452, 451f, 452f

Thermotolerance, 447–448, 448f, 508

6-Thioguanine (6-TG), 353, 377, 381–382
  resistance to, 399
  structure of, 382f
Thrombospondin-1 (TSP-1), 213, 214t
Thrombus formation, and metastases, 229
Thymidine, tritiated, 145–146, 509
Thymidine labeling, 145–146, 148, 150, 152, 159, 354
Thymidine monophosphate (dTMP), 377
Thymidine phosphorylase (tP)/platelet-derived endothelial cell growth factor (PD-ECGF), 210t
Thymidine suicide method, 146, 157
Thymidylate synthase inhibitors, 365, 382–383
  structure of, 383f
  toxicity of, 383
Thymine
  chemical carcinogenesis and, 173f
  structure of, 379f
Thymine-psoralen, 174
Thyroid cancer, metastatic, 222t
Thyroid hormone receptor, 269f
Tiam-1 gene, 234t
tie-1 receptor, 211, 212t
tie-2/tek receptor, 211, 212t
TILs (tumor-infiltrating lymphocytes), 427, 509
Time trade-off method (in utilities), 488–489
TIMPs (tissue inhibitors of metalloproteinases), 4, 212, 214t, 508
  and metastases, 233
Tin ethyletiopurpurin, 456t
Tirapazamine, 340, 359
  structure of, 341f
Tissue factor molecule, 212t
Tissue inhibitors of metalloproteinases (TIMPs), 4, 212, 214t, 508
  and metastases, 233
Tissue in situ hybridization, 43–46
T lymphocyte(s). See T cell(s)
T-lymphocyte anaplastic large-cell lymphoma, 126
TNF-α. See Tumor necrosis factor α
TNM classification system, 476
TNP-470 (AGM1470), 214t
Tobacco, as risk factor for cancer, 8, 12, 13, 14, 17t, 17–18, 18f, 21, 182, 182f. See also Smoking

Tolerance, 240, 508–509
  central, 244
  peripheral, 245
Tomudex, 382–383, 383f
Topoisomerase, 387, 402t, 405f, 405–406, 406f, 509
  resistance to, 397t
Topotecan, 387–388, 406
  structure of, 387f
Toremifine, 283
Toxicity of drugs. See Drug toxicity
TPA (12-O-tetradecanoyl-phorbol-13-acetate), 168, 168f, 193
T_{POT} (potential doubling time of tumor), 146, 148, 158, 158t, 344, 505
Transactivation, 509
Transactivation response element (TAR), 91–92
Transcription factors, 509
  abnormalities of, 127–128
  activation of, 115, 116f, 300
Transduction, 509
Transfection, 509
  assays of, 98, 99
Transformation, 93, 93f, 175–177, 185–187, 509
Transforming growth factor α (TGF-α), 108t, 210t, 211, 252, 509
  and breast cancer, 273, 274t
  radiation and, 301
Transforming growth factor β (TGF-β), 107, 108t, 138, 153, 210t, 211, 212t, 242, 259, 509
  and breast cancer, 273, 274t
  and cell cycle, 138–139, 139t
  extracellular matrix and, 199
  and metastases, 234
  radiation and, 327
Transgenic mice, 3, 39–41, 40f, 81, 509
  breast cancer models, 278–279
  for chemical carcinogen assays, 177, 177t
Translocation, 509. See also Chromosomal translocation
Transplantation, immunity and, 248–249
Transport, active, 493
Transport proteins, 250, 251f
TRAs (tumor-rejection antigens), 420–421, 421t, 422, 422f, 433–434, 434f, 436
TR-4 cell line, 449
Treatment allocation, 479–480

Treatment studies. See also Clinical trials
  choice and assessment of outcomes, 480–481
  clinical decision making, 488–489, 489f
  economic analyses, 489–490
  guide to, 477–490
  meta-analysis, 486, 487f
  purpose of, 477–478
  quality of life assessment, 487–488
  statistical issues in, 484–486, 485t
  survival curves, 481–484, 482t
Trichloroethylene, 179, 179f
Trichothiodystrophy (TTD), 59t, 60, 69
Trifluoperazine, 403
Trisomy, 43
Tritiated thymidine, 145–146, 509
trkA gene, 93t, 98
trkB gene, 98
trkC gene, 98
Tropisetron, 364
TSP-1 (thrombospondin-1), 213, 214t
TTD (trichothiodystrophy), 59t, 60, 69
Tumor analysis, 41–46
Tumor angiogenesis. See Angiogenesis, tumor
Tumor angiogenesis factor (TAF), 208–209, 209f
Tumor antigens, 257–258, 509. See also Tumor-rejection antigens
Tumor cells
  genetically modified, 436–438, 437f
  immunotherapy with, 436
Tumor control curve, for radiotherapy, 323–325, 324f
Tumor cure, remission of tumor vs., 393, 394f
Tumor dormancy, 209
Tumor formation assay, 93, 93f
Tumor growth, 3–4, 153f, 153–155, 154f, 155t
  clonality and, 155–157
  decelerating, 155
  measurement of, 153f, 153–155, 154f
  stem cells and, 155–157
Tumor immunity, 257–260
Tumor-infiltrating lymphocytes (TILs), 427, 509
Tumor markers, 495, 502
Tumor necrosis factor α (TNF-α), 117, 119, 210t, 241, 249, 250, 258, 259f, 427–428, 437–438, 439
  radiation and, 301, 327

Tumor progression. *See* Progression of tumors
Tumor promoters, chemical, 168, 168f
Tumor-rejection antigens (TRAs), 420–421, 421t, 422, 422f, 433–434, 434f, 436. *See also* Tumor antigens
Tumor remission, cure vs., 393, 394f
Tumor suppressor genes, 3, 52, 53t, 54–55, 73–74, 79, 80, 100–102, 257, 509
  and cell survival after radiation, 316–317
  chromosomal location of, 53t
  and gene therapy, 426
  and loss of heterozygosity, 100
  loss or inactivation of, 80
  and metastases, 232, 233
  p53. See p53 gene
TUNEL (TDT-mediated dUTP nick-end labeling) assay, 141–142, 142f, 509
"Two-hit" model of tumorigenesis, 55, 74–75
Type I error, 484, 493, 509
Type II error, 484, 494, 509
Tyrophostins, 366
Tyrosinase antigen, 421, 421t
Tyrosine, phosphorylation of, 202
Tyrosine kinase, 509. *See also* Receptor protein tyrosine kinases
  activity of, 202
  chemotherapy research and, 366
Tyrosine kinase receptors, 107, 109f, 151

UDP-glucuronosyltransferases, 183
Ulceration from chemotherapy, 363, 379
Ultraviolet (UV) light, 295–296, 296f, 299. *See also under* Radiation
  and carcinogenesis, 17t, 20, 167, 186, 192–193
  genetic sensitivity to, 60, 61f, 62, 64f, 67, 192
Uncertainty (test), 466–467
Univariable analysis, 475
Uracil, 379f
Urokinase, 235
Utility (in studies), 488
UV light. *See* Ultraviolet light
Uvomorulin, 205
uvrA gene, 401f

v-*abl* gene, 127. *See also bcr/abl* gene
Validity (in studies), 488
Vascular cell adhesion molecule (V-CAM), 206
Vascular endothelial growth factor (VEGF), 5, 209–211, 213, 509
  abnormalities of, 124t, 125
  characteristics of, 209–211, 210t
  function of, 212t
  and metastases, 232, 234
  receptors for, 210t, 211
Vascular hot spots, 215
Vascular permeability factor (VPF). *See* Vascular endothelial growth factor (VEGF)
Vasculature of tumors, 208, 357. *See also* Angiogenesis, tumor
  cell proliferation and, 159
  hyperthermia and, 450, 450f
  and metastasis, 221, 228, 230, 230f
Vasectomy, prostate cancer and, 279, 279t
V-CAM (vascular cell adhesion molecule), 206
Vector, 509
VEGF. *See* Vascular endothelial growth factor
VEGFR1 receptor, 209
VEGFR2 receptor, 209
Verapamil, 403
v-*fms* gene, 126
VHL gene, 53t, 102
Videomicroscopy, intravital (IVVM), of metastases, 225f, 225–226, 229–230, 231
Vinblastine, 351, 353, 354, 354f, 358, 385–386
  structure of, 385f
Vinca alkaloids, 351, 351f, 385–386. *See also individual drugs*
  pharmacology of, 385–386
  resistance to, 397t, 402t
  structure of, 385f
  toxicity of, 386
Vincristine, 351, 353, 354, 354f, 358, 385–386
  structure of, 385f
Vinorelbine, 386
Vinyl chloride
  cancer and, 19
  structure of, 167f
Viral oncogenes, 92–100, 93t. *See also* Oncogenes
Viral vectors, 37, 509

Viruses. *See also individual viruses*
  acute transforming, 493
  and cancer, 17t, 20, 52–53
  chronic tumor (slowly transforming), 88–89, 496
  DNA tumor, 79, 80–86
  Epstein-Barr virus, 17t, 21, 84–85, 127, 498
  Friend leukemia virus, 52–53
  for gene transfer, 423–425, 425t
  hepatitis B virus, 85–86
  herpes simplex virus type 2, 84
  human adenoviruses, 37, 83
    for gene transfer, 424, 425t
  human herpesviruses-8, 92
  human papillomaviruses, 17t, 20, 53, 83–84, 84f, 504
  human T-cell leukemia virus 1, 89–90, 90t, 91f, 102
  human T-cell leukemia virus 2, 90–91
  polyomavirus, 80–83
  provirus, 87, 506
  retroviruses. *See* Retroviruses
  simian sarcoma virus, 124
  simian virus 40, 80–83, 81f, 82f
Vitamin C (ascorbic acid), 183
Vitamin D analogues, 366
Vitamin D3 analogues, 214t
Vitamin D receptor, 269f
Vitamin E (α-tocopherol), 183
Vitaxin, 214t
V(D)J recombination, 253
VM-26. *See* Teniposide
v-*myc* gene. *See myc* gene
Volume doubling time of tumor, 3, 146, 153f, 153–155, 154f, 155t
Volume of drug distribution, 370
v-*onc* genes. *See* Oncogenes
Vorozole, 285
VP-16. *See* Etoposide

WAP (whey acidic protein promoter), 278
Warfarin, antimetastatic activity of, 235
Western blot, 32, 402–403, 510
Whey acidic protein promoter (WAP), 278
Wilcoxon test, 483
Wilms' tumor, 48, 73, 100
WT-1 gene, 53t, 73, 100, 102, 124t, 128
Wy-14,643, 168
  structure of, 168f

Xenobiotic, 510
Xenograft studies, 504, 510
    of chemotherapy, 355
Xeroderma pigmentosum (XP), 23,
        363, 510
    clinical and cellular characteristics
        of, 58–60, 59t, 69
    genetics of, 51t, 58–59, 59t, 60

X-linked clonal markers, 156,
        156f
x-ray(s), 295–296, 296f
    exposure to. *See* Ionizing
        radiation carcinogenesis
x-ray crystallography, 510
    in chemotherapy research,
        365

yes gene, 93t
Ytrium 90 radioisotope, 432

ZAP-70 (p70 zeta-associated protein
        kinase), 123
Zinc-finger transcription factors, 115,
        116f, 127–128, 268, 269f, 510

ISBN 0-07-105484-7

90000

9 780071 054843

TANNOCK/BASIC SCIENCE
OF ONCOLOGY